Internal Organs

THIEME Atlas of Anatomy

Fourth Edition

Thieme

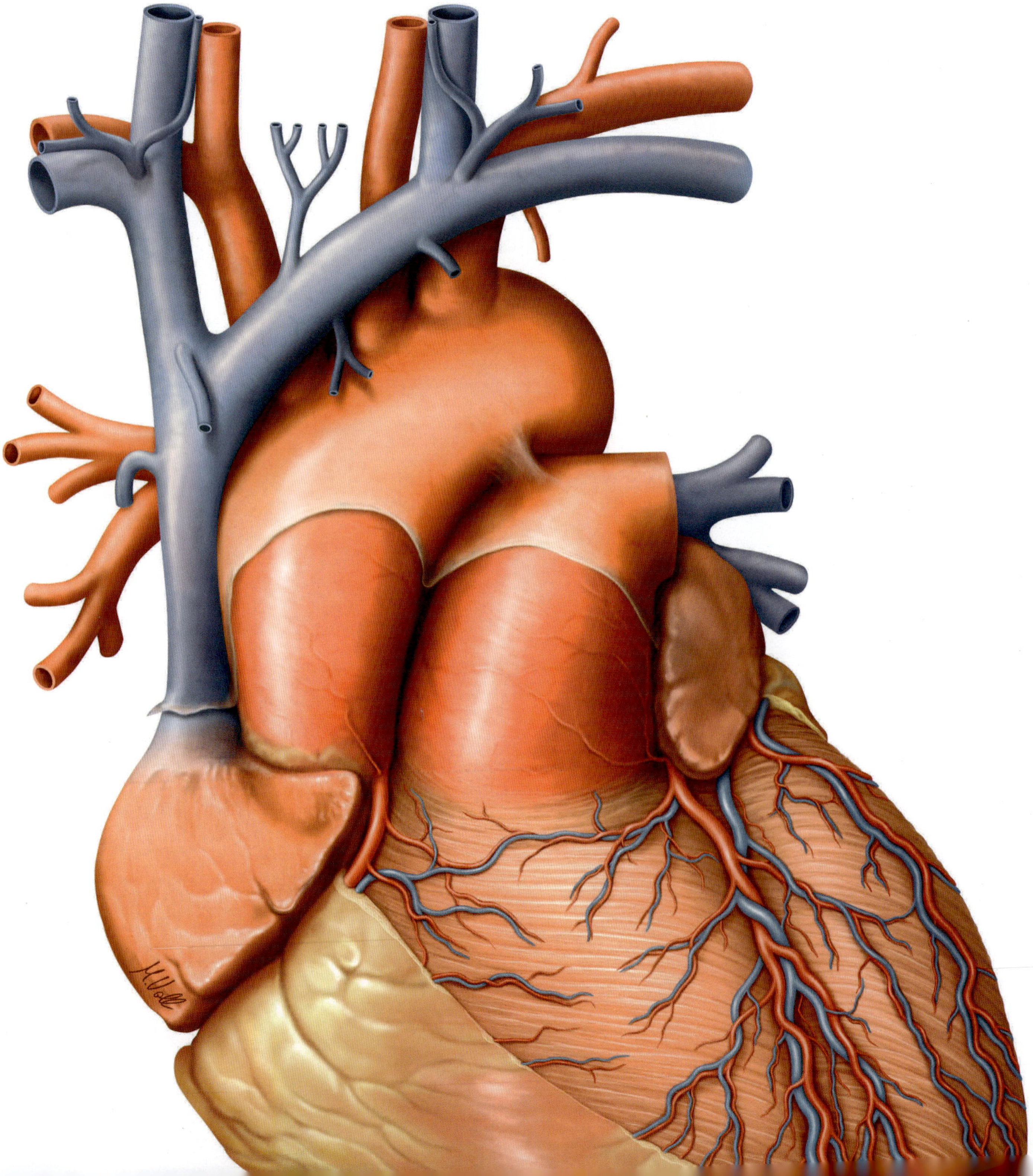

Internal Organs

THIEME Atlas of Anatomy

Fourth Edition

Authors

Michael Schuenke, MD, PhD
Institute of Anatomy
Christian Albrechts University, Kiel

Erik Schulte, MD
Institute of Functional and Clinical Anatomy
Johannes Gutenberg University, Mainz

Udo Schumacher, MD
FRCPath, CBiol, FIBiol, DSc
MSB Medical School, Berlin

Consulting Editor

Wayne A. Cass, PhD
Department of Neuroscience
University of Kentucky College of Medicine
Lexington, Kentucky

Illustrations by
Markus Voll
Karl Wesker

1437 Illustrations

Thieme
New York • Stuttgart • Delhi • Rio de Janeiro

Translators: Terry Telger, John Grossman, and Judith Tomat
Illustrators: Markus Voll and Karl Wesker
Compositor: DiTech Process Solutions

Library of Congress Cataloging-in-Publication Data is available from the publisher.

Thieme Medical Publishers, Inc.
Thieme Publishers New York
333 Seventh Avenue, New York, NY 10001 USA
+1 800 782 3488, customerservice@thieme.com

Typesetting: DiTech Process Solutions

Printed in India by Replika Press Pvt. Ltd. 5 4 3 2 1

DOI: 10.1055/b000001062
ISBN: 978-1-68420-591-2
Also available as eBook:
eISBN (PDF) 978-1-68420-592-9
eISBN (epub) 978-1-68420-593-6

Foreword

Each of the authors of the single volume *Thieme Atlas of Anatomy* was impressed with the extraordinary detail, accuracy, and beauty of the illustrations that were created for the *Thieme* three-volume series of anatomy atlases. We felt these images were one of the most significant additions to anatomic education in the past 50 years. The effective pedagogical approach of this series, with two-page learning units that combined the outstanding illustrations and captions that emphasized the functional and clinical significance of structures, coupled with the numerous tables summarizing key information, was unique. We also felt that the overall organization of each region, with structures presented first systemically — musculoskeletal, vascular, and nervous — and then topographically, supported classroom learning and active dissection in the laboratory.

This series combines the best of a clinically oriented text and an atlas. Its detail and pedagogical presentation make it a complete support for classroom and laboratory instruction and a reference for life in all the medical, dental, and allied health fields. Each of the volumes — *General Anatomy and Musculoskeletal System, Internal Organs*, and *Head, Neck, and Neuroanatomy* — can also be used as a stand-alone text/atlas for an in-depth study of systems often involved in the allied health/medical specialty fields.

We were delighted when *Thieme* asked us to work with them to create a single-volume atlas from this groundbreaking series, and we owe a great debt to the authors and illustrators of this series inasmuch as their materials and vision formed the general framework for the single volume *Thieme Atlas of Anatomy*.

We thank the authors and illustrators for this very special contribution to the teaching of anatomy and recommend it for thorough mastery of anatomy and its clinically functional importance in all fields of health care-related specialties.

Lawrence M. Ross, Brian R. MacPherson, and Anne M. Gilroy

Preface of the Authors and Illustrators

When Thieme started planning the first edition of this atlas, they sought the opinions of students and instructors alike in both the United States and Europe on what constituted an "ideal" atlas of anatomy—ideal to learn from, to master extensive amounts of information while on a busy class schedule, and, in the process, to acquire sound, up-to-date knowledge. The result of our work in response to what Thieme had learned is this atlas. The *Thieme Atlas of Anatomy*, unlike most other atlases, is a comprehensive educational tool that combines illustrations with explanatory text and summary tables, introducing clinical applications throughout, and presenting anatomic concepts in a step-by-step sequence that includes system-by-system and topographical views.

For the first edition we had hoped that our *Atlas of Anatomy* would help the medical student to understand the anatomical basis of clinical medicine. This indeed was accepted by the students all over the world and soon a second edition had to come on the market in Germany, which was extensively extended and revised, followed by further third, fourth, fifth, and sixth editions. More and more information has been added over these editions, including spreads on important foundational information on the common imaging planes for plain film, MRI, and CT scans, the structure of and function of muscle fasciae, the structure and chemical composition of hyaline cartilage, and the regeneration of peripheral nerves, bone marrow, and paraganglia, as well as new graphical summaries in neuroanatomy and new sections describing internal female genitalia and surgical interventions with respect to female genitalia. This atlas takes special care to cover variants in human anatomy such as blood vessels whose courses deviate from the "norm," or anomalous positions of organs. Hence the sixth German edition looks ever more distinctly different from the first one. Of course, we have also checked, corrected, and updated all of the information in this atlas.

We are grateful to the American branch of Thieme that they have made this fourth English edition possible. We hope that this updated version will serve the medical students and practitioners of medicine alike in helping them to understand human morphology which is indispensable for diagnosis and therapy.

Michael Schünke, Erik Schulte, Udo Schumacher,
Markus Voll, and Karl Wesker

Acknowledgments

First we wish to thank our families. This atlas is dedicated to them.

Since the publication of the first volume of the *Thieme Atlas of Anatomy* in 2006, we have received numerous suggestions for refinements and additions. We would like to take this opportunity to express our sincere thanks to all those who through the years have helped us to improve the *Thieme Atlas of Anatomy* in one way or another. Specifically, this includes Kirsten Hattermann, Ph.D.; Runhild Lucius, D.D.S.; Prof. Renate Lüllmann-Rauch, M.D.; Prof. Jobst Sievers, M.D.; Ali Therany, D.D.S.; Prof. Thilo Wedel, M.D. (all at the Anatomic Institute of Christian Albrecht University of Kiel); as well as Prof. Christoph Düber, M.D. (University of Mainz Medical School); Christian Friedrichs, D.D.S. (Practice for Tooth Preservation and Endodontics, Kiel); Prof. Reinhart Gossrau, M.D. (Charité Berlin, Institute of Anatomy); Prof. Daniel Haag-Wackernagel, Ph.D. (Basel); Johannes-Martin Hahn, M.D., (Tübingen); Prof. Stefan Müller-Hülsbeck, M.D. (DIAKO Krankenhaus gGmbH Flensburg); Róbert Késmárszky, M.D.; Prof. Susanne Klutmann (UKE Hamburg); Michael Kriwat (Kiel); Prof. Paul Peter Lunkenheimer, M.D. (Westphalian Wilhelm University Münster); Dr. Janos Mester, professor (UKE Hamburg); Dr. Jörg Detlev Moritz, associate professor (Klinik für Radiologie und Neuroradiologie Kiel); Dr. Thomas Müller, associate professor (University of Mainz Medical School); Dan mon O'Dey, M.D., associate professor (Luisenhospital Aachen); Dr. Kai-Hinrich Olms, Fußchirurgie Bad Schwartau, Daniel Paech, M.D., M.S. (physics) (Deutsches Krebsforschungszentrum Heidelberg); Dr. Thilo Schwalenberg, senior physician (Urologische Klinik des Universitätsklinikums Leipzig); Hans-Peter Sobotta, M.D. (Stiftung Herzogin Elisabeth Hospital Braunschweig); Dr. Katharina Spanel-Borowski, professor emeritus (University of Leipzig); Dr. Jürgen Specht (Orthopaedicum Frankfurt); Prof. Christoph Viebahn, Ph.D. (Georg-August-Universität Göttingen); Imke Weyers, M.D. (Univ. Lübeck).

For extensive corrections, especially in the first edition, we thank Gabriele Schünke, M.S. biology; Jakob Fay, M.D.; as well as medical students Claudia Dücker, Simin Rassouli, Heike Teichmann, Susanne Tippmann, and dental student Sylvia Zilles; also, Julia Jörns-Kuhnke, M.D., especially for her assistance with the figure labels.

We extend special thanks to Stephanie Gay and Bert Sender, who prepared the layouts. Their ability to arrange the text and illustrations on facing pages for maximum clarity has contributed greatly to the quality of the atlas.

We particularly acknowledge the efforts of those who handled this project on the publishing side:

Jürgen Lüthje, M.D., Ph.D., executive editor at Thieme Medical Publishers, has "made the impossible possible." He not only reconciled the wishes of the authors and artists with the demands of reality but also managed to keep a team of five people working together for years on a project whose goal was known to us from the beginning but whose full dimensions we only came to appreciate over time. For this he has earned our deepest heartfelt gratitude. Since Dr. Jürgen Lüthje retired in 2018, Dr. Jochen Neuberger has taken over and has shown great initiative in continuing and further developing the *Thieme Atlas of Anatomy*.

Sabine Bartl, developmental editor, became a touchstone for the authors in the best sense of the word. She has, as a humanities scholar, not a doctor, reviewed the text and, in connection with the illustrations, was able to determine whether a beginning student, and thus one who is not (yet) a physician, could clearly appreciate the logic of the presentation. Based on her suggestions topics were also reformulated and redesigned. It is not only the authors who are indebted to her, but also the reader benefits from her didactic talent.

We owe a great debt of thanks to Martin Spencker, who was at the time of publication of the first edition managing director of Educational Publications at Thieme, especially to his ability to make quick and unconventional decisions when dealing with problems and uncertainties. His openness to all the concerns of the authors and artists and the transparency and fairness in all discussions gave the project momentum and established conditions for a cooperative partnership. We also owe him a huge debt of gratitude.

We are grateful to Antje Bühl, who was there from the beginning as project assistant, working "behind the scenes" on numerous tasks such as repeated proofreading and helping to arrange the figure labels.

We are also indebted to Yvonne Strassburg, Michael Zepf, and Laura Diemand who saw to it that the *Thieme Atlas of Anatomy* was printed and bound on schedule, and that the project benefited from the best practical expertise throughout the entire process of publication. We also thank Susanne Tochtermann-Wenzel and Anja Jahn for their assistance with technical issues involving every aspect of the illustrations; Julia Fersch who ensured that the *Thieme Atlas of Anatomy* is also accessible via eRef; Almut Leopold and Dr. Wilhelm Kuhn for the exceptional index; Marie-Luise Kürschner and Nina Jentschke for the appealing cover design; as well as Dr. Thomas Krimmer, Liesa Arendt, Birgit Carlsen, Stephanie Eilmann, Marion Hamm, and Anne Döbler, representing all those now and previously involved in the marketing, sale, and promotion of the *Thieme Atlas of Anatomy*.

The authors, August 2022

As consulting editor I was asked to review the English translation of *Thieme Atlas of Anatomy: Internal Organs*, Fourth Edition. My work involved reviewing and editing the translation and nomenclature conversion of the German text to currently used English terms. In addition, some minor changes in presentation were made to reflect commonly accepted approaches in North American educational programs. This task was facilitated by the clear organization of the original text and the exceptional work of the translators. Throughout this process I have tried to remain faithful to the intentions and insights of the authors and illustrators, whom I thank for this outstanding revision. I would also like to thank the entire team at Thieme Medical Publishers who worked on this edition. In particular I would like to give special thanks to Andrew Moyer, Executive Content Portfolio Manager, for inviting me to work on this atlas and for his continued support, Torsten Scheihagen, Senior Content Service Manager, for his support and help throughout the process of completing this atlas, and translator John Grossman for his work with the new and altered text.

Wayne A. Cass

The people behind the Thieme Atlas of Anatomy

A work such as the *Thieme Atlas of Anatomy* can only arise when the people involved in the project work hand in hand. The integrated educational and artistic work you now hold in your hands is the product of an intensive discourse between anatomy professors Michael Schünke, Erik Schulte, and Udo Schumacher and anatomic illustrators Markus Voll and Karl Wesker.

Creating learning units that comprehensively treat a topic on a two-page spread is a challenge in itself. The authors must carefully select the content, assemble it, and add explanatory legends. Yet how this content is presented in the atlas, how appealing and memorable it is, depends largely on the illustrations. And the *Thieme Atlas of Anatomy* now includes a good 5,000 of them. In creating them, Markus Voll and Karl Wesker drew on many years of experience in anatomic illustration, visited anatomic collections, studied specimens, and immersed themselves in old and new works of anatomy. This was the foundation on which the *Thieme Atlas of Anatomy* arose.

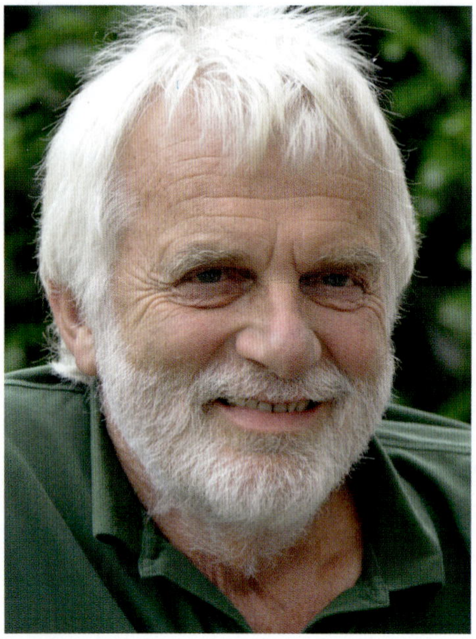

Photo: private

Michael Schuenke, MD, PhD, professor

Institute of Anatomy of the University of Kiel; studied biology and medicine in Tübingen and Kiel; extensive teaching of medical students and physical therapists; author and translator of other textbooks.

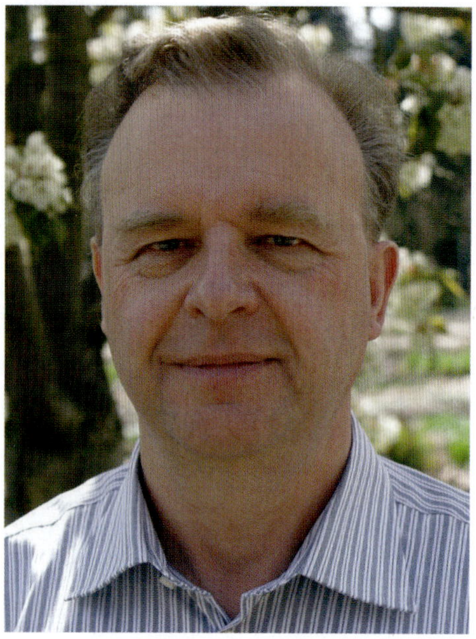

Photo: Kristina Schäfer

Erik Schulte, MD, professor

Institute of Functional and Clinical Anatomy of the Johannes Gutenberg University of Mainz; studied medicine in Freiburg; extensive teaching of medical students; award for excellence in teaching in Mainz.

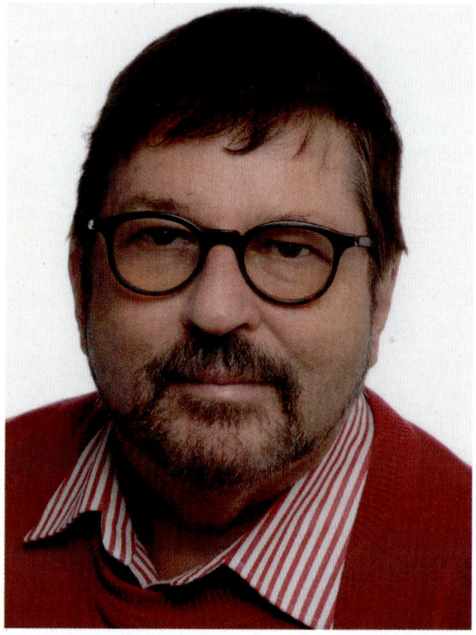

Photo: private

Udo Schumacher, MD, professor

MSB Medical School Berlin; studied medicine in Kiel, and a one-year sojourn at the Wistar Institute of Anatomy and Biology, Philadelphia; intensive experience in teaching medical students, physical therapists, and specialty candidates (FRCS). Spent several years in Southampton and gained experience in integrated interdisciplinary instruction.

It guides the reader through anatomy step by step, revealing what a crucial role anatomy will later play in medical practice. This was a particularly important consideration for the authors. Whether performing bowel surgery for a tumor, puncturing the tympanic membrane in a middle ear infection, or examining a pregnant patient, no physician lacking knowledge of anatomy is a good physician.

Even the *Thieme Atlas of Anatomy* cannot spare you the effort of learning, yet the authors and illustrators can assure you that it will make it a lot more pleasant.

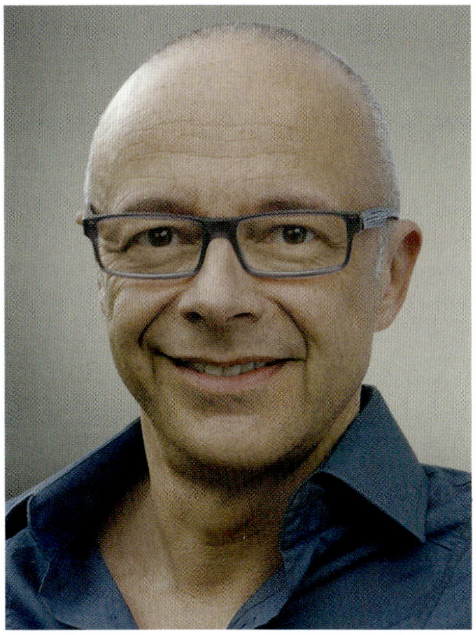

Photo: private

Markus Voll

Freelance illustrator and graphic artist in Munich, trained as an artist at the Blocherer School of Design in Munich, studied medicine at the University of Munich. He has decades of experience as a scientific illustrator for numerous book projects.

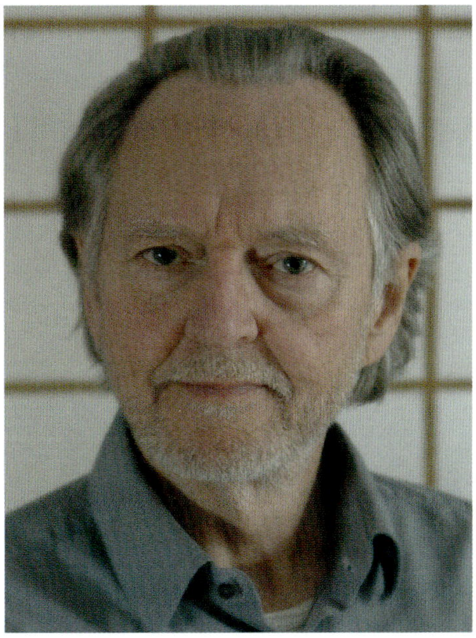

Photo: private

Karl Wesker

Freelance painter and graphic artist in Berlin. Apprenticeship as a plate etcher and lithographer, studied visual communication at the University of Applied Sciences in Münster and at the Berlin University of the Arts and art science at the Technical University of Berlin. He has worked for decades as a freelance painter and graphic scientific artist, including book projects in anatomy.

Contents

A Structure and Development of Organ Systems

B Thorax

C Abdomen and Pelvis

D Neurovascular Supply to the Organs

E Organ Fact Sheets

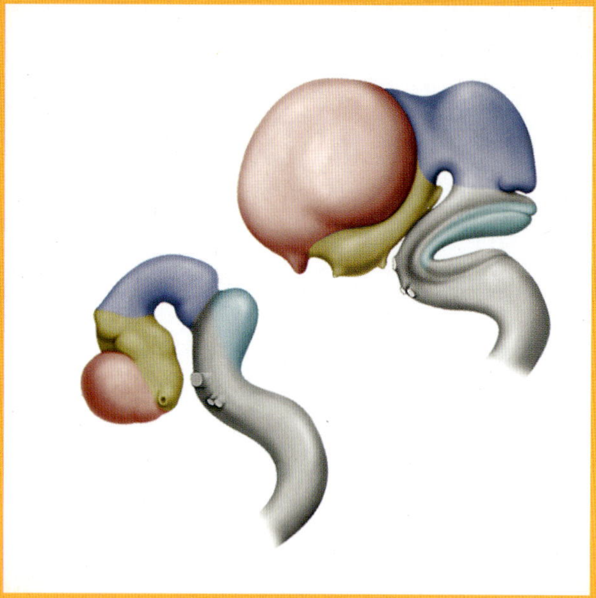

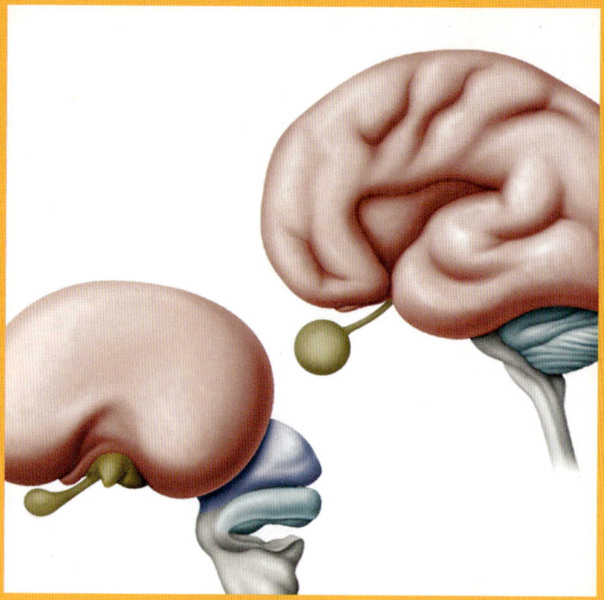

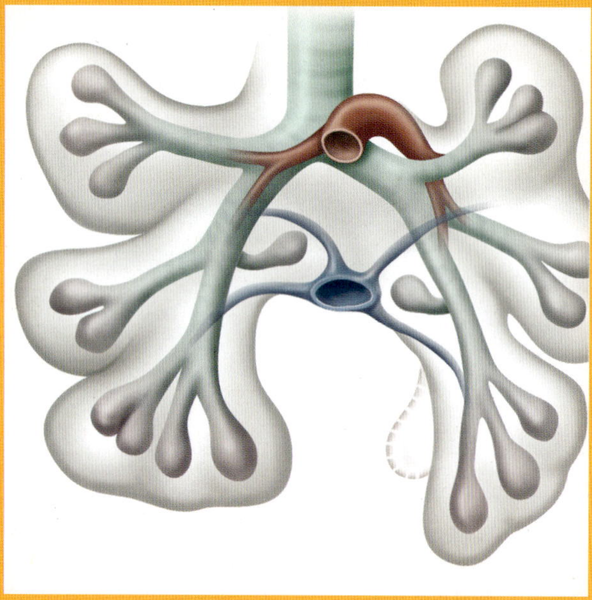

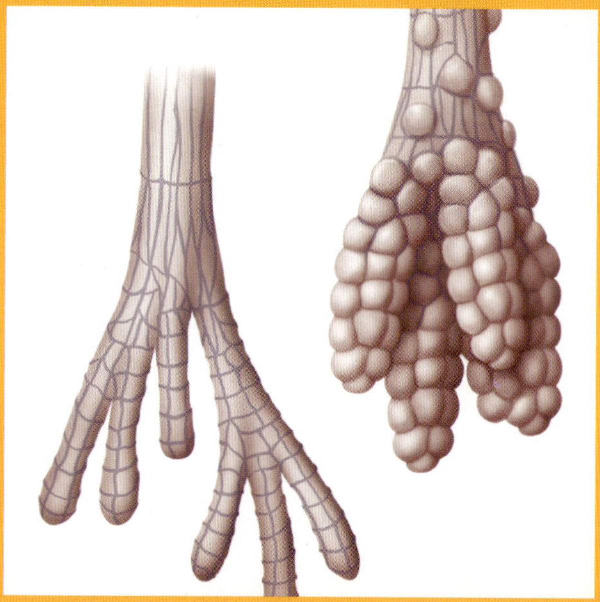

A Structure and Development of Organ Systems

1.1 Definitions, Overview, and Evolution of Body Cavities

Definitions
The human body, similar to all higher organisms, is organized into a hierarchy of different levels:

- A **cell** is the smallest unit of life, that in principal can survive on its own.
- A **tissue** consists primarily of cells from the same origin, and the extracellular matrix they form. A tissue is an ensemble of cells, organized to do a specific job.
- An **organ** is a structural unit composed of different tissues. Thus, it combines the functions of the various tissue components.
- An **organ system** is made up of organs that function together to perform a specific function. For example, the digestive organs make up the *digestive system*. For the most part, the individual organs are related to each other morphologically.
- An **organism** is composed of several organ systems.

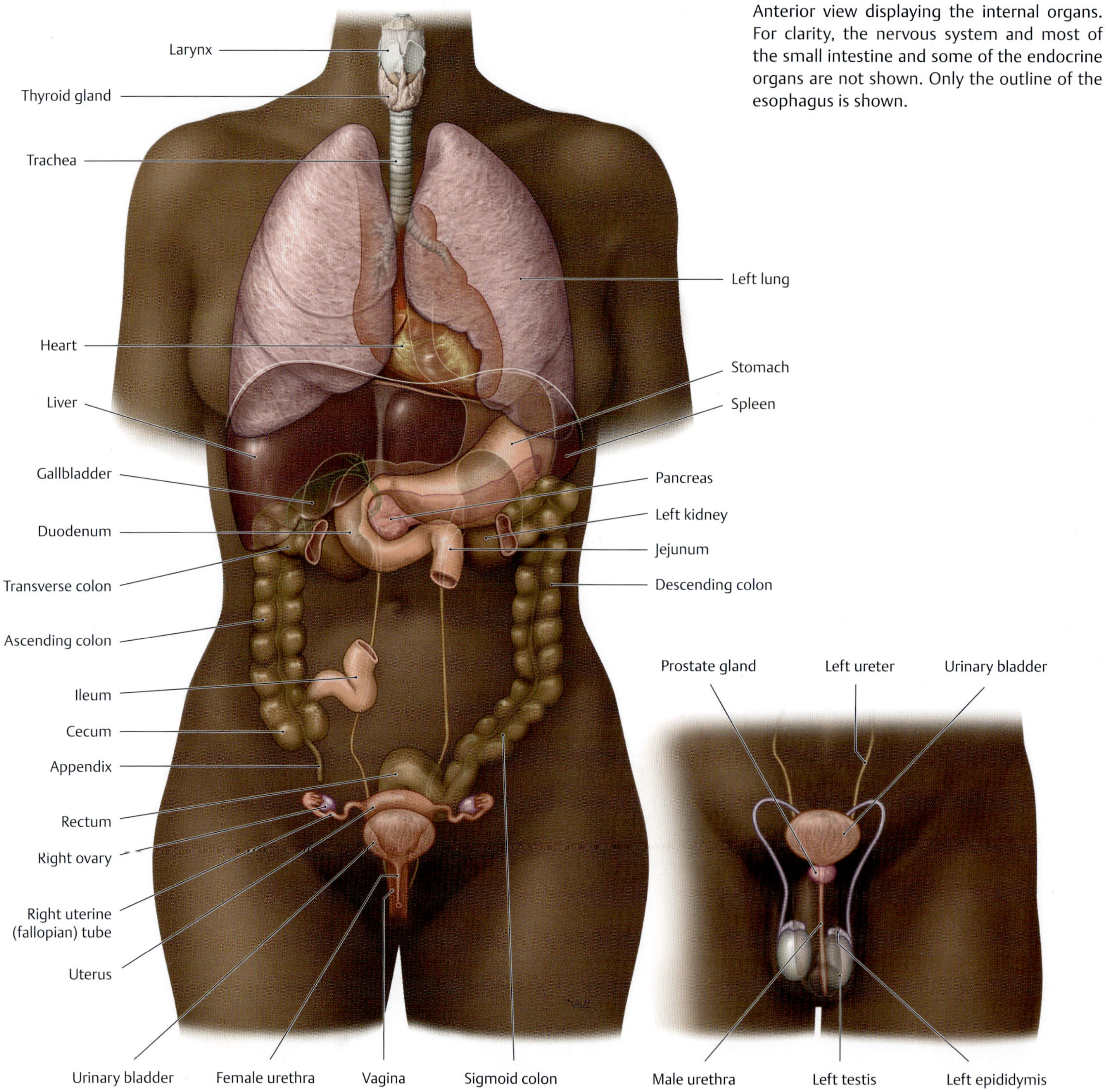

A Overview of the internal organs
Anterior view displaying the internal organs. For clarity, the nervous system and most of the small intestine and some of the endocrine organs are not shown. Only the outline of the esophagus is shown.

B Overview of organ systems

Since, by definition, every structural unit composed of different tissues is referred to as an organ (according to this definition, every muscle is an organ), the term is commonly used for structures in the skull, neck, and body cavities. The organs situated inside the body cavities are referred to as internal organs or viscera. This atlas is a study aid for learning gross anatomy. Thus, the individual organs are discussed with respect to their topography. However, since groups of individual organs form morphological and functional systems, which due to evolutionary processes don't conform to topographical anatomy, those organ systems along with their embryology will be discussed first. This overview will aid in understanding the location, shape and function of the internal organs in the developing organism.

Note: Peripheral nerves, bone marrow, and blood are usually not referred to as "organs." For the sake of completeness, they will also be discussed since they are part of whole organ systems.

* Organs that are highlighted in italics are located in the neck or skull and thus will not be discussed here.

System	Organs*
Digestive system	*Oral cavity with teeth and salivary glands, pharynx,* esophagus, stomach, small intestine, large intestine, rectum, pancreas, liver, and gallbladder
Respiratory system	*Nasal cavity and paranasal sinuses, larynx,* trachea, lungs
Urinary system	Kidneys, ureters, bladder, urethra
Reproductive system	♀ Uterus, uterine tubes, ovary, vagina, Bartholin's glands ♂ Testicles, epididymis, ductus deferens, seminal vesicles, prostate, Cowper's gland
Circulatory system	Heart, vessels, blood, *and bone marrow*
Immune system	*Bone marrow, tonsils,* thymus, spleen, lymph nodes, thoracic duct
Endocrine system	*Thyroid, parathyroid glands,* suprarenal (adrenal) glands, paraganglia, pancreas (islet cells), ovaries, testicles, *pituitary gland, hypothalamus*
Nervous system	*Brain, spinal cord,* peripheral nervous system (with *somatic* and autonomic components)

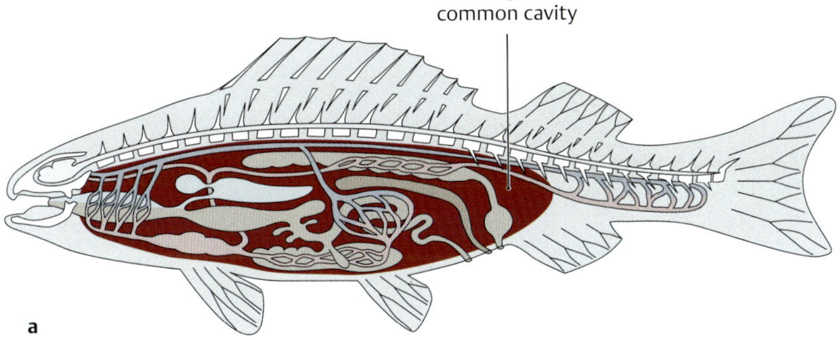

a

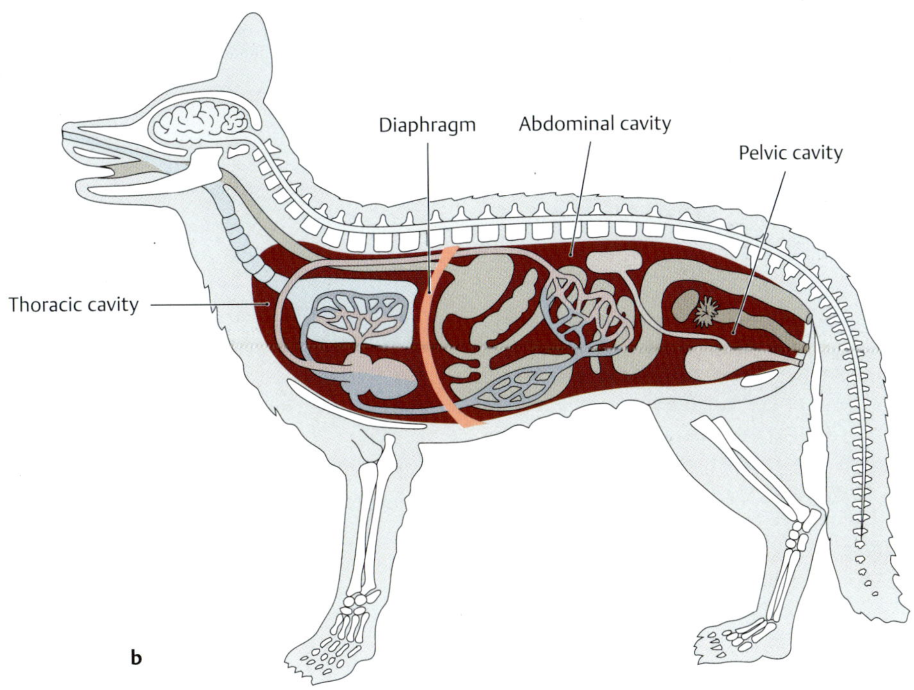

b

C Evolution of body cavities

While in fish (**a**) all internal organs are situated in a single common body cavity, in mammals (**b**), the diaphragm separates the thoracic cavity from the abdominal cavity. Due to shared evolutionary history, the structures of these two body cavities are basically identical. The different anatomical terms used for similar structures (e.g., pleura – peritoneum) are functionally meaningless. In mammals, there is no physical structure that separates the abdominal cavity from the pelvic cavity. They form a continuous space that in terms of Its topographical anatomy is divided only by the superior border of the bony pelvis. The anatomical unit of the abdominal and pelvic cavities is of clinical significance as there are no anatomical barriers to restrict the spread of inflammation or tumors between these two compartments. The diaphragm acts as a barrier to stop tumors or inflammation from spreading from the abdominal to the thoracic cavity and vice versa.

1.2 Organogenesis and the Development of Body Cavities

A Differentiation of the germ layers

After the formation of the trilaminar embryonic disc at the end of the third week (see **B**) the primordia (precursor cells destined to become a specific tissue or organ) of the different tissues and organs are arranged according to the body plan. In the subsequent embryonic period (weeks 4 to 8), the three germ layers (ectoderm, mesoderm, and endoderm) give rise to all major external and internal organs (organogenesis). At the same time, the trilaminar embryonic disc begins to fold, resulting in major changes in body form and internal structure. By the end of the embryonic stage, the major features of the body are recognizable and the organs have moved into their eventual position within and outside of the body cavities.

Germ layer	Primordium		Derivatives
Ectoderm	Neural tube		Brain, retina, spinal cord
	Neural crest	Neural crest of the head	Sensory and parasympathetic ganglia, intramural nervous system of the bowel, parafollicular cells, smooth muscle, pigment cells, carotid body, bone, cartilage, connective tissue, dentin and cementum of the teeth, dermis, and subcutaneous tissue of the head
		Neural crest of the trunk	Sensory and autonomic ganglia, peripheral glia, suprarenal medulla, pigment cells, intramural plexuses
	Surface ectoderm	Ectodermal placodes	Anterior pituitary, cranial sensory ganglia, olfactory epithelium, inner ear, lens
			Enamel of the teeth, epithelium of the oral cavity, salivary glands, nasal cavities, paranasal sinuses, lacrimal passages, external auditory canal, epidermis, hair, nails, cutaneous glands
Mesoderm	Axial	Notochord, prechordal mesoderm	Extraocular muscles
	Paraxial		Spinal column, ribs, skeletal muscle, connective tissue, dermis and subcutis of the back and part of the head, smooth muscle, blood vessels
	Intermediate		Kidneys, gonads, renal and genital excretory ducts
	Lateral plate mesoderm	Visceral (splanchnopleure)	Heart, blood vessels, smooth muscle, bowel wall, blood, suprarenal cortex, visceral serosa
		Parietal (somatopleure)	Sternum, limbs (cartilage, bones, and ligaments), dermis and subcutaneous tissue of the anterolateral body wall, smooth muscle, connective tissue, parietal serosa
Endoderm			Epithelium of the bowel, respiratory tract, digestive glands, pharyngeal glands, pharyngotympanic (auditory) tube, tympanic cavity, urinary bladder, thymus, parathyroid glands, thyroid gland

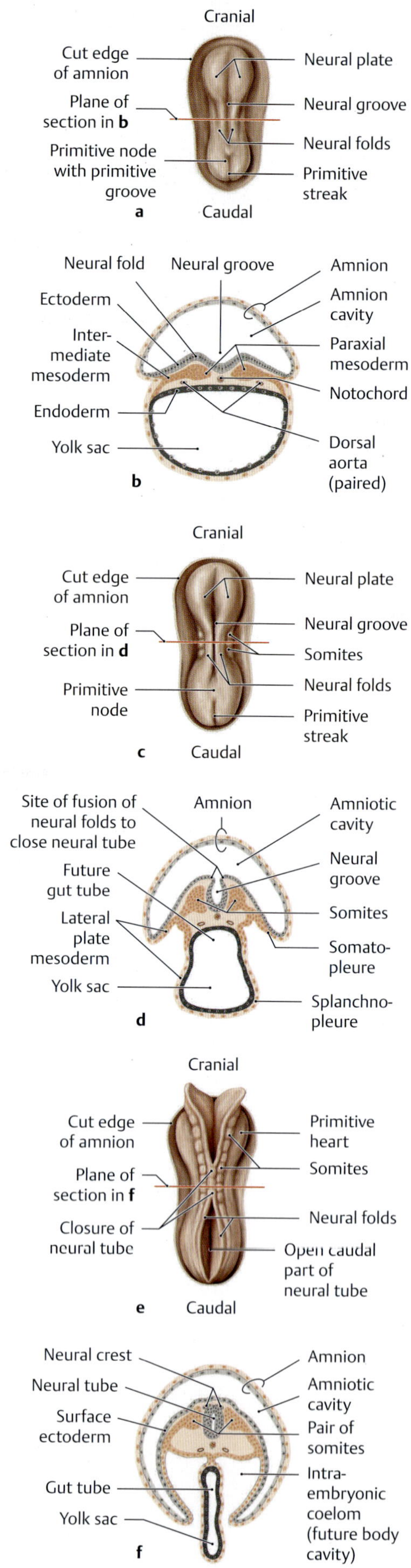

B Neurulation and Somite Formation

a, c, and **e** Dorsal views of the embryonic disc after removal of the amnion;
b, d, and **f** Schematic cross-sections of the corresponding stages at the planes of section as marked in **a, c,** and **e**; Age is in postovulatory days.
During neurulation (formation of the neural tube from the neural plate), the neuroectoderm differentiates from the surface ectoderm, due to inductive influences from the notochord, and the neural tube and neural crest cells move inside the embryo.

a and **b** Embryonic disc at 19 days: The neural groove is developing in the area of the neural plate.

c and **d** Embryonic disc at 20 days: In the paraxial mesoderm, flanking both sides of the neural groove and notochord, the first somites have formed (they contain cellular material assigned to form the spinal column, muscles, and subcutaneous tissue). Immediately lateral to the paraxial mesoderm is the intermediate mesoderm, and lateral to that is the lateral plate mesoderm. The neural groove is beginning to close to form the neural tube and the embryo begins to fold.

e and **f** Embryonic disc at 22 days: Eight pairs of somites are seen flanking the partially closed neural tube which is sinking below the ectoderm. In the lateral plate mesoderm, the intraembryonic coelom, or future body cavity, arises. It will later develop both a parietal and a visceral layer (somatopleure and splanchnopleure). On the side facing the coelom, a mesothelial lining develops from the somato- and splanchnopleure. It later forms the serous membranes lining the pericardial, pleural, and peritoneal cavities. The neural tube migrates deeper into the mesoderm, and the somites differentiate into sclerotome, myotome, and dermatome.

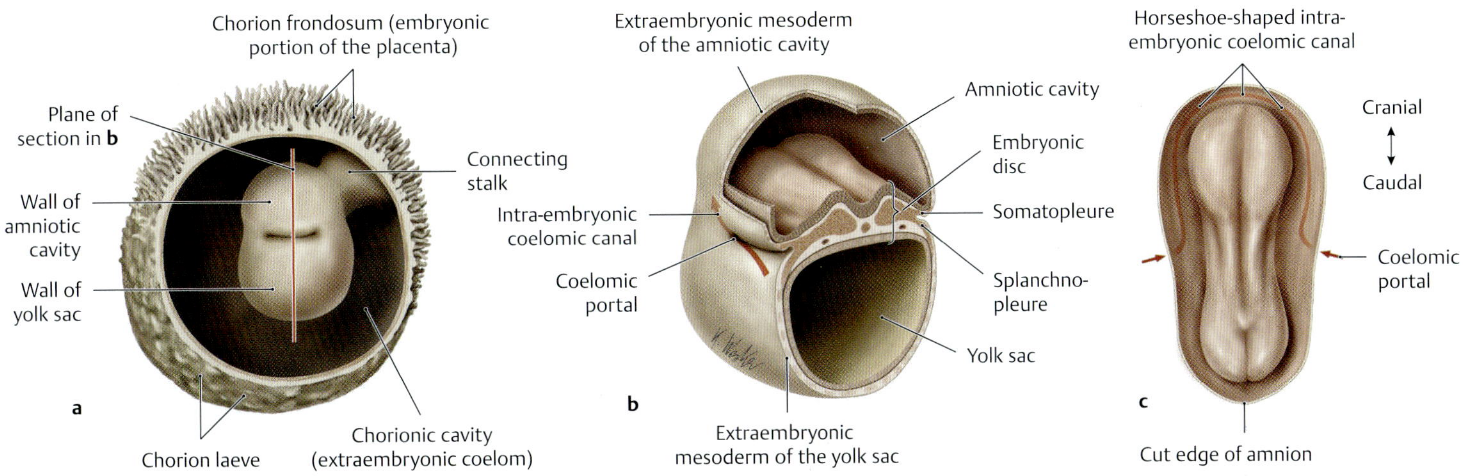

C Formation of the intraembryonic coelom

a View into the chorionic cavity (extraembryonic coelom); **b** Cut through the amnionic cavity, embryonic disc and yolk sac (the chorionic cavity has been removed); **c** View of the embryonic disc (the intraembryonic coelomic canal has been highlighted in red).

The eventual definitive serous cavities (pericardial, pleural, and peritoneal) arise from the intraembryonic coelom which begins to form in week 4 when intercellular clefts (not shown) appear in the lateral plate mesoderm (see **B**). The intraembryonic coelom divides the lateral plate mesoderm into parietal and visceral layers (*somatopleure* and *splanchnopleure*). At the edges of the embryonic disc, the somatopleure adjacent to the surface ectoderm is continuous with the extraembryonic mesoderm of the amnion. The splanchnopleure adjacent to the endoderm is continuous with the extraembryonic mesoderm of the yolk sac. Thus, the intraembryonic coelom surrounds the opening of the yolk sac like a ring (the *coelomic ring*). In the cranial part of the embryo, the coelomic ring closes off from the extraembryonic coelom (chorionic cavity) and forms a horseshoe shaped intraembryonic *coelomic canal*, which is visible when viewed from above. The caudal intra- and extraembryonic coeloms (see **D**) continue to communicate with one another through the *coelomic portals*. Later, as a result of embryonic folding, the caudal intra- and extraembryonic coeloms become separated from each other. During the course of embryonic development, the intraembryonic coelom compartmentalizes with the pericardial cavity arising from the unpaired cranial part of the coelom and the paired pleural and peritoneal cavities arising from the lateral limbs of the coelom.

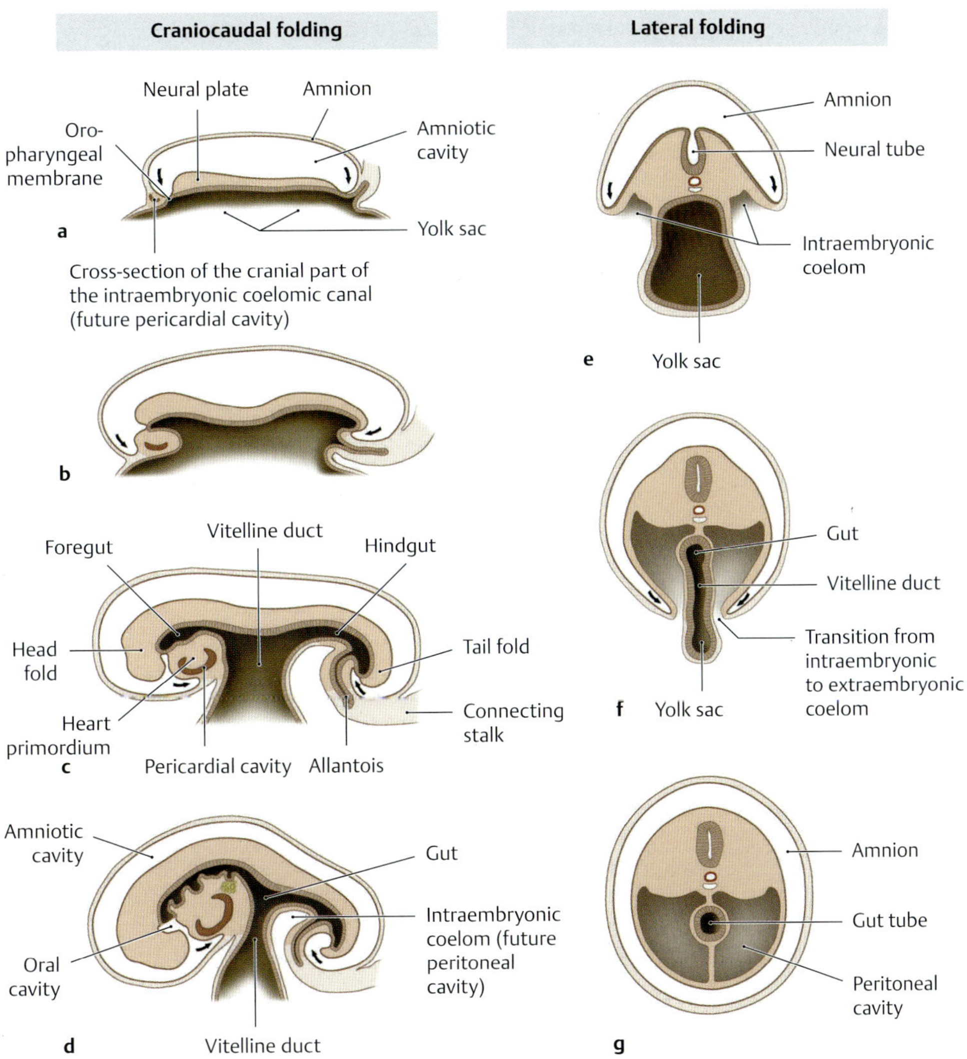

D Embryonic folding

a–d Midsagittal sections; **e–g** Frontal sections at the level of the yolk sac.

During folding the embryo is rapidly growing and it rises up from the surface of the original disc. The neural plate grows rapidly and extends in both the cranial and caudal directions. As a result, the embryo curves upon itself (**a–d**). The formation of somites causes a lateral expansion (lateral folding) of the embryo in the area above the yolk sac (**e–g**). As a result, the intraembryonic coelomic canal shifts ventrally. Due to cranial folding (head fold), the cranial portion of the intraembryonic coelom moves ventral to the foregut and broadens into the pericardial cavity. The folding of the caudal tail moves the connecting stalk (the future umbilical cord) and the allantois to the ventral aspect of the embryo. While lateral folding occurs, the intraembryonic coelom progressively separates from the extraembryonic coelom. These processes result in the junction between embryonic endoderm (primitive gut tube) and yolk sac (future yolk stalk) becoming increasingly narrow. At the same time, the left and right caudal parts of the intraembryonic coelom merge with one another forming a single large coelomic cavity, which is the future peritoneal cavity (for position of pleural cavities see p. 6).

1.3 Compartmentalization of the Intraembryonic Coelom

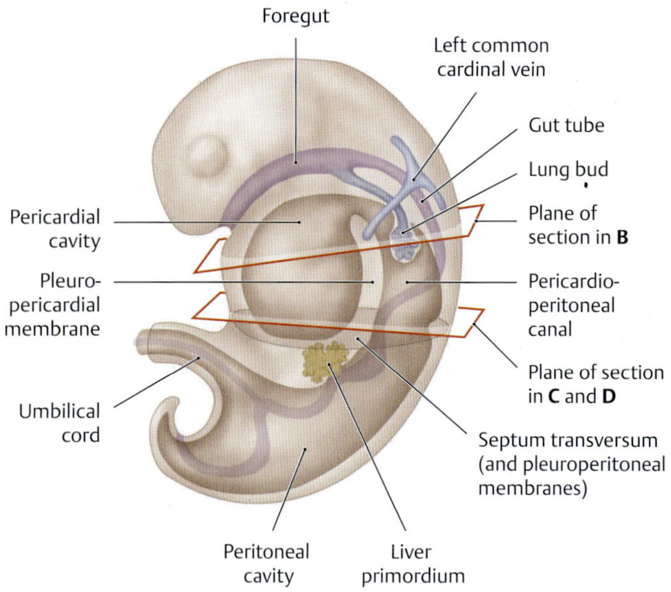

A Overview of the compartmentalization of the intraembryonic coelom

Embryo at 4 weeks (viewed from left side).

Due to cranial folding, the cranial portion of the intraembryonic coelom moves ventral to the foregut and broadens into the pericardial cavity. The pericardial cavity flanking the gut tube communicates with the caudally located peritoneal cavity through the pericardioperitoneal canals. The still unfolded parts of the future peritoneal cavity initially open laterally into the chorionic cavity. The lung buds, which push from the gut tube into the pericardioperitoneal canals, grow into the future paired pleural cavities. Through the formation of partitions, the pleural cavities separate from both the pericardial cavity (pleuropericardial membranes or folds) and the peritoneal cavity (septum transversum and pleuroperitoneal membranes or folds) (see **B**). In the frontal plane the pleuropericardial folds originate on the craniolateral side of the two pericardioperitoneal canals in the area surrounding the common cardinal veins. They fuse with the mesoderm located ventral to the gut tube (the future esophagus). The pleuroperitoneal folds develop in the caudolateral wall of the pericardioperitoneal canals and, together with the dorsal mesentery of the esophagus and the septum transversum, form the future diaphragm (see **D**).

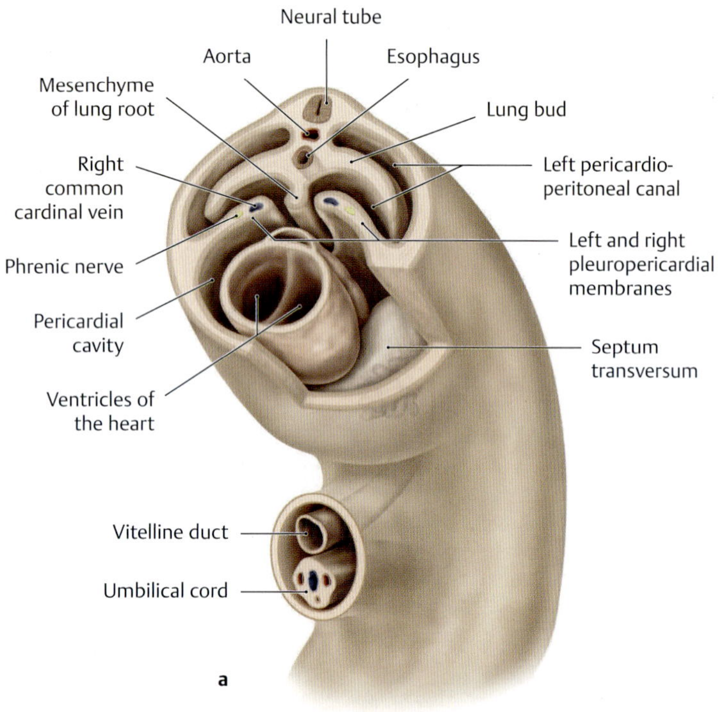

B Separation of the pericardial cavity from the pleural cavities

Embryo at 5 weeks. Frontal section at the level of the future pericardial cavity; for plane of section see **A**.

In the 5th week, at the junction between the unpaired pericardial cavity and the two pericardioperitoneal canals, two thin mesoderm folds (pleuropericardial folds), coming from the lateral direction, grow toward one another. They contain the trunks of the common cardinal veins and the phrenic nerves. The pleural cavities form as a result of the lung buds growing into the pericardioperitoneal canals (see p. 36, development of the lungs). In the course of further development, the pleural cavities further expand and become separate from the pericardial cavity. The separation is complete once both of the pleuropericardial folds have fused with the mesenchyme at the root of the lungs. The anterior cardinal veins merge to form the superior vena cava; and the two pleuropericardial folds give rise to the future fibrous pericardium (see p. 14, development of the heart).

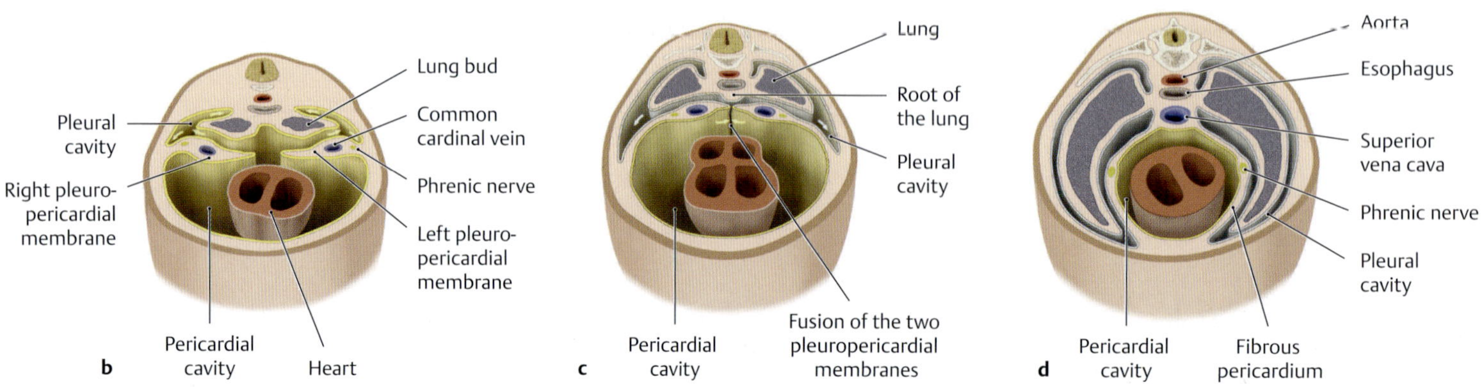

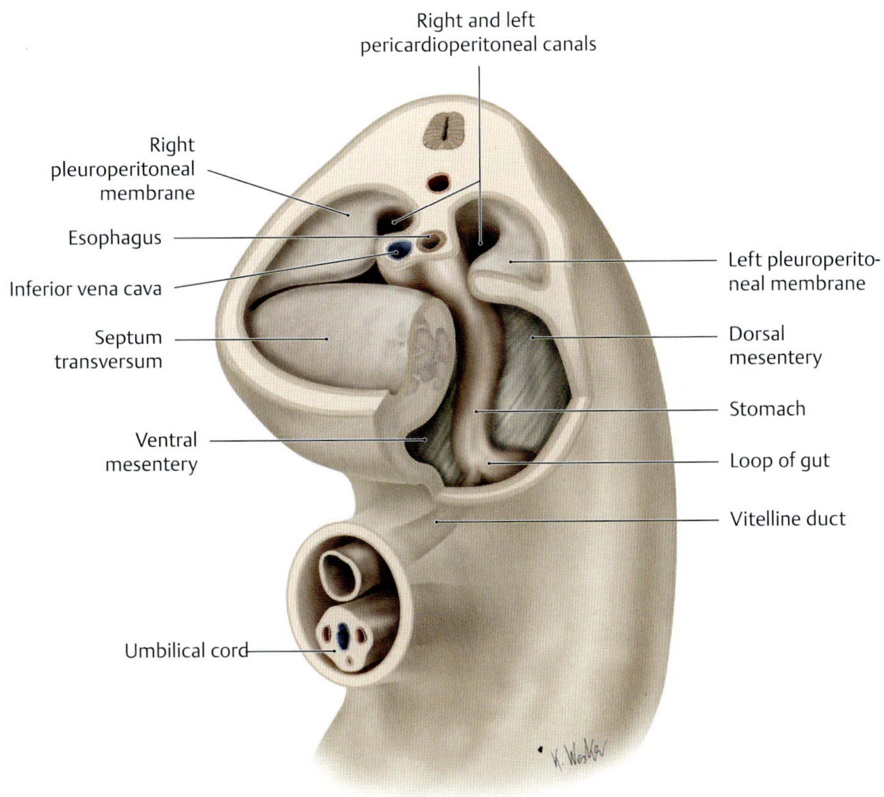

C Separation of the pleural cavities from the peritoneal cavity

After the pleural cavities have separated from the pericardial cavity, they are still temporarily connected to the peritoneal cavity through the pericardioperitoneal canals. They become completely sealed off by the end of the 7th week with the development of the diaphragm, which is formed from several different structures (see **D**). Faulty closure of the pericardioperitoneal canals can lead to a *congenital diaphragmatic hernia* (e.g., Bochdalek hernia) allowing abdominal viscera to enter into the pleural cavities.

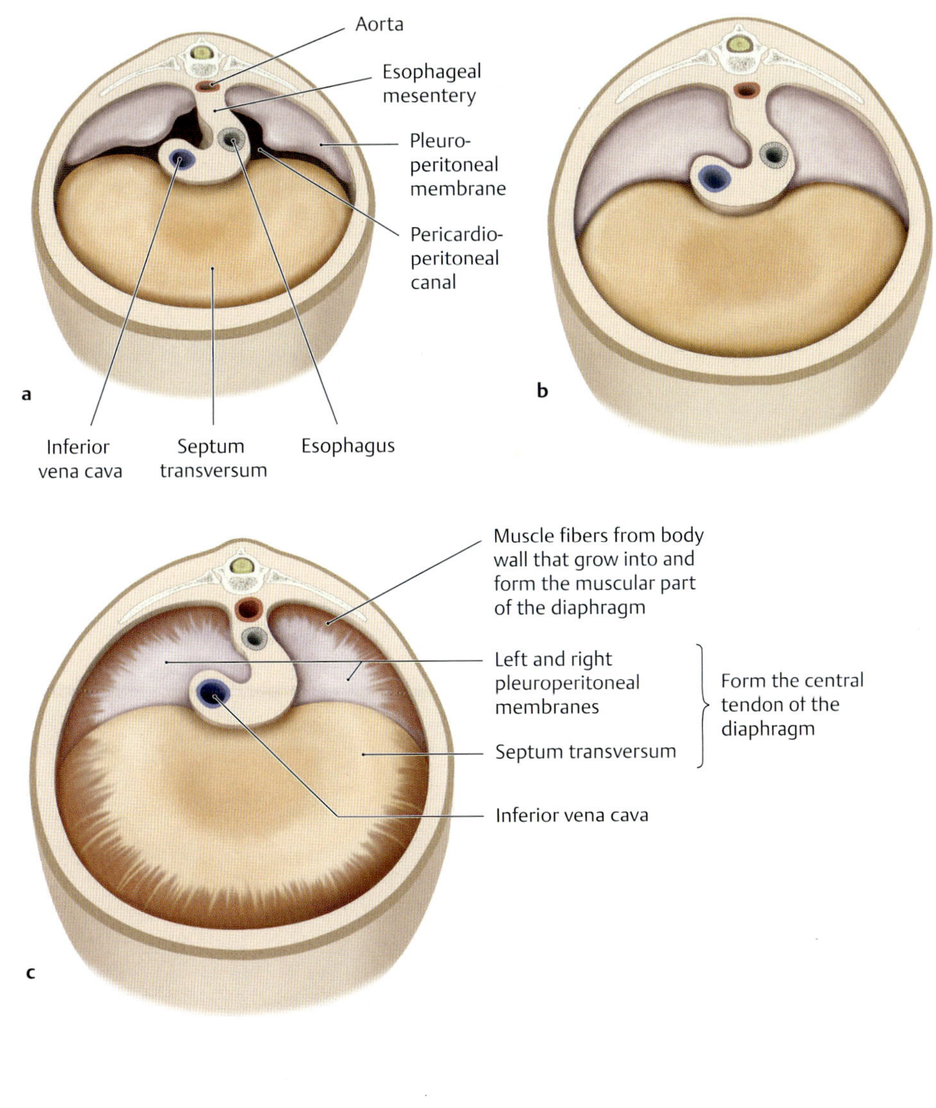

D Development of the diaphragm

The diaphragm is derived from four different structures:

- the septum transversum
- the left and right pleuroperitoneal folds
- the dorsal mesentery of the esophagus
- body wall musculature

In the 4th week the septum transversum develops as a thick mesenchymal plate in the area between the pericardial cavity and yolk stalk. In the 6th week, the septum transversum moves caudally (**a**). The liver forms in the ventral mesentery directly below it. During further development, the septum transversum fuses with both of the pleuroperitoneal folds and forms the future *central tendon* (**b**). The dorsal mesentery of the esophagus and the adjacent body wall musculature give rise to the muscular part of the diaphragm (**c**).

Note: The phrenic nerves (C3, C4 and C5), located in the pleuropericardial folds directly next to the trunks of the common cardinal veins, provide motor innervation to the diaphragm. The striated muscle of the diaphragm (from somites), as well as the septum transversum, are originally from cervical regions. This explains why the nerve supply to the diaphragm (the phrenic nerves) comes from cervical spinal cord levels.

1.4 Organization and Architecture of Body Cavities

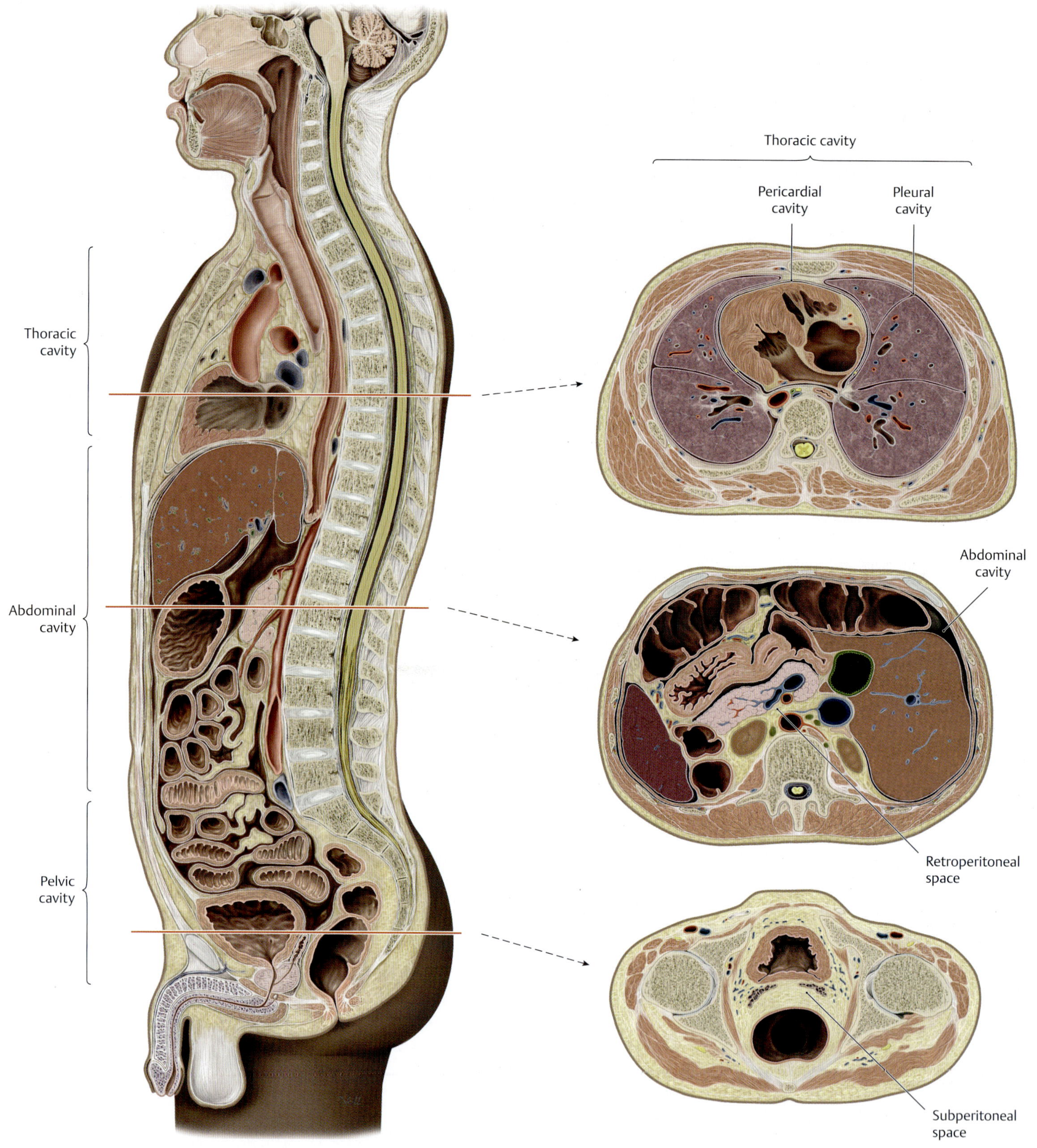

A Organization of the body cavities
Midsagittal section, viewed from the left side. Three large body cavities can be identified. From the top down they are as follows:

- thoracic cavity
- abdominal cavity
- pelvic cavity

These body cavities are completely surrounded by parts of the body wall. The majority of the walls consists of muscle and connective tissue. In addition, the thorax is surrounded by ribs, and the pelvis by the pelvic bone. At its upper end, the connective tissue space of the thoracic cavity is continuous with the connective tissue space of the neck. The pelvic floor muscles close off the inferior pelvic aperture. Depending on their location in one of the three cavities, organs are referred to as thoracic, abdominal or pelvic organs (see **C**).

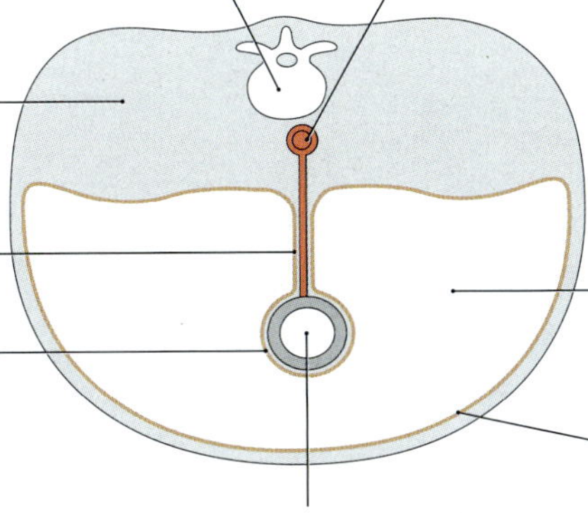

B Structure of the body cavities
Highly schematic cross-section of a human body; superior view. Every body cavity can be divided into two differently structured spaces:

- A **hollow space**: A smooth, moist epithelial layer, the serous membrane or serosa, lines the inner wall of the cavity and the adjacent outer wall of the organs. The portion of the serosa that covers the organ is called the *visceral layer* (viscera refers to internal organ). The portion lining the walls of the cavity is called the *parietal layer* (parietal refers to wall). The organs located in the cavity are movable. They are attached to the connective tissue space (see below) by a connective tissue bridge covered by a serous membrane (a mesentery).
- A **connective tissue space** within which run the pathways leading to and from the organ. Organs situated in these spaces are surrounded by connective tissue and are more or less immovable.

While this general structure applies to all three body cavities, the terms for the individual regions vary (see **C**):

- In the **thorax**, most of the connective tissue is located in the central compartment of the thoracic cavity, the mediastinum, in which the pericardial cavity (a hollow space lined with a serous membrane) is embedded. The pleural cavities are located lateral to the mediastinum.
- In the **abdomen**, the connective tissue is situated behind the peritoneal cavity in the retroperitoneal space (an extraperitoneal space).
- In the **pelvis**, the connective tissue is situated both behind and below the peritoneal cavity in the retroperitoneal and subperitoneal spaces (extraperitoneal spaces).

Correspondingly, all organs in the thorax, abdomen, and pelvis can be organized according to their location in the connective tissue space or in one of the serous-membrane lined cavities (see **C**).
Note: While the partition between the thoracic and abdominal cavities is clearly defined by the diaphragm, the separation between the abdominal and pelvic cavities is often only demarcated by bony reference points on the body wall. Thus, the abdominal and pelvic cavities essentially remain a single cavity, and therefore form a single region where disease processes can spread from one cavity to the other.
A mesentery is a layer of connective tissue covered by peritoneum. Within it run the organ's neurovascular supply (blood and lymph vessels, nerves). With reference to organs, the mesentery is often identified with the prefix "meso" (e.g., transverse mesocolon).

C Spaces and body cavities and their respective organs in the thorax, abdomen, and pelvis

Body cavity and the organs it contains	Serous cavities and the organs they contain	Serous membrane	Connective tissue spaces and their embedded organs
Thoracic cavity (thorax) Thoracic organs	• Paired pleural cavities with lungs: *Intrapleural organs* • Pericardial cavity with heart: *Intrapericardial organ*	• Visceral and parietal pleura • Visceral and parietal pericardium	• Mediastinum (middle section of the thoracic cavity) between the pleural cavities as well as behind the unpaired pericardial cavity with the mediastinal organs: esophagus, trachea, and thymus as well as vessels and nerves: – *Mediastinal organs*
Abdominal cavity (abdomen) Abdominal organs	• Abdominal peritoneal cavity with stomach, parts of the small and large intestine, spleen, liver, gallbladder and cecum with vermiform appendix: *Intraperitoneal organs*	• Visceral and parietal peritoneum	• Extraperitoneal space behind the abdominal peritoneal cavity (retroperitoneal) with kidneys, ureters, pancreas and parts of the duodenum, large intestine, and rectum: – *Extraperitoneal organs*
Pelvic cavity (pelvis) Pelvic organs	• Pelvic peritoneal cavity with fundus and body of uterus, ovaries, uterine tubes and upper rectum: *Intraperitoneal organs*	• Visceral and parietal peritoneum	• Extraperitoneal spaces behind and below the pelvic peritoneal cavity (retroperitoneal and subperitoneal) with urinary bladder and adjacent portions of the ureters, prostate, seminal vesicles, uterine cervix, vagina, and parts of the rectum: – *Extraperitoneal organs*

2.1 Overview and Basic Wall Structure

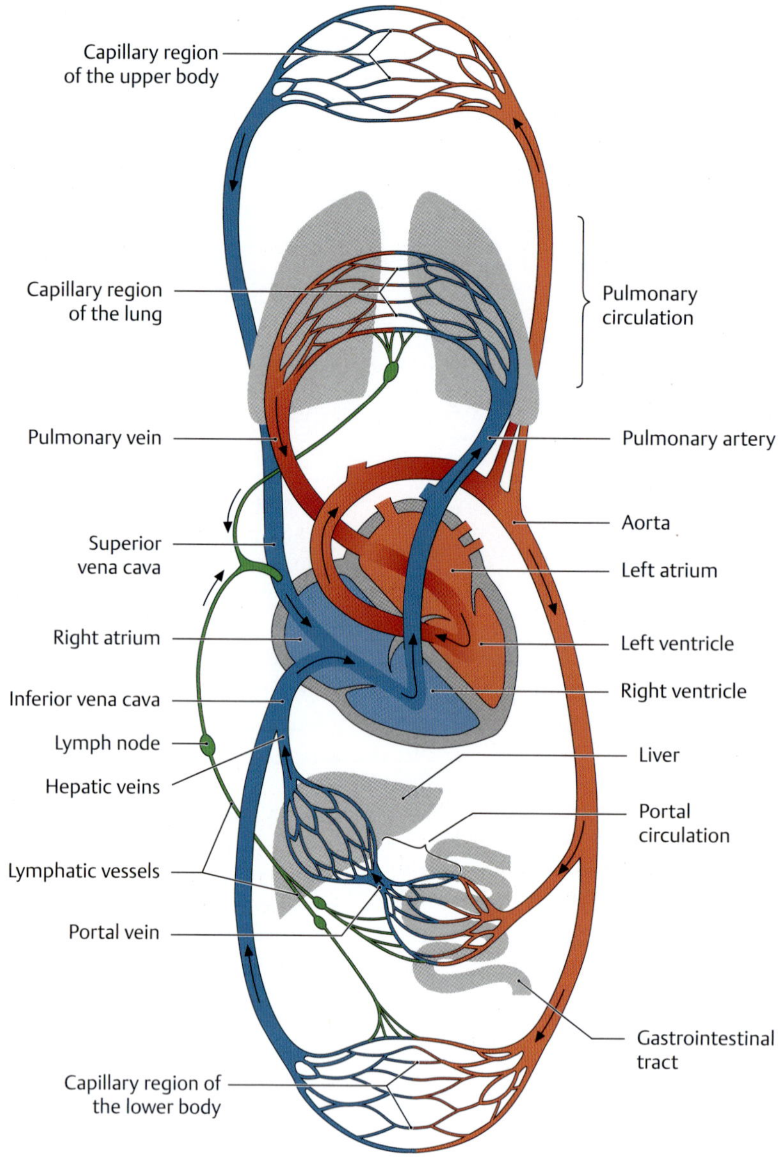

A Overview of the cardiovascular system

The **cardiovascular system** is a closed system of vessels through which the blood is transported. This circulation is necessary to supply the organs with oxygen, nutrients, and hormones and to carry carbon dioxide and other metabolic waste products away to the excretory organs. Additionally, cells and proteins of the immune system travel through the bloodstream. Using blood as a transport medium, they "patrol" the body by constantly looking out for pathogens. The blood can also transport heat, so that circulation helps to regulate body temperature. In addition to these functions, the blood also helps to seal off leaks. It contains clotting factors that are activated when vessels gets damaged. The circulation is powered by the heart which functions as a pressure pump.

The circulatory system can be divided into two main circuits:

- the systemic circulation (high-pressure system, average blood pressure of 100mmHg in the major arteries) and
- the pulmonary circulation (low-pressure system, average blood pressure of 12mmHg; the difference in pressure from the systemic circulation is almost a factor of 10).

Regarding the vessels and pump, both circulatory systems can be divided into four parts:

- arteries and arterioles: they lead away from the heart and distribute blood to the organs
- capillaries: they connect arterioles to venules and enable the exchange of substances in organs
- venules and veins: receive blood from the capillaries and carry it back to the heart
- heart: functions as a circulation pump and transports the blood back to the arteries

The **lymphatic system** is an additional vascular system that carries fluid away from the organs. It begins with lymphatic capillaries in the organs and transports lymph back to the venous system.

Note: A vessel is designated an "artery" or "vein" solely according to the direction of blood flow. In this book, arteries are usually shown in red and veins usually in blue. However, figure **A** depicts blood oxygenation regardless of the direction of flow and shows *oxygenated* blood in red and *deoxygenated* blood in blue to illustrate the transport of oxygen. Hence, in the diagram, the pulmonary artery contains oxygen-low blood (blue), while the pulmonary vein contains oxygen-rich blood (red).

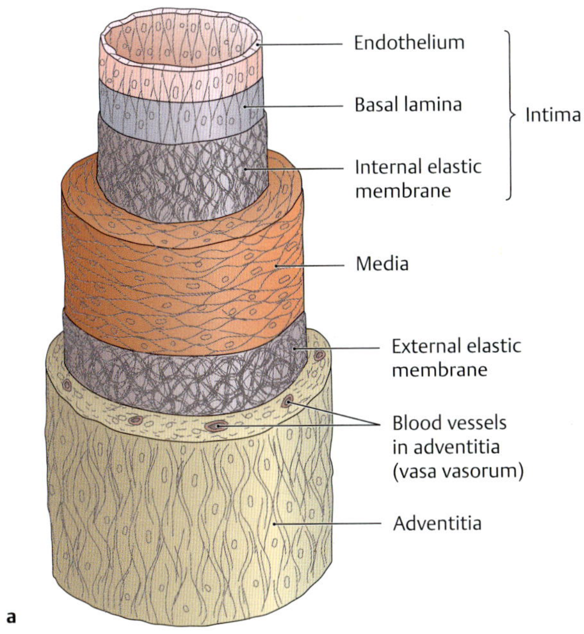

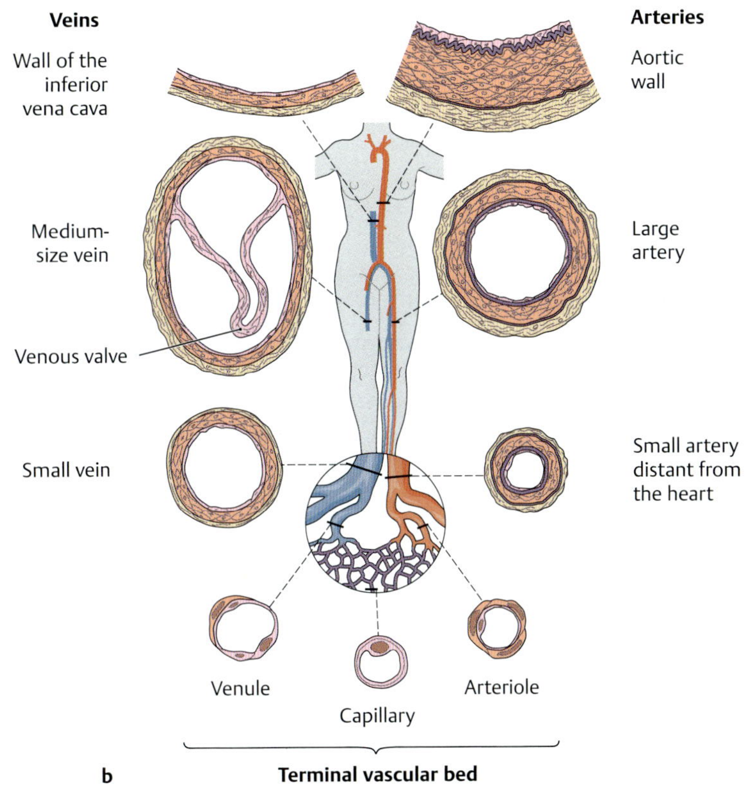

B Basic wall structure of large blood vessels

a The major blood vessels (arteries and veins) generally consist of three layers:

- The tunica intima (intima): an endothelium consisting of a single layer of squamous epithelial cells, with the cells elongated in the direction of blood flow, and a thin a layer of subendothelial connective tissue
- The tunica media (media): consisting of a circular arrangement of smooth muscle cells, and elastic fibers of the *internal* elastic membrane (which separates the intima from the media) and *external* elastic membrane (which separates the media from the adventitia)
- The tunica adventitia (adventitia): consisting mainly of loose connective tissue, which integrates the blood vessel into its surroundings and allows for movement of vessels with organ movements. It can contain blood and lymphatic vessels as well as nerves.

b (from Frick/Leonhardt/Starck) While veins have a similar three-layered structure as arteries, they have fewer and less dense layers of smooth muscle cells, giving the media of veins a looser structure. These structural characteristics are the result of lower venous blood pressure compared to arterial blood pressure. The peripheral veins in limbs contain valves to help direct blood flow back to the heart. The small exchange vessels, the capillaries, have no muscle tissue and consist only of endothelium and basement membrane.

C Blood pressure in different regions of the cardiovascular system (from Siegenthaler)

The function and structure of the cardiovascular system are closely interconnected, as higher blood pressure leads to the thickening of blood vessel walls and lower blood pressure allows walls to thin. Thus, knowledge of blood pressures is important when interpreting morphology. In the heart and major arteries closest to the heart, blood pressure fluctuates substantially with each cardiac cycle. While blood pressure in the left ventricle reaches 120 mmHg during systole, during diastole it drops to 0 mmHg. Due to the vessel wall properties of the arteries close to the heart, blood pressure fluctuations in them during the cardiac cycle are less extreme. Resistance vessels further help regulation so that capillary pressure remains constant. Pressure is lowest in the central veins closest to the heart. Because of their thin walls, they can expand and store blood.

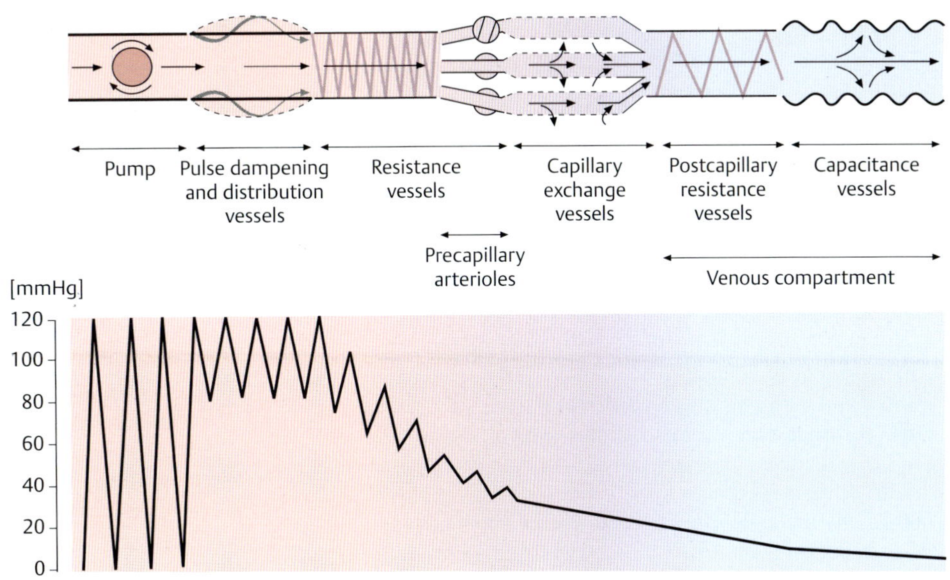

Note: The different regions of the vascular system are assigned specific functions, which are described in the illustration above.

2.2 Terminal Vessels and Overview of the Major Blood Vessels

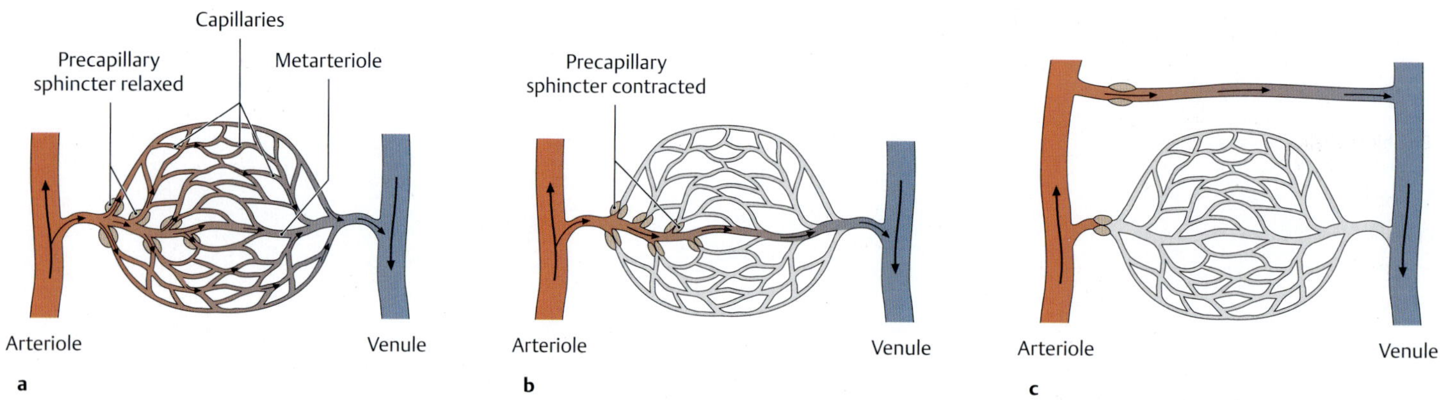

A Terminal vessels

a The primary function of the arteries and veins is to transport blood. Terminal vessels are concerned with the exchange of substances between blood and tissue. This is often called the *microcirculation*. The terminal vascular bed consists of

- Arterioles
- Capillaries
- Venules

b It is important to point out that capillary perfusion can vary within organs. Precapillary sphincters, which consist of smooth muscle cells, help to regulate perfusion in *one* capillary. Terminal vessel perfusion within a specific organ is related to the organ's function and varies from organ to organ.

c Additionally, arteriovenous anastomoses help regulate the circulation in a group of neighboring capillaries that have formed one functional unit. Thus, entire capillary beds can be shut down. Disruption of the fine regulation of the microcirculation is a major problem when patients go into shock because blood can pool in capillaries.

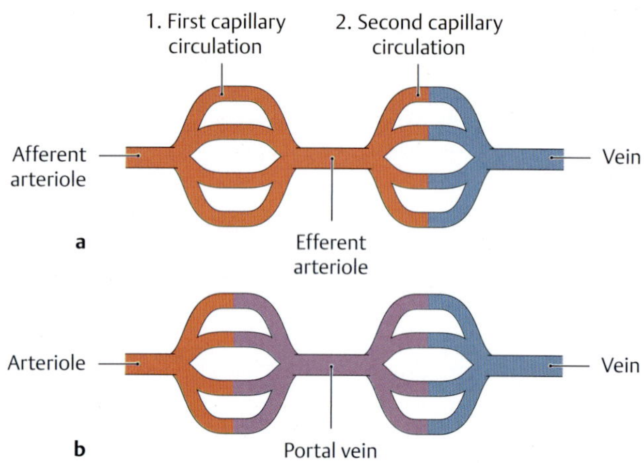

B Vascular relationships

In addition to the above mentioned descriptions of typical organ circulation: artery – capillary – vein, there are additional blood flow patterns in some organs.

a Flow of arterial blood through two serially connected capillary beds: Two serially connected capillary beds are found in the kidney where arterial blood initially flows through the renal corpuscles (glomeruli) and then into the capillaries of the renal medulla.

b Flow through two venous circuits (portal venous system): Venous blood flowing through two serially connected capillary beds is known as a portal venous system. For clarification, the blood in the first capillary bed is colored purple because it is not yet completely deoxygenated. Such a portal venous system exists in the digestive tract, where the portal vein collects the venous blood from the unpaired abdominal organs (stomach, intestines, spleen). From there it flows to the capillaries of the liver.

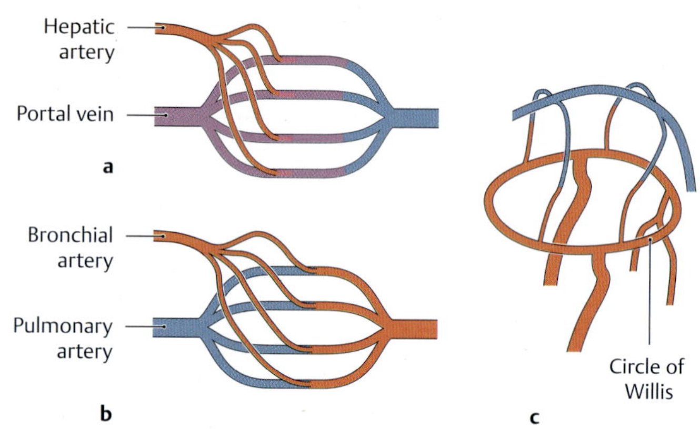

C Dual organ circulation

The liver receives its blood supply from the hepatic artery and the hepatic portal vein (**a**). The vessel responsible for suppling oxygenated blood to the liver tissue is the hepatic artery. The vessel that contains the blood with the substances to be metabolized in the liver is the portal vein. The **lungs** also have a dual arterial supply (**b**). Here, the pulmonary arteries contain deoxygenated blood and the bronchial arteries contain oxygenated blood. Another pattern of multiple blood supply can be found in the **brain**. Four arteries form a closed ring (the circle of Willis) from which other vessels supply the brain (**c**). All three forms of blood supply through multiple vessels allow for a certain degree of compensation in case one of the supplying vessels fails.

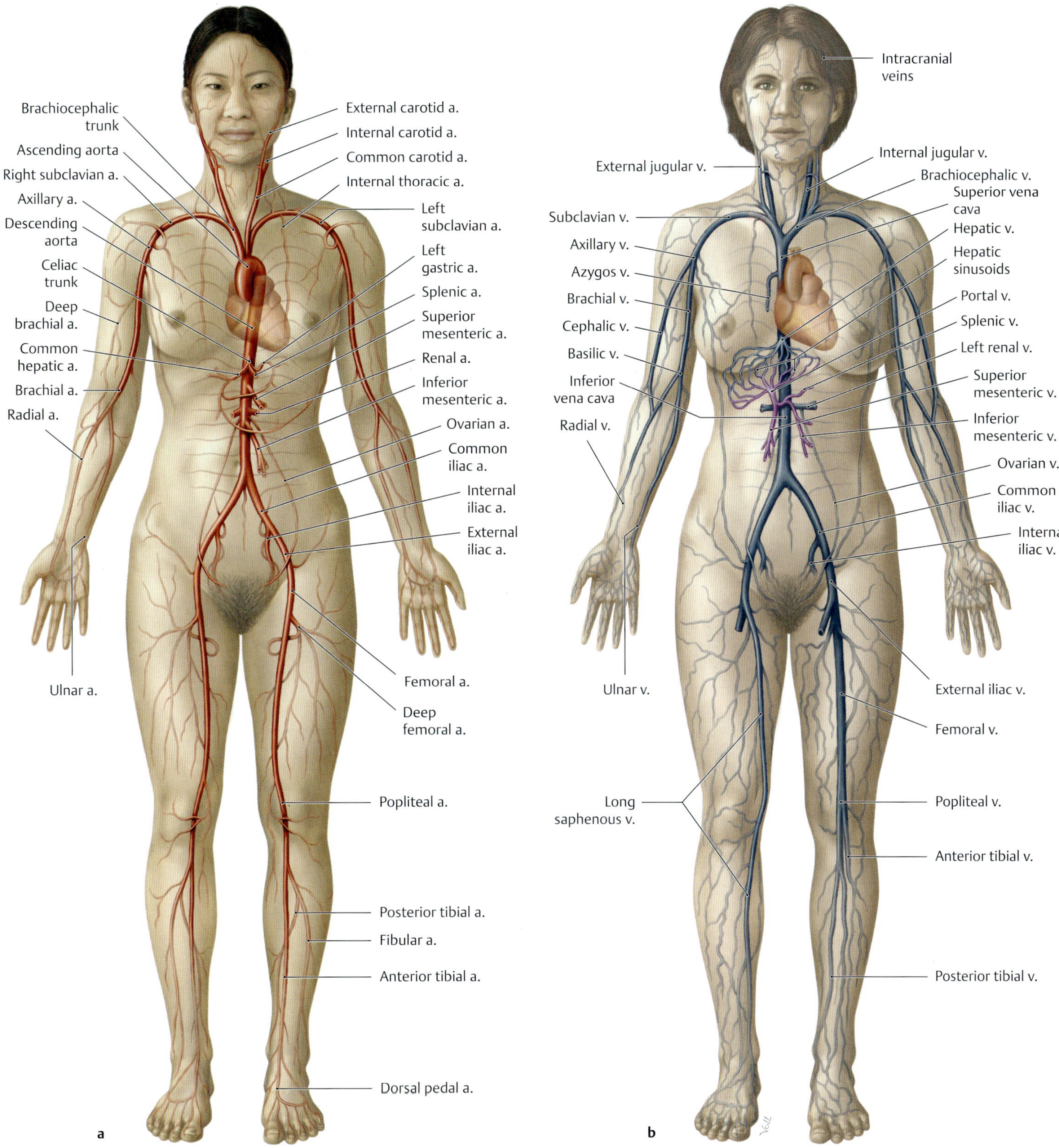

D Major blood vessels

This overview depicts the major arteries (**a**) and veins (**b**). In the following organ descriptions, knowledge of the major vascular trunks is assumed, and the smaller organ-supplying vessels will be discussed with the respective organs.

2.3 Cardiogenic Area, Development of the Heart Tube

Characteristics

In many respects, the cardiovascular system is extraordinary. It is the *first system to function* in the human embryo; it is already functional by the end of the third week (first contractions of the primitive heart tube). Additionally, the cardiac loop (see below) is the body's *first asymmetrical structure*. Since the human embryo is poorly supplied with yolk, which ensures nutrition by diffusion for a limited time only, it depends on extraembryonic circulation from a very early stage. While the yolk sac circulation appears earlier, it is the *placental circulation* that ultimately provides nutrients and removes waste over the course of embryonic and fetal development (see **D**).

A Origins of the cardiac tissue (cardiogenic area)

Dorsal view of the embryonic disc from the amniotic cavity. During the third week of development (presomite stage), the cardiogenic mesoderm, from which the heart develops, forms a horseshoe-shaped area (cardiogenic area) that consists of a thickened layer of mesenchymal cells. It lies anterolateral to the neural plate. At this stage in development, the mesenchyme is still located under the similarly horseshoe-shaped intraembryonic coelomic cavity. The cardiogenic area is composed of splanchnopleure (the layer of lateral plate mesoderm facing the viscera) and it borders the future pericardial cavity (see **Be**). During craniocaudal and lateral embryonic folding, the cardiogenic area, which originally lies in the anterolateral portion of the embryonic disc, moves ventrally under the developing foregut along with the adjacent coelomic cleft (see **Bc**).

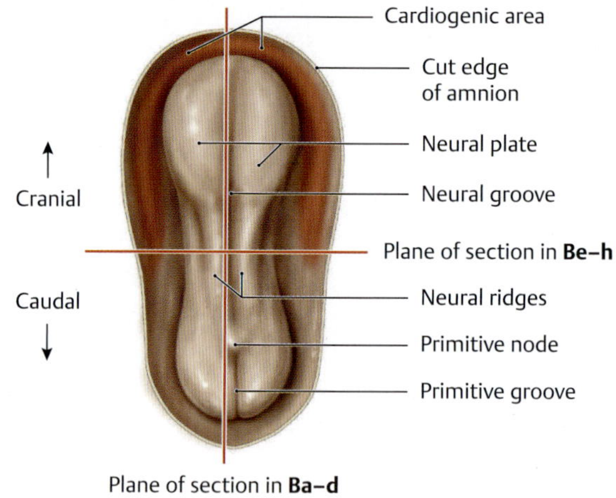

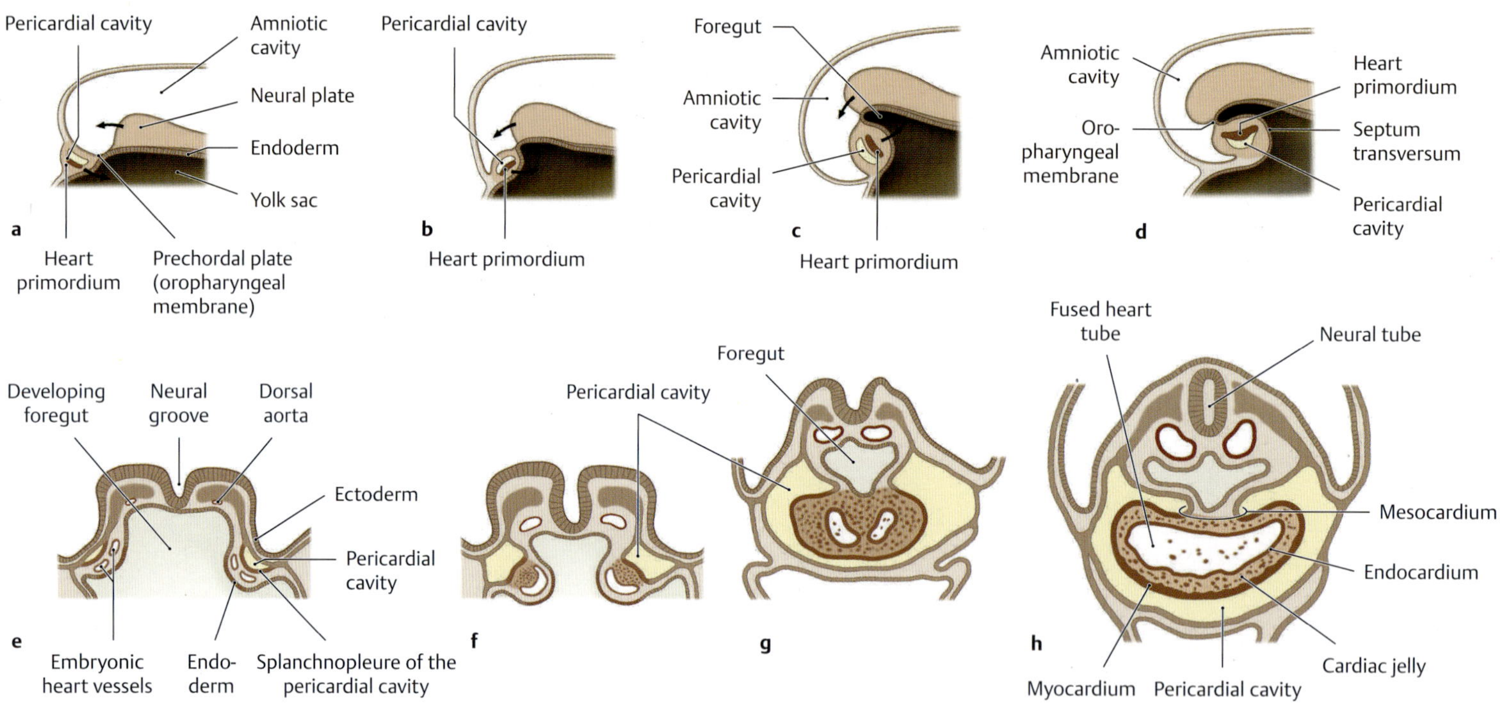

B Formation of the heart

a–d Sagittal sections; **e–h** Cross-sections (21–23 days / 4–12 somites); Lateral (**a–d**) and rostral (**e–h**) views; For location of the respective plane of section see **A**.

As a result of craniocaudal folding (**a–d**) the heart primordium and the adjacent pericardial cavity rotate 180 degrees and move under the foregut (descent of the heart). The prechordal plate (the future site of the oral cavity), which previously was located caudally, is now rostral to the developing heart. The septum transversum (future central tendon of the diaphragm) also moves caudally under the heart and pericardial cavity. During the slightly delayed process of lateral folding (**e–h**) the initially paired heart primordia fuse to form the unpaired heart tube (**h**). During this fusion, endothelial-lined embryonic vessels (endocardial tubes) that developed from angioblasts in the cardiogenic area fuse to form a single cavity in the heart tube. After fusing with the opposite side, the adjoining splanchnopleure thickens and develops into cardiac muscle (*myocardium*). Between the endocardial and myocardial layers develops a basement membrane-like structure consisting of a gelatinous extracellular matrix (cardiac jelly). Thus, the fused embryonic heart tube consists of three layers—from inside to outside: endocardium, cardiac jelly, and myocardium. The visceral layer of the pericardium, the *epicardium*, develops from progenitor cells in the area around the sinus venosus, which then overgrow the myocardium.

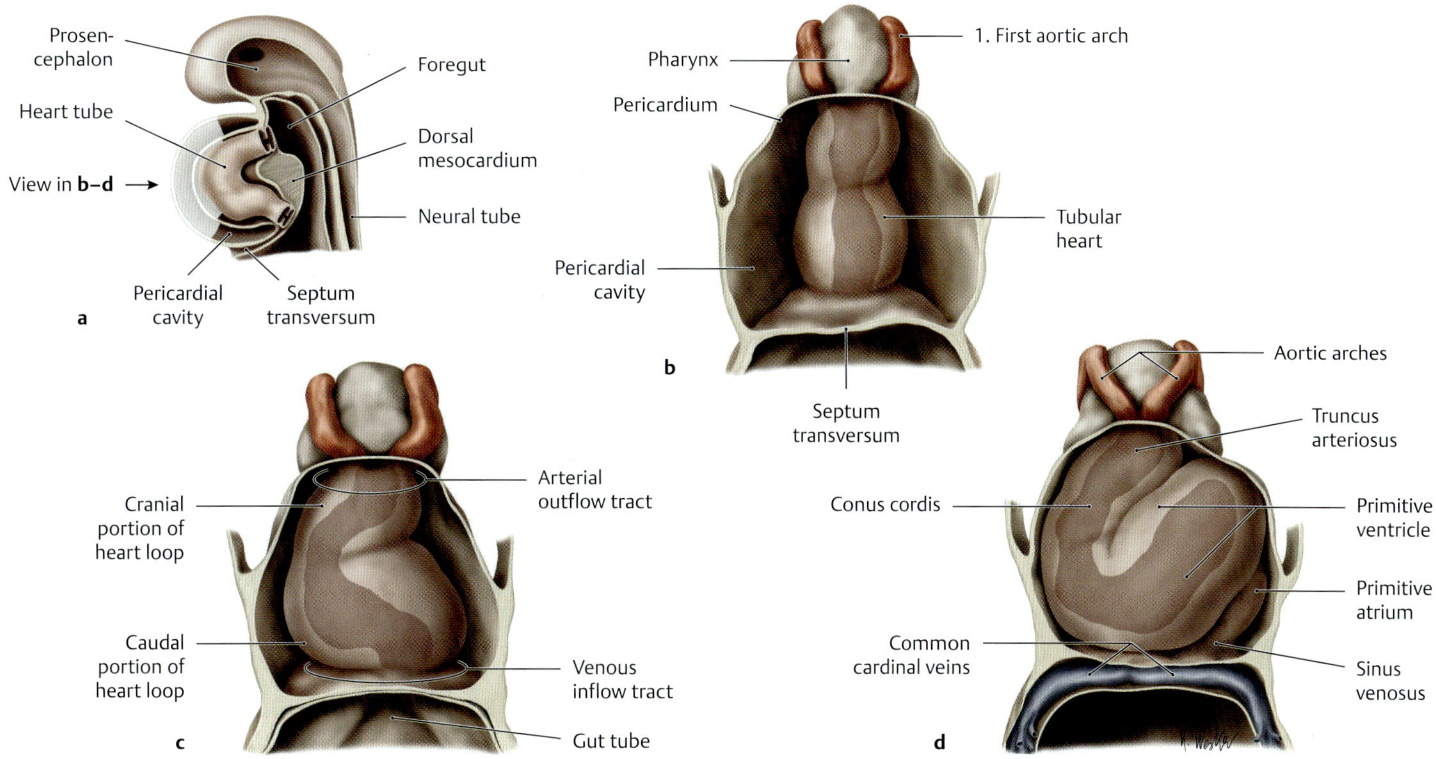

C Formation of the cardiac loop

a Left lateral view; **b–d** Anterior view (with the pericardial cavity opened).

During cranial embryonic folding, the developing heart and pericardial cavity shift in a ventral and caudal direction. With the start of the fourth week, the heart tube elongates and curves to form the *cardiac loop*, which at this stage is attached by a dorsal mesocardium to the posterior wall of the pericardial cavity. Over the course of development, this connection regresses (allowing formation of the *transverse pericardial* sinus), so that only the venous inflow and arterial outflow tracts attach the heart tube to the pericardium (see **c**). During formation of the cardiac loop, the cranial portion of the heart tube shifts ventrocaudally and to the right, while the caudal portion moves dorsocranially and to the left (**d**). Thus, the venous inflow tract lies dorsal and the arterial outflow tract ventral. At the same time, the cardiac loop subdivides into multiple portions as a result of constriction and expansion, forming the following regions:

- truncus arteriosus
- conus cordis
- primitive ventricle
- primitive atrium
- sinus venosus

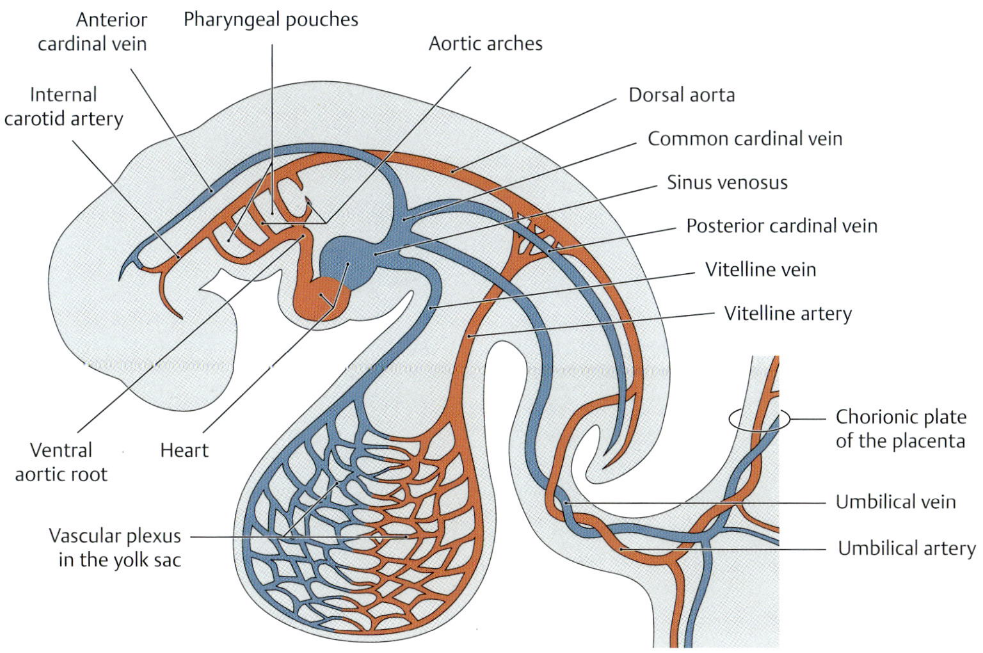

D Early embryonic circulation

Lateral view. The cardiovascular system of a 3- to 4-week-old embryo consists of a contractile muscular cardiac tube and three distinct circulatory systems:

- An **intraembryonic systemic circulation** (ventral and dorsal aorta, branchial arch and aortic arches, anterior and posterior cardinal veins)
- An **extraembryonic vitelline circulation** (omphalomesenteric arteries and veins)
- A **placental circulation** (umbilical arteries and veins).

The partially oxygenated blood (yolk sac or placenta) in the six major venous trunks (two vitelline or omphalomesenteric veins, two umbilical veins, and two common cardinal veins) flows into a common, venous cavity close to the heart called the sinus venosus. It then flows through the heart tube and out the paired, dorsal aorta to enter the systemic circulation, yolk sac or placenta (for development of the sinus venosus see p. 17).

2.4 Development of the Inner Chambers of the Heart and Fate of the Sinus Venosus

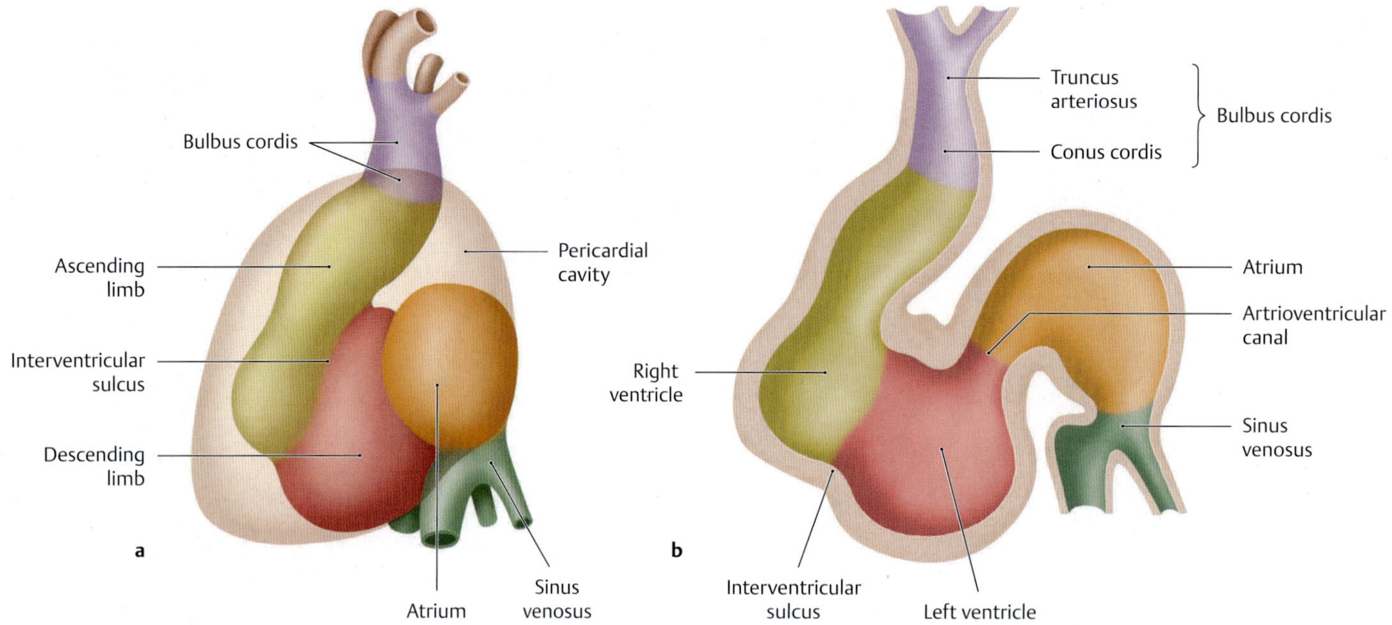

A The cardiac loop and the parts of the heart that develop from it
a Cardiac loop, left lateral view; **b** Sagittal section of the cardiac loop. By the end of the 3rd or beginning of the 4th week, the precursors of the definitive parts of the heart are clearly visible:

- The bulbus cordis (truncus arteriosus and conus cordis) differentiates into the smooth-walled *outflow tract* of the left and right ventricle as well as the proximal portion of the ascending aorta and pulmonary trunk.
- The ascending limb of the cardiac loop forms the right ventricle.
- The descending limb of the cardiac loop forms the left ventricle.
- The interventricular sulcus marks the boundary between the definitive left and right ventricles.
- The future atrioventricular valves will form at the level of the atrioventricular canal.

Between the 27th and 37th day of development, a complex series of steps occurs in the cardiac loop to form septa in the atrium, ventricle and outflow tract (see p. 18) to divide the heart into right and left sides.

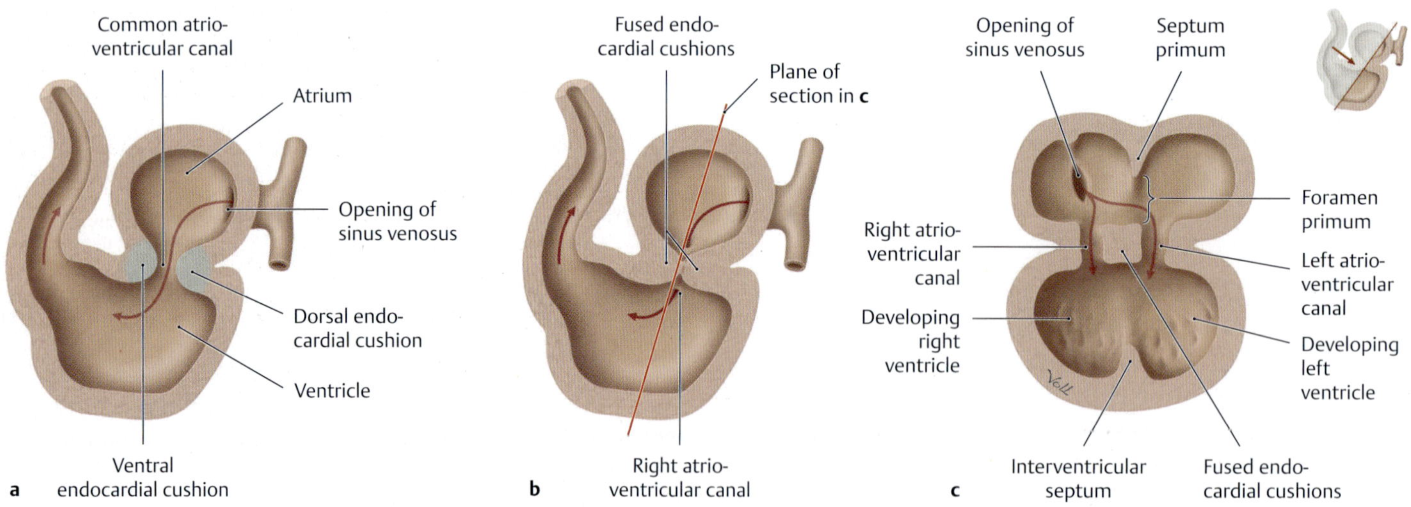

B Formation of the endocardial cushions and development of the heart's internal chambers
a and **b** Sagittal section of the cardiac loop; **c** Anterior view at the level of the endocardial cushions (for plane of section see **b**).
During the 4th week, the heart tube narrows at the junction of the atrium, ventricle and atrioventricular canal (AV canal). This narrowing is a result of the formation of dorsal and ventral endocardial cushions. These are thickened areas of mesenchyme that develop in the region of the cardiac jelly. The cushions fuse, and with continued development divide the AV canal into right and left sides (right and left atrioventricular canals). Later, the fused endocardial cushions give rise to the atrioventricular valves (tricuspid and mitral valves), which separate the atria from the ventricles. Simultaneously, the atrium begins to separate into two chambers (see p.18).

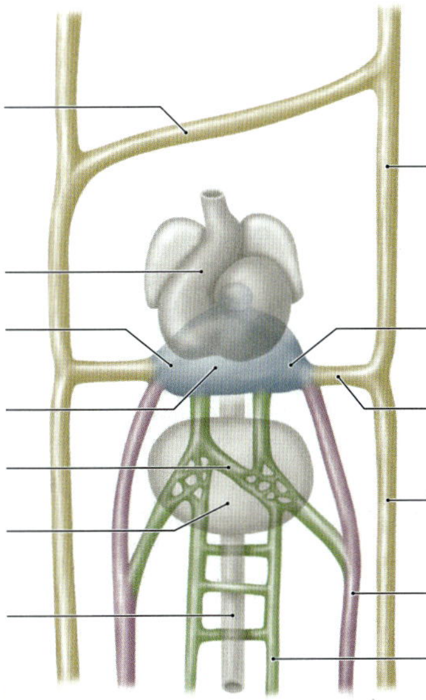

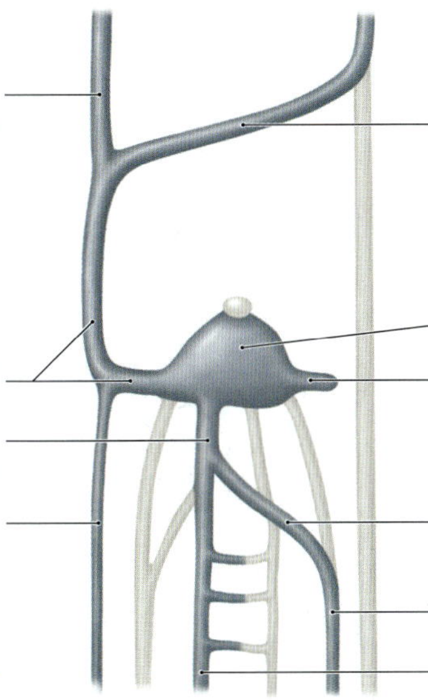

C Fate of the sinus venosus and the veins opening into it

a 4th week; **b** 3rd month; ventral view.

By the beginning of the 4th week, the sinus venosus is a separate part of the heart at the opening of the venous inflow tract. It opens into the still undivided atrium. Three large paired veins open into each side of the atrium through the left and right horns of the sinus venosus. These are the vitelline veins, umbilical veins, and common cardinal veins. Through two *left-right circuits* (see below), the inflow tract increasingly shifts to the right side of the body. On the left side, the majority of these veins disappear (see **E**):

1. **Left-right circuit:** Blood flowing from the placenta passes through the left umbilical vein and ductus venosus and enters the liver on the right side. From there it passes through the proximal portion of the right *vitelline vein* (future *inferior* vena cava) and then to the right sinus horn.
2. **Left-right circuit:** Both of the anterior cardinal veins become connected by an anastomosis. Blood flowing through the systemic circulation enters the right sinus horn through the right *common cardinal vein* (future *superior* vena cava). The right sinus horn enlarges and is gradually incorporated into the right atrial wall (**b**). The *left sinus horn*, however, increasingly regresses and forms the coronary sinus.

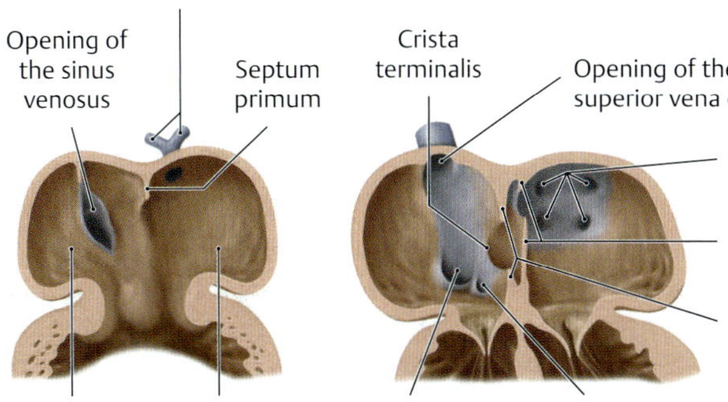

D Transformation of the atria

The separation of the common atrium into left and right atria begins in the 5th week with the formation of the *septum primum* (see p. 18). Around the same time the chambers of the atria enlarge by incorporating venous wall tissue. On the right side, parts of the right sinus horn are incorporated into the atrial wall. On the left side, a large part of the left atrium develops by incorporating the primitive pulmonary veins. The origins of the parts of the atria are still detectable in the mature heart:

- The smooth-walled portions of the atria developed from venous wall tissue (sinus venosus, pulmonary veins).
- The trabecular portions (mainly the left and right auricles) developed from the former common atrium.

In the right atrium, the border between the smooth-walled and trabecular portions is demarcated by a vertical ridge, the crista terminalis. Its cranial portion is the former right sinus valve; its caudal portion is the valves of the inferior vena cava and coronary sinus.

E Transformation of the sinus venosus and veins opening into it by the end of the 4th week (see also **Cb**)

Sinus venosus and veins opening into it through the 4th week	Structures that remain on the right side of the body after the 4th week	Structures that remain on the left side of the body after the 4th week
Right and left sinus horn	Smooth-walled portion of the right atrium	Coronary sinus
Right and left common cardinal veins	Right vein develops into part of the superior vena cava	Left vein becomes part of the coronary sinus
Right and left anterior cardinal veins	Right vein also develops into part of the superior vena cava	Left vein regresses
Right and left posterior cardinal veins	Right vein develops into the azygos vein	Left vein regresses
Right and left umbilical veins	Right vein regresses	Left distal portion remains until birth
Right and left vitelline veins	• Proximal portion of the right vein develops into part of the inferior vena cava • Distal portion of the right vein develops into the hepatic portal vein	Left vein regresses

2.5 Cardiac Septation (Formation of Atrial, Interventricular, and Aorticopulmonary Septa)

Development of cardiac septa—the basics
Cardiac septation begins at the end of the 4th week and is completed over the next three weeks. Over this period, the embryo grows in length from 5 mm to 17 mm. As a result of the development of the various cardiac septa, the heart tube separates into two sides with a circuit for the left heart and another for the right heart. The two circuits are completely separated from one another at the time of birth with the closure of the foramen ovale (see p. 20). This closure is due in part to increased blood flow to the infant's lungs and the resulting decrease in pressure in the right heart circuit.

Note: Septation defects play a key role in many heart malformations (e.g., atrial and ventricular septal defects, transposition of large vessels, tetralogy of Fallot, see p. 21). The incidence rate of heart malformations among newborns is 7.5/1000 making them the most frequent congenital diseases. In Germany, 6,000 children are born with a heart defect every year.

A Atrial Septation (formation of the atrial septum)
a, c, e, g, i, k Frontal sections, ventral view; **b, d, f, h, j** Sagittal section, viewed from the right side.

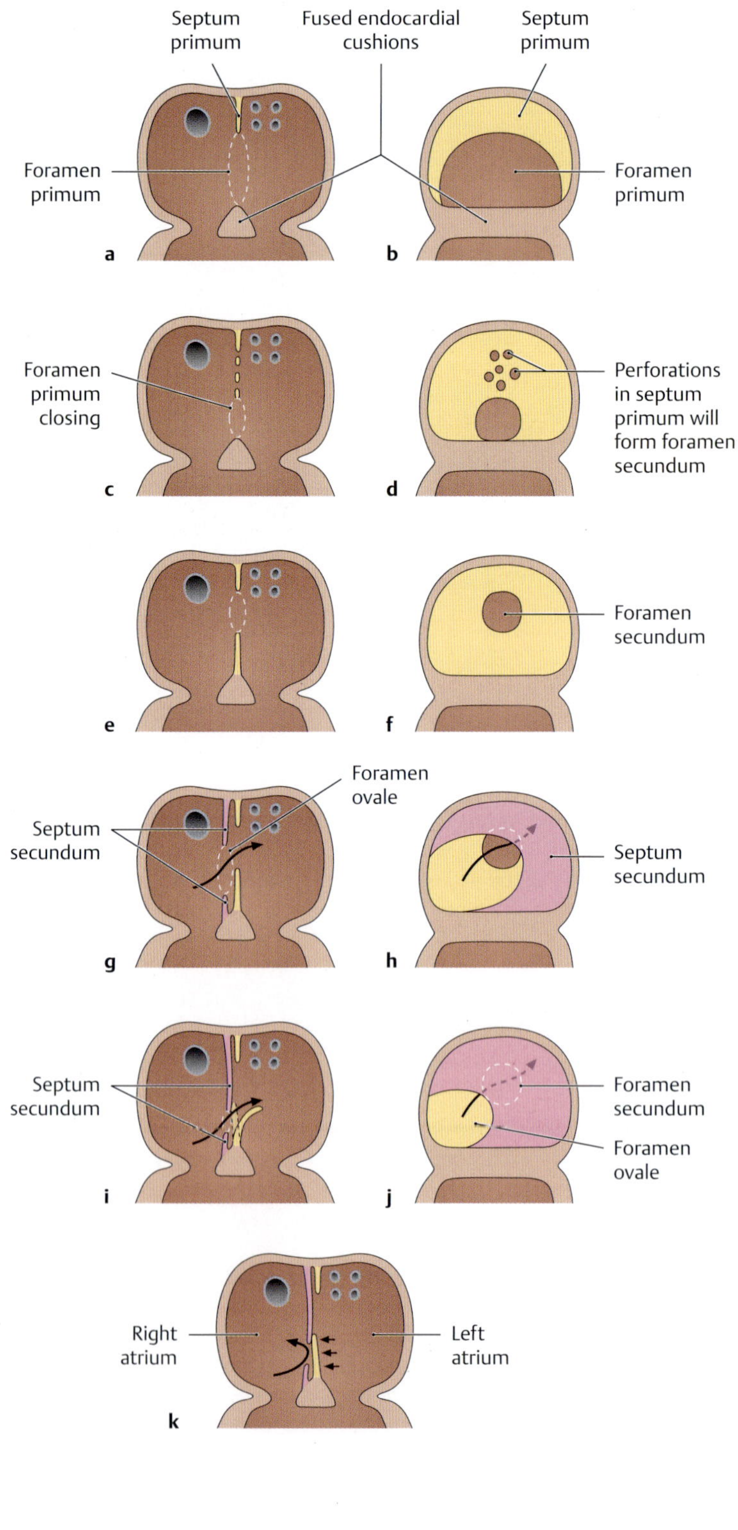

Septum primum and foramen secundum: After the 4th week the common atrium gradually gets divided into two chambers. From the roof of the still undivided atrium, the crescent-shaped *septum primum* grows and extends toward the already fused endocardial cushions of the atrioventricular canal (**a** and **b**). Between the margin of the septum and the endocardial cushion remains an opening, the *foramen primum*. It becomes progressively smaller and finally disappears as the septum primum continues to grow. At the same time, perforations produced by apoptosis appear in the central part of the septum primum. The perforations coalesce to form a new, large opening between the two atria, the *foramen secundum* (**c** and **d**). From now until birth, this new opening ensures continuous flow of oxygenated blood from the right to the left atrium.
Septum secundum and foramen ovale: By the end of the 5th week, a second crescent-shaped septum called the septum secundum grows from the ventrocranial wall of the right atrium toward the fused endocardial cushions (**g** and **h**). The *septum secundum* does not completely reach the endocardial cushions and an opening, the *foramen ovale*, remains in the septum. The extending septum secundum progressively overgrows the *foramen secundum* in the *septum primum* (**i** and **j**). However, blood can continue to flow from the right atrium to the left atrium due to differing blood pressures in the two sides. Before birth, pressure in the right atrium is higher than in the left atrium and blood entering the right atrium from the inferior vena cava passes into the left atrium. This is because the blood pressure is sufficient to push the septum primum aside and open it like a door. In this way, blood can pass through the foramen ovale, into the gap between the septum secundum and septum primum, and through the foramen secundum to enter the left atrium (**i** and **j**).
Closure of the foramen ovale and the definitive separation of the atria: Due to changes in the pulmonary circulation at birth, blood pressure in the left atrium increases. As a result, the septum primum is pushed against the septum secundum. The foramen ovale closes and the two atria are separate from one another (**k**). The septum primum forms the future fossa ovalis, and the free edge of the septum secundum develops into the limbus (border) of the fossa ovalis. Once these two septa fuse the foramen ovale remains permanently closed.
Note: Failure of the septa to fuse results in the foramen ovale remaining open (patent foramen ovale [PFO]). However, this is of little significance due to the pressure differences in the atria (see p. 21). The higher pressure in the left atrium pushes the septum primum firmly against the septum secundum.

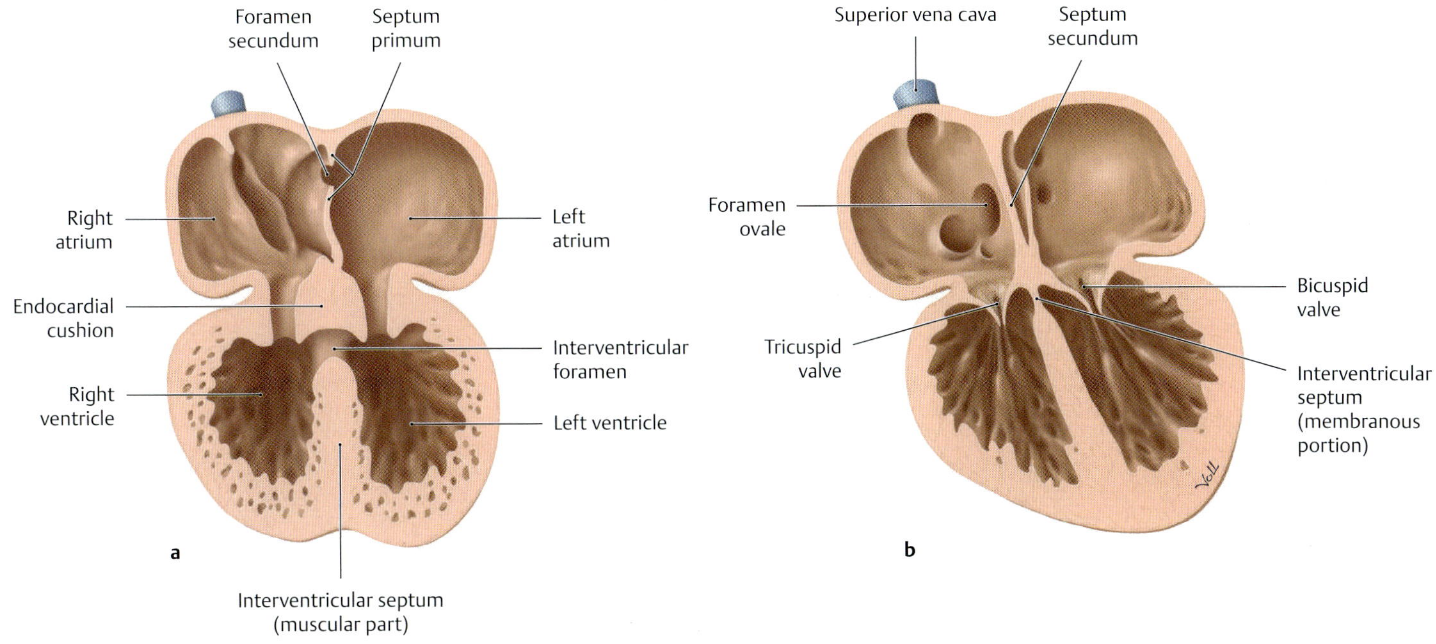

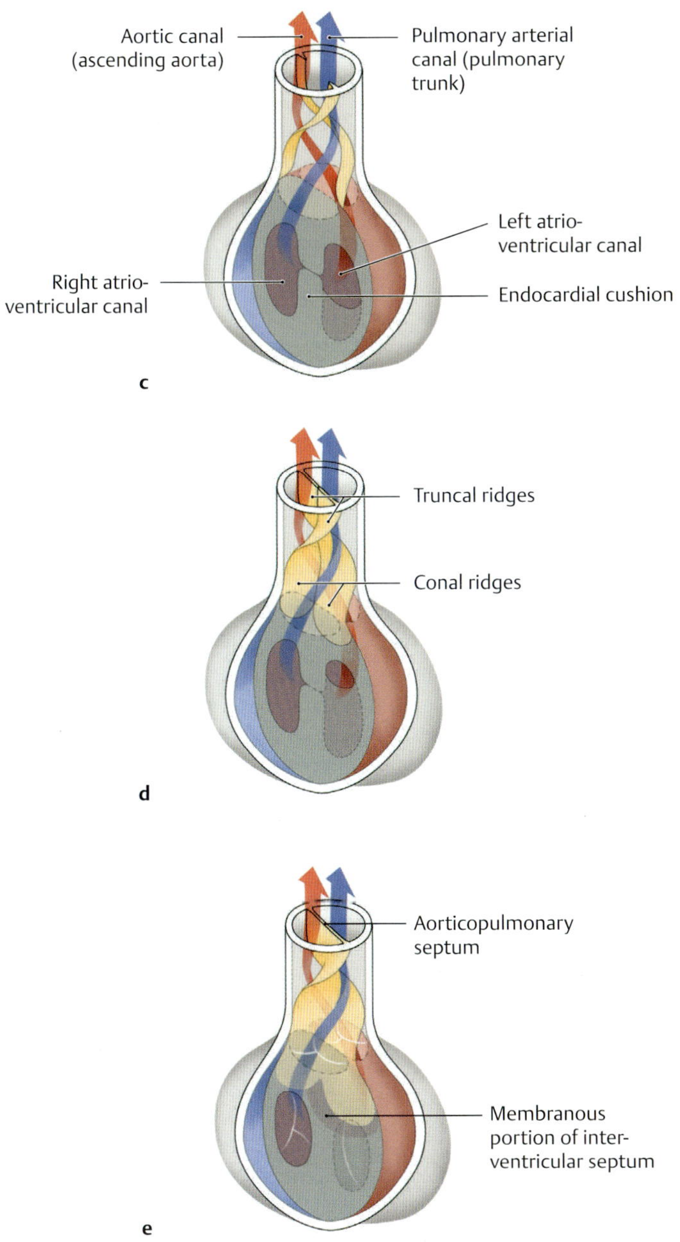

B Septation of the ventricles and the outflow tract (formation of the interventricular and aorticopulmonary septi)

Ventricular septation also begins by the end of the 4th week with the formation of a myocardial wall between the ascending and descending limbs of the cardiac loop.

Ventricular septation (a and b): A crescent-shaped muscular ridge called the muscular part of the *interventricular septum* develops from the wall of the ventricle and projects into the ventricular lumen. With continued development, its two limbs fuse with the endocardial cushions of the atrioventricular canal (however, the bottom of the crescent-shaped ridge does not fuse with the cushions). The remaining opening between the two ventricles is called the *interventricular foramen*. In the 7th week, it is completely closed by the *membranous portion* of the interventricular septum, which comes from the endocardial cushions and the proximal end of the conal ridges (see below).
Outflow tract septation (c–e): While the interventricular septum forms, the common outflow tract of both ventricles (bulbus cordis) begins to differentiate into the *ascending aorta* and *pulmonary trunk*. This is the result of the formation of two opposite longitudinal ridges in the lower (conus cordis) and upper (truncus arteriosus) parts of the outflow tract. These conal and truncal ridges develop through increased proliferation of mesenchyme. Their progenitor cells migrated from cranial neural crest cells in the pharyngeal arches.
Note: Neural crest cells give rise to most of the peripheral nervous system, but also contribute to cardiovascular development. Thus, cranial neural crest cells are of central importance for the normal development of the cardiac outflow tract.
Over the course of septum formation, the conal and truncal ridges complete a rotation of 180 degrees. This pattern of fusion leads to the formation of the spiral-shaped *aorticopulmonary septum*, which separates the common outflow tract of the two ventricles.
Heart valve formation: Formation of the aortic and pulmonary semilunar valves is related to formation of the *aorticopulmonary septum*. The valves develop from three subendocardial ridges (endocardial cushions) located at the junction of the conus cordis and truncus arteriosus (thus at the root of the aorta and pulmonary trunk).

2.6 Pre- and Postnatal Circulation and Common Congenital Heart Defects

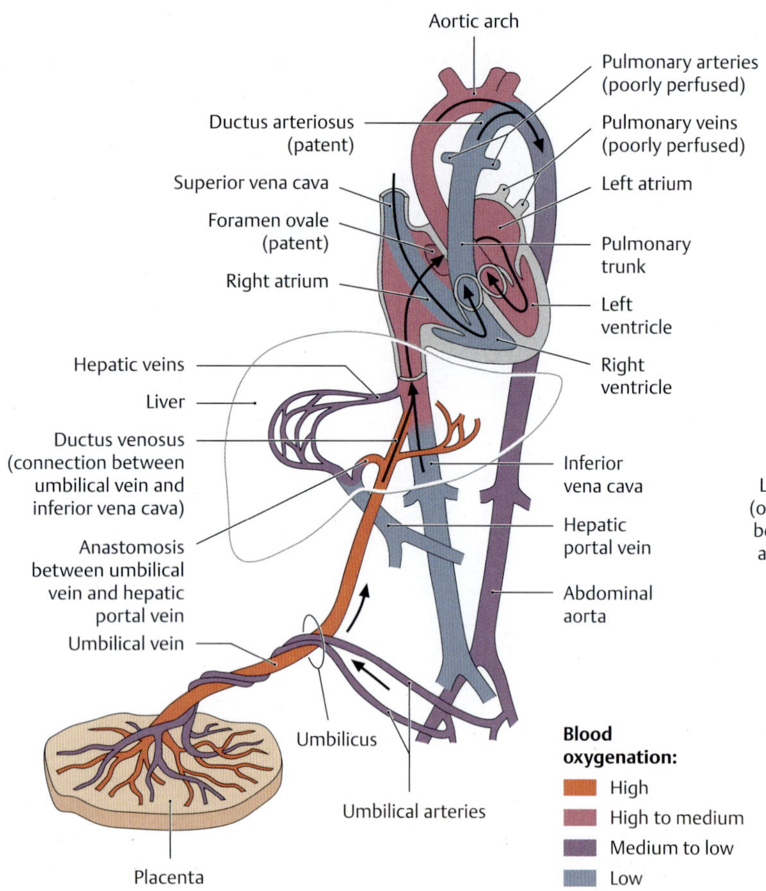

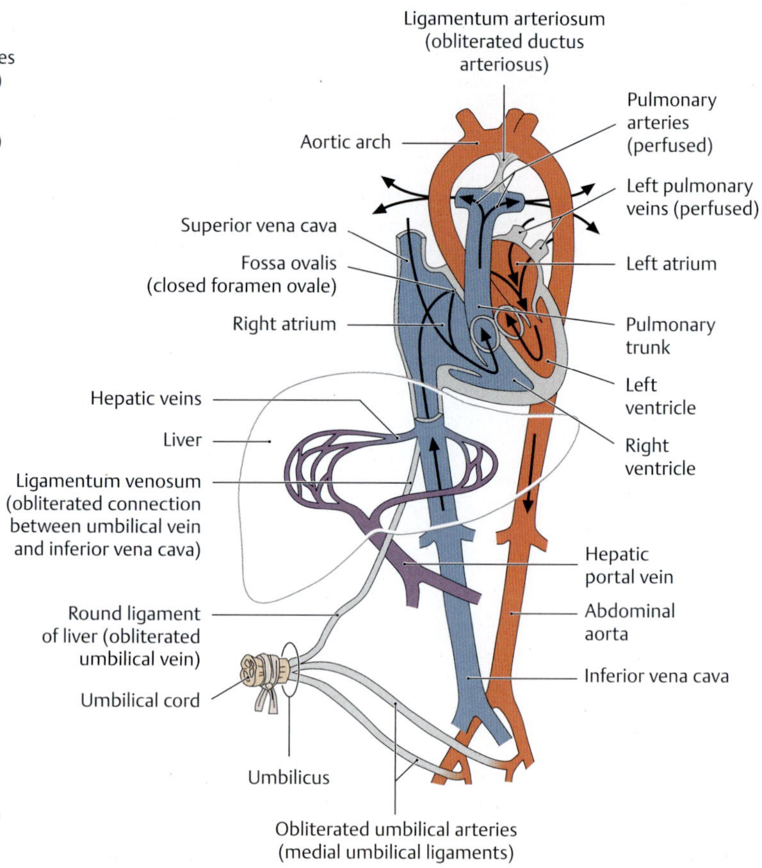

A Prenatal circulation (after Fritsch and Kühnel)
The prenatal circulation is characterized by the following:

- Very little pulmonary blood flow
- Gas exchange in the placenta
- Delivery of oxygen and nutrients to the fetus through the placenta
- A right-to-left shunt in the heart

The fetal **lungs** have not yet expanded, are not aerated and have minimal blood flow. Consequently exchange of O_2 and CO_2 takes place outside the fetus in the placenta. Oxygenated and nutrient-rich fetal blood from the placenta passes to the fetus through the unpaired umbilical vein. Near the liver, the umbilical vein empties into the inferior vena cava through the ductus venosus (a venovenous anastomosis). There, oxygen-rich blood (from the umbilical vein) mixes with oxygen-poor blood (from the inferior vena cava). At the same time, the umbilical vein passes nutrient-rich blood, via another venous anastomosis, to the hepatic portal vein which transports it to the liver for metabolic processing.
Blood flow in the **heart** is characterized by a right-to-left shunt. Blood from both venae cavae flows into the right atrium. Blood from the *inferior* vena cava passes into the left atrium through the foramen ovale (see p. 18). The blood from the *superior* vena cava passes through the right atrium to the right ventricle and then enters the pulmonary trunk. However, it does not enter the unexpanded fetal lungs but passes via the ductus arteriosus (an arterioarterial anastomosis) into the aorta and then to peripheral fetal vessels. Blood returns to the placenta through the paired umbilical arteries (branches of the internal iliac arteries). Since the pulmonary circulation is greatly reduced, very little blood is returned to the left atrium through the pulmonary veins.

B Postnatal circulation (after Fritsch and Kühnel)
At birth, gas exchange and blood flow undergo a radical change. The postnatal circulation is characterized by the following:

- Loss of the placental circulation
- Pulmonary respiration with pulmonary gas exchange
- Functional occlusion of the right-to-left shunt and all fetal anastomoses

When respiration begins, the lungs are expanded, aerated and become responsible for gas exchange. Vascular resistance in the expanded lungs drops abruptly. The sudden drop in blood pressure in the right atrium (pressure in the left atrium is now higher than in the right atrium) causes the foramen ovale to close (see p. 18). Contraction of vascular smooth muscle in the ductus arteriosus functionally closes that anastomosis. Later it closes completely by scarring and forms the ligamentum arteriosum. The right ventricle pumps blood through the pulmonary arteries into the expanded lungs. Blood from the left ventricle is distributed through the aorta to all body regions and returns to the right atrium through the superior and inferior venae cavae. Both sides of the heart are now hemodynamically separate. The umbilical vein is no longer perfused and the ductus venosus connecting it to the inferior vena cava occludes and eventually scars to form the ligamentum venosum. The umbilical vein also becomes occluded and fibrous over its entire length, forming the round ligament of the liver. The proximal portions of the umbilical arteries remain patent, while the distal portions become occluded and form the medial umbilical ligament on each side.

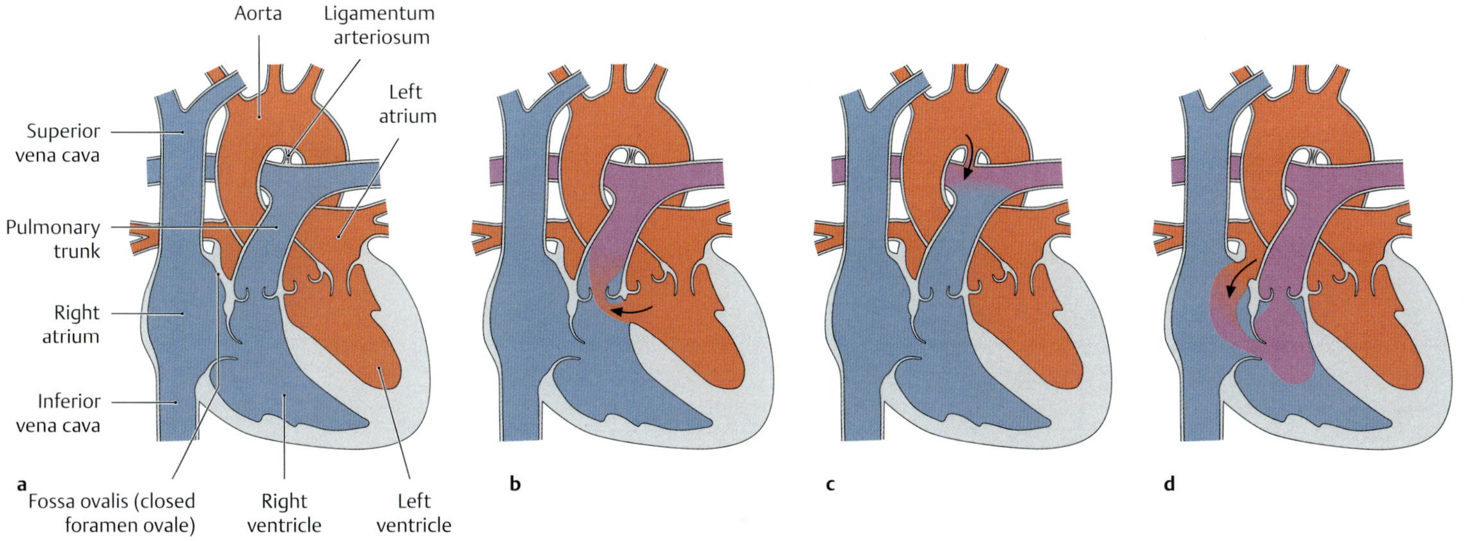

C Congenital heart defects

Heart defects are the most common birth defects (incidence in liveborn infants is 7.5/1000). The factors are usually genetic (trisomy 21) or exogenous (e.g., virus infections/rubella, alcohol, medications, cytostatics, ionizing radiation).

Note: The heart is most sensitive to teratogen exposure between the 4th and 7th weeks, a time period in which a woman may not know yet that she is pregnant.

Thanks to enormous progress in diagnosis and therapy, more than 85% of children born today with congenital heart disease survive and reach adult age. Among the most common congenital heart defects are acyanotic heart defects (cyanosis: bluish discoloration of the skin/mucosae due to low oxygen saturation). They are ventricular septal defects (31%), atrial septal defects (10%) and patent ductus arteriosus (9%), in which a non-physiological connection exists between the left and right sides of the heart. Since blood always flows from high pressure to low pressure, and the left side of the heart has the higher pressure in postnatal circulation, the heart abnormalities described are characterized by an initial left-to-right shunt. The shunt leads to higher pressure in the right side of the heart. In response to the increased pressure, the walls of the right ventricle and pulmonary arteries thicken which results in continuously increasing resistance and pressure in the pulmonary circulation (pulmonary hypertension). Over time the pressure in the pulmonary circulation becomes higher than the pressure in the systemic circulation, which leads to a shunt reversal (now right-to-left shunt [Eisenmenger reaction]) and decompensated right-sided failure. As less blood flows through the pulmonary arteries, the oxygen saturation decreases leading secondarily to cyanosis. During childhood, acyanotic heart defects are usually well tolerated and become symptomatic only later in life. If a patent ductus arteriosus is surgically closed (e.g., using an endoscopic catheter) before complications occur, life expectancy is normal.

- **a Normal postnatal heart:** The foramen ovale closes, the ductus arteriosus atrophies, and systemic and pulmonary circulation are completely separated.
- **b Ventricular septal defect (VSD):** VSDs are usually located in the membranous portion of the interventricular septum and arise from failure of fusion of the muscular portion of the interventricular septum with the proximal aorticopulmonary septum. As a result, the interventricular foramen remains open, and with each contraction blood from the left ventricle enters the right ventricle. Ventricular septal defects are frequently associated with an asymmetric septation of the outflow tract such as a narrowed pulmonary trunk (stenosis), an "overriding" aorta on the ventricular septum, and right ventricular hypertrophy caused by the pulmonary stenosis (*tetralogy of Fallot*, the most common cyanotic heart defect. An infant's mucous membranes, lips and fingers have a bluish color because too little blood is pumped through the pulmonary circulation for adequate oxygenation).
- **c Patent ductus arteriosus (PDA):** frequently occurs in premature infants (75% will spontaneously close within one week). Symptoms are the result of increased backflow of aortic blood into the pulmonary trunk, which leads to volume overload on the pulmonary circulation (see above). If the ductus arteriosus is closed (e.g., using an endoscopic catheter), life expectancy is normal.
- **d Atrial septal defects (ASD):** depending on location, these defects are subdivided into three types: primum atrial septal defects (ASD I), secundum atrial septal defects (ASD II) and sinus venosus atrial septal defects (SV). The most common type is the secundum atrial septal defect (75% of all cases), characterized by the excessive resorption of septum primum tissue at the site of the foramen ovale (foramen secundum is too large) or inadequate growth of the septum secundum (foramen secundum is not sufficiently covered, see p. 18). As a result, in postnatal circulation, blood flows from the left atrium to the right atrium which, depending on the shunt volume, leads to volume overload in the pulmonary circulation. Significant symptoms can occur later in life once the shunt has reached a certain size. Thus, ASD II defects are corrected even though patients have not yet shown symptoms. Closure of secundum atrial septal defects is generally performed by using an interventional approach with a stent and a self-expanding double-umbrella device made of a nickel titanium alloy.

Note: Failure of the septum primum to fuse with the septum secundum after birth leads to an anatomically open (through which a probe could be passed) foramen ovale ("probe" patent foramen ovale [PFO]). Due to the valve mechanisms and the existing pressure differences, it is clinically insignificant (see p. 18) and thus is not a true heart defect but rather a normal variant (almost 30% of adults are affected). Pathological conditions, (e.g., resulting from an acute hemodynamically relevant pulmonary embolism) can lead to the formation of a right-to-left shunt. As a result, blood clots (thrombi), which are usually filtered out in the lungs, can enter the systemic circulation causing an ischemic stroke (a paradoxical or crossed embolism). Even smaller clots can be potentially life-threatening. Even routine activities (lifting heavy loads, coughing, etc.) can lead to quick changes in intrathoracic pressures so that a PFO can temporarily cause a right-to-left shunt.

3.1 Blood: Components

A Composition of blood

Blood is a unique tissue in that it is liquid. Yet like every other tissue it consists of an extracellular matrix (plasma) and cellular components (red and white blood cells as well as platelets). A transport and communication organ, it is contained within a closed vascular system that interconnects all organ systems. Its functions are accordingly diverse: transport of gases and substances, protection, thermoregulation, regulation of pH value, and coagulation. Coagulation prevents all of the blood from draining out of the cardiovascular system when its walls have been damaged.

A protein-containing fluid (plasma) accounts for 50–63% of the blood volume; 37–50% is blood cells. The ratio of the volume of red blood cells to the total volume of blood is referred to as hematocrit. **Plasma** is obtained by centrifuging whole blood which has been prevented from coagulating by the addition of a substance such as heparin. Serum is obtained by initially allowing the blood to coagulate and then centrifuging it. Serum is thus plasma minus clotting factors. About 90% of plasma consists of water; the rest includes proteins, electrolytes, and low-molecular-weight substances of metabolism and metabolic regulation (hormones). Most plasma proteins are synthesized by the liver. Accounting for a full 99% of the hematocrit, the vast majority of **blood cells** (see p. 24) are the *non-nucleated red blood cells*. Their cytoplasm is filled with hemoglobin, which serves to transport oxygen and buffer the blood. The white blood cells have a protective function; the platelets promote blood coagulation. All blood cells come from stem cells of the red bone marrow (see p. 27) where they are constantly produced.

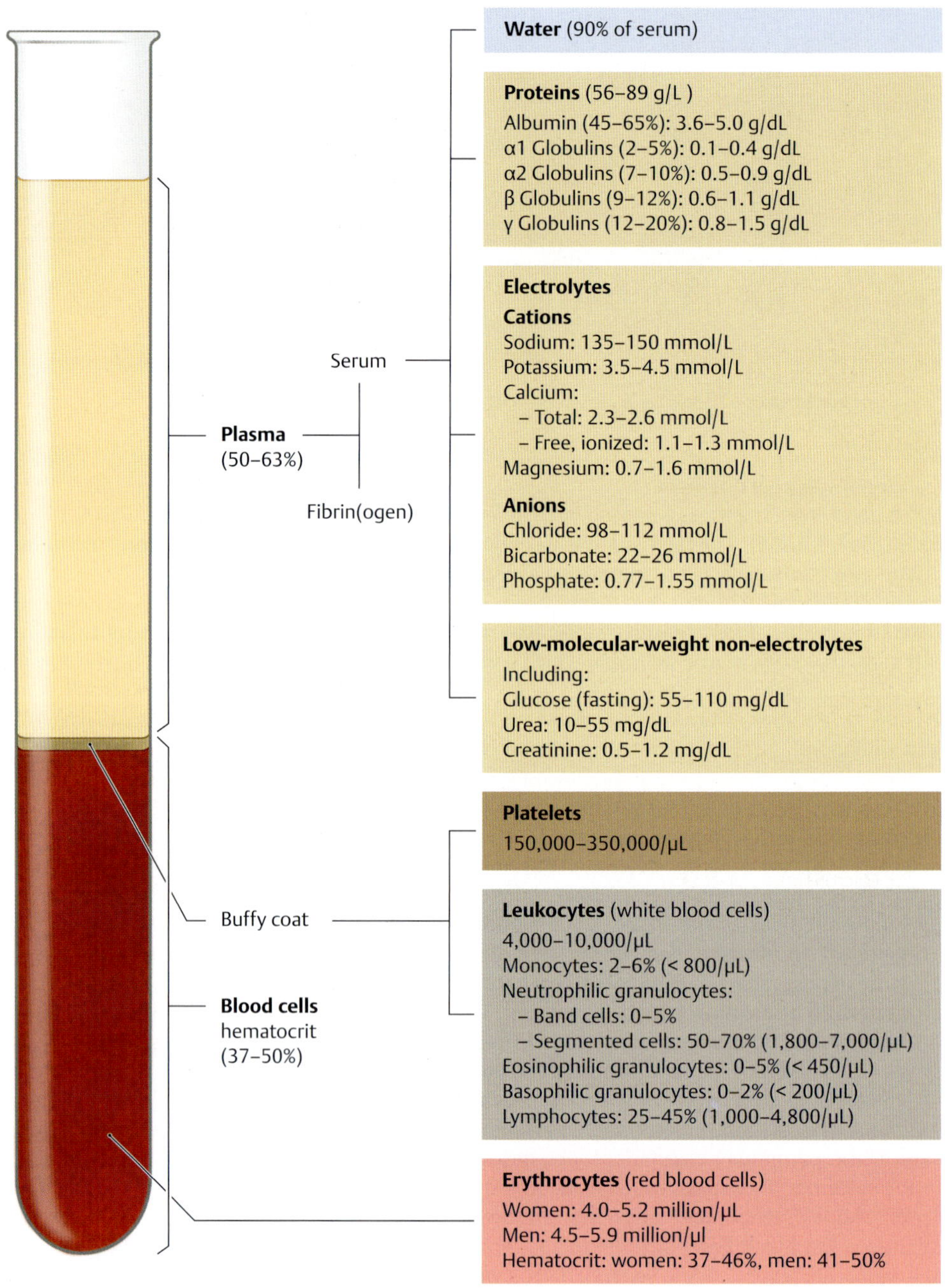

B Phases of blood formation during development

Blood is required before birth even prior to the development of red bone marrow. As a result, blood is initially formed elsewhere: in the yolk sac (insular), in the liver (hepatic), in the spleen (splenic), and finally in the secondary bone marrow (medullary). Malignant systemic diseases of the blood and the immune system "remember" these sites that provide favorable conditions for growth, and certain forms of these diseases then colonize the liver and spleen.

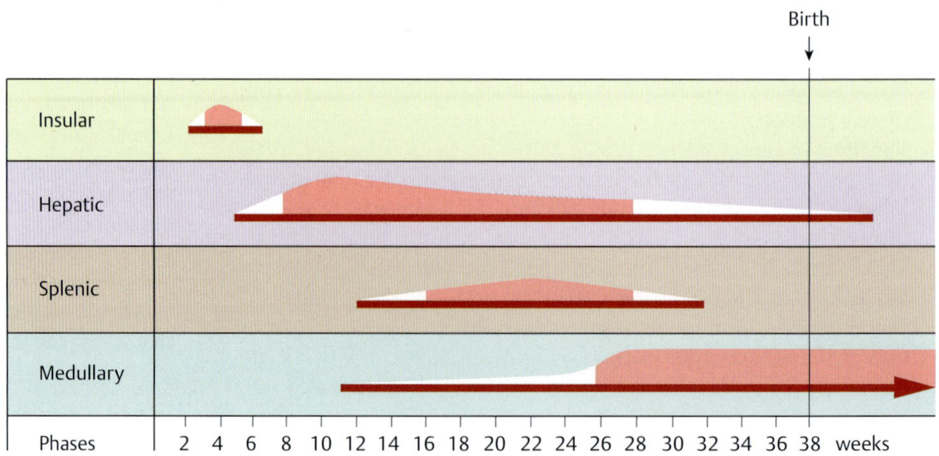

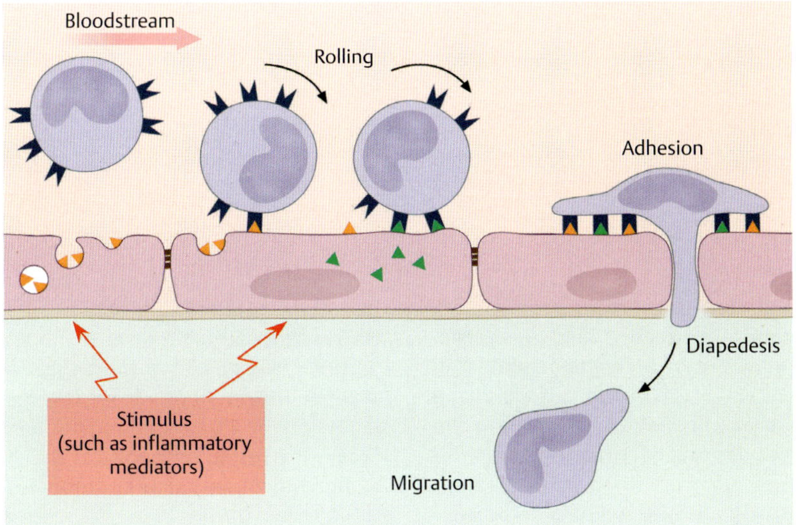

C Blood as a transport medium for blood cells (modified from Lüllmann-Rauch)

White blood cells circulate through the blood and as a result are distributed throughout the body. They constantly migrate out of the blood stream and into the connective tissue of the organs where they attack bacteria or cancer cells. Migration (diapedesis) occurs via the *leukocyte adhesion cascade*. Upon receiving a stimulus, endothelial cells express cell adhesion molecules on their luminal surface. These molecules either come to the surface immediately through vesicles in the cytoplasm or they are synthesized in response. Ligands on the cell membrane of the leukocytes bind to these molecules. This binding (keying) causes the leukocytes to roll along the endothelium. Sometimes they come to a stop and sometimes they disconnect and rejoin the bloodstream. When they stop, the endothelial cells reduce their intercellular cohesion to allow the leukocytes to pass through the gap between them.

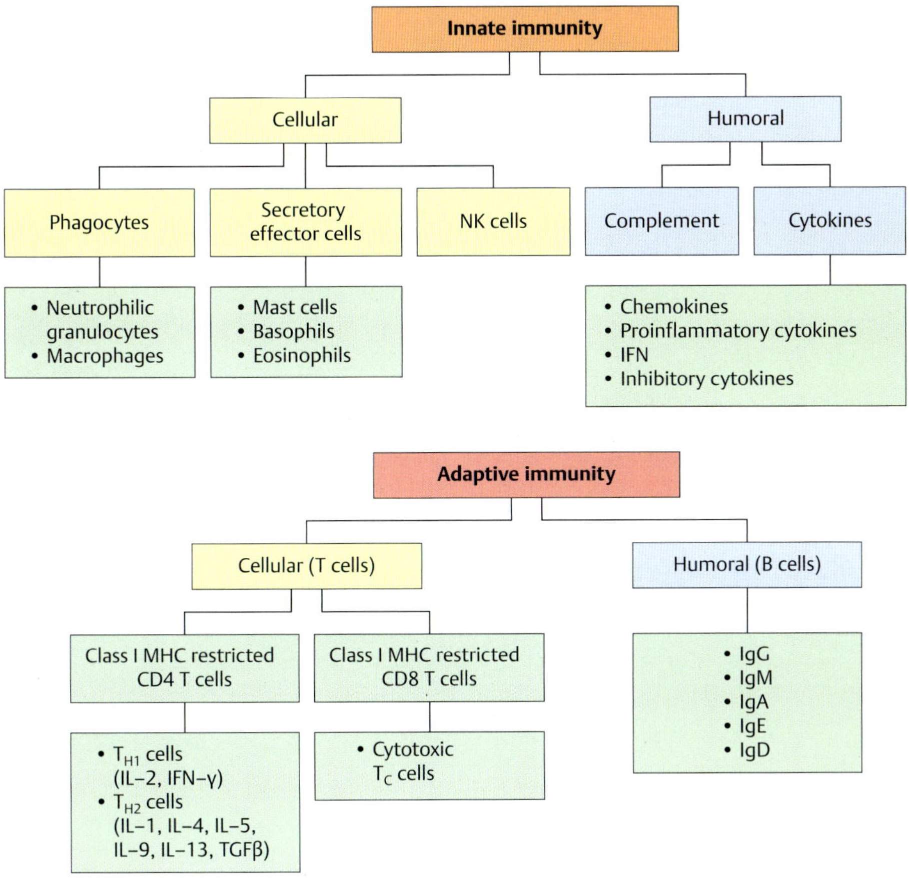

D Innate and adaptive immunity

As the blood has access to all organs, it plays an important role in the immune system in defending against infections and malignant cells. The immune system and the blood are thus tightly integrated. The innate immune system responds immediately to an appropriate stimulus and is nonspecific as it must respond to many possible attacks. Cellular components (cells are transported by the blood) and humoral components are differentiated. Humoral ("liquid") components include complement and cytokines in the blood. Adaptive immunity is specific and is directed toward a specific noxious agent such as a certain virus. The adaptive immune system includes T and B cells, which also circulate in the blood. T cells kill cancer cells or cells infected by viruses by direct contact (cellular immunity); B cells secrete various classes of antibodies (humoral immunity).

E Lifespan facts of certain blood cells

Type of cell	Retention time in blood	Lifetime in interstitium	Creation of new cells in bone marrow
Erythrocyte	120 days	–	About 8 days
Platelet	10 days unless consumed earlier	–	About 8 days
Neutrophilic granulocyte	< 1 day	1–2 days	About 8 days
Monocyte	About 1–3 days	Months (as a macrophage)	About 8 days

3.2 Blood: Cells

This unit discusses the cells of the blood that can be morphologically distinguished in a normal blood smear. The classic blood smear is colored with Pappenheim stain. Red and white blood cells as well as platelets are readily identifiable. See p. 22 for their normal values in blood.

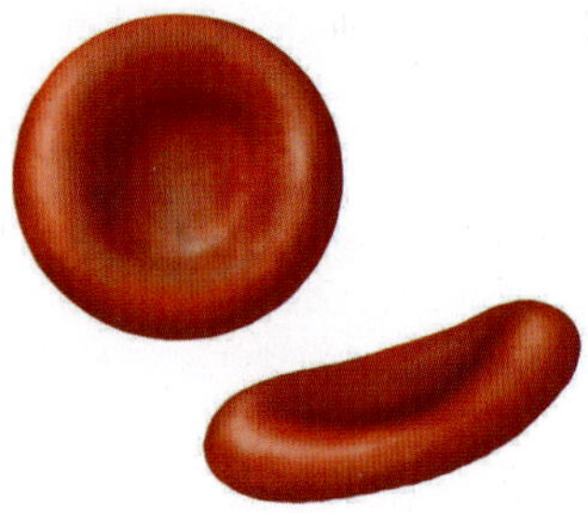

A Red blood cells (erythrocytes)
Erythrocytes (approx. 5 million/μL) are large, biconcave cells measuring about 7.5 μm in diameter. In mammals they contain no nucleus or cytoplasmic organelles. Their lack of organelles and their specially reinforced cell membrane allow erythrocytes to adapt particularly well to different flow characteristics in blood so that they can even squeeze through narrow capillaries. This adaptability allows them to survive in the blood about 120 days. After this, erythrocytes are eliminated by macrophages in the liver and spleen. Because they lack mitochondria, they must obtain their energy from anaerobic glycolysis. As a result they are dependent on glucose as a source of energy. Ninety-five percent of the interior of erythrocytes is filled with the protein hemoglobin, which binds O_2 and, to a lesser extent, CO_2. Erythrocytes are created in a series of morphologically distinct stages from a precursor cell containing a nucleus (see page 27). Reticulocytes represent the stage immediately preceding mature erythrocytes. They can be demonstrated with Cresyl violet stain. This stain binds to the RNA of the rough endoplasmic reticulum of erythrocytes, whose precursor cells ejected their nuclei 1–2 days previously and still contain residual traces of the endoplasmic reticulum. About 2.5 million reticulocytes leave the bone marrow per second. They mature into erythrocytes within a day. About 1% of erythrocytes are reticulocytes. As a result, reticulocytes are particularly suitable for monitoring erythropoiesis. When the number of reticulocytes increases, as can occur after acute bleeding, it is referred to as a reticulocyte crisis. This indicates that the bone marrow has responded to the blood loss by increasing the production of new erythrocytes. Here, the term crisis is used in a positive sense to indicate the regenerative output of the bone marrow.
Note: As the average diameter of erythrocytes is a reliably constant 7.5 μm, it can be used in histologic sections as an intrinsic scale for the size of a histologic structure.

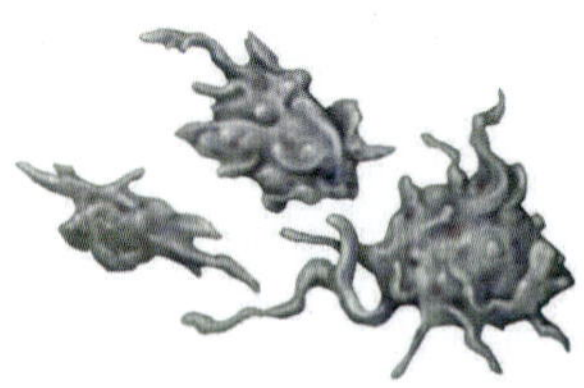

B Platelets (thrombocytes)
Platelets (about 250,000/μL) are non-nucleated fragments of megakaryocytes, multinuclear giant cells that reside in the bone marrow. They survive in blood for about 10 days after which they are phagocytized by macrophages in the liver and spleen, so new cells must be generated constantly. In flowing blood they assume the shape of a biconcave disk measuring 2.5 μm in diameter. Platelets are an essential component of blood coagulation. Increases, decreases, and anomalies of platelets can be diagnosed in blood smears. Below 30,000/μL fine capillary hemorrhaging known as petechial bleeding occurs. Below 10,000/μL life-threatening bleeding occurs. A change in the platelet count is a sensitive indicator of bone marrow function. A decreased platelet count can be an early indicator of worsening bone marrow function. Conversely, an increased platelet count can be an early indicator of increased bone marrow function.

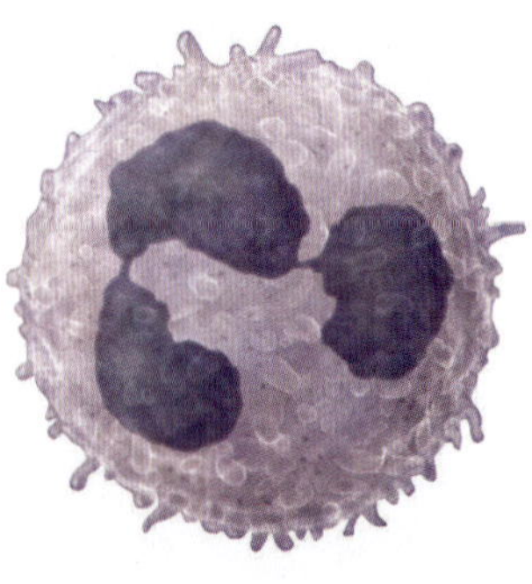

C Neutrophilic granulocytes
Neutrophils (the commonly used short form of neutrophilic granulocytes) represent the largest share of leukocytes in blood (4,000–10,000/μL), accounting for about 60%. A neutrophil measures 10–12 μm in diameter and remains in the blood for less than a day. It is characterized by a cell nucleus consisting of 3–4 segments connected to one another by narrow nucleic bridges. As a result it is also referred to as polymorphonuclear. Granulocytes take their respective name from how their granules stain with Pappenheim dye. The term *neutrophilic* comes from the fact that their cytoplasmic granules (< 1 μm) don't stain well with either basophilic dyes or eosinophilic dyes. They are therefore neutral. Neutrophils belong to the nonspecific immune system and phagocytize bacteria (microphages) in particular. Therefore, a large share of their granules are lysosomes in which phagocytized bacteria are broken down. Neutrophils are generated in the bone marrow and are released from there into the peripheral bloodstream when acutely needed (as is the case in bacterial infection). In such cases, a blood smear will reveal increased numbers of neutrophil precursors ("juvenile" cells) with unsegmented or less clearly segmented nuclei. Thus, a reactive increase in neutrophils in a blood smear can suggest a bacterial infection.

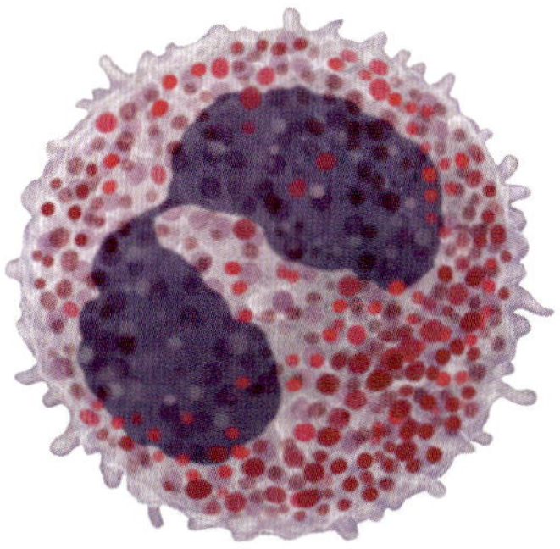

D Eosinophilic granulocytes

Eosinophils (12 μm in diameter) have a bilobed nucleus. They contain eosinophilic granules measuring 1.5 μm which represent modified lysosomes that release their contents to the extracellular matrix in degranulation. The anionic dye eosin binds to the cationic proteins in the granules (such as major basic protein, and eosinophil cationic protein). Eosinophils defend against worms in particular (small eosinophils cannot completely phagocytize large multicellular parasites), which is why their blood count is increased in parasitic diseases. They frequently migrate from the blood into the mucosa of the gastrointestinal tract and lungs. Their numbers are also increased in allergic disorders.

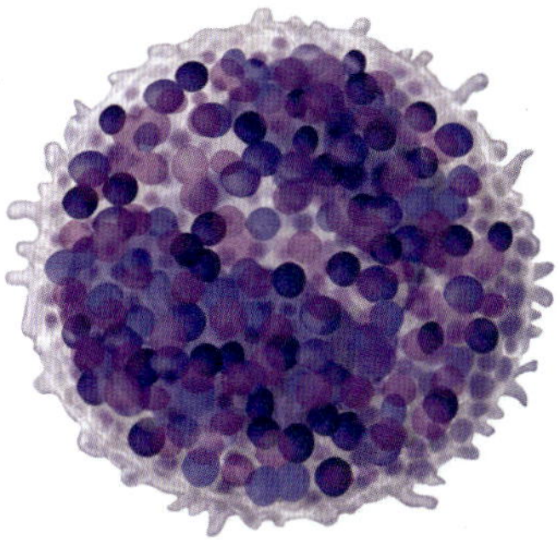

E Basophilic granulocytes

The lobulated nucleus of basophils is often undetectable as it is obscured by granules, which measure 1 μm and stain intensely bluish-violet. The polyanionic heparin contained in the granules takes up cationic dyes (methylene blue, azure). The granules also contain histamine, which is released in an allergic reaction. Although basophils resemble mast cells in their morphology and function, the two are separate types of cells that arise from different stem cells and they do not merge with each other.

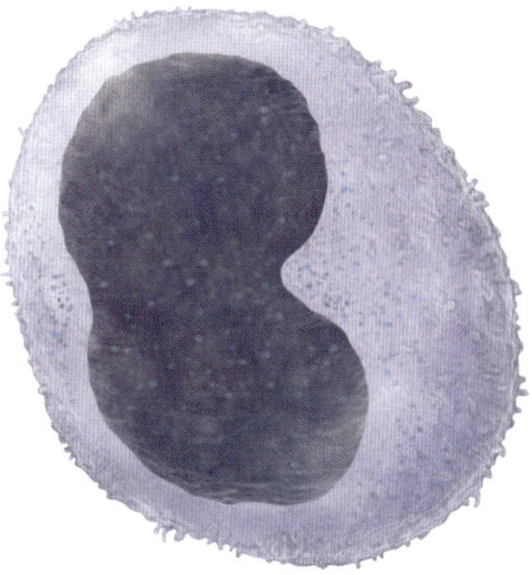

F Monocytes

Measuring 20–40 μm in diameter, monocytes are the largest cells in the blood. They exhibit a pale grayish blue cytoplasm and an indented bean-shaped nucleus that also can assume other shapes. This means that monocytes are the most variable type of cell in a blood smear. Small, barely discernible azure granules may be found in the cytoplasm, especially in the indentation of the nucleus. These represent lysosomes.

Monocytes leave the bloodstream after about a day and migrate into the connective tissue of the organs, where they differentiate into macrophages. Macrophages are monocytes that have become resident and in which a number of differentiation processes occur. The number of lysosomes in particular increases greatly. The mononuclear phagocytic system (MPS) is a generic term introduced by van Furth which includes all of these cells.

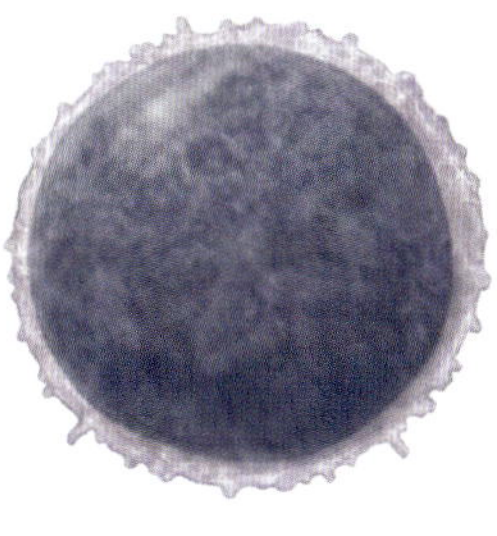

G Lymphocytes

Lymphocytes are characterized by a round nucleus rich in heterochromatin. In small lymphocytes (4–7 μm in diameter), the nucleus is surrounded by a narrow ring of cytoplasm; in medium-sized lymphocytes (up to 15 μm) this ring is wider and can contain granules (see **H**). Lymphocytes are part of the adaptive or specific immune system and occur in two main forms, B lymphocytes and T lymphocytes, which are indistinguishable in a blood smear. They are analyzed with the aid of monoclonal antibodies in flow cytometry (important in AIDS patients). B lymphocytes ultimately differentiate into plasma cells that produce antibodies; T lymphocytes aid in providing specific cell-mediated immunity. Lymphocytes only use the bloodstream for a short time (approximately 1 hour) as a transport medium to enter the lymphatic organs and the interstitium of other organs. Lymphocytes have a similar appearance to monocytes, which is why the two are often grouped together as mononuclear cells. These are distinguished from the granulocytes (polymorphonuclear cells). Reactively increased numbers of lymphocytes in the blood occur often in viral disorders.

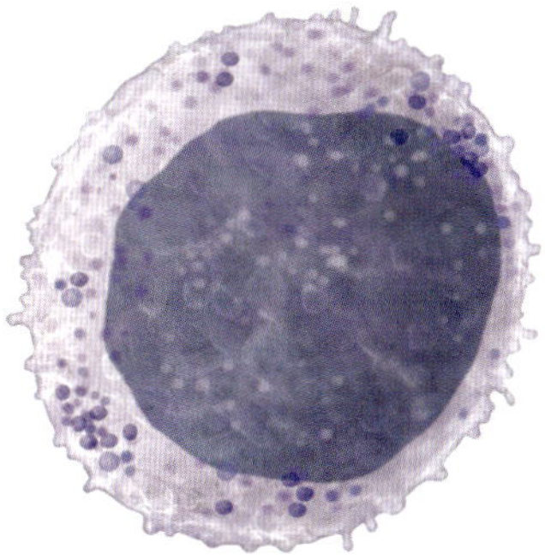

H Azurophilic granulated lymphocytes

Azurophilic granulated lymphocytes are a special form of large lymphocyte distinguishable by their large ring of cytoplasm and their azurophilic granules (large granular lymphocytes or LGL). They represent the natural killer cells (NK cells) that form part of the nonspecific immune system. They react immediately upon contact with virus-infected cells or bloodborne cancer cells and usually destroy these target cells after direct contact.

3.3 Blood: Bone Marrow

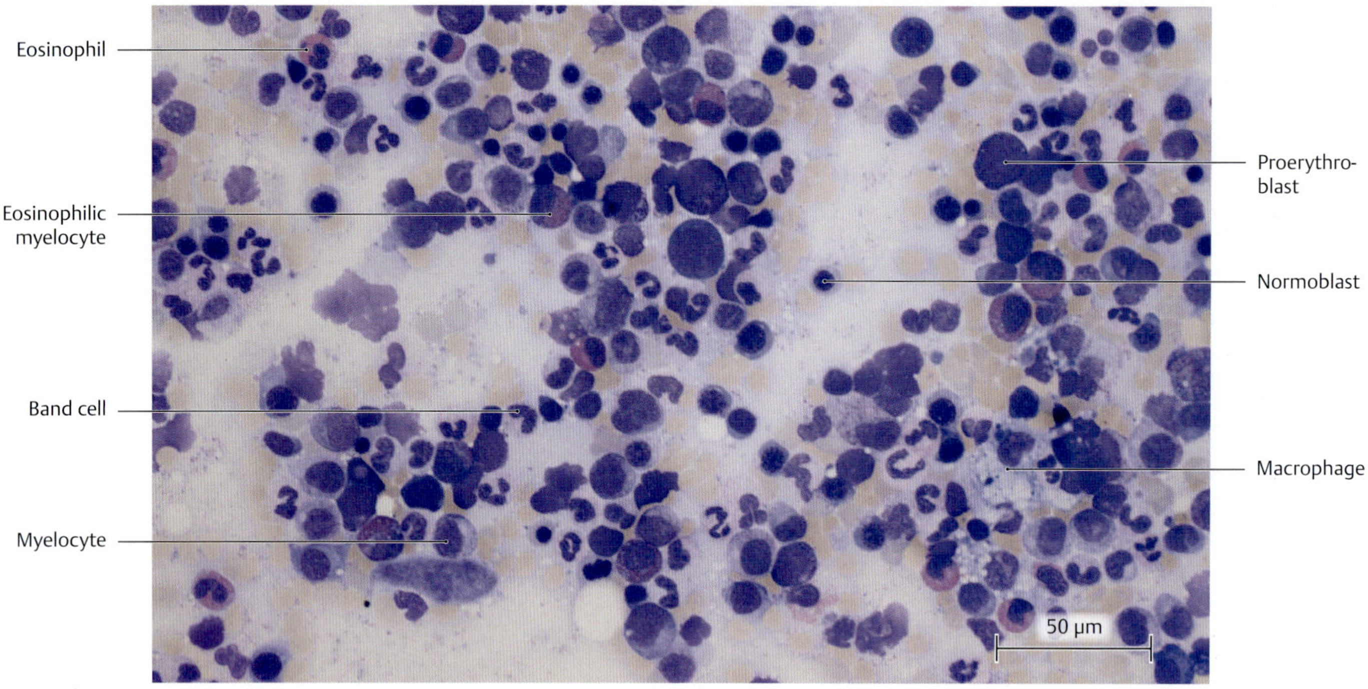

A Bone marrow cytology

Normal bone marrow contains a bewildering variety of cells. The reason for this is that starting from a single pluripotent stem cell, erythropoiesis, granulopoiesis, and lymphopoiesis all occur simultaneously and produce several different morphologically distinct intermediate stages. A few of the cell types that occur are shown here (see **D** for the classification of cell types in the various lines). In bone marrow cytology, the cells of hematopoiesis from the aspirate are spread out on a slide and are viewed as a single layer of spread out cells. Because the cells are spread out in a single layer in their entirety, cellular details are far more readily discernible than in bone marrow histology where cells may be only partially sectioned because of their size.

(Specimen provided by Prof. Hans-Peter Horny, Munich)

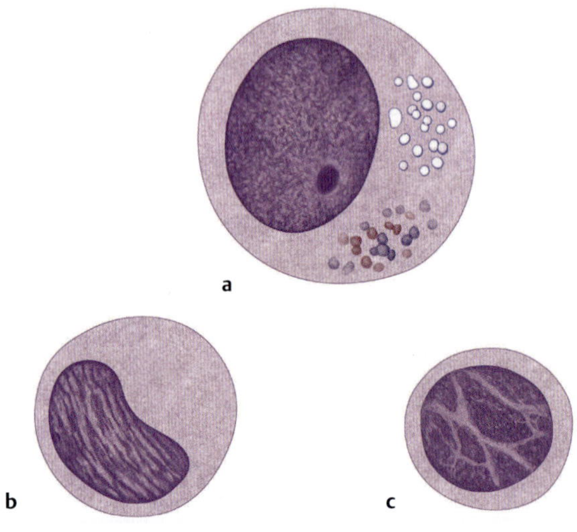

B Cytologic evaluation criteria for bone marrow aspirates

The various different chromatin structures allow us to identify different cell types: **a** myeloblast through promyelocyte; **b** myeloblast through band cell; **c** lymphocyte; clumped chromatin structure. Aside from the structure of the chromatin in the cell nucleus, the structure of the cytoplasm and its granules are evaluated. When granules are present, their affinity for dye allows their classification within a certain series of cells, such neutrophils (granules that do not easily stain) or eosinophils (red stained granules).

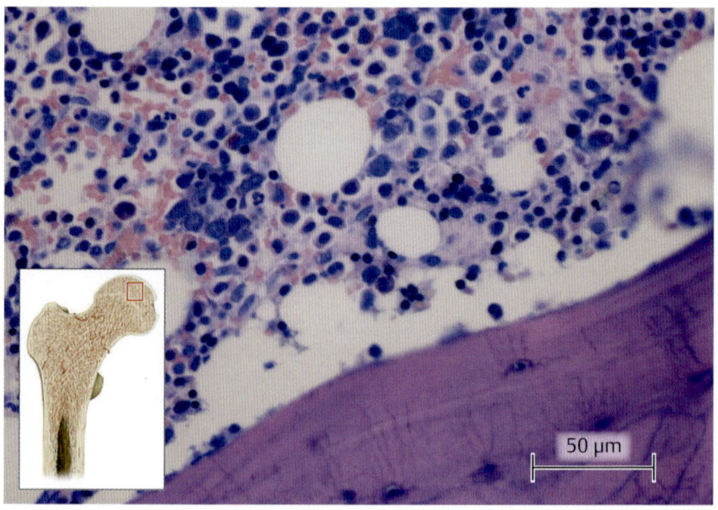

C Bone marrow histology

To obtain a histologic specimen, one removes a section of red bone marrow from the femur (in living patients via a biopsy of the posterior superior iliac spine). The cells of the red marrow fill the spaces between the trabeculae. In contrast to bone marrow cytology, histology allows local classification of the cells of hematopoiesis among themselves and with respect to the trabeculae of the bone marrow. This precise classification can be helpful in certain lines of inquiry.

(Specimen provided by Prof. Hans-Peter Horny, Munich)

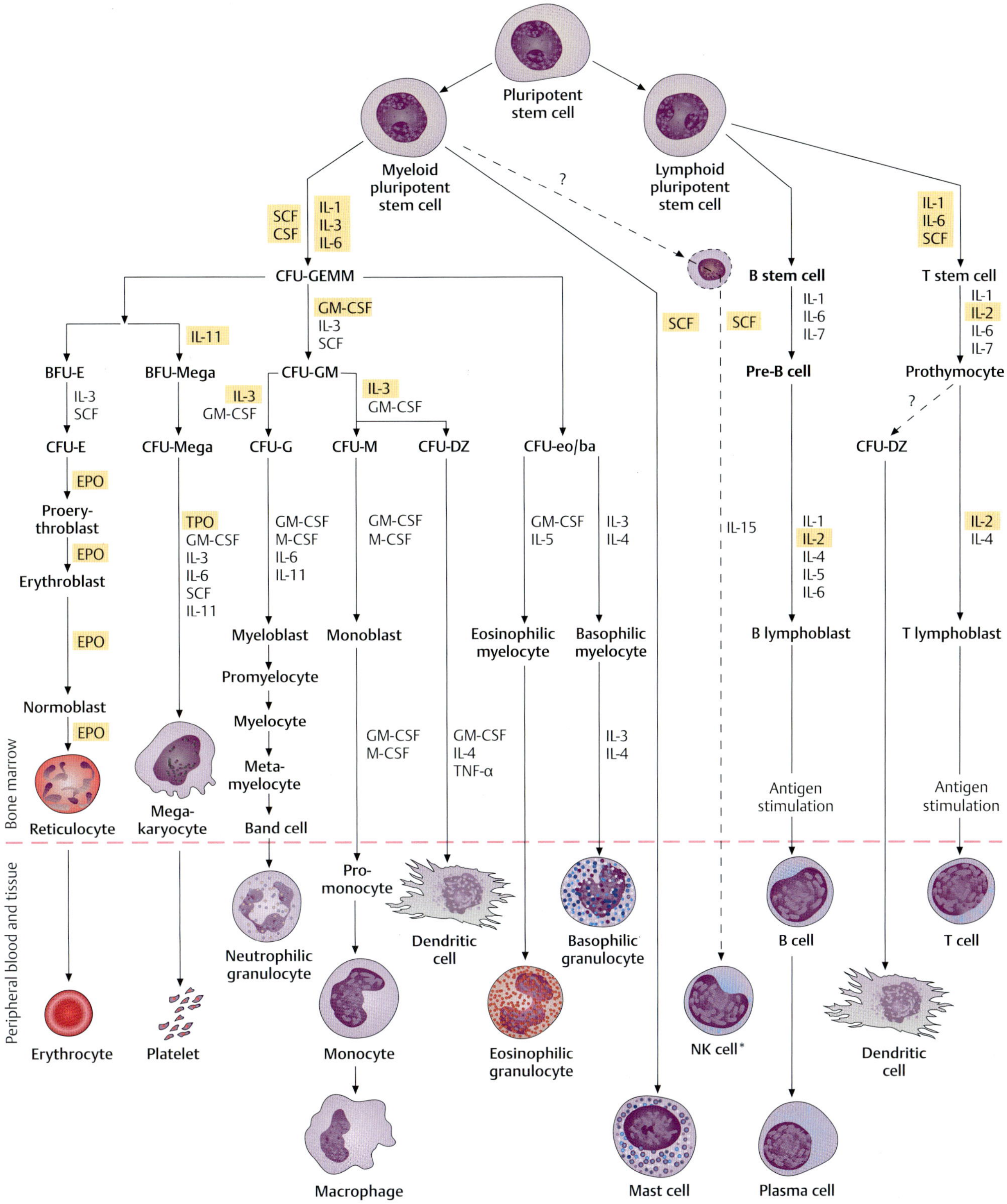

D Hematopoiesis

The yellow highlighted growth factors are the most important hematopoietic growth factors for cell differentiation.

All cells in the blood are descended from the pluripotent stem cell. It gives rise to two other cells also referred to as pluripotent stem cells: the lymphoid (right) and the myeloid (left). The various stem cell populations are morphologically indistinguishable from one another. The stem cells that descend from the two pluripotent stem cells are determined; they are stem cells only for the cell populations that follow them. The hematopoietic system requires such a complex hierarchy of stem cells because cells of the most widely varied functions and lifetimes (an erythrocyte that lives 120 days, a neutrophil that lives only a few days) must be constantly produced at a single location (bone marrow). Additionally, increased numbers of erythrocytes must be produced when there has been blood loss, and increased numbers of neutrophils in a bacterial infection. This means the system needs a high degree of flexibility in order to produce cells that function differently and have different lifetimes. The various stem cell populations ensure this flexibility. The morphology of the various normal cells of hematopoiesis is used as the basis for classifying leukemic cells (malignant degenerative cells), for example promyelocytic leukemia or erythroleukemia. This hierarchical scheme of a stem-cell-containing tissue was then applied to other types of tumors, including solid ones (concept of the malignant stem cell).

* The exact classification of the natural killer cells with respect to stem cells has not yet been fully clarified.

4.1 Overview of the Lymphatic System

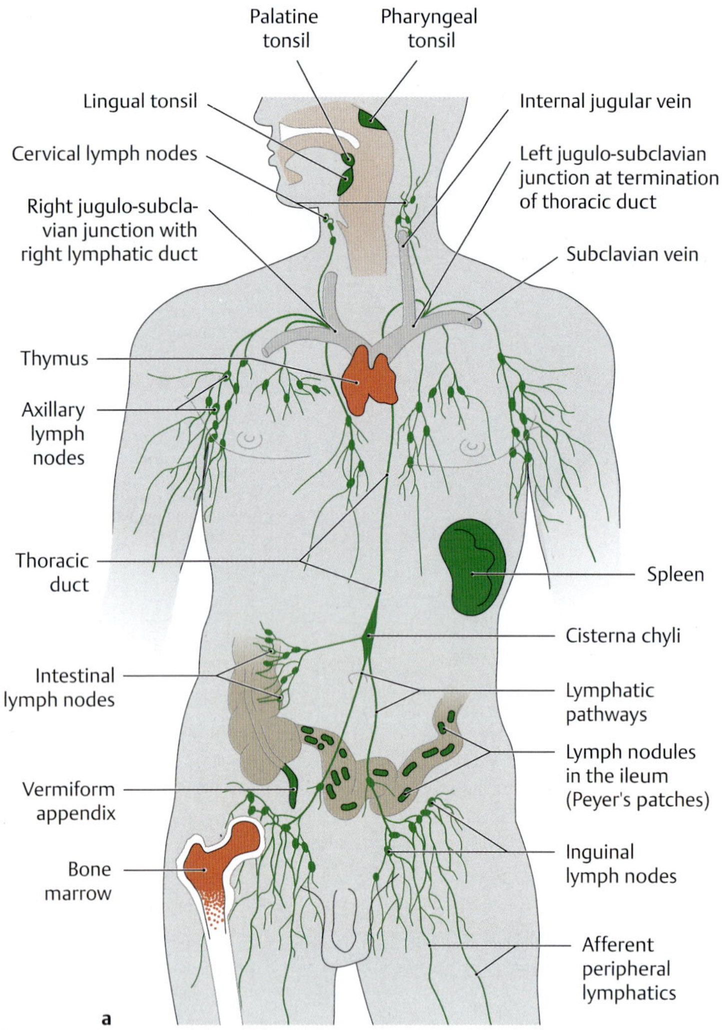

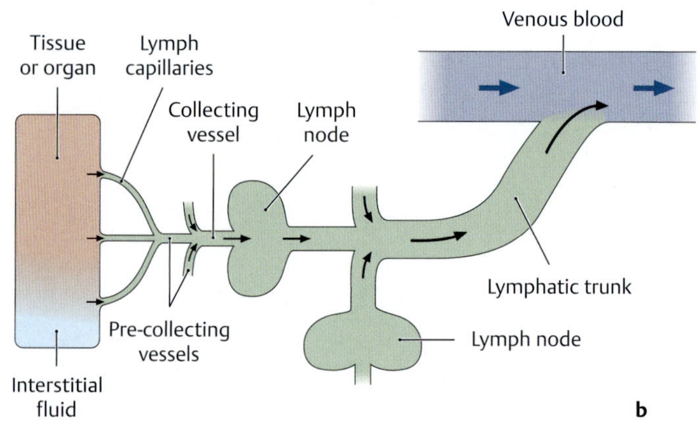

A Lymphatic organs and vessels
The lymphatic system, which is widely distributed throughout most of the body, consists of lymphatic organs and lymphatic vessels. It has three main functions:

- Immunological defense (lymphatic organs and vessels). The main function of the immune response is to distinguish "self" from "nonself" (or foreign) substances (such as pathogens, or transplanted tissues) and destroy the "nonself" substances.
- Transport of interstitial fluid to venous blood (lymphatic vessels)
- Removal of lipids from the small intestine while bypassing the hepatic portal system. This allows triglycerides to avoid liver metabolism and to be transported directly to organs that can utilize them.

a Lymphatic organs: All lymphatic organs have a stroma that is populated by lymphocytes that originated in bone marrow. They are directly or indirectly responsible for eliminating antigens (immune response). Antigens are molecules (proteins, carbohydrates, lipids), which the immune system recognizes as foreign and mounts a defense against. There are two types of *lymphocytes*, which can be further subdivided. (For more details see immunology textbooks).

- B lymphocytes ("B" stands for bone marrow, where the cells are produced) differentiate into plasma cells, which produce antibodies. Antibodies are essential components of the *humoral immune response*. Humoral immunity refers to antibodies dissolved in blood and interstitial fluid that bind to antigens. Thus, the plasma cells are not directly involved in the immune response.
- T lymphocytes ("T" stands for thymus, where the cells mature) attack and destroy foreign substances (e.g., virus-infected cells) on direct contact (*cellular immune response*).

There are both *primary* (red organs in **a**) and *secondary* (green organs in **a**) *lymphatic organs*:

- In the primary lymphatic organs, lymphocytes derived from stem cells mature and become immunocompetent cells (meaning they are capable of distinguishing between self and nonself substances).
- From these primary lymphatic organs, lymphocytes migrate to the secondary lymphatic organs where they continue to proliferate and mature. They are then able to fulfill their specific roles in the immune response. Lymphocytes can leave an organ and enter the bloodstream.

The structure and function of the individual lymphatic organs will be discussed in the respective organ chapters.

b Lymphatic vessels: Lymphatic vessels (green in **a**) are part of a tubular system that is distributed to all parts of the body (except for the CNS and renal medulla). The vessels are responsible for absorbing fluid from the interstitial spaces (it is now called lymph) and transporting it to the venous blood. Lymphatic vessels start out as tiny, thin-walled capillaries, which drain into larger pre-collecting and collecting vessels (**b**). These eventually coalesce into lymphatic trunks. These trunks join to form two larger ducts that end at each of the two venous angles (the junction of the internal jugular vein and subclavian vein) (see p. 30). Lymph nodes are incorporated into the system of peripheral lymphatic vessels. Lymphatic vessels converge in the lymph nodes, where the lymph is filtered and checked for pathogens as it passes through.

B Overview of the lymphatic pathways

Lymphatic pathways play a clinically significant role in the classification of tumors and their cells that metastasize to lymph nodes. Since lymph node metastases are sometimes discovered before the primary tumor, the organ where the cancer initiated can be determined from the affected lymph nodes. Thus it is crucial to know the lymphatic pathways of organs and regions. The classification of lymph vessels and the lymph nodes associated with them is illustrated below. If one follows the pathway the lymph travels from the site of origin until it flows into the venous blood stream, the basic classification becomes apparent:

- Lymph is formed by ultrafiltration from capillaries in the connective tissue (**C**).
- There is a superficial and deep lymphatic network (**D**).
- 5 major lymphatic trunks drain lymph from all areas of the body (see p. 30).
- The lymph nodes incorporated into the lymphatic system can be classified according to their location (see p. 31)

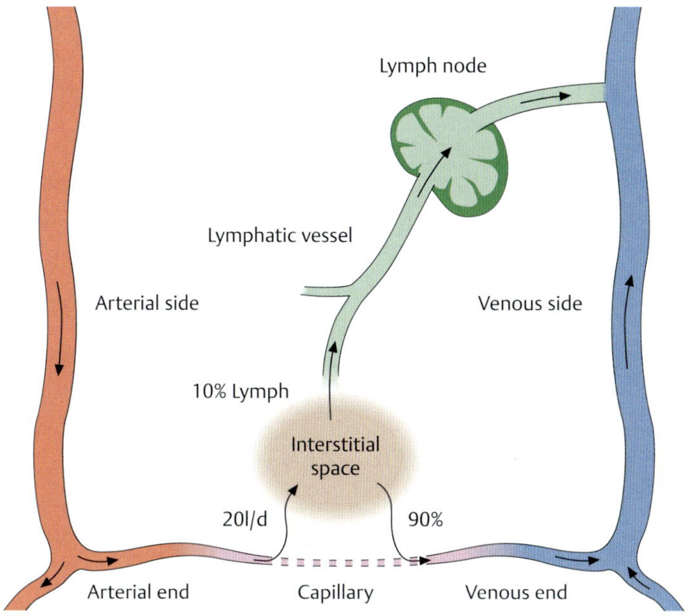

C Lymph formation

Lymph forms as a clear fluid in the capillaries by blood ultrafiltration. Blood passes through capillaries from the arterial to the venous side of the circulatory system. The internal capillary blood pressure is greater than the colloid osmotic pressure in the capillary. As a result, 10% of the fluid from the capillaries remains as interstitial fluid in the interstitial space. This 1.8–2 liters of interstitial fluid (over 24 hours) that is not returned to the blood capillaries is absorbed by lymph capillaries (see **Ab**), and then collected into larger lymphatic vessels and trunks before it drains into venous blood. Eventually all the lymph in the body drains into two lymphatic trunks (thoracic duct and right lymphatic duct, which drain into the left and right venous angles, respectively, at the junction of the neck and thorax [see page 28, Fig. **Aa**]). The lymphatic vessels direct lymph through lymph nodes, and the nodes check the lymph for germs and toxins. In cases of purulent inflammation caused by bacteria, reddened superficial lymphatic pathways are visible, which in layman terms is referred to as "blood poisoning."

Note: After a fat-rich meal, lymph from the small intestine is rich in emulsified lipoprotein particles (chylomicrons) and thus has a milky appearance. Lymph flowing from the small intestine is called chyle and the lymph vessels of the small intestine are sometimes referred to as chyle vessels.

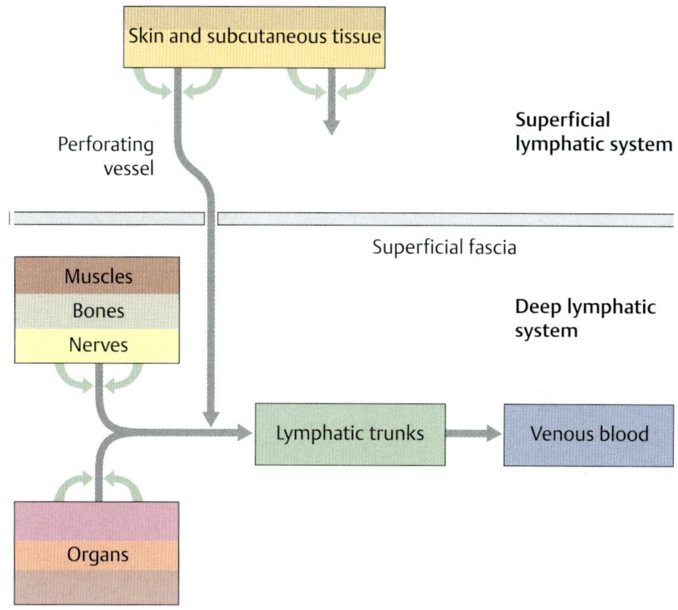

D Superficial and deep lymphatic systems

There are both superficial and deep lymphatic systems.

- The superficial lymphatic system is located in and above the superficial fascia and collects lymph from the skin and subcutaneous tissue.
- The deep lymphatic system lies underneath the superficial fascia and collects lymph from the organs, muscles, bones, and nerves.

Only the deep lymphatic system has direct contact with the major lymphatic trunks (see p. 30). The superficial lymphatic system transports lymph to the deep lymphatic vessels through perforating vessels (which penetrate the superficial fascia). The connection between superficial lymphatic vessels and deep lymphatic vessels is very pronounced in three spots:

- the sides of the neck
- the armpit
- the groin

Lymph nodes are also particularly numerous in these sites, where they can be readily palpated during clinical examinations.

4.2 Lymphatic Drainage Pathways

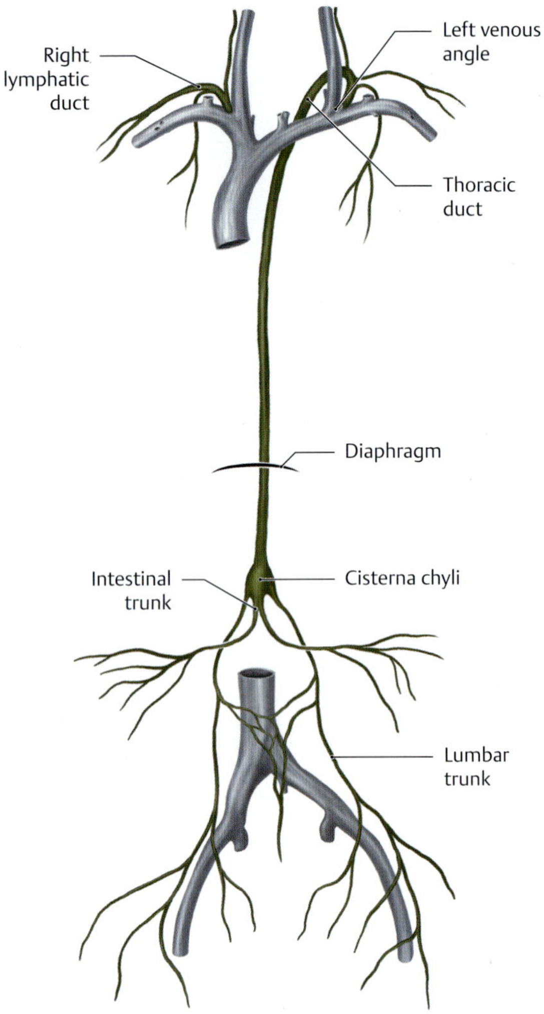

A The major lymphatic trunks
There are 5 major lymphatic trunks, most of them paired, which drain lymph from the various regions of the body. Table **B** lists all the trunks and the regions they drain. Generally, all trunks drain into either the *thoracic duct* or the *right lymphatic duct*, both of which empty into the venous system. The 3 major lymphatic trunks for the abdomen, pelvis, and lower limbs (the intestinal trunk and the two lumbar trunks) merge just beneath the diaphragm into a dilated collecting sac, the *cisterna chyli*. The **long thoracic duct** originates from the cisterna chyli, traverses the diaphragm through the aortic hiatus, ascends through the thoracic cavity and eventually drains into the left venous angle. On its way it usually receives the left bronchomediastinal trunk as well as the left jugular and left subclavian trunks. However, all these trunks may empty separately into the venous system.
The right bronchomediastinal trunk, right jugular trunk, and right subclavian trunk merge to form the **very short right lymphatic duct**. The right lymphatic trunk drains into the right venous angle.
Note: Except for the intestinal trunk, all lymphatic trunks are paired, corresponding with the organization of the body regions they drain. The intestinal trunk drains the unpaired abdominal viscera (see **B**). Although it is unpaired, it can often be divided into multiple (not individually named) sub-trunks, which in the nomenclature are collectively referred to as intestinal trunks–plural.

B Organization of the lymphatic trunks and the regions they drain
Summary of the lymphatic trunks and the body regions they drain.

Lymphatic trunk	Drainage area
Head, neck, and upper limbs	
• Left and right jugular trunks • Left and right subclavian trunks	• Left and right sides of the head and neck • Left and right upper limbs
Thorax	
• Left and right bronchomediastinal trunks	• Organs, internal structures, and walls of the left and right thorax
The trunks located on the right side merge to form the right lymphatic duct. The trunks located on the left side drain into the thoracic duct (see below).	
Abdomen, pelvis, and lower limbs	
The thoracic duct collects most of the lymph circulating throughout the body. The duct is formed by the convergence of	
• The intestinal trunk	• Unpaired abdominal viscera (digestive tract and spleen)
• The left and right lumbar trunks	• Paired abdominal viscera (kidneys, suprarenal glands) • All pelvic viscera • Left and right abdominal walls • Left and right pelvic walls • Left and right lower limbs
The thoracic duct drains all lymph from areas below the diaphragm and from the left side of the body above the diaphragm. The right lymphatic duct only drains the lymph from the right side of the body above the diaphragm. Accordingly, it is possible to divide the body into 4 lymphatic drainage quadrants (see **C**).	

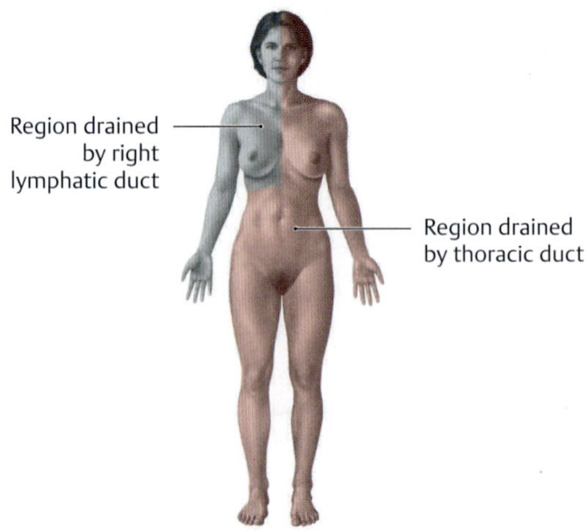

C Organization of the body into lymphatic drainage quadrants
The lymphatic drainage of the body is not symmetrical. Rather, it is organized by quadrants. The right lymphatic duct drains the right upper quadrant, and the thoracic duct drains the other three quadrants (see **B**).

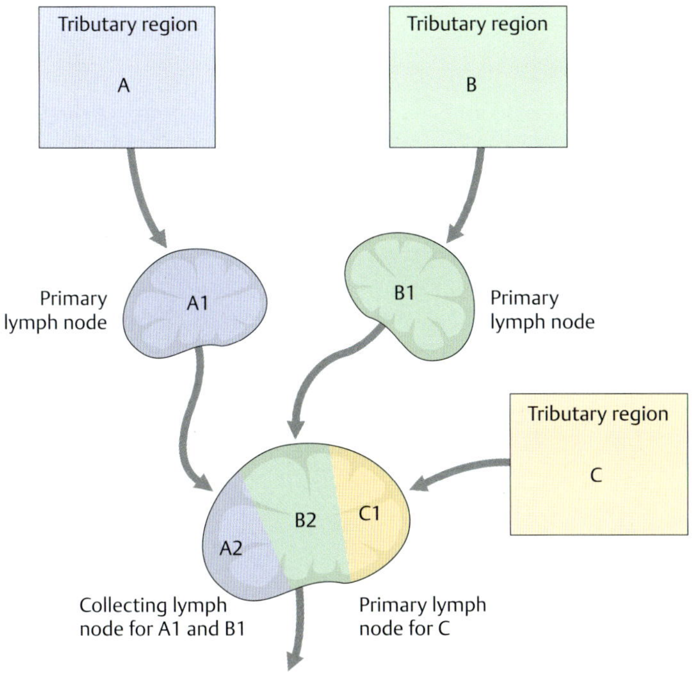

D Classification of lymph nodes

Groups of lymph nodes can be classified in different ways. One classification is based on the direction of lymph flow, and another is based on their location relative to the internal organs.

Classification based on direction of lymph flow: If lymph is classified based on the direction it flows (from peripheral tissue to the venous system), it usually passes through several serially connected groups of lymph nodes. These nodes are referred to as primary, secondary, and tertiary lymph nodes:

- Primary lymph nodes (regional lymph nodes) take up lymph directly from a circumscribed area of the body (organ; limb; part of trunk). The area that passes its lymph to a particular group of primary lymph nodes (blue or green node, A1 or B1) is called the tributary region of the specific group of nodes (in the figure labeled A–C).
- Once the lymph leaves the primary lymph nodes, it can be passed to subsequent (secondary or tertiary) lymph nodes. Since secondary lymph nodes often collect lymph from multiple groups of primary lymph nodes, they are also referred to as collecting lymph nodes (in the figure marked as a multicolored node).

Note: A group of primary lymph nodes for one tributary region can, at the same time, be the secondary or collecting lymph nodes for another region. Thus, the three-colored lymph node is a primary node for tributary region C (yellow), while at the same time it is also a collecting node for primary nodes A1 and B1 (blue and green).

Classification based on location relative to the internal organs: Lymph nodes in the abdomen and pelvis are classified as parietal or visceral depending on their relationship to major vessels and organs:

- Parietal lymph nodes of the abdomen and pelvis are located either directly adjacent to the major vessels (abdominal aorta, inferior vena cava or iliac vessels) or close to the abdominal wall.
- Visceral lymph nodes of the abdomen are related to the unpaired abdominal viscera, which are supplied by the three major unpaired arterial trunks. Groups of visceral lymph nodes are also located next to the organs in the pelvis. These lymph nodes pass their lymph primarily to the (parietal) iliac lymph nodes, which would then be considered as collecting lymph nodes for the visceral group.

Lymph node group	Parietal group	Visceral group
Abdominal	• Left, right, and intermediate lumbar lymph nodes • Inferior epigastric lymph nodes • Inferior phrenic lymph nodes	• Named after organ (see p. 238)
Pelvic	• Internal, external, and common iliac lymph nodes	• Named after organ (see p. 239)

E Embryonic development of lymphatic organs and vessels

The lymphatic organs and vessels are derived mostly from mesoderm.

Note: Growth and development of the thymus is not complete until after birth. While the other organs develop in the given time frame, they mature in function only around the time of birth (when the immune cells can make the immunologically important distinction between "self" and "nonself").

Lymphatic structure	Parietal group	Developmental process
Lymphatic vessels	Approx. weeks 5–9	Endothelial buds of the cardinal veins form sac-like, enlarged vessels, which are connected to a lymphatic plexus close to the dorsal body wall. The major ducts develop from this plexus.
Tonsils	Approx. weeks 12–16	Epithelial invagination of the 2nd pharyngeal pouch
Spleen	Approx. weeks 5–24	Proliferation of mesenchymal cells in the dorsal mesogastrium. As part of stomach rotation, the spleen moves to the left upper quadrant.
Thymus	Approx. weeks 4–16	Epithelial invagination of the ventral endoderm and ectoderm in the 3rd pharyngeal pouch

5.1 Overview of the Respiratory System

Introduction and overview

The respiratory organs are the site of gas exchange between the organism and the atmosphere (external respiration vs. internal respiration = cellular respiration). Additionally, respiratory organs contribute to voice production.

Inhaled air reaches the lung alveoli through a network of finely branched tubes (the trachea, bronchi and bronchioles). *Gas exchange* takes place in the alveoli. In the air passages, incoming air is warmed, moistened and filtered. Blood is transported to the lungs through a similarly finely branched network, the pulmonary arteries and their branches. *Carbon dioxide*, an end product of cellular metabolism, is carried with the blood to the lungs. During respiration, *oxygen* is absorbed from the air, and then binds with hemoglobin. At the same time, carbon dioxide is excreted. Carbon dioxide in the blood is a component of the bicarbonate buffering system. Thus, respiration influences the body's acid-base balance by releasing CO_2. The gas exchange between air and blood occurs by diffusion, driven by the differences in partial pressure of the two gases (the difference in the pressure of the gas between the blood and air). Blood does not come into direct contact with the air; they are separated by the blood-air barrier. From the lungs, blood is pumped through the pulmonary veins back to the heart, and from there it reenters the systemic circulation.

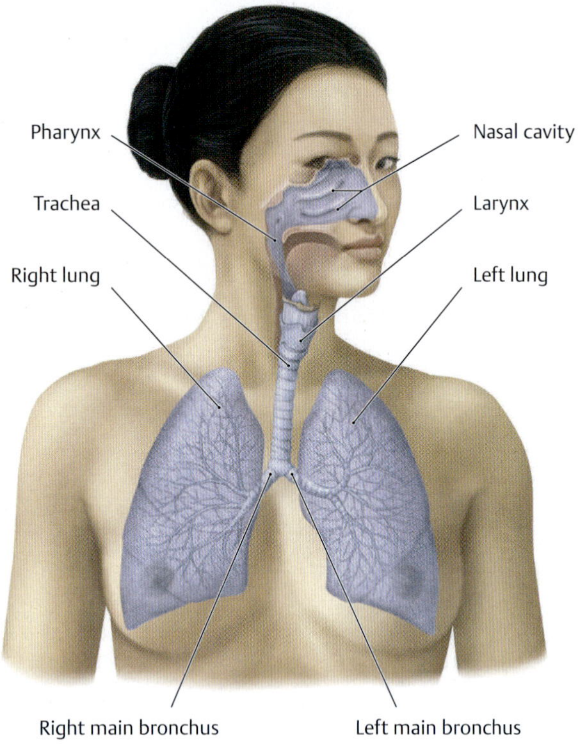

A Structure of the air passages

The respiratory system is divided into an upper and lower respiratory tract:

- **The upper air passages include**
  - the external nose and nasal cavity,
  - the paranasal sinuses,
  - the pharynx (only the upper portion, the nasopharynx, is exclusively a part of the respiratory tract. In the middle portion of the pharynx the respiratory and digestive tracts cross each other).
- **The lower air passages include**
  - the larynx, which serves to temporarily close the air passages during swallowing, and also contributes to voice production;
  - the trachea, which divides into the two main bronchi;
  - the two main bronchi, which then progressively subdivide;
  - the alveoli, located at the end of the network of progressively narrowing tubes. They are the site of gas exchange.

The histology of the different parts of the respiratory tract will be further discussed in the organ chapters.

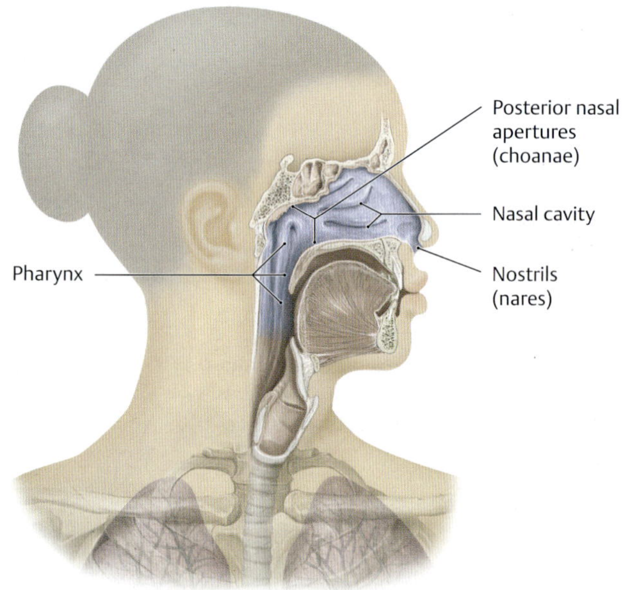

a

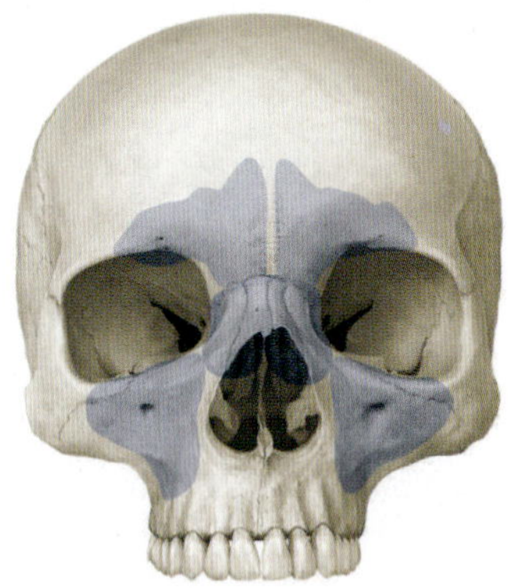

b

B Upper air passages: nose, nasal cavity, and pharynx

a Main nasal cavity and pharynx viewed from the right side with the head turned left; **b** Bony skull, anterior view of the paranasal sinuses.

Air is inhaled through the nostrils (nares) into the nasal cavity. It then passes through the posterior aperture of the nose (choana) into the pharynx, and then to the larynx. Narrow openings connect the paranasal sinuses to the main nasal cavity.

Note: In addition to conducting air, the main nasal cavity is also involved in odor perception.

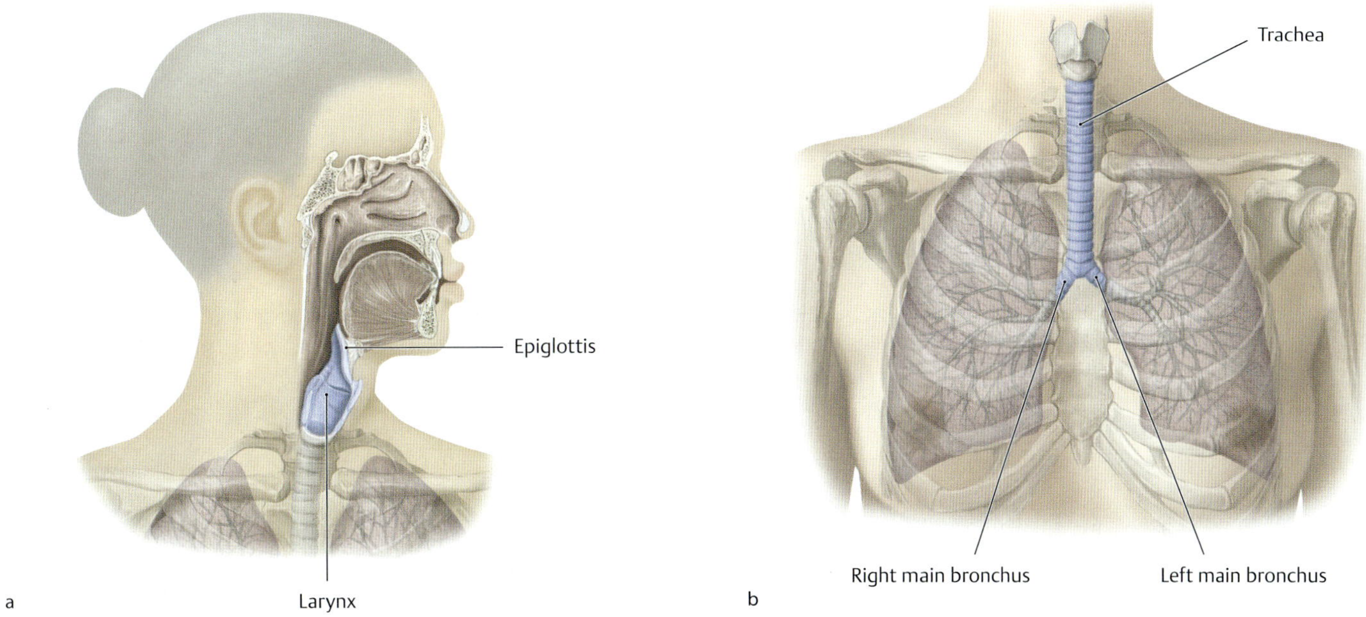

C Lower air passages: larynx and trachea

a Larynx viewed from the right side; **b** anterior view of the trachea.

The larynx marks the entrance to the lower air passages. The epiglottis, which is part of the larynx, can temporarily close the entrance to the airways during swallowing. This helps to prevent food from entering the lower respiratory passageways (which could lead to choking). Additionally, the larynx contributes to voice production. The trachea is the continuation of the larynx. It is located in the neck and thorax and divides into the two main bronchi, which carry air to each lung. Cartilage is an important structural component of the larynx and trachea.

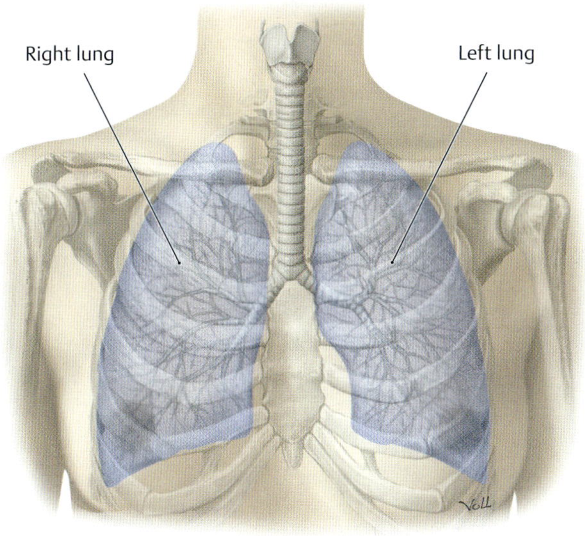

D Lower air passages: bronchial tree and lungs

Anterior view of the bronchial tree and lungs. On the right side, the two main bronchi divide into three lobar bronchi, and on the left side into two lobar bronchi. They further subdivide over several more steps with the final respiratory bronchioles ending in alveoli, where gas exchange takes place. The bronchial tree provides the structural framework of the lungs. Each lung is located in a separate pleural cavity, which is lined by a pleural membrane. The function of the bronchial tree is to conduct air to and from the lungs.

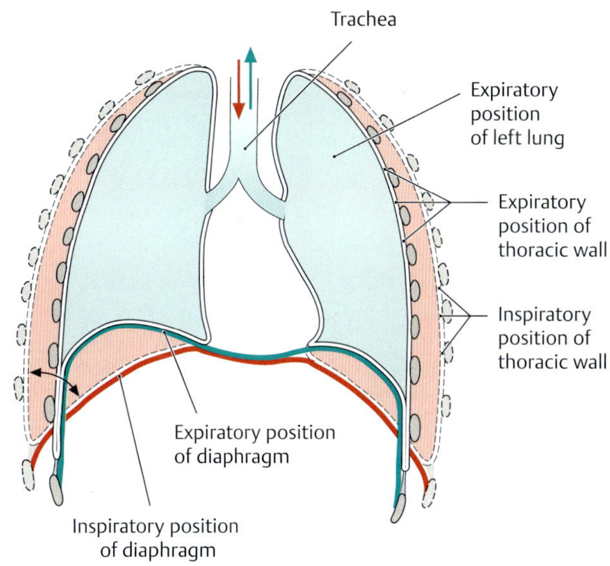

E Breathing mechanics

Anterior view of the lungs (schematic frontal section). The rhythmic activity of the respiratory muscles causes the thoracic cavity to expand (upward, downward, and laterally) and contract. The change in thoracic volume also causes the lungs to rhythmically expand, and then retract due to their elasticity. Thus, the bony and muscular structures of the thoracic wall and diaphragm, which surround the lungs, function like a pair of bellows.

5.2 Development of the Larynx, Trachea, and Lungs

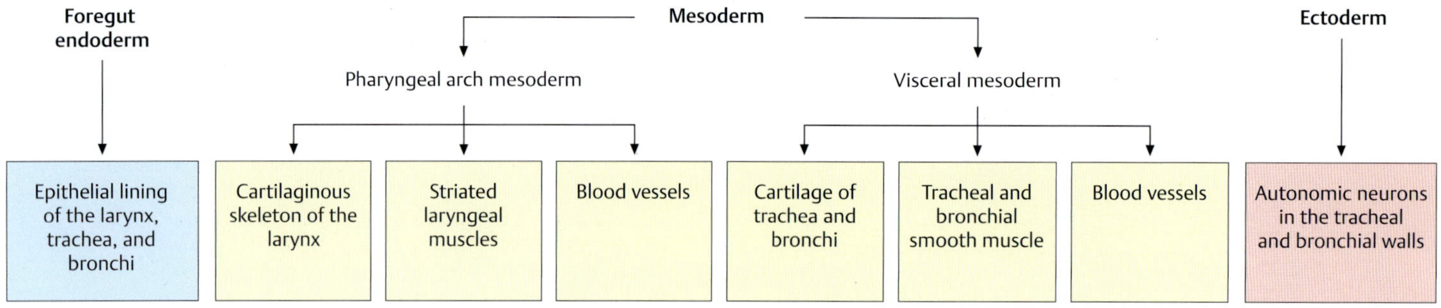

A Development of the respiratory tract from the three germ layers

All three germ layers are involved in the embryonic development of the larynx, trachea, and bronchial tree. A protrusion from the foregut in the area around the esophagus gives rise to the trachea and bronchial tree. While the cartilage, muscle, vessels, and nerves of the larynx are mostly derived from the 4th–6th pharyngeal arches, the laryngeal epithelium is derived from the foregut.

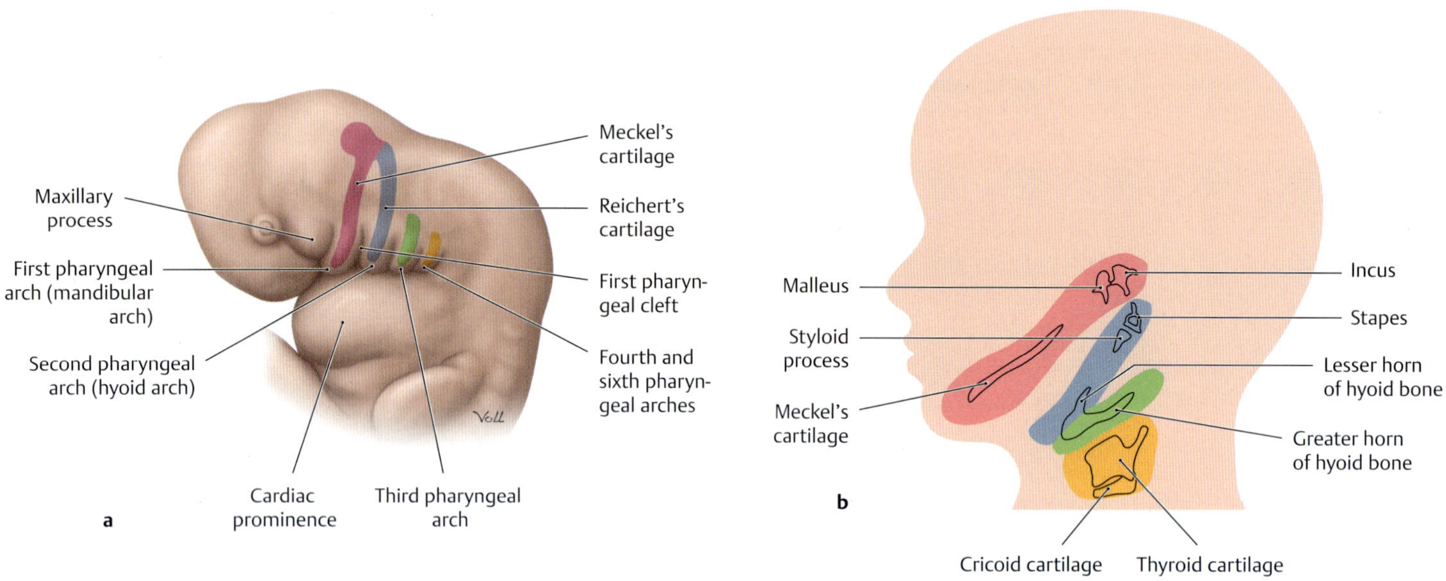

B Embryonic development of the larynx

a Embryo, viewed from the left side; **b** Location of structures derived from the cartilaginous elements of the pharyngeal arches, viewed from the left side; **c** Dorsal view of the pharyngeal arches in an embryo at 6 weeks, frontal section.

In **a**, the embryonic pharyngeal arches are visible. The visceral cranium is derived from pharyngeal arches 1 and 2. Arch 3 gives rise to most of the hyoid bone. The cartilaginous skeleton of the larynx and the laryngeal muscles are from arches 4 and 6. Corresponding to their embryonic origin, the striated laryngeal muscles are innervated by a cranial nerve (the vagus nerve).

Note: The laryngeal epithelium is derived from foregut endoderm, like that of the trachea and bronchi, and not from the pharyngeal arches.

The dorsal view of the pharyngeal arches of an embryo at 6 weeks (**c**) shows the developing entrance into the larynx adjacent to pharyngeal arches 4 and 6. This is where the passageways for food and air divide and continue in the caudal direction as two separate systems (see **C**).

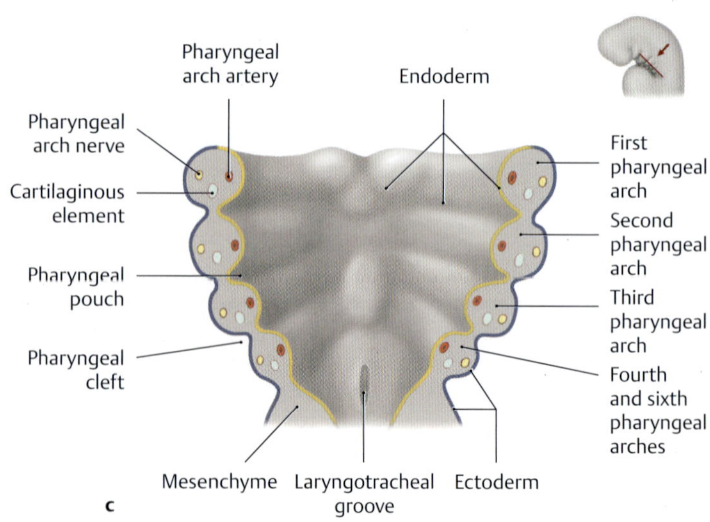

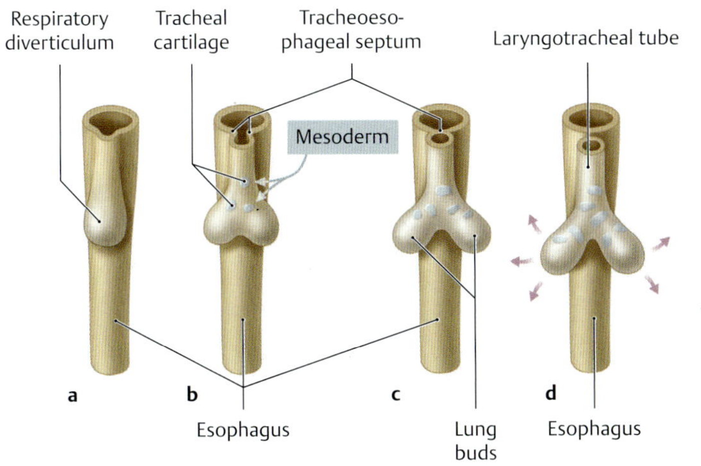

C Development of the trachea and lungs: laryngotracheal tube and lung buds
Ventral aspect of the foregut. The respiratory diverticulum (**a**) develops as a protrusion on the ventral aspect of the foregut toward the end of the 4th week of embryonic development. It later elongates into the laryngotracheal tube. This tube is initially open to the foregut. However, the tracheoesophageal septum (**b** and **c**), which develops from two lateral folds, soon separates the laryngotracheal tube almost completely from the foregut. This divides the foregut in a ventrodorsal direction into two portions (**d**):

- the developing respiratory tract, located ventral to the septum; and
- the developing esophagus, located dorsal to the septum (for the location of the foregut see p. 40).

Only the cranial end of the laryngotracheal tube—the area around the future entrance to the larynx—is in open communication with the foregut (see **b**). At the caudal end of the tube, a smaller left and a larger right lung bud forms (**c**). The lung buds are the primordia for the two lungs, and they continue to grow downward while at the same time expanding laterally (**d**). The right lung bud gives rise to the right main bronchus and the left lung bud to the left main bronchus.

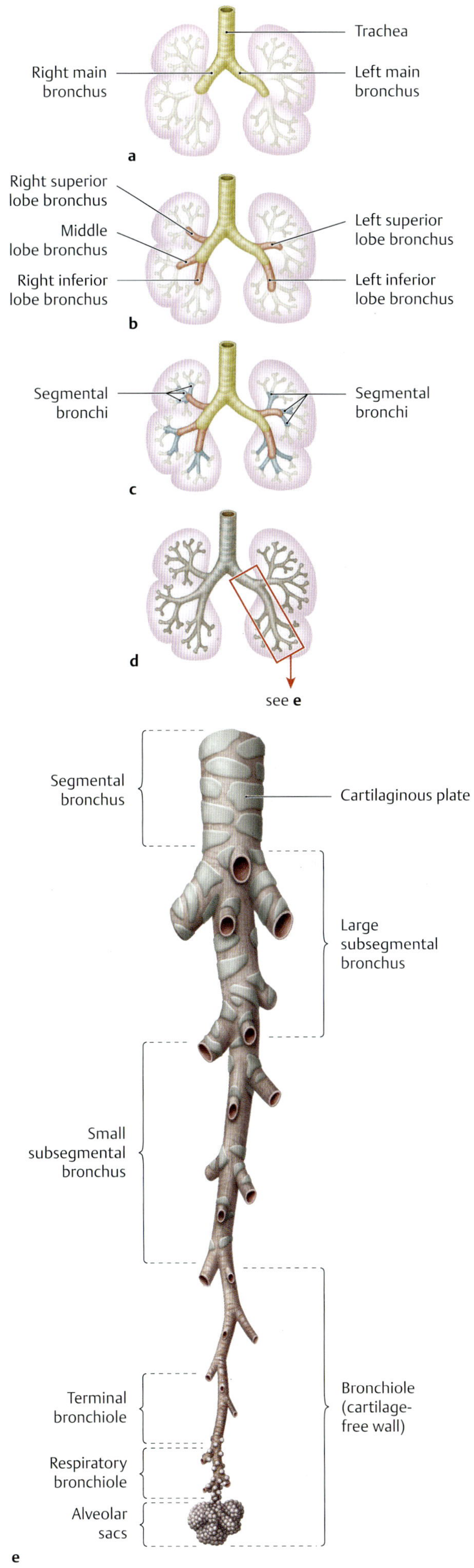

D Development of the trachea and lungs: the bronchial tree
Bronchial tree at 5 (**a**), 6 (**b**), and 8 (**c**) weeks of embryonic development, ventral view; **d** fully developed bronchial tree; **e** detail of **d**.
The lung buds initially form the right and left main bronchi. These give rise to three lobar bronchi on the right side and two on the left side, corresponding to the lobes of the lungs. These future lobar bronchi further elongate and subdivide into segmental bronchi that supply the segments of the lung (10 segments in the right lung and usually only 9 in the left lung). Further subdivisions lead to subsegmental bronchi, which decrease in size, and finally to the terminal bronchioles (**e**). The laryngotracheal tube undergoes about 23 dichotomous divisions, beginning with the lung bud. The first 17 divisions take place before birth and lead to the formation of simple alveoli, mainly in the form of alveolar sacs (see p. 37). The remaining 6 divisions take place after birth, resulting in dramatically enlarged lungs due to the high number of newly formed mature alveoli. The maturation of the lungs begins in their cranial segments and ends in their caudal segments 8 to 10 years after birth.

5.3 Lung Development and Maturation

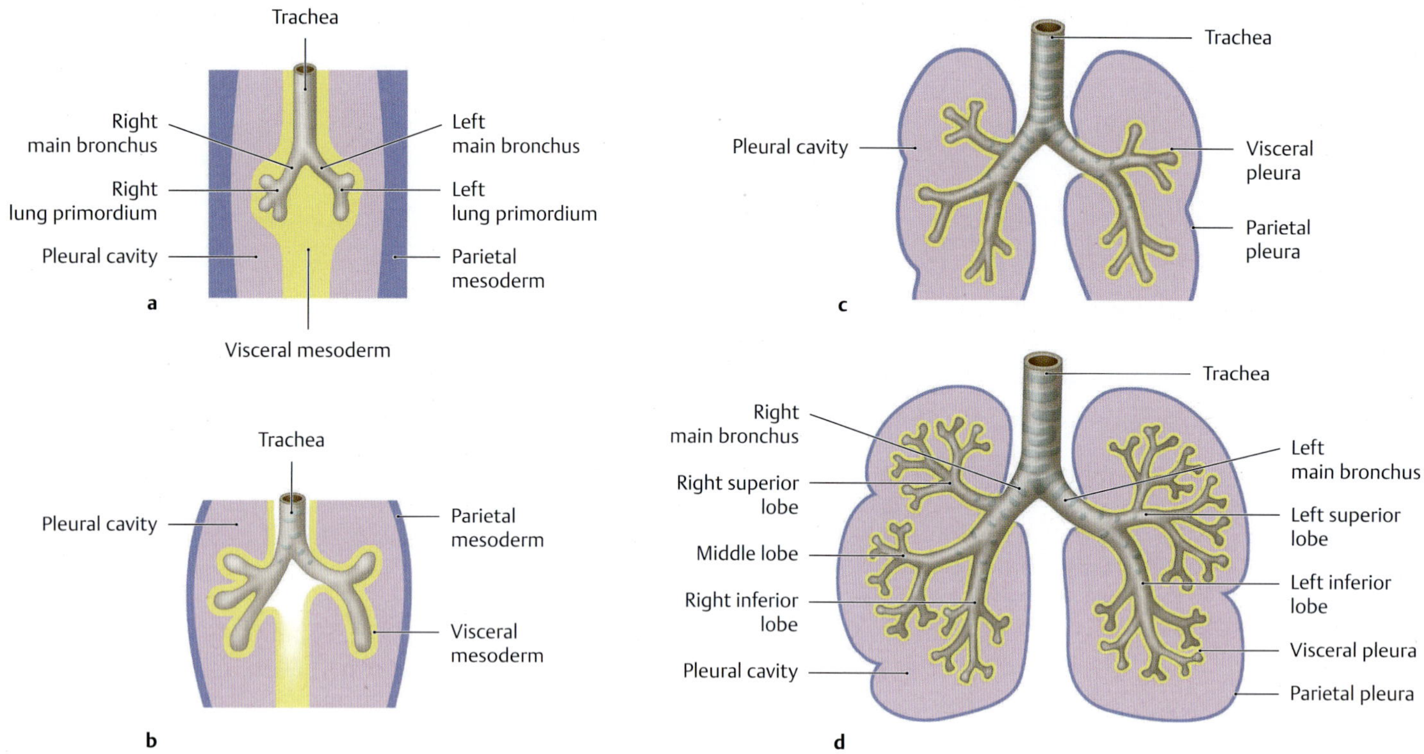

A Development of the trachea and lungs: the pleural cavities
Schematic view of the pleural cavities at 5 (**a**) and 6 (**b**) weeks; Ventral view of bronchial tree.
As part of the branching described above, the bronchial tree grows laterally and caudally toward the abdominal cavity expanding against the visceral mesoderm (**a**), until it almost touches the parietal mesoderm (**b**). The visceral pleura develops from the visceral mesoderm near the lung buds, and the parietal pleura, which lines the inside of the body cavity, develops from the parietal mesoderm. Thus, the expanding lung tissue, covered by visceral pleura, progressively fills up the parietal pleura lined body cavity (**c** and **d**). Due to its channel-like appearance, the still undivided cavity is referred to as the pericardioperitoneal canal since it connects the pericardial cavity (above) with the peritoneal cavity (below). Two folds, the pleuropericardial membranes, grow medially and fuse with each other and connect with the central compartment of the thoracic cavity (the future mediastinum, see p. 79) thus separating the now paired pleural cavities from the pericardial cavity which contains the heart (see p. 6). The septum transversum (the future diaphragm, not shown) separates the pleural cavities from the abdominal cavity, resulting in the complete partitioning of the initially single body cavity.

B Overview of the phases of lung development
The development of the lungs can be roughly divided into four phases: pseudoglandular, canalicular, terminal sac, and alveolar. The first three stages end before or at birth (see **C**).
Note: The phases can overlap.

Phase of development	Before birth (weeks of development)	Developmental stages
• Pseudoglandular phase	5–17	Division of the bronchial tree up to the terminal bronchioles. Respiratory bronchioles and alveoli have not yet formed.
• Canalicular phase	16–25	Division of the terminal bronchioles into respiratory bronchioles, which subdivide into alveolar ducts with alveoli.
• Terminal sac phase	24 until birth	Primitive alveoli form and are in contact with capillaries. Epithelial cells begin to differentiate into specialized type I and II cells. Lungs are capable of a limited degree of respiration.
	After birth	
• Alveolar phase	Around birth until 8 to 10 years after birth	Large increase in the number of alveoli as a result of further divisions. Differentiation of mature alveoli and formation of the blood–air barrier.

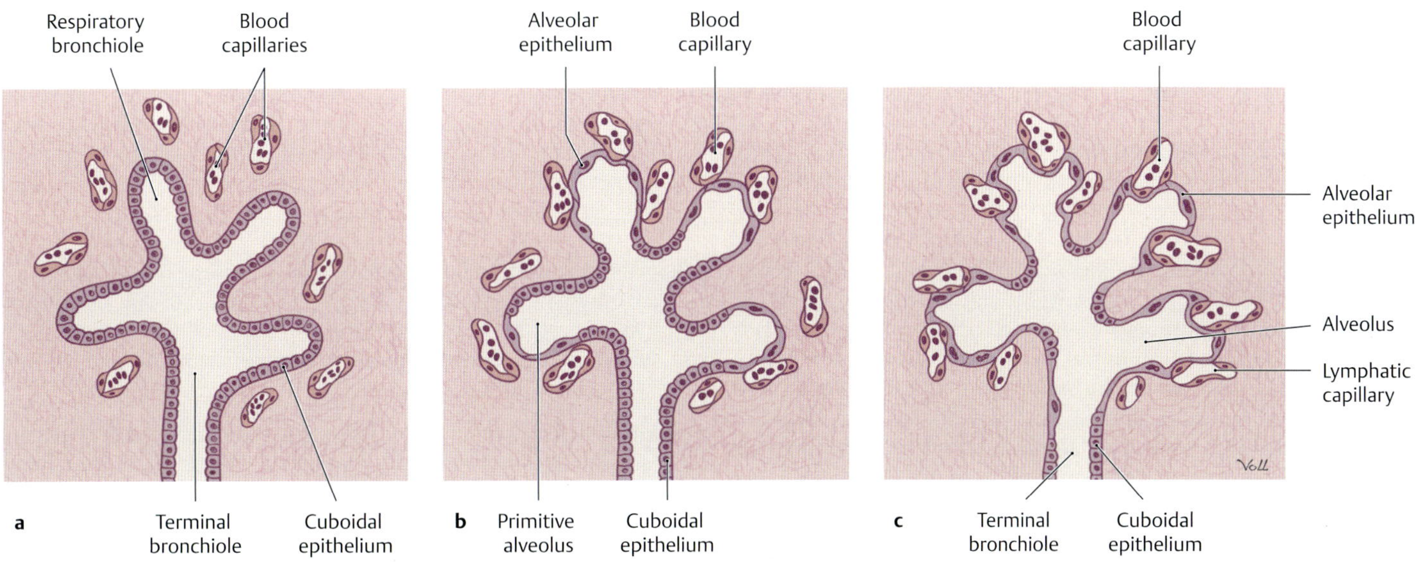

C Development of the lungs: alveolar formation and lung maturation

Alveolar development occurs simultaneously with the previously mentioned stages in lung development (see **B**). From the formation of the lung buds around the 5th week to the formation of the terminal bronchioles around the 17th week, the primitive lungs resemble an endocrine gland (thus, the *pseudoglandular phase*, see **B**). The alveoli are still unexpanded and resemble an acinous gland with an exit duct. During the subsequent *canalicular phase*, the bronchial tree subdivides repeatedly into progressively smaller branches, with the respiratory bronchioles being the smallest bronchi that exhibit alveolar precursors. Cuboidal epithelial cells of the respiratory bronchioles proliferate to form flat alveolar epithelial cells, which make contact with the capillaries (**b**; morphological correlate to the blood–air barrier). This process results in the formation of *primitive alveoli* (**b**). By the end of the 7th month, sufficient numbers of alveoli guarantee that a premature infant is capable of breathing on its own. In the last two months before birth (*terminal sac phase*), the lungs enlarge as a result of continuous branching of the bronchial tree and an increasing number of respiratory bronchioles and alveoli. The first *alveolar sacs* form (see **D**, p. 35), and blood capillaries protrude into the alveolar spaces (**c**). In the alveoli, the epithelium further differentiates into type I and type II epithelial cells (see p. 157). The type II alveolar epithelial cells produce surfactant, a phospholipid, that reduces surface tension in alveoli, thus enabling the lungs to expand with the newborn's first breath. At the time of birth, only 15–20% of the eventual number of alveoli have formed! There are around 300 million alveoli in a mature lung. The remaining 80–85% develop over the next 8–10 years as the lungs continuously produce new alveoli through differentiation (the *alveolar phase*).

Note: Fetal lungs contain fluid (amniotic fluid and bronchial secretions). When the newborn takes its first breath, air replaces this fluid. The expansion of the lungs is the result of air replacing lung fluid, not enlargement or distension of the lungs. Surfactant lowers the surface tension to such a degree that the ventilated alveoli can expand and remain open. Congenital absence of surfactant leads to *respiratory distress syndrome* (RDS), which is life threatening. In cases of RDS, surfactant is administered therapeutically by direct intrapulmonary application. Despite these measures, lung development and maturation is still a critical phase in embryonic development: Failure of the lungs to develop properly is among the most common causes of death in newborns.

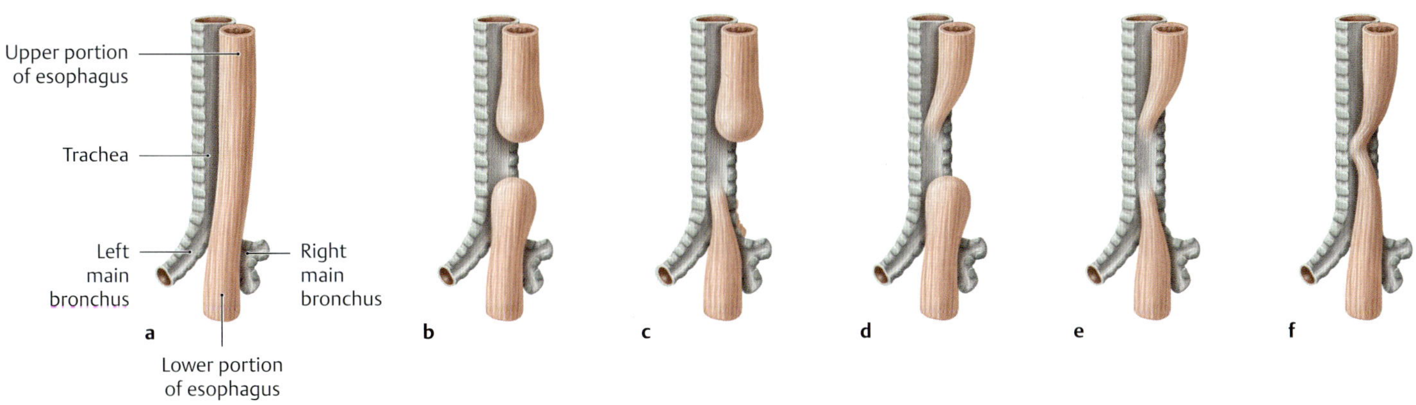

D Development of the trachea and lungs: abnormalities

Left posterior view: **a** Normal case; **b–f** Abnormalities.

Abnormalities in the development of the trachea, including irregular separation from the foregut, lead to various malformations that may or may not involve communications between the trachea and esophagus. Often, the upper portion of the esophagus ends blindly (**b** and **c**). This requires immediate corrective surgery because the infant is unable to ingest milk into its stomach. If the esophagus remains in communication with the trachea it is called a tracheoesophageal fistula. There are several types (**c–f**), and they can lead to aspiration ("breathing in") of milk resulting in constant inflammation of the trachea and lungs (the infant coughs after drinking milk). Tracheoesophageal fistulas must be surgically corrected.

6.1 Overview of the Digestive System

Introduction

Function, localization, and terms: the digestive organs break down ingested solids and fluids, absorbs their nutrients, and excrete the remaining substances that the body can't use (*digestion*). The organs form a continuous tube from the head to the lesser pelvis, and thus traverse the body cavities in the thorax, abdomen, and pelvis. The entire system is also referred to as the *digestive apparatus*, and the portions that are contained in the body cavities are called the *gastrointestinal tract*. In addition to the usual terms of location and direction, the terms *oral* and *aboral* are used when discussing the digestive system. They refer to direction along the longitudinal axis of the tract: "oral" = "toward the mouth" (os = mouth), "aboral" = "away from the mouth."

Structure of the digestive apparatus and processing of food: the digestive system is made up of a continuous series of tube-like organs that transports a bolus of food in an oral to aboral direction. In the first portion of this tube system (oral cavity to stomach), food is broken up into small pieces. The next, and longest, portion (small intestine to colon) is responsible for absorption of nutrients and water. The terminal portion (rectum and anal canal) is responsible for temporary storage and controlled excretion (defecation) of feces. In the digestive system:

- *Solid food* is broken up, mixed with water and converted into a bolus (chyme). Enzymes in the stomach and small intestine digest the food into absorbable components. Most of the nutrients are absorbed through the epithelial cells lining the small intestine and into blood capillaries. They are then transported by the portal vein to the liver where they are further metabolized. Fats, however, are absorbed directly into lymphatic vessels, and they bypass the portal venous system and liver metabolism.
- *Water* is mostly absorbed by the intestinal wall and into blood or lymph capillaries. As part of the regulation of the osmotic pressure of blood, the kidneys also control water excretion and resorption (see urinary organs, p. 50).

Additional factors that aid digestion: The stomach and portions of the intestinal tract are in constant motion in order to churn the bolus and propel it along the digestive tract. The movement of the bolus in the aboral direction toward the rectum is called *peristalsis*. The *enteric nervous system*, which is the gastrointestinal tract's intrinsic nervous system, controls peristalsis. *Glands*, which are either attached to the tube system or located directly in the system's walls, secrete hydrochloric acid, enzymes, and other substances that mix with the bolus and water to aid digestion. *Parts of the lymphatic system* (tonsils and lymph follicles in the intestinal wall) are also located in the gastrointestinal tract and play an important role in the body's immune system.

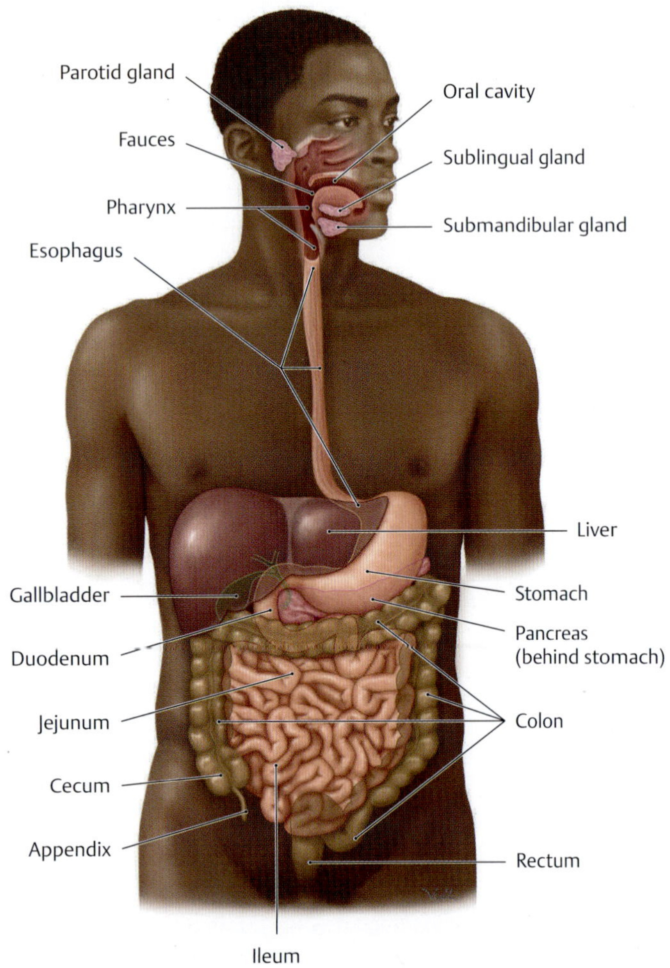

A Regional organization of the digestive organs

Digestive organs and associated structures are are located in the following regions:

In the **head** and **upper part of the neck**:
- Oral cavity with fauces at the transition between mouth and pharynx

In the **middle** and **lower part of the neck**, and in the **thorax**:
- Oropharynx and laryngopharynx
- Esophagus with cervical and thoracic parts

In the **abdomen**:
- Abdominal part of esophagus
- Stomach
- Small intestine with duodenum, jejunum, and ileum
- Large intestine with cecum, appendix, and colon (ascending, transverse, descending, and sigmoid).

In the **pelvis**:
- Large intestine with rectum and anal canal.

Glands involved in digestion and their locations:
- Salivary glands (submandibular, sublingual, and parotid as well as small salivary glands in the oral cavity)
- Pancreas in the abdomen
- Liver with gall bladder in the abdomen

Numerous small glands are present in the walls of the digestive organs from the esophagus to the rectum.

B Oral cavity, fauces, pharynx, esophagus, and stomach

In the **oral cavity** the teeth, tongue, and salivary glands chop food into small pieces and moisten it with saliva. The three large paired salivary glands, sublingual, submandibular, and parotid, secrete saliva into the oral cavity through their ducts.

Fauces and pharynx: The oral cavity connects to the pharynx through the fauces. The pharynx, which is also a part of the respiratory system, is divided into three sections. The lower portion of the pharynx, the laryngopharynx, connects to the esophagus. In some textbooks, the *entire pharynx* is considered part of the neck.

Esophagus and stomach: The pharynx is continuous with the esophagus, which traverses the thorax and diaphragm and ends in the stomach. The function of the esophagus is to transport fluids and food to the stomach, where the food bolus is further broken down by the stomach's churning. The bolus is mixed with acids to help denature proteins, and enzymatically digested. Over time the bolus is parceled out into the small intestine through the pyloric orifice.

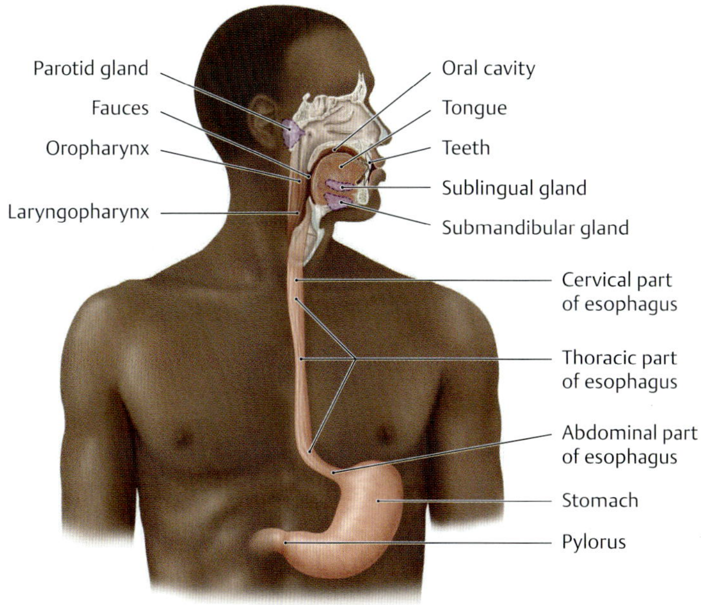

C Small intestine, large intestine, and abdominal glands (liver, gallbladder, and pancreas)

Small and large intestine: the upper portion of the small intestine, the *duodenum*, is a C-shaped structure located behind and beneath the liver. The subsequent parts of the small intestine, the *jejunum* and *ileum*, are difficult to distinguish from one another. Their multiple loops are located behind the anterior abdominal wall and are surrounded by the large intestine. While nutrients are absorbed along the entire length of the *small intestine*, the *large intestine* absorbs primarily water and electrolytes. Stool is evacuated from the rectum.

The **liver** is located in the right upper quadrant of the abdomen (**a**). The liver metabolizes the nutrients and other compounds that are brought to it from the small intestine through the venous portal system (see p. 13). The liver produces bile, which it delivers to the duodenum via the bile duct. Bile, which emulsifies fats to ease their absorption, is stored in the gallbladder located beneath the liver. The **pancreas** (**b**) is located in the craniodorsal part of the abdomen close to the duodenum and consists of two glands:

- An exocrine gland, which discharges a watery, enzyme-rich secretion into the duodenum through the pancreatic duct. These enzymes aid in the digestion of substrates.
- An endocrine gland (the "islet cells"), which produce several compounds including the hormones insulin and glucagon which regulate blood sugar levels.

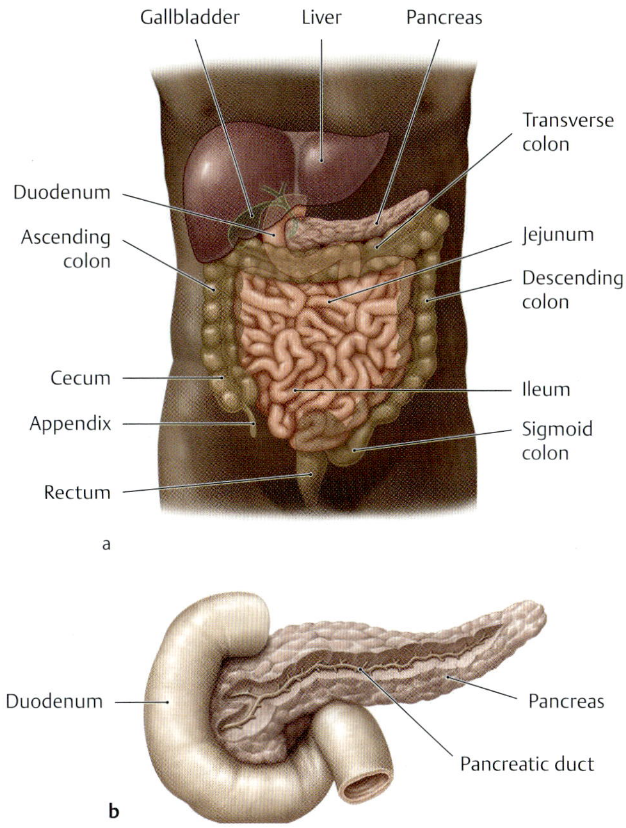

D Schematic cross-section illustrating the histology of the gastrointestinal tract

All segments of the gastrointestinal tract are divided into four layers:

- Mucosa: an epithelial layer surrounding the lumen.
- Submucosa: a layer of connective tissue surrounding the mucosa; contains blood and lymphatic vessels and autonomic nerves.
- Muscularis: the layer surrounding the submucosa; consists of an inner circular and an outer longitudinal layer of smooth muscle.
- Adventitia or serosa (depending on its location in the gastrointestinal tract): the outermost layer that attaches the gastrointestinal tract to its surroundings.

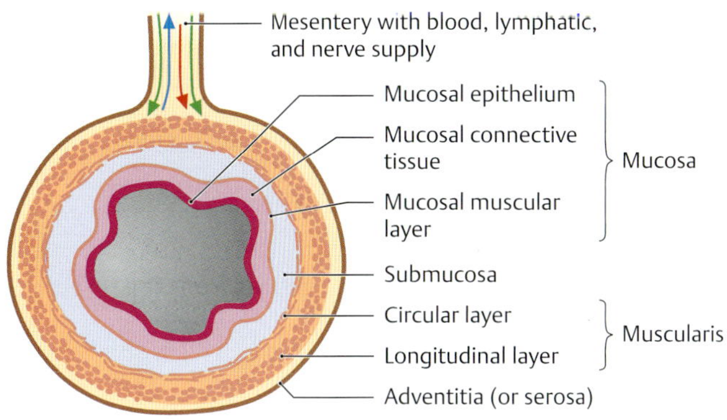

6.2 Development and Differentiation of the Gastrointestinal Tract

Introduction

The digestive organs are located in the head, neck, and major body cavities. Their complex development influences the structure of the body cavities, and thus their development will be discussed in relation to that of the body cavities. When development is complete there is a continuous tube extending from the oral cavity ("entrance") to the anus ("exit"). The liver and gallbladder, and the pancreas, discharge their secretions into this tube in the abdomen.

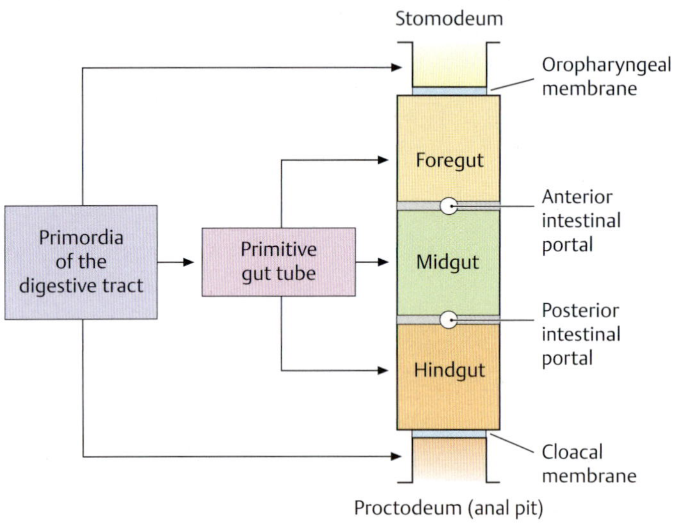

a

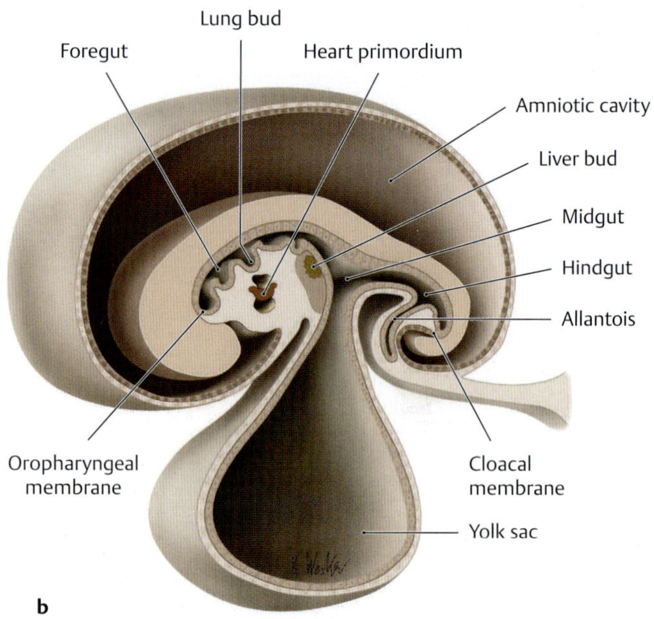

b

A Development of the gastrointestinal tract: Overview

a Overview; **b** Midsagittal section of an embryo at the beginning of the 5th week.

The primitive gut tube is derived from the dorsal part of the yolk sac, which is incorporated into the body of the embryo. The formation of two intestinal portals divides the primitive gut tube into three sections:

- The cranially located *foregut*
- The *midgut* (the longest portion of the gut)
- The caudally located *hindgut*

Cranially and caudally the primitive gut tube ends blindly. The cranial end of the foregut is closed by the *oropharyngeal membrane* and the caudal end of the hindgut by the *cloacal membrane*. The two membranes lie in contact with two ectodermal depressions. The depression at the cranial end is called the *stomodeum* and at the caudal end it is called the *proctodeum*. At first, the initially very short midgut is in direct communication with the yolk sac along its entire length. During embryonic folding additional portions of the yolk sac become incorporated into the developing midgut. The midgut is a continuation of the foregut at the *anterior intestinal portal*, and the hindgut is a continuation of the midgut at the *posterior intestinal portal*. The hindgut is connected to the allantois, which is an outpouching of the caudal wall of the yolk sac in the early embryo (see **b**).

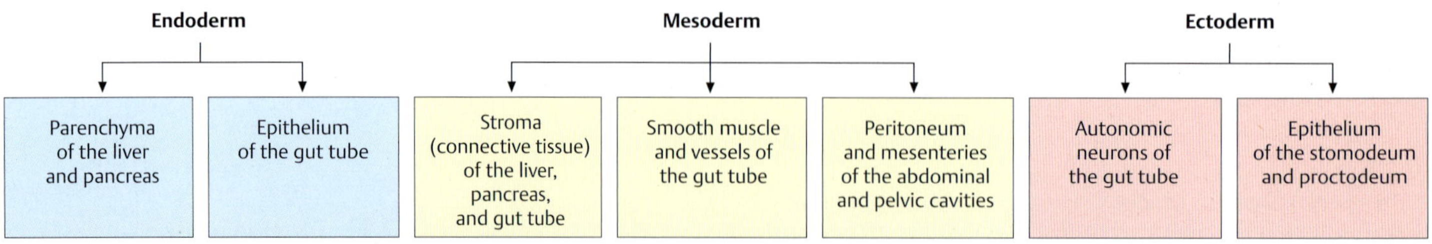

B Development of the gastrointestinal tract from the three germ layers

The organs of the gastrointestinal tract are derived from the three germ layers.

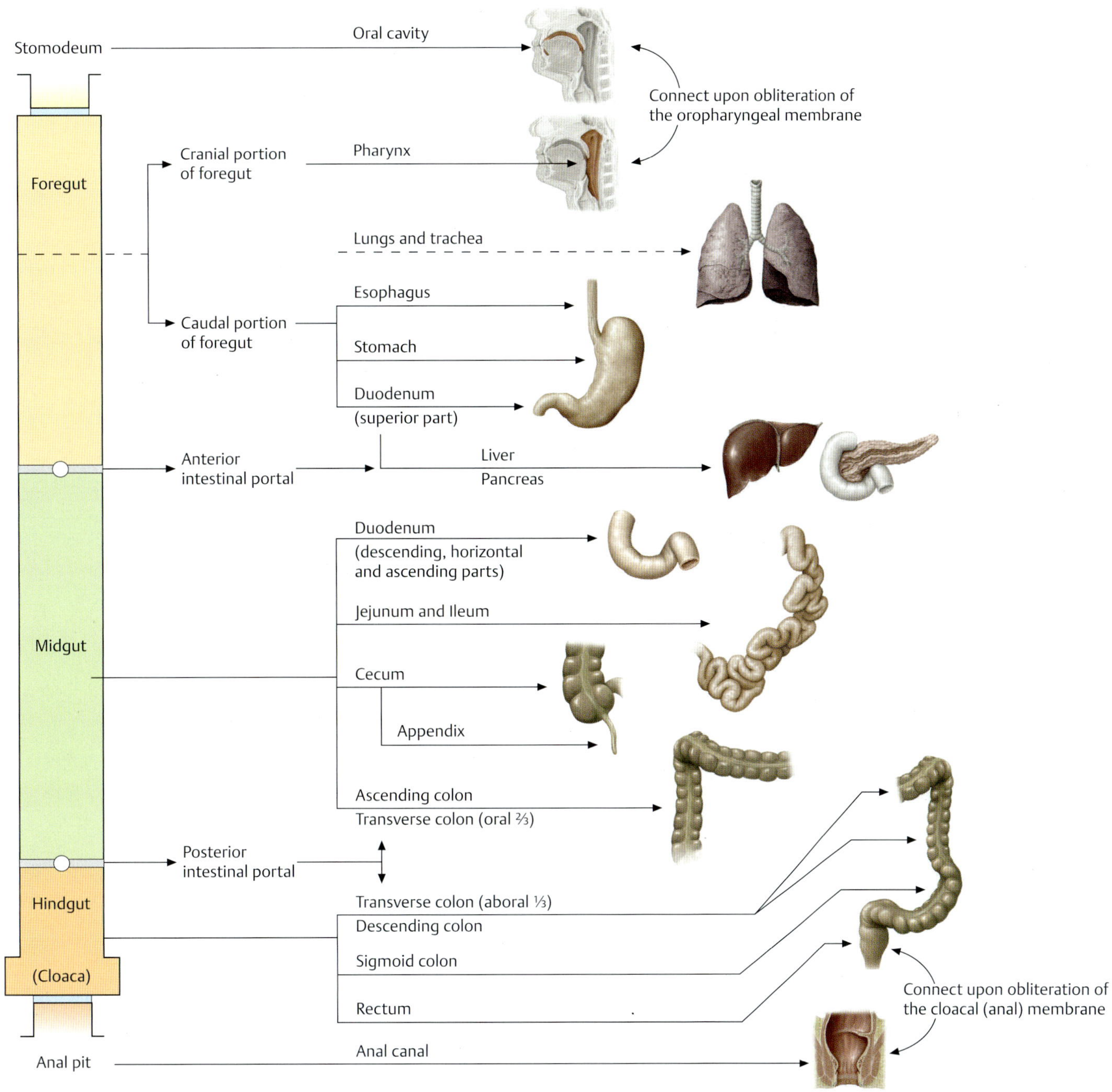

C Differentiation of the gastrointestinal tract

The primitive gut tube gives rise to all parts of the digestive tract. The epithelium of the gut tube is derived from *endoderm* (see **B**). The oropharyngeal membrane and cloacal membrane, which are lined on the outside with ectoderm, break down later in development to allow the gut tube open access to the external environment (see p. 47).

- The **foregut** divides into a *cranial portion*, which gives rise to the pharynx, and a *caudal portion*, which gives rise to the esophagus, stomach, and the superior part of the duodenum (see p. 42). The respiratory diverticulum, which will develop into the trachea and lungs, marks the boundary between the two portions of the foregut (see p. 35).
- The **midgut** gives rise to the remainder of the small intestine as well as the ascending colon and oral ⅔ of the transverse colon.
- The **hindgut** gives rise to the remainder of the colon and the rectum. The expanded caudal end of the hindgut is called the *cloaca*. Both the rectum and part of the urogenital system develop from the cloaca.

The **anterior intestinal portal** marks the border between the foregut and midgut. It is located along the duodenum and it gives rise to the liver, gallbladder, and pancreas. The junction between the midgut and hindgut is called the **posterior intestinal portal** and it lies between the oral ⅔ and aboral ⅓ of the transverse colon. This region, also referred to as the Cannon-Boehm point, plays a significant role in the arrangement of the colon's autonomic innervation. The **stomodeum** develops into the oral cavity and the **proctodeum** gives rise to the anal canal. The epithelial lining of both structures is derived from ectoderm and is continuous with the outer lining of the oropharyngeal and cloacal membranes. At these two sites, the endodermal and ectodermal epithelium are adjacent to each other. The obliteration of the oropharyngeal and cloacal membranes results in the primitive gut tube becoming open to the embryo's external environment.

6.3 Mesenteries and Primordia of the Digestive Organs in the Caudal Foregut Region; Stomach Rotation

Introduction
Two processes are crucial for the embryological development of the digestive organs:

- The rotation of the stomach in the *caudal foregut* (see p. 44)
- The rotation of the intestinal loop (the loop-shaped fetal gut tube, see p. 46) in the *midgut* and *hindgut*.

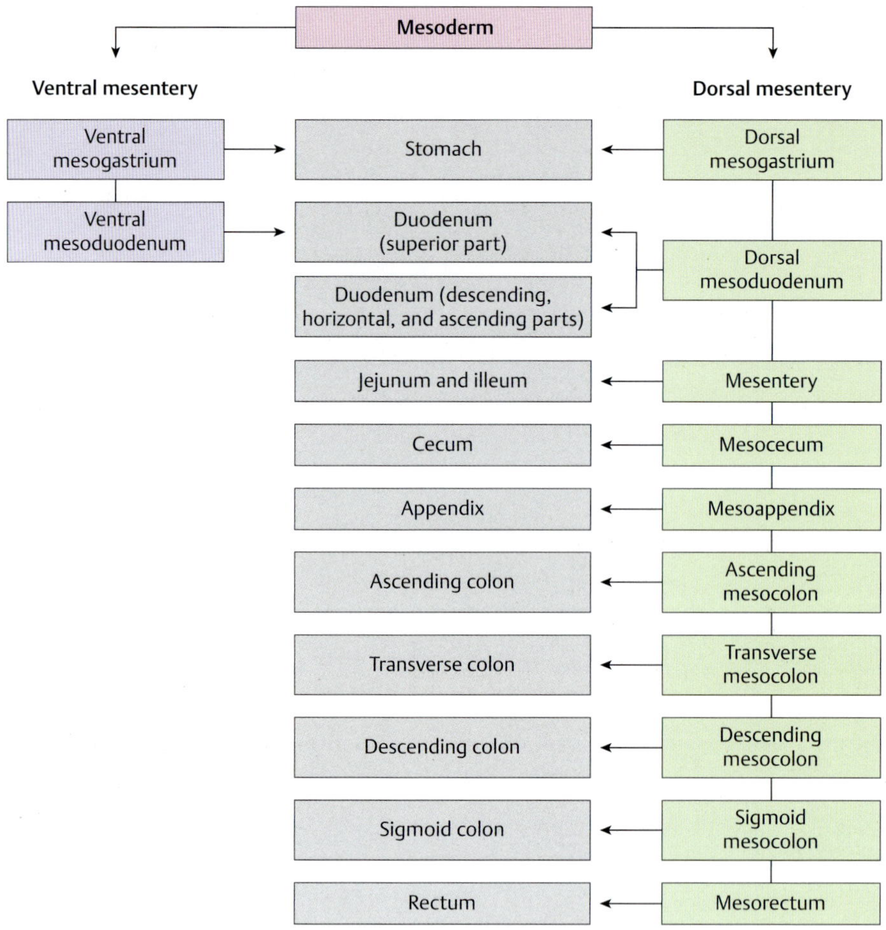

A Mesenteries of the gut tube in the embryo (overview)
The esophagus, stomach, and superior part of the duodenum originate from the caudal portion of the foregut. Like all organs of the digestive system in the abdomen and pelvis, they have a dorsal mesentery (a passageway extending from the posterior wall of the peritoneal cavity to the posterior wall of the organ). In the area surrounding the stomach and the superior part of duodenum, there is also a ventral mesentery. It arises from the anterior wall of the peritoneal cavity and attaches to the anterior wall of the organs. The umbilical vein carries oxygenated blood from the placenta to the liver and inferior vena cava of the embryo through this ventral mesentery. Due to this additional mesentery, the peritoneal cavity at the level of the stomach and duodenum is divided into a left and a right half (see p. 44).

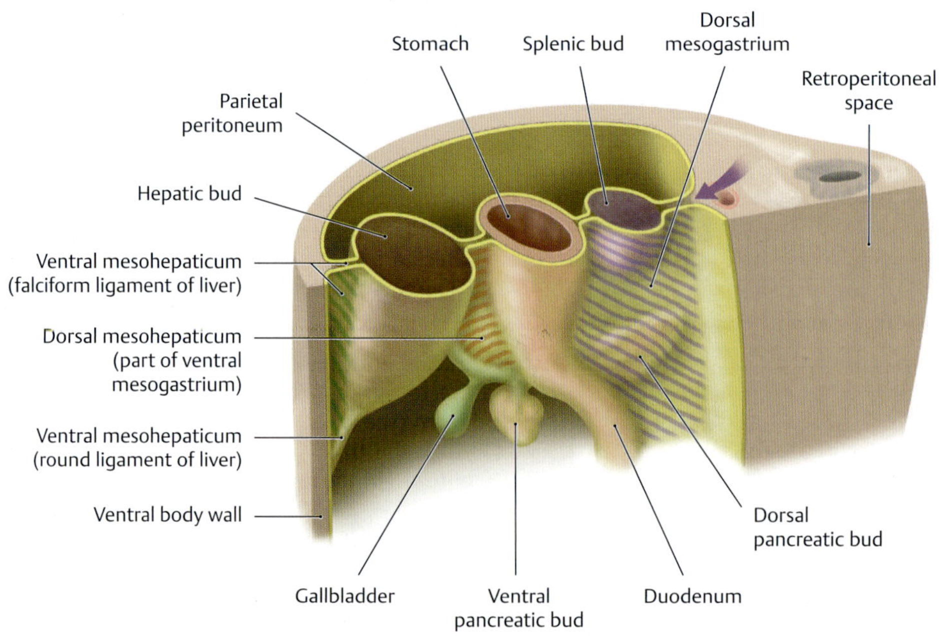

B Mesenteries of the caudal foregut in the embryo
The following organs arise from the duodenal epithelium and grow into the mesenteries of the duodenum and stomach (see **A**):

- The liver and bile ducts grow into the area between ventral meso*duodenum* and ventral meso*gastrium*.
- The ventral pancreatic bud and dorsal pancreatic bud grow into the *ventral* mesoduodenum and *dorsal* mesoduodenum, respectively.

In the 5th week, the spleen, a lymphatic organ, migrates from mesenchyme in the retroperitoneal space located dorsal to the peritoneal cavity, to the dorsal mesogastrium. Thus, both the spleen and dorsal pancreatic bud are located in the dorsal mesentery. During stomach rotation (see **D**), the mesenteries shift along with the organs they contain (see p. 44). The terminology for the mesenteries in the mature organism are indicated in **E**.

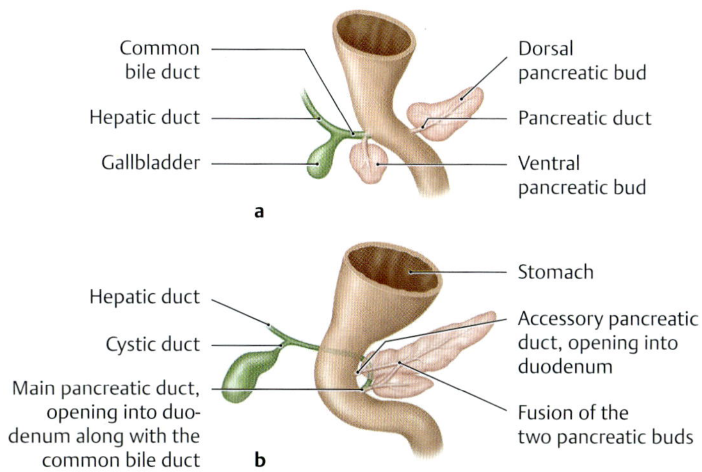

C Fusion of the dorsal and ventral pancreatic buds

Simplified schematic view of the left side of the gastrointestinal tube of the stomach with the primordial bile ducts and pancreas. The two pancreatic buds (**a**) form as outgrowths from the duodenal epithelium and migrate into the ventral and dorsal mesogastrium at the junction with the mesoduodenum (see **B**). The ventral pancreatic bud develops in close proximity to the primordium of the bile duct. It migrates with the primordium of the bile duct around the right side of the duodenum toward the dorsal pancreatic bud, eventually coming to rest in the dorsal mesoduodenum (**b**) (for the effect of stomach rotation on the ventral pancreatic bud see p. 44). Both pancreatic buds fuse and their ducts anastomose.

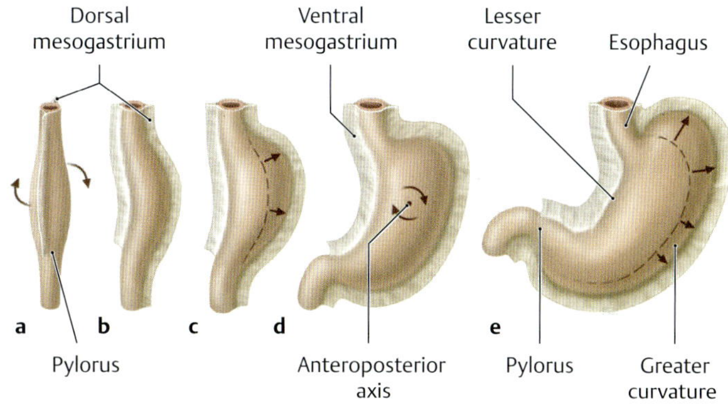

D Stomach rotation

Ventral view. At the beginning of the 5th week, the stomach (viewed from above) rotates clockwise 90 degrees around its longitudinal axis (**a**). At the same time, it widens asymmetrically with the left wall (original dorsal wall) growing significantly faster than the right wall (original ventral wall) (**b** and **c**). Finally, the entire stomach rotates clockwise around an anteroposterior axis and now sits obliquely in the abdomen. The greater curvature (original dorsal wall) now points to the left and downward, and the lesser curvature (original ventral wall) points to the right and upward (**d**). The two *mesenteries* of the stomach (ventral and dorsal mesogastrium) also participate in this rotation, asymmetrical growth, and tilting of the stomach: the ventral mesogastrium shifts to the right (and upward), and the dorsal mesogastrium shifts to the left (and downward, **e**).

E Mesentery terminology in the caudal foregut: Comparison of embryonic and mature organisms

As a result of the rapid growth of the liver and spleen in the embryo, both mesenteries of the stomach, the dorsal and ventral mesogastrium, are further subdivided into a ventral and dorsal mesohepaticum (hepar = liver) and a ventral and dorsal mesosplenicum (splen = spleen). In the mature organism, these mesenteries are referred to as omenta and ligaments.

Term in the embryonic organism	Term in the mature organism
Ventral mesogastrium with subsections	
• Dorsal mesohepaticum (“in the back of the liver”)	• **Lesser omentum**; connection from liver to lesser curvature of the stomach and superior part of duodenum; divided into – hepatoesophageal ligament (liver to esophagus, only very small) – hepatogastric ligament (liver to stomach) with flaccid and hard portions – hepatoduodenal ligament (liver to duodenum)
• Ventral mesohepaticum (“at the front of the liver”)	• Connection between liver and anterior trunk wall; divided into – falciform ligament – round ligament of the liver (contains the obliterated umbilical vein)
Dorsal mesogastrium with subsections	• **Greater omentum**; connection between the *greater* curvature of the stomach and the fundus of the stomach on one hand and the spleen and transverse colon and posterior wall of the peritoneal cavity on the other hand, as well as several ligaments:
• *At the level of the splenic bud* – ventral mesosplenicum (“at the front of the spleen”) – dorsal mesosplenicum (“in the back of the spleen”)	– gastrosplenic ligament (part of greater omentum, stomach to spleen) – phrenicosplenic ligament (diaphragm to spleen) – splenorenal ligament (spleen to kidney and posterior wall of peritoneal cavity)
• *Above the splenic bud* (no anatomical terms for the embryonic organism)	– gastrophrenic ligament (part of greater omentum, stomach to diaphragm)
• *Below the splenic bud* (no anatomical terms for the embryonic organism)	– gastrocolic ligament (part of greater omentum, stomach to transverse colon) – phrenicocolic ligament (posterior wall of peritoneal cavity to left colic flexure)

Note: In the mature organism, all structures arising from the dorsal mesogastrium are often referred to as greater omentum.

6.4 Stomach Rotation and Organ Location in the Caudal Foregut Region; Formation of the Omental Bursa

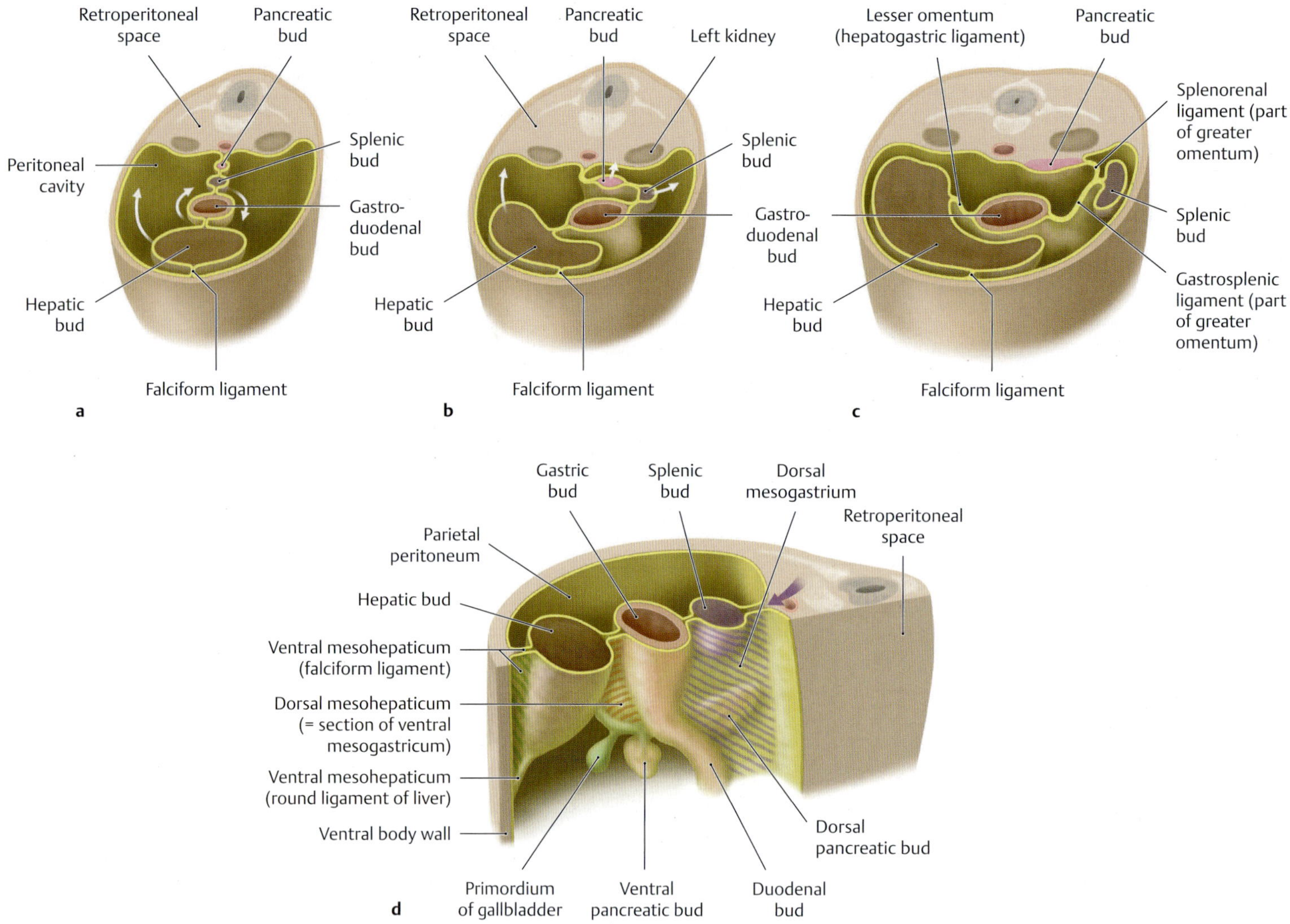

A Effects of stomach rotation on its mesenteries and on the position of organs in the caudal foregut region

Schematic spatial representation of the embryonic abdomen in successive stages. Anterosuperior view (**a–c**) and left superior view (**d**). The white arrows indicate the direction of rotation and organ migration.

Duodenum: Stomach rotation moves the duodenum to the right and slightly up. By the time stomach rotation ends, the duodenum is bent into a C-shape with the open side facing left. As the duodenum rotates to the right its ventral mesoduodenum rotates with it. This affects the position of the ventral pancreatic bud that is developing in the mesoduodenum. In addition to its migration as illustrated on page 43, this rotation moves the ventral pancreatic bud toward the dorsal pancreatic bud.

Pancreas: The ventral and dorsal pancreatic buds fuse as the duodenum rotates clockwise. Initially they lie in the abdomen in an oblique position, but rotation further shifts the fused buds toward the posterior wall of the peritoneal cavity. The *visceral* peritoneum of the pancreas and duodenum then fuse with the *parietal* peritoneum on the posterior wall of the peritoneal cavity. Thus, the pancreas and duodenum are *secondarily* retroperitoneal, and the *anterior side* of both organs is covered by *parietal* peritoneum.

Liver: Since the developing liver lies in the ventral mesogastrium, it is shifted to the right and upward along with the mesogastrium. Its peritoneal membrane is attached to the peritoneum covering the diaphragm. As the liver grows it contacts the diaphragm and the peritoneum of both the liver and diaphragm disintegrates at the area of contact. The portion of the liver not covered by peritoneum is referred to as the bare area. The portion on the diaphragm is called the hepatic surface of the diaphragm. The rest of the liver remains intraperitoneal. However, due to its rapid growth, it moves dorsally and closer to the right kidney, which keeps the right kidney slightly more inferior than the left.

Bile ducts: The portion of the bile duct adjacent to the liver will form the hepatic ducts. The portion of the bile duct that opens into the duodenum runs through the lateral edge of the lesser omentum (the hepatoduodenal ligament). The extrahepatic bile ducts are thus largely intraperitoneal, but portions become secondarily retroperitoneal after coursing through the pancreas to join with the pancreatic ducts close to the duodenum.

Spleen: Stomach rotation moves the spleen bud, which lies in the dorsal mesogastrium, to the left. It remains intraperitoneal within the mesogastrium.

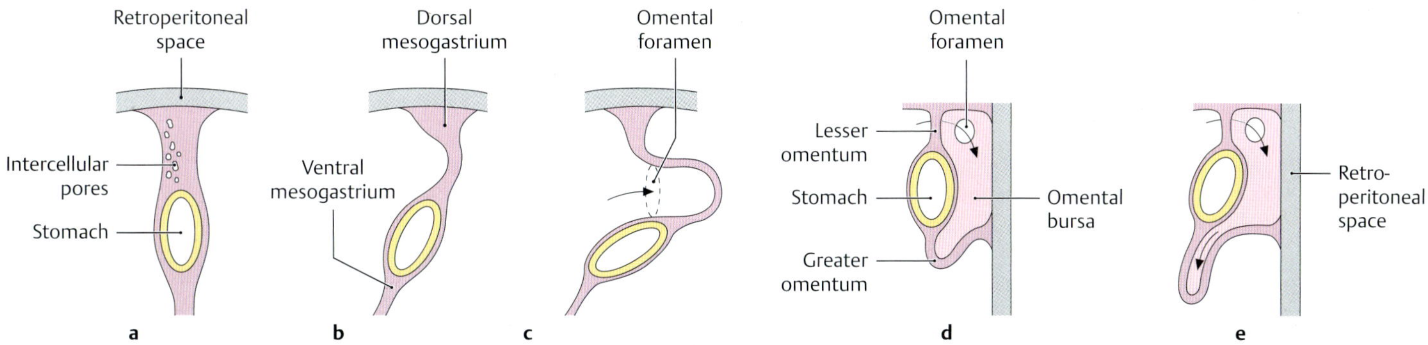

B Development of the omental bursa
Stomach and mesogastria; **a–c** Horizontal sections of the abdomen, superior view; **d** and **e** Sagittal sections, viewed from the left. The upper arrows in **c–e** point to the omental foramen, which is the only physiological opening into the omental bursa. The lower arrow in **e** shows the deepening pouch formed by the greater omentum.
As the stomach and mesogastria rotate, the originally right wall of the stomach is shifted posteriorly, and the left wall of the stomach anteriorly. The dorsal and ventral mesogastria are still holding stomach in place, and as a result of the rotation, the original right side of the peritoneal cavity becomes enclosed posterior to the stomach. This space is called the omental bursa, and its borders are demarcated:

- posteriorly by the posterior wall of the peritoneal cavity (anterior to the already retroperitonealized pancreas, see **Ac**),
- anteriorly by the posterior wall of the stomach and both of the mesogastria,
- to the right by the liver,
- to the left by the spleen,
- superiorly by the diaphragm (diaphragm not visible here),
- inferiorly by an outpouching of the dorsal mesogastrium (between layers of the greater omentum).

C Development of the caudal region of the foregut: Summary and peritonealization
The following processes are crucial for the formation of mature structures. They overlap in time, but are presented here in chronological order to aid clarification.

Organ primordia; stomach rotation and mesenteric rotation

The stomach and upper duodenum have both dorsal and ventral mesenteries. Thus, at the level of these organs, the peritoneal cavity is divided into left and right halves.

↓

Organ primordia develop in both mesenteries:
- ventral: liver, bile ducts and ventral pancreas;
- dorsal: spleen and dorsal pancreas.

↓

Viewed from above, the stomach rotates 90 degrees clockwise. The duodenum follows the stomach in a clockwise rotation while acquiring its C-shaped loop.

↓

The two mesenteries follow this rotation with the ventral mesentery being pulled right and the rapidly growing dorsal mesentery pulled left.

→

Tilting of the stomach; shifting of the pancreas, liver and spleen

The ventral and dorsal pancreatic buds move toward each other. This is partially due to the duodenum shifting right which causes the *ventral* pancreatic bud to move slightly dorsally. The two pancreatic buds fuse.

↓

Viewed from the front, the developing stomach tilts clockwise and grows asymmetrically: the greater (left) and lesser (right) curvatures form with the dorsal and ventral mesogastria still attached.

↓

The rotation and tilting of the stomach shifts the developing liver to the right and upward where it becomes attached to the diaphragm. The splenic bud shifts left and remains intraperitoneal.

↓

The developing duodenum and the fused pancreatic buds associated with it move dorsally along with their dorsal mesentery and become secondarily retroperitoneal.

→

Differentiation of the mesenteries; peritoneal membranes of the organs

The dorsal mesogastrium (along the greater curvature) becomes the greater omentum. The rapid growth of the liver divides the ventral mesogastrium into a ventral and a dorsal mesohepaticum.

↓

The dorsal mesohepaticum becomes the lesser omentum (connects the liver to the stomach and duodenum). The ventral mesohepaticum becomes the falciform and round ligaments of the liver (connects the liver to the anterior abdominal wall).

↓

The splenic bud divides the upper portion of the dorsal mesogastrium into a ventral mesosplenicum (becomes the gastrosplenic ligament) and a dorsal mesosplenicum (becomes the phrenicosplenic ligament).

↓

The omental bursa, a separated portion of the peritoneal cavity, forms posterior to the stomach and omenta. The liver, gallbladder, spleen and stomach remain intraperitoneal. The pancreas and most of the duodenum become secondarily retroperitoneal.

6.5 Rotation of the Intestinal Loop and Development of Midgut and Hindgut Derivatives

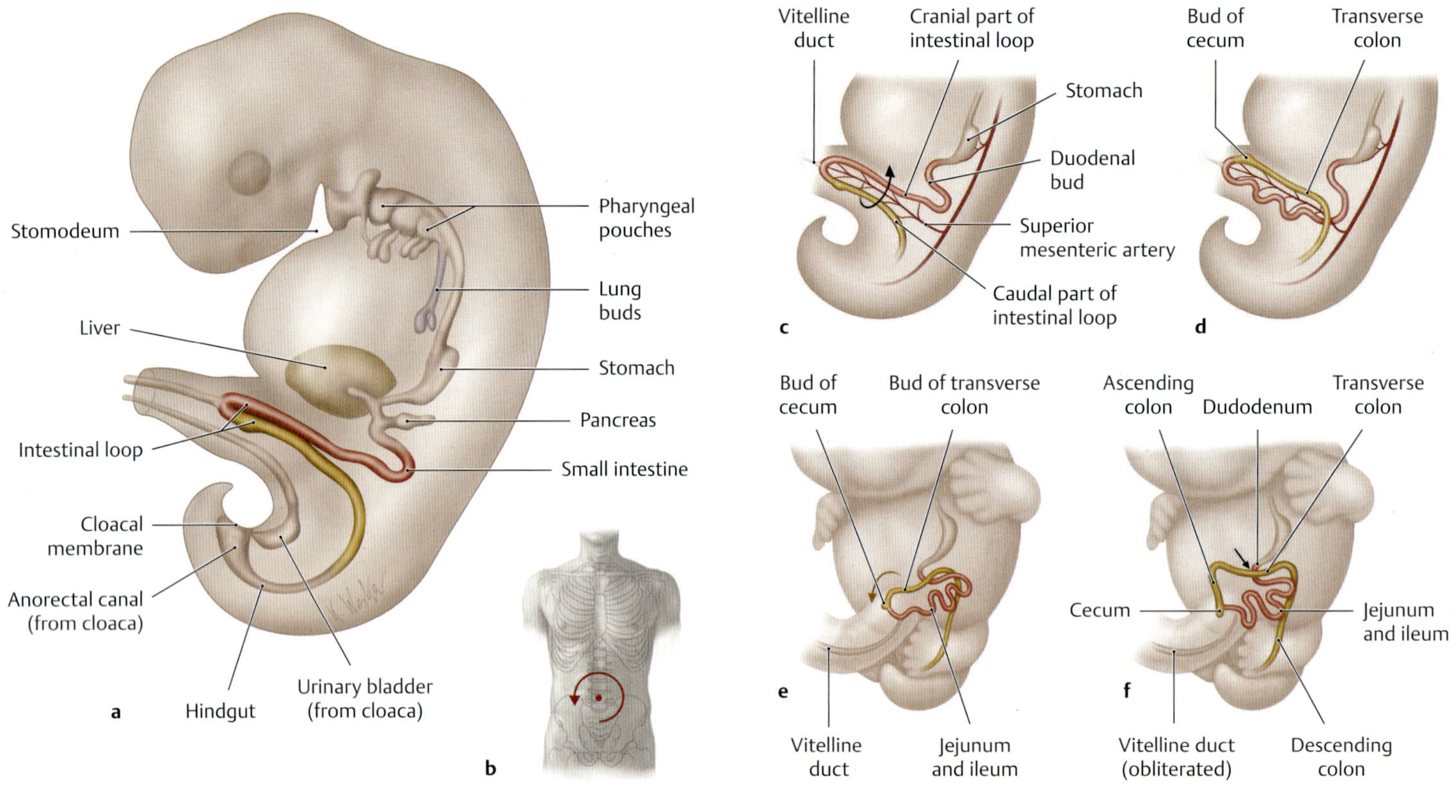

A Rotation and differentiation of the intestinal loop

a Overview of the intestinal loop: embryo viewed from left side, 5th week of embryonic development; **b** Direction of rotation of the intestinal loop: anterior view of abdomen; **c–f** Rotation of the intestinal loop, viewed from left side (**c** and **d**: the stomach has *not yet rotated*); **e** and **f** Position of the small and large intestine after the rotation of the intestinal loop is complete, left anterior view.

In the midgut and hindgut (at the level of small and large intestine) a second rotation occurs between the 6th and 11th week of embryonic development, the "rotation of the intestinal loop." The entire intestinal loop rotates along an axis formed by the superior mesenteric artery and the vitelline (omphaloenteric) duct (**c**). Viewed from the front, the rotation is *counter*clockwise (**d** and **e**). The loop rotates 270 degrees as the gut tube elongates. The initially cranial portion of the intestinal loop grows rapidly into the coiled jejunum and ileum (**e** and **f**). The caudal portion grows into the terminal portion of the ileum, the cecum, and vermiform appendix (see **B**), and the large intestine, which encloses the coils of the small intestine (**f**). Thus, rotation of the intestinal loop can be divided into three phases:

- the cranial and caudal parts of the intestinal loop rotation 90 degrees counterclockwise (**c**),
- the rotated loops shift to the right upper quadrant and rotate an additional 180 degrees (**d** and **e**);
- the region of the ileocecal junction and ascending colon descends into right lower quadrant (**f**).

Note: The first phase in the rotation of the intestinal loop (the first 90 degrees) occurs outside the abdominal cavity in the extraembryonic cavity in the umbilical cord at the start of the 6th week (**c**). This rotation outside of the body cavity is referred to as physiological umbilical herniation. Later, in the 10th week, the intestinal coils return back to the abdominal cavity.

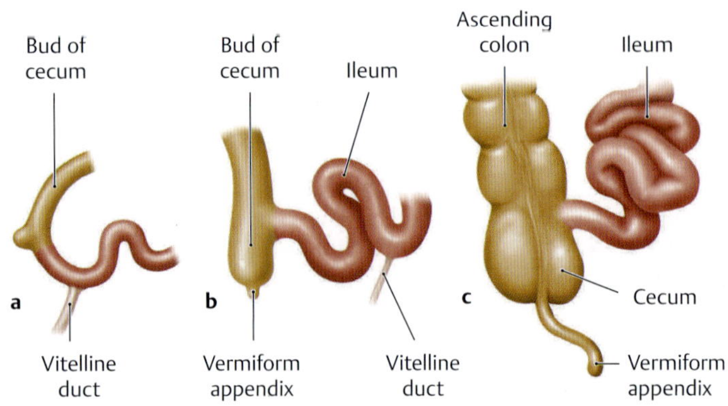

B Development of the cecum and vermiform appendix

In the 6th week of development the cecum starts to form in the caudal limb of the intestinal loop at the junction of the small intestine and large intestine (**a**). Between the 7th and 8th weeks, as the cecum is enlarging, the worm-like vermiform appendix begins to form (**b**). The cecum develops into a blind sac at the beginning of the ascending colon (**c**). The ileum opens perpendicularly into the junction of the cecum and ascending colon. The development of the cecum occurs outside of the abdominal cavity, and it is the last part of the intestinal tube to return to the abdominal cavity.

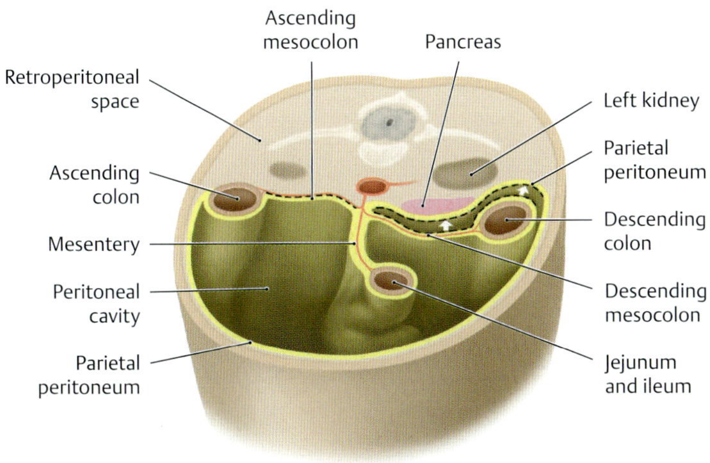

C Retroperitonealization of the ascending and descending colon
Horizontal sections of the abdomen, anterosuperior view.
Following rotation of the intestinal loop, the ascending and descending colon lie on the right and left sides of the abdominal cavity. They are in direct contact with the posterior wall of the peritoneal cavity, and they fuse to the posterior wall along with their mesenteries. Thus, the ascending and descending colons become secondarily retroperitoneal. The *ascending* colon (on the right in the body) and its ascending mesocolon have already fused. The *descending* colon (on the left in the body) still remains within the peritoneum and is soon to become fused (arrows). The *transverse* colon (not shown), like the jejunum and ileum, also remains within the peritoneum (see **D**).

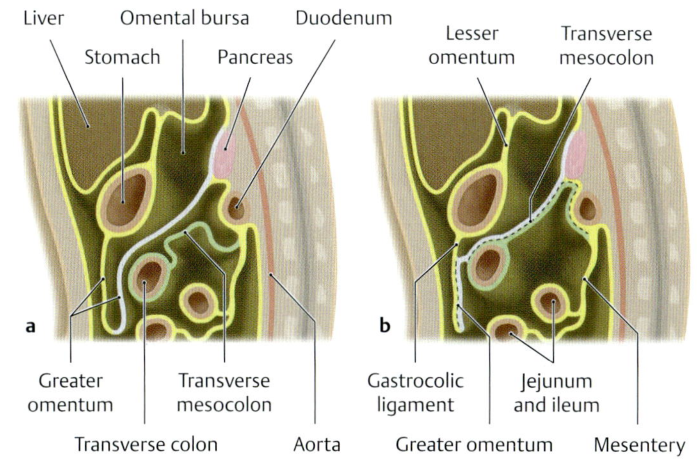

D Fusion of the greater omentum
Sagittal sections of the abdomen, viewed from the left. The greater omentum (derived from the dorsal mesogastrium, see p. 45) extends down from the greater curvature of the stomach. As it grows downward, its two layers partially fuse with one another and with the transverse colon and the transverse mesocolon (**a**). This forms a pouch-like space between the bottom part of the stomach and the upper part of the transverse colon (**b**), which marks the inferior boundary of the omental bursa (see p. 47). The fused part of the greater omentum, which connects the stomach with the transverse colon, is called the gastrocolic ligament.

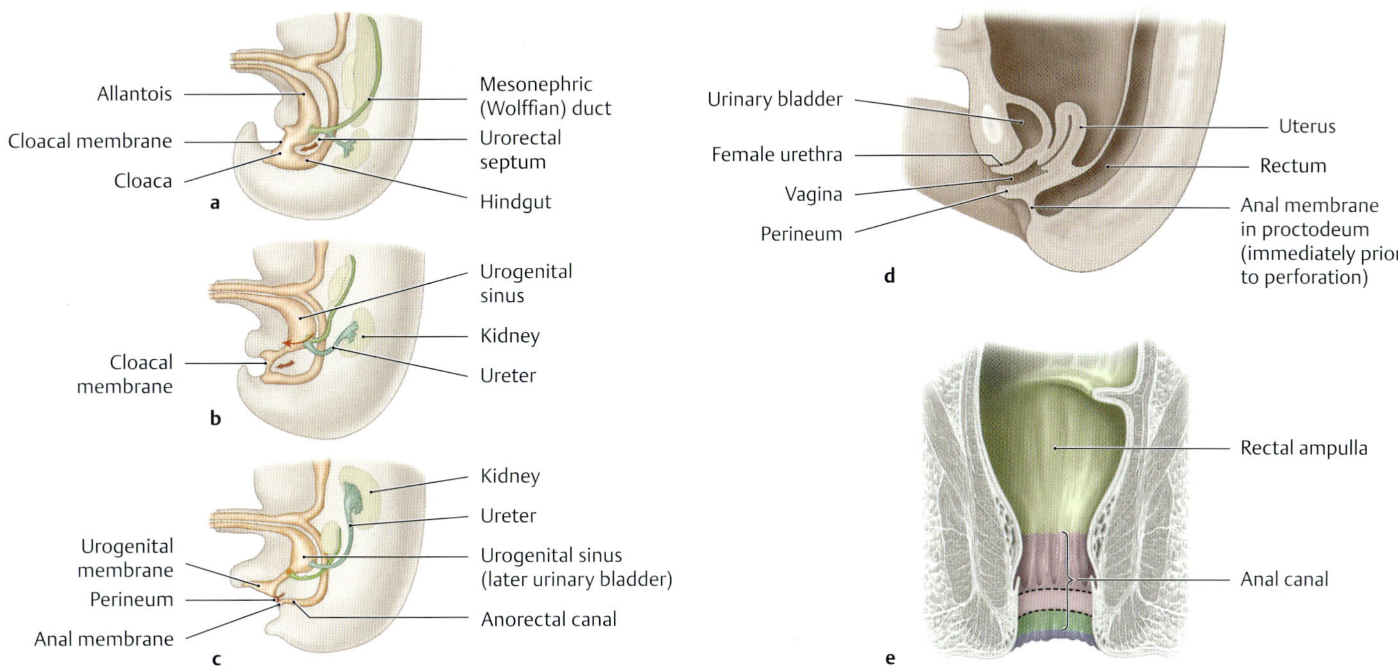

E Development of the cloaca
a–d Pelvic viscera of the fetus, viewed from the left side; **e** Anterior view of the mature anorectal canal.
Together with the urinary tract, the terminal portion of the hindgut enters into the cloaca. A transverse ridge of mesenchyme called the urorectal septum grows toward the cloacal membrane (which is closing off the cloaca) (**a** and **b**). In about the 7th week of development the urorectal septum divides the cloaca into an anterior urogenital sinus, which gives rise to parts of the urogenital system, and posterior anorectal canal (**c**). Both are still closed by the cloacal membrane, which is now divided into an anterior urogenital membrane and a posterior anal membrane. The perineal body forms at the junction of urogenital and anal membranes. Mesenchymal swellings form at the margins of the anal membrane and, as a result, the anal membrane lies in a depression called the anal pit (proctodeum) (**d**). By the end of the 9th week, the anal membrane ruptures and the rectum is in open communication with the body's exterior (**e**). Thus, the rectum consists of two parts: the upper portion that develops from the hindgut, and the lower portion that develops from the cloaca.

6.6 Summary of the Development of the Midgut and Hindgut; Developmental Anomalies

A Development of the midgut and hindgut: Summary and peritonealization

The development of the midgut and hindgut can be divided into two processes: "rotation of the intestinal loop" and "peritoneal relationships and formation of the cloaca."

Rotation of the intestinal loop

The intestinal loop rotates around a virtual axis formed by the superior mesenteric artery and the vitelline duct. As it rotates, it continues to grow and differentiate.

↓

Viewed from the front, the intestinal loop undergoes a 270 degree counterclockwise rotation. The first 90 degrees take place outside of the body cavity during physiological umbilical herniation. The intestinal coils retract back into the abdomen by the 11th week.

↓

The cranial part of the intestinal loop elongates rapidly forming the numerous coils of the jejunum and ileum. They remain attached to the posterior wall of the peritoneal cavity by their mesentery.

↓

As the loop rotates, its caudal limb forms a frame around the coils of the jejunum and ileum, thereby dividing the colon into individual sections, which assume their definitive position in the abdomen.

↓

A lateral protrusion forms in the caudal (large intestinal) limb of the intestinal loop close to the axis of the superior mesenteric artery. This protrusion differentiates into the cecum, and the vermiform appendix develops from it.

↓

When rotation is complete, the small and large intestines have reached their definitive position, with the large intestine forming a frame around the small intestine. The subsequent retroperitonealization determines the final peritoneal relationships of the gut tube.

Peritoneal relationships and formation of the cloaca

Rotation of the loop moves the cecum to the lower right quadrant, and the ascending and descending colons move dorsally and become secondarily retroperitoneal. The transverse colon and sigmoid colon remain intraperitoneal with a mesocolon.

↓

The transverse colon and transverse mesocolon fuse and become attached to the greater omentum, which originally was the dorsal mesogastrium (along the greater curvature of the stomach). Thus, the omental bursa, located behind the stomach, is almost completely closed off.

↓

The urorectal septum divides the enlarged end of the hindgut, the cloaca, into an anterior urogenital sinus and a posterior anorectal canal. The septum grows caudally until it contacts the cloacal membrane.

↓

The division of the cloaca leads to the division of the cloacal membrane into an anterior urogenital membrane and a posterior anal membrane. Mesenchymal tissue surrounding the anal membrane proliferates and forms a depression called the anal pit.

↓

The anal pit deepens toward the hindgut and gives rise to the anal canal. As the anal membrane ruptures in the 9th week, the rectum, which is derived from the cloaca, becomes open to the outside of the body.

↓

The rectum lies deep within the pelvis. It moves posteriorly and becomes retroperitonealized along most of its length. The anal canal derived from the proctodeum does not have any peritoneal relationships.

B Summary of the rotational motion of the gut tube and peritoneal relationships

Organ rotation	Leads to the following organ positions	Which results in the following peritoneal relationships
Rotation of the stomach along with its ventral and dorsal mesogastria	• Liver and gallbladder in the right upper quadrant • Spleen in the left upper quadrant • *Most* of the duodenum and the *entire* pancreas become attached to the posterior wall of the peritoneal cavity	• Intraperitoneal with lesser omentum, falciform ligament and round ligament of the liver • Intraperitoneal • Secondarily retroperitoneal
Rotation of the intestinal loop along with its mesenteries	• Cranial portion of the loop forms two segments of the small intestine, the jejunum and ileum, along with their mesenteries • Caudal portion forms the large intestine and rectum along with their mesocolon and mesorectum: the large intestine and rectum form a frame around the small intestine • Ascending colon, descending colon, and rectum become attached to the posterior wall of the peritoneal cavity	• Mesentery remains and the jejunum and ileum are intraperitoneal • Transverse colon and sigmoid colon retain their mesocolons and remain intraperitoneal • Ascending colon, descending colon, and rectum lose their mesenteries and are secondarily retroperitoneal

C Developmental anomalies of the gastrointestinal tract

The anomalies listed here, some of which are quite rare except for Meckel's diverticulum, vary considerably in their pathological significance. A complete occlusion or extreme narrowing of the lumen in the gastrointestinal tract is usually fatal without treatment. Mild degrees of narrowing can remain asymptomatic. The twisting of intestinal segments can cause obstructions that often lead to life-threatening conditions.

Duodenal atresia	Solid duodenum without lumen
Duodenal stenosis	Narrowing of the duodenal lumen (e.g., by an annular pancreas)
Biliary atresia	Congenital or acquired obstruction of some or all extrahepatic bile ducts
Annular pancreas	Duodenal stenosis (see above) caused by a circle of pancreatic tissue
Omphalocele	Extracorporeal protrusion of the small intestine at the umbilicus due to failure of the rotated intestinal loop to retract
Malrotation	Abnormal or failed rotation of the intestinal loop (see **E**)
Volvulus	Twisting of intestinal segments caused by failure of fixation of the mesentery; risk of getting ileus
Intestinal stenosis	Narrowing of the intestinal lumen
Intestinal atresia	Complete occlusion of the intestinal lumen, if not treated this is incompatible with life
Meckel's diverticulum	Failure of regression of the vitelline duct with potential ileal diverticulitis (see **D**)

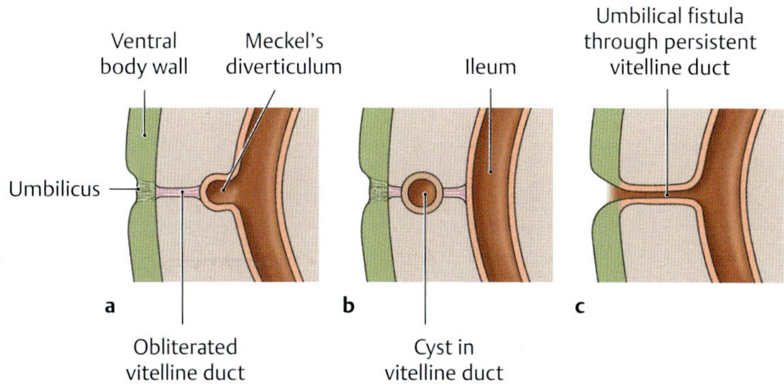

D Remnants of the vitelline duct

The vitelline duct, initially patent in the embryo, usually is completely obliterated and lost as a connection between the ileum and trunk wall. Occasionally, however, the obliteration is incomplete or leaves a cord of connective tissue that attaches the ileum to the anterior trunk wall. This can have various manifestations:

- **a** The wall of the ileum is partially outpouched and a fibrous cord remains. A **Meckel's diverticulum** forms (usually located 40–60 cm cranial to the ileocecal valve), which is subject to inflammatory changes and often contains ectopic gastric or pancreatic tissue.
- **b** A cyst remains within the fibrous cord. This cyst may cause complaints and must be differentiated from a tumor.
- **c** The vitelline duct remains patent over its entire length, resulting in an **umbilical (or vitelline) fistula**. In extreme cases, portions of the small intestine may herniate at the umbilicus and become inflamed. If a remnant of the vitelline duct persists as a fibrous cord between ileum and umbilicus, mobile small intestinal loops may wrap around it and become strangulated (intestinal paralysis, or ileus, which is often fatal if untreated).

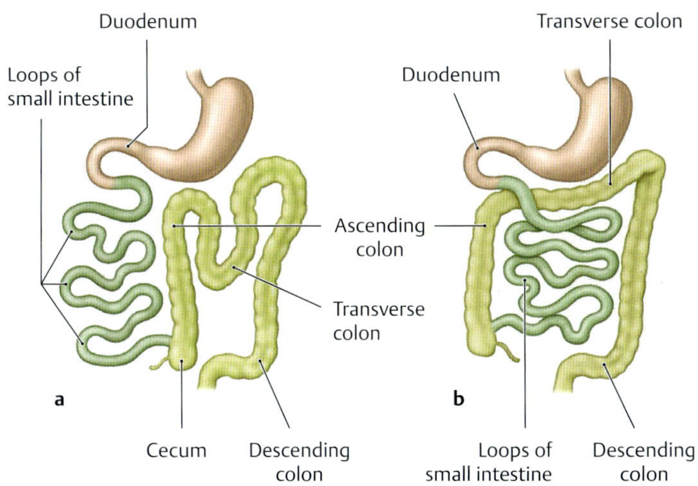

E Developmental anomalies of the gastrointestinal tract: malrotation

Ventral view. As long as the intestinal segments do not become twisted and do not lose gastrointestinal motility (see **C**, volvulus), the following types of malrotations may remain asymptomatic.

- **a** Rotation of only 90 degrees instead of 270. The large intestine remains to the left of the small intestine and doesn't form a frame around the small intestine.
- **b** Clockwise rotation (viewed from the front), here 90 degrees. The initially caudal part of the loop comes to lie behind the cranial part and the transverse colon crosses posterior to the small intestine.

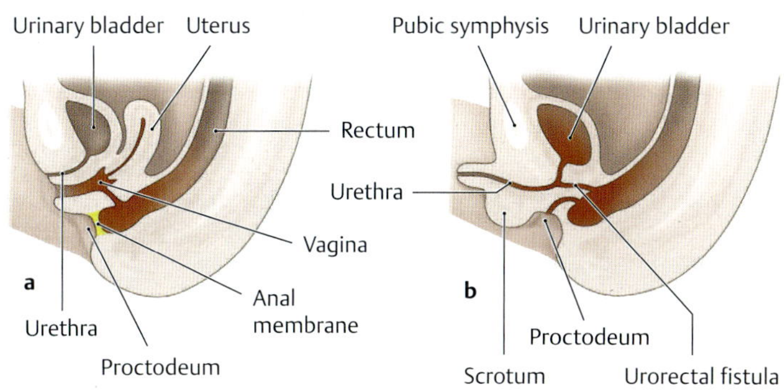

F Malformation of the anal canal

Pelvic viscera, viewed from the left side. In 1 out of 5000 births, the anal membrane fails to rupture. As a result, the rectum is not connected to the outside environment. The two most frequent developmental anomalies are presented below:

- **a** Imperforate anus: The anal canal is present yet the anal membrane fails to break down and persists. A rectovaginal fistula has developed as well; see **b**.
- **b** Anorectal atresia (with fistula formation): Malformations of the urorectal septum, with the anal canal missing, may create a nonphysiological fistula between the rectum and the perineum or the urogenital system.

Both of these conditions require surgical correction.

7.1 Overview of the Urinary System

Introduction
The urinary organs extend from the abdomen through the pelvis. Since they are closely related to the genital organs, both groups of organs are often referred to collectively as *urogenital organs*. For didactic reasons, both systems will be discussed separately in the following chapters.
The urinary organs help regulate the level of water and minerals in the body, and thus help regulate osmotic pressure. They excrete end products of body metabolism and harmful substances into a watery fluid, the *urine* (the excreted metabolites are dissolved in the water component of urine). By regulating the amount of water in the body, the kidneys also influence blood pressure. Through excreting or retaining sodium, potassium, calcium and chloride ions, they are involved in regulating the level of these important electrolytes in blood. In addition, the blood's acid-base balance is influenced by the excretion or retention of hydrogen ions. Many pharmaceutical substances are excreted through the kidneys. The kidneys also influence blood pressure by producing the enzyme renin, and the formation of red blood cells by producing the hormone erythropoietin. Lastly, they also play an important role in vitamin D metabolism.

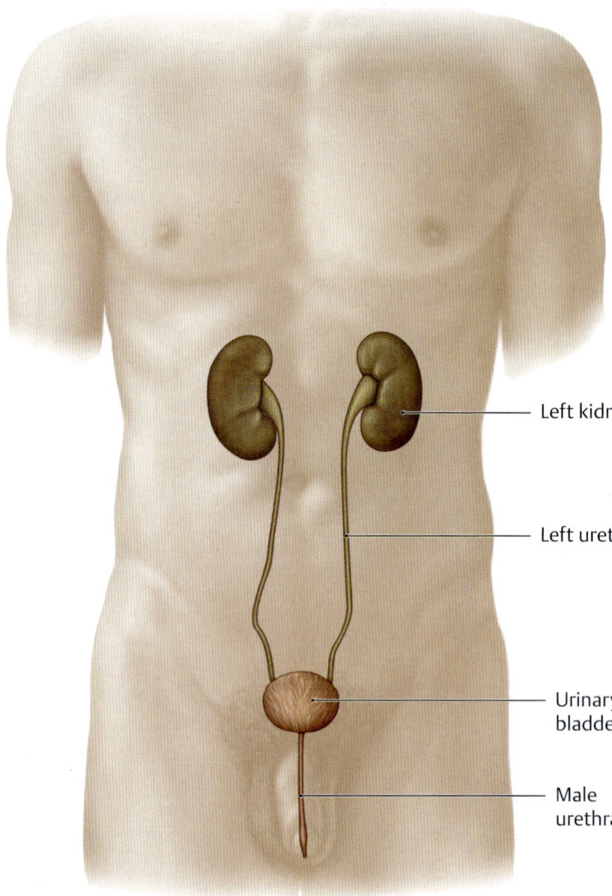

A Overview of the urinary organs
Male urinary organs, anterior view. The urinary system consists of the following organs:

- the paired kidneys, which continuously produce urine;
- the paired ureters, which transport urine from the kidneys to the urinary bladder;
- the unpaired urinary bladder, which temporarily stores and discharges urine in a controlled manner; and
- the unpaired urethra. In women it is called the female urethra and it is solely a urinary organ, whereas in men it is called the male urethra and it is also a genital organ. In the urinary system, the urethra is involved in discharging urine from the urinary bladder to the outside of the body. In men it is also serves as a passageway for sperm.

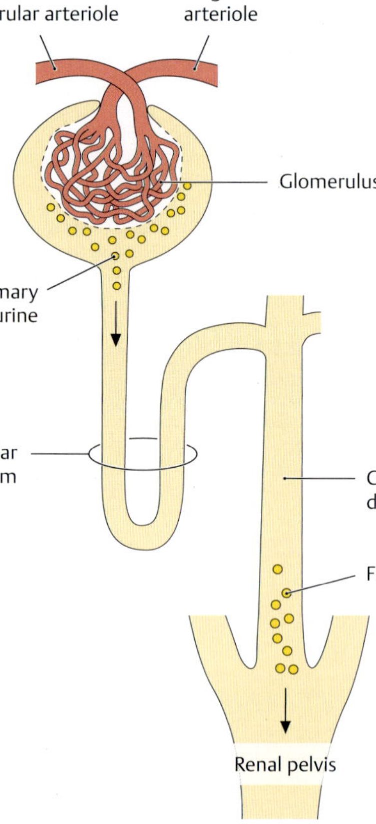

B Basics of urine production
The nephron, illustrated above, is the smallest functional unit of the kidney (see p. 54).
In the glomeruli, richly branched capillary loops, which are supplied by branches of the renal arteries, drain an ultrafiltrate of blood called primary urine into a system of tubules. Adults produce approximately 170 liters of *primary urine* in 24 hours. However, in the tubular system, the primary urine is concentrated to 1% of its volume (by reabsorption of electrolytes and water back into the blood), and based on its composition, further modified with electrolytes and hydrogen ions. The volume of *final urine* formed in 24 hours is 1–2 liters. The final urine drains through collecting ducts into the renal pelvis and then it is carried by the ureters to the urinary bladder.

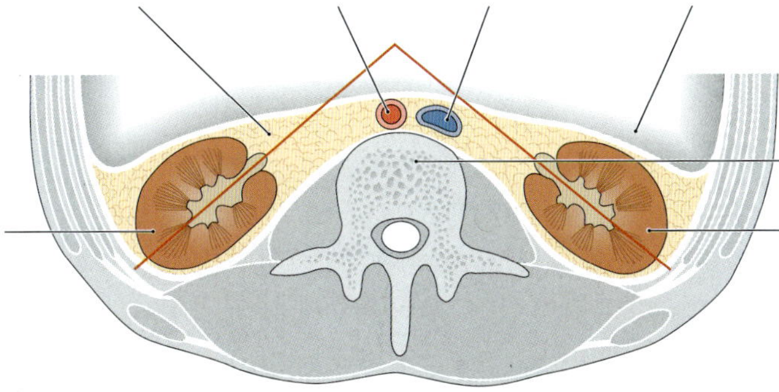

C Location of the kidneys and ureters
Horizontal section of the body at the level of the first lumbar vertebra, viewed from above. Both kidneys are embedded in a fatty, connective tissue capsule. They are located in the retroperitoneal space with one on either side of the vertebral column. The retroperitoneal space also contains the ureters (not visible in this section), which extend downward to the lesser pelvis to reach the urinary bladder. The hilum of each kidney faces medially and anteriorly (red axes).

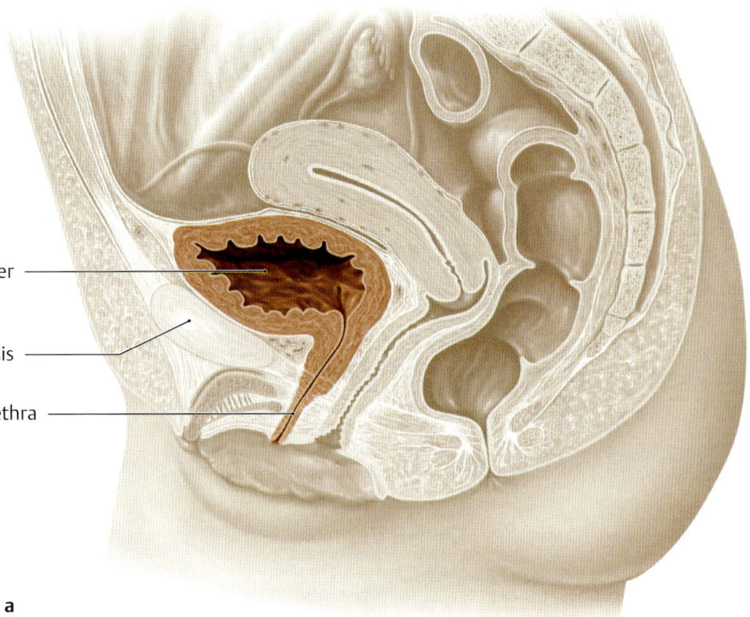

a

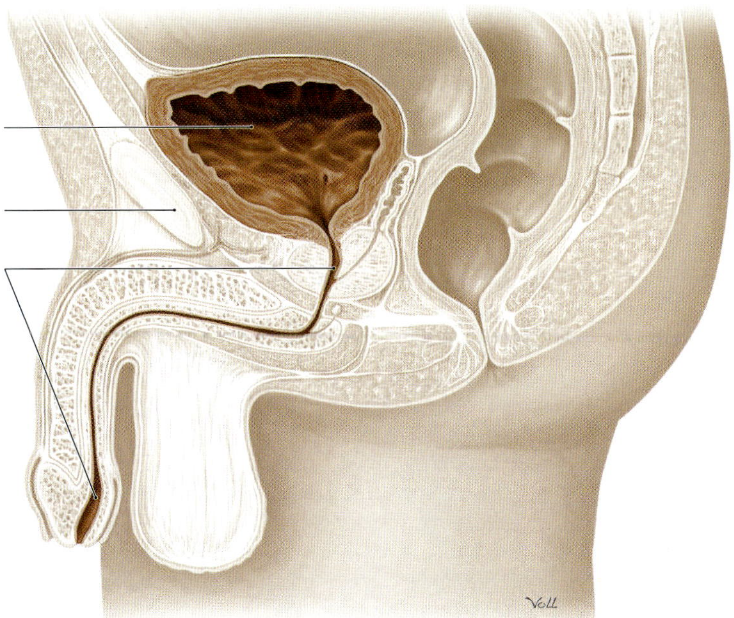

b

D Location of the urinary bladder and urethra
Midsagittal section of a female (**a**) and male (**b**) pelvis, each viewed from the left side.
In both sexes, the urinary bladder is located in the lesser pelvis behind the pubic symphysis. In females it is situated in front of both the vagina and the uterus, and in males it is in front of the rectum. Depending on its degree of distension, the urinary bladder is flattened or spherical. The female urethra is straight and short, while the male urethra traverses the penis and bends multiple times along its course.

7.2 Development of the Kidneys, Renal Pelvis, and Ureters

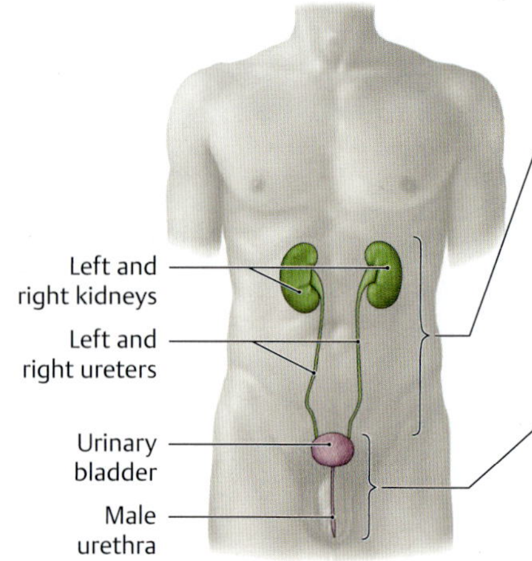

Paired primordia
Intermediate mesoderm: (specifically: metanephric mesoderm) → kidneys **Mesonephric duct:** → ureter (genital system: → ductus deferens)

Unpaired primordia
Cloaca → (digestive ↓ system → anal canal) **Urogenital sinus:** → urinary bladder and urethra (genital system → male urethra)

A Overview of the embryonic development of the urinary organs
The embryonic development of the urinary organs is complex and overlaps with the development of the genital and digestive organs:

- overlap with the genital system: the development of some parts of the male reproductive system (see p. 62) is closely related to the development of the mesonephric ducts, ureters, and urogenital sinus.
- overlap with the digestive system: the anal canal is derived from the cloaca.

The development of the urinary system can be divided into the development of the *paired* kidneys and ureters, and development of the unpaired urinary bladder and urethra. The kidneys and ureters arise from the intermediate mesoderm. The urinary bladder and urethra develop from the urogenital sinus, which formed from the ventral portion of the cloaca in the region of the future pelvic floor (see p. 47). The urogenital sinus is derived from endoderm. Thus, the urinary organs are derived from two germ layers. Over the course of development the two sets of urinary organs will connect with each other.

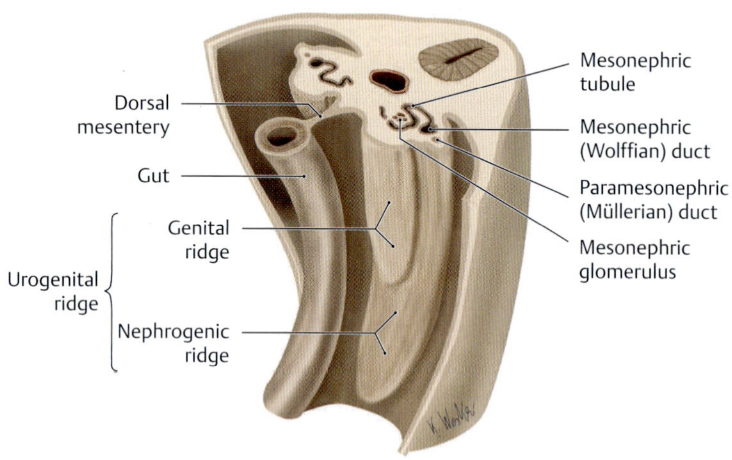

B The urogenital ridge
Posterior body wall of the embryo, viewed from the front and above. The renal and internal genital primordia border each other. They bulge ventrally into the body cavity in the form of two ridges: the nephrogenic ridge and the genital ridge ("urogenital ridge"). The developing gonads lie anteromedially to the developing kidney systems. The paramesonephric (Müllerian) ducts, which in females develop into the uterine tubes and uterus, lie anterolaterally to the renal primordia.

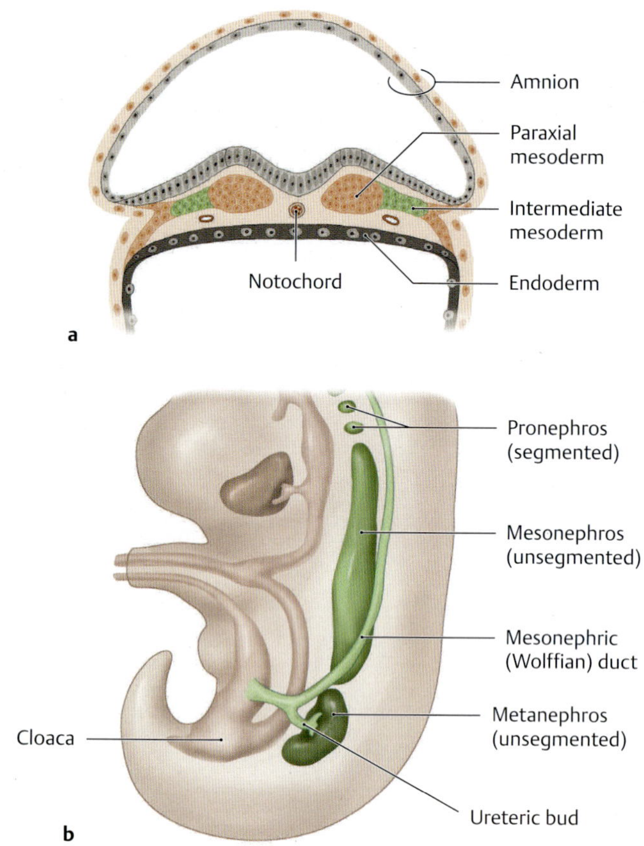

C Renal primordia in the intermediate mesoderm
a Cross-section of an embryo, approx. 19 days, cranial view; **b** Embryo viewed from the left (unlike **a**, this figure does not depict a stage in the embryonic development but rather shows the location of the developing renal primordia and what it would look like if they all existed in the embryo at the same time).
The kidneys develop as pairs in a specialized region of the mesoderm, the intermediate mesoderm, which becomes further differentiated in the posterior body cavity. In cervical and upper thoracic regions it becomes segmented and forms nephrotomes. It remains unsegmented in lower thoracic and abdominal regions and forms nephrogenic cords. Renal development within the mesoderm proceeds in three successive steps. From cranial to caudal the three systems formed are as follows:

- Pronephros in the cervical and upper thoracic regions
- Mesonephros in the lower thoracic and abdominal regions
- Metanephros in the abdominal and pelvic regions

The pronephros is nonfunctional and completely degenerates while the mesonephros is developing. During development, the mesonephros produces urine for a short period. Most of the mesonephros system also degenerates. The portions that remain are the mesonephric tubules, which form the efferent ductules of the testis (see p. 64), and the mesonephric duct (Wolffian duct). Initially, the mesonephric duct develops adjacent to the pronephros, but soon becomes associated with the mesonephros. While the pronephros is still degenerating, the caudally located metanephros develops. Together with part of the mesonephric duct it forms the definitive kidney.
Note: The definitive kidney, which in adults sits just below the diaphragm, develops in the pelvic region and ascends only secondarily (ascent of the kidneys, see **D**).

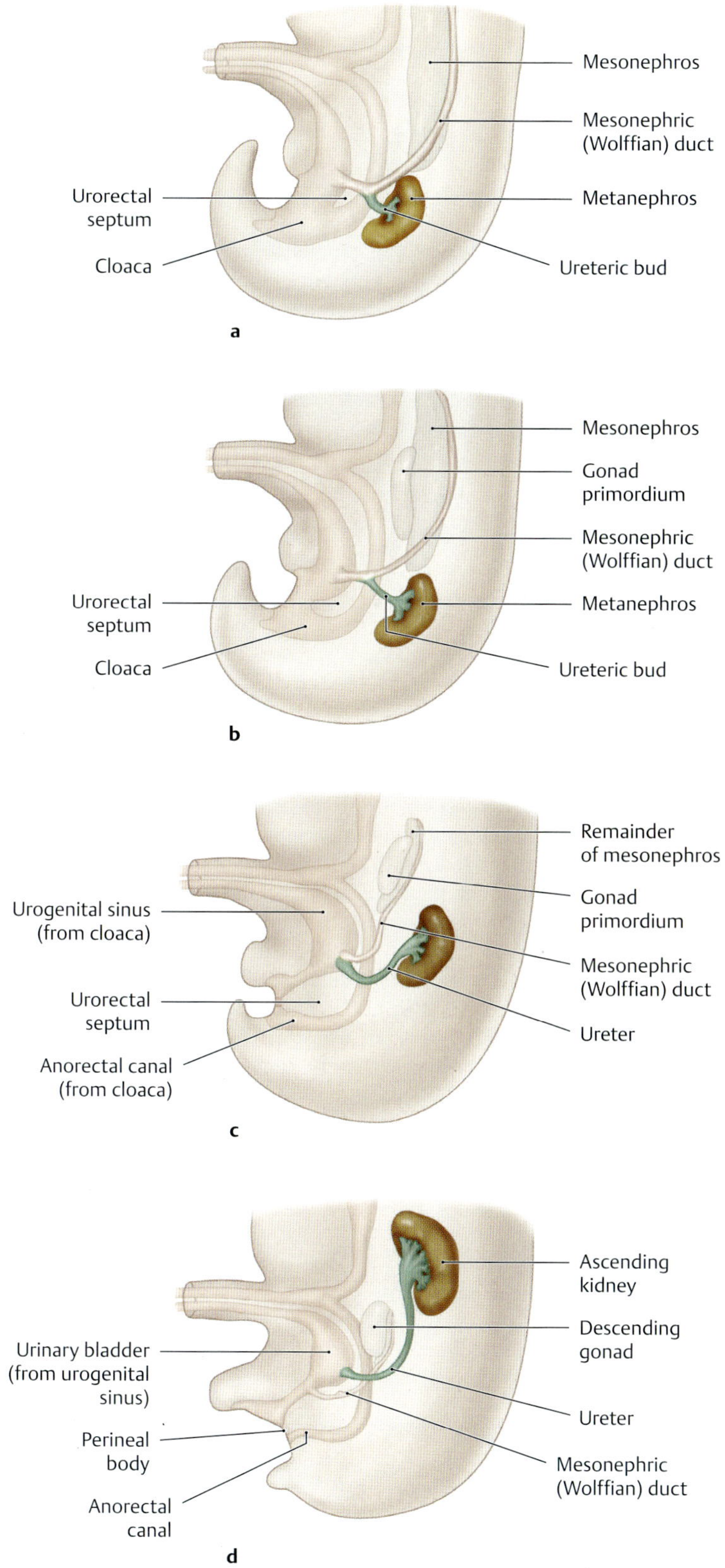

D Development of the ureter and kidney
Ureteric bud and metanephros (**a**), as well as ascent of the kidneys (**b–d**), viewed from the left side; **e–h** Further development of the metanephros (for location of the urogenital ridge see **B**).

a The metanephros develops during the 5th week in the most caudal portion of the intermediate mesoderm. It is also called the *metanephric blastema*. The *ureteric bud* sprouts from the mesonephric duct adjacent to the blastema and grows into the metanephros. The initially short stalk of the ureteric bud elongates further and develops into the *ureter*. The tip of the bud, which has entered into the metanephros, differentiates into components of the definitive kidney (the *renal pelvis* with its calyces, and the collecting duct system) (**e–h**). *Note:* At this stage, the ureter is not in direct contact with the cloaca, which gives rise to the urinary bladder. Rather, the ureter opens indirectly into the cloaca via the mesonephric duct. However, the other end of the ureter is already connected to the kidney.

b–d The metanephros and ureteric bud grow from the pelvic region in a cranial direction and later come to lie just below the diaphragm (ascent of the kidneys). This ascent is partially the result of a reduction of bending and increased growth of the sacro-lumbar region of the embryo. If a kidney fails to ascend the result is referred to as a pelvic kidney (see p. 55). While the kidneys are ascending, the gonads descend along with the remnants of the mesonephri (descent of the gonads).

e–h The ureteric bud enlarges after invading the metanephros and develops into the renal pelvis with 2–3 major renal calyces (**f**). In the course of continuous branching into numerous tubules, the bud enters deeper into the metanephros (**g**). Within the kidney, the "tubules" form collecting ducts (**h**), which converge into groups close to the calyces and empty into them through papillae. The last generation of collecting ducts does not divide further. Thus, the ureteric bud gives rise to the following:

- Ureter
- Renal pelvis
- Renal calyces
- Papillae with ducts
- Collecting ducts with connecting tubules (see p. 54)

Note: The metanephric blastema forms the urine producing part of the definitive kidney, and the ureteric bud forms the collecting system.

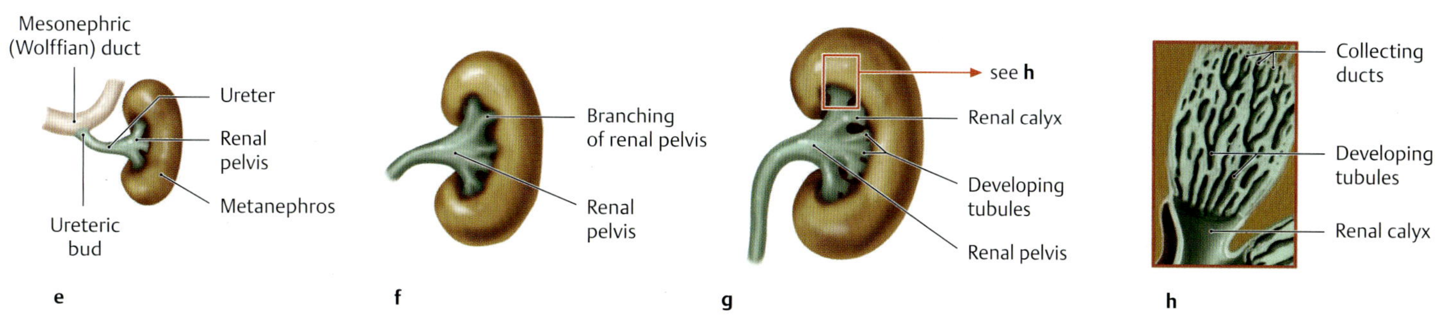

7.3 Development of Nephrons, and the Urinary Bladder and Ureters; Developmental Anomalies

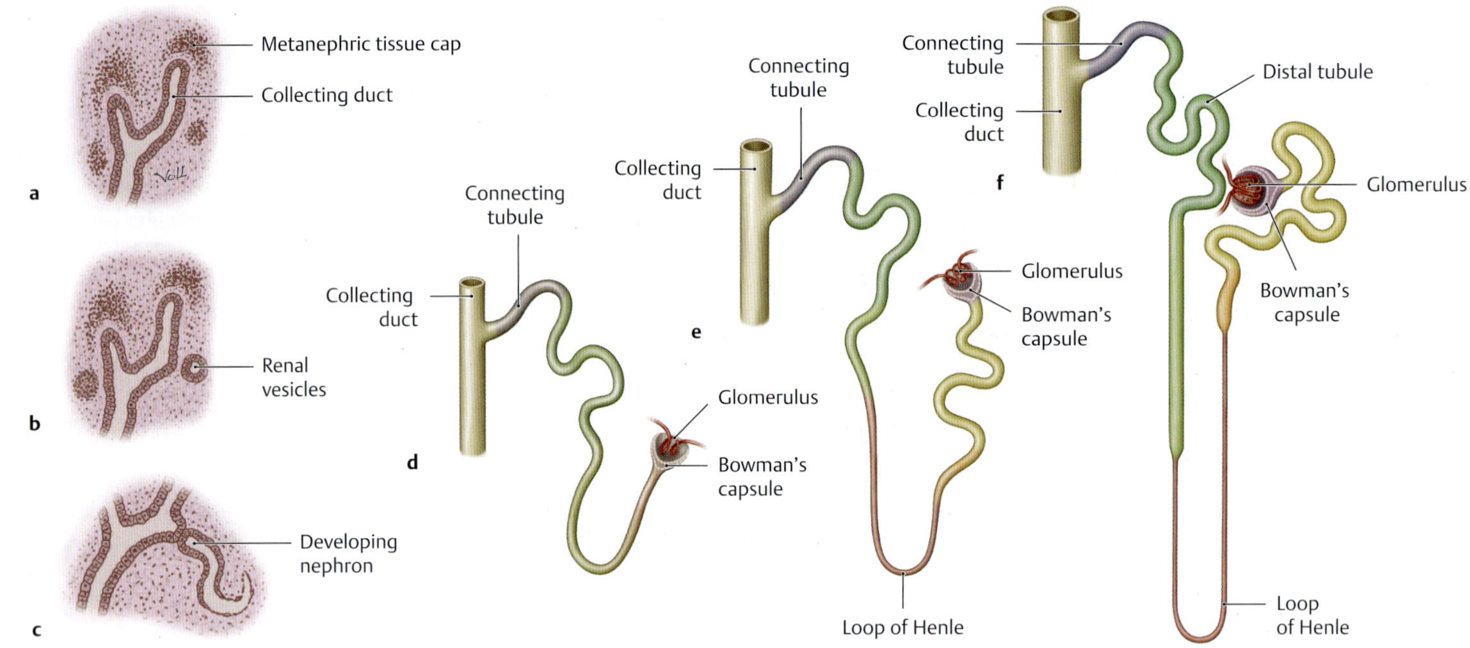

A Development of nephrons

The nephron is the smallest functional unit of the kidney. It consists of a capillary tuft, through which primary urine is discharged into the renal tubular system in a process called ultrafiltration. Within this tubular system, primary urine is concentrated into secondary or final urine through reabsorption of electrolytes and water (see p. 50). Nephron development is the final step necessary for the metanephros to become functional and proceeds in two stages:

- A vascular system is connected to the renal tubular system (for urine formation.)
- The tubular system is connected to the collecting duct system (for urine discharge).

Nephron formation is induced by branching of the ureteric bud, with each terminal collecting duct being covered by a *metanephric tissue cap* (**a**). Cells of the tissue cap move laterally and develop into renal vesicles (**b**). Each vesicle gives rise to a *small S-shaped tubule* (**c**). While segments of the tubule continue to differentiate and elongate, its distal end, the junctional (connecting) tubule, connects it to a collecting duct (**d**). Its proximal end (*Bowman's capsule*) becomes invaginated by a tuft of capillaries (the *glomerulus*), which is supplied by a branch of the renal artery (**e**): Continuous lengthening and differentiation of the tubules result in the formation of the *tubular system* including the *loop of Henle* (**f**). The loop of Henle helps to concentrate primary urine (approximately 170 liters of primary urine is produced in 24 hours) to 1% of its volume to produce the final urine. At the start of the 13th week, almost 20% of nephrons are functional and can form urine.

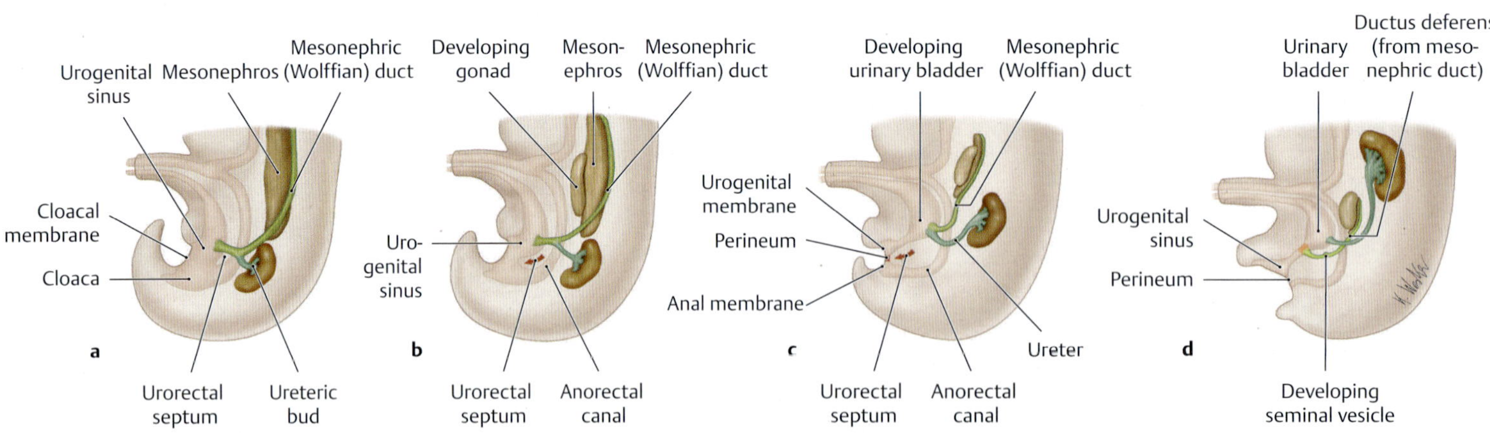

B Development of the urinary bladder and urethra

Embryo viewed from the left side at 5 (**a**), 7 (**b**) and 8 weeks (**c**), **d** approx. 10 weeks.

The development of the urinary bladder and urethra leads to a system concerned with the temporary storage and release of urine. Both structures are derived from the *cloaca*, the common excretory organ of the urinary and digestive systems. The *urorectal septum*, a wedge of caudally-growing connective tissue, completely divides the cloaca into two parts; an anteriorly located *urogenital sinus* and a posteriorly located *anorectal canal* (**a–c**). As the *urorectal septum* grows caudally it fuses with the cloacal membrane, dividing it into an anteriorly located *urogenital membrane* and a posteriorly located *anal membrane*. The point of fusion becomes the *perineal body*. As the urogenital and anal membranes disintegrate, the urogenital sinus and anorectal canal become connected to the outside of the body. The cranial part of the urogenital sinus gives rise to the urinary bladder, and the pelvic part to the urethra (**d**).

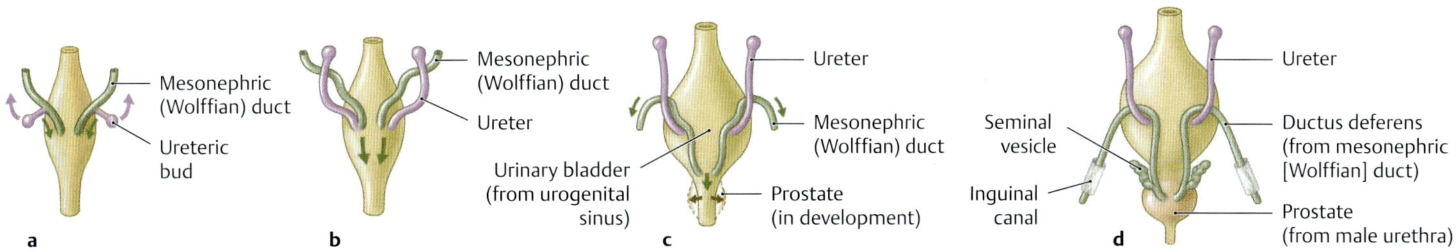

C Development of the connection between the ureters and urinary bladder

Dorsal view of the urinary bladder and mesonephric ducts. Initially, the ureters are not in direct contact with the cloaca but open into it via the mesonephric ducts (**a**). As the urinary bladder further differentiates and grows, the caudal portions of the mesonephric ducts get incorporated into the wall of the bladder as they continue to move caudally. For a short period of development, the mesonephric ducts and ureters share a common opening into the urinary bladder (**b**). After further incorporation of the mesonephric ducts into the wall of the urinary bladder, the mesonephric ducts and ureters are no longer in contact, and the ureters open into the posterior wall of the urinary bladder through their own connection. The mesonephric ducts continue to move caudally until they reach the region of the urethra (**c**). In males the *prostate* arises as an outgrowth of the urethra in the region of the mesonephric ducts (**d**), and the mesonephric ducts differentiate into the *ductus deferens* (see **E** and p. 62 and 64). In females, the mesonephric ducts regress after the ureters have become embedded in the wall of the urinary bladder, and only two remnants, the epoophoron and paroophoron, remain (see p. 62 and 64).

Note: The incorporation of the mesodermal mesonephric ducts and ureters into the posterior wall of the urinary bladder takes place over a broad, triangular area. As a result mesodermal tissue grows into the endodermally-lined bladder.

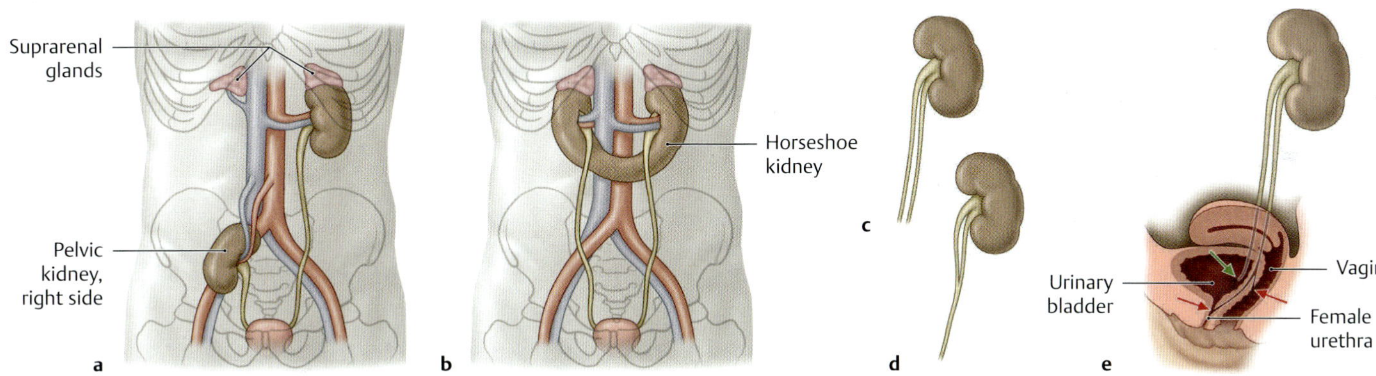

D Developmental anomalies of the urinary system

a A kidney fails to ascend resulting in a pelvic kidney.

Note: The suprarenal glands develop in the upper retroperitoneal space, and the ascending kidneys stop just below the suprarenal glands. Thus, in this figure, the right kidney remains in the pelvis, and the right suprarenal gland is in its correct location.

b The two nephrogenic cords fuse resulting in a horseshoe kidney; **c** and **d** *Split* ureter with complete (**c**) or partial (**d**) duplication of the ureter (there is only one ureteric bud, and the ureter splits along its course; **e** *accessory* ureter (there are *two separate* ureteric buds on the mesonephric duct). The accessory ureter atypically drains into the urethra or vagina (shown here).

These developmental anomalies may lead to the following conditions:

- *Bacterial pyelonephritis.* The flow of urine can be obstructed which leads to bacteria migrating from the urinary bladder to the renal pelvis.
- *Nonbacterial* inflammation, for example vaginitis due to the continuous release of urine from an accessory ureter draining into the vagina. The vaginal epithelium does not tolerate the hypertonic urine. This initially *nonbacterial* inflammation can develop into *bacterial* inflammation as bacteria migrating up the ureter may lead to bacterial pyelonephritis.

E Summary: Development of the urinary organs

Summary of the embryonic structures and the definitive body parts and organs they give rise to. Only functionally relevant structures are listed.

Embryonic structure	Definitive structure in the male	Definitive structure in the female
Metanephric blastema	Definitive nephron	Definitive nephron
Mesonephric duct	Renal pelvis, calyces, collecting ducts, ureters	Renal pelvis, calyces, collecting ducts, ureters
	Epididymis Ductus deferens Ejaculatory ducts Seminal vesicles	
Mesonephric tubules	Efferent ductules	–
Urogenital sinus	Urinary bladder	Urinary bladder
	Male urethra Prostate Bulbourethral glands	Female urethra Greater vestibular glands
	Urethral glands	Urethral glands

8.1 Overview of the Genital System

Introduction

Function and terms: The genital organs, which in humans are sex-specific, are responsible for producing offspring. In mammals, including humans, the primary function of the reproduction system in males and females is to produce haploid cells in specialized organs (the *gonads*), which then fuse in the female organism to form a diploid zygote. During *sexual intercourse*, male gametes are propelled out of the male's reproductive tract and into the female reproductive tract where they fuse with the female gametes (*conception*). The initially single-celled organism, the *zygote*, is transported to the uterus where further embryonic development takes place. At the end of pregnancy (*gestation*), the baby is delivered through the birth canal. In mammals, the male is only involved in conception, whereas the female reproductive system helps create optimal conditions for the fetus to grow and to ensure a timely delivery. In both sexes, gender-specific hormones (sex hormones), which are produced in the gonads, control these functions. These hormones determine the development and function of both the reproductive organs and the secondary sex characteristics of the individual organism.

Classification: The organization of the male and female reproductive systems can be classified in various ways:

- Topographically (see **A**): the *internal* genital organs (within the body cavity) and the *external* genital organs (outside of the body cavity).
- Functionally (**B** and **C**): as organs responsible for producing gametes and hormones (the gonads), as organs involved in transport (of gametes), as organs involved with incubation and copulation, and as glands associated with the organs.
- Ontogenetically (see p. 4).

Functional differences between male and female genital systems: Both sexes produce gametes, which in males are referred to as *spermatozoa* and in females as *oocytes*. While spermatozoa are continuously produced from primordial germ cells (spermatogonia) from puberty until old age (several dozen millions per day), the number of oocytes is already determined at birth (they can only differentiate into fertilizable germ cells—one egg ripens each menstrual cycle). The production of spermatozoa, and thus offspring, in males is possible from puberty until old age. In females the ability to reproduce is limited to a period ranging from the differentiation of the first ovum in her first menstrual cycle (menarche, onset around ages 13–14) to the differentiation of the last ovum (menopause, onset varies considerably, approx. between ages 40–60). It is important to keep in mind that mature eggs released in one of the first or last menstrual cycles may be less fertilizable.

A Male and female internal and external genitalia*

	Male	Female
Internal genitalia	Testis Epididymis Ductus deferens Prostate Seminal vesicle Bulbourethral gland	Ovary Uterus Uterine tube Vagina (upper portion)
External genitalia	Penis and urethra Scrotum and coverings of the testis	Vagina (vestibule only) Labia majora and minora Mons pubis Greater and lesser vestibular glands Clitoris

* The *female* external genitalia (pudenda) are known clinically as the *vulva*.

B Functions of the male genital organs

Organ	Function
Testis	Germ-cell production Hormone production
Epididymis	Reservoir for sperm (sperm maturation)
Ductus deferens	Transport organ for sperm
Urethra	Transport organ for sperm and urinary organ
Accessory sex glands (prostate, seminal vesicles, and bulbourethral glands)	Production of secretions (semen)
Penis	Copulatory and urinary organ

C Functions of the female genital organs

Organ	Function
Ovary	Germ-cell production Hormone production
Uterine tube	Site of conception and transport organ for zygote
Uterus	Organ of incubation and parturition
Vagina	Organ of copulation and parturition
Labia majora and minora Clitoris	Copulatory organ
Greater and lesser vestibular glands	Production of secretions

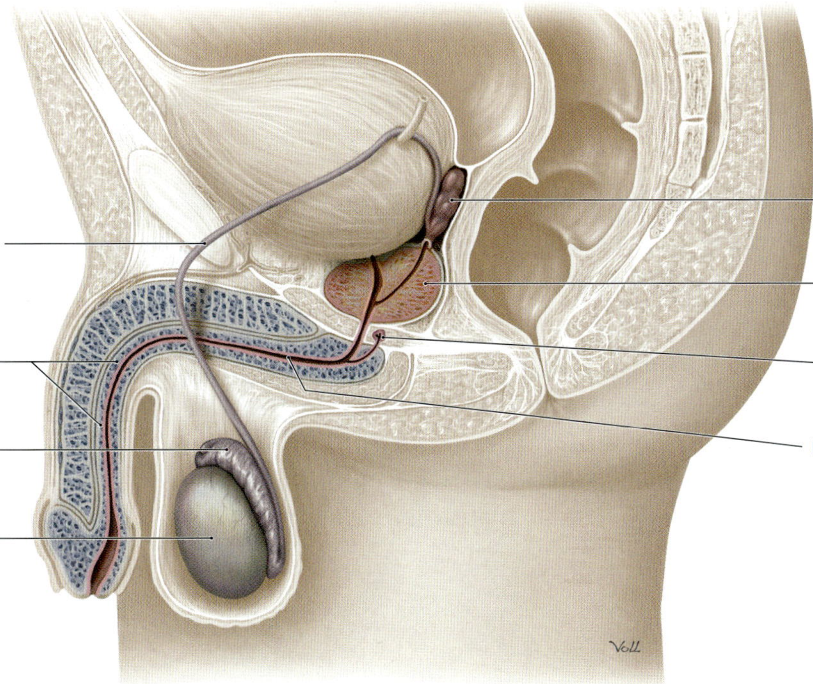

D Overview of the male genital organs
Schematic representation of the male genital organs, viewed from the left side.

Note: The male urethra is part of both the male urinary system and the male reproductive system. The male gonads, the testes, lie outside the body cavity in a pouch of skin called the scrotum.

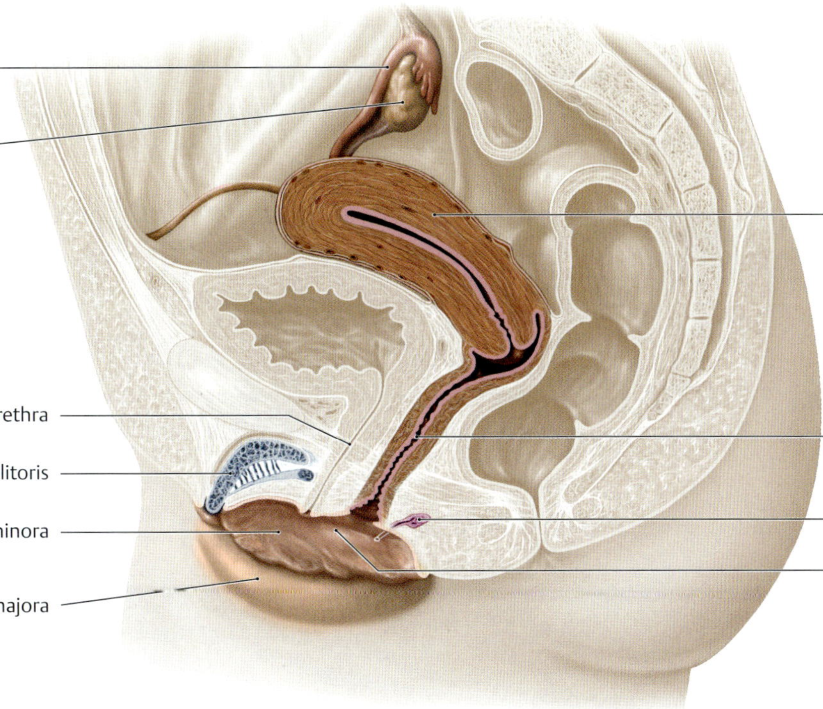

E Overview of the female genital organs
Schematic representation of the female genital organs, viewed from the left side.
Note: The female urethra opens into the vestibule of the vagina. However, unlike in males, the female urethra is not part of the female reproductive system. The female gonads, the ovaries, are located in the cavity of the lesser pelvis.

8.2 Development of the Gonads

Ontogeny-based classification of the genital organs

Embryological structures involved in the formation of male and female genital organs:

- Derivatives of the gonadal primordia: They give rise to the gonads and develop from coelomic epithelium and mesoderm in the genital ridge (see **A–C**).
- Derivatives of the mesonephric and paramesonephric ducts (see p. 60). They give rise to major parts of the genital tracts:
  - in males the mesonephric duct gives rise to the ductus deferens;
  - in females the paramesonephric ducts gives rise to the uterine tubes, uterus and part of the vagina.
- Derivatives of the perineal region: The genital tubercles, folds, and swellings give rise to the external genitalia (see p. 65).
- Derivatives of the urogenital sinus adjacent to the perineal region:
  - in both sexes the urogenital sinus gives rise to the urethra. In males the urethra and the associated prostate gland are also part of the genital system;
  - in females the urogenital sinus gives rise to part of the vagina.

Note: In males and females, the development of both the gonads and the duct system initially pass through an indifferent stage in which gender is not morphologically distinguishable. Over subsequent stages, only one gender-specific duct system fully develops in each sex, while the other regresses. In some people, nonfunctioning remnants of the regressed duct system can become clinically significant (e.g., Gartner's duct cyst, see p. 64).

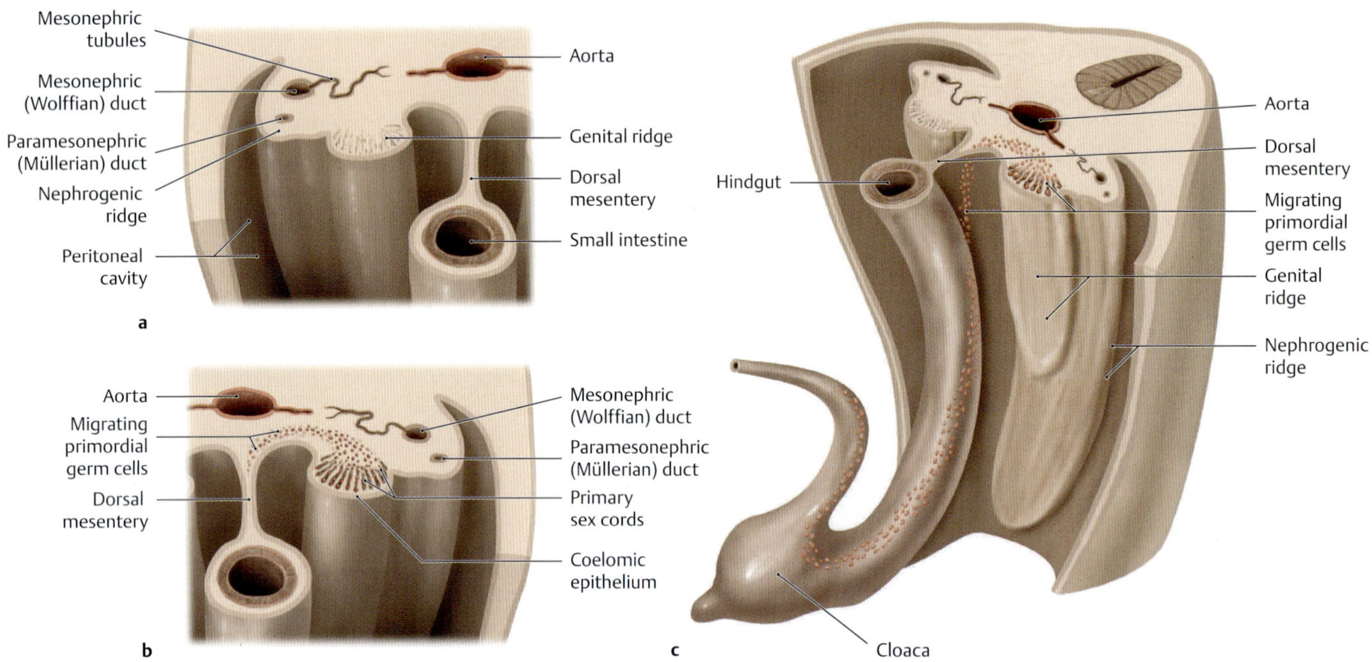

A Development of the genital ridges and gonad primordia; germ cell migration

Schematic horizontal section of an embryo (**a** and **b**; superior view) and in spatial representation (**c**; left superior view).

a and **c** **Genital ridge and gonad primordia:** The primordia of the gonads, which will develop into testes in males and ovaries in females, are initially present as paired, morphologically indifferent organs (*indifferent gonad primordia*) in the *genital ridge*. However, their future differentiation as male or female has already been genetically determined. These indifferent primordia lie along the posterior wall of the body cavity medial to the mesonephric region of the nephrogenic ridges. Together, the nephrogenic ridges and genital ridges protrude from the posterior body wall into the body cavity as the *urogenital ridge*.
Note: These gonad primordia do not yet contain any germ cells. They migrate secondarily from the wall of the yolk sac starting in the 6th week of embryonic development (see **b** and **c**).

b and **c** **Development of the gonads and migration of germ cells:** After the 3rd week of embryonic development, the gonads in the genital ridges start to develop. This is the result of proliferation of the coelomic epithelium (see **b**) and the underlying embryonic connective tissue called mesenchyme. The epithelial cells invade the mesenchyme and form primary sex cords, which in both males and females are still in contact with the coelomic epithelium. In the 6th week, the *primordial germ cells* in the wall of the yolk sac migrate to the gonad primordia by way of the dorsal hindgut mesentery. Germ cell migration (**b** and **c**) leads to the formation of the indifferent gonads in males and females. At the start of the 7th week, the morphological differentiation of the gonads becomes apparent as they begin to develop into testes (male embryo) or ovaries (female embryo, see **C**).

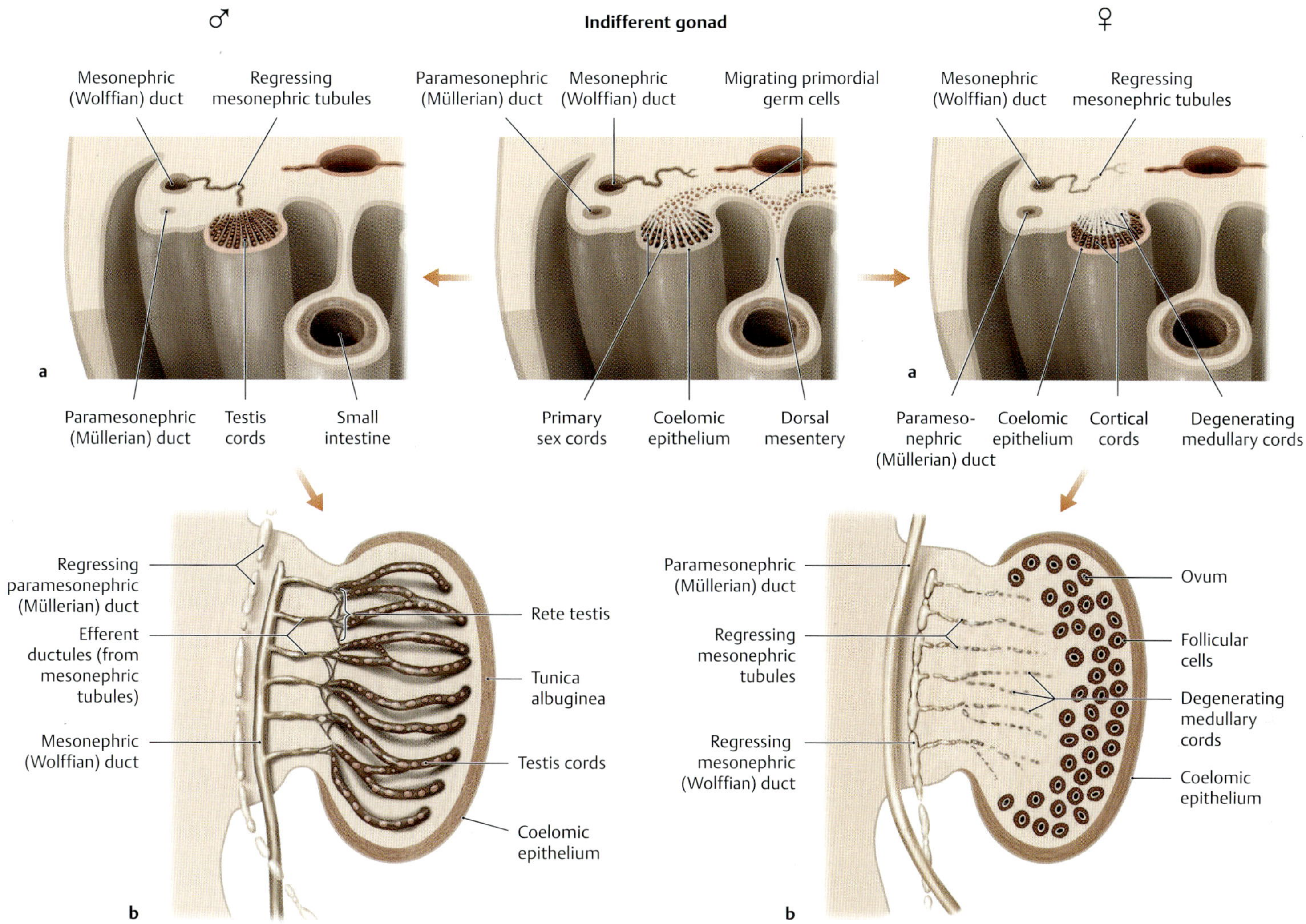

B Development of the testes

Cross-section of the developing testis and genital ducts in the male embryo, viewed from above (**a**) and from the front (**b**).

The primary sex cords continue to grow and extend into the medulla of the gonadal primordia where they form the *testis* (or *medullary*) *cords*. The cords adjacent to the hilum anastomose to form a network of tubules, the future *rete testis*. The testis cords lose contact with the coelomic epithelium and are separated from it by a connective tissue layer called the tunica albuginea. Around the 4th month, the ends of the testis cords opposite from the hilum form horseshoe-shaped loops, which become continuous with the rete testis at the hilum. The solid testis cords are now composed of spermatogonia (from the primordial germ cells) and Sertoli cells (from the surface epithelium of the gonadal primordium). Around the 7th–8th week, Leydig cells in the interstitial mesenchyme between the cords start producing the gender-specific hormone testosterone. The testosterone induces the gender-specific development of the genital ducts. The testis starts to descend from its position high up in the abdominal cavity, through the inguinal canal and into the scrotum. Its location in the scrotum indicates mature development in the male newborn. At the onset of puberty (around age 12–13) the testis cords become canalized and are now called seminiferous tubules. The seminiferous tubules are now connected to the rete testis, which in turn connect with the efferent ductules (remnants of the mesonephric tubules). The efferent ductules open into the ductus deferens, which was derived from the mesonephric duct (induced by testosterone).

C Development of the ovary

Cross-section of developing ovary and genital ducts in a female embryo; viewed from above (**a**) and from the front (**b**).

Primary sex cords also grow into the ovary. Ingrowths of mesenchyme penetrate the cords and divide them into cell clusters of various sizes. The cell clusters shift to the center of the ovary and are replaced by a highly vascularized tissue, which will form the ovarian medulla. Around the 7th week, epithelial extensions from the coelomic epithelium of the ovarian primordia again penetrate into the ovarian mesenchyme and form a second generation of cords called the *cortical cords*. These cords, unlike the primary sex cords, remain closer to the surface. In the 4th month, the cortical cords are divided by ingrowths of mesenchyme into single, smaller cell clusters. These cell clusters then surround one or more germ cells. The germ cells become *oogonia*, and the surrounding layer consisting of cortical cord epithelial cells develops into the *follicular cells* (**b**). Surrounding mesenchyme forms the theca folliculi around the follicles. Over the course of development, the ovary descends into the lesser pelvis to its definitive position. The mesonephric tubules and duct located close to the hilum of the ovary largely degenerate (the nonfunctioning remnants form the paroophoron and epoophoron, see p. 64).

8.3 Development of the Genital Ducts

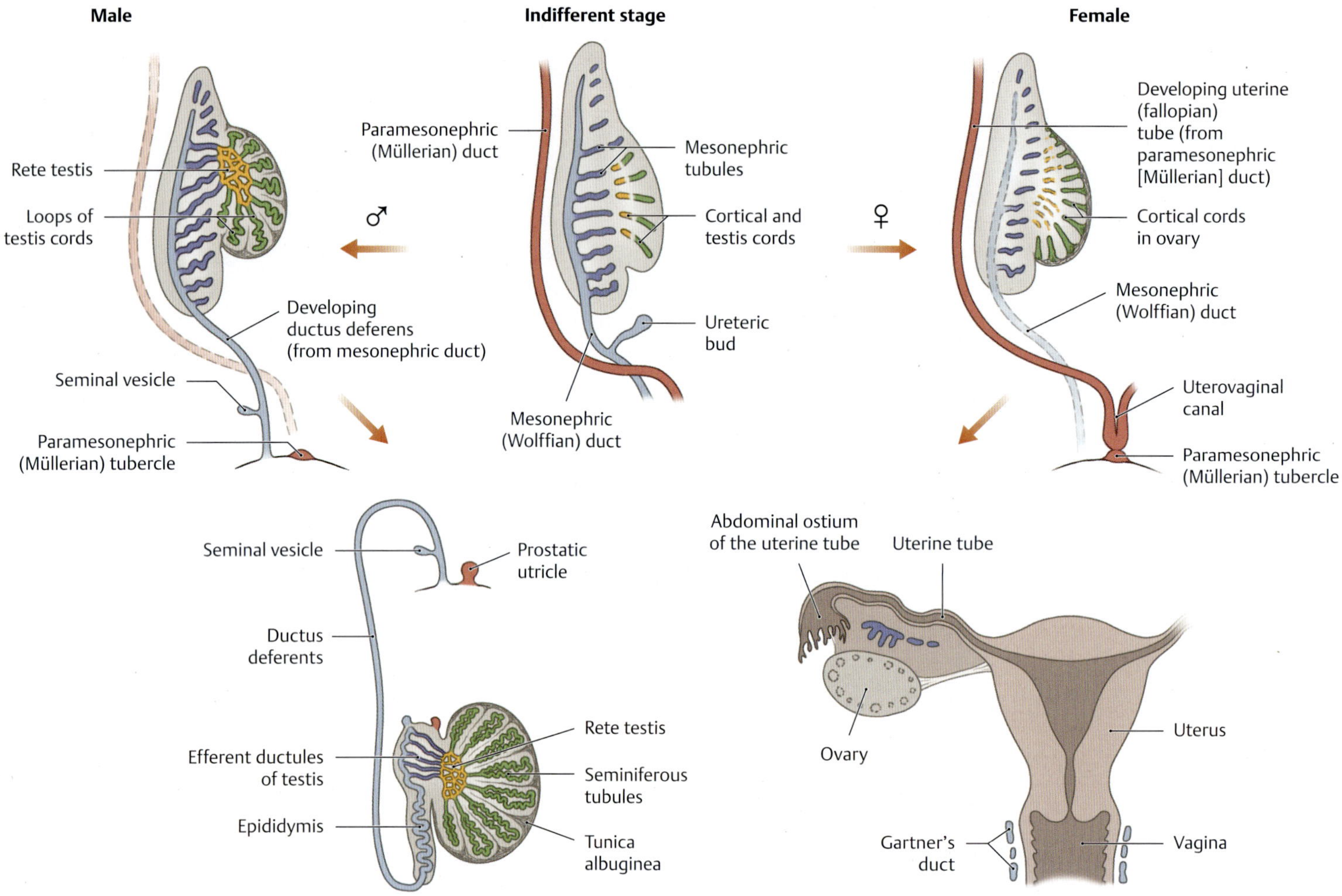

A Differentiation of the mesonephric and paramesonephric ducts
Cross-section of the developing gonads and genital ducts, viewed from the front.
Similar to the gonads, the genital ducts pass through an indifferent stage. The embryo has two pairs of ducts: the mesonephric (Wolffian) ducts and the paramesonephric (Müllerian) ducts, both of which develop in the urogenital ridge. Both ducts eventually connect with the wall of the urogenital sinus. The *mesonephric duct* is a derivative of the intermediate mesoderm, while the *paramesonephric duct* develops from a longitudinal invagination of the coelomic epithelium. Two hormones from the developing testis, testosterone and anti-Müllerian hormone (AMH), largely determine the fate of both ducts. In male fetuses, testosterone stimulates the differentiation of the mesonephric ducts, while AMH causes degeneration of the paramesonephric ducts. Absence of these hormones leads to degeneration of the non-urinary portions of the mesonephric ducts, and to persistence of the paramesonephric ducts.
Note: In both male and female embryos the mesonephric ducts give rise to the ureters.

Male embryo

- Medullary (testis) cords form the rete testis.
- *Some* mesonephric tubules connect with the rete testis.
- The *remaining mesonephric tubules* degenerate. Remnants form the nonfunctioning paradidymis.
- The mesonephric duct gives rise to the ureter, and to the epididymis and ductus deferens (which gives rise to the seminal vesicle and ejaculatory duct).
- The prostate develops from urethral epithelium (not shown).The ductus deferens and seminal vesicle connect with the excretory duct of the prostate. The seminal colliculus is a remnant of the paramesonephric tubercle, the prostatic utricle is a remnant of the paramesonephric duct.
- AMH causes degeneration of the paramesonephric ducts.

Female embryo

- Medullary cords degenerate.
- Mesonephric tubules *don't connect* with other structures.
- *All* mesonephric tubules degenerate. Remnants form the nonfunctioning epoophoron and paroophoron.
- The mesonephric duct gives rise to the ureter, and the *remaining parts of the duct degenerate*. Nonfunctioning remnants may persist adjacent to the vagina in the form of a Gartner's duct.
- Parts of the paramesonephric ducts fuse: the upper portions form the paired uterine tubes, the lower portions form the uterus (see **C**).
- The *mesonephric ducts* degenerate in the *absence of testosterone*.

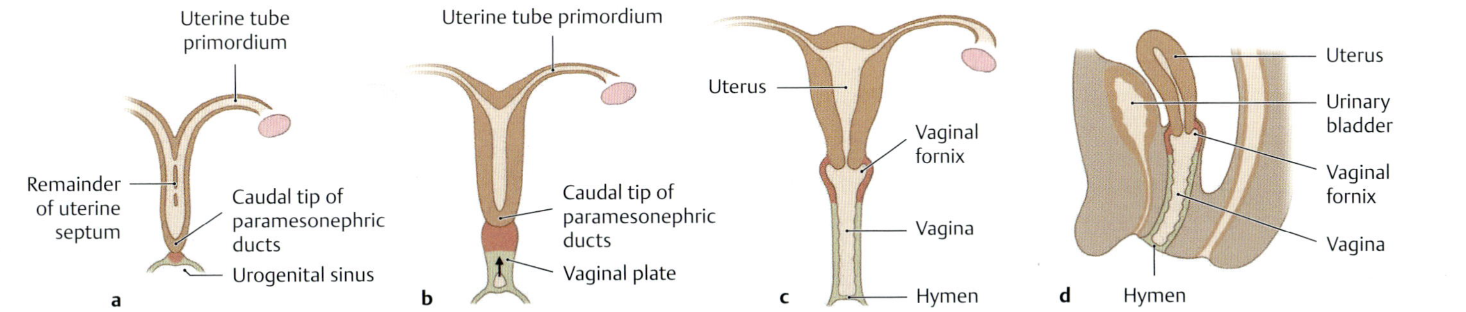

B Development of the genital ducts in the female embryo: Development of the uterus, uterine tubes, and vagina

Anterior view (**a–c**) and view from the left side (**d**) of the developing uterine tubes, uterus and vagina.

As development continues, the upper part of the paramesonephric ducts become horizontal in position while the lower parts remain in vertical. The horizontal parts remain separated and develop into the uterine tubes. The end of the upper part of the paramesonephric duct retains its open connection with the coelomic cavity (which later becomes the peritoneal cavity). This distal opening is called the abdominal ostium and it projects toward the ovary. The lower parts of the ducts fuse, forming the uterovaginal canal. The septum that initially separated the ducts resorbs resulting in a single uterine cavity. The lower part of the fused ducts further grows caudally toward the urogenital sinus. Shortly before reaching it, they merge with a cranial evagination of the urogenital sinus called the sinovaginal bulbs. The sinovaginal bulbs form the solid vaginal plate (**b**). The vaginal plate continues to extend upward. Canalization of the vaginal plate proceeds from the caudal end toward the cranial end and is completed by the 5th month (**b**). As a result of the upward growth, the distance between the developing uterus and urogenital sinus increases. The vaginal plate forms the lower vagina, and the paramesonephric ducts form the upper vagina. A thin membrane of connective tissue called the hymen separates the vagina from the urogenital sinus (**c**, **d**). Failure of the paramesonephric ducts to fuse completely, or of the septum between them to degenerate completely, results in a double uterine cavity or septate uterus (for possible variations see **D**). Failed canalization of the vaginal plate leads to partial or complete vaginal atresia.

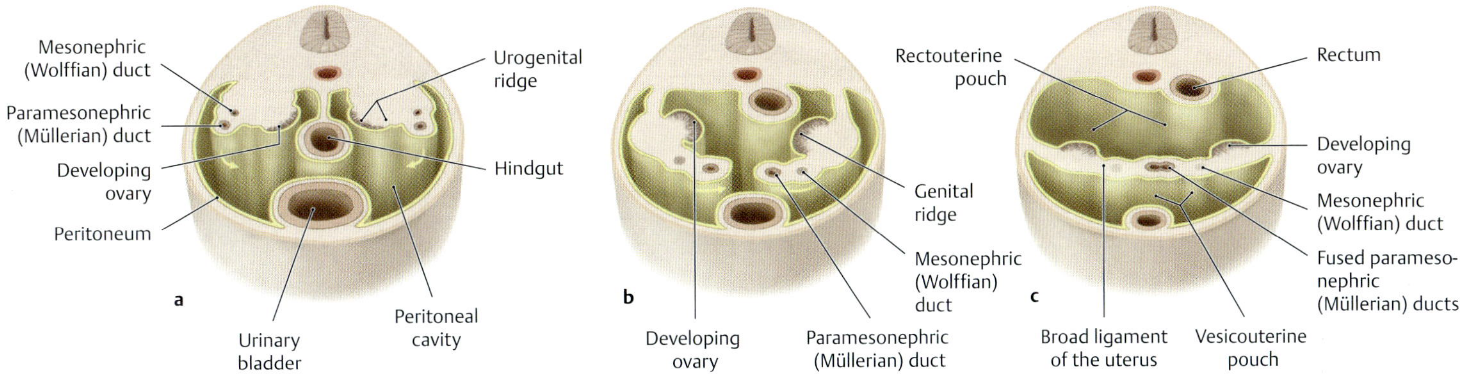

C Fusion of the urogenital ridges in the female embryo

Horizontal sections of the abdomen in a female embryo, viewed from above. **a** Protruding urogenital ridges; **b** Urogenital ridges approaching each other; **c** Fusion of the urogenital ridges.

As a result of continuous proliferation of mesodermal tissue, the urogenital ridges protrude into the coelomic cavity. At the same time, both paramesonephric ducts shift medially until they are in contact with each other. The paramesonephric ducts fuse to form the uterovaginal canal, which together with the fusion of the urogenital ridges results in a layer of connective tissue located in the lesser pelvis. This sheet of connective tissue extends laterally from the developing uterus and is called the broad ligament of the uterus. The broad ligament divides the peritoneal cavity in the lesser pelvis into anterior and posterior pouches:

- Anterior to the uterus (and posterior to urinary bladder): the vesicouterine pouch
- Posterior to the uterus (and anterior to rectum): the rectouterine pouch.

Note: As the urogenital ridges shift position, the developing ovaries shift from an anterior position to a medial position and finally to a posterior position. Thus the definitive ovaries lie in the posterior aspect of the broad ligament.

The paramesonephric ducts originally develop lateral to the mesonephric ducts (see p. 59). As a result of the shifting urogenital ridges and the fusion of their caudal portions, the fused paramesonephric ducts lie medial to the mesonephric ducts in the lower part of the coelomic cavity. The mesonephric ducts give rise to the ureters, which thus traverse the broad ligament on their way from the kidneys to the urinary bladder.

D Developmental anomalies

Anterior view of the developing uterus and vagina. Several defects can arise from failed fusion of the paramesonephric ducts. Incomplete fusion (**a–c**) with double uterus (and/or double vagina); rudimentary horn on one side of the uterus (**d**); atresia of the cervix (**e**); vaginal atresia (**f**). Developmental defects of the developing vagina, mainly atresia, may result from anomalies of the urogenital sinus.

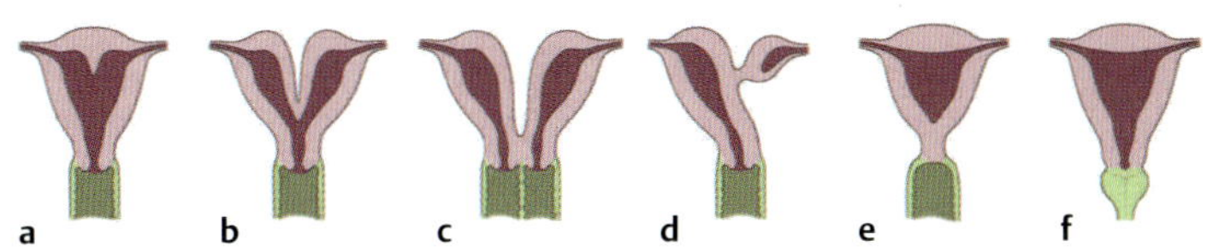

8.4 Comparison of Gender Differences and Relationship to the Urinary System

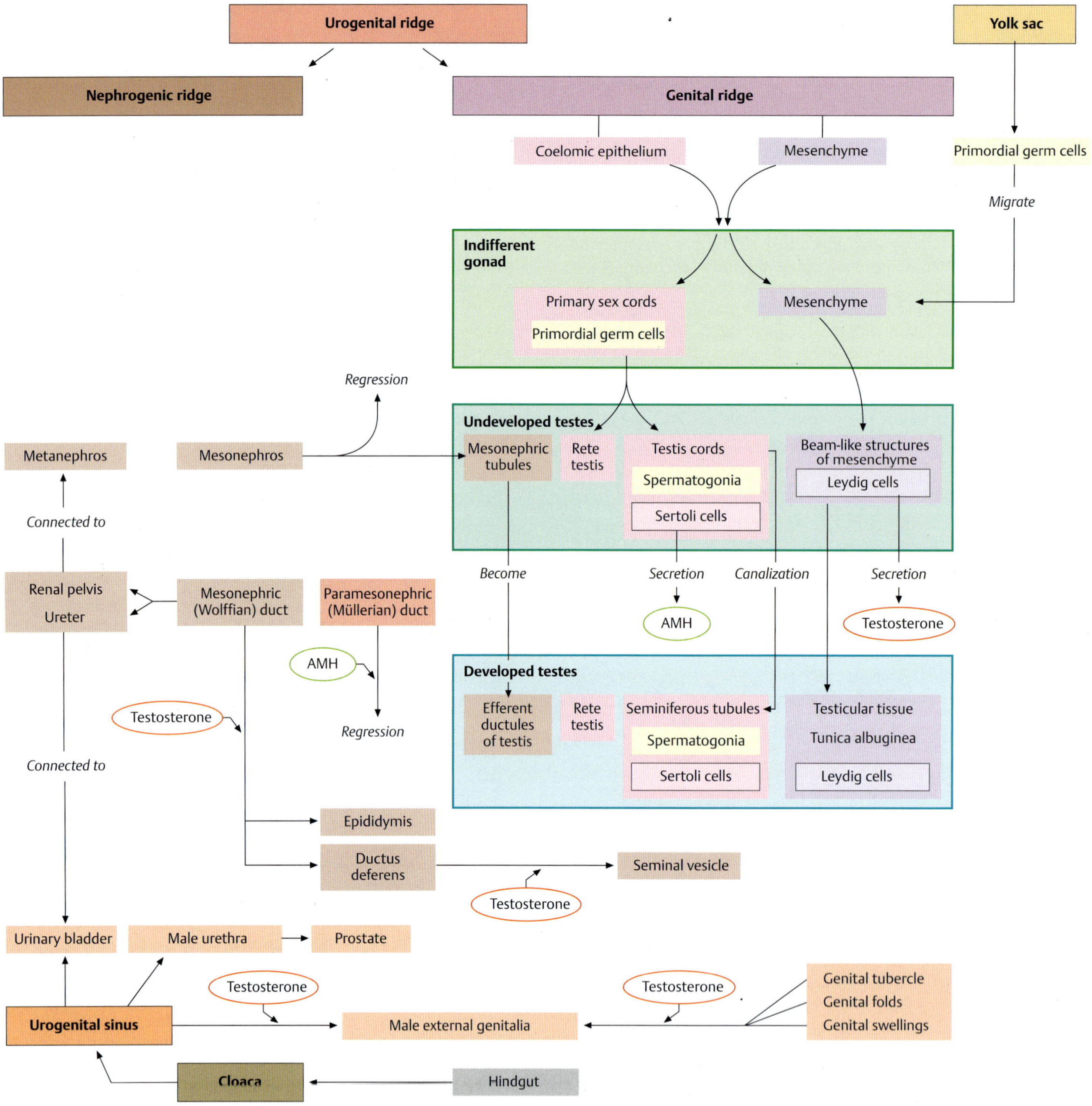

a

A Comparison of genital development in both sexes, and relationships to the urinary system

Schematic representation of the development of the male (**a**) and female (**b**) genital systems. Nonfunctioning embryonic remnants are not shown here (see **A**, p. 64). The relationship of the genital system to the urinary system, which is similar in both sexes, is shown here to illustrate the close relationship between the two systems.

Note: Primary sex cords develop in both the male and female gonadal primordia. They degenerate in females and are replaced by secondary cords, the cortical cords, which are involved in the development

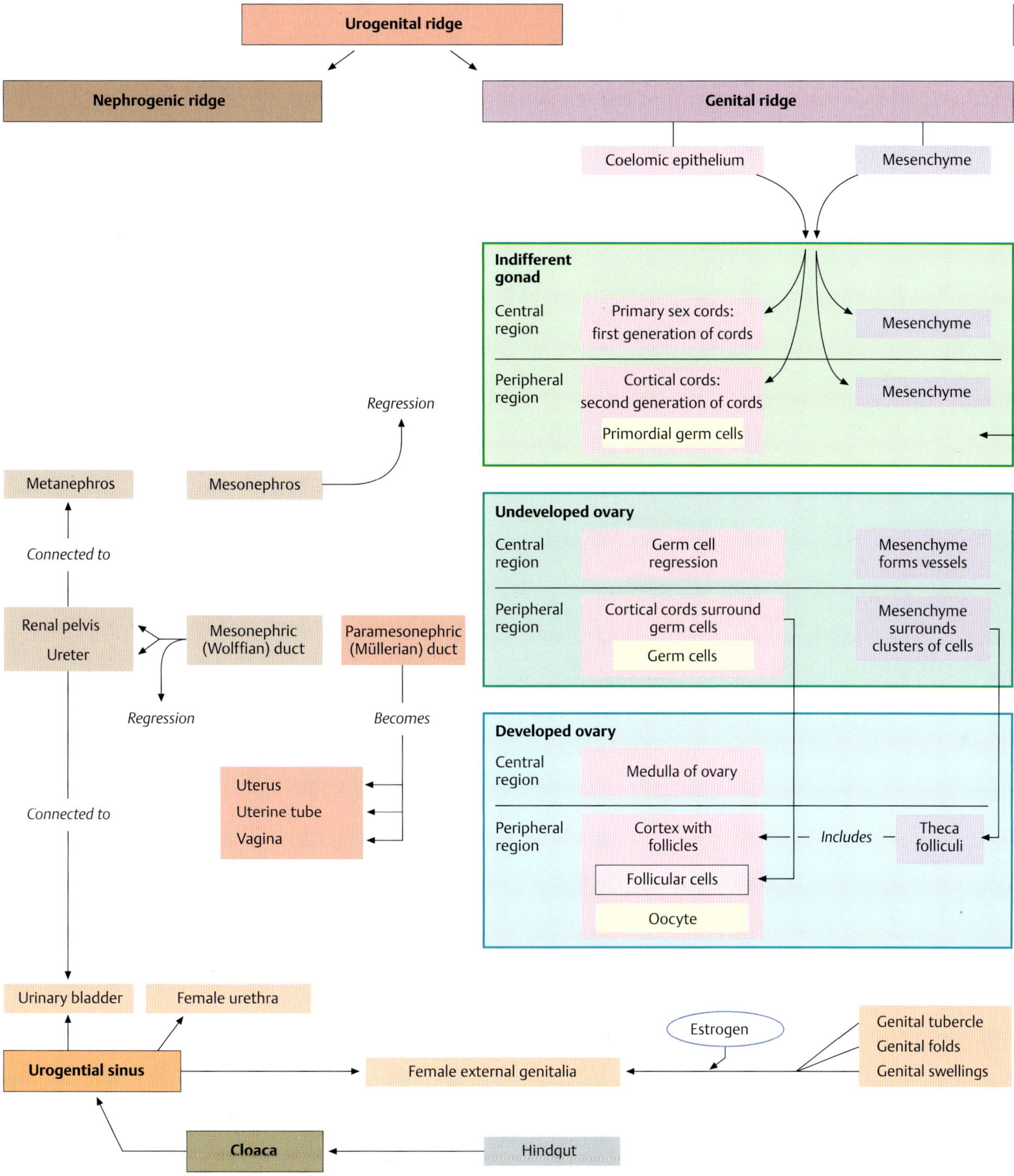

b

of follicles. In males, the primary sex cords become testis (medullary) cords, which develop into the seminiferous tubules. Cortical cords don't develop in the testes. Development of a male phenotype requires testosterone (development of the male genital ducts) and anti-Müllerian hormone (AMH, causes regression of the paramesonephric ducts). If these two hormones are absent—or the ducts don't respond to them due to a lack of hormone receptors—a female phenotype develops even in the absence of estrogen.

8.5 Comparison of Embryonic and Mature Structures

A Comparison of embryonic and mature structures
Overview of development in both sexes. Some embryonic structures develop into *functionally active* mature structures, while others form *nonfunctioning remnants*. A male vs. female comparison of the structures listed in the following table is illustrated on the following page.

Embryonic promordium	Definitive structure in the male	Definitive structure in the female	Nonfunctioning remnants in the male	Nonfunctioning remnants in the female
Indifferent gonad with • Cortex • Medulla	Testis with • Seminiferous tubules • Rete testis	Ovary with • Follicles • Ovarian stroma		
Mesonephric tubules	Efferent ducts		Paradidymis	Epo- and paroophoron
Mesonephric (Wolffian) duct	• Epididymis • Ductus deferens • Ejaculatory duct • Seminal vesicle • *Ureter* • *Renal pelvis and calyces, collecting ducts*	• *Ureter* • *Renal pelvis and calyces, collecting ducts*	Appendix of epididymis	Gartner's duct
Paramesonephric (Müllerian) duct		• Uterine tube • Uterus • Superior portion of vagina	• Appendix of testis • Fibromuscular part of prostatic utricle	Hydatid of Morgagni
Urogenital sinus	• Prostate • Bulbourethral gland • *Urinary bladder* • *Male urethra*	• Inferior portion of vagina • Greater and lesser vestibular glands • *Urinary bladder* • *Female urethra*	Epithelium of prostatic utricle	
Genital tubercle (phallus)	Corpus cavernosum of penis	• Body of clitoris with ascending and descending parts • Angle of clitoris • Crura of clitoris		
Genital folds	• Corpus spongiosum of the penis • Glans of penis	• Labia minora • Vestibular bulb • Glans of clitoris • Infracorporeal residual spongy part (RSP)		
Genital swellings	Scrotum	Labia majora		
Gubernaculum		• Proper ovarian ligament • Round ligament of uterus	Gubernaculum of testis	
Paramesonephric tubercle			Seminal colliculus	Hymen

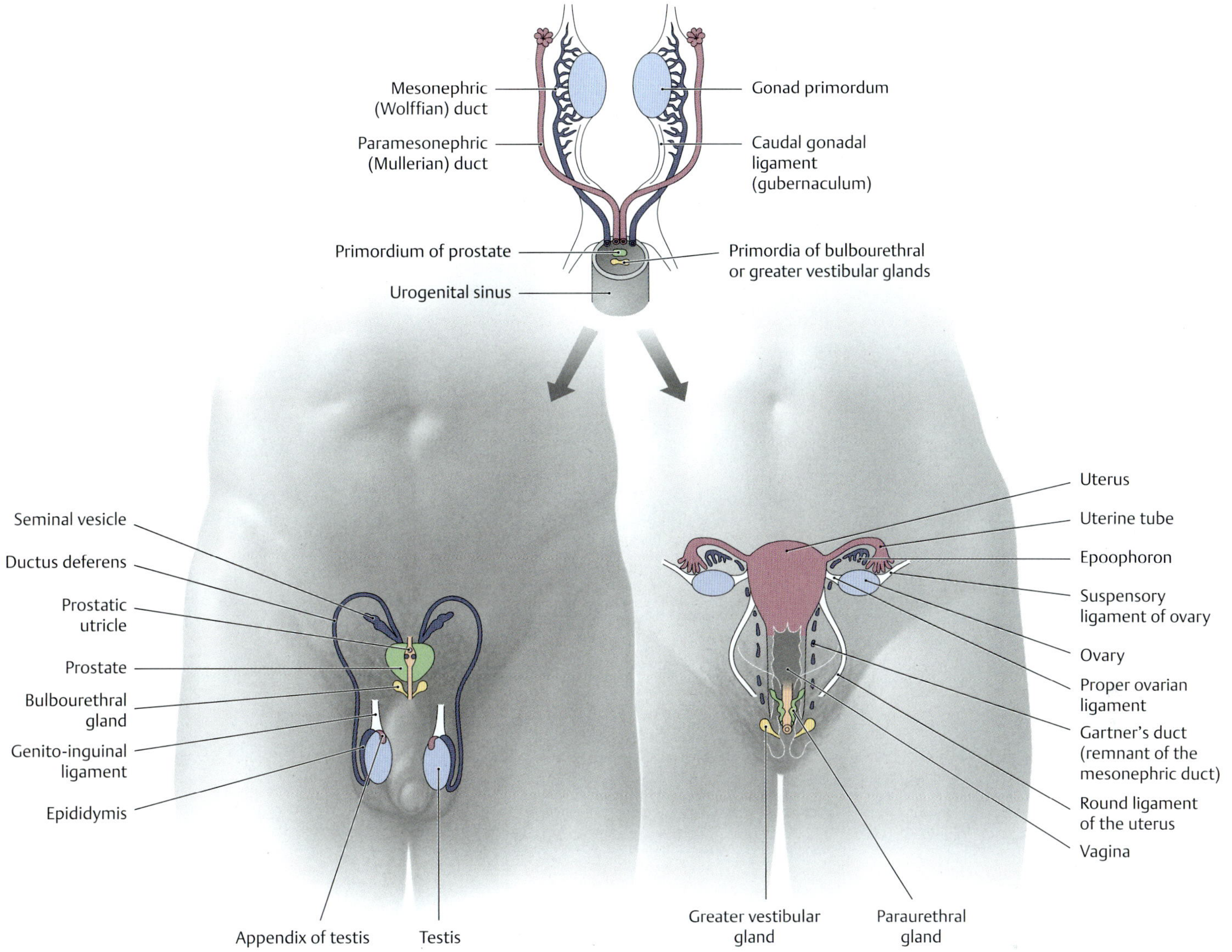

B Development of the internal genitalia

Embryonic primordia of the genital organs, and the mature organs, anterior view. For clarity, the representation of the primordia and the mature organs does not correspond with their actual sizes.

Note: The internal genital organs are located in the lesser pelvis or outside the body in the scrotum. With the descent of the gonads, the genital tracts, which develop from the mesonephric ducts in males and the paramesonephric ducts in females, move downward as the gonads descend. Thus, the ducts shift from a craniocaudal orientation to a horizontal position (the uterine tube in females) or to an almost upside-down position (the ductus deferens in males).

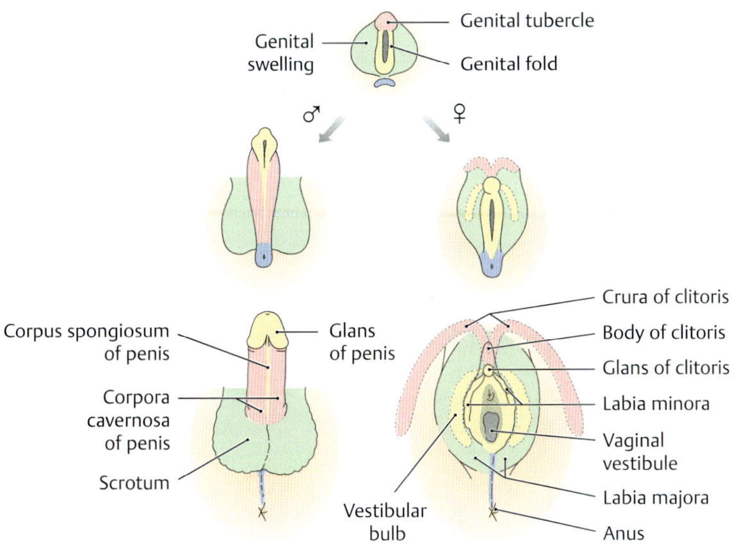

C Development of the external genitalia

Schematic representation of the developing external genitalia, inferior view.

In both sexes, the urethra develops from the urogenital sinus. In the male the urethra becomes part of both the urinary and reproductive systems. In the female the urethra is solely a urinary organ and is located directly superior to the vagina. Its opening in the vaginal vestibule lies between the vaginal introitus and the glans of the clitoris. The female internal and external genitalia are completely separated from the urinary organs; however, due to their close topographical relationship, developmental anomalies of one system may affect the other (such as a urethral-vaginal fistula where there is an abnormal connection between the urethra and vagina).

9.1 Overview of the Endocrine System

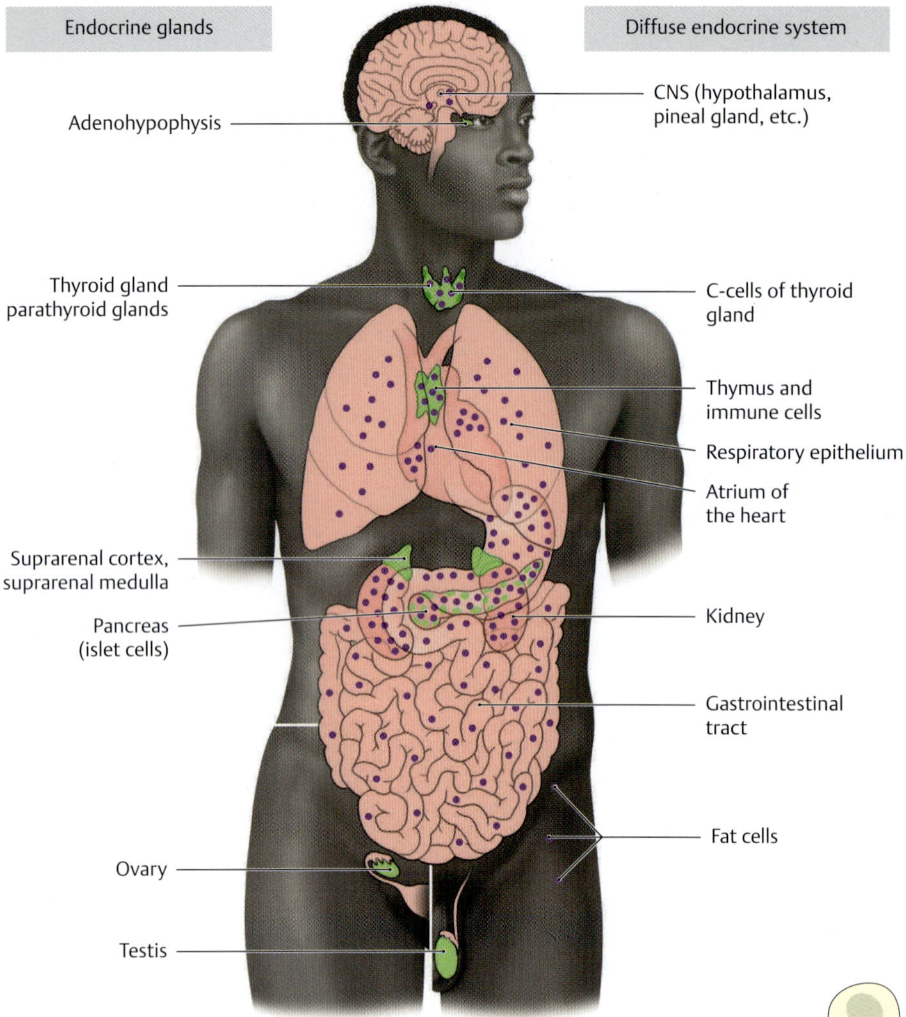

A The endocrine system

By secreting hormones, the endocrine system enables cells to communicate with other cells and coordinates bodily functions. Thus, the endocrine system is closely related to the nervous system, which has a similar coordinating function. The endocrine system includes the classic endocrine glands, which are visible *macroscopically* (left). Additionally, it includes individual cells or small groups of cells, which also secrete hormones, but are only visible *histologically*. These cells constitute the diffuse endocrine system (right), and they are located in a number of organs, including the endocrine glands.

The hormones produced by endocrine organs affect other cells in very low doses, and the organs themselves are usually small and difficult to dissect. In addition, they are difficult to classify histologically because they produce a number of different types of hormones (see **C**). Thus, this chapter will focus on the functional and biochemical aspects of the endocrine system.

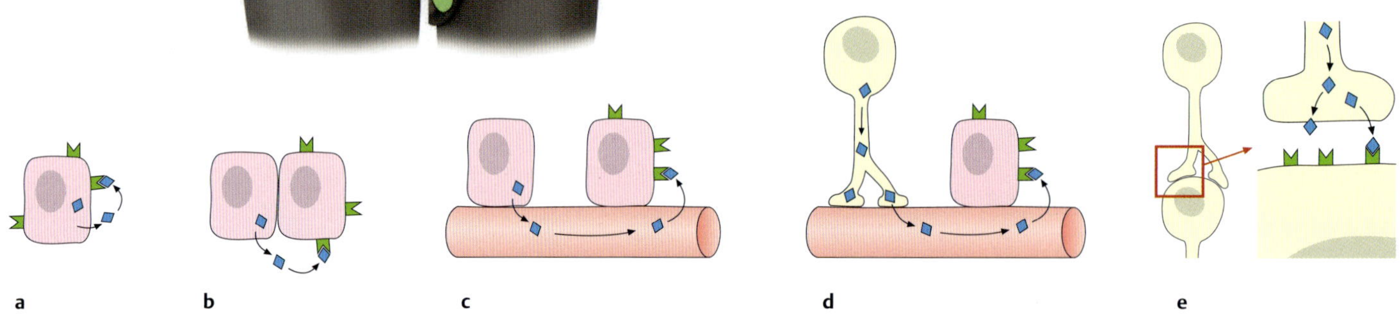

B Types of hormonal communication

In hormonal communication a cell secretes a hormone, and a receptor recognizes the hormone and triggers a signal transduction cascade leading to changes in the cell that bears the receptor. There are several types of hormonal communication.

- **a Autocrine secretion:** the hormones are synthesized and secreted by the same cells that possess the receptors. Thus, the cell stimulates itself. Autocrine secretion plays a particularly important role in tumor development.
- **b Paracrine secretion:** the hormones are released into the interstitial fluid and diffuse to neighboring cells that have the hormones' receptors. This is the most primitive form of hormonal effect; it developed early in evolution and it still plays a major role in the human endocrine system. Diffuse endocrine cells (see above) act this way, and the immune system uses paracrine signaling with interleukins to enable communication between cells.
- **c Endocrine secretion:** the secreting cell releases the hormone into the blood, where it is transported to the receptor-bearing cells. All major endocrine glands utilize this mechanism.
- **d Neurosecretion:** the secreting cell, a neuron, releases its neurotransmitter, which acts as a hormone, directly into the blood stream. Neurosecretion is a transitional type of communication between endocrine signaling and synaptic transmission. It illustrates the close relationship between nervous system and endocrine system.
- **e Synaptic transmission** (neurocrine secretion): Synaptic transmission is a special form of paracrine signaling. The neurotransmitter (hormone) is released by a neuron from its presynaptic membrane. The transmitter diffuses across the synaptic cleft to receptors on the postsynaptic membrane.

C Classification of hormones as lipophilic or hydrophilic molecules (after Karlson)

Hormones can be either lipophilic or hydrophilic, which helps explain the substantial differences in their synthesis and function. Lipophilic hormones such as the steroid hormones are synthesized in smooth endoplasmic reticulum, while hydrophilic hormones such as the protein hormones are synthesized in rough endoplasmic reticulum. These differences in synthesis are reflected in the varying amounts of the organelles in hormone-producing cells.

	Lipophilic hormones	Hydrophilic hormones
Signaling molecule	• Steroid hormones • Thyroid hormones • Retinoic acid	• Amino acids and their derivatives • Peptide hormones • Protein hormones
Plasma transport	Bound	Mostly unbound
Half-life	Long (hours to days)	Short (minutes)
Receptors	Intracellular	Membranous
Effect	Transcription control	Intracellular signaling cascades via membrane proteins

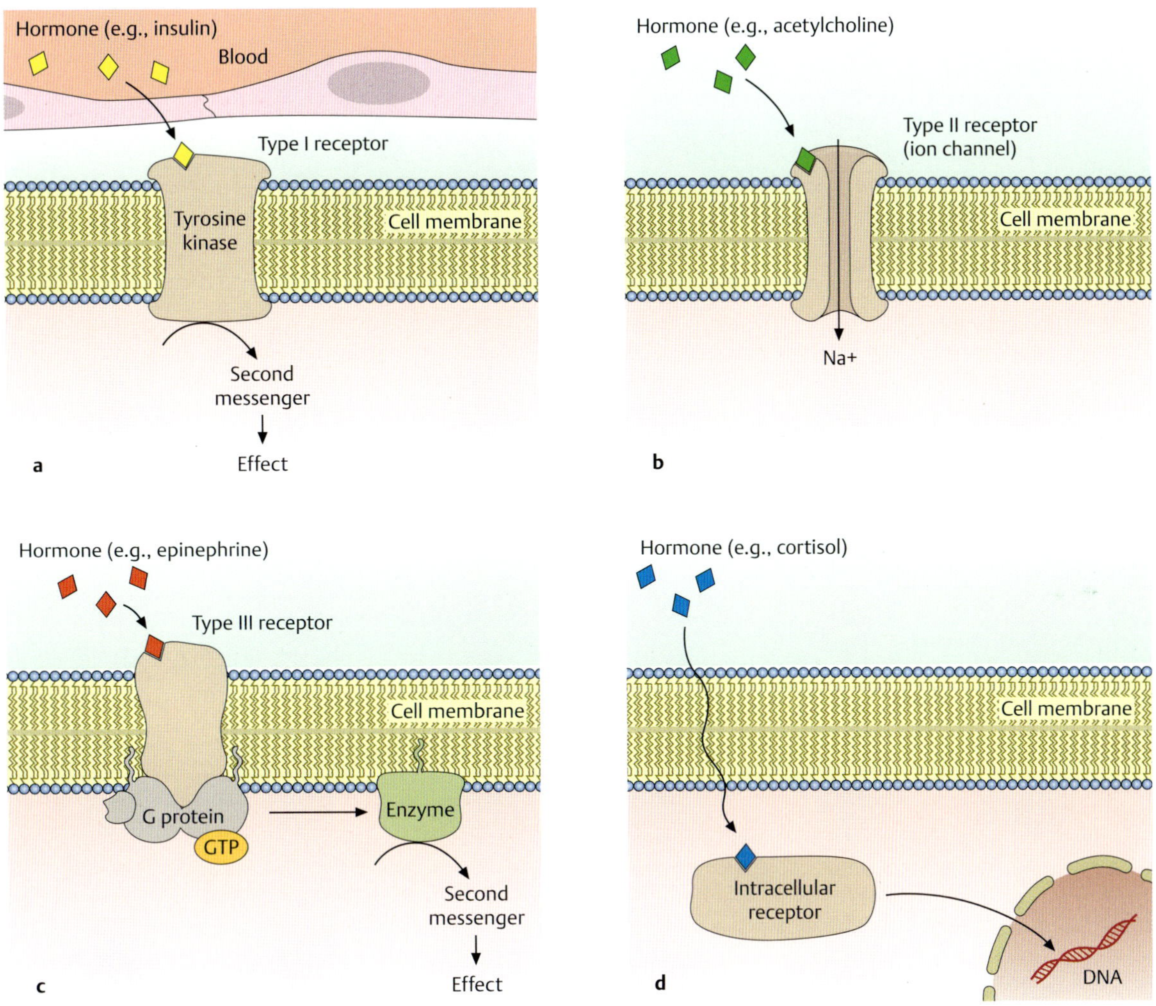

D Types of hormone receptors

There are 4 general types of hormone receptors.

- **a Type I receptors:** The receptor protein, which is an enzyme, is embedded in the lipid bilayer of the cell membrane. The hormone binds to cell-surface receptors. However, the enzymatic reaction occurs on the cytoplasmic side of the membrane, where the substrate-binding site for the enzymatic reaction is located. Generally, the enzyme is a tyrosine kinase that phosphorylates substrates when activated. *Example: insulin receptors.*
- **b Type II receptors:** The receptors are ion channels, which change their conductance depending on ligand-binding. *Example: Acetylcholine receptors* in neurons (another example of the close relationship between the endocrine and nervous systems).
- **c Type III receptors:** The hormone receptors activate G proteins (guanine nucleotide-binding proteins), which in turn activate intracellular proteins (indirect activation). This is the largest group of hormone receptors. *Example: epinephrine receptors.*
- **d Intracellular receptors:** Lipophilic hormones pass directly through the cell membrane and activate intracellular receptors. The primary function of these receptors is regulation of gene expression. *Example: cortisol receptors.*

  Note: The hormonal effects regulated by gene expression are characterized by a slower response compared to the fast effects regulated by type II receptors.

9.2 Metabolism and Feedback Loop Regulation in the Endocrine System

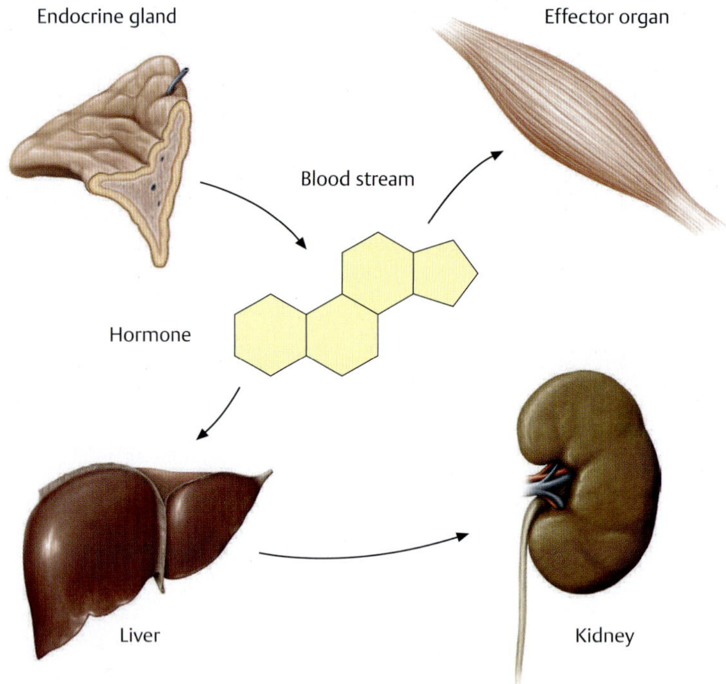

A Metabolism of hormones
The hormone is produced by the cells of an endocrine gland (in this example a steroid hormone from the suprarenal cortex) and released into the blood as needed. The hormone is transported in the bloodstream to the effector organ (here: skeletal muscle), where it binds to receptors that mediate the cellular effects of the hormone. The hormone is broken down in the liver and the metabolites are excreted via the kidneys.

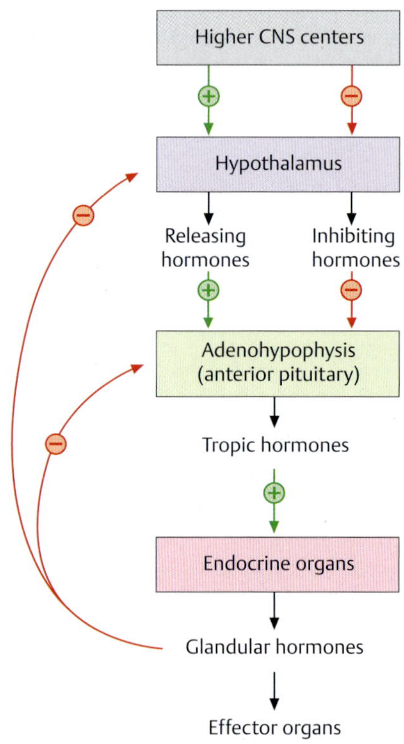

B Feedback loops in the endocrine system
Inhibitory (red) and stimulatory (green) pathways from higher centers of the brain modulate the hypothalamus, which is part of the diencephalon and serves as a master control center for a large part of hormone regulation. A preponderance of inhibitory input leads to the release of inhibiting hormones and a preponderance of stimulatory input leads to the release of releasing hormones. If releasing hormones outweigh inhibiting hormones, the adenohypophysis (anterior pituitary) will release a glandotropic hormone (a hormone that affects a peripheral endocrine gland, e.g., suprarenal gland or thyroid). This hormone stimulates the gland to release its hormones, which stimulate the effector organ. At the same time the hormone inhibits the adenohypophysis and hypothalamus, which leads to a reduction in further hormone production and release (a negative feedback loop). Thus, in the regulation of hormone production and release, multiple hormones can be thought of being serially connected in a chain with a feedback mechanism incorporated into the links.

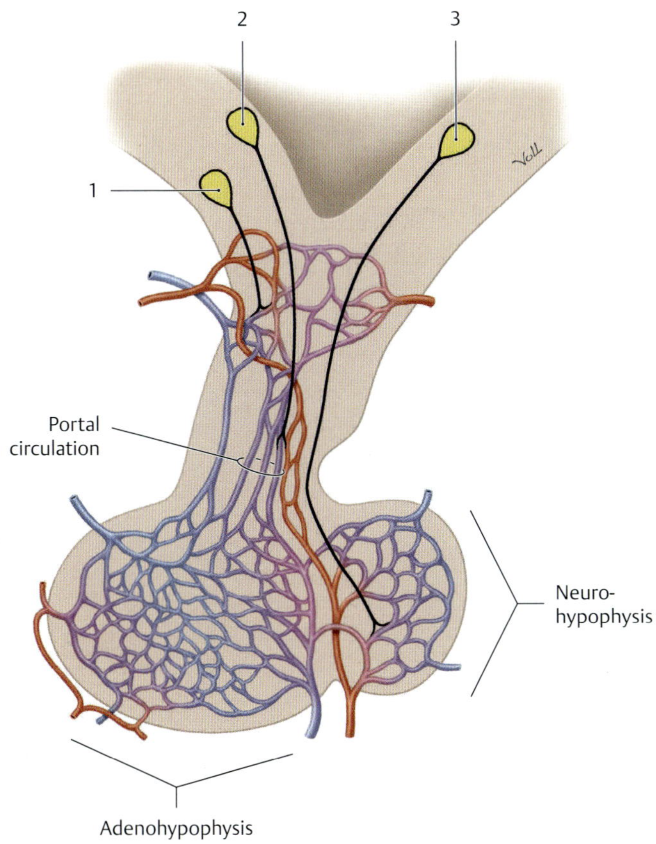

C The hypothalamic-pituitary axis and hormone regulation

The hypothalamus and pituitary gland function as higher control centers for hormone release by other endocrine glands. They are connected to each other through the pituitary stalk by a venous portal system and a long axon system:

- Regulation via the portal system: Neuronal cell bodies in the hypothalamus (neurons 1 and 2) synthesize releasing and inhibiting hormones, and, via short axons, release them into the portal blood vessels. They are then transported in the vessels to cells in the *anterior* pituitary (*adenohypophysis*). These cells then produce hormones, which are released into the systemic circulation. The first neurons (neurons 1 and 2) are called neuroendocrine transducers because they transform neural information into hormonal information by releasing their transmitters into the portal circulation. They do not terminate at other nerve cells.
- Regulation via *long* axons: Neurons located in the hypothalamus (neuron 3) project to the *posterior* pituitary (*neurohypophysis*), where they release their hormones directly into the blood vessels of the neurohypophysis (neurosecretion). This system bypasses the portal circulation, and the neurons themselves (neuron 3) are the neuroendocrine transducers. The hormones oxytocin and vasopressin (ADH) are released in this way.

Note: The secretions of the disseminated endocrine cells in the digestive and respiratory tracts is not regulated by the hypothalamic-pituitary axis.

D Principal sites where hormones and hormone-like substances are formed

Hormones are vitally important chemical messengers that enable cells to communicate with one another. Usually, very small amounts of these messengers act on metabolic processes in their target cells. Different hormones can be classified on the basis of their

- site of formation,
- site of action,
- mechanism of action, or
- chemical structure.

Examples are steroid hormones (e.g., testosterone, aldosterone), amino acid derivatives (e.g., epinephrine, norepinephrine, dopamine, serotonin), peptide hormones (e.g., insulin, glucagon), and fatty acid derivatives (e.g., prostaglandins).

Principal sites of formation	Hormones and hormone-like substances
Classic endocrine hormonal glands	
Pituitary gland (anterior and posterior lobes)	ACTH (adrenocorticotropic hormone, corticotropin) TSH (thyroid-stimulating hormone, thyrotropin) FSH (follicle-stimulating hormone, follitropin) LH (luteinizing hormone, lutropin) STH (somatotropic hormone, somatotropin) MSH (melanocyte-stimulating hormone, melanotropin) PRL (prolactin) ADH (antidiuretic hormone or vasopressin) Oxytocin (formed in the hypothalamus and secreted by the posterior pituitary)
Pineal gland	Melatonin
Thyroid gland	Thyroxine (T4) and triiodothyronine (T3)
C cells of the thyroid gland	Calcitonin
Parathyroid glands	Parathyroid hormone
Suprarenal glands	Mineralocorticoids and glucocorticoids Androgens Epinephrine and norepinephrine
Pancreatic islet cells (Langerhans cells)	Inulin, glucagon, somatostatin, and pancreatic polypeptide
Ovary	Estrogens and progestins
Testis	Androgens (mainly testosterone)
Placenta	Chorionic gonadotropin, progesterone
Hormone-producing tissues and single cells	
Central and autonomic nervous system	Neuronal transmitters
Parts of the diencephalon (e.g., the hypothalamus)	Releasing and inhibitory hormones
System of gastrointestinal cells in the GI tract	Gastrin, cholecystokinin, secretin
Cardiac atria	Atrial natriuretic peptide
Kidney	Erythropoietin, renin
Liver	Angiotensinogen, somatomedins
Immune organs	Thymus hormones, cytokines, lymphokines
Tissue hormones	Eicosanoids, prostaglandins, histamine, bradykinin

10.1 The Sympathetic and Parasympathetic Nervous Systems

The autonomic, or visceral, nervous system innervates the internal organs. It is divided into three parts: the sympathetic, parasympathetic, and enteric nervous systems. For didactic reasons these systems are discussed separately; however, they represent one functional unit.

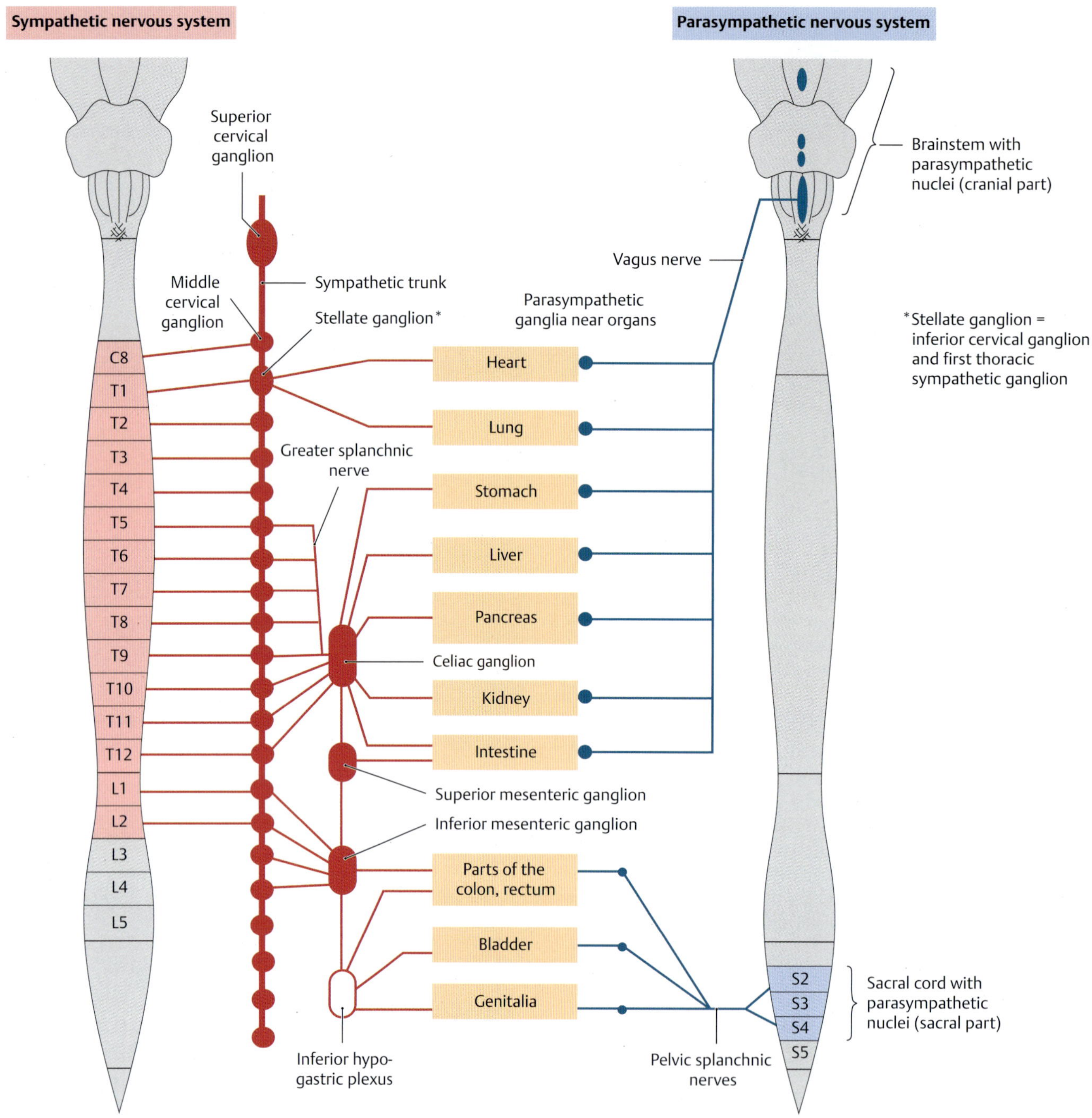

A Structure of the sympathetic (red) and parasympathetic (blue) nervous systems

Both the sympathetic and parasympathetic systems utilize a two-neuron pathway between the CNS and their targets. The first neuron is called the preganglionic neuron, and the second neuron is the postganglionic neuron. The preganglionic sympathetic neurons are located in the lateral horn of lower cervical, thoracic, and upper lumbar regions of the spinal cord. The preganglionic parasympathetic neurons are located in cranial nerve nuclei and the sacral region of the spinal cord. The vagus nerve, a cranial nerve, contains the preganglionic parasympathetic neurons that will innervate cervical, thoracic, and abdominal viscera. In both the sympathetic and parasympathetic nervous systems, the preganglionic neurons of the CNS synapse with the postganglionic neurons in ganglia of the peripheral nervous system (see **C** and **D**).

- In the sympathetic nervous system, the preganglionic neuron synapses with the postganglionic neuron in ganglia of the sympathetic trunk (for trunk and limbs), in prevertebral ganglia (for viscera) or directly in the organs (only suprarenal glands).
- In the parasympathetic nervous system, the vagus nerve terminates at ganglia close to or in the walls (intramural ganglia) of the organs.

According to Langley (1905), the terms sympathetic and parasympathetic nervous system originally referred only to efferent neurons and their axons (visceral efferent fibers, as shown above). It has now been shown that the sympathetic and parasympathetic nervous systems contain afferent fibers (visceral afferent fibers, pain and stretch receptors not shown here, see p. 72).

B Synopsis of the sympathetic and parasympathetic nervous systems

1. The sympathetic nervous system can be considered the excitatory part of the autonomic nervous system that prepares the body for a "*fight or flight*" response.
2. The parasympathetic nervous system is the part of the autonomic nervous system that coordinates the "*rest and digest*" responses of the body.
3. Although there are separate control centers for the two divisions in the brainstem and spinal cord, they have close anatomic and functional ties in the periphery.
4. The principal transmitter at the target organ is *acetylcholine* in the parasympathetic nervous system and *norepinephrine* in the sympathetic nervous organ.
5. Stimulation of the sympathetic and parasympathetic nervous systems produces the following different effects on specific organs:

Organ	Sympathetic nervous system	Parasympathetic nervous system
Heart	Increased heart rate	Decreased heart rate
Lungs	Bronchodilation and decreased bronchial secretions	Bronchoconstriction and increased bronchial secretions
Gastrointestinal tract	Decreased secretions and motor activity	Increased secretions and motor activity
Pancreas	Decreased endocrine and exocrine secretions	Increased exocrine secretions
Male genitalia	Ejaculation	Erection

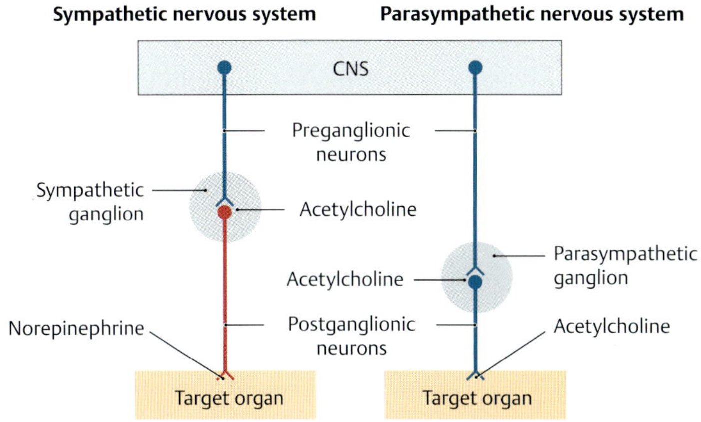

C Circuit diagram of the autonomic nervous system

In both the sympathetic and parasympathetic nervous systems the first neuron lies in the CNS (*central* neuron). Switching between the first neuron and second neuron (*peripheral* neuron) always occurs in a ganglion (sympathetic or parasympathetic ganglion, respectively). In both cases, the first neuron uses *acetylcholine* as a transmitter for switching *in the ganglion* (*cholinergic* neuron, shown in blue). In the parasympathetic nervous system, the second neuron also uses *acetylcholine* as a transmitter (also cholinergic). In contrast, the transmitter of the second *sympathetic* neuron is norepinephrine (adrenergic neuron, shown in red).

Note: Various types of receptors for acetylcholine (neurotransmitter sensors) are located in the membrane of the target cells. As a result, acetylcholine can produce a range of effects depending on the receptor type.

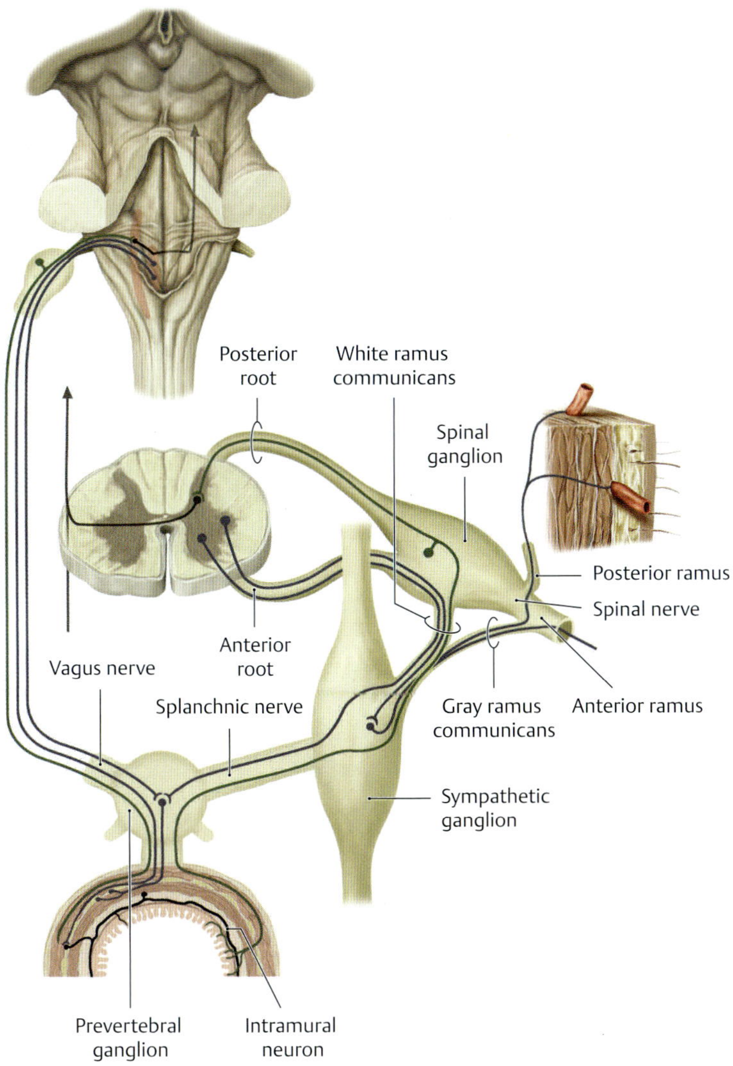

D Circuitry of the autonomic nervous system

Although the sympathetic and parasympathetic nervous systems emerge from two different regions of the CNS (see **A**), they form a close structural and functional unit close to the organs. The perikarya of the preganglionic **sympathetic** neurons are located in the lateral horn of the spinal cord. Their axons exit the spinal cord through the anterior root and travel in the white rami communicans (white because they are myelinated) to the sympathetic chain ganglia. The axons synapse with the postganglionic neurons at three different levels:

- For the sympathetic fibers going to the limbs and trunk wall, the preganglionic sympathetic neurons synapse with the postganglionic neurons in the sympathetic chain ganglia. The postganglionic fibers travel in the gray rami communicans (gray because they are unmyelinated) back to the spinal nerves.
- For the sympathetic fibers going to the viscera, the preganglionic sympathetic fibers usually pass through the sympathetic chain ganglia as splanchnic nerves. They synapse with the postganglionic sympathetic neurons in ganglia close to the organs (prevertebral ganglia). From there, the postganglionic fibers travel to the organs. The sympathetic nervous system also influences the enteric nervous system, which is referred to as the third part of the autonomic nervous system (see p. 73). In the colon, for example, sympathetic fibers will contact intramural neurons of the enteric system.
- For the sympathetic fibers going to the suprarenal medulla, the preganglionic sympathetic fibers terminate on the cells of the medulla (not shown here).

The preganglionic **parasympathetic** neurons of the viscera located in the body cavities originate from brainstem nuclei of the vagus nerves or from sacral spinal cord levels (not shown). They synapse in ganglia that are either very close to or embedded in the organ (intramural ganglia). Afferent pain fibers (marked in green) accompany both sympathetic and parasympathetic nerve fibers. The axons of these fibers originate in pseudounipolar neurons, which are located either in spinal ganglion or in ganglia of the vagus nerves (see p. 72).

10.2 Afferent Pathways of the Autonomic Nervous System and the Enteric Nervous System

A Pain afferents from the viscera conducted by the sympathetic and parasympathetic pathways

a Sympathetic pain fibers, **b** Parasympathetic pain fibers.

Both nervous systems also carry axons of afferent pain fibers, which run parallel to the efferent pathways. They only make up about 5% of all afferent pain fibers and thus, quantitatively, they play a minor role and become active mainly in response to organ lesions.

a The pain conducting (nociceptive) axons from the viscera run along with the splanchnic nerves to the sympathetic ganglia and reach the spinal nerves by way of the white rami communicans. They then run in the posterior roots of the spinal nerves to the spinal ganglia, where their perikarya are located. From the ganglia, their axons pass through the posterior roots to the posterior horn of the spinal cord, where they synapse and establish connections with ascending pain pathways.
Note: Unlike the efferent system, the afferent nociceptive fibers do not synapse in peripheral ganglia.

b The perikarya of the pain-conducting pseudounipolar neurons in the *cranial part* of the parasympathetic nervous system are located in the inferior or superior ganglia of the vagus nerves. Those of the *sacral part* of the parasympathetic system are located in spinal ganglia of sacral spinal cord levels S2–S4. Their fibers run parallel to the efferent vagal, or spinal, fibers and establish a central connection with the pain-processing systems.

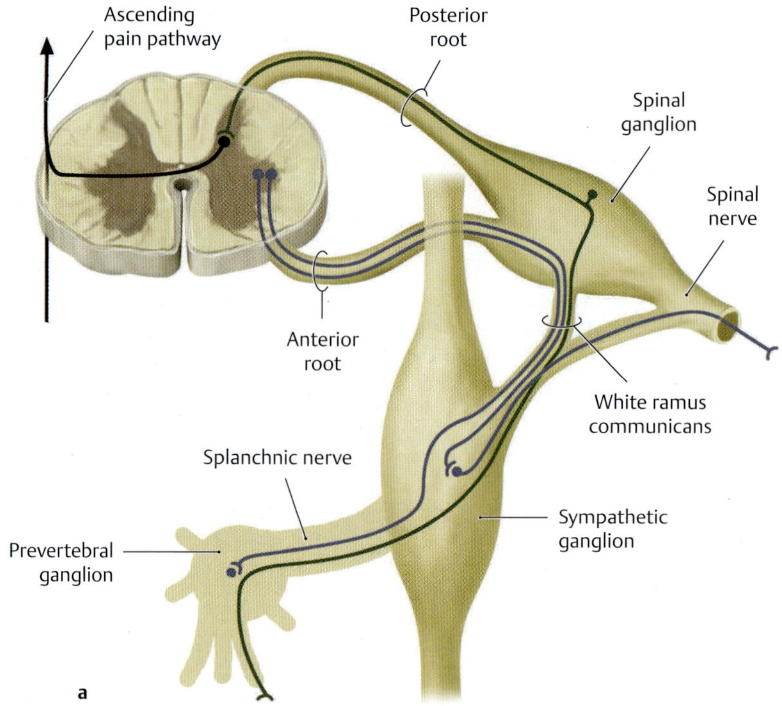

a

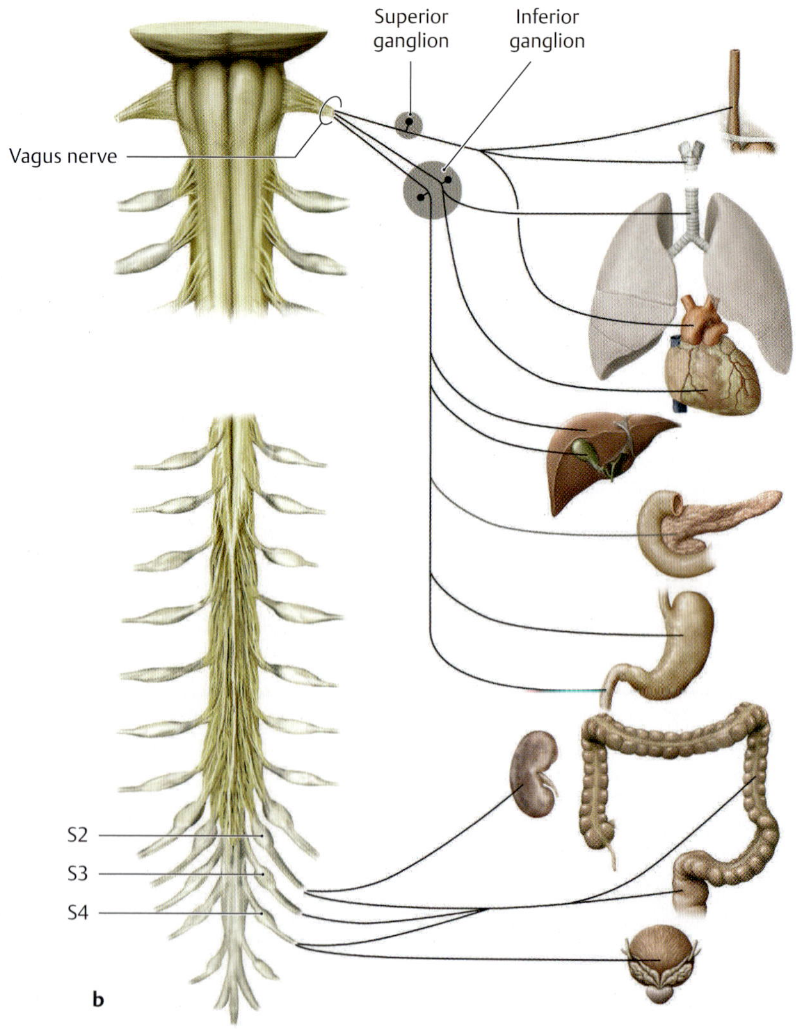

b

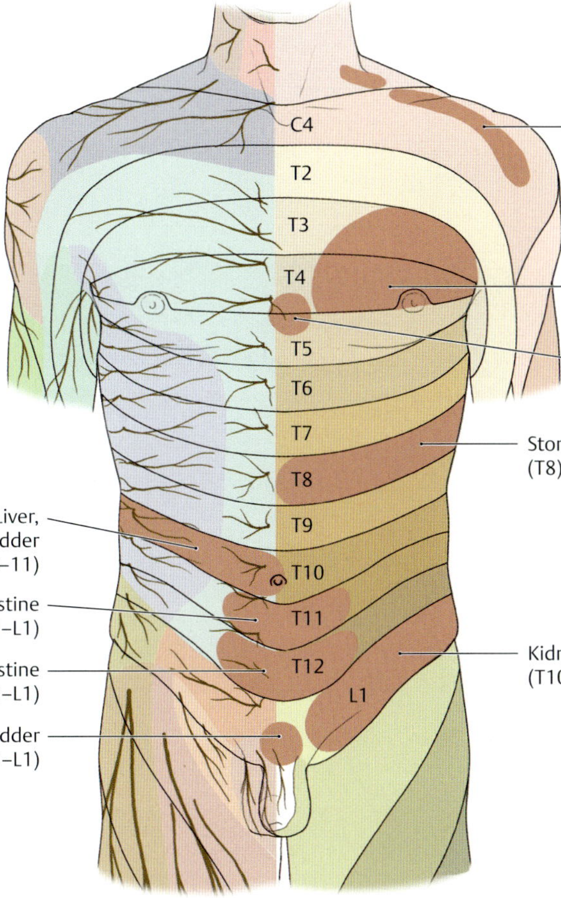

B Referred pain

Pain afferents from the viscera (visceral pain) and dermatomes (somatic pain) terminate at the same pain processing neurons in the posterior horn of the spinal cord. The convergence of visceral and somatic afferent fibers confuses the relationship between the pain's origin and its perception. Thus, the cortex may register pain impulses from the stomach as coming from the abdominal wall. This phenomenon is known as referred pain. The pain impulses from a particular internal organ are consistently projected to the same well-defined skin area (see dermatome levels on figure). Thus, the area of skin that the pain is projected to provides crucial information regarding what organ is affected. The skin areas to which a particular internal organ projects its pain are referred to as Head-zones, named after their discoverer, the English neurologist Sir Henry Head. This model considers only the peripheral processing of impulses, which the cortex perceives as pain. It is not clear why somatic pain is not perceived as visceral pain.

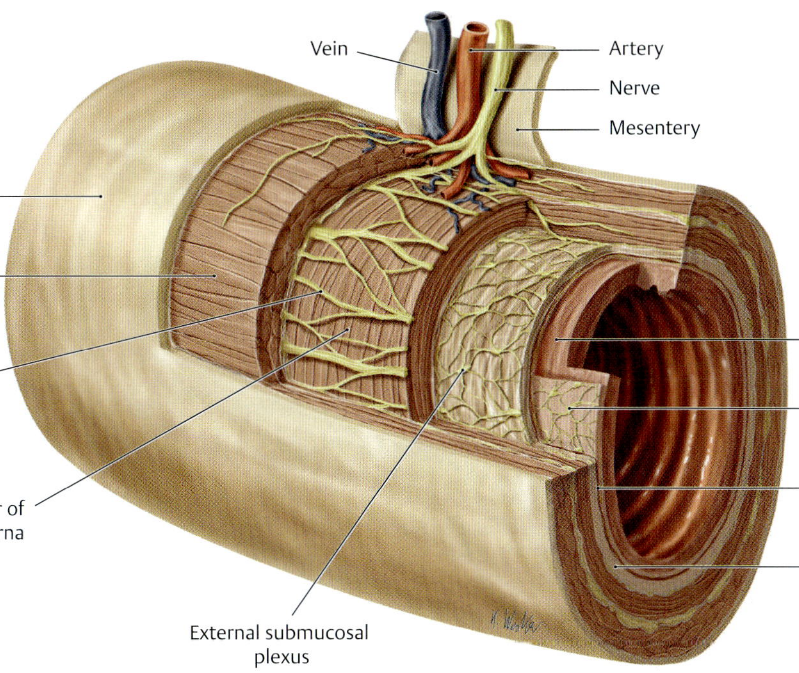

C The enteric nervous system in the small intestine

The enteric nervous system is considered a third and independent part of the autonomic nervous system ("The gut as a small brain"), and thus it is discussed separately after the sympathetic and parasympathetic nervous systems. The enteric nervous system consists of small groups of neurons that form interconnected, microscopically visible ganglia in the wall of the gut tube. The enteric system is organized into two plexuses: the *myenteric plexus* (Auerbach's), located between the longitudinal and circular muscle layers of the muscularis externa, and the *submucosal plexus* (in the submucosa), which is subdivided into an external plexus (Schabadasch's) and an internal plexus (Meissner's). (For more details on the structure of the enteric nervous system see histology textbooks.) These networks of neurons form the basis for autonomic reflex pathways. In principle, they can function without external innervation but their activity is greatly influenced by the sympathetic and parasympathetic nervous systems. Activities regulated by the enteric nervous system include gastrointestinal motility, secretions into the gut tube and local blood flow.

10.3 Paraganglia

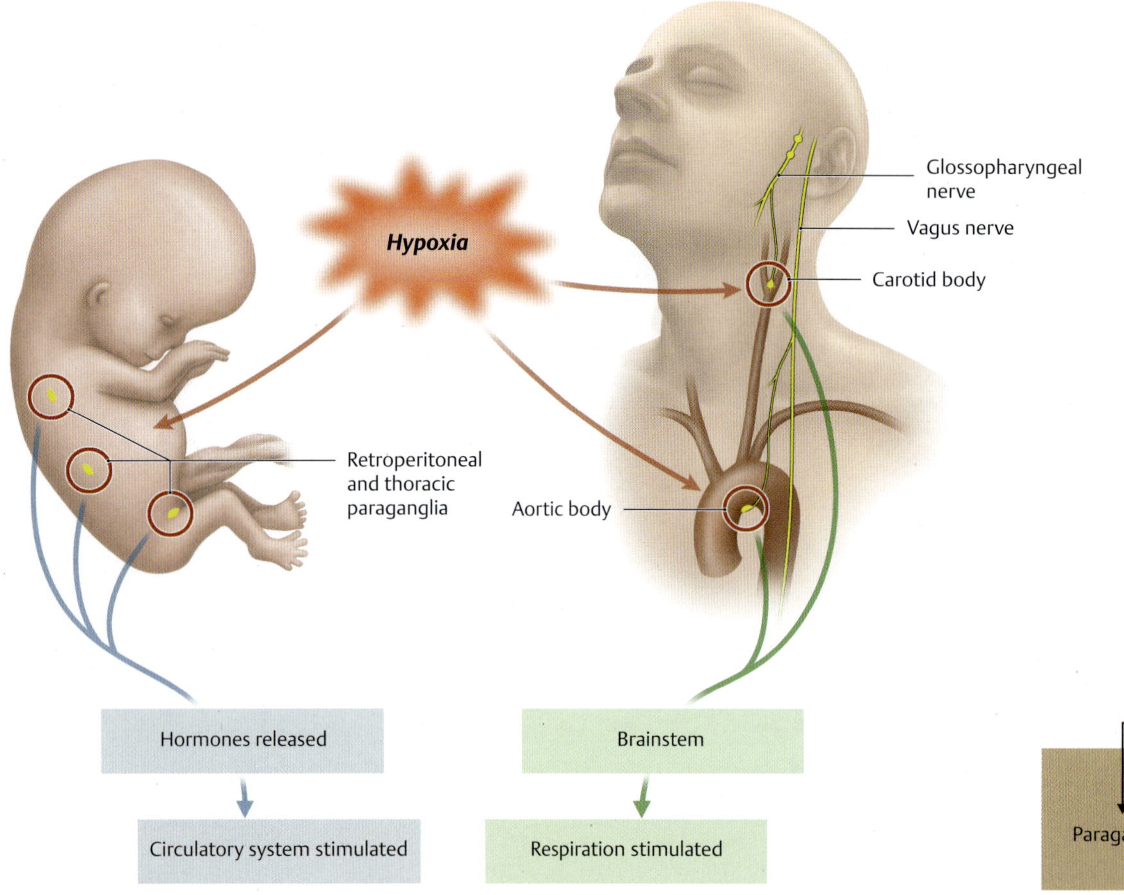

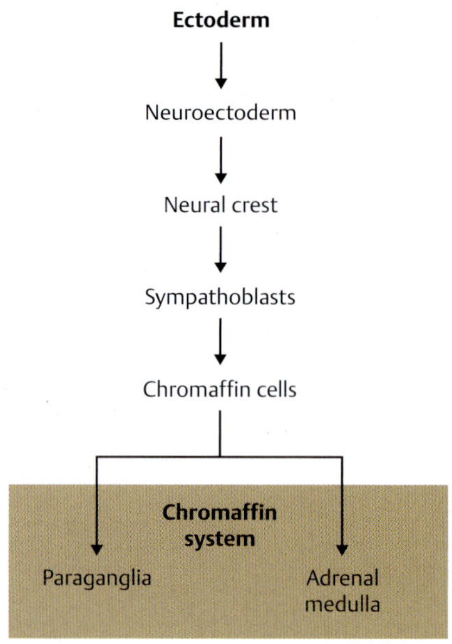

A Definition, function, and classification of paraganglia

Ganglia are aggregations of nerve cell bodies in the peripheral nervous system. Paraganglia are aggregations of specialized neurons in the peripheral nervous system which in part have an endocrine function. As such they are between the nervous system and the hormone system. Measuring only a few millimeters in size, the paraganglia act as an "early warning and control system" for lack of oxygen in arterial blood (hypoxia). They continuously measure the intra-arterial partial pressure of O_2 and CO_2 as well as the pH value. Thus they act as *chemosensors*. In the fetus, paraganglia respond to hypoxia by releasing hormones that increase circulatory activity. In the fully developed body after birth, certain paraganglia respond to hypoxia by transmitting a signal to the brainstem via nerves. The brainstem reflexively increases respiration, improving the supply of oxygen. This means that paraganglia are of paramount importance for regulating the supply of oxygen in the body. Two types are differentiated according to their location in the body:

- *Retroperitoneal ganglia*: In the embryo and small child they are found in large numbers in the thorax and in the *retroperitoneal* space of the abdomen next to (= *para*) the ganglia of the sympathetic trunk. Such ganglia are also found in the genital region. Their number decreases markedly in the adult. In the fetal period and at birth, they respond to hypoxia by secreting the hormone norepinephrine, which increases the unborn child's blood pressure and pulse rate. Their functional significance in adults is the subject of discussion. A comparatively large group of paraganglia ususally located at the level of the origin of the inferior mesenteric artery where it arises from the abdominal aorta are known as the *organs of Zuckerkandl*.
- *Glomus bodies* (especially the *carotid body* and the *aortic body; glomus = ball*): These extravascular structures lie at the bifurcation of the common carotid artery (*carotid body*; at the level of the C4 vertebra, one on each side) and at the aortic arch (usually multiple *aortic bodies* are present). Functionally, they are directly associated with the ninth cranial nerve (*glossopharyngeal nerve; carotid body*) and the tenth cranial nerve (*vagus nerve; aortic bodies*) through which their signal reaches the brainstem. The hypoxia signal of the glomus bodies leads to increased respiratory activity. In unborn fetuses, which do not yet have independent respiration, they have no functional significance.
- A *jugular body* lying near the base of the skull along the internal jugular vein is occasionally observed. Little is known about its function. It is not shown here.

B Origin of the paraganglia

Paraganglia arise from the neural crest and thus from the neuroectoderm. They share a key histologic characteristic with the adrenal medulla, which also arises from the neural crest: so-called "chromaffin cells" (see **C**). *Chromaffin cells* contain granules (*chromaffin granules*) in which catecholamines (adrenaline, norepinephrine, dopamine) are stored as hormones or neurotransmitters. If one histologically fixes such cells with chromic salts, the granules (and thus indirectly the cells) stain grayish brown. The histophysiologic term *chromaffin cell* is a synonym for *catecholamine-synthesizing cell*. As both the adrenal medulla and the paraganglia synthesize catecholamines and their cells contain chromaffin granules, both of them are histologically classified as belonging to the *chromaffin system*. Chromaffin cells arise in the embryo from a special neuroectodermal cell, the *sympathoblast*. Because of their embryonal relationship and their common histochemical characteristics, the adrenal medulla is generally understood to be a special form of paraganglia, although the literature is not consistent in this regard.

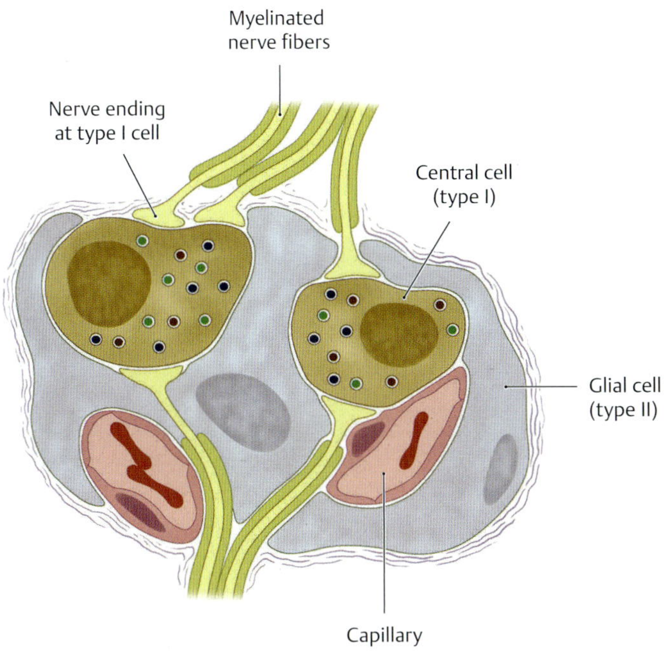

C Structure of the paraganglia
Schematic diagram of a glomus body. Paraganglia contain at least two types of cells:

- *Central cells* = type I cells (brown): They store catecholamines (especially dopamine), serotonin, and enkephalins in small granules and secrete the *neurotransmitter* dopamine. Functionally, they are the true chemosensors and morphologically they are the *chromaffin* cells. As secondary sensory cells, they have no axons but directly contact the afferent fibers of the glossopharyngeal or vagus nerves.
- *Glial cells* = type II cell (blue): They envelop the type I cells and are regarded as part of the peripheral glia. They are not chemosensitive but are thought to aid in signal transmission from the central cell to the nerve cell.

Glomus bodies contain numerous sensory nerve endings (yellow) of the glossopharyngeal and vagus nerves and are connected via the *inferior ganglion of the glossopharyngeal nerve (carotid body)* or the *vagus nerve (aortic body)* to the *nucleus of the solitary tract* which in turn projects onto neurons of the respiratory center of the medulla oblongata (see **D**). Glomus bodies are highly vascularized with a *fenestrated* epithelium. Their relative perfusion is 25 times as high as that of the brain. This extreme perfusion ensures that representative quantities of blood can continuously be evaluated for their O_2 and CO_2 content.

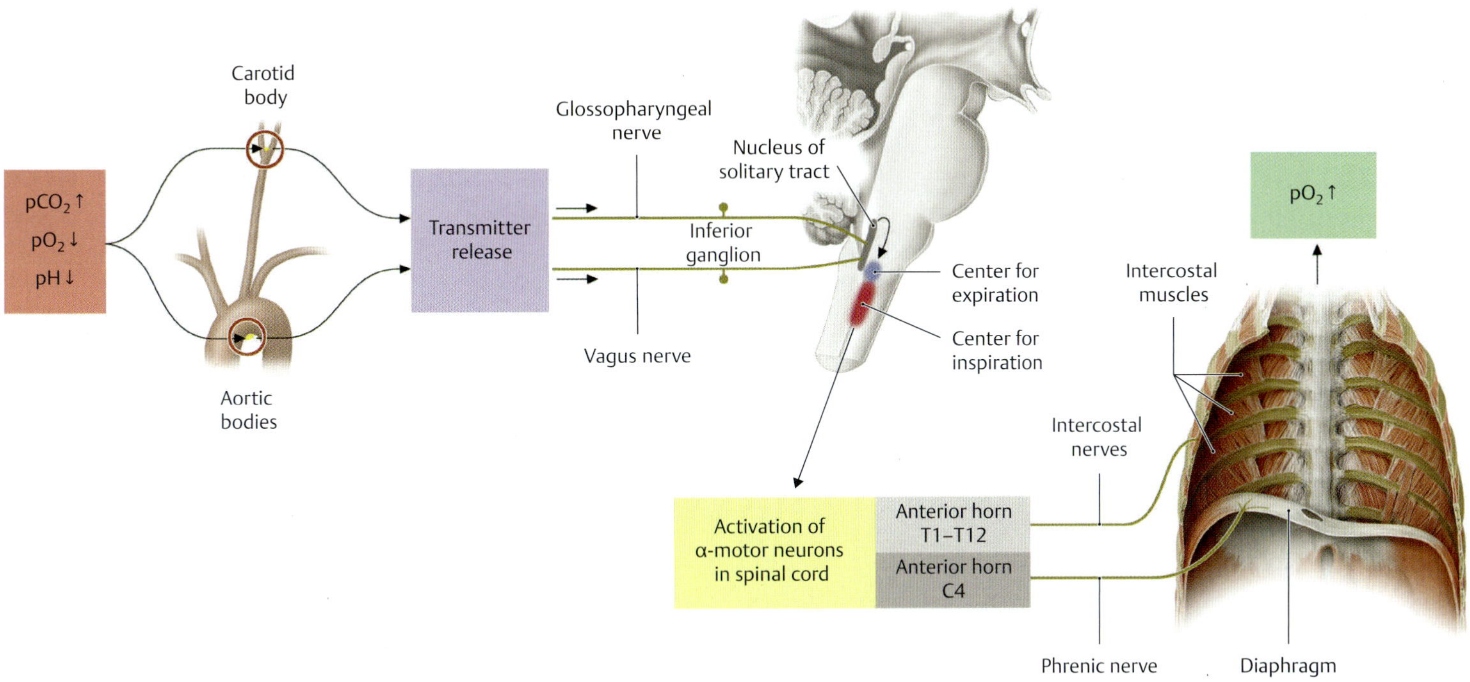

D Functional synopsis of the glomus bodies
Type I cells detect a drop in intra-arterial O_2 partial pressure (actual value is below target value), a drop in the pH value, or an increase in intra-arterial CO_2 partial pressure. They then release the neurotransmitter *dopamine* from their granules. Afferent fibers of the glossopharyngeal nerve (carotid body) or the vagus nerve (aortic bodies) project via the inferior ganglion of the respective cranial nerves to the nucleus of the solitary tract which in turn activates respiratory centers in the medulla oblongata. These act on α-motor neurons in the spinal cord. The respiratory musculature is activated via the phrenic nerves. The increased respiratory activity then leads to an increase in O_2 partial pressure and a decrease in CO_2 partial pressure.

Retroperitoneal paraganglia in the embryo stimulate the circulatory system because it is not possible to increase respiration in an embryo (see **A**). Little is known about the function of the retroperitoneal paraganglia in the fully developed body.
Clinical note: Similar to the adrenal medulla, tumors can also arise from the paraganglia (*pheochromocytomas* or *paragangliomas*). Their spontaneous release of catecholamines can lead to episodic blood pressure crises. The clinical course of such tumors in children is usually unfavorable.
It is also thought that spontaneously occurring "incorrect readings" of the oxygen content of the blood reported by the glomus bodies can lead to a sensation of asphyxiation and panic attacks.

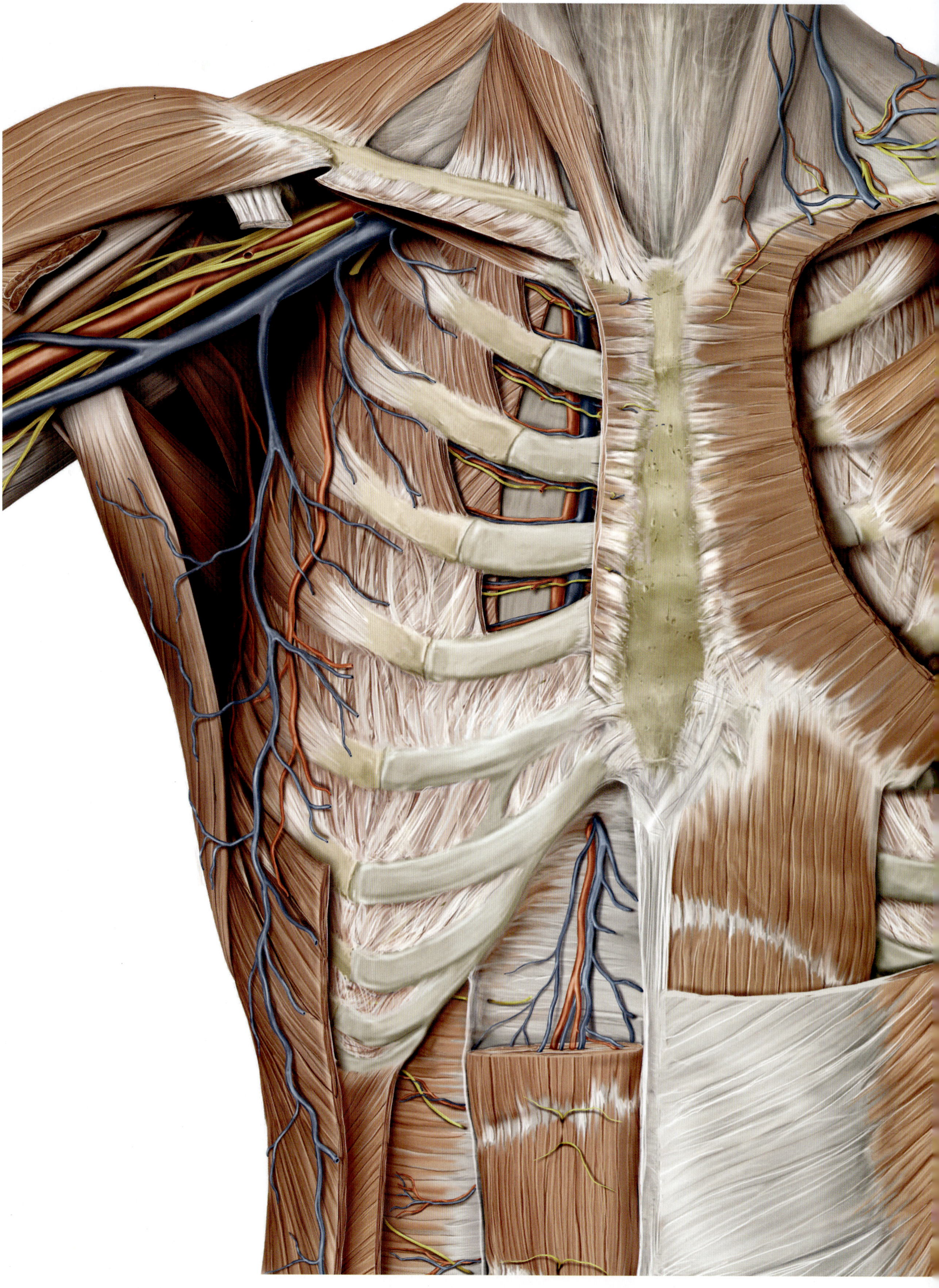

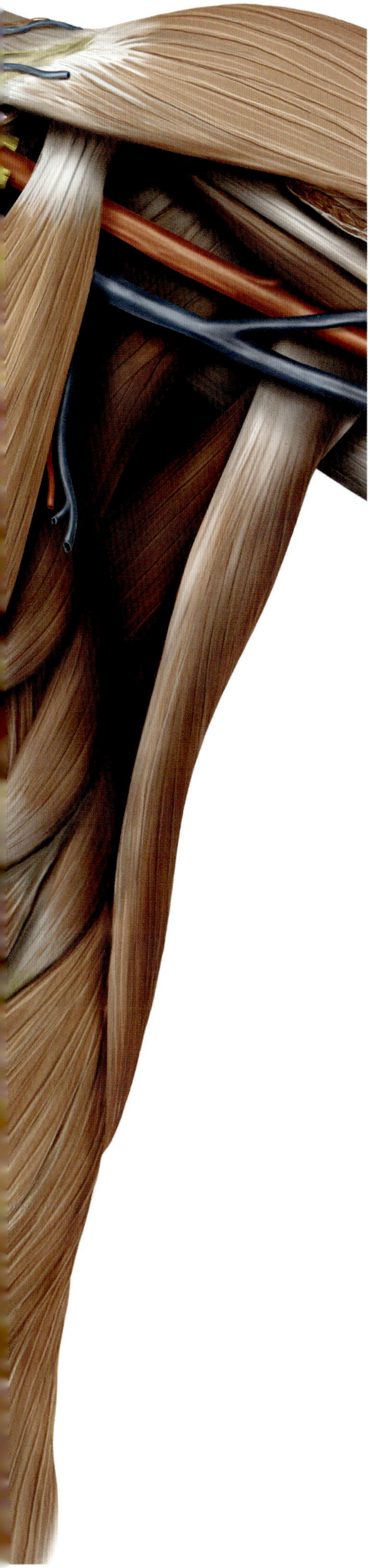

B Thorax

1.1 Divisions of the Thoracic Cavity and Mediastinum

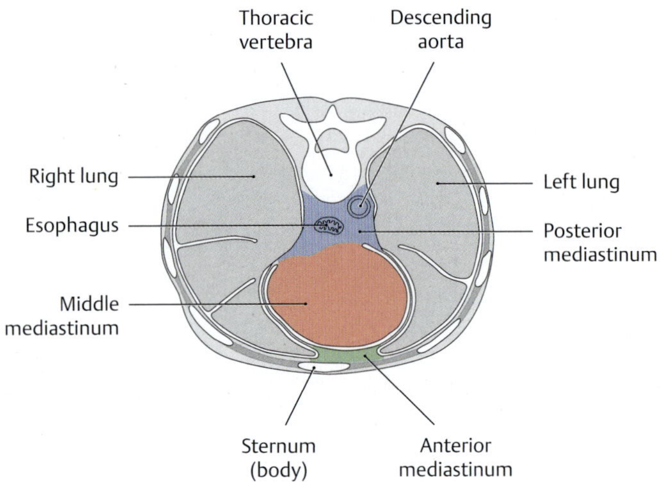

A Divisions of the thoracic cavity and mediastinum
Transverse section, superior view.
The thoracic cavity is divided into three large spaces:

- The **mediastinum**, in the midline, is divided into an upper, smaller *superior mediastinum* and a lower, larger *inferior mediastinum* (see **B**). The inferior mediastinum is further subdivided, from front to back, into the *anterior*, *middle*, and *posterior mediastinum*. The anterior mediastinum is an extremely narrow space between the sternum and pericardium, containing only small vascular components (see table, **C**).
- The **paired pleural cavities** on the left and right sides of the mediastinum are lined by serosa (parietal pleura) and contain the left and right lungs. They are completely separated from each other by the mediastinum. The mediastinum extends further to the left than to the right owing to the asymmetrical position of the heart and pericardium. Because of this, the pleural cavity (and lung) is smaller on the left side than on the right. The pleural cavities terminate blindly at their upper end, but the mediastinum is continuous with the connective tissue of the neck.

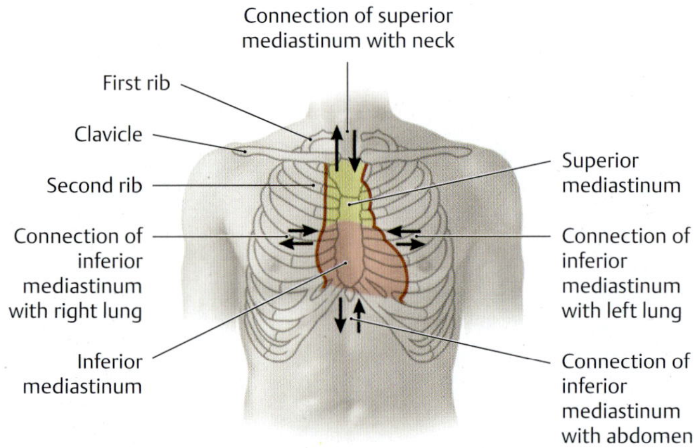

B Principal neurovascular structures that enter and leave the mediastinum
Superior mediastinum (borders the neck, yellow):

- The vagus and phrenic nerves, veins (tributaries of the superior vena cava), esophagus, and trachea enter the superior mediastinum from the neck.
- Arterial branches from the aortic arch and the cervical part of the sympathetic trunk leave the superior mediastinum to enter the neck.

Inferior mediastinum (borders the abdomen and pleural cavities, red):

- The thoracic duct and ascending abdominal lumbar veins (the azygos vein on the right side, the hemiazygos vein on the left side) pass through the diaphragm to enter the inferior mediastinum.
- The vagus and phrenic nerves, portions of the sympathetic nervous system, the aorta, and the esophagus descend from the inferior mediastinum and pass through the diaphragm to enter the abdomen.

Pulmonary arteries and veins, lymphatic vessels, autonomic nerves (pulmonary plexus), and the main bronchi connect the mediastinum to the lungs (and vice versa).

C Contents of the mediastinum (for divisions see **A**)

	Superior mediastinum	Inferior mediastinum		
		Anterior mediastinum	*Middle mediastinum*	*Posterior mediastinum*
Organs	• Thymus • Trachea • Esophagus	• Thymus (in children)	• Heart • Pericardium	• Esophagus
Arteries	• Aortic arch • Brachiocephalic trunk • Left common carotid artery • Left subclavian artery	• Smaller arteries	• Ascending aorta • Pulmonary trunk and its branches • Pericardiacophrenic arteries	• Thoracic aorta and its branches
Veins and lymphatic vessels	• Superior vena cava • Brachiocephalic veins • Accessory hemiazygos vein • Thoracic duct	• Smaller veins and lymphatic vessels • Smaller lymph nodes	• Inferior vena cava • Azygos vein • Pulmonary veins • Pericardiacophrenic veins	• Azygos vein • Hemiazygos vein • Thoracic duct
Nerves	• Vagus nerves • Left recurrent laryngeal nerve • Cardiac nerves • Phrenic nerves	–	• Phrenic nerves	• Vagus nerves • Sympathetic trunk

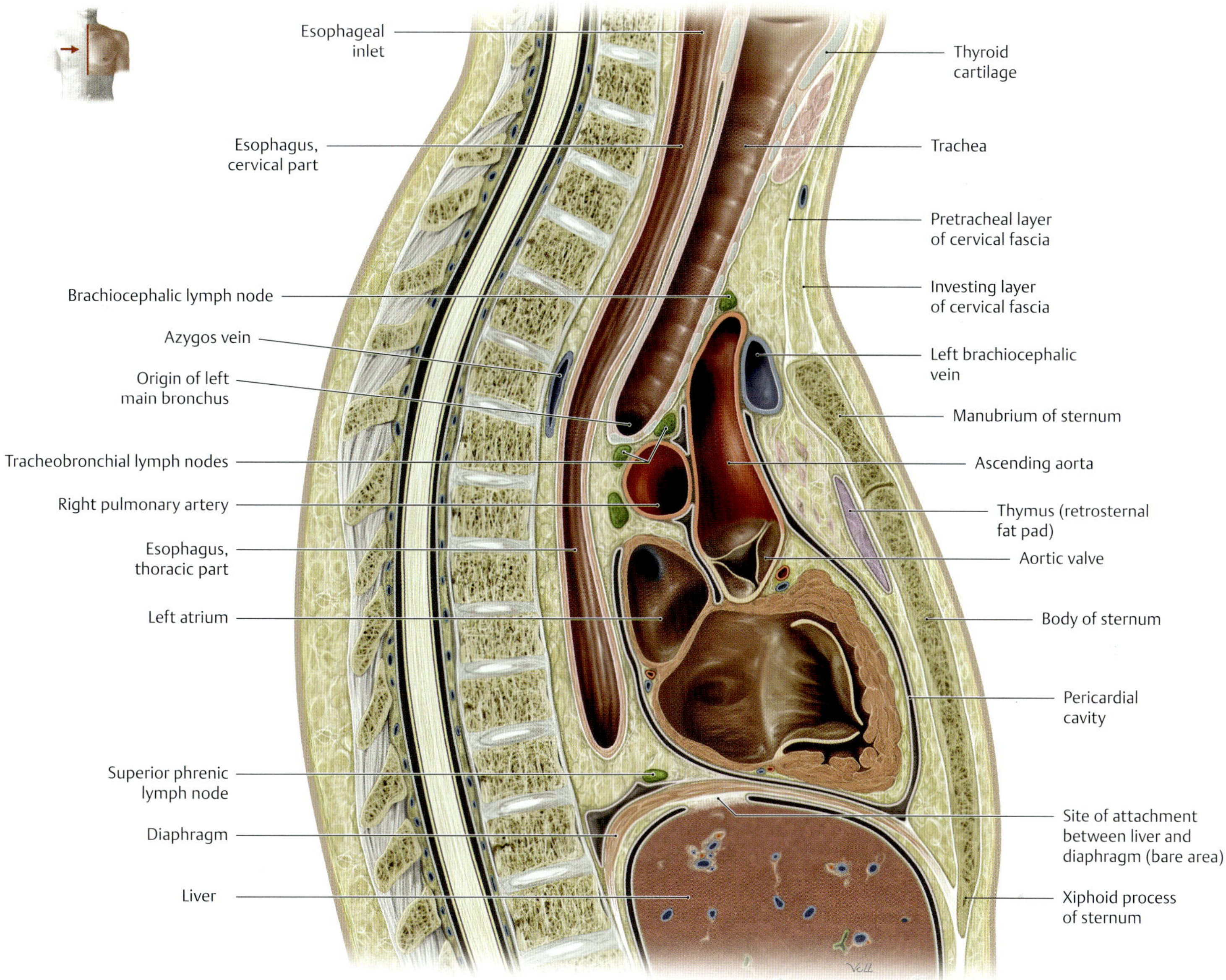

a

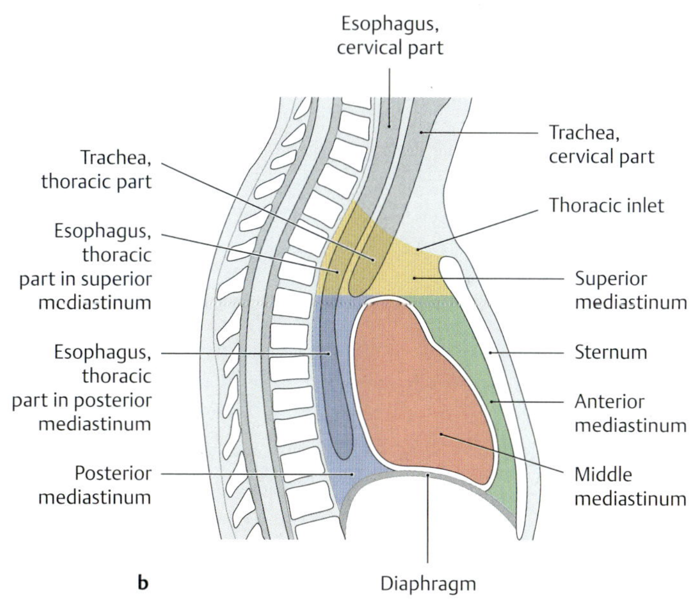

b

D Subdivisions of the mediastinum
Midsagittal sections viewed from the right side.

- **a Detailed view:** simplified drawing of the pericardium, heart, trachea, and esophagus in midsagittal section. This lateral view demonstrates how the left atrium of the heart narrows the posterior mediastinum and abuts the anterior wall of the esophagus. Because of this proximity, abnormal enlargement of the left atrium may cause narrowing of the esophageal lumen that is detectable by radiographic examination with oral contrast medium. Radiologists call the area between the images of the heart and vertebral column the *retrocardiac space*.
- **b Schematic view:** subdivisions of the mediastinum (described in **A**, with contents listed in **C**).

Note: Single diagrams cannot adequately show the components and configuration of the mediastinum, because of its asymmetry and extensions in all three axes. The anatomical relations in this space are best appreciated when viewed from multiple directions, at different planes (see p. 192ff).

1.2 Diaphragm: Location and Projection onto the Trunk

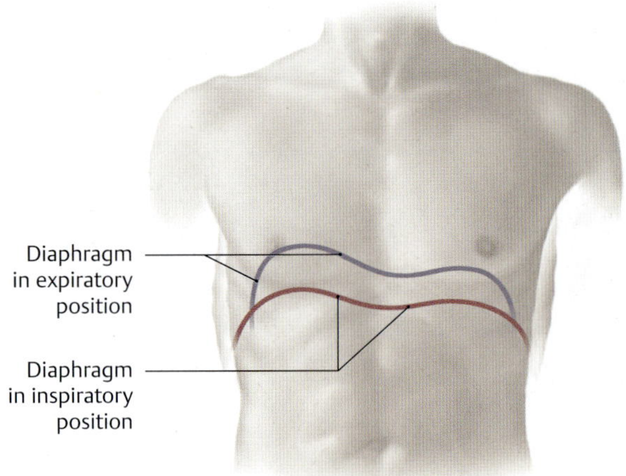

A Projection of the diaphragm onto the trunk
Anterior view. The positions of the diaphragm in expiration (blue) and inspiration (red) are shown. The right hemidiaphragm rises as high as the fourth rib during expiration, and the diaphragm may fall almost to the level of the seventh rib at full inspiration.
Note:

- The exact position of the diaphragm depends on body type, sex, and age.
- The left diaphragm leaflet is lower than the right due to the asymmetrical position of the heart.
- Inspiration is marked by an overall depression of the diaphragm and also by a flattening of the diaphragm leaflets.
- The diaphragm is higher in the supine position (pressure from the intra-abdominal organs) than in the standing position.
- The degree of diaphragmatic movement during inspiration can be assessed by noting the movement of the hepatic border, which is easily palpated.
- The diaphragm in a cadaver occupies a higher level than the expiratory position in vivo due to the loss of muscular tone.

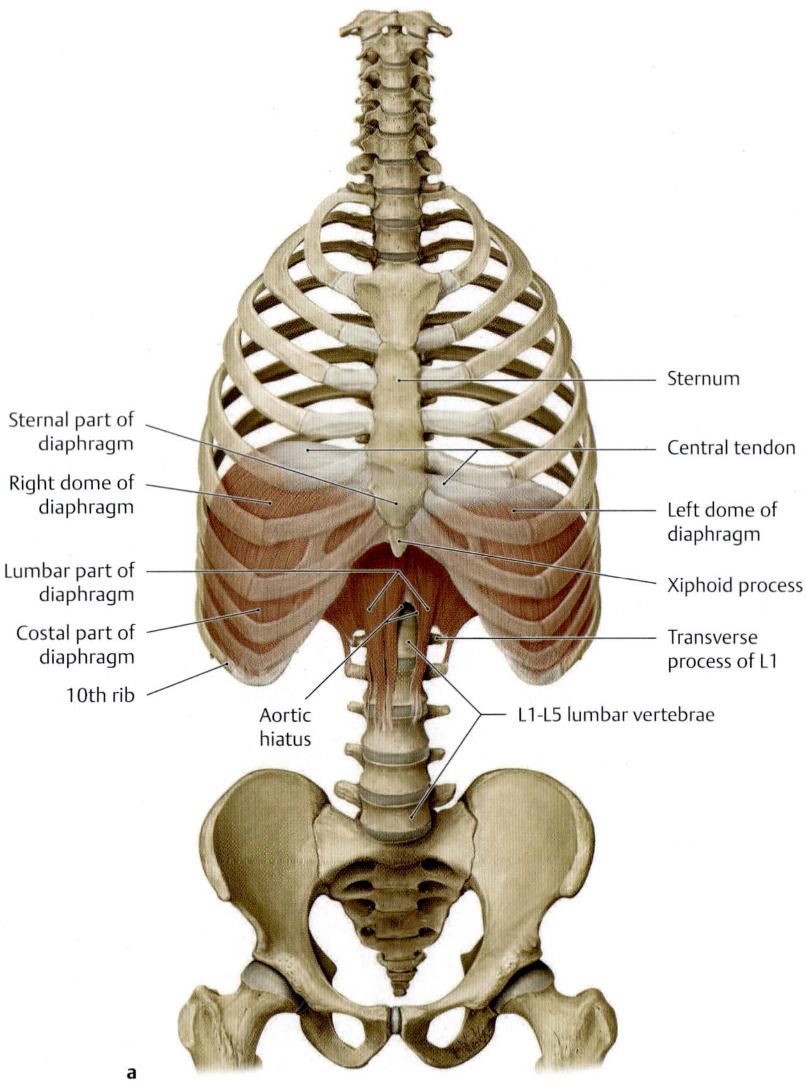

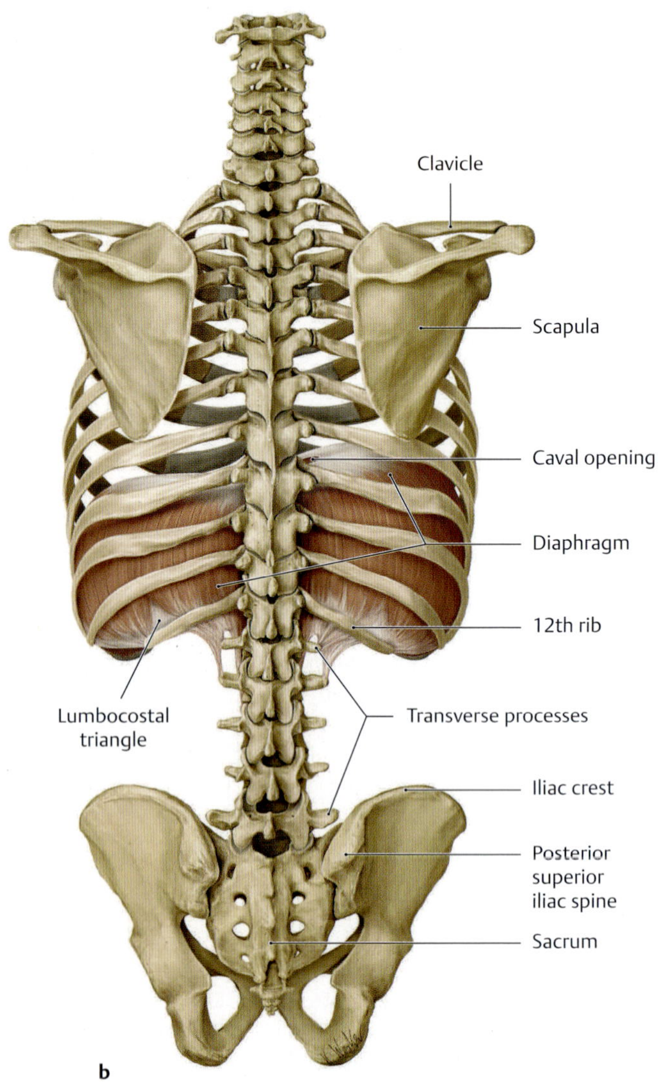

B Anterior (a) and posterior (b) views of the diaphragm
In **a**, the *anterior* rib segments in front of the diaphragm are shown transparent to demonstrate the location of the diaphragm; in **b** the *posterior* rib segments are not shown transparent.

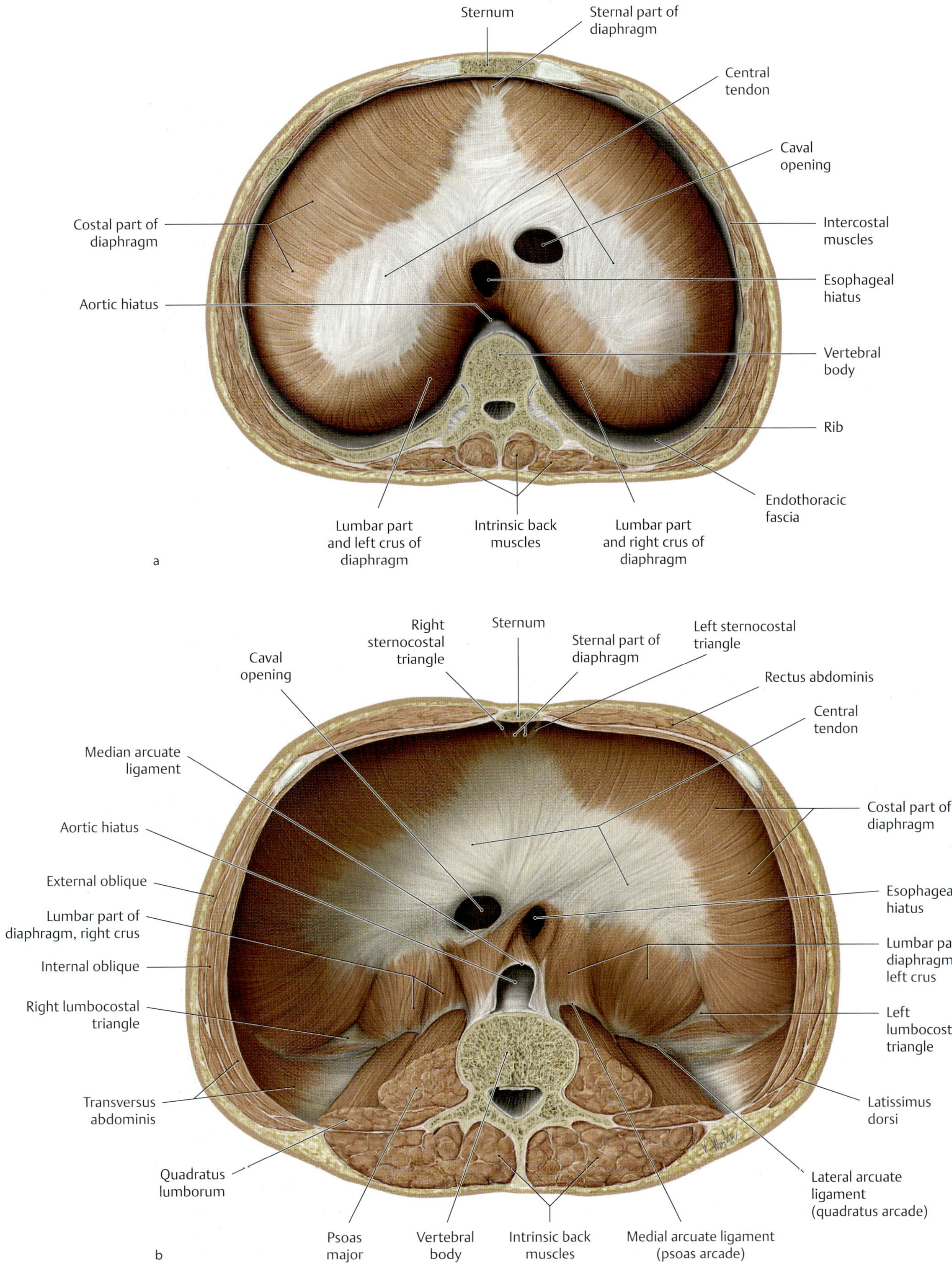

C Superior (a) and inferior (b) views of the diaphragm

Fascias and serous membranes lining the superior and inferior surfaces of the diaphragm have been removed.

The muscular diaphragm closes the inferior thoracic aperture. It completely separates the thoracic and abdominal cavities and has three openings for the esophagus, aorta, and inferior vena cava.

Both the sternocostal trigone (left, "Larrey's cleft"; right, "Morgagni's cleft") and the lumbocostal trigone (both sides also referred to as "Bochdalek's triangle") represent places of lower mechanical resistance as connective tissue-filled muscle gaps in the diaphragm (*locus minoris resistantiae*, the place of least resistance). In these places, hernias can form from the abdomen into the thoracic cavity. Hernias are often referred to by proper names based on their anatomical location (e.g. "Bochdalek hernia").

1.3 Diaphragm: Structure and Main Openings

A Shape and structure of the diaphragm
a Inferior view; **b** Frontal section of the diaphragm, anterior view; **c** Midsagittal section with diaphragm in intermediate position.
The diaphragm is divided into three parts, here color coded for clarity: the costal, lumbar, and sternal parts. For details about the origin of these three parts see **C**. For details about the location of the openings in the diaphragm see next page. Sections (**b** and **c**) show the location of the diaphragm between the thoracic and abdominal cavities and illustrate the diaphragm's distinct dome-shaped structure: Recesses along the sides (**b**) and anterior and posterior margins (**c**) of the diaphragm vary in depth (Recesses, see p. 143 and 185). Flattening of the diaphragmatic domes and recesses play a central role in respiratory mechanics.

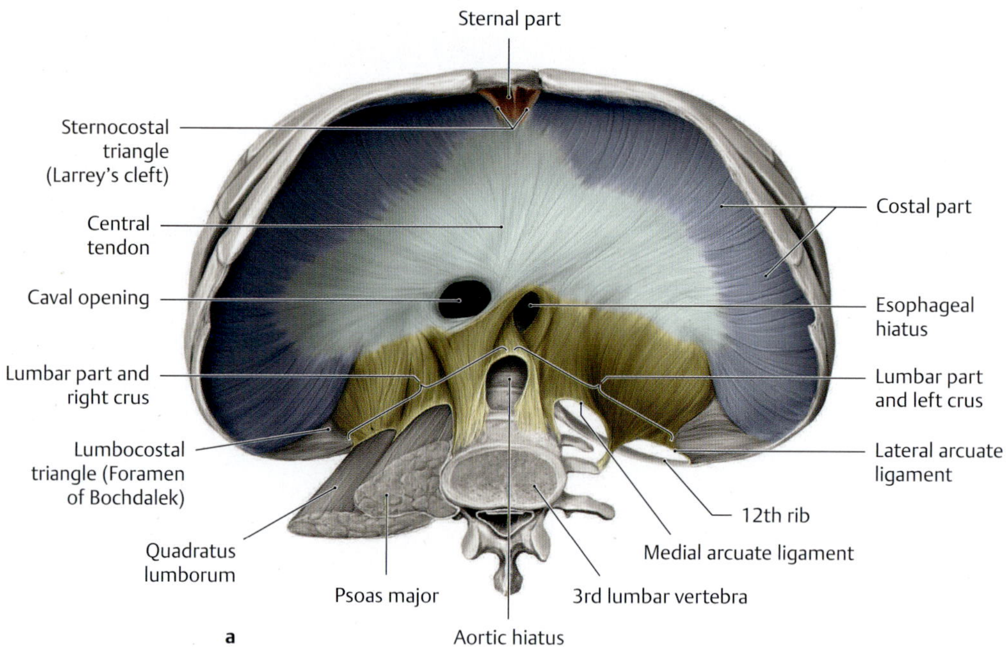

a

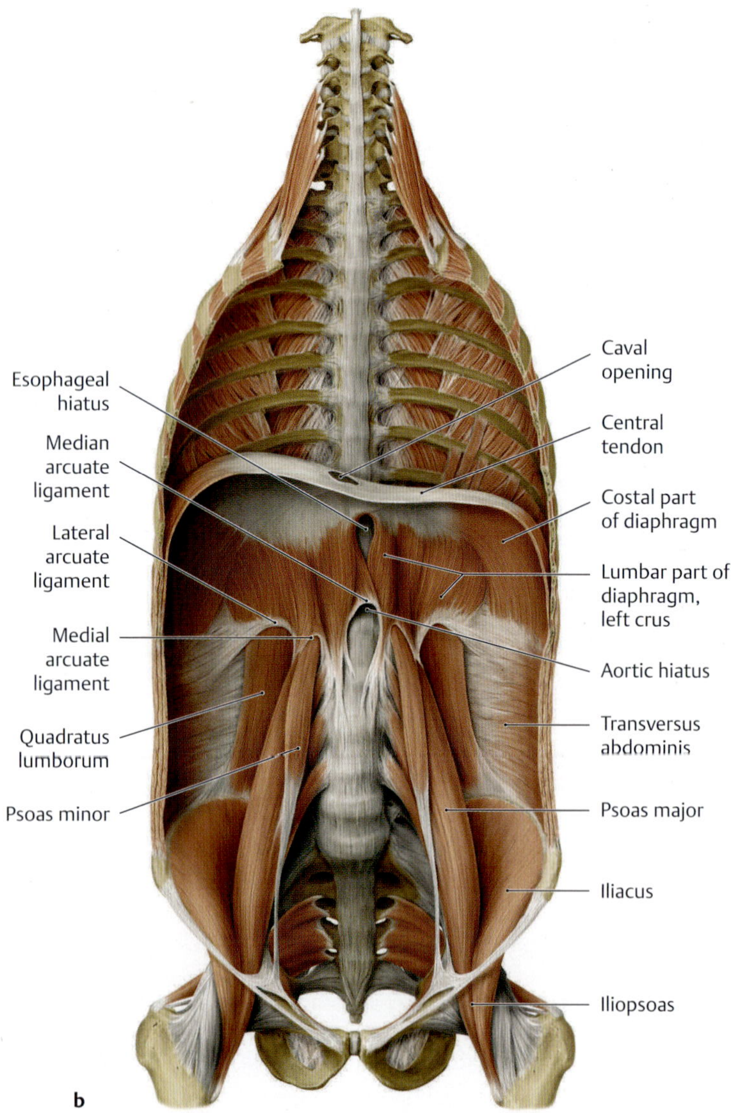

b

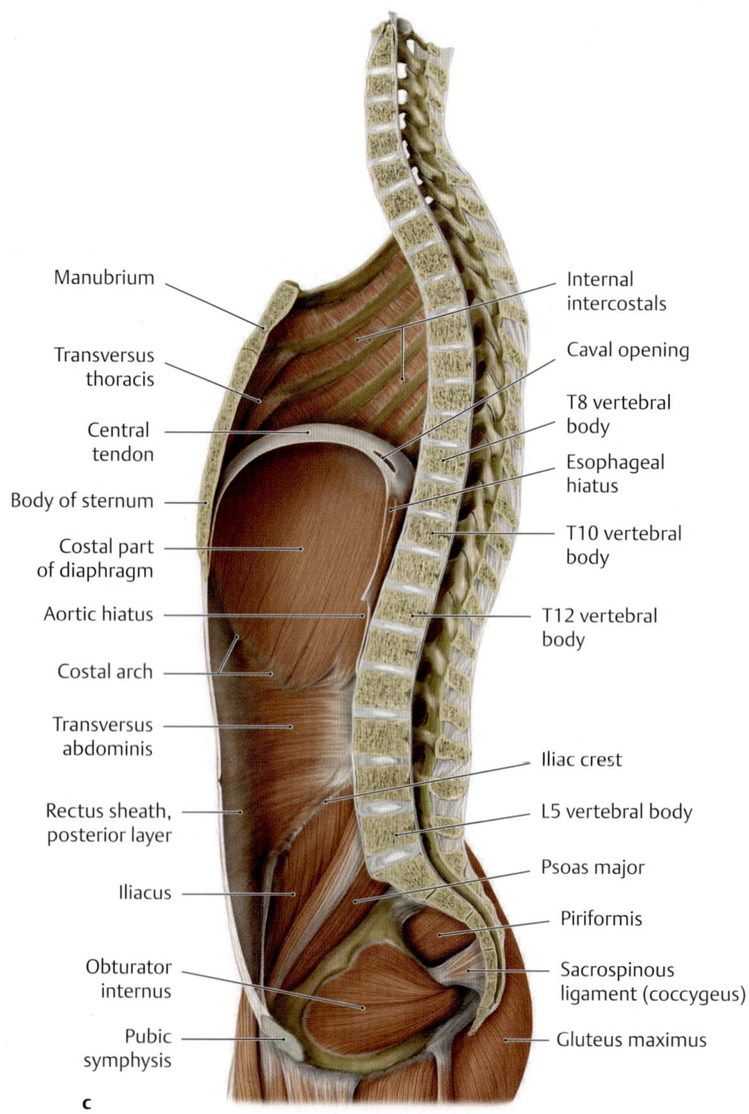

c

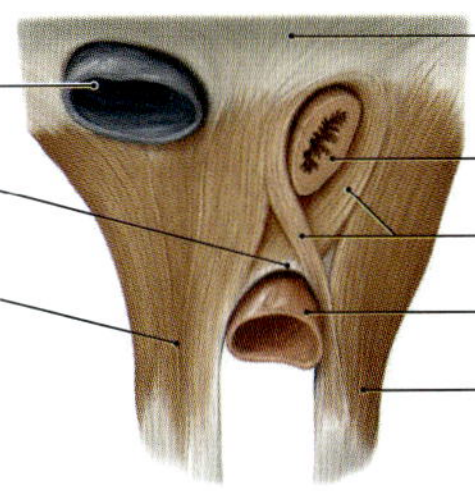

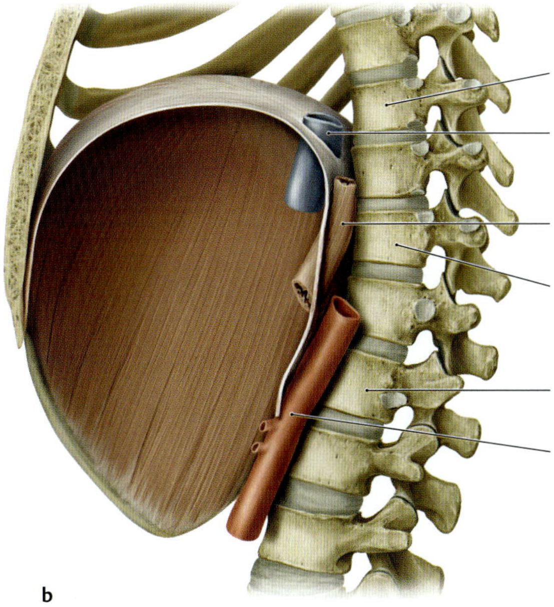

B Openings and gaps in the diaphragm and their clinical significance

a Anterior view of lumbar part and portion of the central tendon; location of the openings; **b** opened thorax viewed from the left side with diaphragm in resting expiratory position; projection of the openings onto the inferior thoracic spine: caval opening at T8, esophageal hiatus at T10, and aortic hiatus at T12.

Openings and gaps in the diaphragm develop

- because the esophagus and large neurovascular structures pass through the muscle tissue and tendinous center of the diaphragm (central tendon) and extend from the thorax to abdomen or vice versa (*functional openings*, see above) and
- because gaps between the different parts of the diaphragm are closed only by connective tissue (e.g., apertures in the medial crus that allow passage of neurovascular structures [splanchnic nerves; ascending lumbar veins]).

The larger ones of these physiological gaps are weak spots through which abdominal organs can herniate into the thorax (diaphragmatic hernia, see **D**).

C Overview of the diaphragm

Origin:	• Costal part: inferior border of the ribs (inner surface of ribs 7 through 12) • Lumbar part (including right and left crura): – medial part: L1–L3 vertebral bodies and intervertebral disks, anterior longitudinal ligament – lateral parts: medial arcuate ligament (from L2 vertebral body to the respective transverse process); lateral arcuate ligament (from the transverse process of L2 to the tip of the 12th rib) • Sternal part: posterior surface of the xiphoid process
Insertion:	Central tendon
Function:	Principal muscle of inspiration (diaphragmatic or abdominal breathing); involved in regulating abdominal pressure
Innervation:	Phrenic nerve from the cervical plexus (C3–5)

D Openings in the diaphragm and transmitted structures

Openings	Transmitted structures
Caval opening (at the level of the T8 vertebra)	Inferior vena cava Phrenicoabdominal branch of right phrenic nerve (the left phrenicoabdominal branch pierces the muscle)
Esophageal hiatus (at the level of the T10 vertebra)	Esophagus Anterior and posterior vagal trunks (on the esophagus)
Aortic hiatus (at the level of the T12/L1 vertebrae)	Descending aorta Thoracic duct
Openings	**Transmitted structures**
Apertures in the medial crus	Azygos vein, hemiazygos vein, greater and lesser splanchnic nerves
Apertures between the medial and lateral crura	Sympathetic trunk, lesser splanchnic nerve (common variant)
Sternocostal triangle	Internal thoracic artery and vein, superior epigastric artery and vein

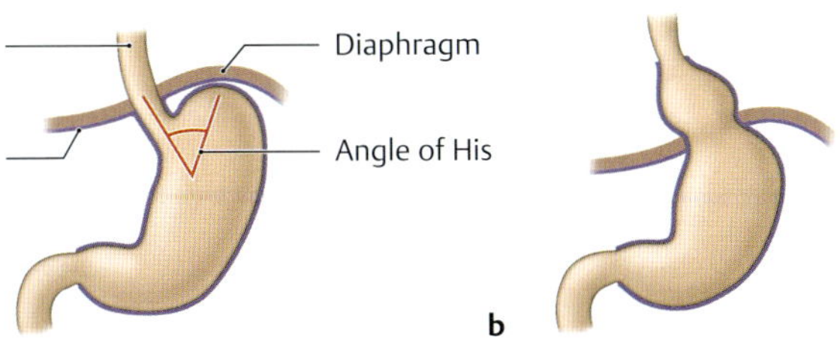

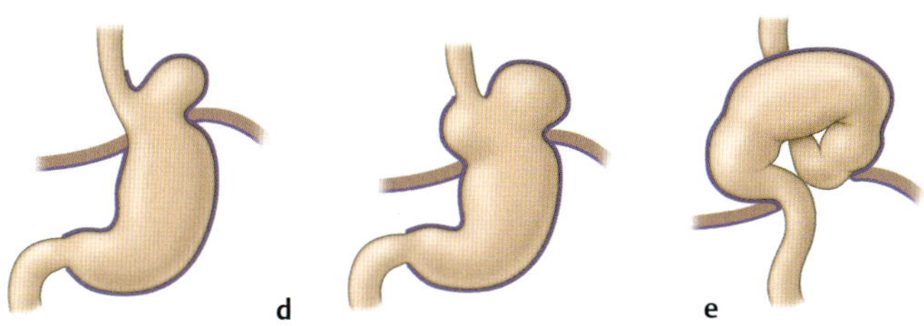

E Hiatal hernias

a Normal findings; **b** axial hiatal hernia; **c** paraesophageal hernia; **d** mixed hernia (partial displacement of the stomach into the thorax); **e** upside down stomach (displacement of the stomach into the thorax).

The most common site of herniation of abdominal organs into the thoracic cavity is the esophageal hiatus (hiatal hernia, 90% of all cases). Usually the end of the esophagus and the cardia (entrance) of the stomach slide through the esophageal hiatus into the thorax (axial hernia or sliding hernia, approximately 85% of all hiatal hernias). Typical complaints range from heartburn, belching, and pressure behind the sternum to nausea, vomiting, shortness of breath, and functional heart problems.

1.4 Diaphragm: Innervation, Blood, and Lymphatic Vessels

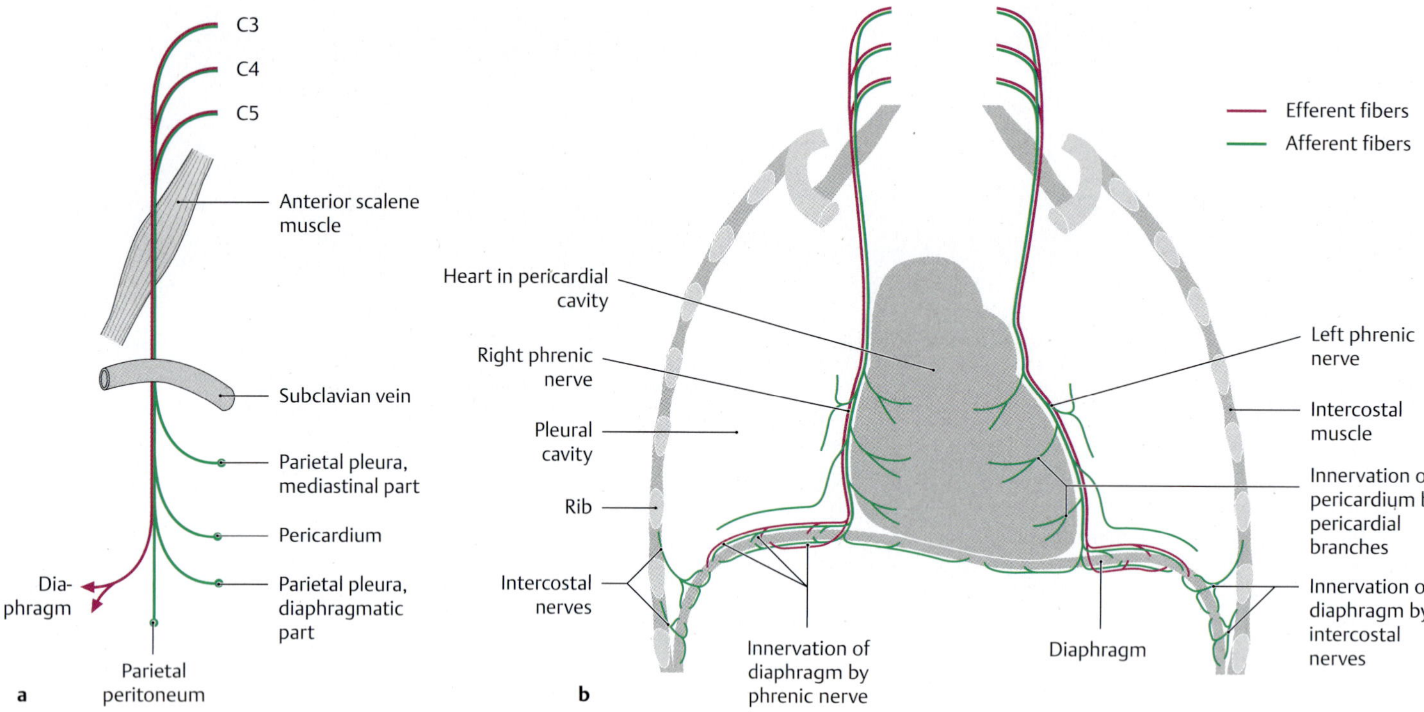

A Innervation

The diaphragm is largely innervated by the phrenic nerve, a somatomotor and somatosensory nerve that arises from the cervical plexus, specifically cervical spinal cord segments C3–C5 (mainly C4, see **a**). The phrenic nerve descends while giving off branches to the mediastinal pleura and the pericardium (pericardial branches, see **b**). It contains more efferent (motor) than afferent (sensory) fibers; the latter being responsible for pain conduction from the serous membranes (diaphragmatic pleura and parietal peritoneum) that cover the diaphragm. A phrenicoabdominal branch passes through the diaphragm to the peritoneum on its inferior surface. The serous membranes covering the diaphragm near the ribs also receive somatosensory innervation from the tenth and eleventh intercostal nerves (see **b**) and from the subcostal nerve (T12, not shown). Occasionally, an accessory phrenic nerve (not shown here) is observed as fibers from C5 (C6) join with the phrenic nerve via the subclavian nerve. Similar to other blood vessels, those of the diaphragm receive an autonomic innervation.

Note: Bilateral disruption of the phrenic nerve (e.g., due to a high transection of the cervical spinal cord) leads to bilateral paralysis of the diaphragm. Because the diaphragm is the dominant muscle of respiration, bilateral diaphragmatic paralysis is usually fatal.

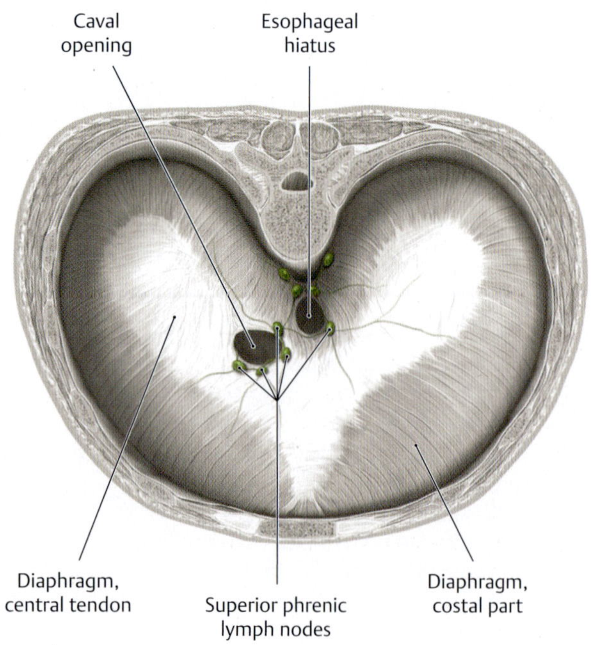

B Lymph nodes and lymphatic drainage of the diaphragm

Superior view. The lymph nodes of the diaphragm are divided into two groups based on their location:

- Superior phrenic lymph nodes on the superior surface of the diaphragm.
- Inferior phrenic lymph nodes on the inferior surface of the diaphragm.

The **superior phrenic lymph nodes** are *thoracic* lymph nodes that collect lymph from the diaphragm, lower esophagus (see p. 174), lung, and also from the liver (by a transdiaphragmatic route, see p. 91). The superior lymph nodes on the right side are involved in hepatic drainage. The superior lymph nodes drain to the bronchomediastinal trunk. The **inferior phrenic lymph** nodes are *abdominal* lymph nodes; they collect lymph from the diaphragm and usually convey it to a lumbar trunk (see p. 239). They may also collect lymph from the lower lobes of the lungs.

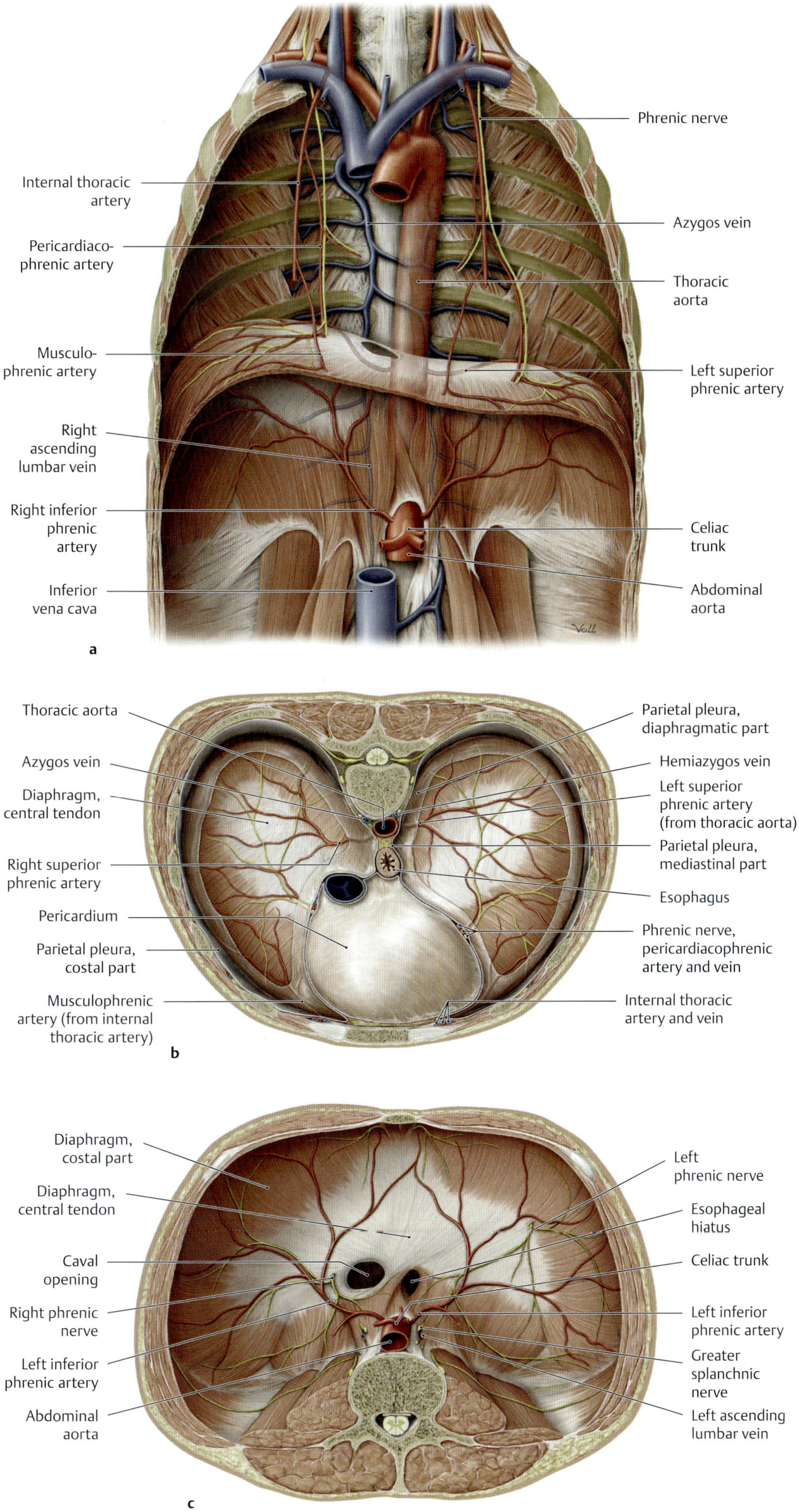

C Arteries of the diaphragm

a Anterior view of the opened thorax; organs, internal fascias, and serous membranes have been removed. The phrenic nerve (for more details see p. 99) along with the pericardiacophrenic artery run lateral to the pericardium, which has been removed here. The long course of the pericardiacophrenic artery through the entire mediastinum is clearly visible.

b Superior surface of the diaphragm viewed from above. The parietal pleura (diaphragmatic part) has been removed over a broad area, leaving the pericardium in place. Three (pairs of) arteries supply the superior surface of the diaphragm:

- Superior phrenic artery: arises from the thoracic aorta just above the diaphragm and supplies the largest area of the diaphragm.
- Pericardiacophrenic artery: arises from the internal thoracic artery, runs close to the pericardium, and gives off branches to the diaphragm.
- Internal thoracic artery: supplies the diaphragm by direct branches or via the musculophrenic artery.

c Inferior surface of the diaphragm viewed from below. The parietal peritoneum has been completely removed. The inferior surface of the diaphragm is supplied by the paired inferior phrenic arteries, the highest branches of the abdominal aorta.

The **diaphragmatic veins** (not shown here) mainly accompany the arteries:

- Inferior phrenic veins: open into the inferior vena cava.
- Superior phrenic veins: usually open into the azygos vein on the right side and into the hemiazygos vein on the left side.

2.1 Arteries: Thoracic Aorta

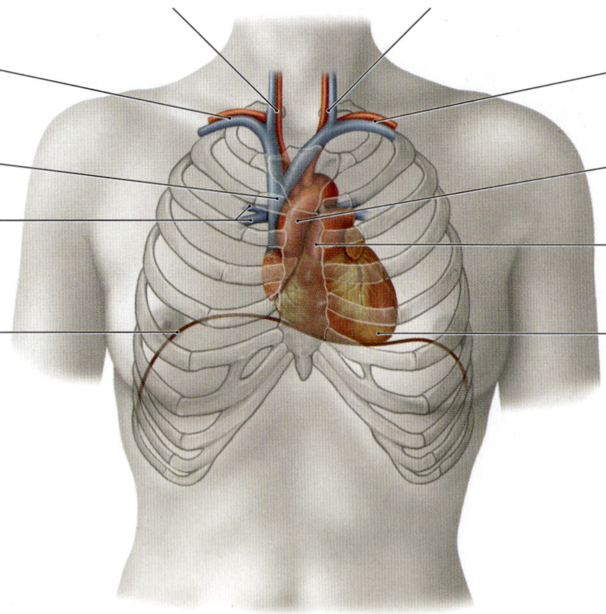

A Projection of the heart and vessels onto the chest wall

Anterior view. The two great arterial vessels in the thorax are the *aorta* and the *pulmonary trunk*. Because the pulmonary arteries run a very short distance before entering the lungs, they are discussed under the heading of the pulmonary vessels (see p. 152f).

The *ascending* aorta is "in the shadow" of the sternum on the PA chest radiograph, while the aortic arch ("aortic knob") forms the superior left portion of the left heart border (see **B**). The *descending* aorta is hidden by the heart itself.

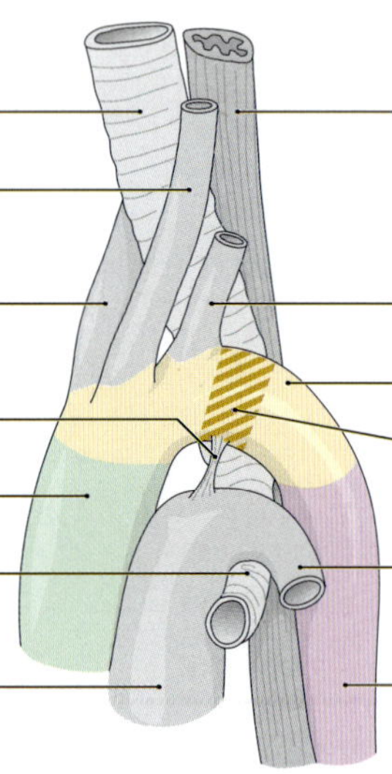

B Parts of the aorta and their relationship to the trachea and esophagus

Left lateral view. The aorta consists of three main parts:

- Ascending aorta: arises from the left ventricle, is dilated near the heart to form the aortic bulb (not visible here).
- Aortic arch: the arched portion of the aorta between the ascending and descending parts, runs posteriorly and to the left. A constriction may persist as an embryonic remnant in this part of the aorta, the aortic isthmus (see crosshatched area in the figure and p. 200).
- Descending aorta: consists of the thoracic and abdominal portions of the aorta (see **D**).

C Functional groups of arteries that supply the thoracic organs

These are mainly vessels that supply the *organs and internal structures* of the thorax. The intrathoracic branches of the aorta can be divided into four main functional groups:

Arteries to the head and neck or to the upper limb:

- Brachiocephalic trunk with
  - Right common carotid artery
  - Right subclavian artery
- Thyroid ima artery (present in only 10% of the population)
- Left common carotid artery
- Left subclavian artery

Direct aortic branches that supply intrathoracic structures:

- Visceral branches to thoracic organs (heart, trachea, bronchi, and esophagus):
  - Right and left coronary arteries
  - Tracheal branches
  - Pericardial branches
  - Bronchial branches
  - Esophageal branches
- Parietal branches to the internal (mainly posterolateral) chest wall and diaphragm:
  - Posterior intercostal arteries
  - Right and left superior phrenic arteries

Indirect paired branches (not arising directly from the aorta) that are distributed primarily to the head and neck but give off branches, usually small, that enter the chest and supply intrathoracic organs:

- Inferior thyroid artery (from the thyrocervical trunk = branch of subclavian artery) with
  - Esophageal branches
  - Tracheal branches

Indirect paired branches which supply the chest wall (mostly anterior, some inferior), usually in the form of parietal branches, and may give off other branches to intrathoracic organs (visceral sub-branches):

- Internal thoracic artery (from the subclavian artery) with
  - Thymic branches
  - Mediastinal branches
  - Anterior intercostal branches
  - Pericardiacophrenic artery (with branches to the pericardium and diaphragm)
  - Musculophrenic artery (with a branch to the diaphragm)

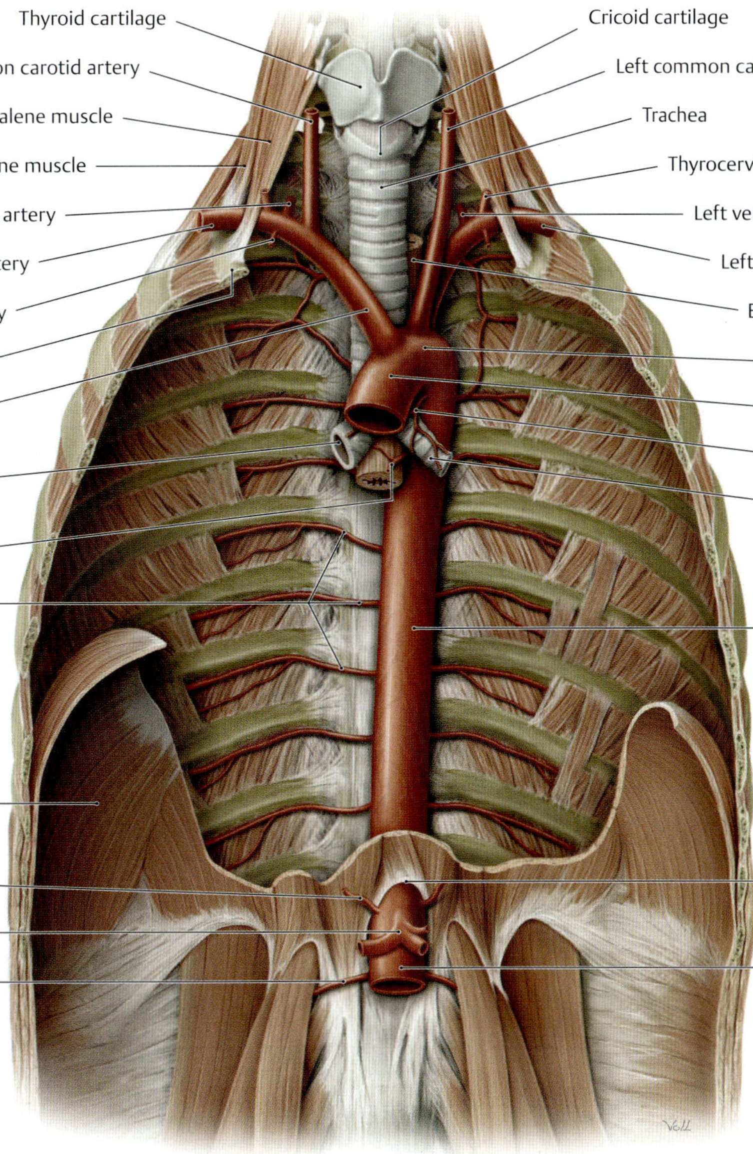

D Position of the aorta in the thorax

Anterior view. The pleura, internal fasciae, and most thoracic organs have been removed, and the diaphragm has been windowed to display more of the thoracic cavity. The branches of the aorta (see **C** and p. 227) supply blood to all the organs, delivering almost 5 liters of blood per minute throughout the body. The thoracic aorta is thick-walled, particularly in its ascending segment and arch, but these walls are also elastic. During the systolic wave of pressure as the left ventricle contracts, these segments of the aorta dilate rapidly and then recoil. This serves to absorb and dissipate the pressure wave to produce a steadier, more even flow of blood in the arteries farther away from the heart. Because the aortic arch runs posteriorly and to the left, the relationship of the aorta to the trachea and esophagus changes as the vessel passes inferiorly through the chest (see also **B** and p. 172). The most anterior part of the aorta is the *ascending aorta*. The *aortic arch* then passes to the left side of the trachea, arching over the left main bronchus. It passes initially to the left of the esophagus but then descends *posterior* to the esophagus and anterior to the vertebral column. Because of this relationship, an abnormal outpouching of the aortic wall (aneurysm) may narrow the esophagus and cause swallowing difficulties (dysphagia). The thoracic aorta pierces the diaphragm at the aortic hiatus (junction of the T11/T12 vertebrae), becoming the abdominal aorta.

Note: In rare cases the aortic arch is constricted behind the ligamentum arteriosum (see **B**). This constriction is normal in the embryonic circulation, but its persistence after birth may produce the clinical manifestations of a *coarctation of the aorta*. This includes hypertension in the head, neck, and upper limbs, insufficient blood flow in the lower extremities, and left ventricular hypertrophy (due to chronic excessive workload and pressure) (see p. 200f).

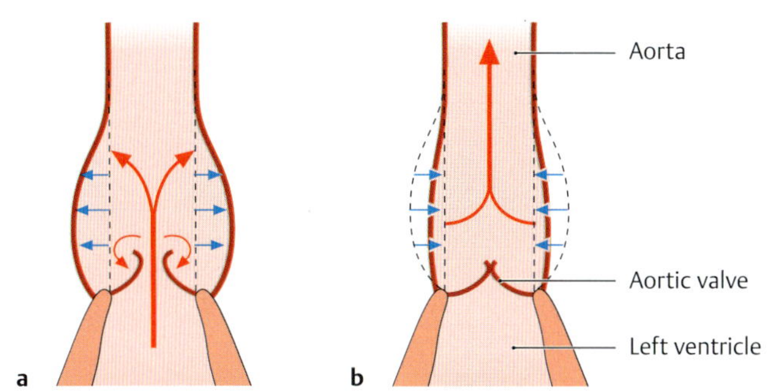

E Aortic Windkessel function

a During systole, part of the ventricular stroke volume is stored in the elastic wall of the aorta (blue arrows pointing outward) and discharged again during diastole (**b**) (blue arrows pointing inward).

2.2 Veins: Vena Cava and Azygos System

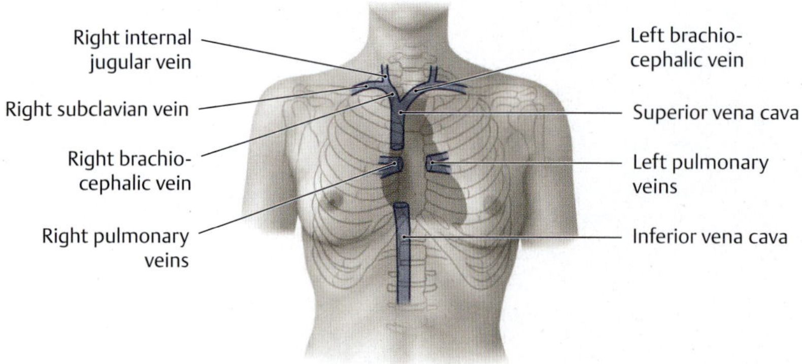

A Projection of the venae cavae onto the skeleton

Anterior view. The *superior vena cava* lies to the right of the midline and appears at the right sternal border on radiographs. Formed by the confluence of the two brachiocephalic veins, the superior vena cava enters the right atrium of the heart from above, forming its border in the PA chest radiograph (see p. 110).

The *inferior vena cava* runs a very short distance within the thorax (approximately 1 cm, not shown here). Immediately after piercing the diaphragm (at the caval opening), it passes through the pericardium and ends by opening into the right atrium of the heart from below. It has no tributaries within the chest (the pulmonary veins are described on p. 152f).

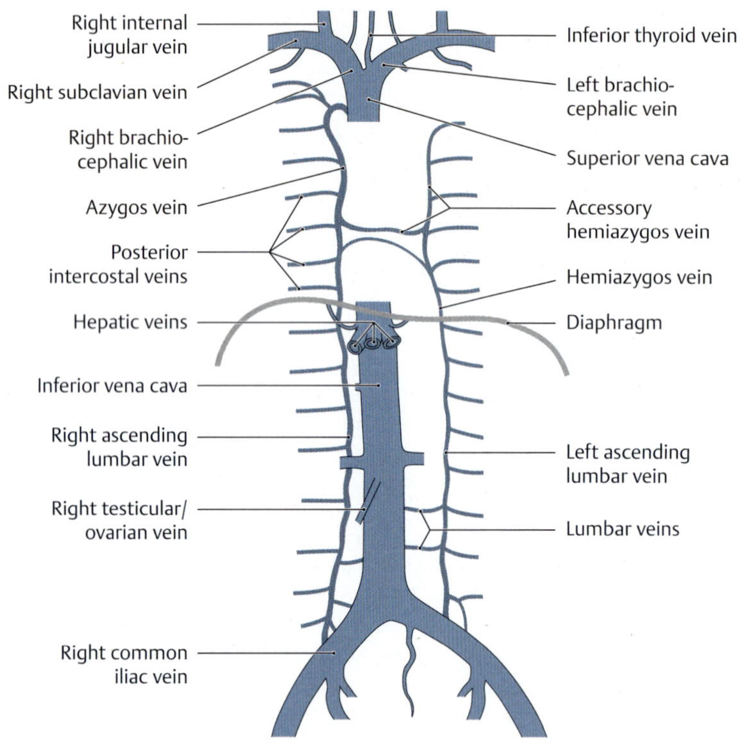

B The azygos system

Anterior view. The venous drainage of the thorax is handled mainly by the long azygos system, which runs vertically through the chest. The *azygos vein* runs to the right of the vertebral column, the *hemiazygos vein* to the left. The hemiazygos vein empties into the azygos vein, which in turn empties into the superior vena cava. An *accessory hemiazygos vein* is frequently present in the upper left thorax; it may open independently into the azygos vein or by way of the hemiazygos vein. The azygos system receives tributaries from the mediastinum and from portions of the chest wall, predominantly in the central and lower thorax.

Note: The azygos vein empties into the superior vena cava, while the ascending lumbar veins on both sides open into the inferior vena cava via the lumbar veins and the common iliac veins. In this way the azygos system creates a shunt between the superior and inferior venae cavae, called the "cavocaval anastomosis." If drainage from the inferior vena cava is obstructed, venous blood can still reach the superior vena cava and enter the right heart by passing through the azygos system (see **D** and p. 234).

C Functional groups of veins that drain the thoracic organs

These are mainly vessels that drain the *organs and internal structures* of the thorax. All of them drain ultimately to the superior vena cava, whose tributaries in the chest can be divided into four main functional groups:

Veins that drain the head and neck or the upper limb:

- Left and right brachiocephalic veins with
  - Right and left subclavian veins
  - Right and left internal jugular veins
  - Right and left external jugular veins
  - Supreme intercostal veins
  - Pericardial veins
  - Left superior intercostal vein

Veins that drain intrathoracic structures (open into the accessory hemiazygos vein or hemiazygos vein on the left side, into the azygos vein on the right side). Blood from both territories is collected in the azygos vein, which empties into the superior vena cava. The tributaries can be grouped as follows:

- Visceral branches that drain the trachea, bronchi, and esophagus:
  - Tracheal veins
  - Bronchial veins
  - Esophageal veins
- Parietal branches that drain the inner chest wall and diaphragm:
  - Posterior intercostal veins
  - Right and left superior phrenic veins
  - Right superior intercostal vein

Indirect paired tributaries of the superior vena cava that descend from the head and neck but receive smaller veins that drain thoracic organs:

- Inferior thyroid vein (tributaries of the brachiocephalic vein) with
  - Esophageal veins
  - Tracheal veins

Indirect paired tributaries of the superior vena cava that mainly drain the anterior chest wall as parietal branches but may also receive tributaries (visceral subbranches) from organs:

- Internal thoracic vein (opens into the brachiocephalic vein) with
  - Thymic veins
  - Mediastinal tributaries
  - Anterior intercostal veins
  - Pericardiacophrenic vein (with tributaries from the pericardium and diaphragm)
  - Musculophrenic vein (with a tributary from the diaphragm)

Note: Structures of the superior mediastinum may also drain directly to the brachiocephalic veins (e.g., via the tracheal veins, esophageal veins, and mediastinal veins).

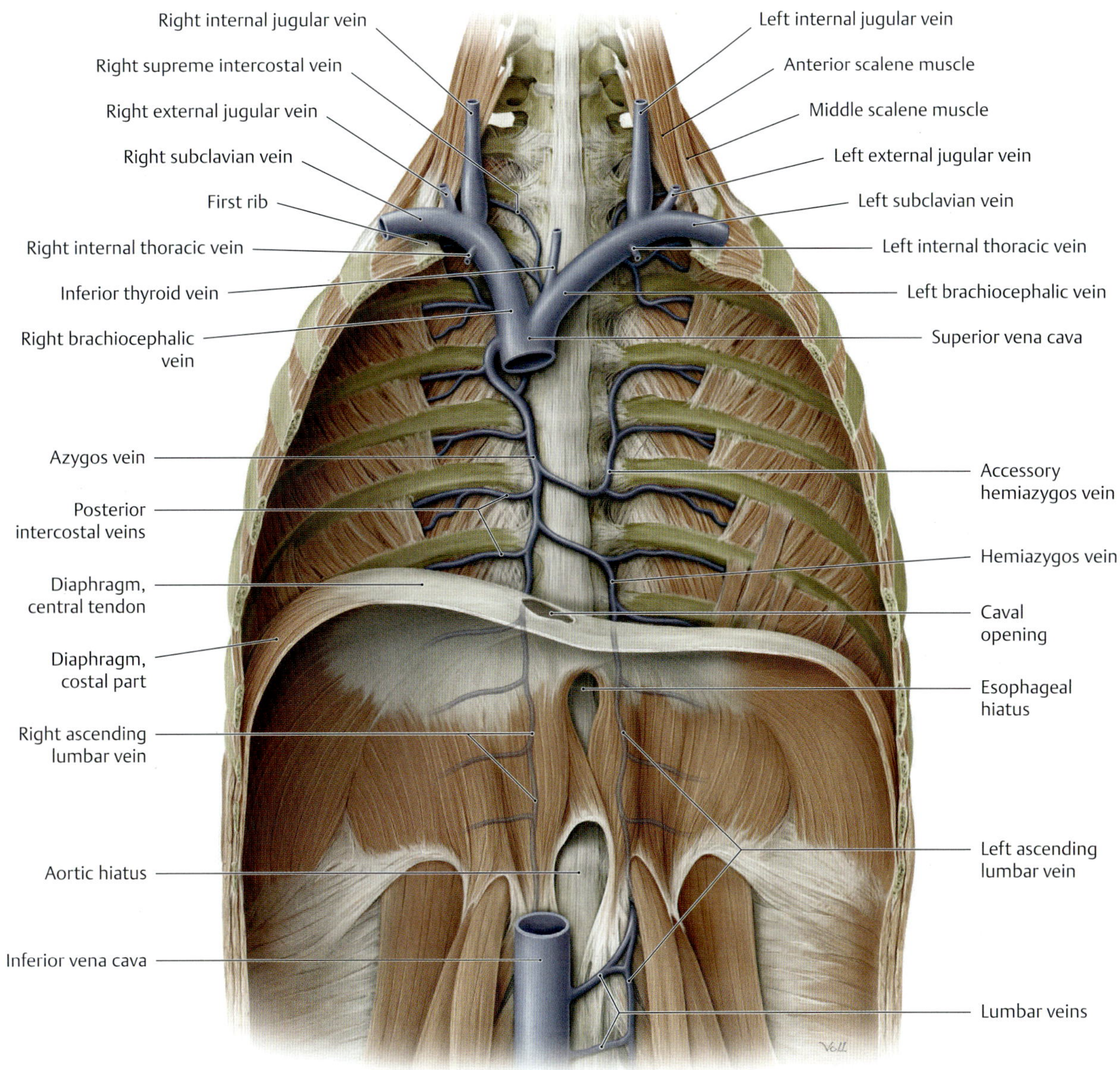

D Superior vena cava and azygos system in the thorax
Anterior view. The thorax has been cut open and the organs, internal fasciae, and serous membranes have been removed. The inferior vena cava has been removed at the level of the L1/L2 vertebrae to display the right ascending lumbar vein. The **superior vena cava** is formed by the confluence of the two brachiocephalic veins at the approximate level of the T2/T3 junction, to the right of the median plane. Each brachiocephalic vein is formed in turn by the union of the internal jugular vein and subclavian vein. The azygos vein ascends on the right side of the vertebral column and opens into the posterior right aspect of the superior vena cava just below the union of the brachiocephalic veins. After the right and left ascending lumbar veins pass through the diaphragm they form the **azygos vein** on the right side and the **hemiazygos vein** on the left side.
At the level of the T7 vertebra, the hemiazygos vein crosses over the vertebral column from the left side and opens into the azygos vein. In this dissection the accessory hemiazygos vein drains separately into the azygos vein after crossing over the vertebral column from left to right. Not infrequently, however, the hemiazygos vein and accessory hemiazygos vein are interconnected by anastomoses.

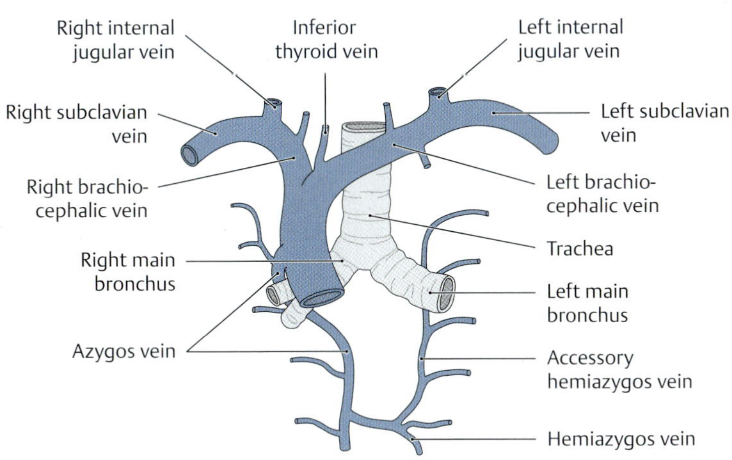

E Relations of the trachea, superior vena cava, and azygos system
The superior vena cava lies to the right of the trachea. The left brachiocephalic vein passes anterior to the trachea from the left side to unite with the right brachiocephalic vein. The azygos vein ascends posterior to the right main bronchus and turns anteriorly to enter the superior vena cava from behind (the azygos vein "rides" upon the right main bronchus). The accessory hemiazygos vein ascends behind the left main bronchus and may open independently into the azygos vein or may join the hemiazygos vein to form a common trunk that opens into the azygos vein.

2.3 Lymphatic Vessels

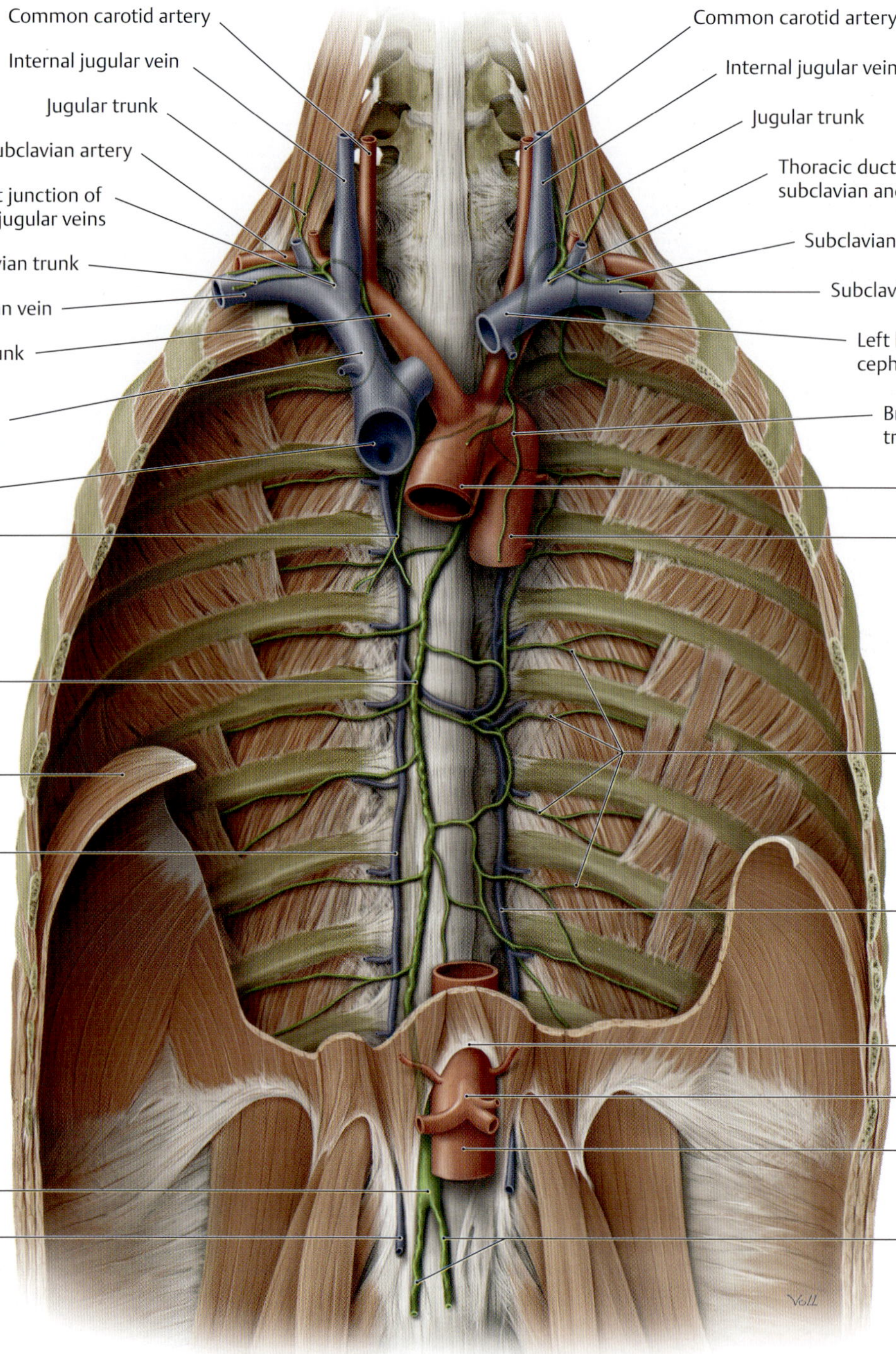

A Lymphatic trunks in the thorax
Anterior view of the opened thorax with the pleura, internal fasciae, and organs removed. The diaphragm has been windowed, and the upper part of the abdomen can be seen. The principal trunks that convey lymph from all body regions to the venous system are the thoracic duct and right lymphatic duct. The **thoracic duct** begins in the abdomen at the upper end of a large sac, the cisterna chyli. It transverses the diaphragm through the aortic hiatus, passing behind the aorta and in front of the vertebral column, and usually ascends just to the right of the midline. Just below the aortic arch it shifts to the left and terminates by opening into the junction of the left subclavian and internal jugular veins. It is joined in the neck by the *left bronchomediastinal trunk*, *left jugular trunk*, and *left subclavian trunk*. A number of small, unnamed lymphatic trunks that collect lymph from smaller groups of lymph nodes convey lymph from the mediastinum and intercostal spaces to the thoracic duct (lymph from the posterior portions of the lower right intercostal spaces usually drains into the thoracic duct rather than the short right bronchomediastinal trunk). The **right lymphatic duct** is a short duct that receives the *right bronchomediastinal trunk*, *right jugular trunk*, and *right subclavian trunk* just before it opens into the junction of the right subclavian and internal jugular veins.

Note: All major lymphatic trunks pass through the thoracic cavity. The intrathoracic pressure undergoes rhythmic variations with breathing, and these pressure changes are transmitted to the lymphatic trunks. These changes act mainly on the relatively large-caliber thoracic duct and have a significant impact on lymphatic return: the fall of intrathoracic pressure during inspiration causes a passive, transient swelling of the thoracic duct, which increases the flow of lymph through that vessel. This principle can be applied therapeutically in lymphedema patients by having the patient perform a slow, deep inhalation to create a sustained negative intrathoracic pressure that will promote lymphatic drainage.

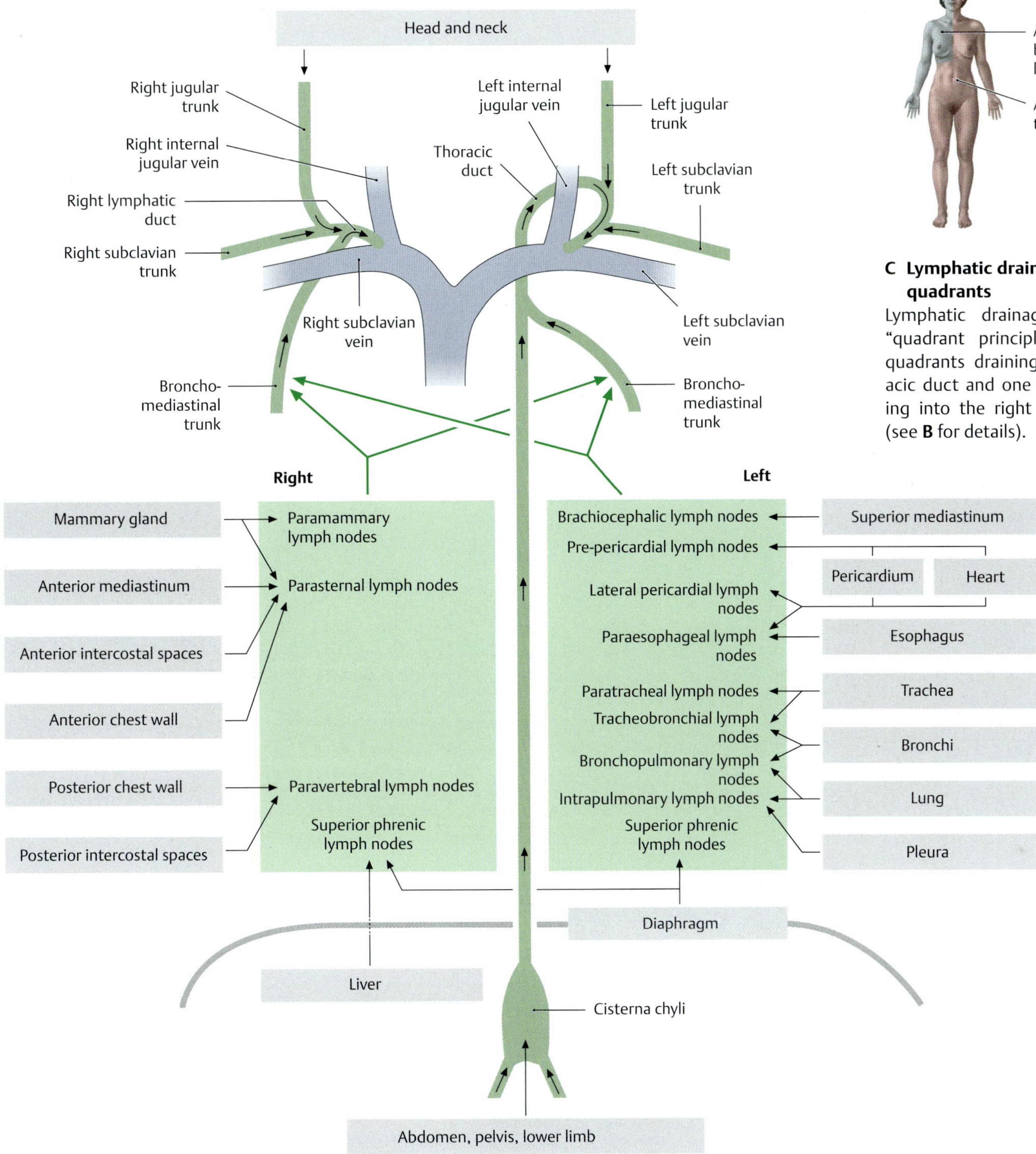

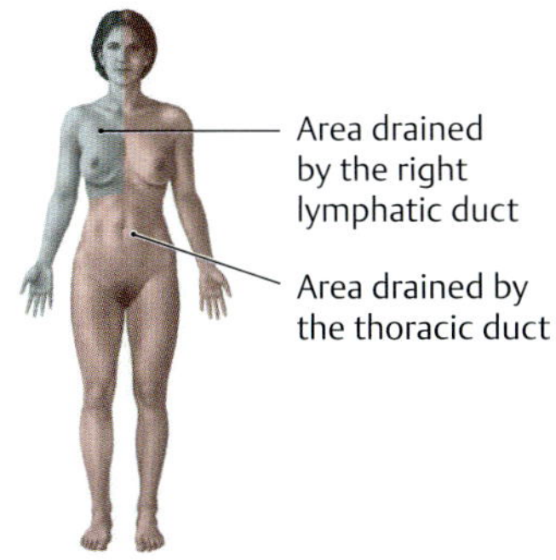

C Lymphatic drainage by quadrants

Lymphatic drainage follows the "quadrant principle," with three quadrants draining into the thoracic duct and one quadrant draining into the right lymphatic duct (see **B** for details).

B Overview of lymphatic pathways in the thorax

The lymph from all body regions is returned to the venous circulation at the junctions of the right and left subclavian and internal jugular veins (sometimes called the right and left "venous angles"). The **thoracic duct** conveys lymph from the abdomen, pelvis, lower limb, left half of the thorax, left upper limb, and left half of the head and neck to the junction of the *left* subclavian and internal jugular veins (corresponding to three of the four quadrants shown in **C**). The **right lymphatic duct** is a short duct (only about 1 cm long) that conveys lymph from the right half of the thorax, portions of the liver, the right upper limb, and the right half of the head and neck to the junction of the *right* subclavian and internal jugular veins (corresponding to one of the four quadrants). Lymph from the posterior portions of the lower intercostal spaces on both sides usually drains into the thoracic duct (see **A**). Both of the main trunks receive thoracic lymph from the **left** and **right bronchomediastinal trunks** and from smaller, unnamed trunks. The **lymph nodes** (see p. 94) may be located close to the chest wall (e.g., the parasternal, paramammary and prevertebral lymph nodes), in the mediastinum (known clinically as the "mediastinal" lymph nodes), or may be closely associated with the bronchial tree and named for their location. Overlapping patterns of lymphatic drainage are common in the chest due to the close topographical relationships of intrathoracic structures. Thus, for example, the paraesophageal lymph nodes collect lymph from the esophagus *and* from the heart.

2.4 Thoracic Lymph Nodes

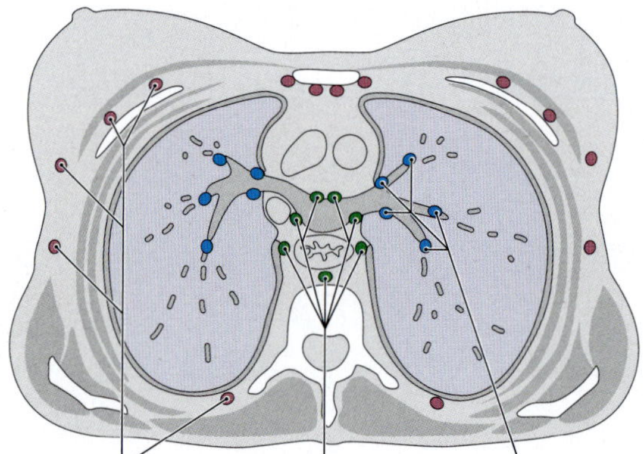

A Overview of the thoracic lymph nodes

Transverse section at the level of the tracheal bifurcation (at approximately T4), viewed from above. Topographically, the thoracic lymph nodes can be divided into three broad groups:

- Lymph nodes in the chest wall (shown here in purple), which drain the chest wall.
- Lymph nodes in the lung and at the divisions of the bronchial tree (intrapulmonary and bronchopulmonary lymph nodes, shown here in blue). This group drains the lung and bronchial tree and conveys its lymph to the next group (see **C** and p. 91).
- Lymph nodes associated with the central structures of the mediastinum (trachea, esophagus, and pericardium, shown here in green).

All lymph nodes shown here connect to the left and right venous angle, mostly via the bronchomediastinal trunks.

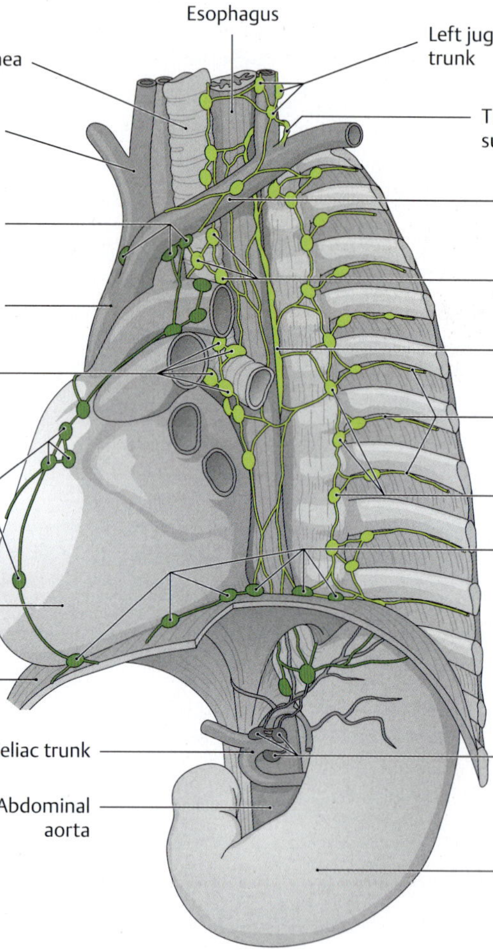

B Thoracic lymph nodes

Schematic, left anterior view (the stomach and brachiocephalic vein are not shown to scale). Part of the diaphragm has been cut away, and the brachiocephalic vein has been retracted posterosuperiorly to display the lymph nodes and the junction of the left subclavian and internal jugular veins. There is no significant functional distinction between parietal and visceral lymph nodes in the thorax (in sharp contrast with the segregated visceral lymphatic flow in the abdomen and pelvis (see p. 238f). The thoracic lymph nodes are grouped in the mediastinum ("mediastinal" lymph nodes) around the pericardium, trachea, esophagus, and bronchi and collect the lymph from these organs.

Note: There may be a transdiaphragmatic connection, varying in different individuals, by which the thoracic lymph nodes communicate directly with abdominal lymph nodes. This connection may allow a direct lymphatic metastasis of malignant tumors (e.g., gastric carcinoma) to the thoracic lymph nodes.

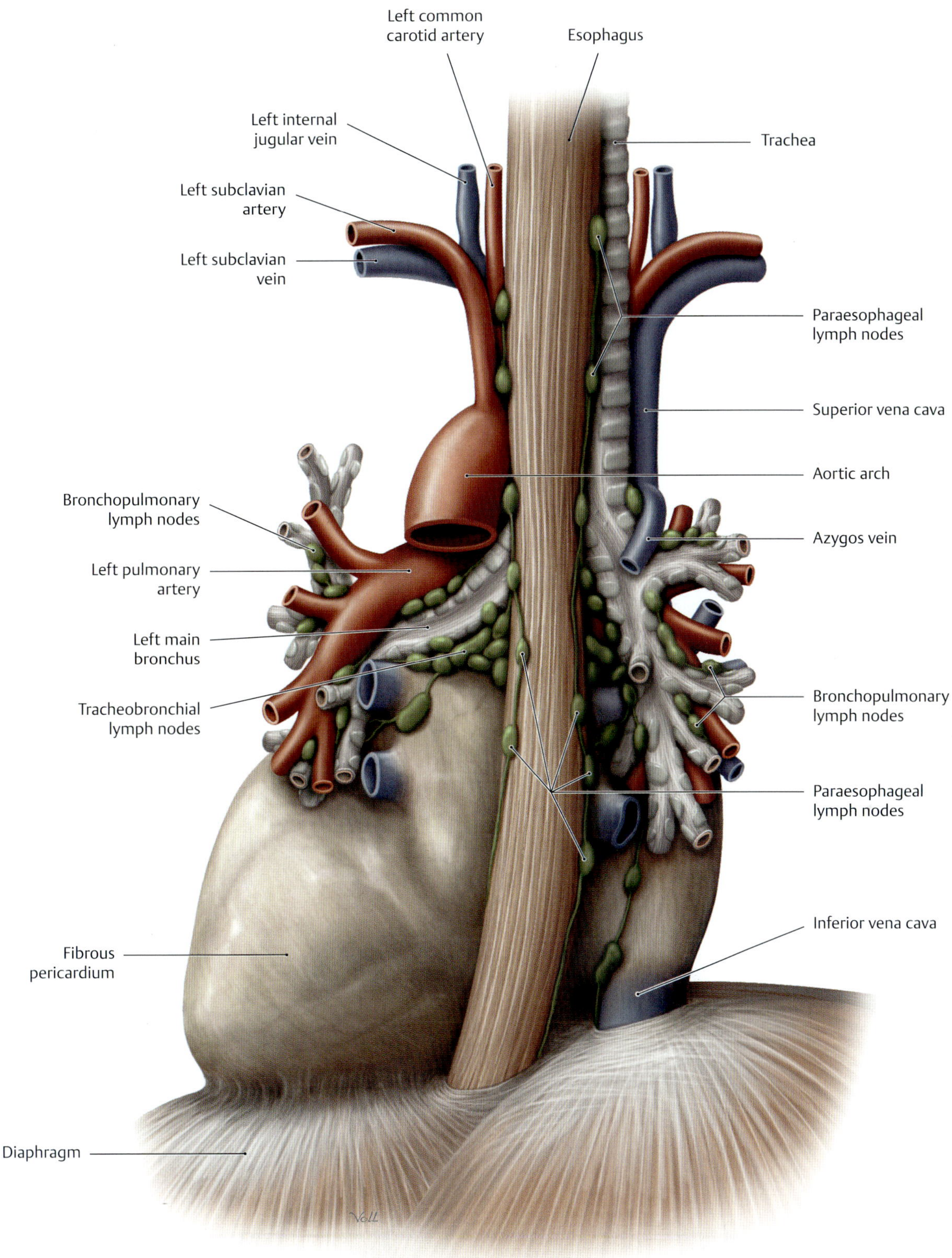

C Thoracic lymph nodes, posterior view
The numerous lymph nodes located at the divisions of the main bronchi into lobar bronchi are often called the "hilar" lymph nodes because they are located in the region of the pulmonary hilum (not shown here). Frequently they are the first group of lymph nodes to be affected by pulmonary disease (tuberculosis, malignant tumors).

2.5 Thoracic Innervation

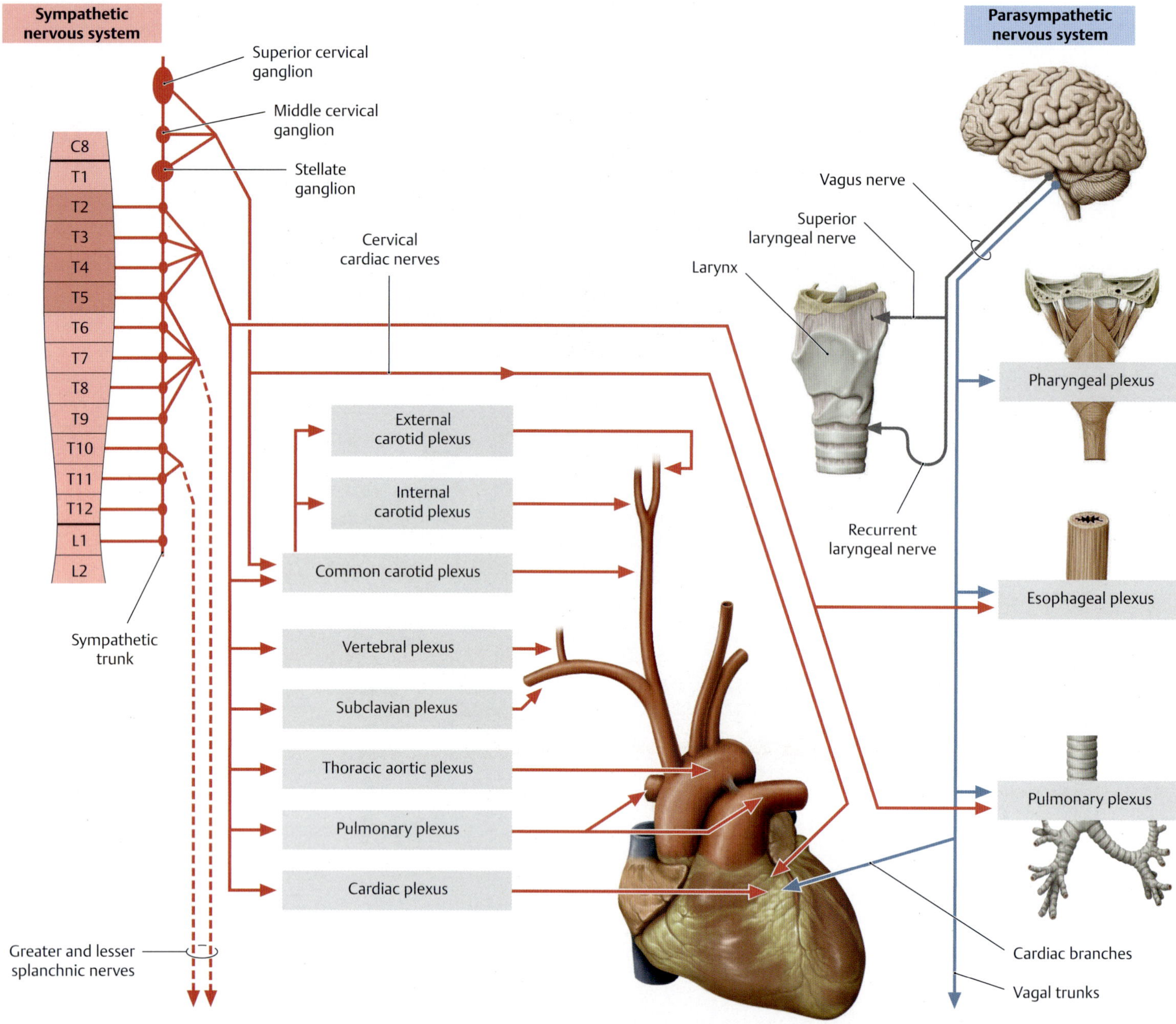

A Organization of the sympathetic and parasympathetic nervous systems in the thorax

With the prominent exceptions of the phrenic nerve and intercostal nerves (**B**), thoracic innervation is largely autonomic, arising from either the paravertebral sympathetic trunks or the parasympathetic vagus nerves.

Sympathetic organization: The peripheral sympathetic system consists of a two-neuron relay, with presynaptic (preganglionic) fibers arising from neurons in the spinal cord. These axons synapse onto neurons in the paired *paravertebral* sympathetic ganglia, which send axons to innervate the thoracic viscera and blood vessels.

The cell bodies of the presynaptic motor neurons are located in the lateral horns of the thoracolumbar spinal cord (T1 to L2); the neurons involved in sympathetic innervation of the thorax are concentrated in upper thoracic levels. Axons from the paravertebral ganglion cells (postsynaptic [postganglionic] fibers) follow several courses: some fibers follow intercostal nerves to innervate blood vessels and glands in the chest wall; others accompany arteries to visceral targets; other groups of postganglionic axons gather in the greater and lesser splanchnic nerves and enter the abdomen (see p. 242).

Parasympathetic organization: The peripheral parasympathetic nervous system has a similar two-neuron relay, but its presynaptic neurons are in the brainstem and the ganglion cells are scattered in microscopic groups in their target organs. The vagus nerve (CN X) carries presynaptic parasympathetic motor axons from brainstem neurons into the thorax and gives off the following branches:

- Cardiac branches to the cardiac plexus (heart)
- Esophageal branches to the esophageal plexus (esophagus)
- Tracheal branches (trachea) and bronchial branches to the pulmonary plexus (bronchi, pulmonary vessels)

The vagus nerves continue beyond these branches, following the esophagus into the abdomen (see p. 243).

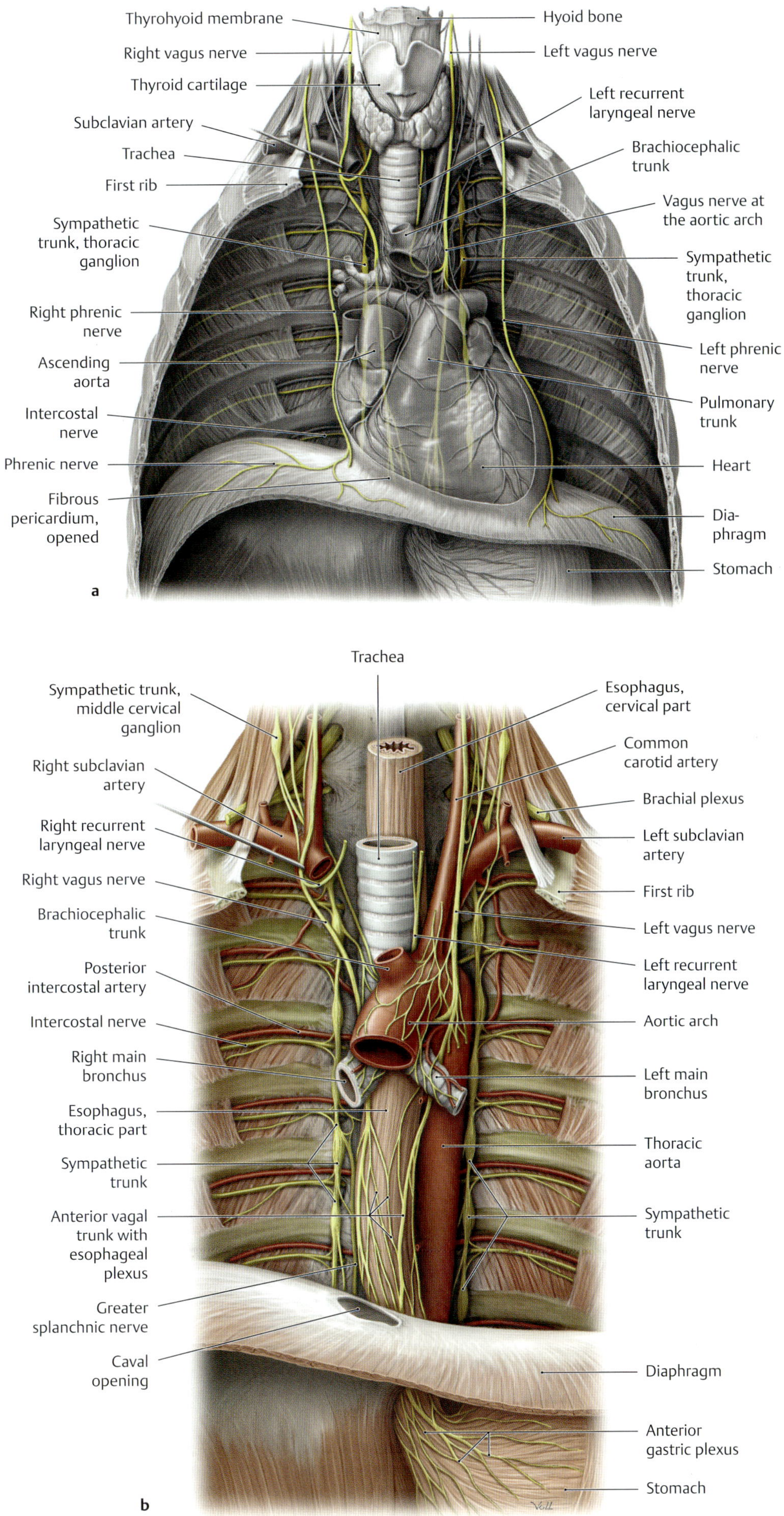

B Overview of nerves in the thorax

Anterior view. **a** The heart and part of the pericardium have been left in place in the middle mediastinum to display the location and course of the phrenic nerves; **b** All organs, except for the esophagus and part of the trachea, and the phrenic nerves have been removed in order to display the sympathetic trunks, intercostal nerves and esophageal plexus.

The **sympathetic trunk** runs alongside the vertebral column in the thorax. Postsynaptic branches of the sympathetic trunk usually accompany the intrathoracic arteries to their target organ in the chest, where they enter the plexus associated with that organ (see p. 94). The **intercostal nerves** are all posterior. They arise from spinal cord segments T1–T12 (the paired nerves arising from segment T12 are called the *subcostal nerves* because they run below the twelfth rib; not shown here) and they emerge below the T1 through T12 vertebra. They initially course with the intercostal vessels along the inferior border of the associated rib. They supply motor innervation to the intercostal muscles and give sensory innervation to the T1–T12 dermatomes. Each intercostal nerve receives postsynaptic sympathetic fibers for the autonomic innervation of glands and vessels in the skin of the dermatomes.

The thoracic portions of the **vagus nerves** initially run in the plane of the trachea, pass posterior to the two main bronchi while giving off branches, and then descend on the esophagus, passing with it through the esophageal hiatus into the abdomen.

Note: The left and right vagus nerves are organized around the esophagus to form the anterior and posterior vagal trunks. Topographically, these trunks are a continuation of the esophageal plexus. Both trunks contain fibers from both vagus nerves: the *anterior* trunk contains more fibers from the *left* vagus nerve, while the *posterior* trunk contains more fibers from the *right* vagus nerve. The left vagus nerve gives off the *left recurrent laryngeal* nerve at the aortic arch, while the right vagus nerve gives off the *right recurrent laryngeal nerve* at the right subclavian artery. Each of these nerves is a recurrent branch of the vagus nerve that ascends into the neck. It is not uncommon for the recurrent laryngeal nerves to run more posteriorly in the neck than shown here, occupying the groove between the trachea and esophagus where they are vulnerable during operations on the nearby thyroid gland. For clarity, the recurrent laryngeal nerves have been retracted slightly forward in this dissection.

Note: The pericardium and diaphragm do not have an autonomic nerve supply (except their blood vessels).

3.1 Location of the Heart in the Thorax

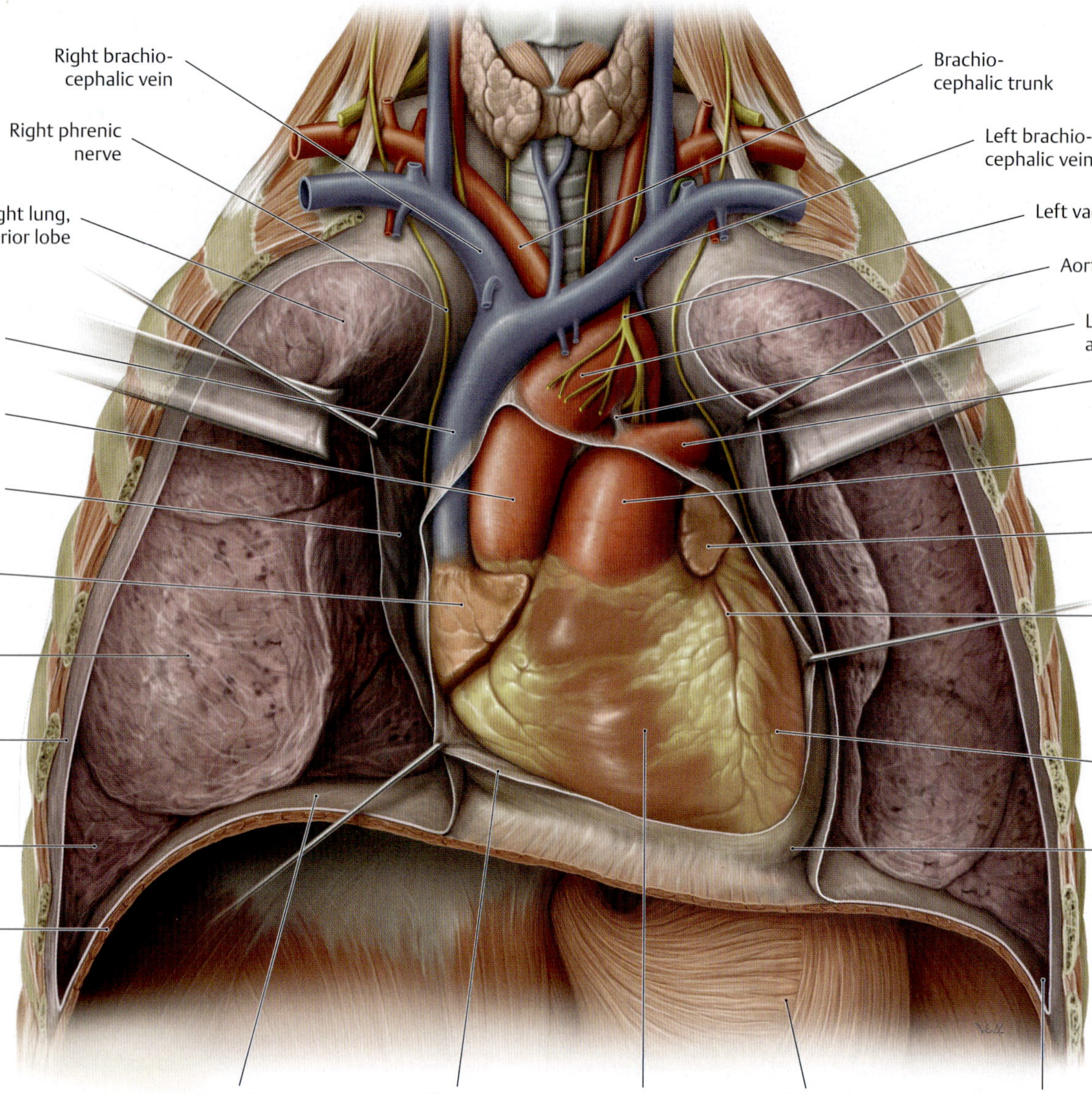

a

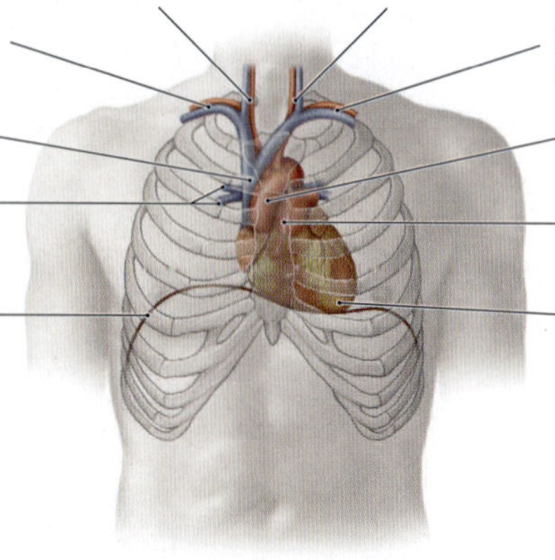

b

A The heart in situ, anterior view

a Simplified illustration. The chest has been widely opened, and the pleural cavities and fibrous pericardium have been cut open. The connective tissue has been removed from the anterior mediastinum to display the heart. Although the pleural cavities have been opened, the lungs are not shown in a collapsed state. **b** Projection of the heart on the bony thorax. The heart lies within the pericardium, which is firmly attached to the diaphragm (see p. 98) but is mobile in relation to the parietal pleura. A longitudinal axis drawn from the base to the apex of the heart demonstrates that this "long axis" is directed forward and downward from right to left. Thus the heart, when viewed from the front, has an oblique orientation and is tilted counterclockwise within the chest. Along this axis it appears slightly "rolled" in a posterior direction. Thus the right ventricle faces forward, as pictured here, while the left ventricle is only partly visible. As a result, all of the great vessels cannot be seen even when the base of the heart is viewed from the front. The short pulmonary veins are covered by the cardiac silhouette because they terminate at the left atrium, which is directed posteriorly. The right and left auricles (atrial appendages) are clearly visible. The cardiac apex points downward and to the left. Most of it is still covered by pericardium in this dissection. Its movement, called the apical beat, is palpable as a fine motion in the fifth intercostal space on the left midclavicular line (see p. 109). The thin serous membrane of the epicardium (see p. 98) gives the surface of the heart a shiny appearance. Under this membrane are clusters of fatty tissue in which the coronary vessels are embedded.

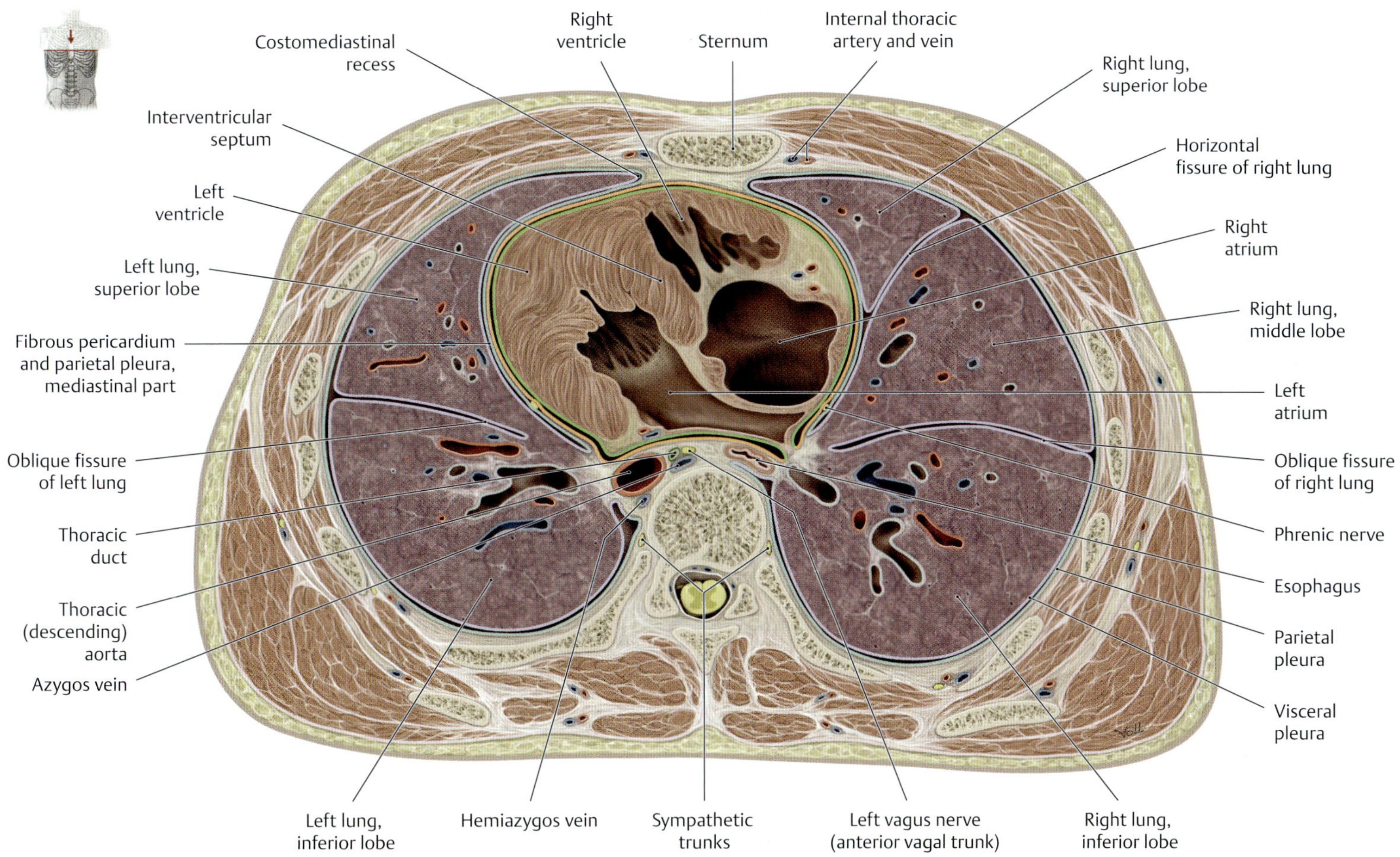

B The heart in situ, superior view

Transverse section through the thorax at the level of T8 vertebra. Viewing the transverse section demonstrates the asymmetrical position of the heart in the middle mediastinum and its slight degree of physiologic counterclockwise rotation: the *left ventricle* faces downward and to the left, while the right ventricle faces forward and to the right. The *right ventricle* thus lies almost directly behind the posterior wall of the sternum (with only the narrow anterior mediastinum intervening, see p. 79). The *left atrium* is in very close relationship to the esophagus. The costomediastinal recess is interposed between the heart and *sternum* on the right and left sides. A relatively small space remains between the heart and *vertebral column* for the passage of neurovascular structures and organs: thoracic aorta, esophagus, thoracic duct, azygos and hemiazygos veins, and portions of the autonomic nervous system. Each lung bears an indentation from the heart called the cardiac impression. This impression is larger in the left lung than in the right lung because of the heart's asymmetric position. The potential spaces between the pleural layers and the serous portions of the pericardium are considerably smaller than pictured here.

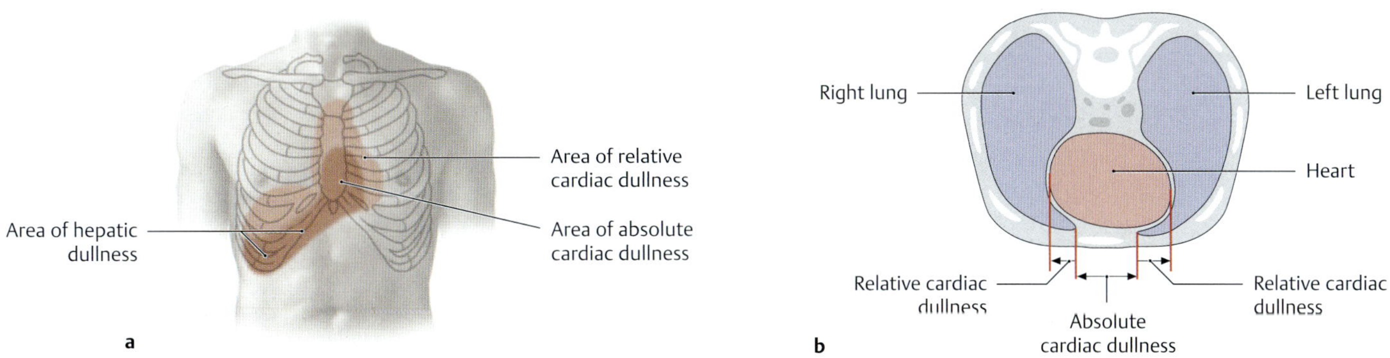

C Cardiac dullness on percussion of the chest

Anterior view (**a**) and transverse section viewed from above (**b**). In contrast to the sonorous sound that is produced by the percussion of *air-filled* lung (see p. 138), the *fluid-filled* heart produces a flat sound on percussion known as *cardiac dullness*. The dullness may be *absolute* (at sites where there is no lung tissue to moderate cardiac dullness) or *relative* (at sites where lung tissue overlies the heart and adds resonance to the percussion sound). Accordingly, the area of absolute cardiac dullness is located between the chest wall and heart while the area of relative cardiac dullness is located over the right and left costomediastinal recesses, which contain small expansions of lung tissue (see **B**).

Note: Cardiac dullness gives way to hepatic dullness in the epigastrium and right hypochondriac region due to the anatomical extent of the liver (see **a**). The boundaries of the heart can be roughly estimated from the area of cardiac dullness because the sound characteristics at the cardiac borders contrast with the more resonant lung sounds.

3.2 Pericardium: Location, Structure, and Innervation

A Location of the pericardium in the thorax, anterior view
The chest has been opened to display the pericardium, which is the dominant structure in the inferior mediastinum. It is attached inferiorly to the diaphragmatic fascia by connective tissue. Anteriorly, it is separated from the posterior surface of the sternum only by connective tissue of the anterior mediastinum (removed here, see p. 79). The pericardium is bounded laterally by the pleural cavities, from which it is separated by mediastinal pleura.

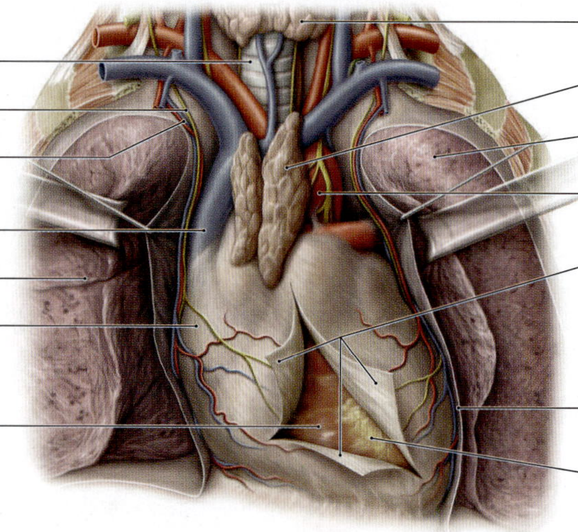

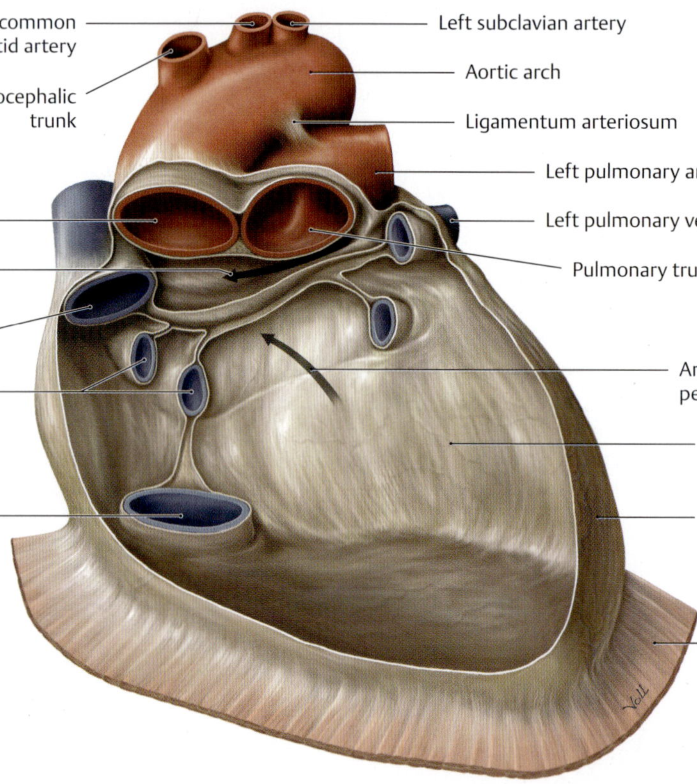

B Pericardial cavity and structure of the pericardium
Anterior view of the empty pericardial sac. The pericardium consists of two **layers**, one within the other, that enclose and protect the heart:

- Parietal layer. The parietal pericardium forms a sac with an outer surface, the *fibrous pericardium*, composed of tough and indistensible connective tissue which is partially attached to the diaphragm. Its inner surface, facing the heart, is lined with a serous membrane.
- Visceral layer (*epicardium*). This is a thin serous membrane which covers, and is firmly adherent to, the heart itself and the proximal parts of the great vessels.

The two serous membranes of the parietal and visceral layers are closely apposed, but move freely over one another, allowing a gliding motion during the heartbeat. These two serous membranes are referred to together as the serous *pericardium*.

In the locations where the parietal layer is folded back onto the visceral layer covering the vessels, two **sinuses** are formed (see arrows):

- The transverse pericardial sinus located between the arteries and veins
- The oblique pericardial sinus located between the left and right pulmonary veins.

Note: Because the pericardium cannot expand significantly, bleeding into the pericardial cavity (e.g., from a ruptured myocardial aneurysm) will place increasing pressure on the heart as the blood accumulates within the sac. This condition, called cardiac tamponade, seriously compromises the ability of the ventricles to fill and pump blood, creating a threat of cardiac arrest. Similar problems may arise from inflammation of the pericardium (pericarditis).

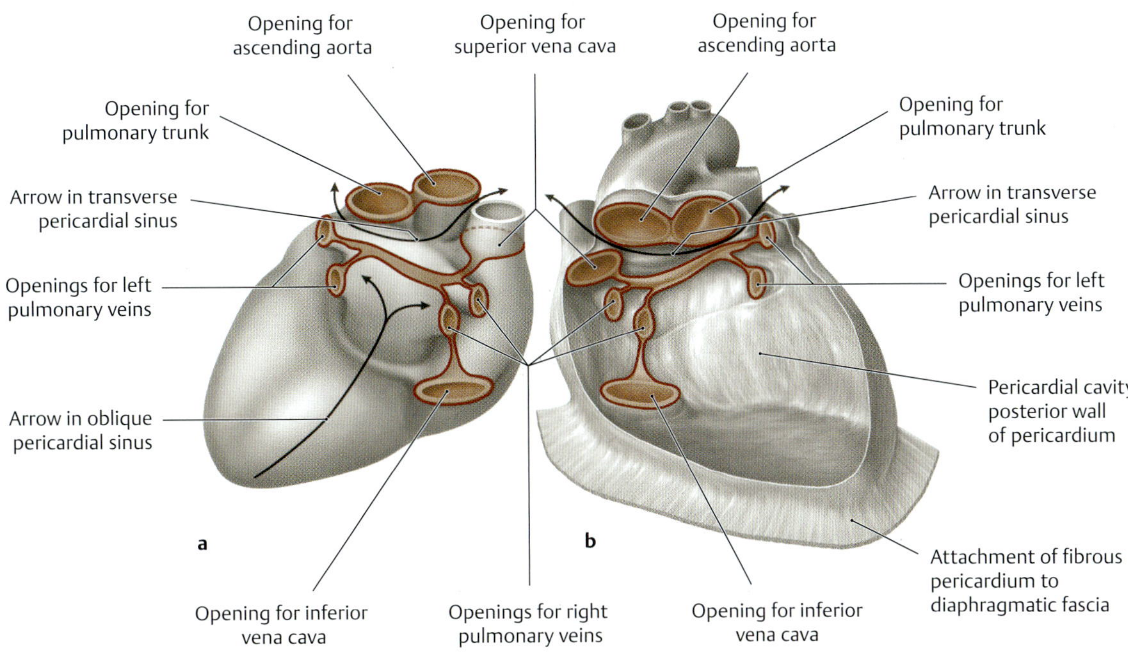

C Openings in the pericardium

a Posterior view of the heart with the epicardium. **b** Anterior view of the "empty" pericardial cavity. An empty pericardium typically has eight openings by which vessels enter and leave the heart:

- One opening for the ascending aorta
- One opening for the pulmonary trunk
- Two openings for the two venae cavae
- Up to four openings for the four pulmonary veins.

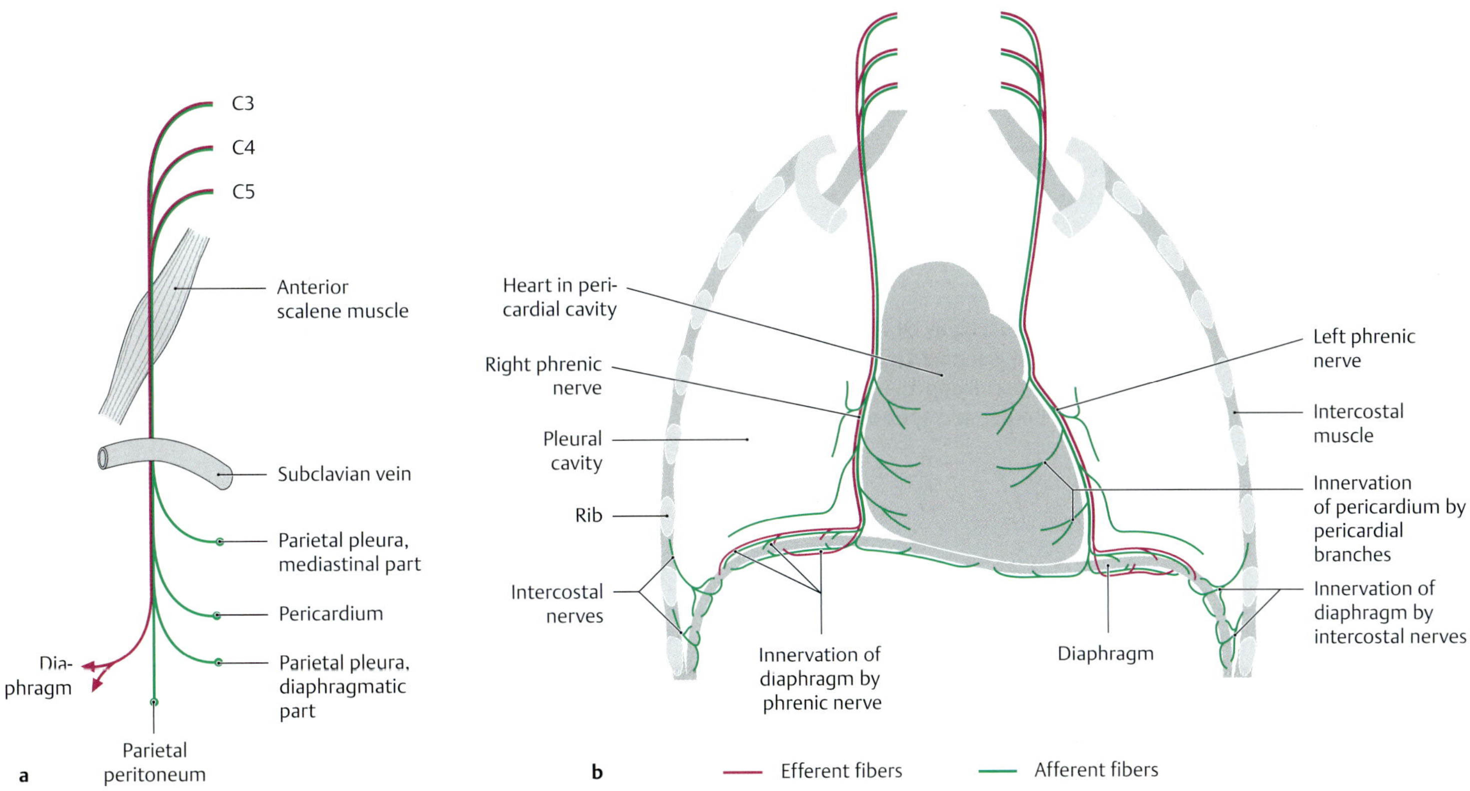

D Innervation of the pericardium

a Somatosensory and somatomotor components of the phrenic nerve

b Sensory and motor distribution of the phrenic nerve

Like the serous membranes of the diaphragm (diaphragmatic pleura and parietal peritoneum), the pericardium (fibrous pericardium and parietal layer of serous pericardium) is innervated by the phrenic nerves, which arise from cervical spinal cord segments C3–5.

3.3 Heart: Shape and Structure

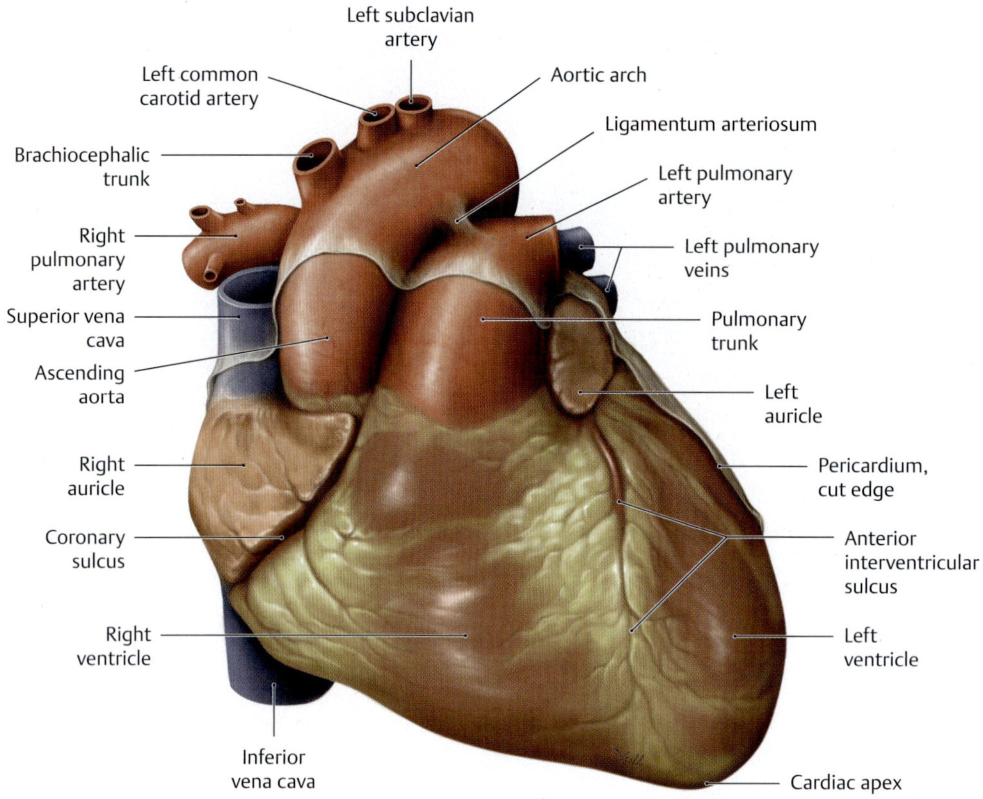

A Heart, sternocostal surface

Anterior view. The heart is a muscular hollow organ shaped approximately like a flattened cone. It consists topographically of a base, apex, and three surfaces:

- The base of the heart, which is occupied by entering and emerging vessels, is directed superiorly, posteriorly, and to the right.
- The apex is directed inferiorly, anteriorly, and to the left.
- The surfaces are described as anterior (sternocostal), posterior, and inferior (diaphragmatic) (see **B**).

The sternocostal surface of the heart is formed chiefly by the right ventricle, whose boundary with the left ventricle is marked by the anterior interventricular sulcus. The left ventricle (occupying the inferior and posterior cardiac surfaces) forms the left border and apex of the heart. The anterior interventricular sulcus contains the anterior interventricular branch of the left coronary artery (see p. 120) and the anterior interventricular (great cardiac) vein. Both vessels are embedded in fat and almost completely occupy the groove, so that the anterior surface of the heart appears nearly smooth. The left and right atria are separated from the ventricles by the coronary sulcus, which also transmits coronary vessels (the intrinsic vessels of the heart, see pp. 120–123). The right auricle lies at the root of the ascending aorta, the left auricle at the root of the pulmonary trunk. The origin of the right pulmonary artery from the pulmonary trunk is hidden by the ascending aorta. For clarity, all three illustrations in this series (**A**, **C**, **D**) show sites where the visceral layer of the pericardium is reflected to form the parietal layer. The pericardium extends onto the roots of the great arteries.

B Surfaces of the heart

Surface	Orientation	Cardiac chambers that form the surface (with vessels)
Anterior (sternocostal) surface	Directed anteriorly toward the posterior surface of the sternum and the ribs	• Right atrium with right auricle • Right ventricle • Small part of left ventricle with cardiac apex • Left auricle • Ascending aorta, superior vena cava, pulmonary trunk
Posterior surface	Directed posteriorly toward the posterior mediastinum	• Left atrium with termination of four pulmonary veins • Left ventricle • Part of right atrium with termination of superior and inferior venae cavae
Inferior (diaphragmatic) surface (clinically: the posterior wall)	Directed inferiorly toward the diaphragm	• Left ventricle with cardiac apex • Right ventricle • Part of right atrium with termination of inferior vena cava

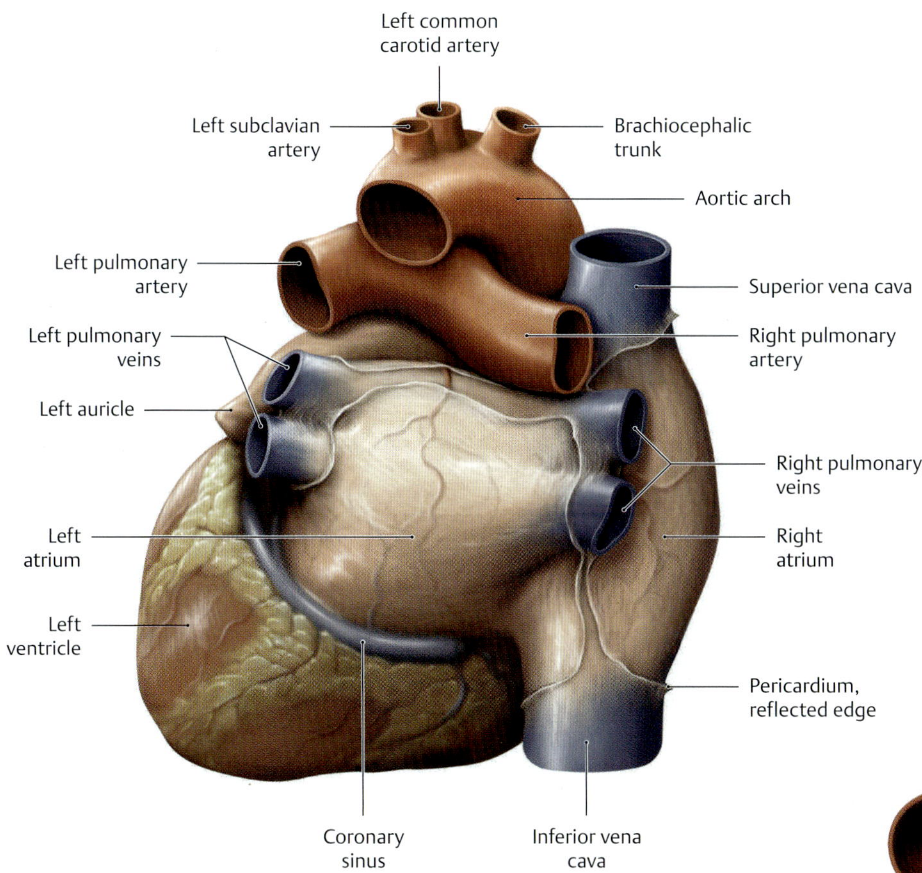

C Heart, posterior surface
Posterior view. This dissection shows how the aortic arch crosses over the pulmonary trunk at the point where the trunk divides into the left and right pulmonary arteries. At that site the aorta gives off the three major arteries to the upper limbs, neck, and head: the brachiocephalic trunk, left common carotid artery, and left subclavian artery. This view also clearly shows the terminations of the pulmonary veins (usually four in number) in the *left* atrium and the terminations of the two venae cavae in the *right* atrium. Note also the coronary sinus in the posterior part of the coronary sulcus, which runs between the left ventricle and left atrium. This sinus is the collecting vessel for venous blood returned from the heart by the cardiac veins.

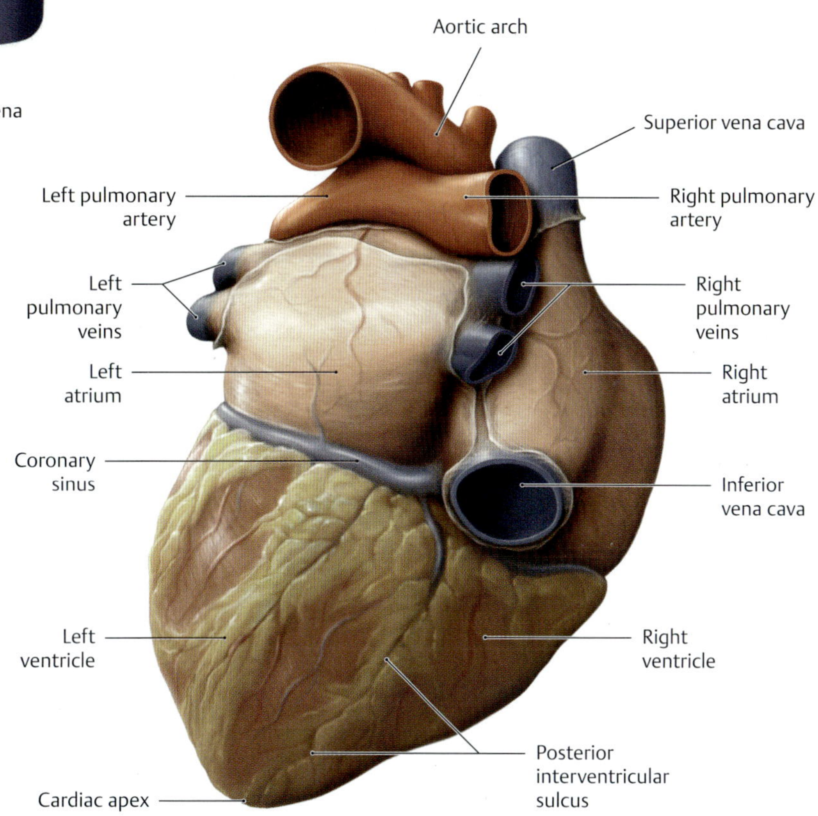

D Heart, diaphragmatic surface
Posteroinferior view. The heart is tilted forward to give a better view of its diaphragmatic surface, which is formed by both ventricles and the right atrium with the termination of the inferior vena cava. If the heart were viewed from below, from the perspective of the diaphragm (not shown here), it would be obvious that both venae cavae are in alignment: Looking into the inferior vena cava, one can see through the terminal part of the superior vena cava.

E Structure of the cardiac wall

Layer	Location	Composition
Endocardium	Innermost layer, lines the cavities of the heart and lines the cusps and pockets of the cardiac valves	Single layer of epithelial cells with a subendothelial layer composed of collagen and elastic fibers; both layers are continuous with the intima of the vessels
Myocardium	Middle layer and thickest part of the heart wall; motor for the pumping action of the heart (see pp. 102 and 103)	Complex arrangement of muscle fibers
Epicardium	Outermost layer of the heart wall; part of the pericardium (see p. 98), forming its visceral layer	Serous membrane (single layer of epithelial cells with underlying layer of connective tissue)

3.4 Structure of the Heart Musculature (Myocardium)

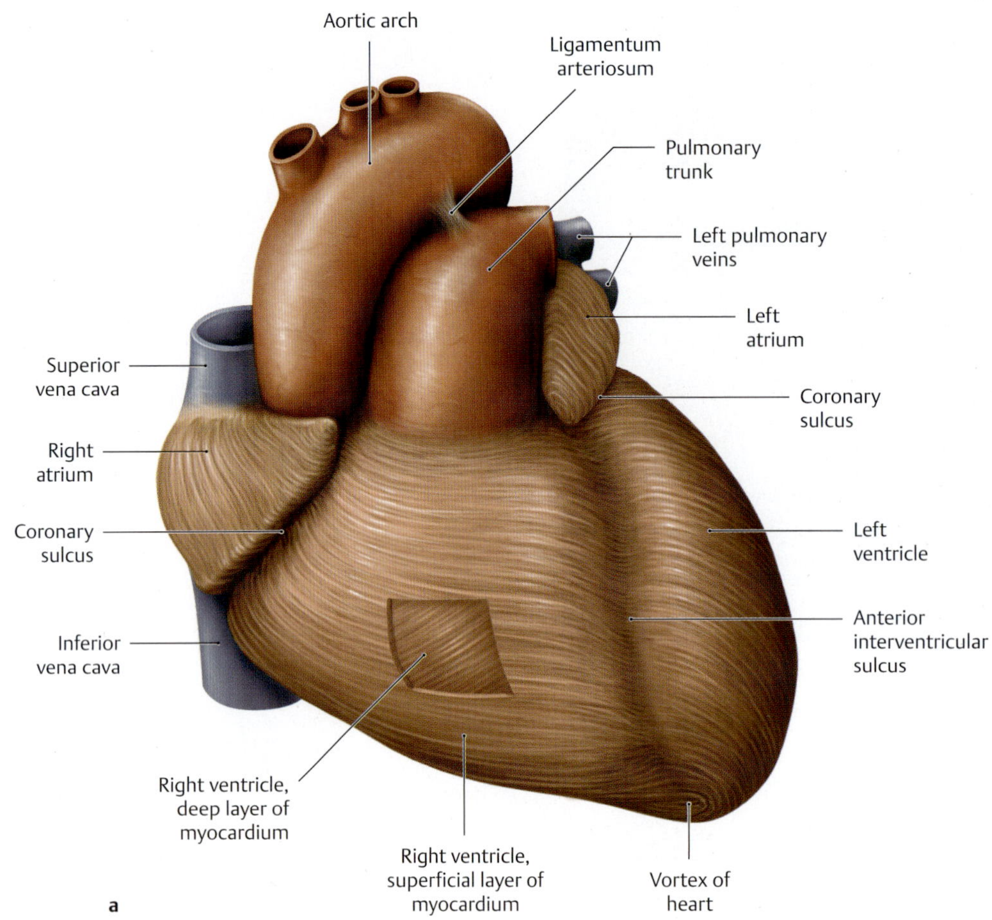

a

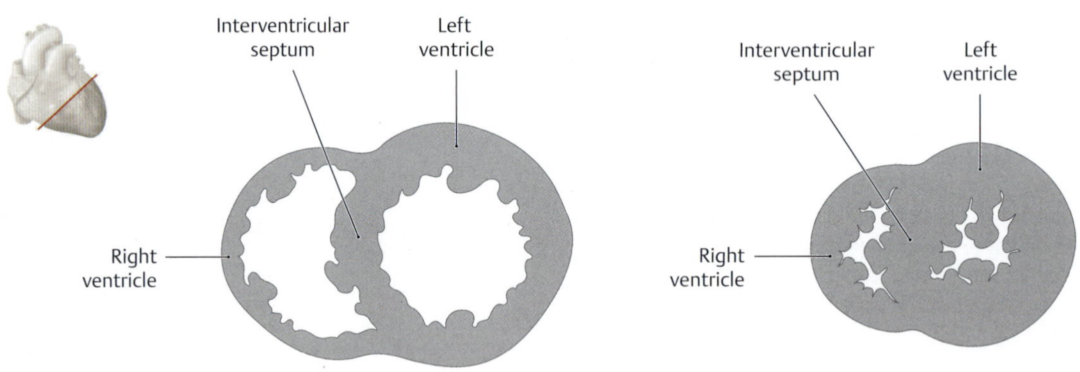

c

A Myocardial architecture

a, b External musculature of the heart, simplified anteroinferior view. The muscular walls of the right and left ventricles have been windowed to display the deeper fibers.

Note: The epicardium has been removed in **a** and **b** along with the subepicardial fat. The coronary vessels are not shown in order to display more clearly the cardiac surface grooves (anterior and posterior interventricular sulci).

The **musculature of the atria** is arranged in two layers, superficial and deep. The superficial layer (shown here) extends over the atria and is common to both, whereas each atrium has its own deep layer. Looped and annular muscle fibers extend down to the atrioventricular boundary and also encircle the venous orifices. The **ventricular musculature** has a complex arrangement, consisting basically of a superficial (subepicardial), middle, and deep (subendocardial) layer. The superficial layer joins apically with the deeper layers to form a whorled arrangement of muscle fibers around the cardiac apex (vortex of the heart). The right ventricle, which is a low-pressure system (see **c**), is less muscular than the left and almost completely lacks a middle layer. The subendocardial layer forms the trabeculae carneae and papillary muscles (see **d** and p. 109).

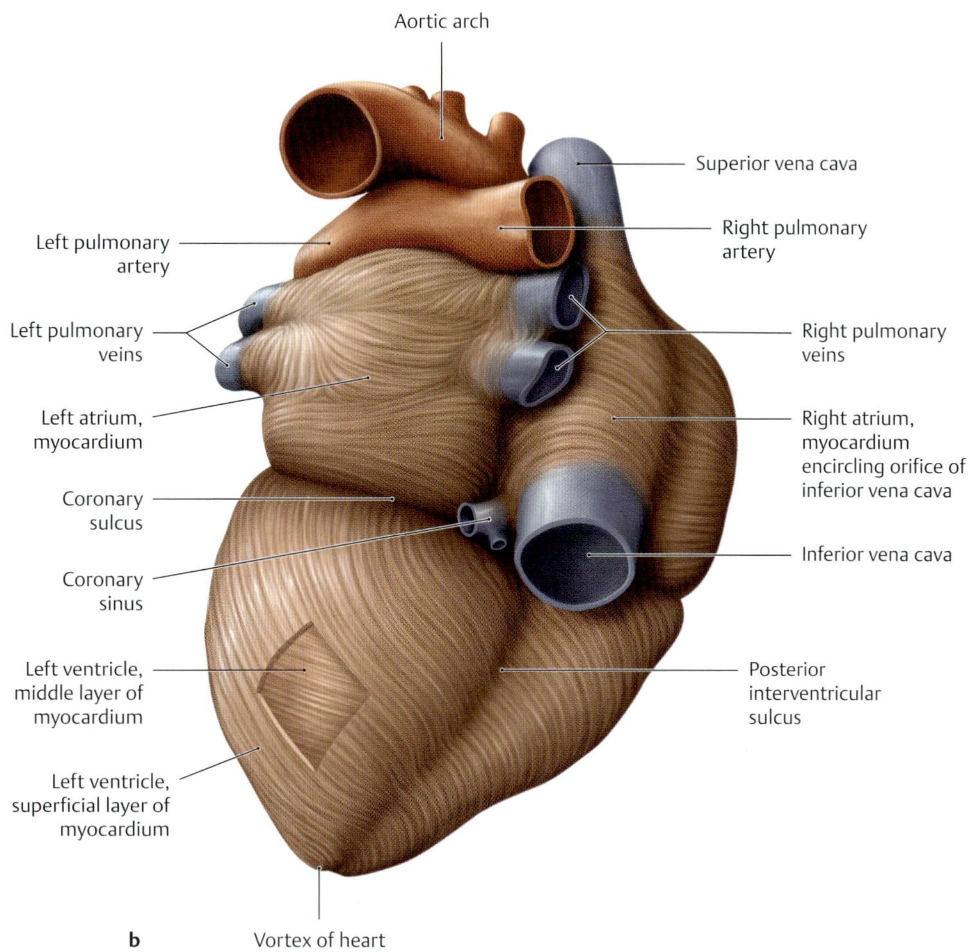

b

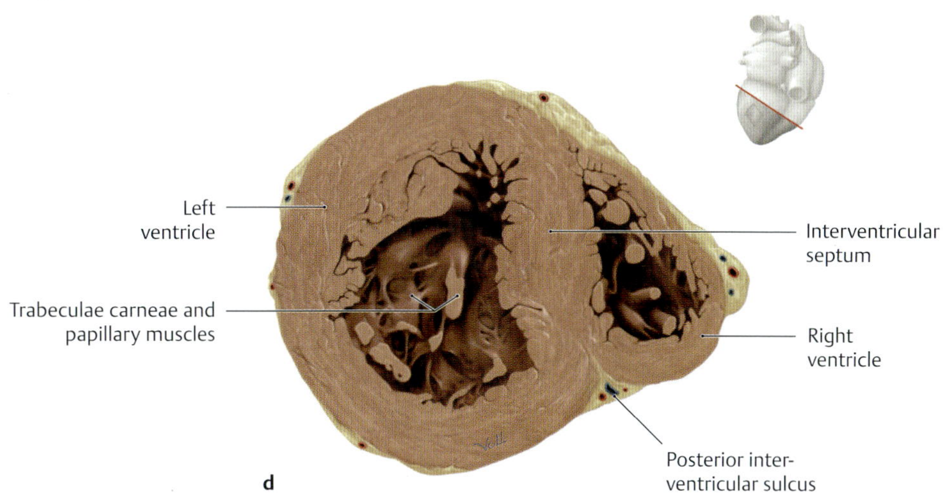

d

The histological unit of the myocardium is the cardiac myocyte, a specialized form of cardiac muscle cell. Unlike their electronically isolated counterparts in skeletal muscle, cardiac myocytes form a syncytium in which membrane depolarization and contraction spread in a wave.

c, d Myocardial axial cross-section perpendicular to the long axis of the heart, viewed from above. **c** Schematic representation: The ventricles in an expanded state (diastole, left figure), and in a contracted state (systole, right figure). **d** Transverse section through a specimen during diastole.

All the sections clearly demonstrate the difference in thickness between the left and right ventricular myocardia: As the left ventricle must generate a significantly higher pressure than the right ventricle when contracting (the left ventricle is part of the high-pressure system during systole), its myocardium is visibly thicker than that of the right ventricle (see **c**), which is always part of the low-pressure system. By comparison, systolic pressure in the left ventricle is 120–140 mmHg, and in the right ventricle 25–30 mmHg.

3.5 Cardiac Chambers

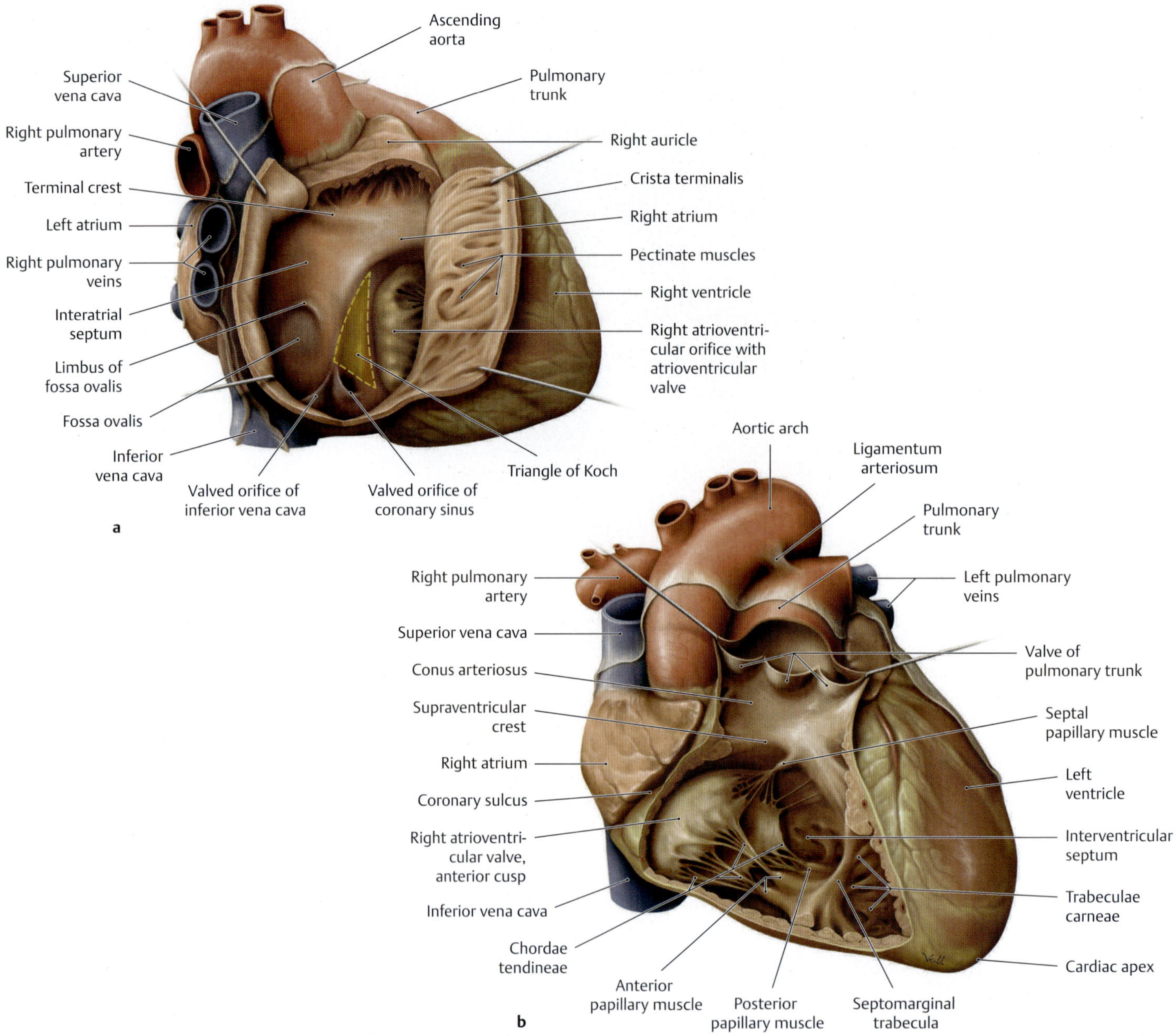

A Chambers of the right heart

a Right view of the atrium. **b** Anterior view of the ventricle. The ventricular and atrial walls have been opened widely, and the heart wall has been cut open to display the internal chambers.

The **right atrium** (see **a**) consists of

- the anterior segment, which comprises the actual atrium with the auricle, and
- the posterior segment with the sinus of the vena cava (not visible here). It bears the orifices of the superior and inferior venae cavae.

The orifice of the coronary sinus, the margin of the septal portion of the tricuspid valve, and the tendon of Todaro define what is known as the *triangle of Koch*, an area on the wall of the right atrium. This is the location of the atrioventricular node. A small valve at the orifice of the inferior vena cava (valve of the inferior vena cava) directs blood in the *prenatal* circulation through the foramen ovale in the interatrial septum. The foramen ovale is sealed shut *postnatally*, becoming the fossa ovalis (surrounded by a rounded margin, the limbus). The orifice of the coronary sinus also bears a small crescent-shaped valve (valve of the coronary sinus). The anterior segment, which comprises the actual atrium with the auricle, is separated from the posterior segment by a ridge, the *crista terminalis*. Small muscular trabeculae, the pectinate muscles, arise from this ridge, giving this segment an irregular wall texture. In contrast, the wall of the posterior segment is smooth.

The **right ventricle** is characterized by two muscular ridges, the supraventricular crest and the septomarginal trabecula. It is also divided into two sections:

- the *inflow tract* posteroinferiorly (with the heart positioned in situ) and
- the *outflow tract* anterosuperiorly (see also p. 119).

The muscular ridges of the trabeculae carneae are visible on the wall of the ventricular inflow tract. Specialized extensions of the trabeculae, the papillary muscles, are attached to the cusps of the right atrioventricular valve by collagenous cords, the chordae tendineae (see p. 109). The *outflow tract* is cone shaped and consists mainly of the conus arteriosus, which has a smooth wall. The right ventricular outflow tract expels blood into the pulmonary trunk, whose orifice is guarded by the pulmonary valve. The wall of the right ventricle is relatively thin (low-pressure system). All of the cardiac chambers are lined with endocardium.

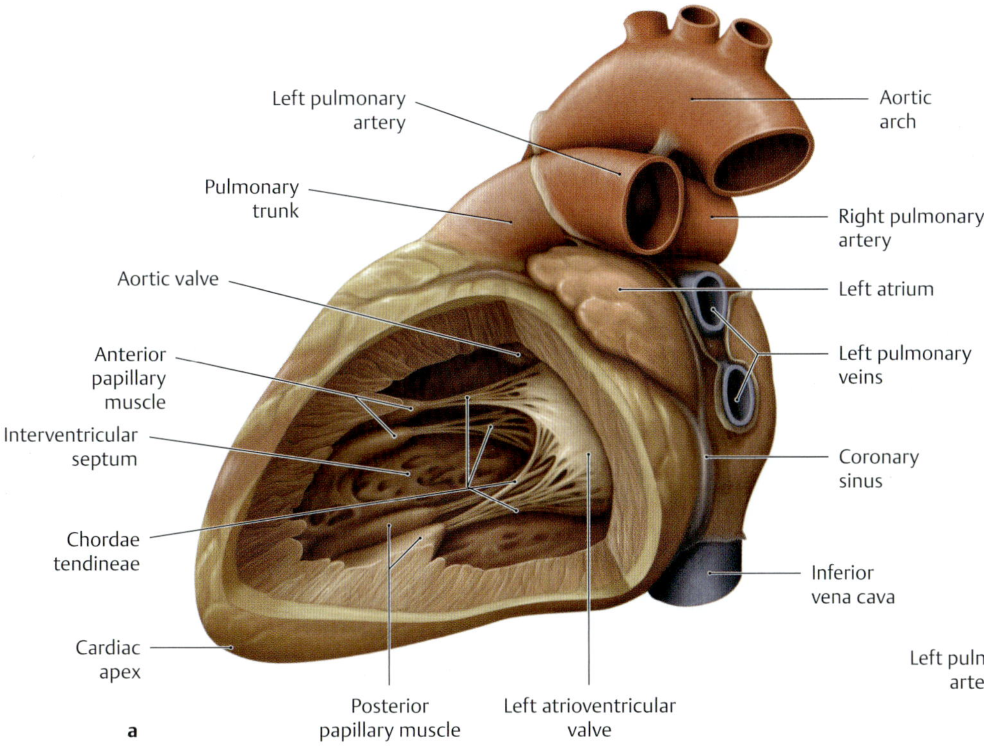

a

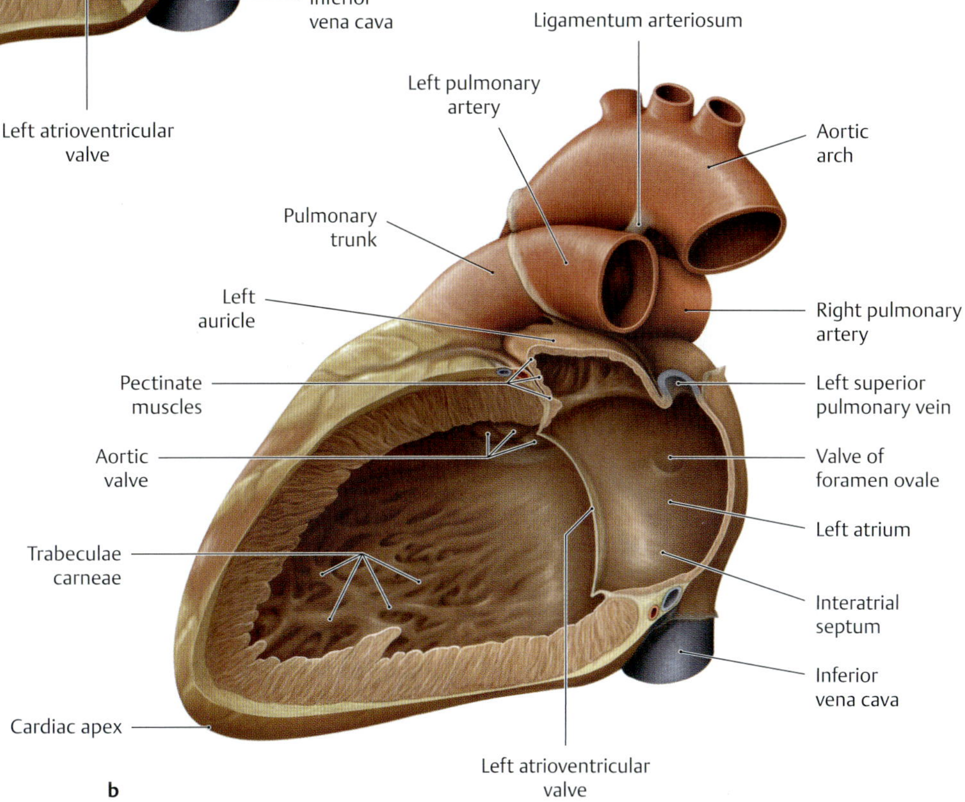

b

B Chambers of the left heart

Left lateral view. **a** Ventricle, **b** ventricle and atrium. The ventricular and atrial walls have been opened.

The **left atrium** is smaller than the right (see **Aa**). Its muscular wall is thin (low-pressure system) and is smooth in areas derived embryologically from the orifices of the pulmonary veins. The rest of the atrium is lined by pectinate muscles. The pulmonary veins, usually four in number, terminate in the left atrium. Occasionally a narrow tissue fold (valve of the foramen ovale) is found on the interatrial septum, formed by a protrusion of the fossa ovalis into the left atrium. It marks the site of fusion between the embryonic septum primum and septum secundum.

The **left ventricle** has an inflow tract and outflow tract. The *inflow tract* begins at the left atrioventricular orifice, which is guarded by the left atrioventricular valve (see p. 107). As in the right ventricle, the wall of the left ventricular inflow tract is studded with trabeculae carneae, and papillary muscles are attached by chordae tendineae to the left atrioventricular valve. The *outflow tract* of the left ventricle has smooth inner walls and lies close to the interventricular septum. It leads to the aorta and is capped by the aortic valve at the root of the ascending aorta (see p. 107). The interventricular septum consists largely of muscle tissue (muscular part), and only a small portion near the aorta consists entirely of connective tissue (membranous part). The placement of the interventricular septum between the cardiac chambers is marked externally by the anterior and posterior interventricular sulci on the cardiac surface. The muscular wall of the left ventricle is significantly thicker than that of the right one, having approximately three times its thickness (see p. 102, Fig. **Ac**). The chambers of the left (and right) heart are lined by endocardium.

3.6 Overview of the Cardiac Valves (Valve Plane and Cardiac Skeleton)

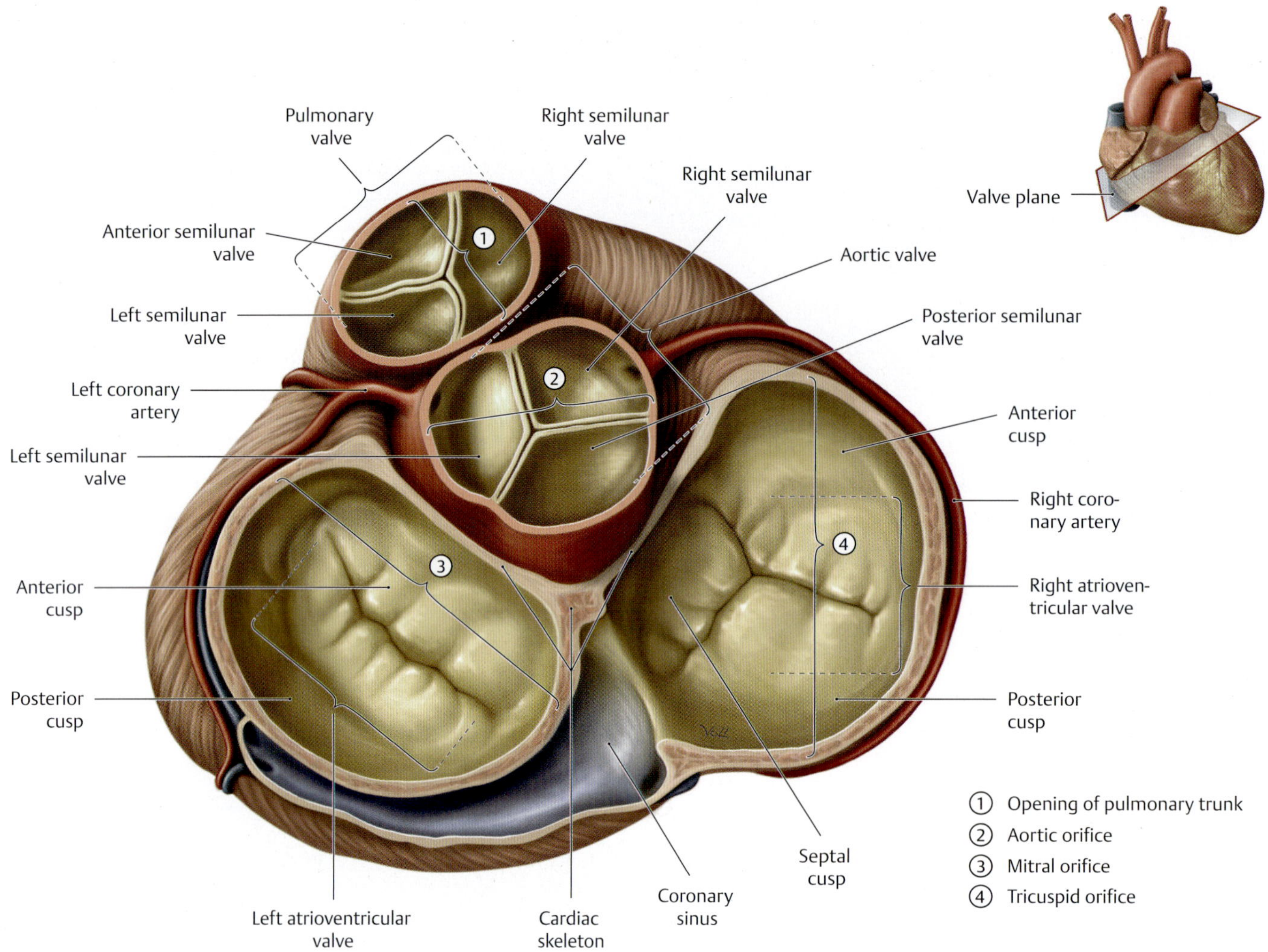

A Overview of the cardiac valves

Plane of the cardiac valves viewed from above. The atria have been removed, and the great arteries have been transected at their roots. The cardiac valves are classified into two types—atrioventricular and semilunar. All heart valves lie in a plane, the valve plane. The cardiac valves function as one-way valves. They ensure the unidirectional flow of blood between the atria and ventricles (left and right atrioventricular valves), and out of the heart (aortic and pulmonary valves).

Atrioventricular valves. Located between the atria and ventricles, the left and right atrioventricular valves are composed of thin, avascular connective tissue covered by endocardium. They are classified mechanically as *sail valves* (see **B**) because the chordae tendineae (see **C**) constrain the movement of each cusp like the tethering ropes on a sail. The function of these valves is to prevent the reflux of blood from the ventricles into the atria.

- The *left atrioventricular valve* has two cusps (*bicuspid valve*): an anterior cusp (anteromedial) and a posterior cusp (posterolateral). The anterior cusp is continuous with the wall of the aorta. The alternate term *mitral valve* is derived from the two major cusps, which are similar in shape to a bishop's miter. Subdivisions in the lateral margins of the otherwise smooth valve have led some anatomists to describe small accessory cusps called the commissural cusps (usually two). These are not true cusps, however, and are not connected to the fibrous anulus of the cardiac skeleton (see **B**). The cusps are tethered by papillary muscles (see **C**).
- The *right atrioventricular valve* has three cusps (tricuspid valve): anterior, posterior, and septal. One or two small accessory cusps may also be found; they do not extend to the fibrous anulus.

Semilunar valves. These valves have three crescent-shaped cusps of approximately equal size placed at the orifices of the pulmonary trunk (pulmonary valve) and aorta (aortic valve). Like the atrioventricular valves, they are composed of thin connective tissue covered by endocardium and seal the aortic orifice and the opening of the pulmonary trunk. The semilunar valves are classified mechanically as *pocket valves* because their cusps pouch into the ventricle like bulging pockets. The wall of the aorta and pulmonary trunk show slight dilations just above the valve (the pulmonary and aortic sinuses). The aortic sinuses expand the cross-section of the aorta, forming the aortic bulb. The right and left coronary arteries branch off the base of the aorta just past the aortic valve (see pp. 120–123 for details).

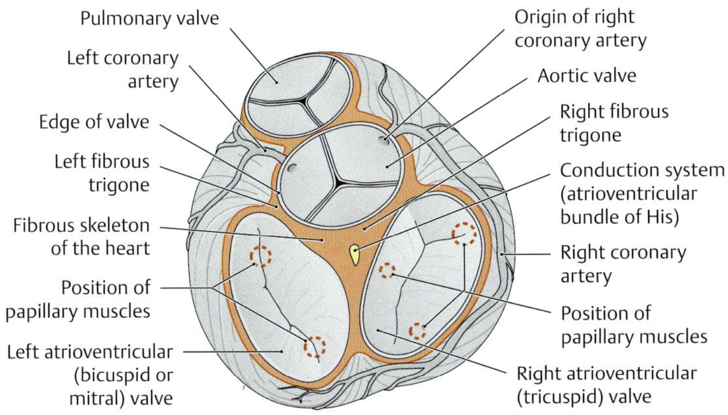

B Skeleton of the heart

The skeleton of the heart is a layer of connective tissue (often with considerable fat) that completely separates the myocardium of the ventricles from that of the atria. The components of the cardiac skeleton in a *narrow sense* are as follows:

- The right and left fibrous anuli and intervening fibrous trigones
- The fibrous ring of the aortic valve, which is connected to both fibrous anuli
- The membranous part of the interventricular septum (not shown here).

In a *broad sense*, the fibrous ring of the pulmonary valve also contributes to the cardiac skeleton. It is connected by a collagenous band (tendon of infundibulum) to the fibrous ring of the aortic valve. The atrioventricular valves are anchored to the fibrous anuli, while the semilunar valves are each attached by connective tissue to their valvular fibrous rings. Thus, the cardiac skeleton in the broad sense provides a mechanical framework for all the cardiac valves. Besides *mechanically stabilizing* the heart, the fibrous skeleton also functions as an *electrical insulator* between the atria and ventricles. The electrical impulses that stimulate cardiac contractions (see p. 116f) can pass from the atrium to the ventricles only through the bundle of His, and there is only one opening in the fibrous skeleton (in the right fibrous trigone) which transmits that bundle.

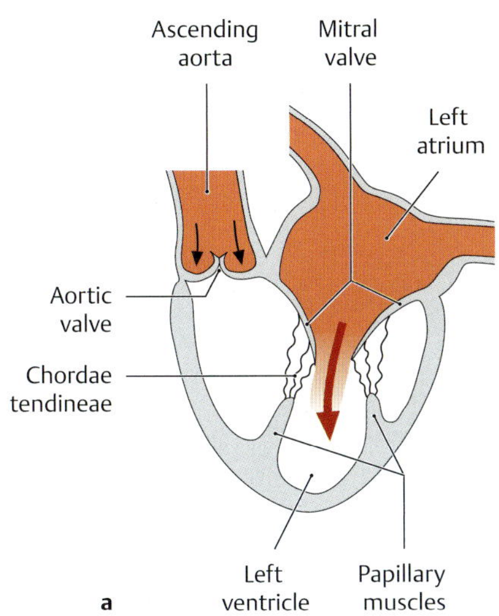

a

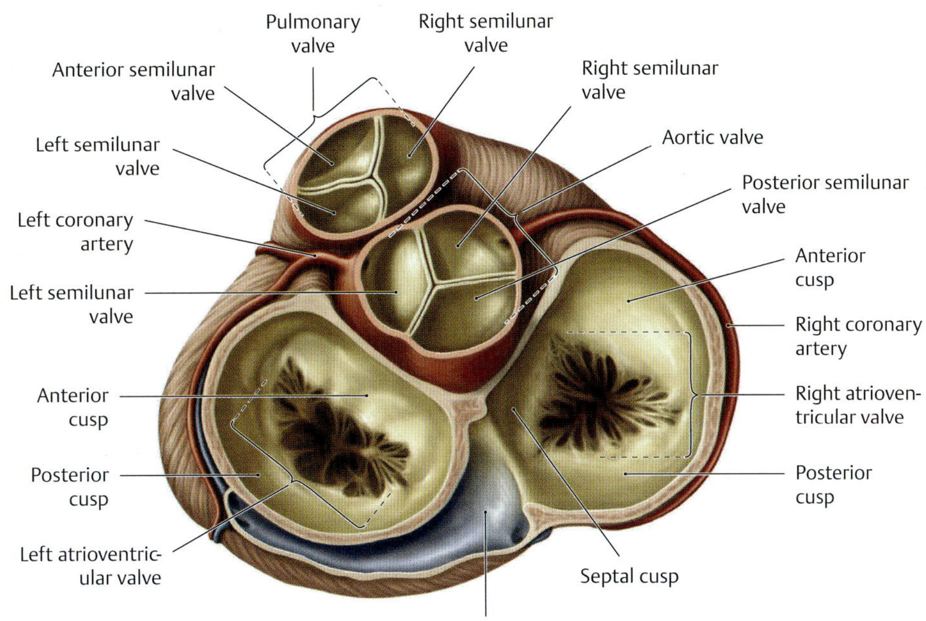

b

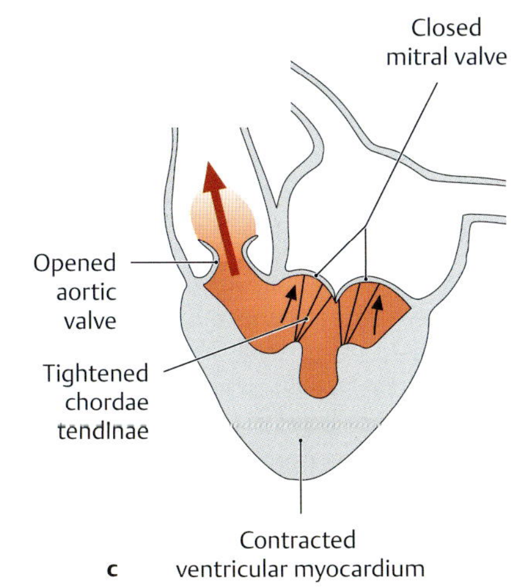

c

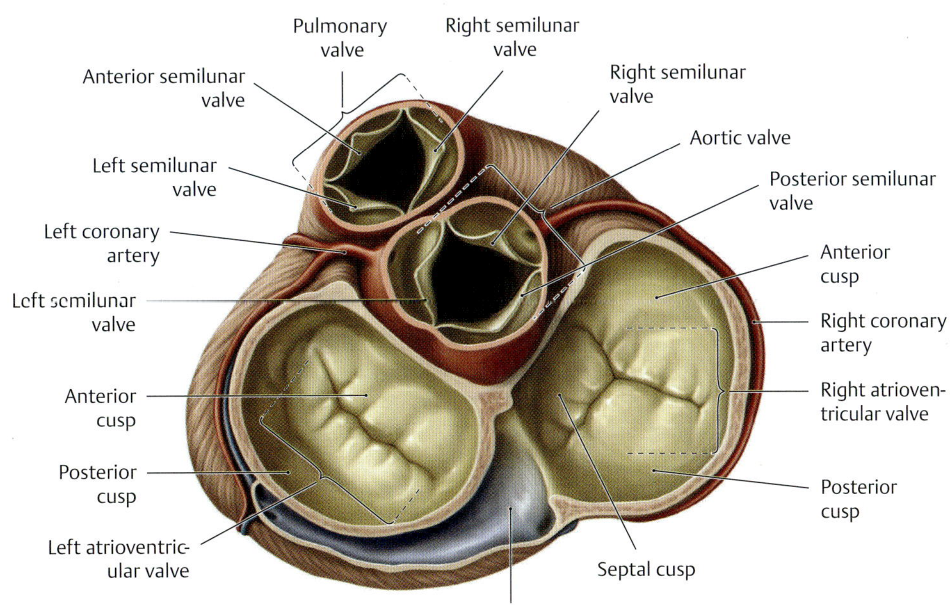

a

C Function of the heart valves during the cardiac cycle

a and **b** Ventricular diastole; **c** and **d** Ventricular systole. **a** and **c** Direction of blood flow in the left heart; **b** and **d** Valve plane viewed from above.

3.7 Cardiac Valves and Auscultation Sites

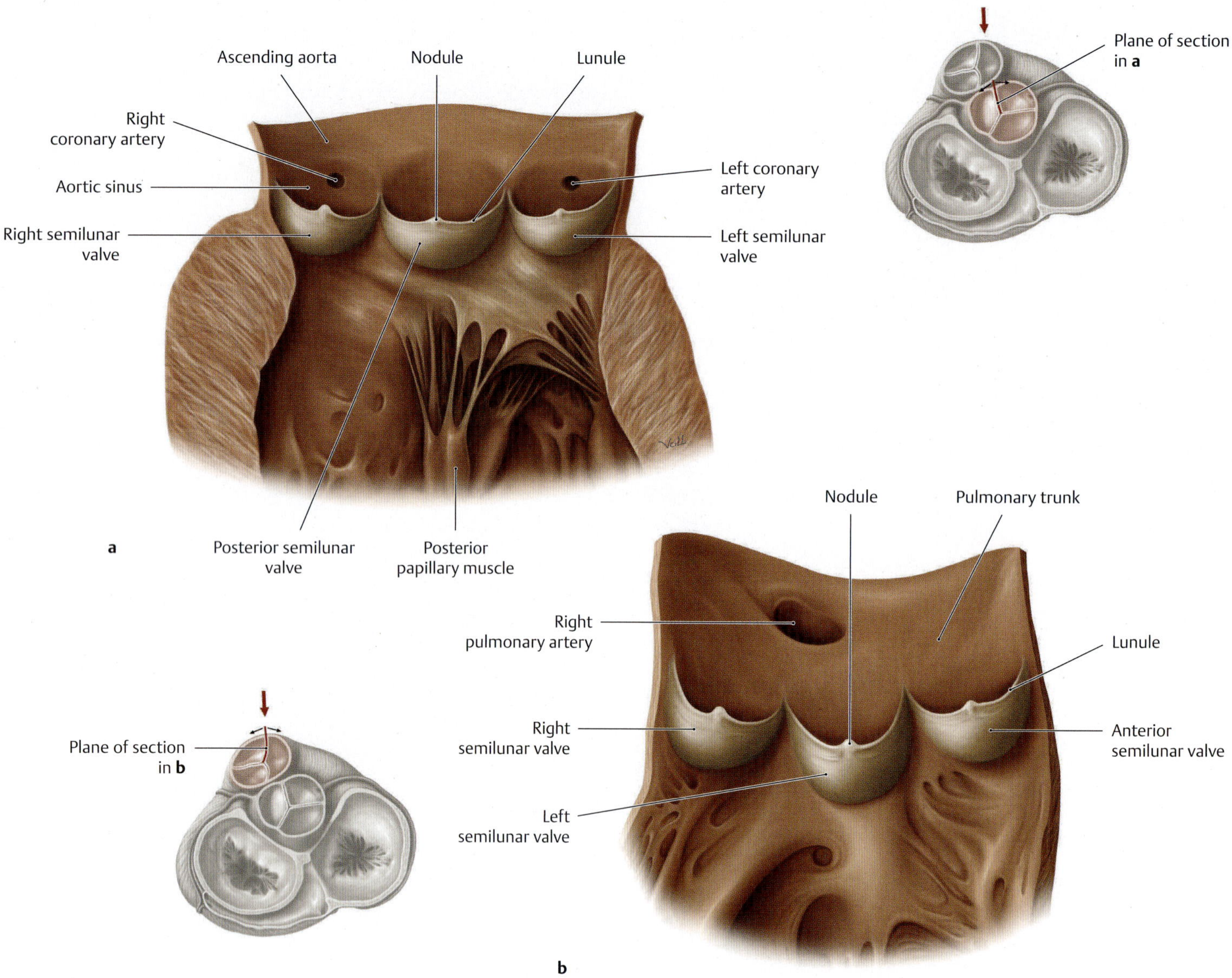

A Semilunar valves of the outflow tracts (aortic and pulmonary valve)

The aortic valve (**a**) and pulmonary valve (**b**) have been displayed by cutting open the ascending aorta and pulmonary trunk and opening them up like a book. The aortic valve and pulmonary valve close the ventricular outflow tracts during diastole:

- The aortic valve closes the left ventricular outflow tract.
- The pulmonary valve closes the right ventricular outflow tract.

These valves almost completely prevent the regurgitation of blood expelled by the ventricles. The origins of the left and right coronary arteries can be clearly identified in the aortic sinuses past the semilunar cusps (**a**), and the origin of the right pulmonary artery can be identified in the pulmonary trunk (**b**). The free margin of each semilunar cusp is thickened centrally to form a valvular nodule, and on each side of the nodule is a fine rim called the lunule. The nodule and lunule ensure that the margins of the cusps appose tightly and completely during valve closure. Both the atrioventricular valves (see p. 106) and the semilunar valves may undergo pathological changes, usually due to inflammation (endocarditis). Inflammation may result in secondary vascularization of the initially avascular valves, causing them to undergo fibrotic changes that stiffen the valves and compromise their function. There are two main abnormalities of valvular mechanics, which may coexist in the same valve:

- Valvular stenosis: *Opening* of the valve is impaired, causing a reduction of blood flow across the valve. Usually this creates a pressure overload on the chamber proximal to the obstruction.
- Valvular insufficiency: *Closure* of the valve is impaired, allowing blood to regurgitate into the chamber proximal to the valve. Such a pathological reflux creates a volume overload on the affected cardiac segments. When the load exceeds a certain magnitude, surgical replacement of the valve may be necessary to prevent further damage to the heart.
- Stenosis and insufficiency may coexist: A valve may become stuck in an intermediate position, unable to open or close completely.

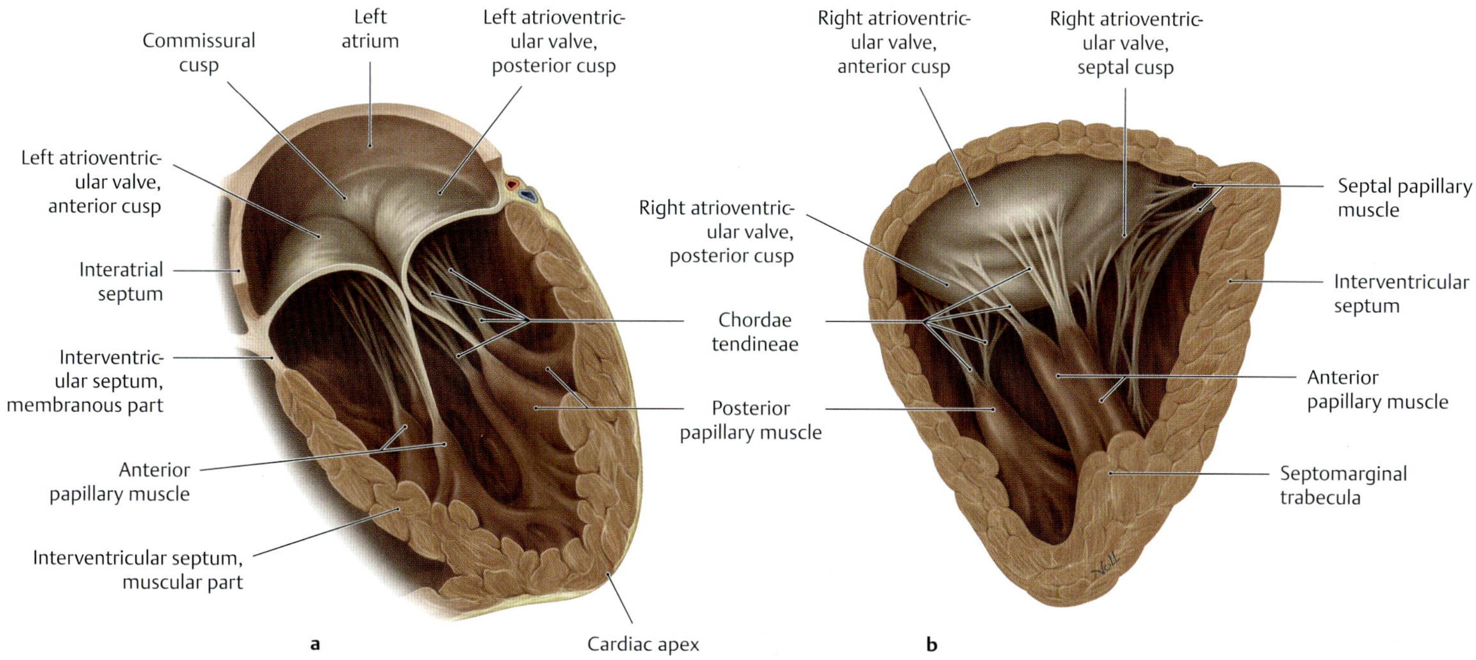

B Atrioventricular valves and papillary muscles

Anterior view of the left (**a**) and right (**b**) atrioventricular valves. The drawings represent a very early phase of ventricular contraction in which the atrioventricular valves have just closed. The papillary muscles are clearly displayed. There are *three* papillary muscles for the *three* cusps of the right atrioventricular valve (anterior, posterior, and septal papillary muscles) and *two* papillary muscles for the *two* cusps of the left atrioventricular valve (anterior and posterior papillary muscles). The papillary muscles (specialized extensions of the trabeculae carneae) are attached to the free margins of the valve cusps by tendinous cords (the chordae tendineae). When the papillary muscles contract (valve closure), the chordae tendineae are shortened to restrict the motion of the valve cusps. This keeps the cusps from opening into the atria during ventricular contraction (systole), thereby preventing the regurgitation of blood back into the atria.

Note: Like other myocardial regions, the myocardium of the papillary muscles may suffer necrosis due to a myocardial infarction, leaving the corresponding cusp prone to prolapse into the atrium. Conversely, pathological shortening of the chordae may also prevent the valve from closing completely. This also would allow blood to regurgitate into the atrium during ventricular systole, producing an audible heart murmur (see p. 118).

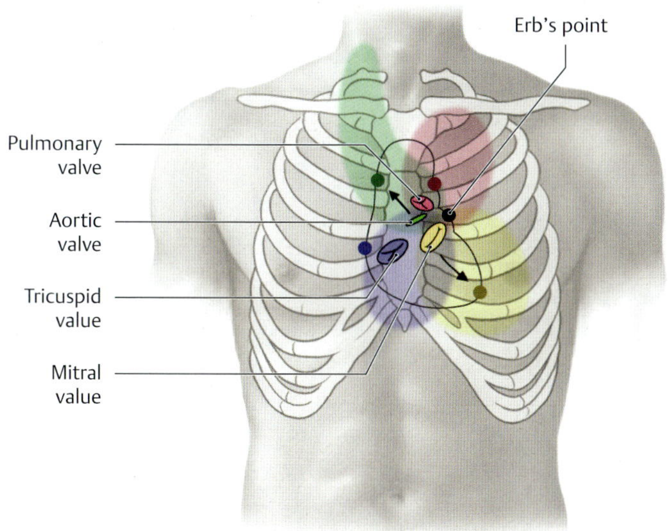

C Auscultation of the cardiac valves

The diagram shows the anatomical projection of the valves onto the thorax and the auscultation sites (the areas to which abnormal heart murmurs of the respective valves are transmitted). In the healthy heart, blood does not generate a perceptible sound as it flows across the cardiac valves (see p. 118 for the physiologic heart sounds). But if the valves are functionally impaired as a result of disease, the blood flow at the cardiac valves becomes turbulent. This type of flow produces audible sounds that are transmitted via the bloodstream. As the thick cardiac wall muffles these sounds, they are not heard best over the anatomical projections of the valves on the chest wall, but are heard more clearly at sites located downstream from the valves (see **D**).

D Anatomical projections and auscultation sites of the cardiac valves

Valve	Anatomical projection	Auscultation site
Aortic valve	Left sternal border at the level of the third intercostal space	Right second intercostal space close to the sternum
Pulmonary valve	Left sternal border at the level of the third rib	Left second intercostal space close to the sternum
Right atrioventricular valve (tricuspid valve)	Sternum at the level of the fifth rib	Right fourth intercostal space close to the sternum*
Left atrioventricular valve (mitral valve)	Left fourth or fifth rib	Left fifth intercostal space in the midclavicular line

* The left lower sternal border is also a common site for auscultation of the right atrioventricular valve.

3.8 Radiographic Appearance of the Heart

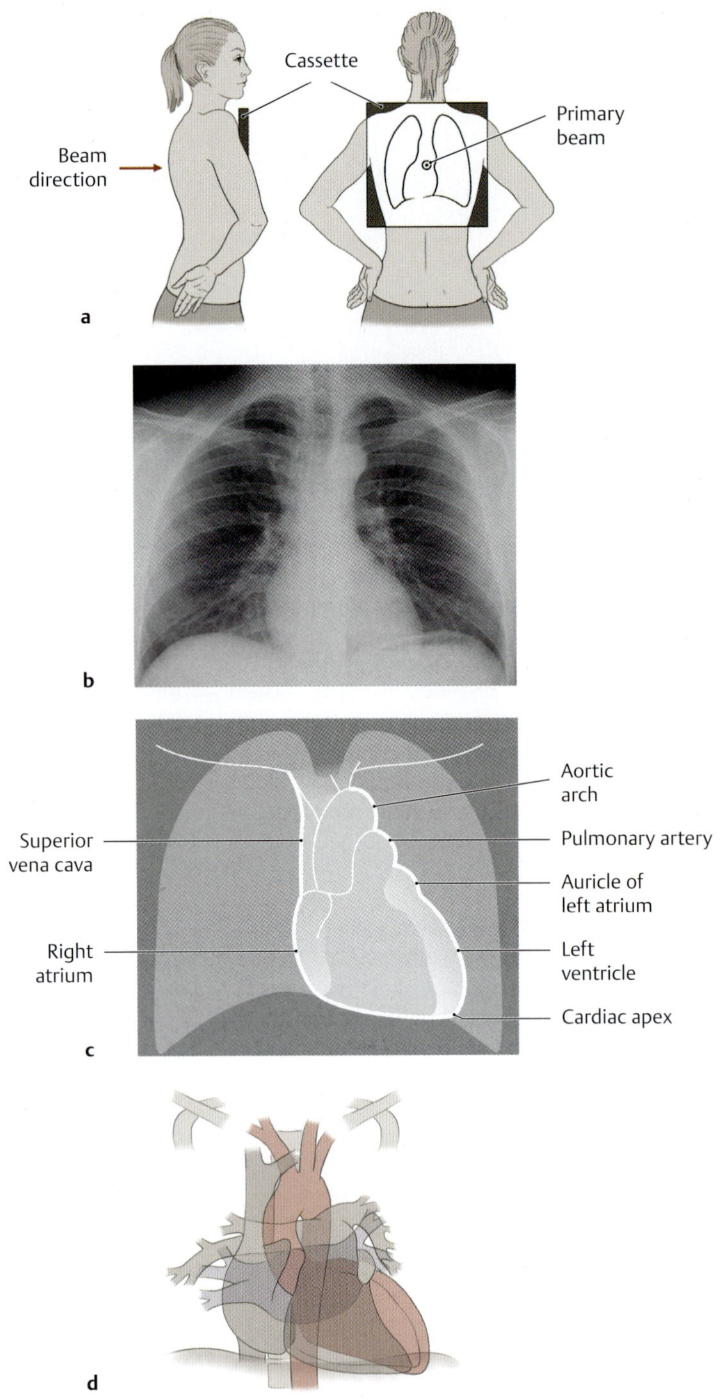

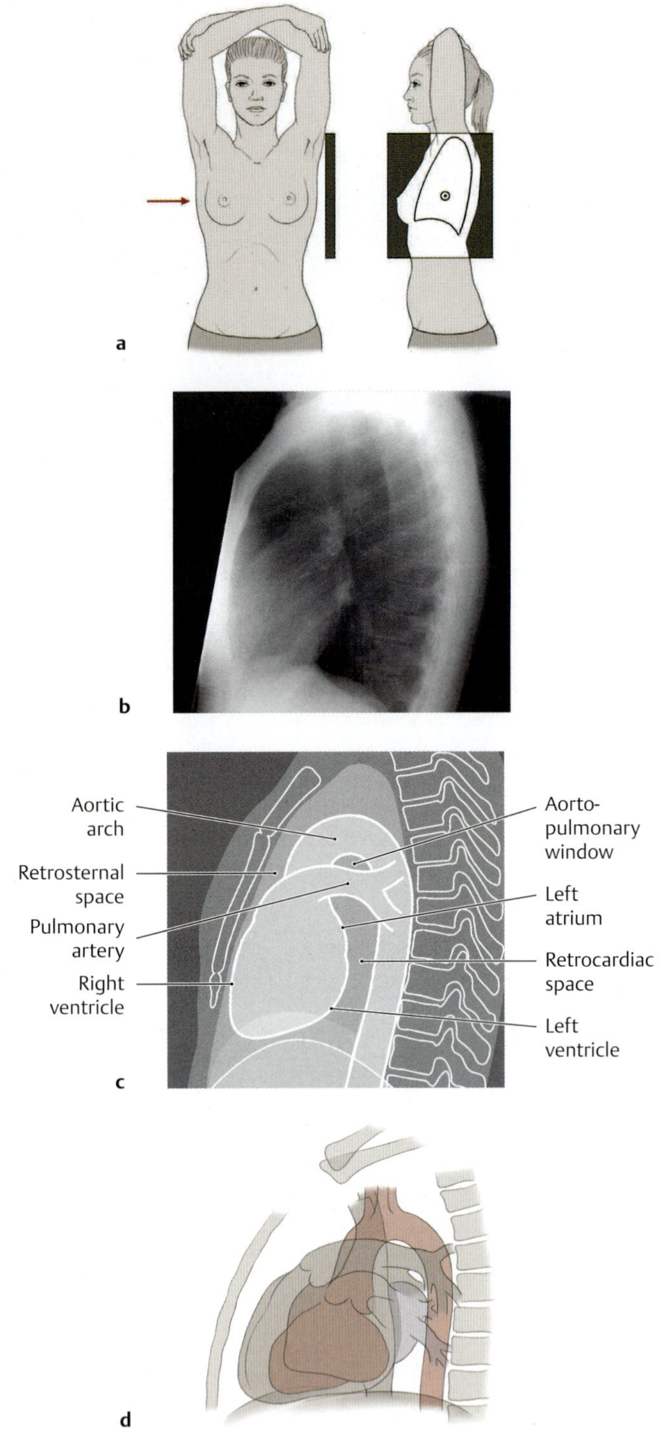

A Posterior-anterior (PA) chest radiograph

a The patient stands with the anterior chest wall on the cassette (the beam "passes" through the patient in a posterior-to-anterior direction with the central beam targeted at the level of the 6th thoracic vertebra). The radiographs are taken with the patient keeping their mouth open, breathing in and holding their breath. The back of the hands are placed on the hips with the elbows turned forward;

b Posterior-anterior radiograph (viewed from an anterior to posterior direction);

c Heart shadow (cardiac silhouette) with structures that form the cardiac borders;

d Topography of the cardiac shadow: right heart with inflow and outflow tract (gray); left ventricle with outflow tract (red), left atrium with inflow tract (blue).

B Lateral chest radiograph

a The patient is standing with his or her left side against the cassette (thus preventing the appearance of an enlarged heart), with the arms raised and crossed above the head. The central beam is targeted a hand's width below the left armpit;

b Left lateral radiograph;

c Heart shadow with structures that form the cardiac borders;

d Topography of the cardiac shadow: right heart with inflow and outflow tract (gray); left ventricle with outflow tract (red), left atrium with inflow tract (blue).

(Radiographs on this page from: Reiser M, Kuhn F, Debus J, eds. *Duale Reihe Radiologie*. 4th ed. Stuttgart: Thieme; 2017.)

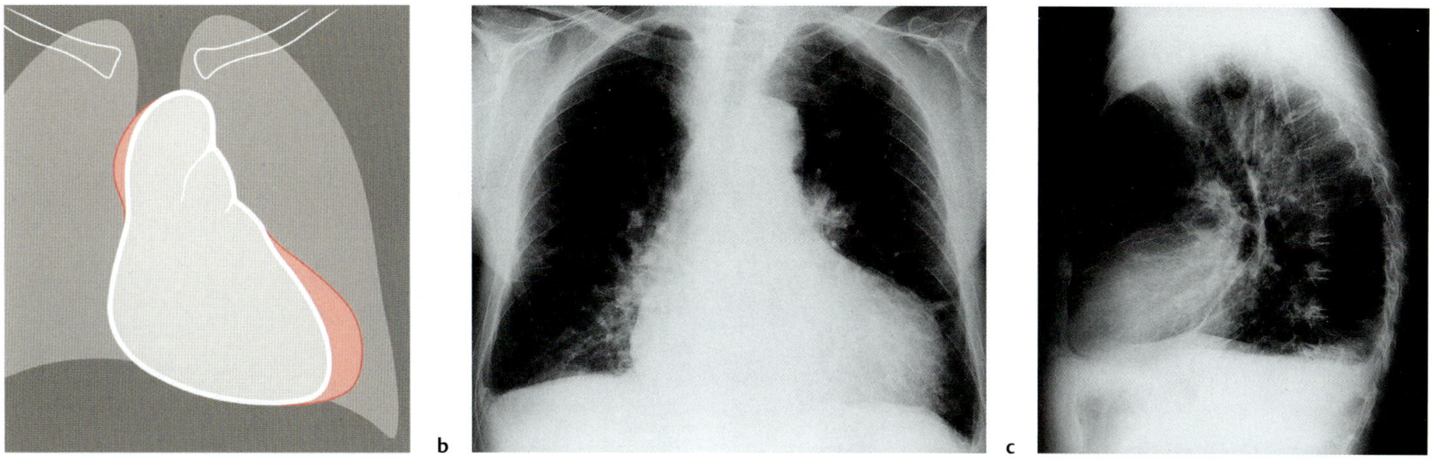

C Conventional diagnostic radiography in aortic valve insufficiency

a Schematic diagram of the heart showing altered cardiac silhouette. *Note* the left ventricular enlargement and the dilation of the ascending aorta due to increased blood volume.

b Posteroanterior (PA) radiograph showing a significantly increased cardiac shadow on the left side and rounding of the apex of the heart. *Note* the demarcating structures in the right superior mediastinal region in the form of an elongated aortic arch instead of the superior vena cava.

c Left lateral radiograph showing significant narrowing of the retrocardial space (see **Bc**).

(Radiographs from: Reiser M, Kuhn F, Debus J, eds. *Duale Reihe Radiologie*. 4th ed. Stuttgart: Thieme; 2017.)

Aortic valve insufficiency results when there is damage to the aortic valve or its root such as can occur in endocarditis. The aortic valve then no longer closes completely (for the function of the cardiac valves, see p. 107). This causes retrograde blood flow back into the left ventricle in the diastolic phase, forcing the ventricle to constantly take in additional blood. This in turn leads to compensatory ventricular enlargement. On clinical examination, valve insufficiency manifests itself as high blood pressure amplitude (high systolic and low diastolic blood pressure; typical diastolic decrescendo murmur). Aortic valve insufficiency may be acute or chronic. Chronic insufficiency occurs primarily in older men (about 70 years and older) and often only becomes symptomatic in the late stage as dyspnea and decreased exercise tolerance. Echocardiography (transthoracic echocardiography or TTE) is the gold standard for confirming the diagnosis.

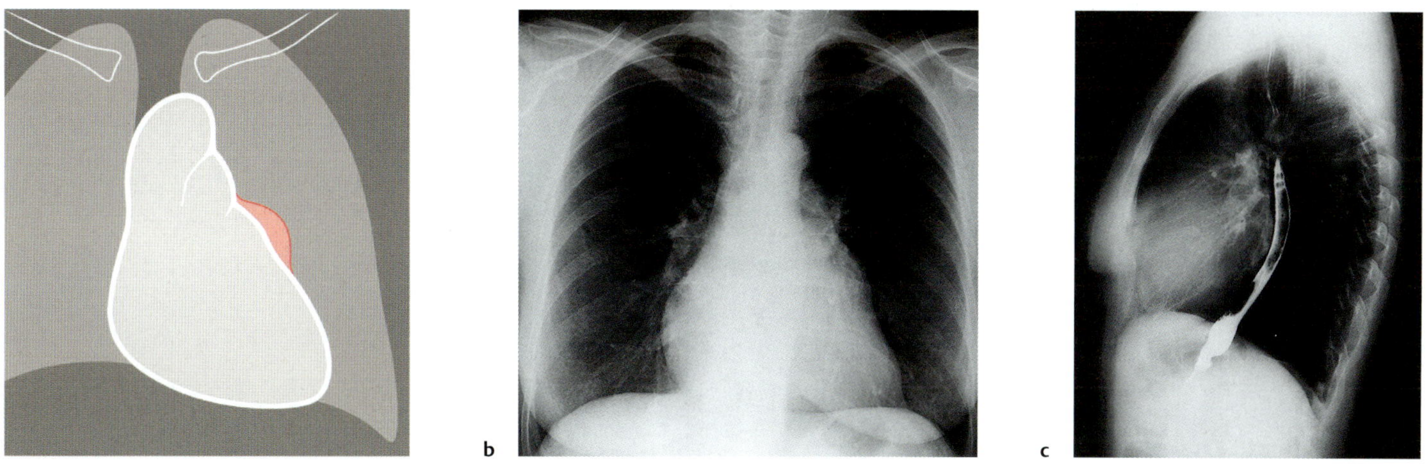

D Conventional diagnostic radiography in mitral valve stenosis

a Schematic diagram of the heart. *Note* the characteristically altered cardiac silhouette with significant enlargement of the demarcating structure at the level of the left atrial appendage (corresponds to the level of the left atrium, shown here in red).

b Posteroanterior (PA) radiograph.

c Left lateral radiograph obtained after a barium swallow to visualize the esophagus and indirectly the left atrium as well. Enlargement of the atrium displaces the esophagus posteriorly, narrowing the retrocardial space.

(Radiographs from: Reiser M, Kuhn F, Debus J, eds. *Duale Reihe Radiologie*. 4th ed. Stuttgart: Thieme; 2017.)

Mitral valve stenosis typically occurs in the setting of rheumatic fever (streptococcal disorder) and leads to calcification of the margins of the valve leaflets with the following effects:

- The area of the opened valve is reduced (in high-grade stenosis down to < 1 cm^2!).
- This means that less and less blood reaches the left ventricle, producing a typical diastolic decrescendo murmur.
- The left atrium becomes enlarged as blood from the pulmonary circuit constantly flows in and progressively less flows out into the left ventricle.

The compensatory atrial enlargement often masks the mitral valve stenosis, and patients may be subjectively asymptomatic for years. The condition becomes symptomatic when the impeded blood flow backs up into the lung. This results in sudden dyspnea with progressively decreased exercise tolerance. Additionally, the atrial enlargement often leads to atrial fibrillation with increased risk of atrial thrombi and arterial embolisms. Electrocardiography is the gold standard for confirming the diagnosis as it simultaneously allows morphological evaluation of the mitral valve as well as quantification of the area of the opened valve and the pressure gradient across the valve.

3.9 Sonographic Appearance of the Heart: Echocardiography

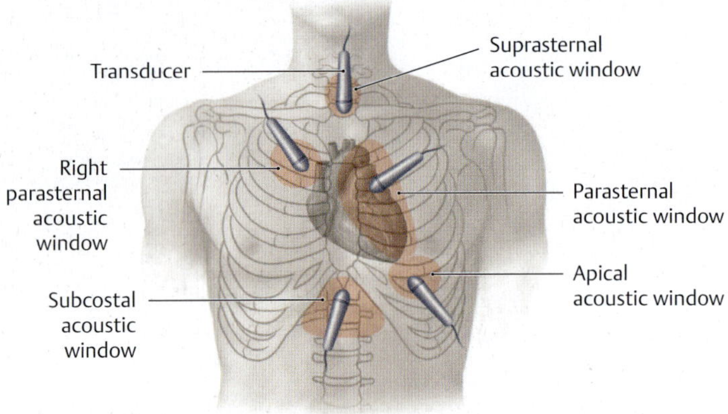

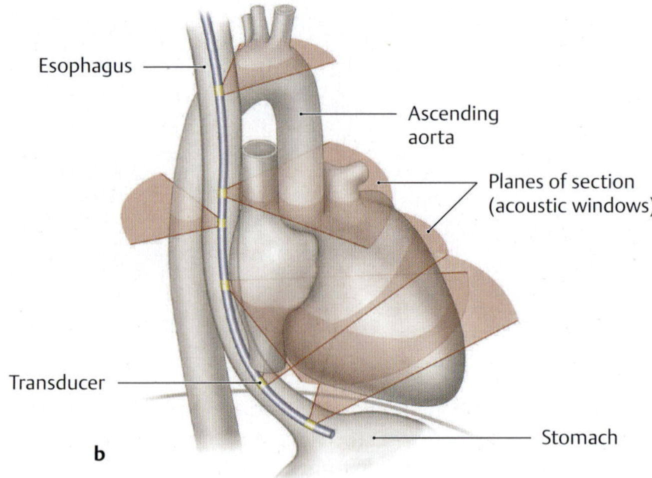

A Transthoracic echocardiography (TTE) and transesophageal echocardiography (TEE)

Echocardiography (cardiac ultrasound) is one of the most common procedures in the diagnosis of heart disease and is considered the most important, noninvasive imaging technique in cardiology. An essential component of every echocardiography device is the transducer. Through its piezoelectric crystals, the transducer generates ultrasonic waves, passes them into the body and receives the reflected ultrasound signal. Modern transducers contain many single crystals, which work in parallel and generate wave fronts resulting in a two-dimensional image (B-mode ultrasound). An echocardiogram is usually done with the patient lying down. The site where the transducer is placed is called the "acoustic window," a place on the body where the passage of sonic waves cannot be impeded by tissue of the lungs or ribs (for example in the intercostal spaces). It is worth noting that the acoustic window is not an exactly determined anatomical landmark but rather refers to an area, within which the optimum transducer location has to be determined individually for every patient. Depending on the acoustic window, one distinguishes between *transthoracic (TTE) and transeophageal (TEE) echocardiography:*

- In **transthoracic echocardiography** (**a**), the acoustic window is located with the patient in the left lateral position (for parasternal and apical acoustic windows), with the patient lying flat on their back (for suprasternal and subcostal acoustic windows), or with the patient in the right lateral position (for the right parasternal acoustic window). In the lateral position, the respective arm is placed under the head to spread the intercostal spaces as much as possible. A disadvantage of this echocardiographic examination is that thoracic and lung structures such as ribs, muscle, fat and even pulmonary diseases (such as emphysema) may impede the diagnosis.
- In contrast to the conventional acoustic windows used in TTE, **transesophageal echocardiography** (**b**) uses part of the esophagus as the acoustic window. Similar to gastroscopy, a miniaturized transducer is inserted through the oral cavity and pharynx and into the esophagus or fundus of the stomach. This places the probe close to the heart. Due to the short distance to the heart and the absence of interference from lung or thoracic structures, TEE provides better image quality than TTE. TEE clearly depicts the dorsal surface of the heart, the cardiac valves, and the descending thoracic aorta. Using a multiplane transducer (which can be rotated throughout 180 degrees), pulling the transducer forward, backward, left and right, allows for a wide variety of sectional planes within the transesophageal acoustic window.

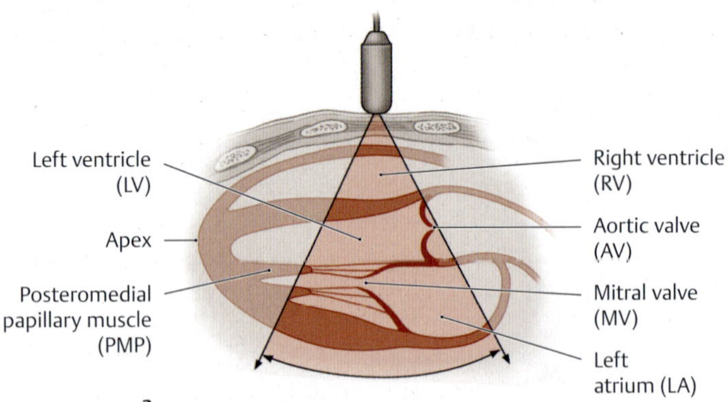

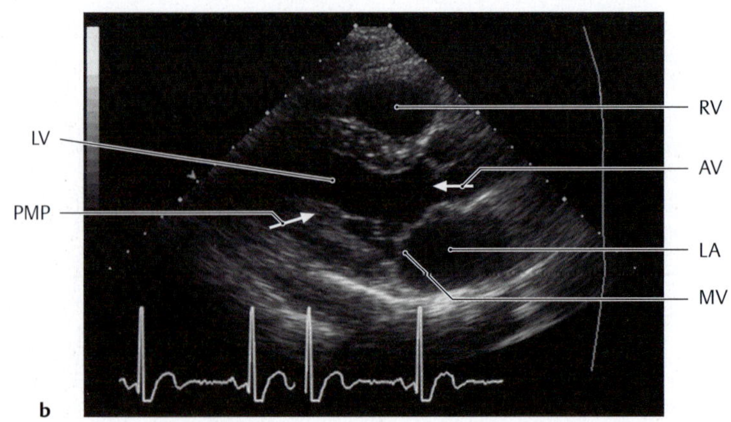

B Transthoracic echocardiography: parasternal acoustic window (long-axis view)

a Schematic representation (*Note*, the apex of the left ventricle is not shown); **b** Parasternal longitudinal view during isovolumic relaxation (from: Flachskampf F. Kursbuch Echokardiografie. 6th ed. Stuttgart: Thieme; 2017).

The echocardiographic examination usually begins with the parasternal *longitudinal view*. It is defined by the appearance of the aortic and mitral valves, the interventricular septum, which runs horizontally, the posterior wall of the left ventricle and part of the right ventricle. Short axis parasternal views of the heart can be obtained by rotating the transducer 90 degrees (see **C**).

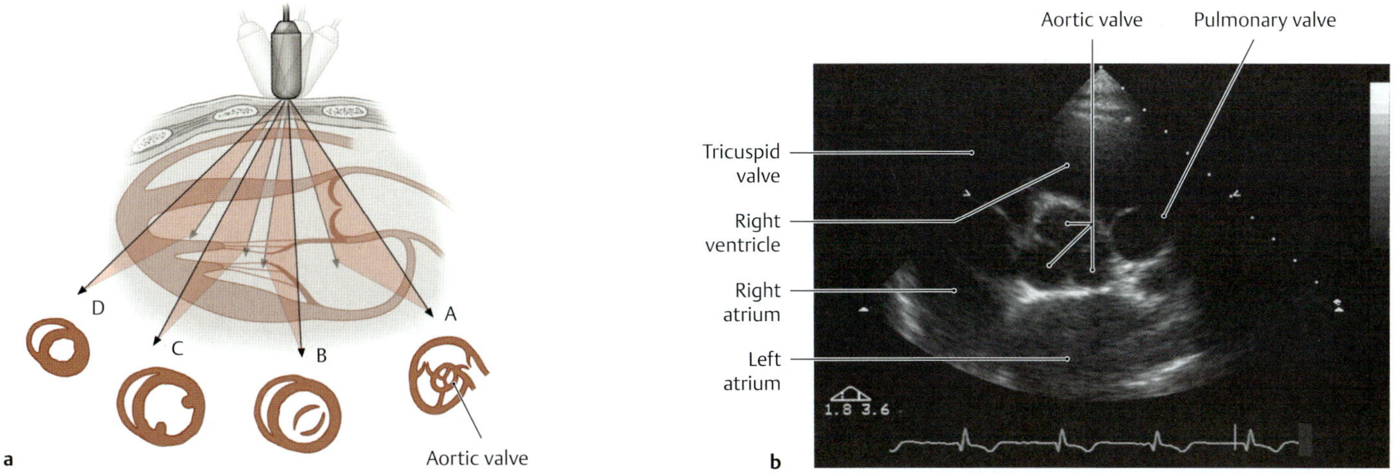

C Transthoracic echocardiography: parasternal acoustic window (short axis view)

a Schematic representation of the major short-axis views (imaging planes A, B, C, and D relative to a long-axis view); **b** Basal short-axis view at the level of the aortic valve (from: Flachskampf F. Kursbuch Echokardiografie. 6th ed. Stuttgart: Thieme; 2017).

This imaging plane shows at its center the aortic valve along with its three cusps (left, right and posterior (non-coronary) cusps, see **B**, p. 130). In this scan, the aortic valve is surrounded by the following structures from clockwise: outflow tract of the right ventricle (12 o'clock), pulmonary valve (2 o'clock), left atrium (5–7 o'clock), right atrium (7–10 o'clock) and tricuspid valve (10 o'clock).

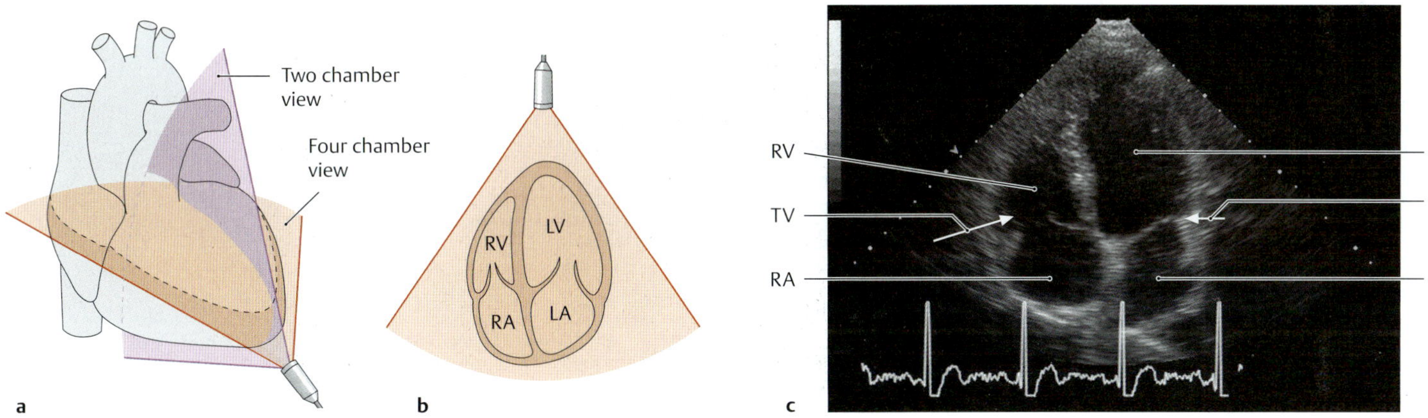

D Transthoracic echocardiography: apical acoustic window (two- and four-chamber views)

a and **b** Schematic representation (four- and two-chamber views are perpendicular to each other); **c** apical four-chamber view at the beginning of systole (from: Flachskampf F. Kursbuch Echokardiografie. 6th ed. Stuttgart: Thieme; 2017).

The apical acoustic window is located approximately at the level of the apical impulse. The apical four-chamber view displays both ventricles (LV, RV), both atria (LA, RA) and the mitral and tricuspid valves (MV, TV). Additionally, this window allows for the visualization of individual structures such as the septum and lateral portions of the myocardium during contraction.

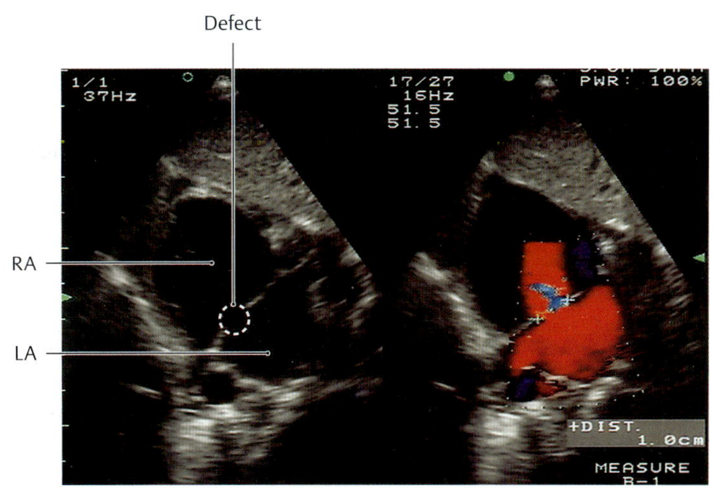

E Transesophageal echocardiogram for atrial septal defect

Color-coded Doppler echocardiography displays a left-to-right shunt, esophageal acoustic window (four-chamber view). The atrial septal defect measures 1 cm in diameter. The Doppler echocardiography allows simultaneous imaging of the two-dimensional ultrasound scan and the color-coded Doppler technique. The blood flow is color-coded according to its direction and velocity. Here the pathological blood flow from the left atrium to the right atrium shown in red is readily discernible. In this way, valve insufficiency and shunting of blood can be detected. (from: Reiser, M. et al.: Radiologie [Duale Reihe], 4th edition. Thieme; Stuttgart: 2017).

3.10 Magnetic Resonance Imaging (MRI) of the Heart

A Examination of cross-sectional images

Examination of **axial** or **transverse** cross-sectional images is done from an inferior view as if the patient is lying flat on his or her back. Thus, the planes of section are displayed with the spinal column, located posteriorly, pointing downward and the thoracic skeleton, located anteriorly, pointing upward. Additionally, anatomical structures located on the right side appear on the left side of the image and vice versa.

The examination of **frontal** or **coronal** cross-sectional images is done as if the patient is standing in front of, and facing, the examiner.

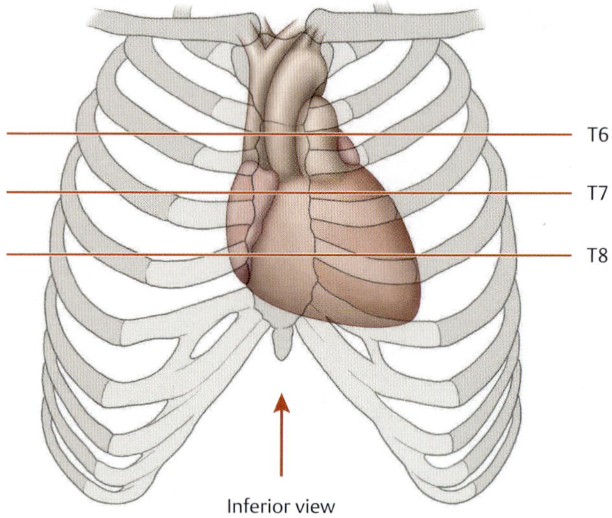

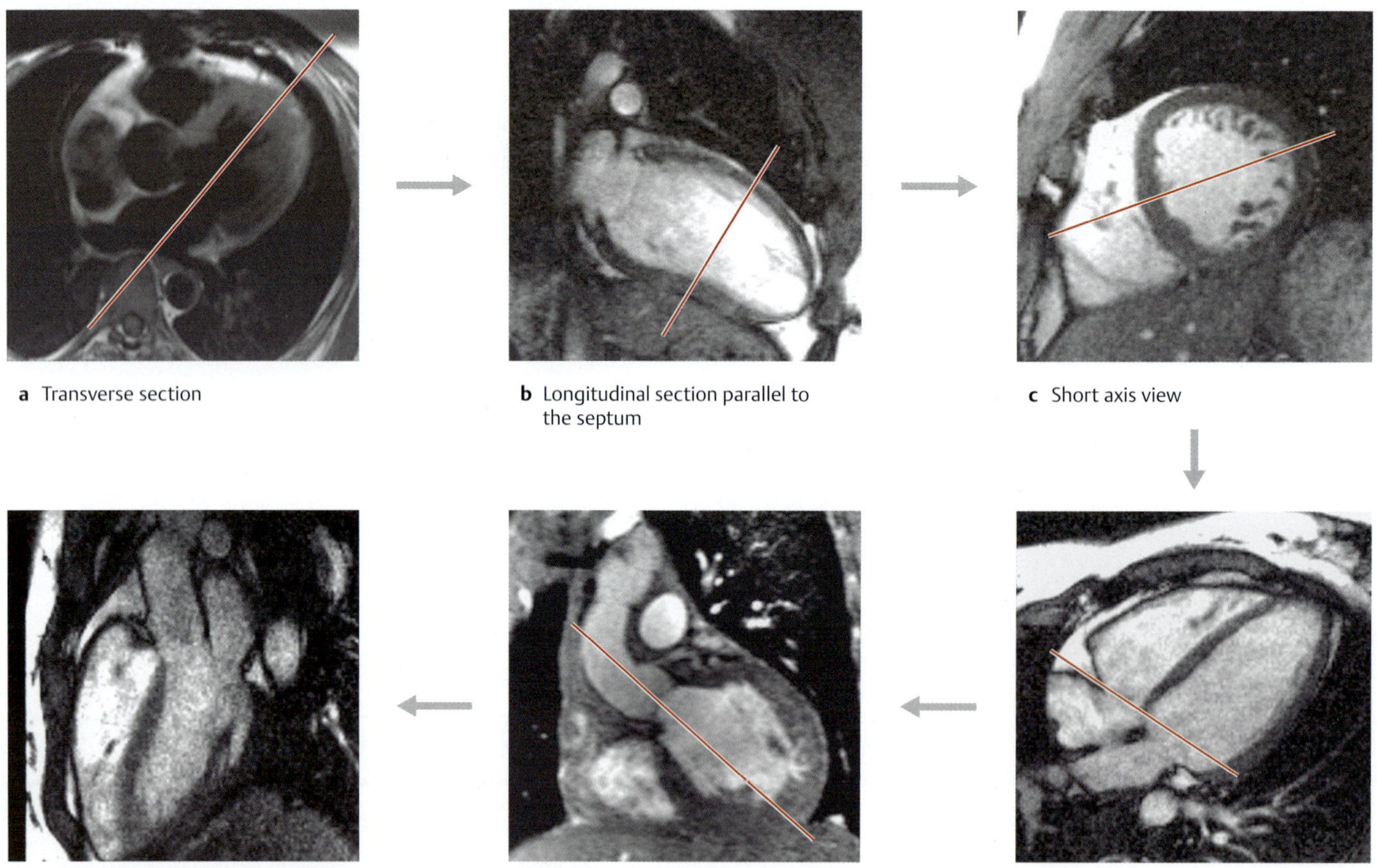

a Transverse section

b Longitudinal section parallel to the septum

c Short axis view

d Four chamber view

e Left ventricular outflow tract

f Left ventricular outflow tract (three chamber view)

B Overview of the standard views of a cardiac MRI

Cross-sectional imaging techniques for diagnosis of the heart use certain standard views obtained in multiple planes (**a–d**). In the single cross-sectional images, the plane of section for the following image has been marked (e.g., **a** shows a transverse section of the heart and the line corresponds to a longitudinal section of the left ventricle parallel to the septum (**b**), etc.).

(All MRIs in this chapter are from Claussen CD et al. *Pareto-Reihe Radiologie*. Herz. Stuttgart: Thieme; 2006.)

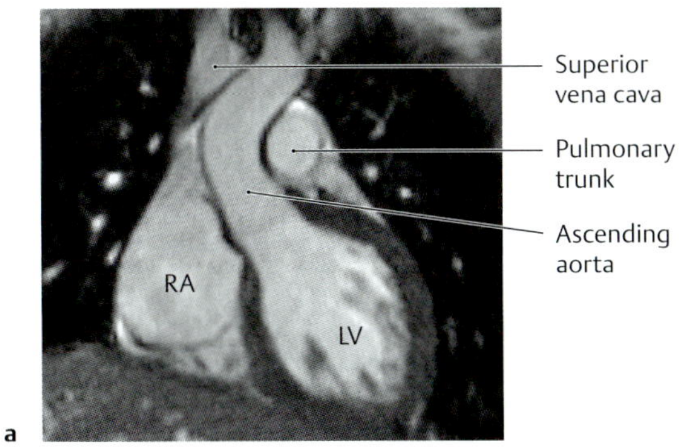

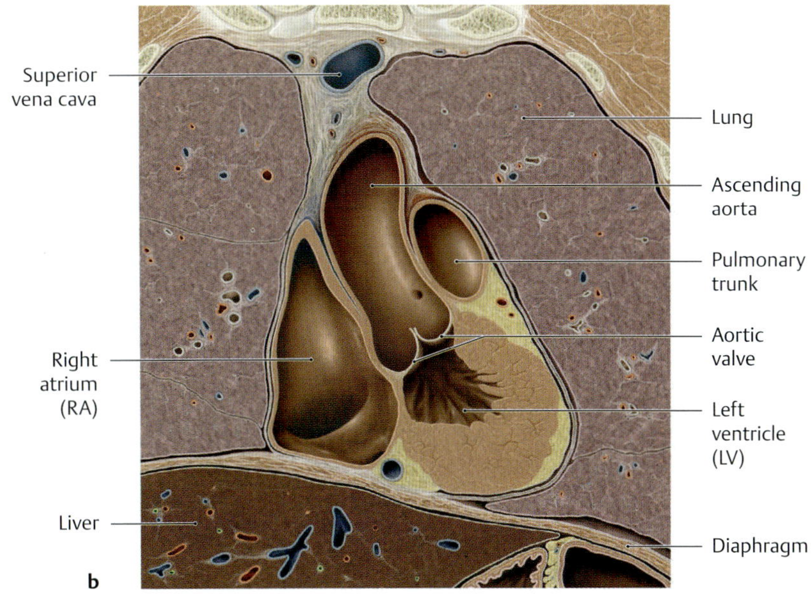

C Coronal MRI of the heart (SSFP sequence)

a Image displays left ventricular outflow tract (LVOT) during diastole.

b Corresponding coronal (frontal) anatomical cross section of the heart, anterior view.

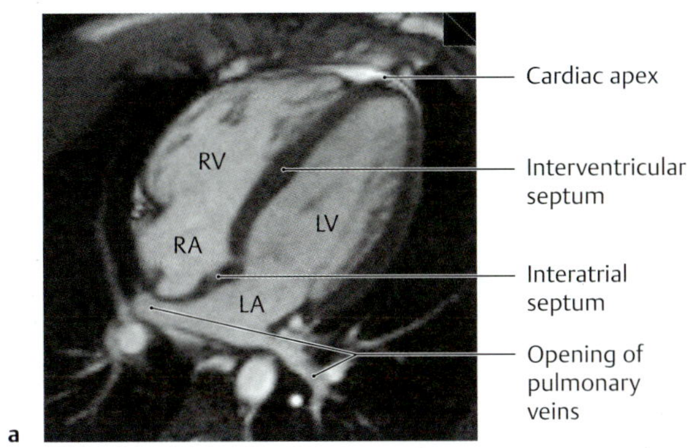

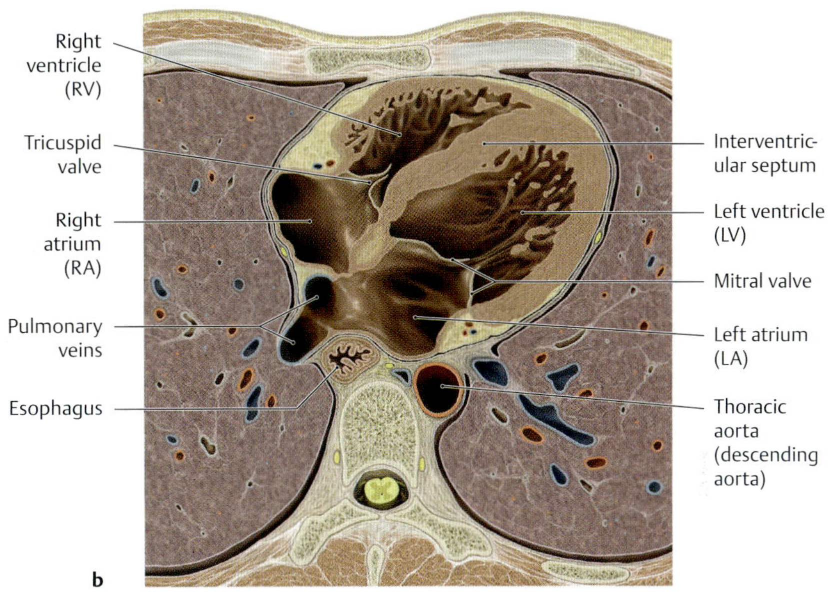

D Axial MRI of the heart (SSFP sequence)

a Image displays the atrioventricular connections of both the right and left sides of the heart during diastole (four-chamber view).

b Corresponding transverse anatomical cross section of the heart, inferior view.

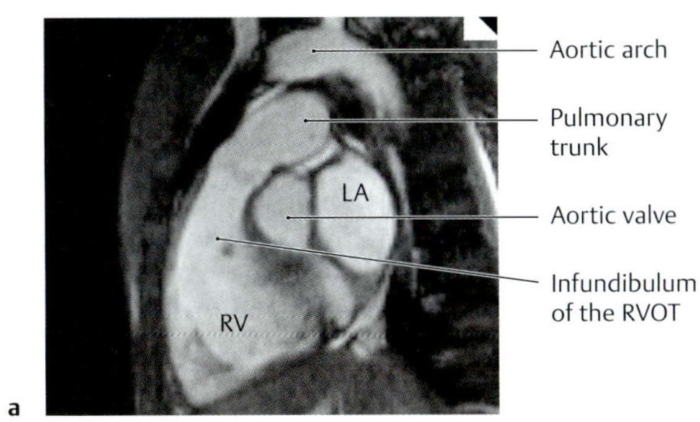

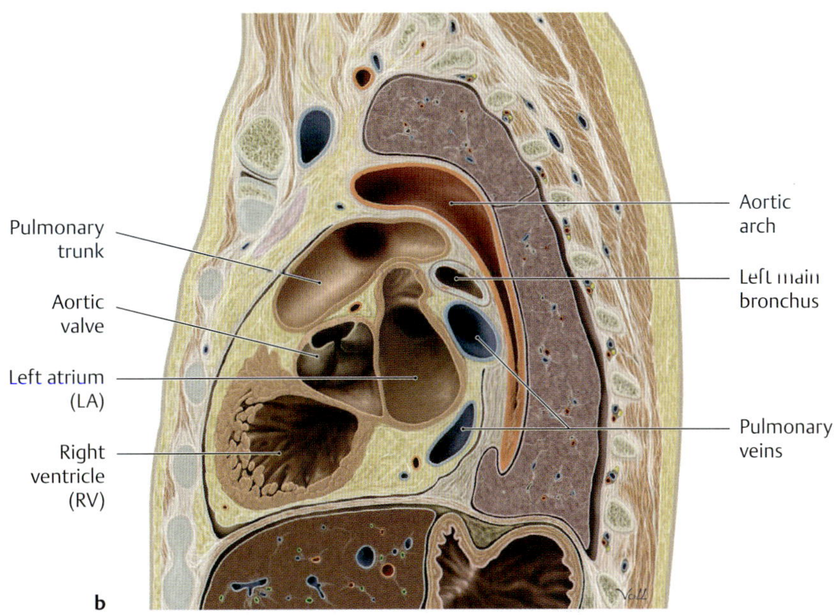

E E Sagittal MRI of the heart (SSFP sequence)

a Image displays the right ventricular outflow tract (RVOT) during diastole.

b Corresponding sagittal anatomical cross section of the heart, viewed from the left side.

3.11 Impulse Formation and Conduction System of the Heart; Electrocardiogram

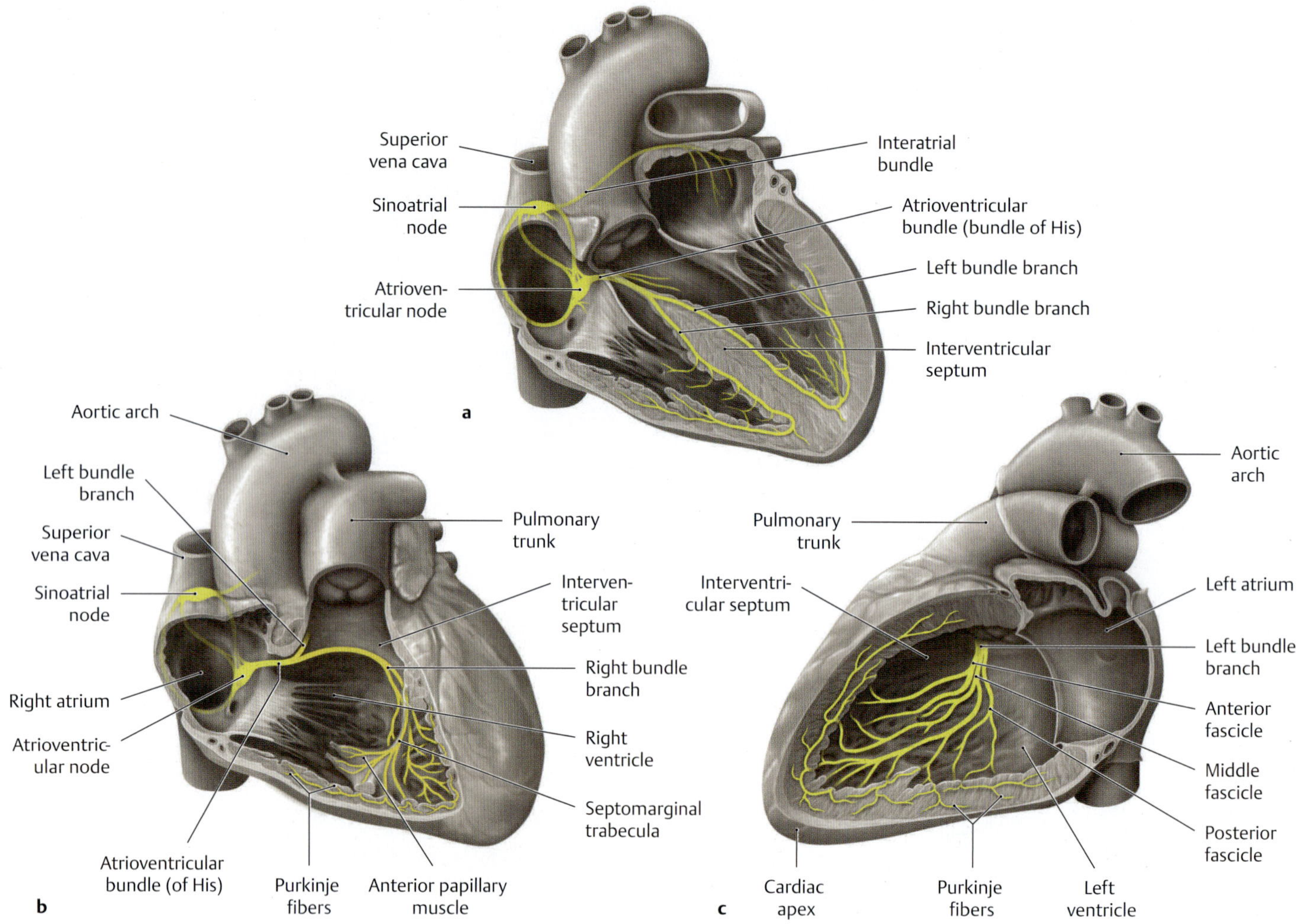

A Overview of cardiac impulse formation and conduction
Anterior view (**a**), right lateral view (**b**), left lateral view (**c**).
Even when the extrinsic nervous control of the heart is completely disrupted, it continues to beat. When supplied with oxygen and nutrients, it can even keep beating after it has been removed from the chest. This is made possible by an intrinsic, independent system that generates and conducts excitatory impulses in the heart. This system consists of specialized myocardial cells and has four main parts:

- Sinoatrial node (SA node, sinus node)
- Atrioventricular node (AV node)
- Atrioventricular bundle (AV bundle, bundle of His)
- Right and left bundle branches

SA node (the "pacemaker" of the heart, approximately 1 cm long). The cardiac impulse begins in the SA node, a subepicardial node located on the posterior side of the right atrium near the orifice of the superior vena cava. The SA node generates salvos of impulses which stimulate the atrial myocardium at a resting rate of 60–70 beats/min. The atrial impulses spread rapidly toward the ventricles (particularly in the crista terminalis and internodal bundles between the SA and AV nodes, as shown by electrophysiologic studies). The impulses travel from the AV node to the bundle of His, which distributes branches to the ventricular myocardium. (Direct impulse conduction from the atrium to the ventricles is normally prevented by the insulating effect of the fibrous skeleton.)
AV node (approximately 5 mm long): located in the interatrial septum near the orifice of the coronary sinus. This node delays impulse conduction to the ventricles, allowing both atria to depolarize before ventricular contraction begins. It can also generate impulses spontaneously, but at a considerably lower rate than the SA node (approximately 40–50 depolarizations/min). Because of its slower rate, the AV node cannot act as a pacemaker for the heart when the SA node is intact.
Atrioventricular bundle (of His) (approximately 2 cm long). The atrioventricular bundle (of His) is subendocardial while still in the atrium. It then passes through the right fibrous trigone (see p. 107) to enter the ventricular septum, where it divides (in the membranous part of the septum) into the right and left bundle branches. The AV bundle conducts impulses from the AV node to the ventricles.
Left bundle branch: branches to the left from the bundle of His and divides into three main fascicles (anterior, middle, and posterior).
Right bundle branch: initially continues in the ventricular septum toward the cardiac apex and is then distributed to the ventricular wall. The main trunk of the right bundle branch enters the septomarginal trabecula, known also as the "moderator band." Finally the impulse is distributed throughout the ventricular myocardium by the Purkinje fibers.
Note: The Purkinje fibers stimulate the ventricular walls in a retrograde direction, proceeding from the cardiac apex toward the atria. Thus the apical myocardium contracts first, pulling the apex of the heart toward the plane of the valves. The papillary muscles, which are stimulated by direct fibers from the bundle branches, contract before the ventricular walls to ensure that the AV valves remain closed during ventricular systole.

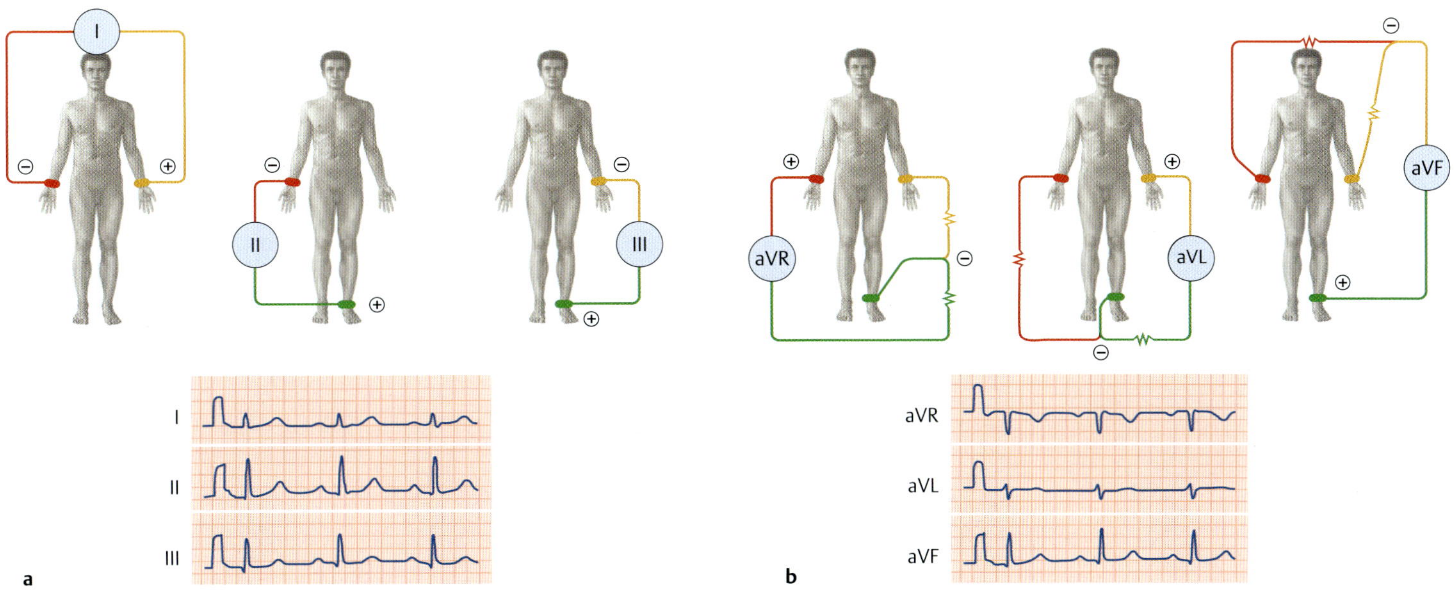

B Electrocardiogram (ECG): standard leads

a Bipolar limb leads after Einthoven; **b** Unipolar limb leads after Goldberger; **c** Chest wall leads after Wilson.

Electrical impulses (called action potentials) generated by the SA node spread across the entire heart via its conduction system (see **A**). The impulses produce an electric field, which is measurable on the body surface. Across this electric field, potential differences of up to 1 mV (1V = 1000 mV) occur between different points on the body surface (e.g., between right arm and left leg) during the spread of cardiac excitation and depolarization. Electrodes are used to record these potential differences on the body surface in the form of lines, spikes and curves (electrocardiogram). In a healthy heart, the spikes and waves show specific shapes and intervals between them, from which one can obtain information about heart rate (and thus cardiac rhythm), the electrical activity of the heart, and especially about the functioning or nonfunctioning of the impulse formation and conduction system of the heart. The standard surface ECG includes recordings from 12 leads: 6 limb leads (I, II, III, aVR, aVL, aVF) and 6 chest wall leads (V_1–V_6).

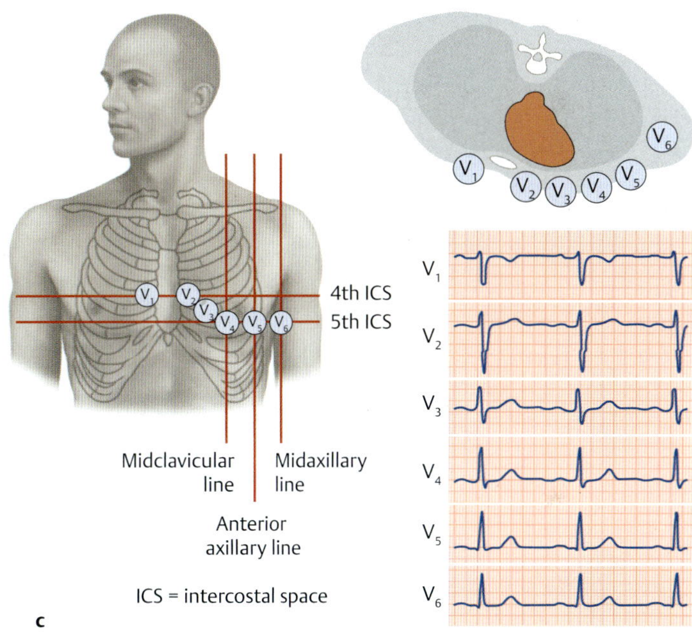

C Names and definition of waves, spikes, and intervals in the ECG

Name	Definition
P wave	Atrial depolarization (< 0.1 s)
Q, R, and S wave (the QRS complex)	Beginning of ventricular excitation (< 0.1 s)
T wave	End of ventricular excitation
PQ interval	Onset of atrial excitation until the onset of ventricular excitation = conduction time = 0.1–0.2 s
QT interval	Q spike until the end of the T wave = time needed for both ventricles for de- and repolarization = 0.32–0.39 s. Varies based on the heart rate of the individual
Cardiac cycle	Interval between two R spikes
Heart rate	60 s/distance between R spikes (s) = beats/minute; e.g., 60/0.8 = 75

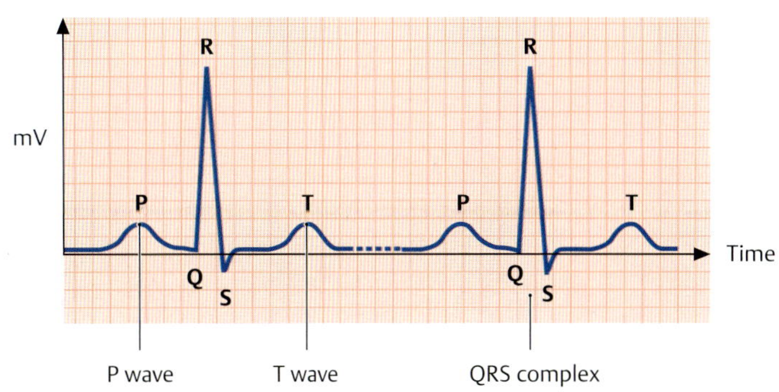

D ECG curve: Excitation cycle (recording of two heartbeats, after Wilson)

The ECG waveform has several spikes and waves, whose names and definitions are indicated in **C**.

3.12 Mechanical Action of the Heart

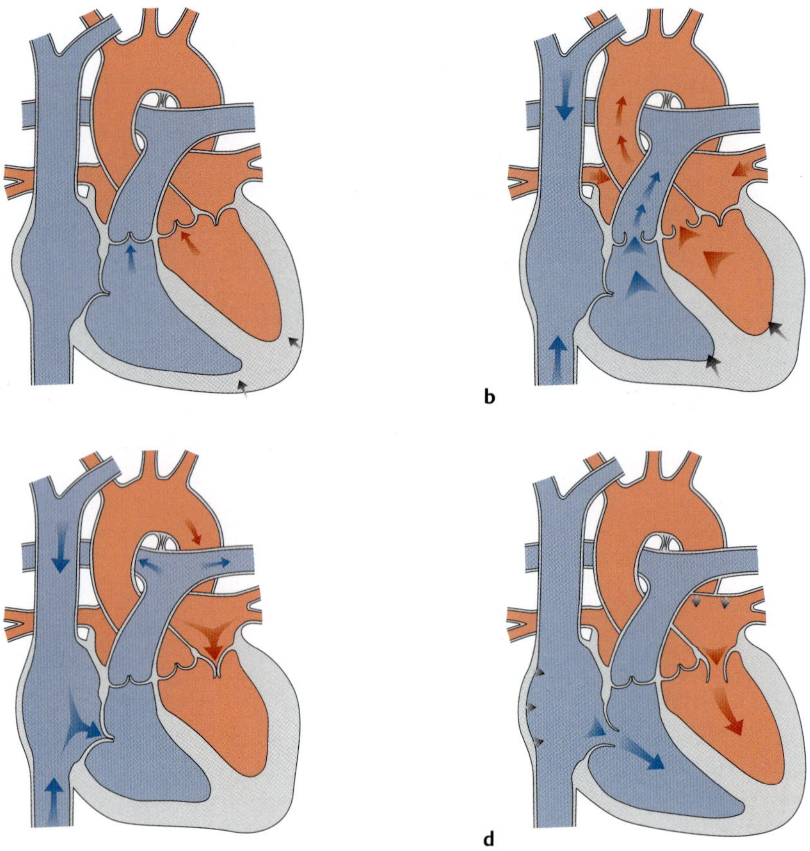

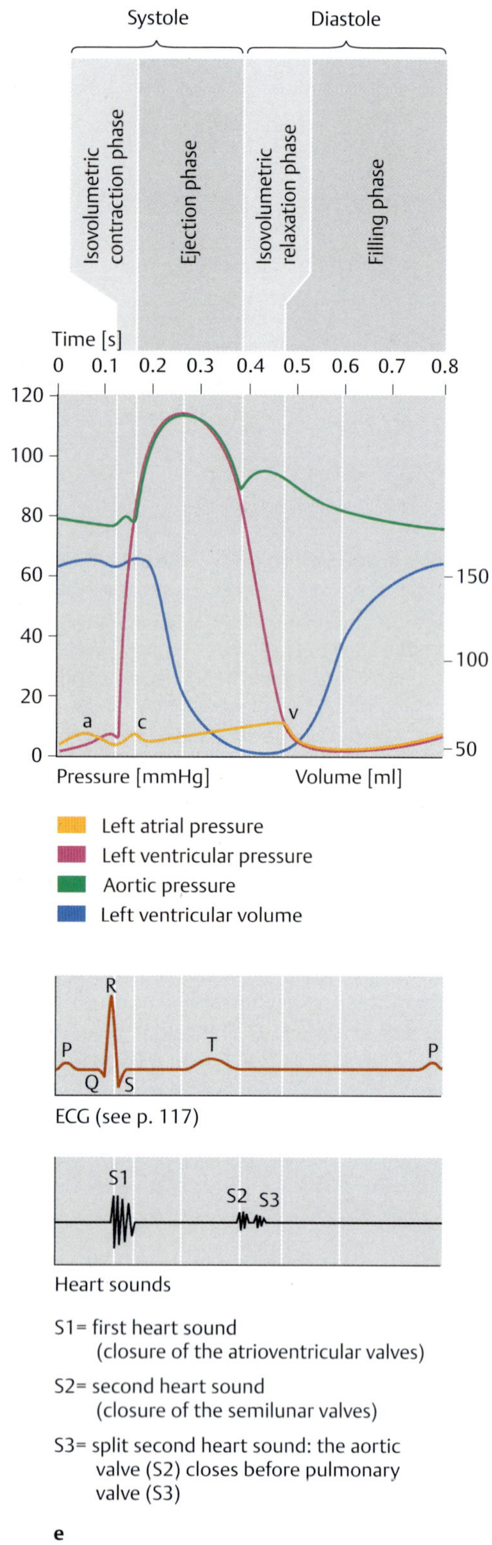

A Phases of the heartbeat

a and **b** Ventricular systole: isovolumetric contraction (**a**) and ejection phase (**b**); **c** and **d** Ventricular diastole: isovolumetric relaxation (**c**) and filling phase (**d**); **e** Correlation between pressure, volume, ECG and heartbeats during systole and diastole. The heartbeat consists of two main phases: contraction (systole) and relaxation (diastole). A total of four phases are distinguished in the contraction and expansion of the ventricles:

Ventricular systole:

- Isovolumetric contraction phase (**a**): The ventricular myocardium contracts and tightens around the blood column within the ventricle. All valves are closed, that is, the AV valves are *already* closed (ventricular pressure exceeds the atrial pressure), and the aortic and pulmonary valves are *still* closed (ventricular pressure is still lower than the intra-arterial pressure). Isovolumetric contraction of the myocardium around the blood column produces a mechanical vibration that is audible as the first heart sound. In fact, it is the closure of the atrioventricular valves, that produces the first heart sound.
- Ejection phase (**b**): The AV valves remain closed and prevent the reflux of ventricular blood into the atria. As the intraventricular pressure exceeds the pressure in the arteries, the aortic and pulmonary valves open, and blood flows into the aorta and pulmonary trunk.

Ventricular diastole:

- Isovolumetric relaxation phase (**c**): The ventricular myocardium relaxes. All valves are closed during this phase: The AV valves are *still* closed, and the aortic and pulmonary valves are *already* closed (to prevent the reflux of ejected blood back into the ventricles). Closure of the aortic and pulmonary valves ("slamming doors") is audible as the second heart sound. Occasionally the arterial valves close at slightly different times, producing a divided second heart sound.
- Filling phase (**d**): The intraventricular pressure is very low, and the arterial valves remain closed. The AV valves open, and blood flows into the ventricles. Ventricular filling results more from the movement of the valve plane than from atrial contraction: The valve plane moves toward the cardiac apex during systole, and it returns very quickly to its initial position during diastole, "throwing itself" over the blood column.

Note: During both the isovolumetric contraction phase and the relaxation phase, there are periods in which all the valves are closed. By contrast, there is no point in the cardiac cycle when all valves are open. *Heart sounds* are normal acoustical phenomena produced by the heart. Abnormal valvular heart sounds (murmurs) are described on p. 109. Although the first heart sound is generated by ventricular contraction itself, that first sound is clinically associated with closure of the atrioventricular valves.

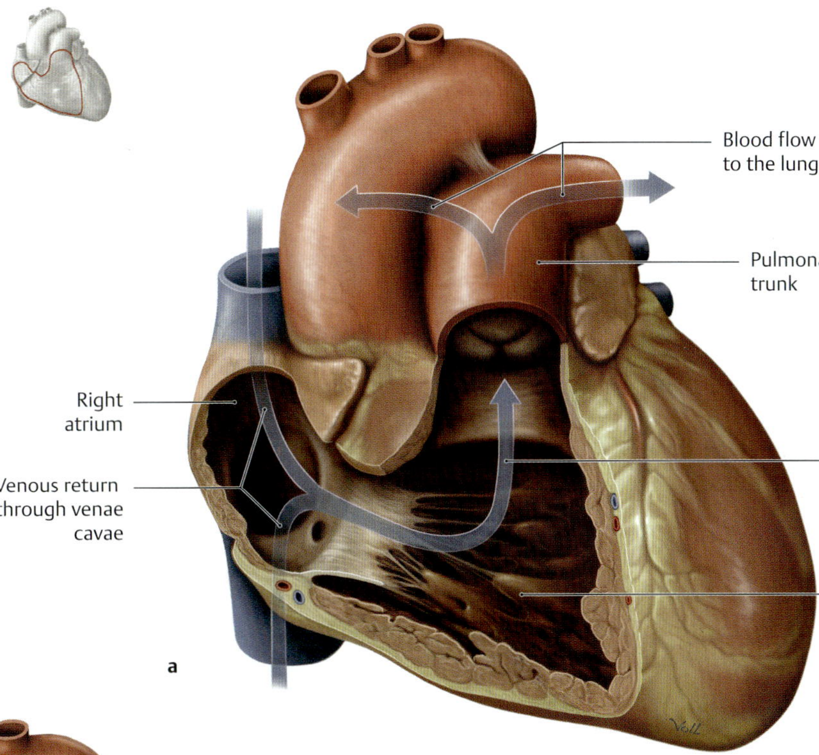

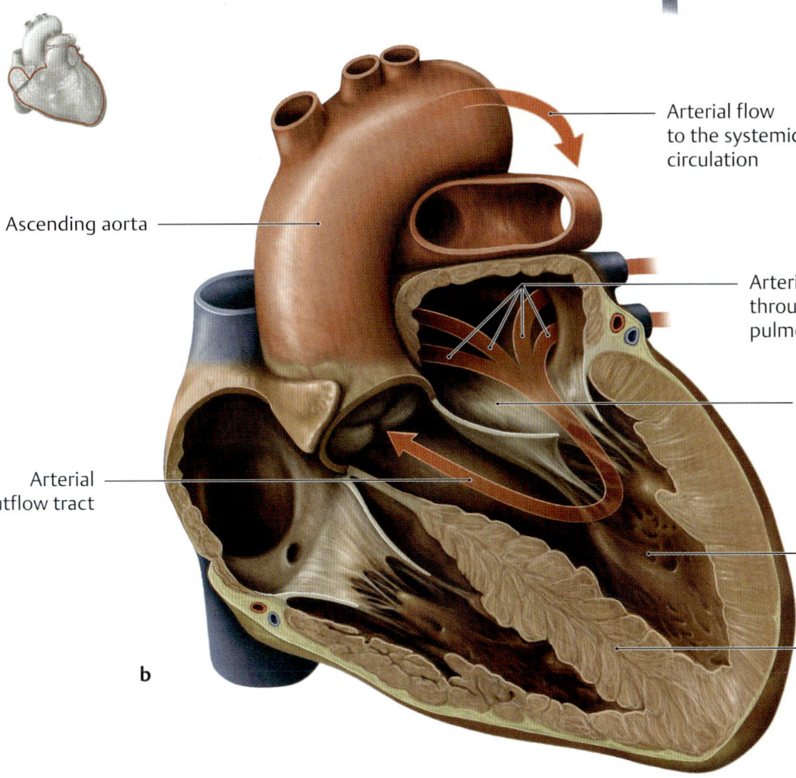

B Blood flow in the heart

The septa between the atria and ventricles functionally divide the heart into two main parts: the right heart and left heart. The cardiac valves define the direction of blood flow through both sides of the heart, enabling the right and left heart to function as finely coordinated tandem pumps.

Blood flow in the right heart (**a**): Anterior view with the right atrium and right ventricle cut open. Venous blood from the superior and inferior venae cavae flows into the sinus venarum and enters the right atrium. From there it flows across the open right atrioventricular valve and passes through the right atrioventricular orifice along the inflow tract into the right ventricle. Inside the ventricle it is redirected into the outflow tract and pumped through the open pulmonary valve (shown closed here) and conus arteriosus into the pulmonary trunk. From there it flows through the pulmonary arteries into the lungs, where it is oxygenated. The right heart pumps blood with a low oxygen tension.

Blood flow in the left heart (**b**): Left anterior view. All of the cardiac chambers have been cut open anteriorly. Oxygenated blood from the lungs flows across the open left atrioventricular valve and through the left atrioventricular orifice along the inflow tract into the left ventricle There it is rerouted into the outflow tract and flows across the open aortic valve (shown closed here) through the aortic orifice into the ascending aorta for distribution throughout the systemic circulation (after first perfusing the coronary arteries). The left heart pumps blood with a high oxygen tension.

3.13 Coronary Arteries and Cardiac Veins: Classification and Topography

A Coronary arteries and cardiac veins

a Anterior view of the sternocostal surface of the heart

b Posteroinferior view of the diaphragmatic surface of the heart

Because the heart functions continuously to pump blood, it has a high oxygen demand. This demand is met by the right and left coronary arteries—intrinsic cardiac vessels that have an extensive capillary network. The coronary arteries spring from small dilations in the aorta (the aortic sinuses) located just above the aortic valve. The main trunk of the **left coronary artery**, which is usually slightly larger, divides into

- Circumflex branch: runs in the coronary sulcus (boundary between the atrium and ventricle) around the *left* side of the heart to the posterior heart wall
- Anterior interventricular branch: runs in the anterior interventricular sulcus (boundary between the ventricles) to the cardiac apex. Each of these vessels gives off smaller branches.

The **right coronary artery**, usually smaller than the left, runs in the coronary sulcus around the *right* side of the heart to the posterior wall, where it forms the posterior interventricular branch. It also gives off numerous branches (see p. 122).

Note: The coronary arteries are functional end arteries because they form anastomoses that are not adequate for reciprocal blood flow. The coronary arteries must efficiently deliver blood to an organ with constant high metabolic demand that is itself at elevated pressure, especially during systole. This difficult requirement is achieved in part by the anatomical relation between the aortic valve and the origin of the coronary arteries, just superior to the valve leaflets. As the left ventricle completes its contraction and the distended aorta begins to recoil, the aortic valve is forced closed by the backflow and a local surge in pressure (a pressure hammer) develops. This pressure hammer drives blood into the coronary arteries. The heart is thus efficiently perfused at the maximum pressure that the cardiovascular system can reach.

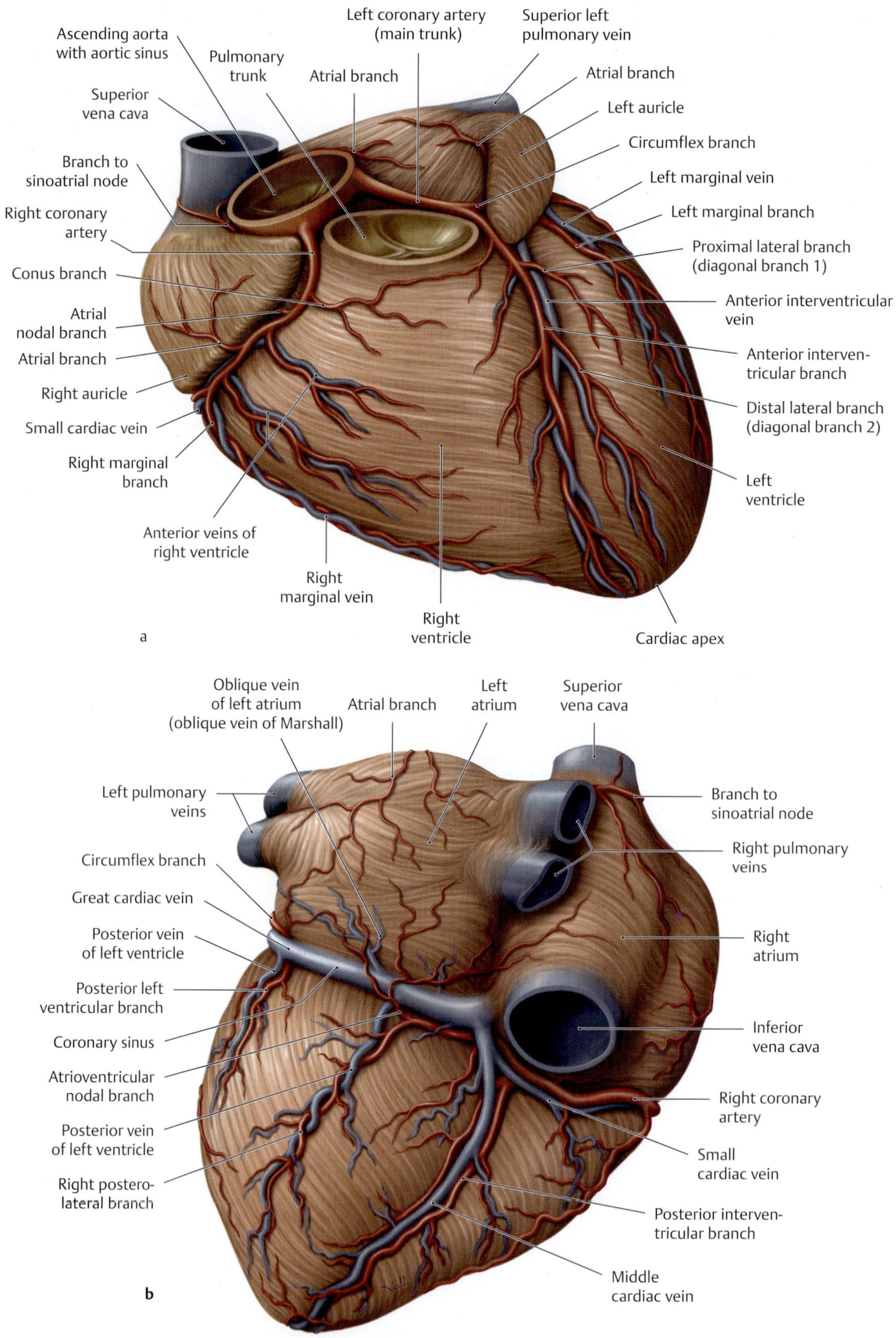

The **cardiac veins** usually course with the coronary arteries and consist of the great, middle, and small cardiac veins. These veins open on the posterior heart wall into the coronary sinus, which empties into the right atrium. Additional smaller veins (smallest cardiac veins, not shown here, Thebesian veins) open directly into the cardiac chambers, mainly the right atrium.

Note: The oblique vein of the left atrium (oblique vein of Marshall) is a remnant of the embryonic left superior vena cava.

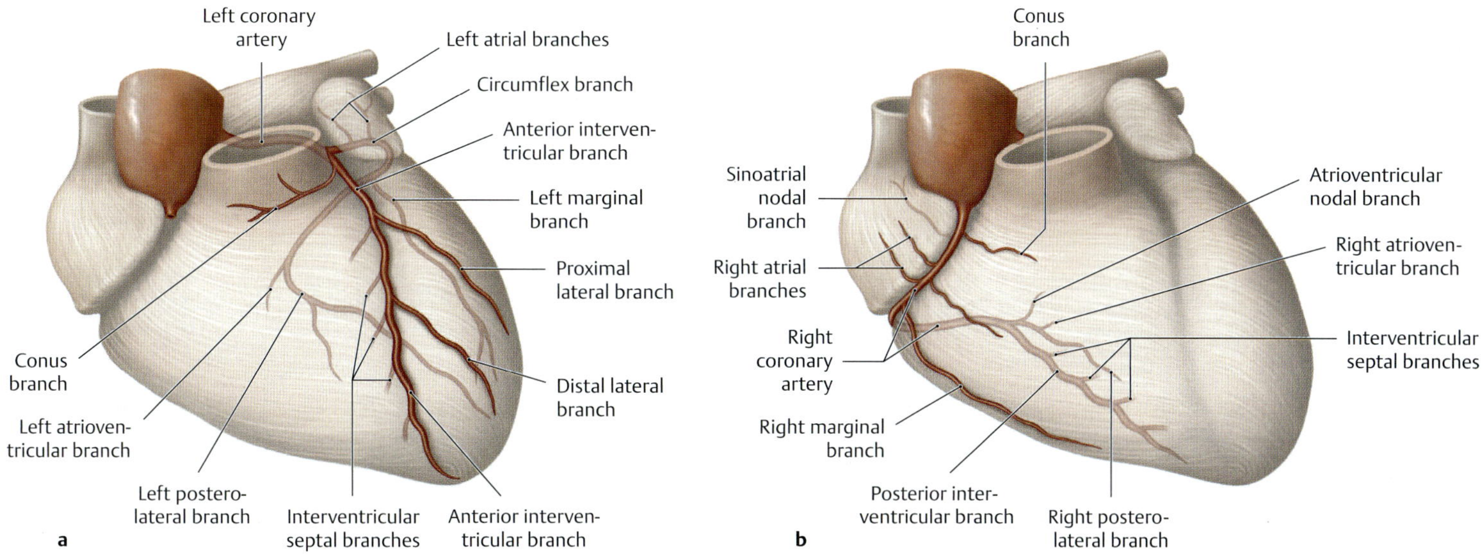

B Classification of the coronary arteries

a Branches of the left coronary artery; **b** Branches of the right coronary artery (anterior views of the sternocostal surface).

The diagram shows the normal or balanced circulation (70% of all cases). In the balanced type, the posterior wall of the heart (diaphragmatic surface; clinically: posterior wall) is supplied equally by the left and right coronary arteries (for details about right or left dominant coronary circulation, see pp. 122 and 123f). Based on a recommendation by the American Heart Association, the individual coronary arteries are divided into segments: right coronary artery (segments 1–4); left coronary artery (segments 5–15). Segment 5 corresponds with the main trunk, segments 6–10 with the anterior interventricular branch, and segments 11–15 with the circumflex branch of the left coronary artery.

C Branches of the coronary arteries*

Left coronary artery (LCA)

Circumflex branch (LCX)

- Left atrial branches
- Left marginal branch (LM)
- Left atrioventricular branch (LAV)
- Left posterolateral branch (LPL or PLA) often also the posterior left ventricular branch

Anterior interventricular branch (AIV or LAD, left anterior descending artery)

- Conus branch
- Proximal lateral branch (diagonal branch 1, D1)
- Distal lateral branch (diagonal branch 2, D2)
- Interventricular septal branches

Right coronary artery (RCA)

- Sinoatrial nodal branch (SAN)
- Right atrial branches
- Conus branch
- Atrioventricular nodal branch (AVN)
- Right marginal branch (RM)
- Posterior interventricular branch (PIV or PDA, posterior descending artery)
- Right atrioventricular branch (RAV)
- Interventricular septal branches
- Right posterolateral branch (RPL or PLA)

* RCA, LCA, LCX and LAD are common medical abbreviations.

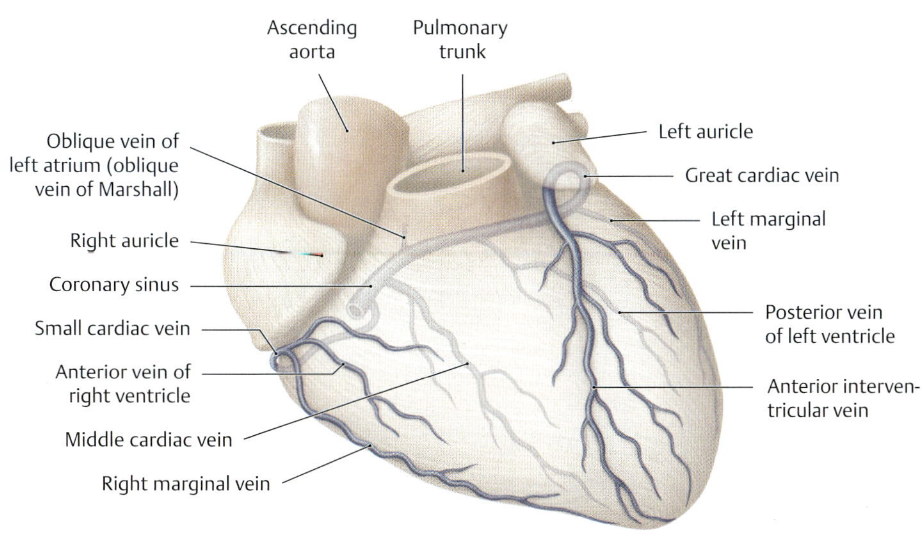

D Classification of cardiac veins

Anterior view of the sternocostal surface.

E Divisions of the cardiac veins

Great cardiac vein

- Left marginal vein
- Anterior interventricular vein
- Posterior vein of left ventricle

Middle cardiac vein (posterior interventricular vein)

Small cardiac vein

- Anterior vein of right ventricle
- Right marginal vein

Note: Venous blood collected by the cardiac veins is largely (75%) carried to the right atrium via the coronary sinus (coronary sinus system). Additionally, venous blood is drained via the transmural (superficial veins, which directly drain into the atrium) and endomural systems (veins from the inner layer of the myocardium, which directly empty into the lumen).

3.14 Coronary Arteries: Coronary Circulation

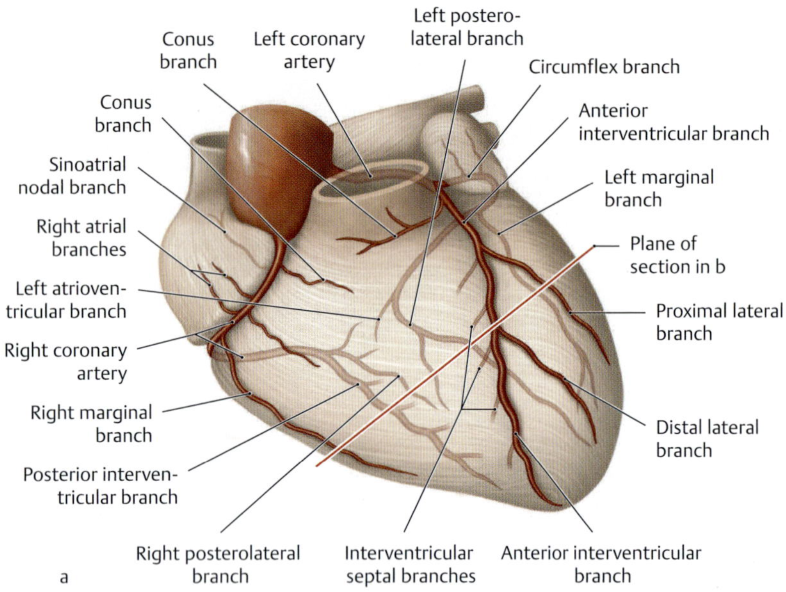

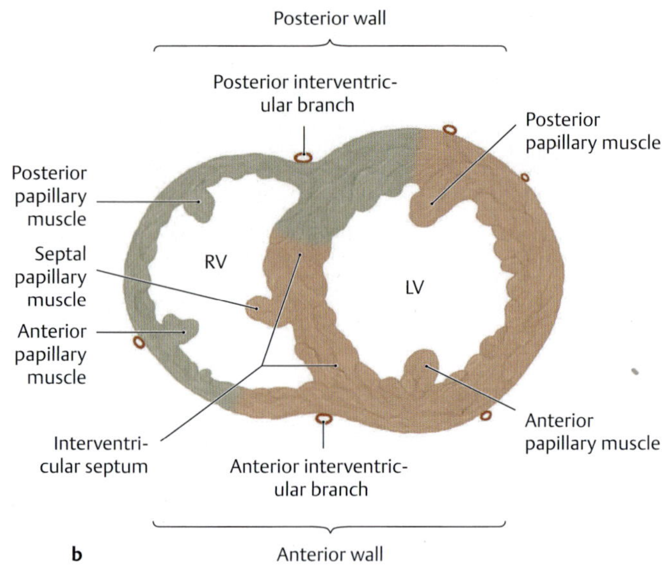

A Balanced (normal) coronary supply
a Course of the right and left coronary arteries (anterior view of the sternocostal surface); **b** Cross-section of both ventricles viewed from above (area supplied by the right coronary artery: colored in green, area supplied by the left coronary artery: colored in red).

In the balanced type of circulation (70%), the posterior wall of the heart is supplied equally by the left and right coronary arteries (the posterior interventricular branch comes off the right coronary artery). It is also referred to as codominant circulation supplying the posterior wall of the heart (diaphragmatic surface) (see **B**).

Note: Since the branches of the right coronary artery also supply major centers of the conduction system (SA node, AV node, AV bundle), a narrowing of the right coronary artery often leads to arrhythmia.

B Distribution of the left and right coronary arteries

Distribution	Left coronary artery	Right coronary artery
Left atrium	Atrial branches and an intermediate atrial branch of the circumflex branch	
Right atrium		Atrial branches and an intermediate atrial branch
Left ventricle • Anterior wall • Lateral wall • Posterior wall	 • Anterior interventricular branch and its proximal and distal lateral (diagonal) branches • Left marginal branch of the circumflex branch • Partly by the posterior left ventricular branch of the circumflex branch	 • Partly by the right posterolateral branch
Right ventricle • Anterior wall • Lateral wall • Posterior wall	 • Strip near the septum by the conus branch and small twigs from the anterior interventricular branch	 • Conus branch with smaller twigs and the right marginal branch • Right marginal branch • Posterior interventricular branch
Interventricular septum	Interventricular septal branches (supply the larger anterior part of the septum)	Interventricular septal branches (supply the smaller posterior part of the septum)
Sinoatrial node (sinus node)		Branch to the sinoatrial node
Atrioventricular node (AV node)		Branch to the atrioventricular node

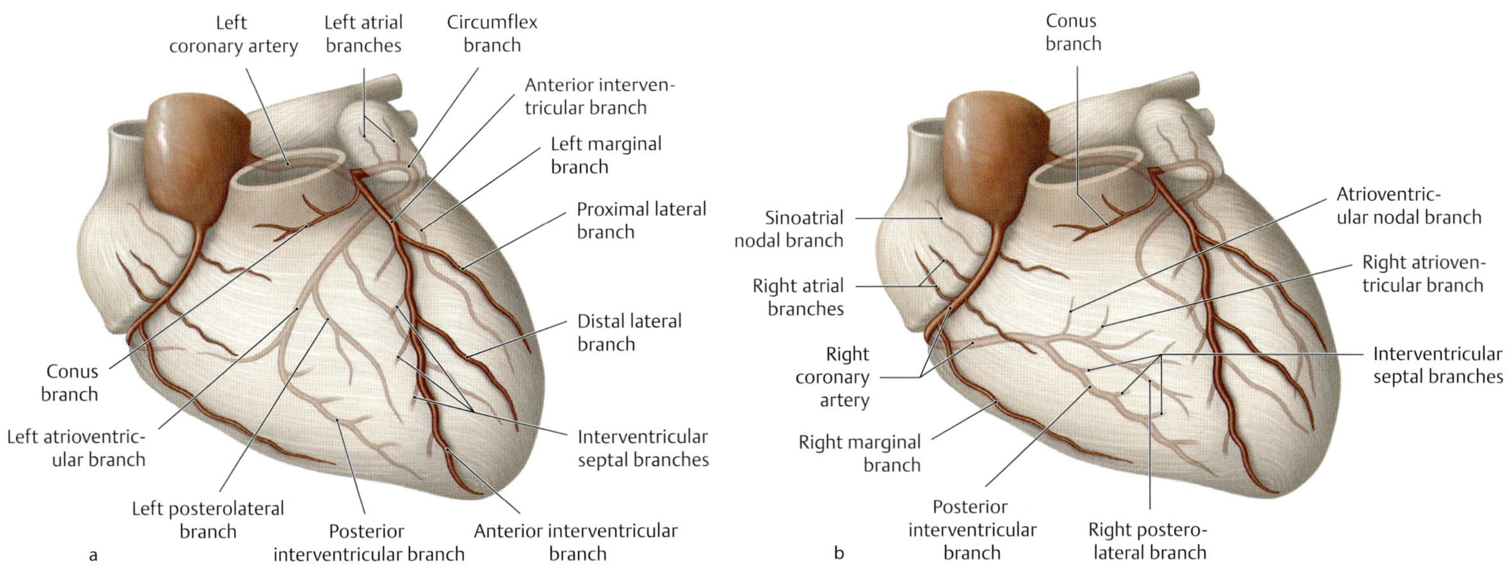

C Left and right dominant coronary circulation

a Left dominant circulation; **b** Right dominant circulation.

Left and right dominant circulations each occur in 15% of hearts. Both types of circulation differ in how the posterior wall of the heart is supplied:

- **Left dominant circulation** (**a**) is dominated by a strong circumflex branch, which ends as the posterior interventricular branch at the posterior wall. In addition to the posterior parts of the interventricular septum, it also supplies parts of the right ventricle.
- **Right dominant circulation** (**b**) is dominated by the right coronary artery, which in addition to the posterior interventricular branch also supplies the largest part of the posterior wall with the help of a strong right posterolateral branch. The circumflex branch of the left coronary artery is weakly developed (for details about the differences between the three types of circulation see also **Da–c**).

Note: Because the posterior interventricular branch is variable in its development and origin, there is also considerable variation in the supply to the left and right ventricles and interventricular septum by the left and right coronary arteries.

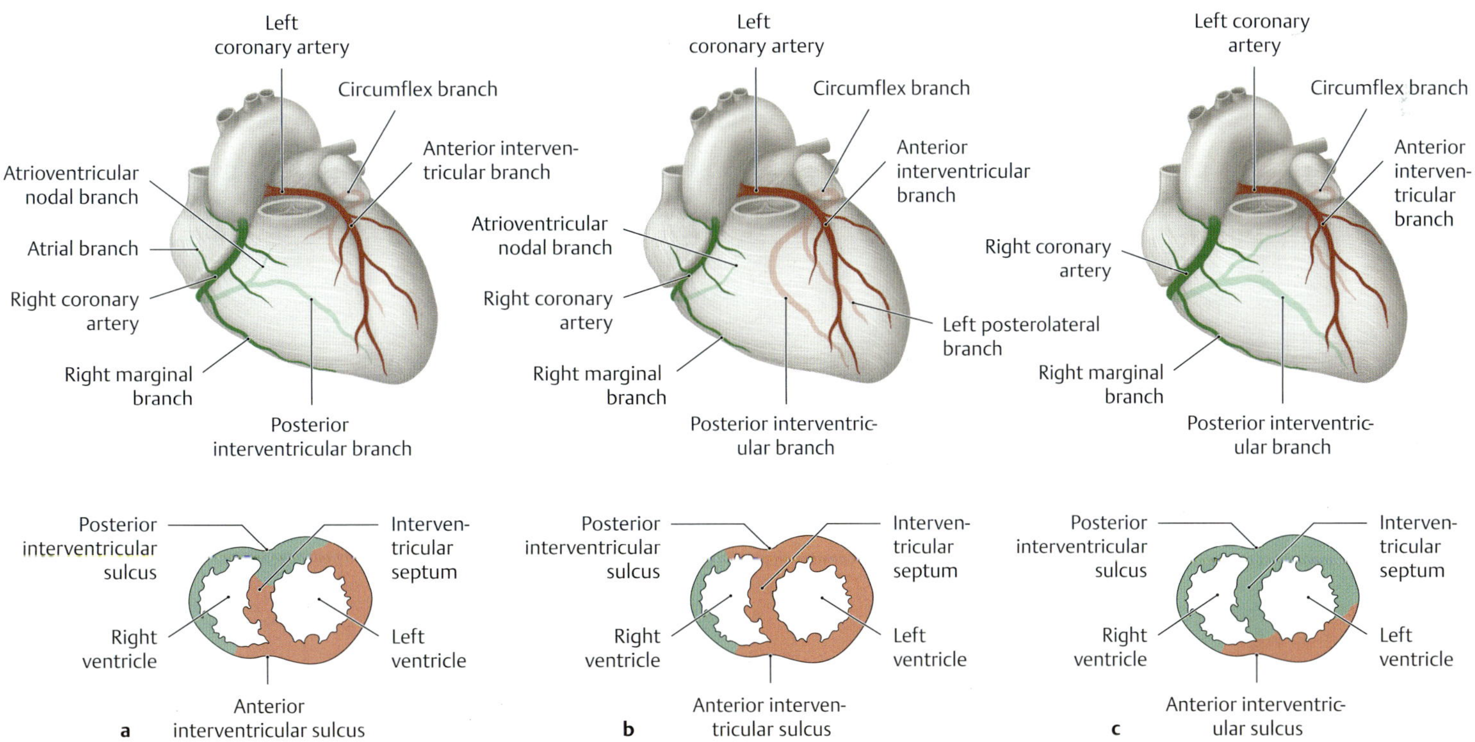

D Comparison of the types of coronary circulation

a Balanced circulation (in 70% of hearts); **b** Left dominant circulation (in 15% of hearts); **c** Right dominant circulation (in 15% of hearts).

Diagrams each show a ventral view and a cross-section of both chambers, viewed from above; left coronary artery and area it supplies colored in red, right coronary artery and area it supplies colored in green.

3.15 Coronary Heart Disease (CHD) and Heart Attack

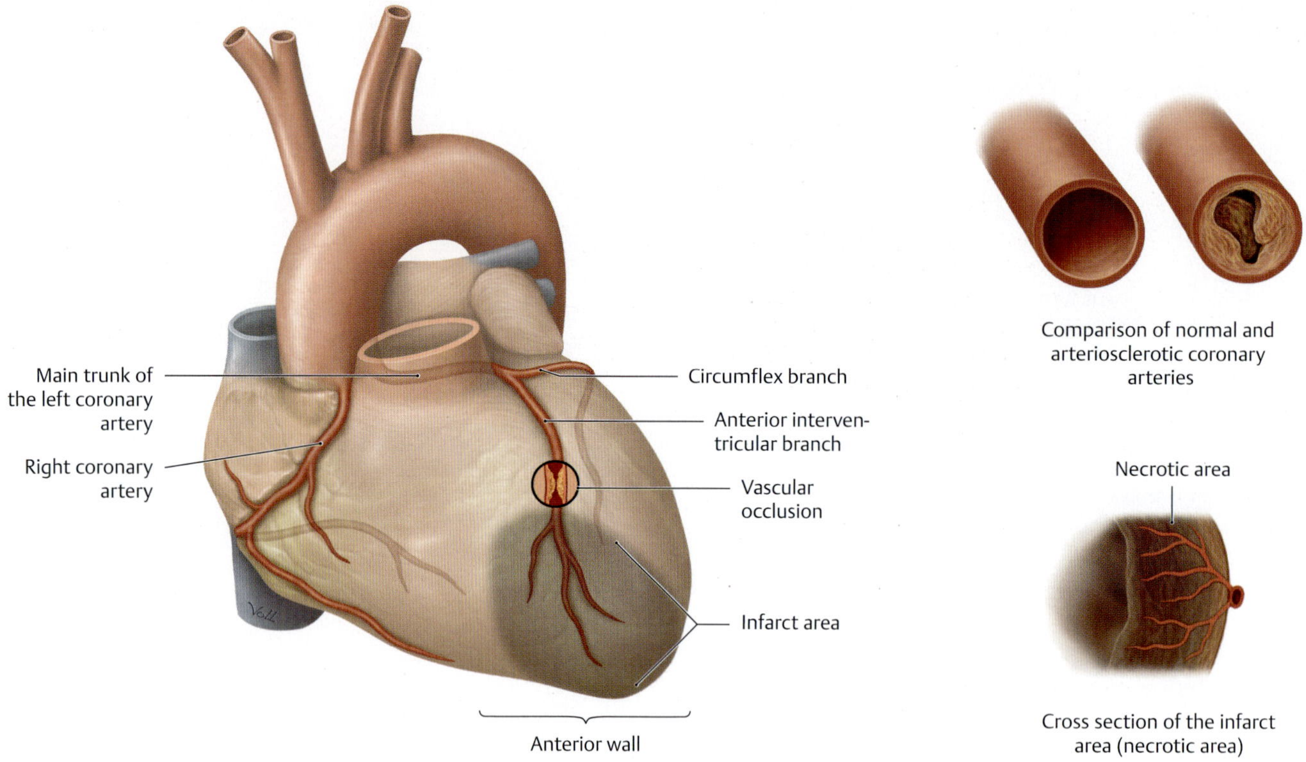

A Acute myocardial infarction

Acute myocardial infarction is characterized by necrosis of myocardial tissue as a result of total occlusion or subcritical impairment of coronary blood flow (incidence rate in Germany 330/100,000 population per year). Acute myocardial infarction is often the result of coronary heart disease (CHD see **C**). Acute myocardial necrosis (myocardial infarction) usually occurs when an arteriosclerotic plaque ruptures (see **D**) which leads to thrombotic occlusion of one or multiple branches of the coronary arteries (known as one-, two-, or three-vessel disease). Myocardial ischemia lasting for 20–30 minutes results in tissue necrosis with the subendocardial layers of the myocardium being damaged first. They are the farthest away from the blood capillaries and have a high rate of oxygen consumption. The damage is the result of the myocardium switching to anaerobic glycolysis, which leads to a reduced ability to produce ATP. The increase in metabolic waste products also inhibits the production of glycolytic ATP. As a result, cells (in particular the cellular membrane, mitochondria, and sarcoplasmic reticulum) are irreversibly damaged. Subsequent intracellular calcium ion overload in turn leads to activation of membrane phospholipases and the formation of inflammatory mediators. As a result, granulocytes and macrophages migrate into the infarct area. The necrotic area is filled in by the formation of granulation tissue. If the patient survives the myocardial infarction, the repair of the necrotic area, in which necrotic tissue is replaced by scar tissue composed of collagen, is usually complete by six weeks.

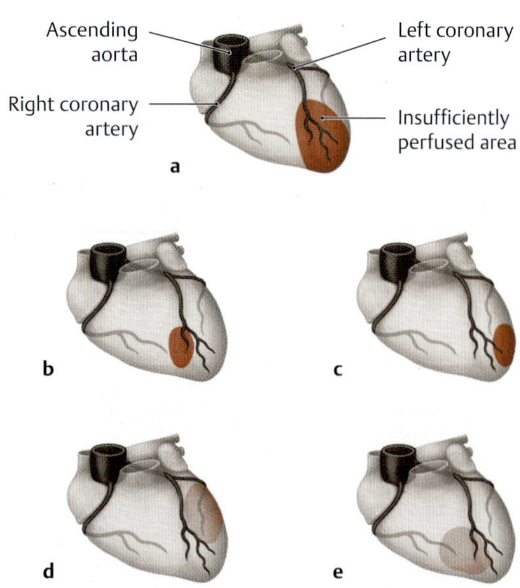

B Infarct localizations and possible complications

The following infarct localizations are based on the location of coronary artery stenosis:

- **a** Anterior wall infarction
- **b** Supra-apical anterior infarction
- **c** Anterior lateral infarction
- **d** Posterior lateral infarction
- **e** Posterior infarction

Blockage of the right coronary artery more frequently leads to arrhythmia because the right coronary artery supplies the sinoatrial node among other structures (see p. 122). Approximately 30% of all patients die within an hour of onset of acute myocardial infarction. The main causes of death include arrhythmia and the ensuing ventricular fibrillation (sudden cardiac death) as well as left ventricular insufficiency and cardiogenic shock. Additional complications include cardiac ruptures (particularly septal perforation) with ensuing pericardial tamponade, mitral insufficiency caused by papillary muscle rupture, and myocardial aneurysm.

C Overview of coronary heart disease (CHD) and myocardial ischemia

Definition: Stenosis of the coronary arteries caused by arteriosclerosis (also known as coronary sclerosis) and the resulting reduced myocardial blood flow (ischemia).

Epidemiology: most common cause of death in Germany; incidence of CHD increases after age 50 (in women mainly after menopause), with men three times more likely to develop CHD than women.

Pathogenesis of myocardial ischemia When the coronary arteries are stenosed as a result of arteriosclerosis (see **D**), they cannot spontaneously transport more blood. Yet this is necessary in order to rapidly supply the myocardium with more oxygen during physical exertion or psychological excitement. The increase in myocardial oxygen demand under stress is mainly due to an elevated heart rate and increased cardiac muscle contractility caused by activation of the sympathetic nervous system. A healthy heart responds by raising the diastolic blood pressure in the aorta and reducing coronary resistance to 20% of the resting value. It can thus increase coronary blood flow under stress to about 5 times the resting level; this is known as the coronary reserve. The ability of sclerotic coronary arteries to dilate is reduced or minimal, leading to insufficient blood supply to the myocardium. The result is ischemia with too little oxygen being supplied to the respective area of the heart muscle. This eventually leads to myocardial tissue necrosis (see **A**). The arteriovenous oxygen difference cannot increase in the heart, because the heart's oxygen consumption from the coronary arteries is maximal even in the resting state.

Clinical symptoms: Symptoms usually occur with a reduction in vascular lumen size of 75 % or greater:

- Cardinal sign: (*angina pectoris*) squeezing, searing pain behind the breast bone (retrosternal), triggered by physical activity and/or psychological stress; pain often spreads to the left side of the thorax and the left arm, and sometimes to the neck, teeth, mouth, and jaw area as well as to the back.
- Accompanying symptoms: sweating, shortness of breath, reduced functional capacity
- Stable angina pectoris: pain vanishes when physical activity or stress has ended.
- Unstable angina pectoris: more frequent bouts of pain, which are more severe and last longer. They don't vanish once physical activity has ended or stress is over; significantly increased risk of heart attack.

Note: 25 % of patients with stable angina pectoris will develop a myocardial infarction within 5 years; patients with unstable angina pectoris will suffer a myocardial infarction within 4 weeks. In more than half of all patients, sudden cardiac death or myocardial infarction are the first "signs" of CHD.

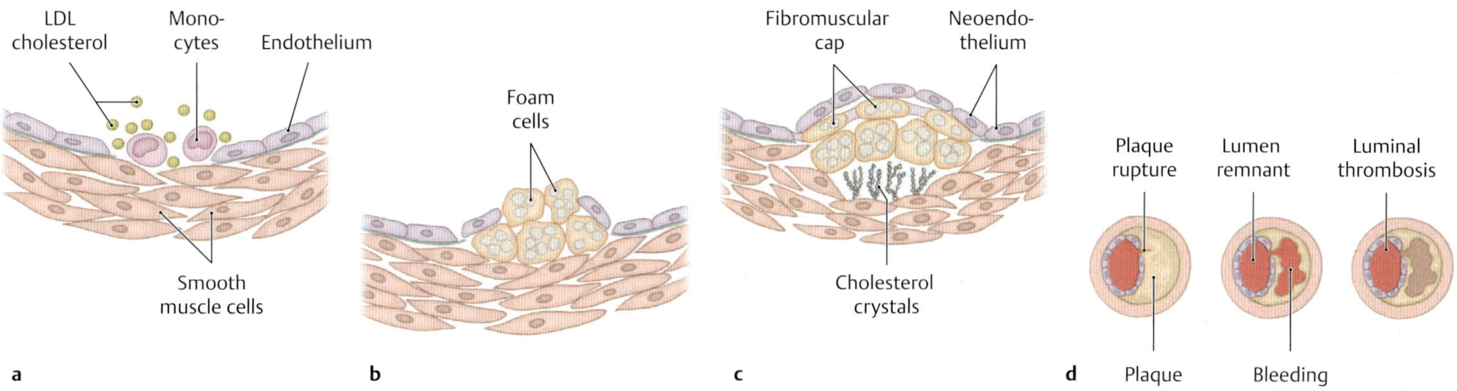

D Pathogenesis of arteriosclerotic changes in the coronary arteries

a Initial lesion; **b** Early lesion; **c** Late lesion; **d** Coronary occlusion.

Predilection sites of arteriosclerotic lesions are the proximal portions of the coronary vessels, particularly in the area where vessels divide as these areas are characterized by increased turbulent blood flow, which is a factor in initiating lesions. Coronary stenosis is caused initially by damage to the endothelium associated with certain risk factors (see **E**). With the help of adhesion proteins, monocytes attach to the sites of initial lesions and migrate as macrophages into the vessel wall. Through accumulation of lipids (mainly oxidized LDL cholesterol), macrophages transform into foam cells. These arteriosclerotic early lesions are also known as fatty streaks. Subsequently, additional cells migrate into the vessel wall. As a result, smooth muscle cells and fibroblasts proliferate forming a fibrous matrix composed of collagen, proteoglycans, calcium, and extracellular lipid deposits. The latter become confluent and are stored in a cavity covered by a fibrous cap and neoendothelium. In this way, complex lesions develop. These fibrous plaques increasingly lead to luminal stenosis. In the course of further progression, particularly lipid-rich plaques may rupture which can lead to intraplaque hemorrhage and formation of thromboses and subsequently to partial or complete coronary occlusion. These plaques, also known as vulnerable plaques, are characterized by high lipid accumulation, increased inflammatory cell activity (macrophages and T -lymphocytes) and high concentrations of tissue-resident coagulation factors.

E Cardiovascular risk factors for arteriosclerosis and CHD

Risk factors for CHD are conditions that occur more frequently in patients with CHD than in healthy subjects. It should be noted that not all cardiovascular events can be explained by the presence of these risk factors. The following risk factors promote arteriosclerosis and thus CHD:

- Arterial hypertension
- Being overweight (BMI > 25kg/m2)
- Lack of exercise
- Hyperlipidemia (particularly lipid metabolic disorder with increased LDL levels and low HDL cholesterol)
- Tobacco abuse
- Diabetes mellitus
- Hereditary disposition

Note: The risk of developing CHD increases disproportionately if multiple risk factors are present.

3.16 Conventional Coronary Angiography (Heart Catheter Examination): Principle and Execution

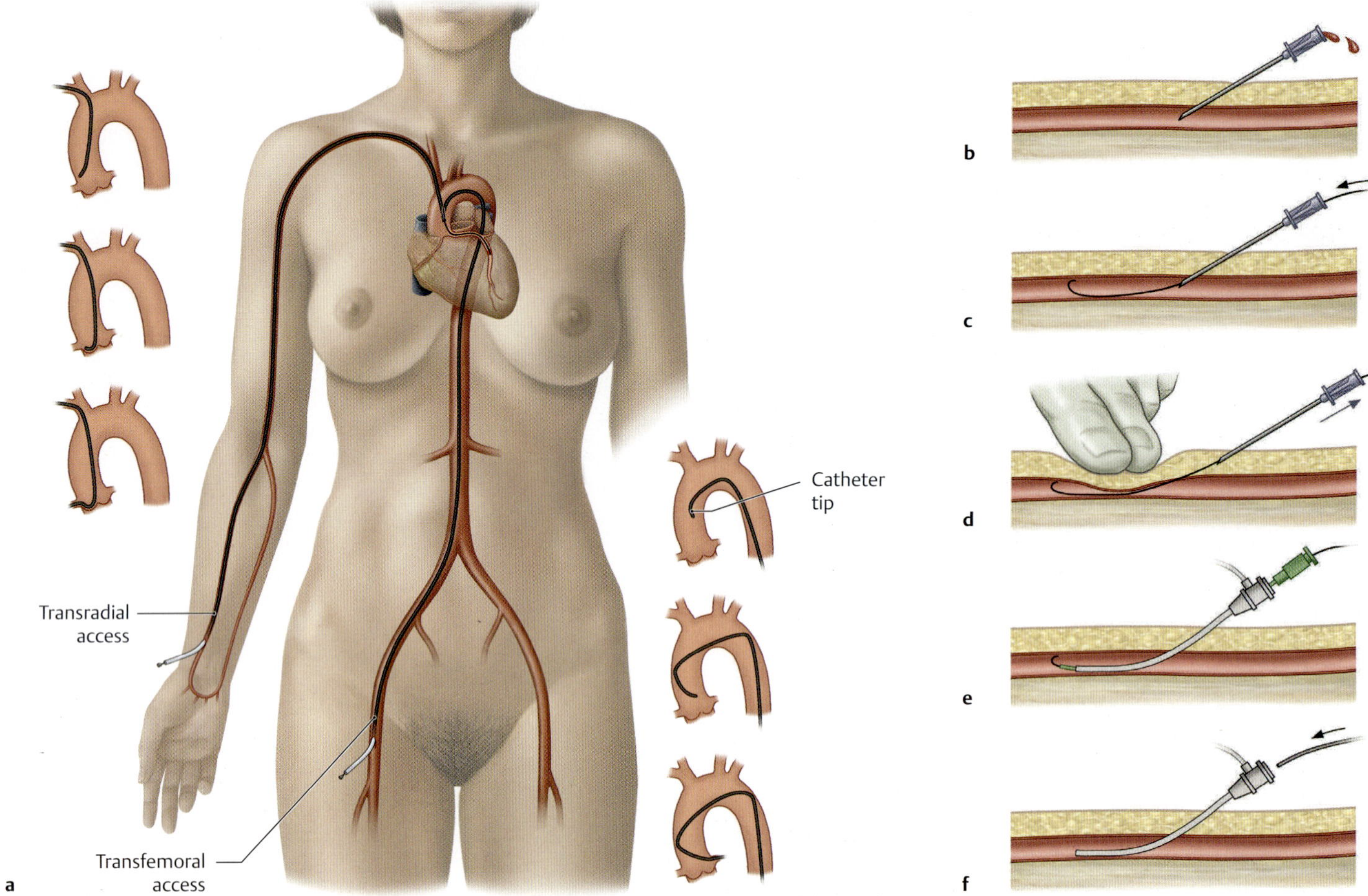

A Principle and execution of selective (conventional) coronary angiography

a Transradial and transfemoral access to the coronary arteries of the heart (see left and right schematic diagrams for the position of the catheter within the aortic arch); **b–f** Arterial puncture and insertion of the catheter sheath.

One distinguishes between left and right heart catheter examinations whereby the left heart catheter examination is significantly more common, for example in the case of suspected coronary artery disease (see p. 124). For the angiographic examination, a water-soluble iodinated contrast agent is injected which then disperses into the coronary arteries. The pattern of dispersion indicates which vessel is affected and to what extent it is stenosed or occluded. The perfusion is documented by fluoroscopy.

Note: As few injections as possible should be performed so as minimize radiation exposure and the volume of injected contrast agent.

In order to advance the catheter carrying the contrast agent into the coronary arteries, access is obtained via the radial artery or femoral artery.

Note: **Access via the radial artery**, approximately 2 finger widths proximal to the wrist, is currently preferred (see **a**). Although it is less straightforward than transfemoral access from a technical standpoint, it offers decisive advantages:

- A significantly lower rate of complications than transfemoral access (no need to immobilize the patient after procedure, no significant bleeding, etc.); there is also minimal risk of nerve injury, and the danger of ischemia is largely excluded as the palmar arch supplies blood from two arteries.
- After the procedure the puncture site is easily closed by applying pressure to the radial artery which here courses superficially.

Execution (b–f):

b After palpating the artery and applying local anesthesia, a percutaneous stab incision is made and the puncture needle is advanced into the artery via the anterior wall (*single wall puncture technique*) until pulsating blood is drawn.

c The guidewire is introduced through puncture needle (the sheath is advanced over the wire into the arterial lumen, see **d**).

d The puncture needle is withdrawn while compression is applied to the puncture site.

e The sheath with the indwelling dilator is advanced over the guidewire.

f After the dilator has been removed, the catheter is introduced into the artery via the sheath.

Note: The catheter is brought into position in retrograde fashion via the ascending aorta. From here the openings of both coronary arteries can be catheterized immediately superior to the aortic valve.

Although conventional coronary angiography is not without risks (sensitivity to contrast agents, vascular damage, cardiac complications), the incidence of severe complications is less than 1% in specialized centers. Other angiographic imaging modalities such as MR and CT angiography are less invasive and therefore significantly safer. These modalities allow detailed visualization of the coronary arteries without invasive arterial puncture and sometimes even without the use of contrast agents (MR angiography). Conventional coronary angiography nonetheless remains the gold standard as it can be combined with interventional therapeutic procedures (such as stent placement, see p. 133). Approximately 700,000 diagnostic procedures and over 290,000 interventional procedures (percutaneous coronary invention) are performed each year in Germany.

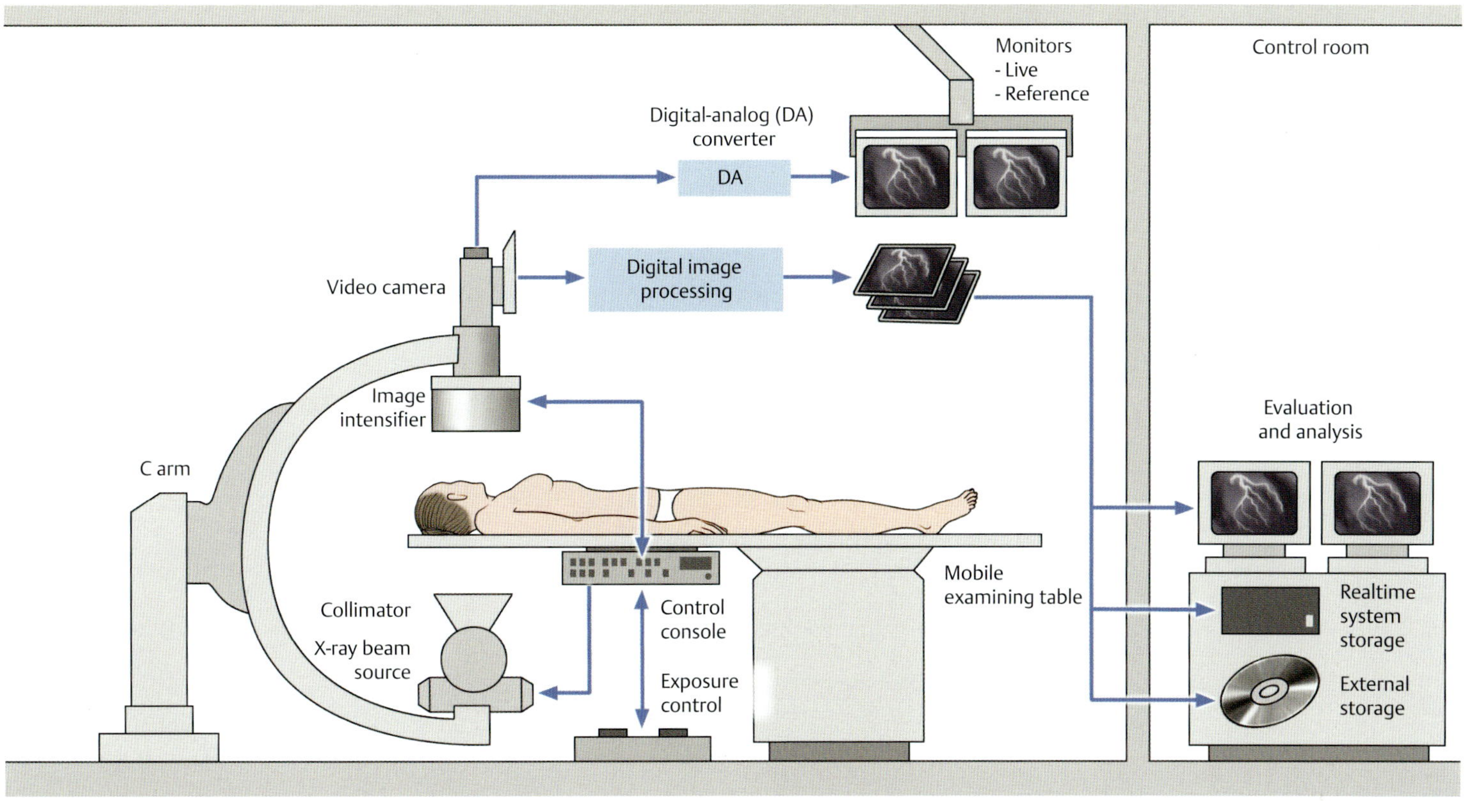

B Design of an angiography system in a heart catheter center
Conventional coronary angiography (see **A**) is performed in heart catheter centers as certain spatial and technological conditions must be met (see guidelines of Deutsche Gesellschaft für Kardiologie):

- Mobile examining table easily accessible from all sides (important in case the patient must be resuscitated);
- Image intensifier system mounted on a C arm that can move freely in three dimensions (important for visualizing the coronary arteries from different positions: rotational range 0–90°, angulation range 0–40°, see **C**).
- X-ray tube and generator for producing a beam. This is located directly opposite the image intensifier.
- Flat panel (not shown here) for digital image acquisition.

Note: As the X-ray beam source is located under the table and the patient is supine, the X-ray beam always travels in a posteroanterior direction. This arrangement minimizes optical distortion.
The German Radiography Ordinance (Röntgenverordnung) defines additional special requirements for a heart catheter center with respect to interventional heart catheter procedures (balloon dilation, placement of stents, etc., see p. 132f). These include such things as enhanced radiation protection at the examining table and the requirement of wearing dosimeters.

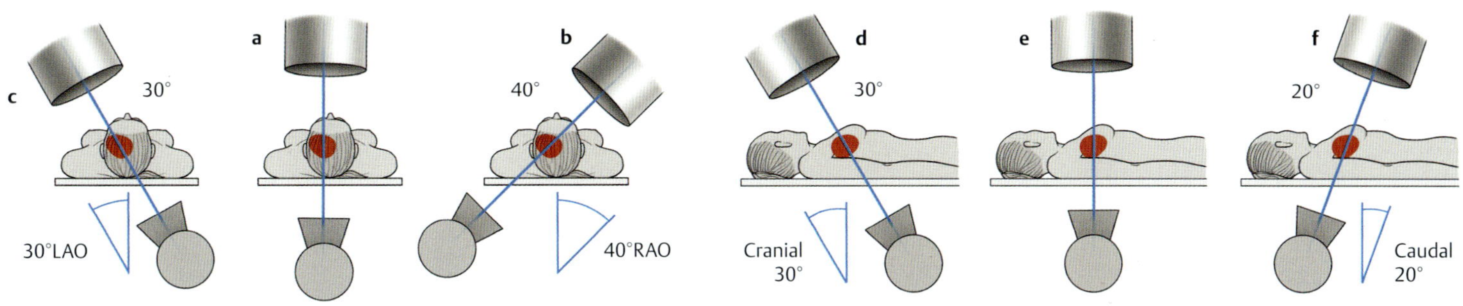

C Projection planes and angulations
a–c Projection planes; **d–f** angulations.
The projection planes are named according to the position of the image intensifier. There are **3 main projections:**

- Anterior projection (anteroposterior, **a**): The image intensifier is located directly above the patient.
- RAO position (right anterior oblique position, **b**): The image intensifier is located to the right of the patient at any desired angle between 0° and 90°.
- LAO position (left anterior oblique position, **c**): The image intensifier is located to the left of the patient at any desired angle between 0° and 90°.

The image intensifier can also be tilted toward the patient's head or feet; that is, angled cranially or caudally.

- Thirty degree cranial angulation (**d**): The image intensifier is tilted toward the patient's head.
- Zero degree position (**e**): The image corresponds to the anteroposterior projection, see **a**, but is shown here from the patient's perspective to better depict the alignment of the image intensifier, which is in the 0° vertical position above the patient.
- Twenty degree caudal angulation (**f**): The image intensifier is tilted toward the patient's feet.

Combining the LAO and RAO projections (**a–c**) with the various angulations allows practically unobstructed visualization of the two coronary arteries and all of their branches.

3.17 Conventional Coronary Angiography: RAO and LAO Projections of the Coronary Arteries

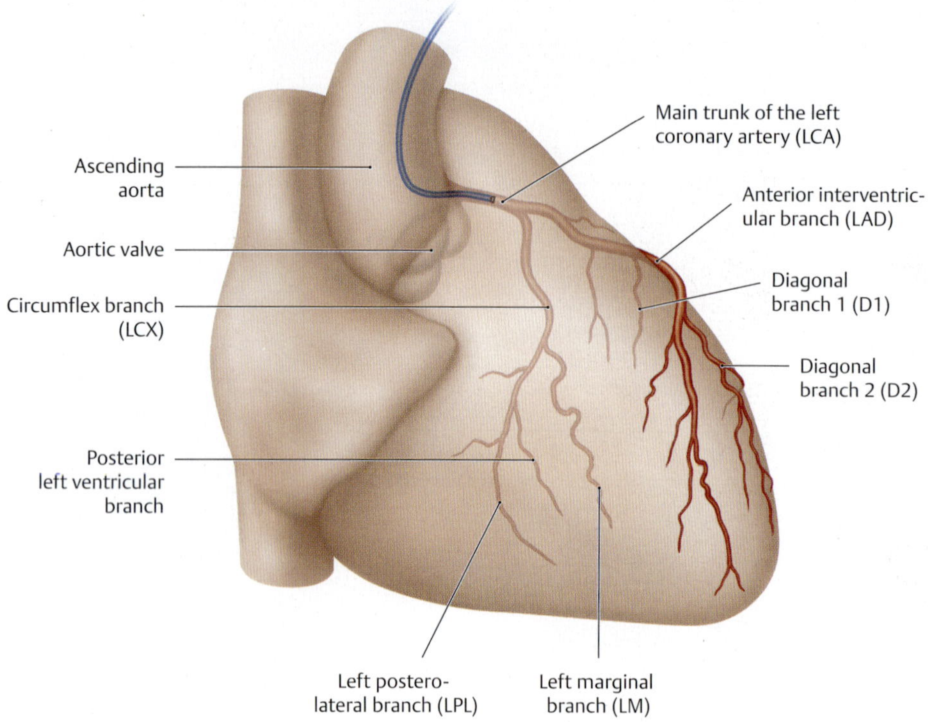

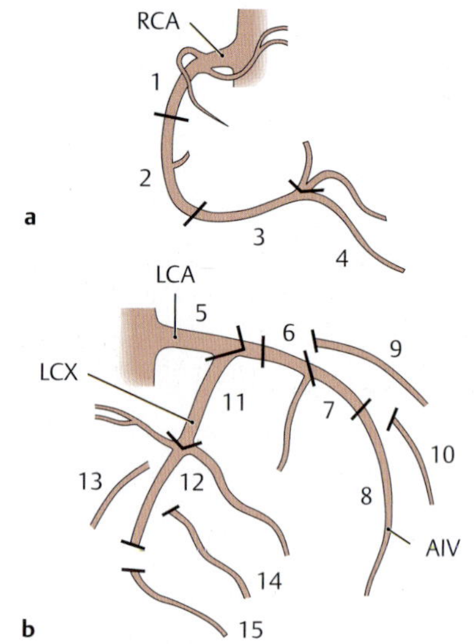

C Segmentation of the coronary arteries
a Right coronary artery (RCA); **b** left coronary artery (LCA) and their respective segments (after a proposal of the American Heart Association, AHA): right coronary artery (segments 1–4); left coronary artery (segments 5–15).

RCA 1 = proximal portion; 2 = mid portion; 3 = distal portion; 4 = posterior interventricular branch (PIV) and right posterolateral branch (RPL)

LCA 5 = main trunk of the left coronary artery

LAD 6 = proximal portion; 7 = mid portion (distal to origin of first diagonal branch, D1); 8 = distal portion (distal to origin of second diagonal branch, D2); 9 = D1; 10 = D2

LCX 11 = proximal portion; 12 = distal portion (origin of left marginal branch, LM); 13 = left atrioventricular branch (LAV); 14 = posterior left ventricular branch; 15 = left posterolateral branch (LPL)

A Topography of the left coronary artery in the RAO projection
Coronary arteries are examined in standard projections that ensure visualization of the entire length of the respective artery unobscured by any overlying structures such as the aorta or spine. This is particularly relevant to visualization of the proximal portions of the vessels such as the main trunk of the left coronary artery. All projections are obtained at maximum possible inspiration to prevent the diaphragm from obscuring the image.

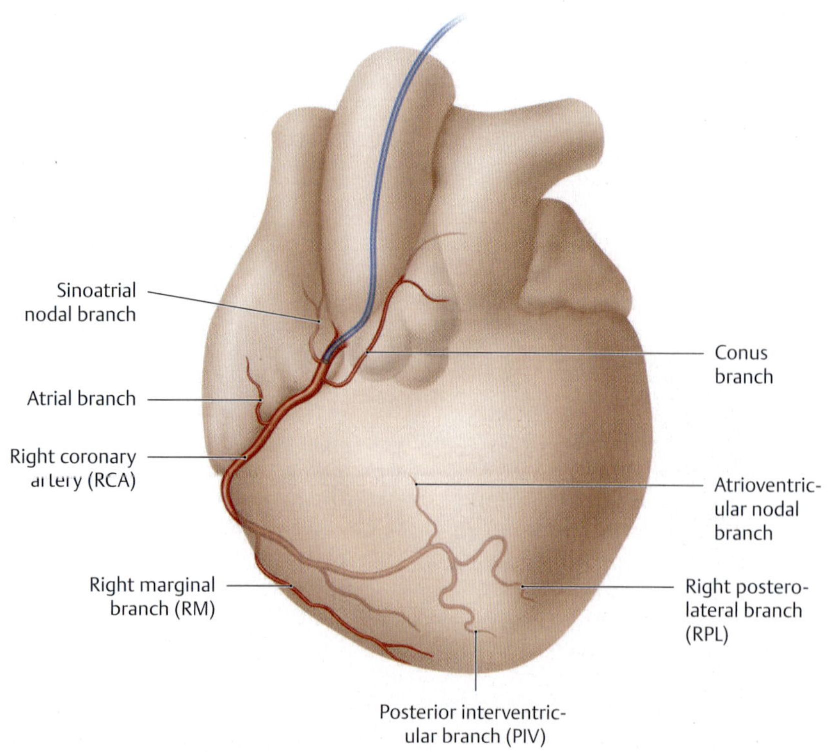

B Topography of the right coronary artery in the LAO projection

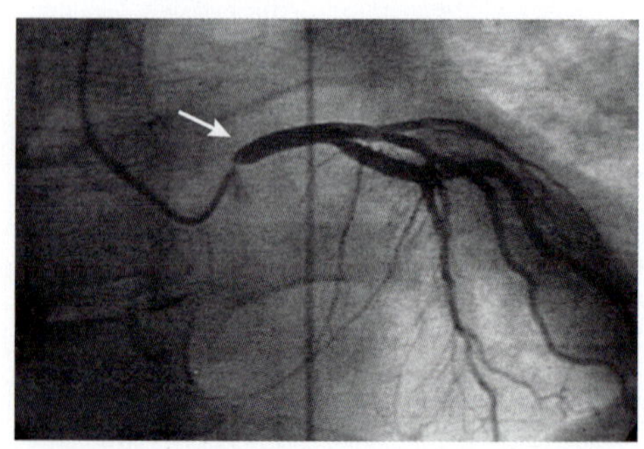

D High-grade stenosis of the main trunk of the left coronary artery
Selective coronary angiography in a 10° RAO projection. The arrow indicates of stenosis more than 90% in segment 5, the main trunk of the left coronary artery (from: Lapp H. Das Herzkatheterbuch. 5th ed. Stuttgart: Thieme; 2019).

E Preferred standard projections for visualizing the left coronary artery

Six standard projections are usually used to visualize the left coronary artery; these three are the most common (from: Lapp H. Das Herzkatheterbuch. 5th ed. Stuttgart: Thieme; 2019).

- RAO 10° (**a**): visualizes the full length of the main trunk of the left coronary artery and permits diagnosis of possible truncal stenosis (see **C**),
- RAO 30° with 20° caudal angulation (**b**): visualizes the full length of the circumflex coronary artery including its marginal branch as well as the posterolateral branch and the proximal third of the anterior interventricular branch (AIV),
- RAO 30° with 20° cranial angulation (not shown): eliminates the overshadowing of the middle portion of the anterior interventricular branch by the first and second diagonal branches.

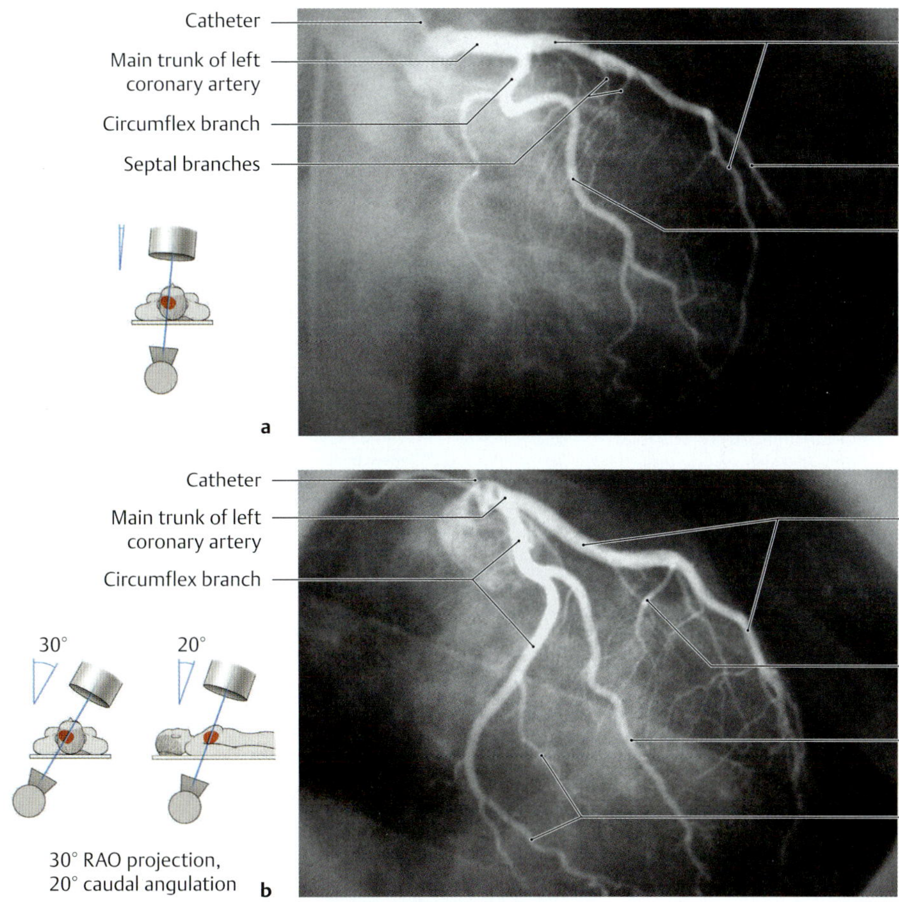

F Preferred standard projections for visualizing the right coronary artery

The following two projections are usually sufficient to visualize the right coronary artery (from: Lapp H. Das Herzkatheterbuch. 5th ed. Stuttgart: Thieme; 2019).

- LAO 60° (**a**): good view of the *right atrioventricular opening* and the long main trunk (but foreshortened visualization of the terminal branches) and
- LAO 45° with 15° cranial angulation (**b**): good view of both *terminal branches*, especially of the *inferior* (*posterior*) *interventricular branch*.

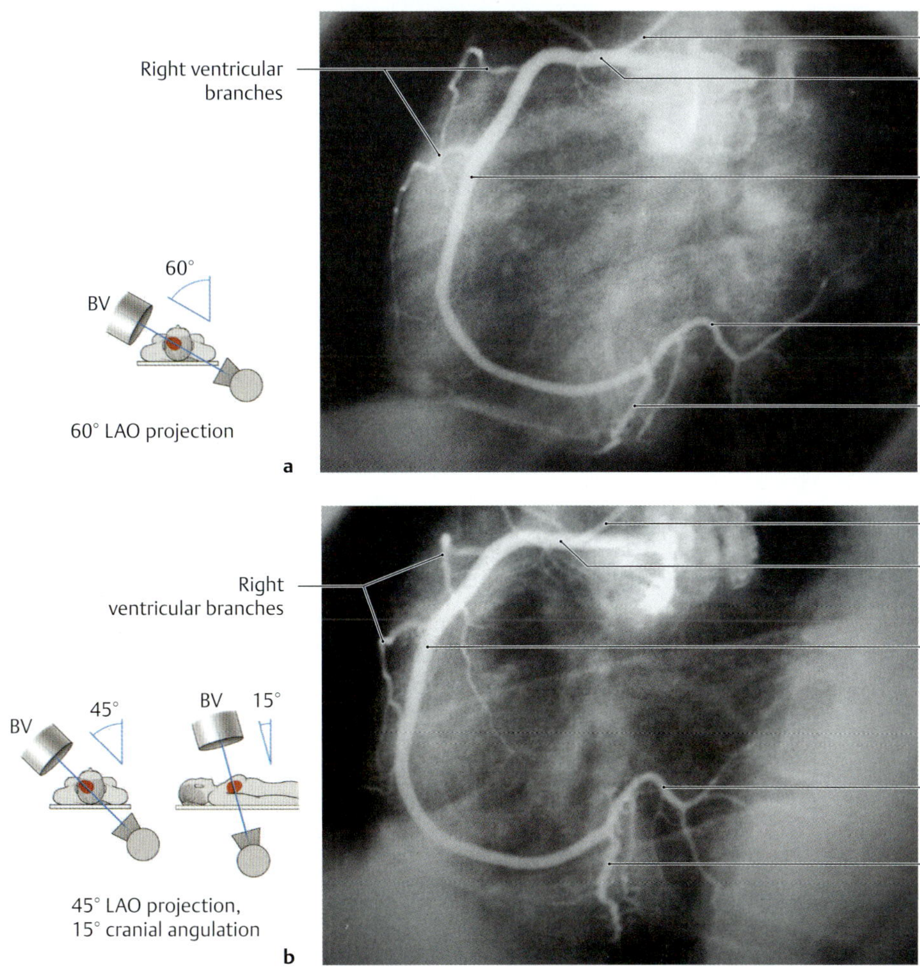

3.18 Multislice Spiral Computed Tomography (MSCT) Coronary Angiography

A Common cardiac imaging planes used in CT

a At the level of the pulmonary trunk; **b** Display of the heart chambers; **c** At the level of the aortic root; **d** Below the left atrium (from Reiser M, Kuhn F, Debus J, eds. *Duale Reihe Radiologie*. 3rd ed. Stuttgart: Thieme; 2011).

Note: Because invasive conventional coronary angiography (see p. 126f) is followed by a coronary intervention (balloon dilatation, stent, see p. 132f) in only 30–40% of cases, less invasive procedures such as MSCT coronary angiography have become an increasingly important tool in the diagnosis of coronary heart disease (CHD, see p. 124f). Nowadays, multislice spiral computed tomography (MSCT) can answer almost all clinically relevant questions regarding diagnostic and interventional radiology. It is possible, for example, to create 0.5 mm thick slices or reconstruct three dimensional images of the heart and coronary vessels with common 64-slice spiral computed tomography without motion artifacts (using ECG synchronization) (see fig. **Ea** and **b**).

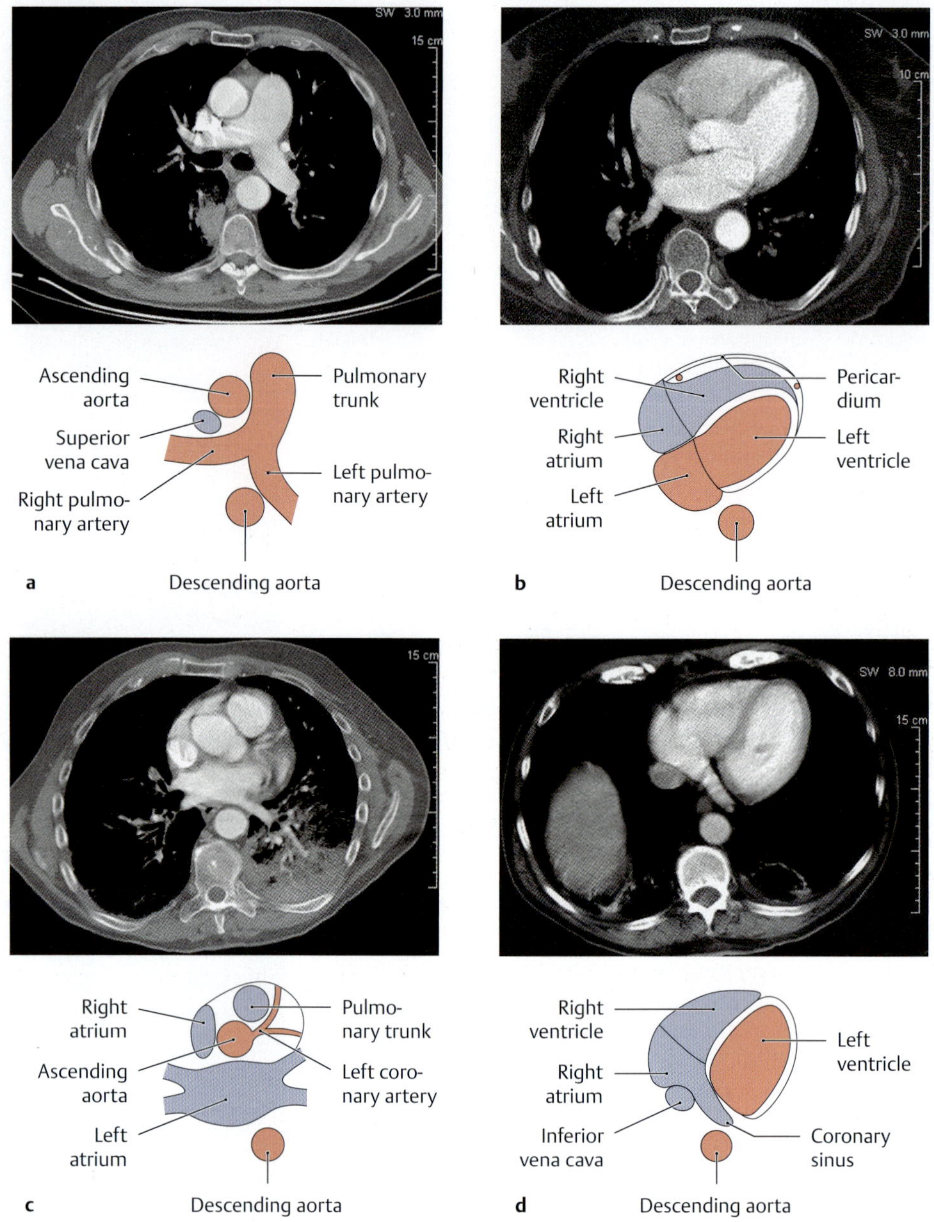

B Representation of the origins of the coronary arteries

Schematic representation of an axial CT section just above the aortic valve (see also sectional plane of **Ac**). In this representation, the aortic root is surrounded by the two atria and the right outflow tract (pulmonary trunk). The location of the left ventricle between the branches of the main trunk of the left coronary artery is indicated.

Note: The aortic valve with its three pocket-like cusps forms three recesses or sinuses, a left-, a right-, and a non-coronary sinus, which are each delimited by their corresponding cusp (left-, right-, and non-coronary cusps). The left coronary artery arises from the left coronary sinus, and the right coronary artery from the right coronary sinus. Coronary anomalies usually involve the origin of the coronary arteries. However, they are rarely encountered in the general population.

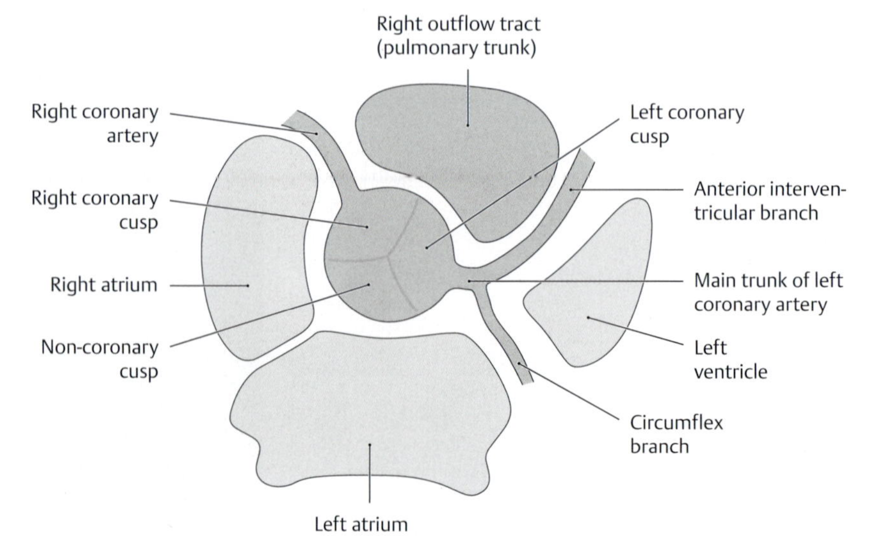

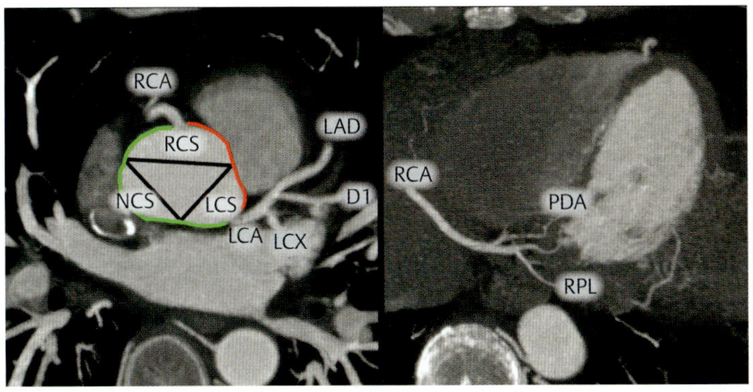

a b

C CT anatomy of the origin of the coronary arteries

a Axial CT section at the level of the origin of the coronary arteries:

LCS, RCS, NCS = left-, right-, and non-coronary sinus,
RCA = right coronary artery,
LCA = main trunk of the left coronary artery,
LCX = circumflex branch,
LAD, left anterior descending artery = anterior interventricular branch,
D1 – diagonal branch 1;

b Course of the right coronary artery (RCA) toward the posterior wall of the heart and branching into a posterior interventricular branch (PDA, posterior descending artery) and a right posterolateral branch (RPL).
(From: Becker C. *CT-Diagnostik der koronaren Herzkrankheit* [Part I: Indikation, Durchführung und Normalbefundung der CT-Koronarographie], Radiologie up2date 1. Stuttgart: Thieme; 2008.)

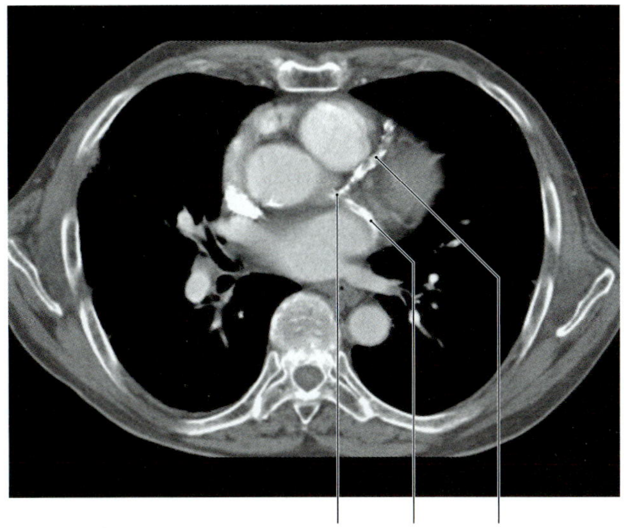

D CT anatomy of coronary sclerosis of the left coronary artery

Transverse (axial) section at the level where the left coronary artery originates.

An important use of cardiac CT technology is in evaluating coronary calcium deposits in arteriosclerotic coronary arteries. This procedure does not require the use of contrast agents. The image shows a diffuse coronary sclerosis of the main trunk of the left coronary artery (LCA) as well as the circumflex branch (LCX) and anterior interventricular branch (LAD) (from: Claussen CD et al. *Pareto-Reihe Radiologie*. Herz. Stuttgart: Thieme; 2006).

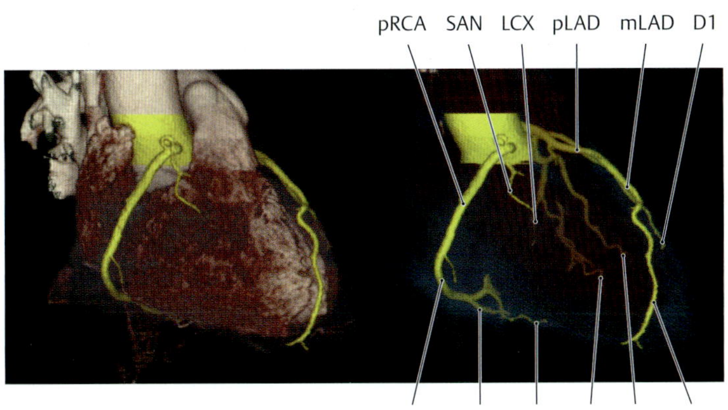

a

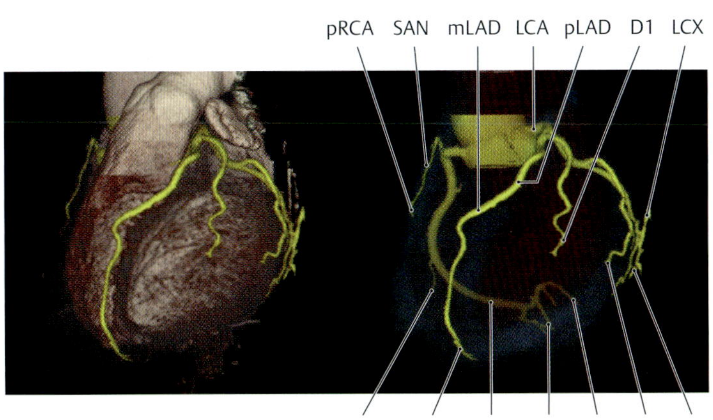

b

E Three-dimensional reconstruction of the heart using CT scan images

a CT anatomy of the heart in a 30-degree RAO projection; **b** Anatomy of the heart in a 60-degree LAO projection.

After the injection of contrast agent, the coronary arteries (or rather the column of contrast medium) can be three-dimensionally reconstructed. Depending on which projection (RAO, right anterior oblique; LAO, left anterior oblique) and angulation was used (30 or 60 degrees), the clarity, with which the course of the coronary arteries can be displayed, varies.

pRCA, mRCA, and dRCA = proximal, middle, and distal portion of the right coronary artery
PDA, *posterior descending artery* = posterior interventricular branch
RPL = right posterolateral branch
SAN = *sinoatrial nodal branch*
LCA = main trunk of the left coronary artery
pLAD, mLAD and dLAD, *left anterior descending artery* = proximal, middle and distal portion of the anterior interventricular branch
LCX = circumflex branch
D1 = diagonal branch 1
LM1 = left marginal branches
LM2 = left posterolateral branches

(From: Becker C. *CT-Diagnostik der koronaren Herzkrankheit* [Part I: Indikation, Durchführung und Normalbefundung der CT-Koronarographie], Radiologie up2date 1. Stuttgart: Thieme; 2008.)

3.19 Balloon Dilatation, Aortocoronary Venous and Arterial IMA Bypass

A Interventional and surgical options for treatment of coronary artery stenosis

The goal of coronary intervention is to improve the prognosis (*prognostic indicators*) and/or symptoms (*symptomatic indicators*) in patients with coronary heart disease (CHD). By restoring sufficient perfusion and oxygenation to the myocardium, myocardial performance is improved. Failure to achieve satisfactory results by treating CHD with drugs indicates the need for interventional (invasive procedure using a catheter advanced along the femoral artery) or surgical treatments (surgery to open the thorax, etc.). Additionally, in cases of acute myocardial infarction, revascularization with aortocoronary bypasses becomes an increasingly important tool. The following procedures are the most commonly performed:

- **Interventional techniques (PCI = percutaneous coronary intervention):**
  - percutaneous transluminal coronary angioplasty (PTCA)
  - percutaneous transluminal stent placement;
- **surgical coronary revascularization techniques:**
  - aortocoronary venous bypass (ACVB)
  - internal mammary artery bypass (IMA bypass).

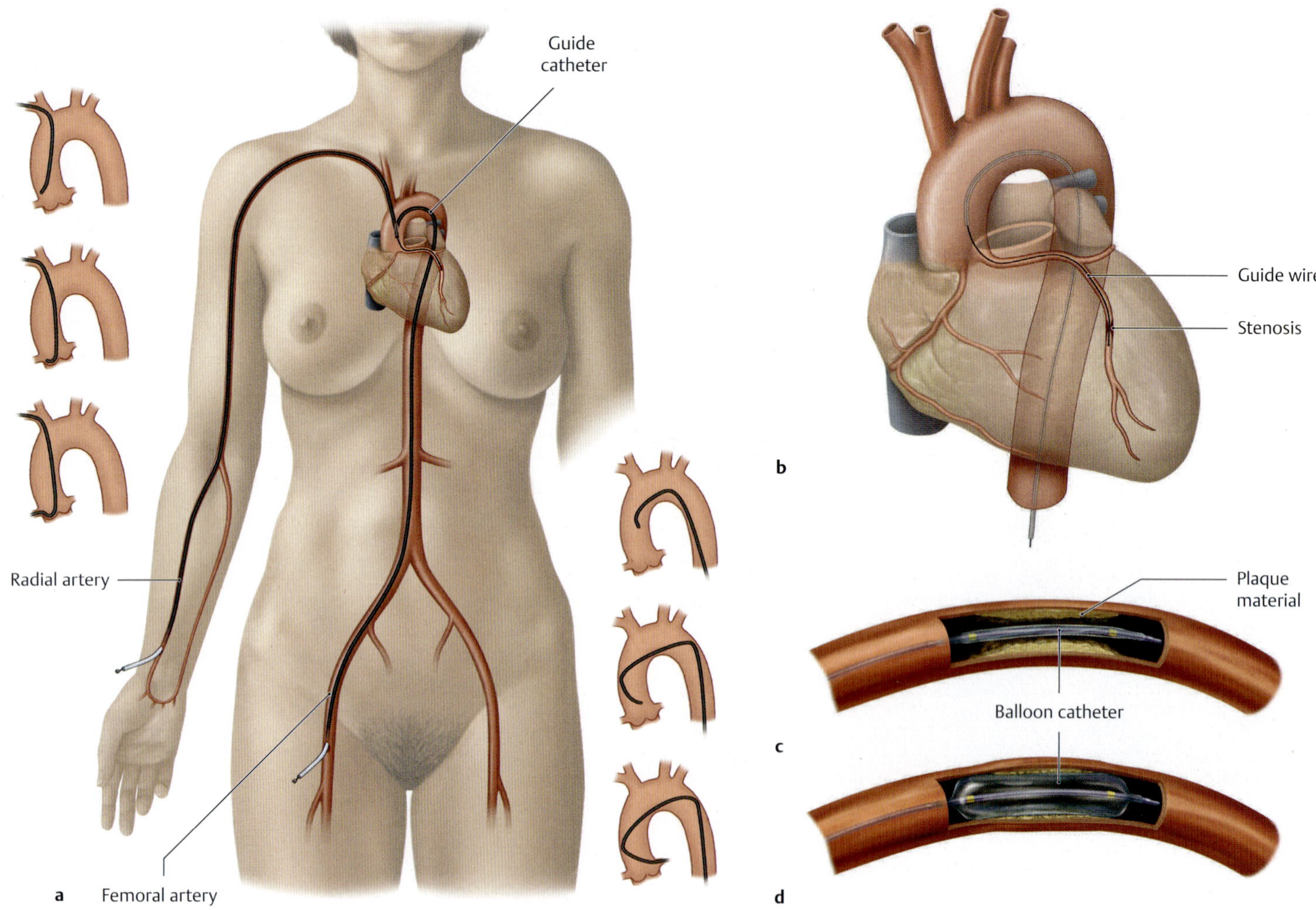

B Percutaneous transluminal coronary angioplasty (PTCA)

a Probing the coronary artery using a guide catheter to insert a guide wire; **b** Passing the stenosis with a guide wire; **c** and **d** Placement of a balloon catheter over the guide wire and dilatation of the stenosis.

The PTCA procedure consists of balloon dilatation of narrowed coronary arteries. The femoral artery or radial artery (**a**) is punctured and a guide wire is used to probe the affected coronary artery. Via the guide wire, a balloon catheter is placed in the narrowed portion of the artery and then inflated in a controlled fashion to 8–20 atm (**c** and **d**), resulting in the compression of plaque material and dilatation of the lumen. Approximately 50–80% of balloon dilatations are successful. However in 15–30% of all cases, a restenosis develops during the first year after the procedure. Contraindications include high-grade stenoses in areas where the coronary arteries branch. Due to possible complications (risk of perforation or occlusion as a result of intimal dissection), coronary dilatations are always performed with cardiovascular surgeons on standby. Since the long-term results (one year post procedure) of dilatations are worse than with bypass surgeries, the use of dilatation methods is currently viewed very critically.

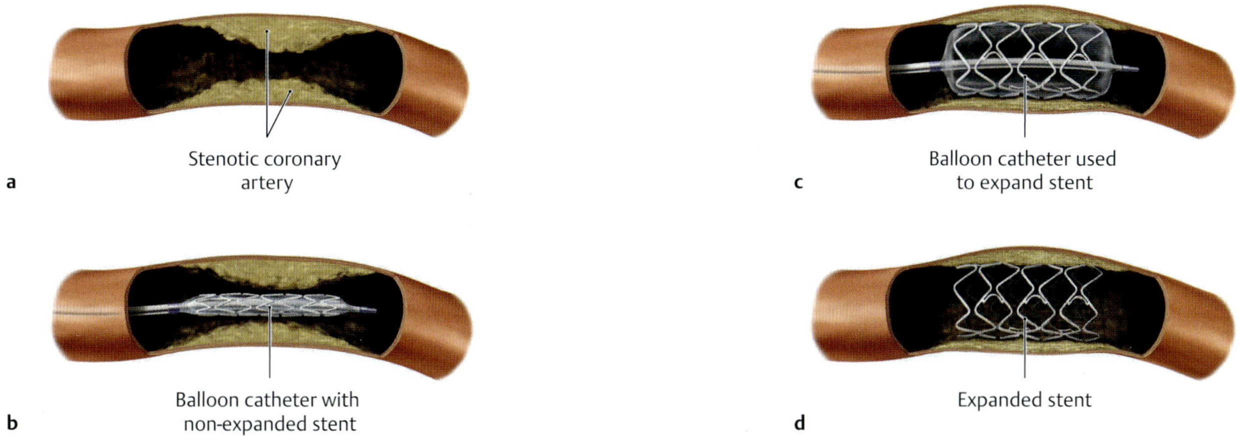

C Stent placement
The placement of wire mesh stents is a standard procedure (80% of all interventions) in PCI. Using balloon catheters, the metal stents are positioned in the affected segment of the coronary artery and expanded by inflation of the balloon catheter (at 12 atm). The dilated segment is supported by the stent and thus kept open. Compared to classic balloon dilatation, stent placement results in a considerably lower rate of restenosis (for example by causing less intimal hyperplasia). Additionally, today's coronary stents are invariably coated with pharmaceuticals.

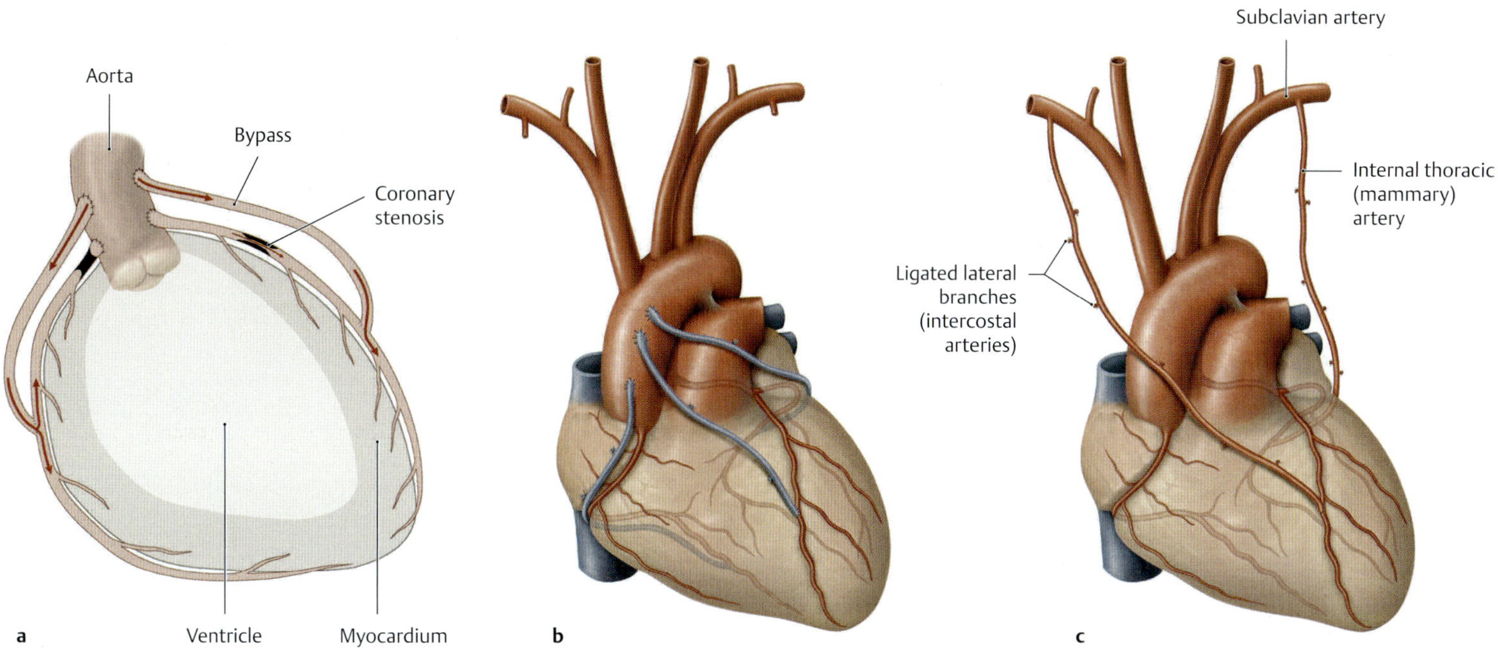

D Surgical coronary revascularization

a Aortocoronary venous bypass (ACVB): In this type of surgical myocardial revascularization one or multiple venous grafts (usually from the great saphenous vein) are placed between the ascending aorta and the post-stenotic segment of the coronary artery. Thus, the grafted vessels bypass the occluded (right) or narrowed (left) segments of the affected arteries. Necessary requirements include a vessel that can be anastomosed post-stenosis and has a diameter of at least 1 mm, and adequate peripheral drainage and functional myocardium in the affected region of the heart. Revascularization with venous bypasses plays an important role in the treatment of acute myocardial infarction.

b Aortocoronary venous bypass in a patient with three vessel disease: In this case, venous grafts are anastomosed to the right coronary artery, and to the anterior interventricular and circumflex branches of the left coronary artery.

c Arterial IMA bypass (IMA = internal mammary artery): In addition to leg veins, arteries are increasingly being used for coronary artery revascularization. Generally, the left and right internal mammary (thoracic) arteries (LIMA; RIMA) are used as in situ grafts, or the radial artery is used as a "free" graft. The distal internal mammary artery is released from its vascular bed and its side branches tied off—up to where it branches from the subclavian artery. The artery is then anastomosed to the post-stenotic coronary artery. The advantage of IMA bypasses over ACVB is a significantly lower occlusion rate. Compared with the patency rate for ACVB of 50% after ten years, 90% of arterial bypass grafts are patent after 10 years. Moreover, cardiac incidents (angina pectoris, myocardial infarction, sudden cardiac death) occur with less frequency following bypass surgery using IMA grafts than after venous bypass surgery.

3.20 Lymphatic Drainage of the Heart

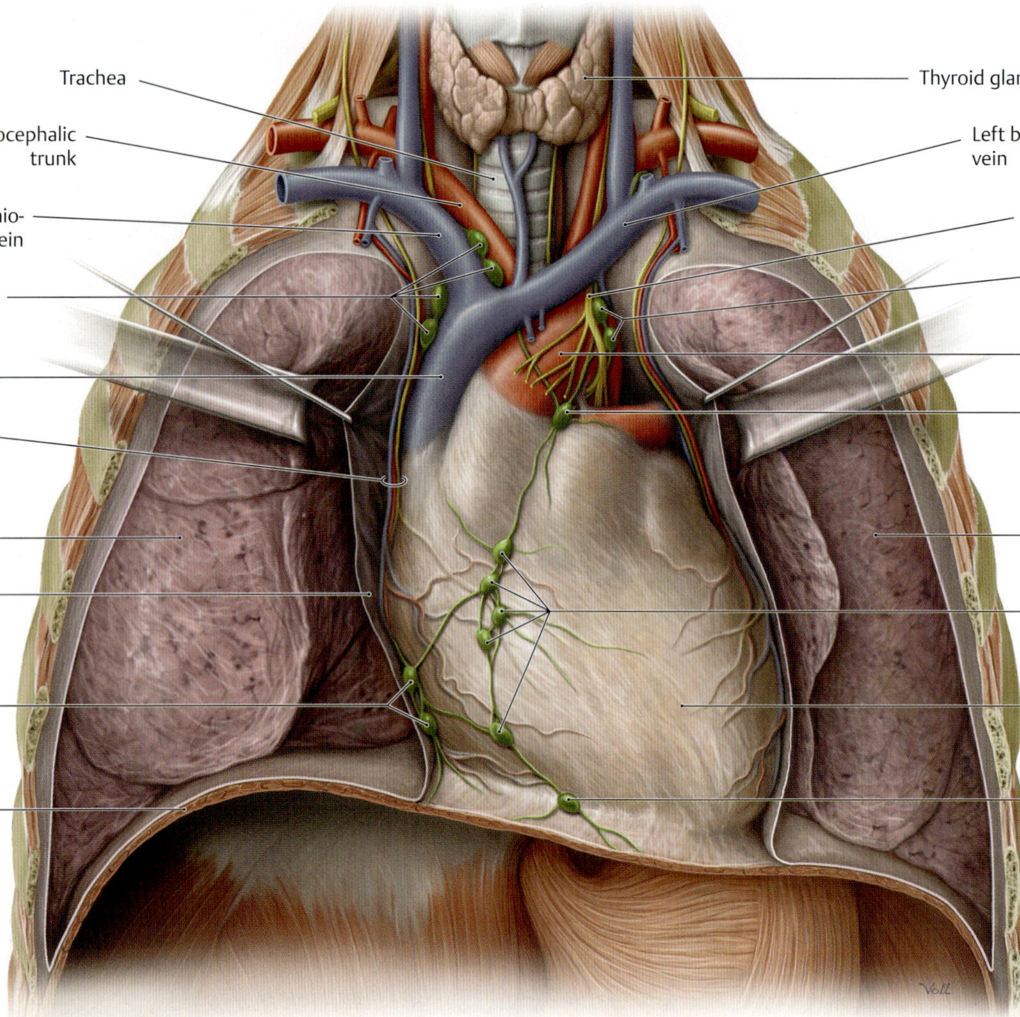

A Lymph nodes and lymphatic drainage of the pericardium
Anterior view of the opened thorax. The pleural cavities have been opened, and the lungs and pleura have been retracted laterally. Due to the close topographical relationship between the heart and pericardium, the lymphatic drainage of the heart and pericardium is discussed together: Both pericardial and cardiac lymph is ultimately conveyed to the bronchomediastinal trunks, but through different primary lymph nodes. Lymph node groups of varying size (prepericardial and lateral pericardial lymph nodes) lie anterior and adjacent to the pericardium and are interconnected by a network of fine lymphatic vessels. These pericardial lymph nodes may drain inferiorly (to the superior phrenic lymph nodes) or cranially (usually to the brachiocephalic lymph nodes). Lymph from the pericardial lymph nodes is ultimately conveyed to the bronchomediastinal trunks (see p. 91), which open at the junction of the right or left subclavian and internal jugular veins.

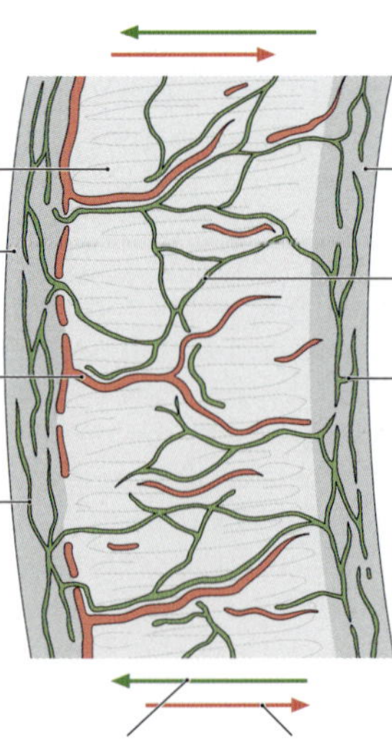

B Lymphatic drainage of the heart wall
Section through the heart wall. There are three networks of densely interconnected lymphatic vessels, corresponding to the three layers of the heart wall:

- Epicardium (visceral layer of the serous pericardium): A subepicardial network collects lymph from the epicardium and from the other two networks. The subepicardial network conveys the lymph to the collecting vessels and lymph nodes of the heart.
- Myocardium: The very extensive myocardial network collects lymph from the myocardium and also from the subendocardial network. Lymphatic vessels of the myocardial network often follow the distribution of the blood capillaries that arise from the coronary arteries. Thus the blood (red arrows) and lymph (green arrows) flow in opposite directions.
- Endocardium: A subendocardial network collects lymph from the endocardium and conveys it to the subepicardial network, either directly or via the myocardial network.

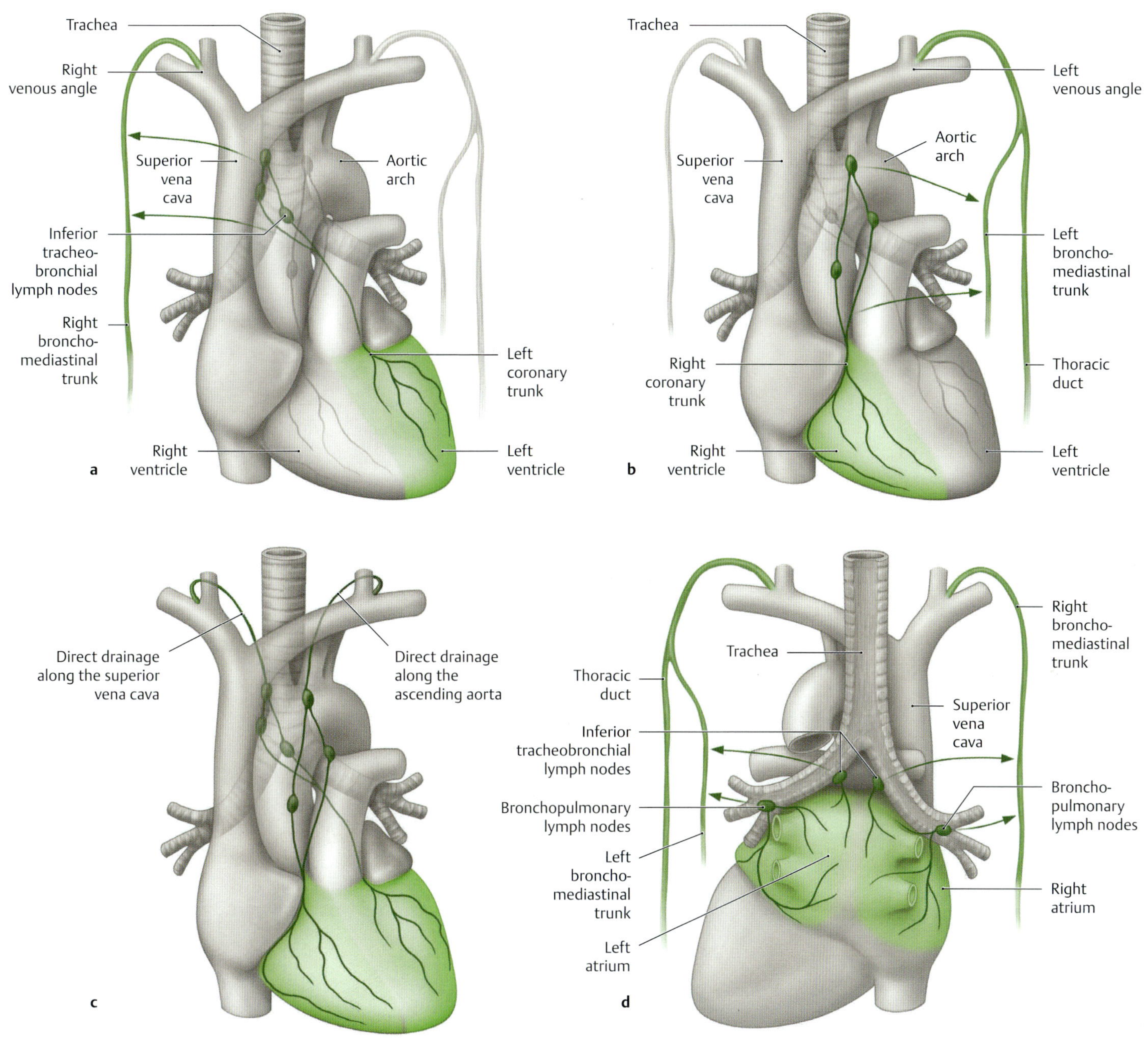

C Lymphatic drainage of the heart

The heart viewed from the anterior aspect (**a**–**c**) and posterior aspect (**d**).

The ventricles and atria have different drainage routes.

Ventricles: The lymphatic drainage of the ventricles (and a small part of the atria) can be roughly divided into two territories referred to as tributary regions (see **a**–**c**):

- The left tributary region (**a**) encompasses the *left* ventricle, a small marginal strip of the *right* ventricle, and small portions of the *left* atrium. It conveys its lymph through a left coronary trunk to the inferior tracheobronchial lymph nodes and from there to the *right* venous angle, either indirectly via the right bronchomediastinal trunk (**a**) or, for a lesser volume, directly via small lymphatic vessels along the superior vena cava (**c**).
- The right tributary region (**b**) mainly encompasses the *right* ventricle and small portions of the *right* atrium. It conveys its lymph through a right coronary trunk to the *left* venous angle, either indirectly via the left bronchomediastinal trunk and the thoracic duct or directly via small lymphatic vessels along the ascending aorta (**c**).

This arrangement creates two "crossed" pathways for lymphatic drainage:

- Left tributary region → left coronary trunk → right venous angle;
- Right tributary region → right coronary trunk → left venous angle.

This "crossed" system of drainage pathways is created during embryonic development by the rotation of the developing heart.

Atria: Lymphatic drainage of the remaining major portions of the atria (**d**): The tributary regions of the two atria are separate from the ventricular pathways; these tributary regions drain to the inferior tracheobronchial lymph nodes or via the ipsilateral bronchopulmonary lymph nodes to the ipsilateral bronchomediastinal trunk and from there to the ipsilateral venous angle.

3.21 Innervation of the Heart

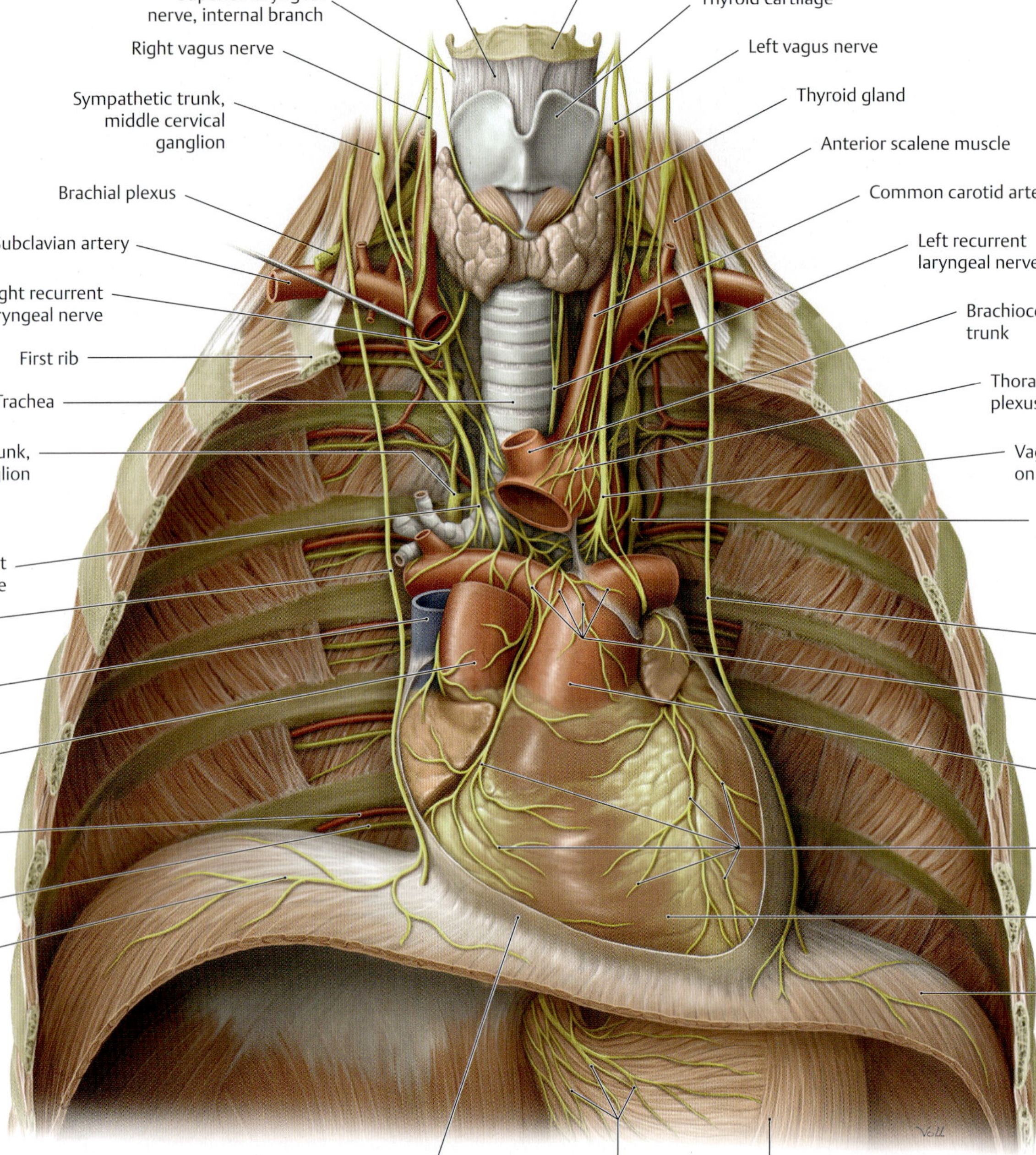

A Autonomic nerves of the heart

Anterior view of the opened thorax with the lungs, pleura, and internal fasciae removed. The pericardium has been broadly opened anteriorly. The vessels surrounding the heart are intact except for a portion of the ascending aorta, which has been removed to display the right pulmonary artery. Part of the upper abdomen is also shown. The cardiac plexus, pulmonary plexus, and thoracic aortic plexus can be clearly identified on the heart and surrounding vessels. These plexuses receive fibers from the vagus nerves and sympathetic trunk. The **right and left vagus nerves** initially run in the anterior part of the superior mediastinum. After giving off branches to the plexuses, they enter the posterior mediastinum (see **B**). **Sympathetic fibers** pass to the cardiac plexus in the form of the cervical cardiac nerves (from the three cervical ganglia) and thoracic cardiac branches (from the thoracic ganglia) (see **B**).

Note: Most of the autonomic fibers in the plexuses are extremely fine, but in this dissection they are shown larger for clarity. The phrenic nerve does not innervate the heart but does give off somatosensory branches to the pericardium (pericardial branches, not shown here) in the middle mediastinum on its way to the diaphragm (see p. 99).

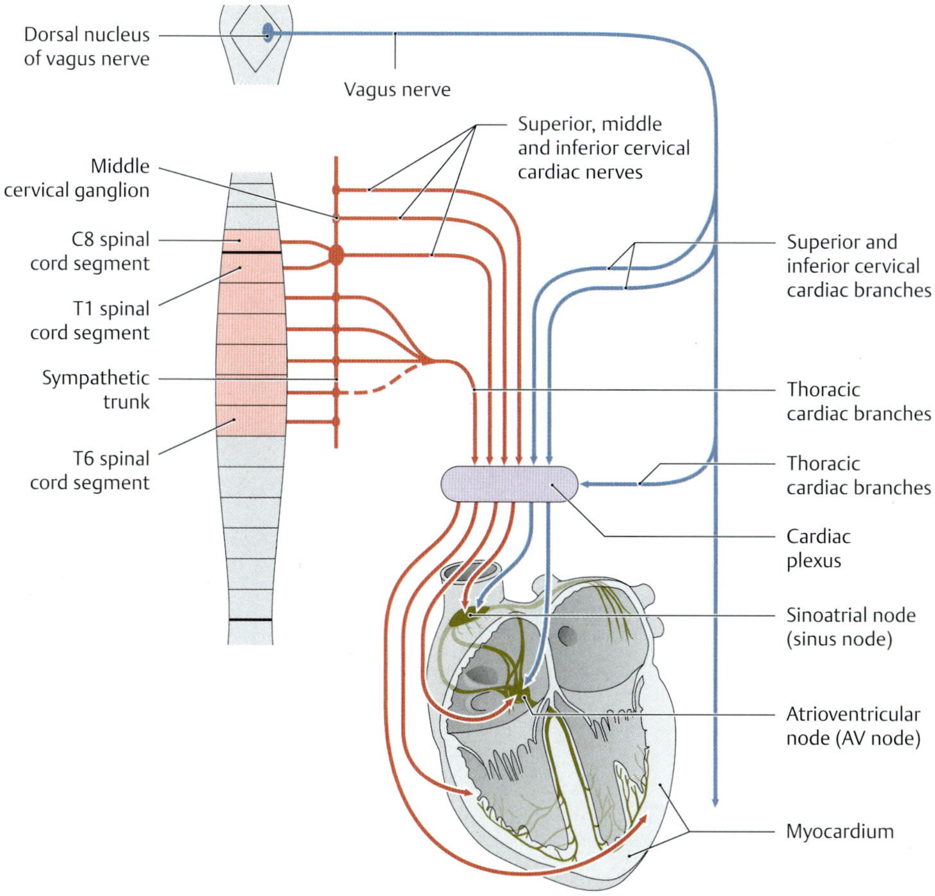

B Autonomic innervation of the heart

Parasympathetic: Vagus nerve fibers from the dorsal vagal nucleus give off the superior and inferior cervical cardiac branches in the neck and the thoracic cardiac branches in the thorax. The cardiac branches pass to the cardiac plexus.

Sympathetic: The three cervical sympathetic ganglia give off the superior, middle, and inferior cervical cardiac nerves, and the thoracic ganglia give off the thoracic cardiac branches. All of the cardiac branches radiate to the *cardiac plexus*, which distributes fibers to the SA node, AV node, myocardium, and coronary vessels. The sympathetic axons, all postsynaptic, innervate all these targets directly, while the parasympathetic axons from the vagus synapse to the SA node, AV node, myocardium, and coronary vessels. The *sympathetic system* increases the rate and force of myocardial contractions and dilates the coronary vessels, while the *parasympathetic system* acts primarily to slow the heart rate. Drugs that act on both systems are used in the treatment of numerous diseases including hypertension, myocardial infarction, and cardiac arrhythmias.

Note: Since the heart has its own pacemaker (see p. 116), the autonomic nervous system does not generate the heartbeat, but instead acts on the SA node to regulate heart rate, and on other areas of the heart to modulate its function under different physiological loads.

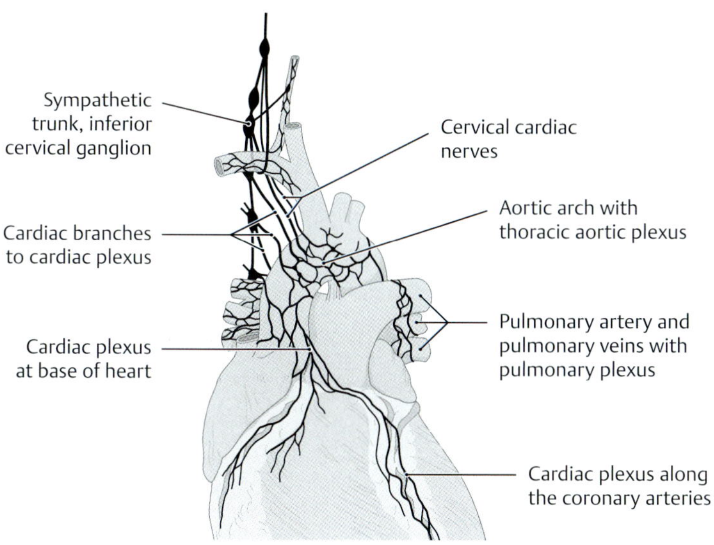

C Autonomic plexuses about the heart

Extensive autonomic nerve plexuses are formed on the heart and surrounding vessels. These plexuses receive fibers from the sympathetic and parasympathetic nervous systems (not shown here):

- Cardiac plexus: located on the heart, especially prominent at the base of the heart and along the coronary vessels (cardiac innervation).
- Thoracic aortic plexus: located about the thoracic aorta (fibers to the heart and other plexuses: pulmonary plexus, esophageal plexus).
- Pulmonary plexus: surrounding the pulmonary arteries (and veins) and the bronchi. The pulmonary plexus is consistently paired, the two parts being connected to each other and to the cardiac plexus (supply the bronchial tree and intrapulmonary vessels).

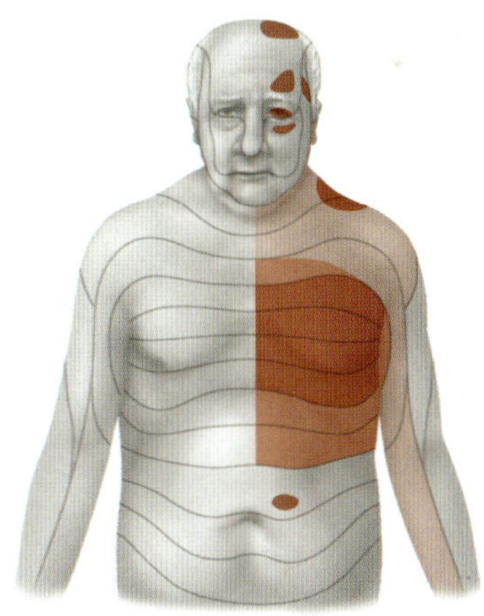

D Referred pain and autonomic reactions associated with heart disease

In patients with heart disease, especially coronary occlusive disease (angina or infarction), the **pain** radiates to characteristic body regions:

- Left shoulder and left arm (particularly the inside of the left arm)
- Left half of the neck and head (jaw pain may present as a "toothache," cranial pain as a "headache")
- Left epigastric region.

Autonomic reactions may be noted in the dermatomes over the heart and in more distant dermatomes: a change in cutaneous blood flow, sweating, piloerection (body hairs "standing on end"), and occasional pupillary dilation (mydriasis) in the left eye.

4.1 Lungs: Location in the Thorax

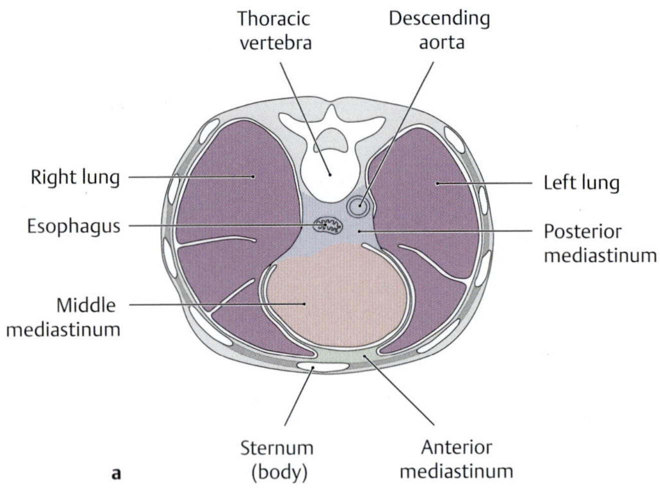

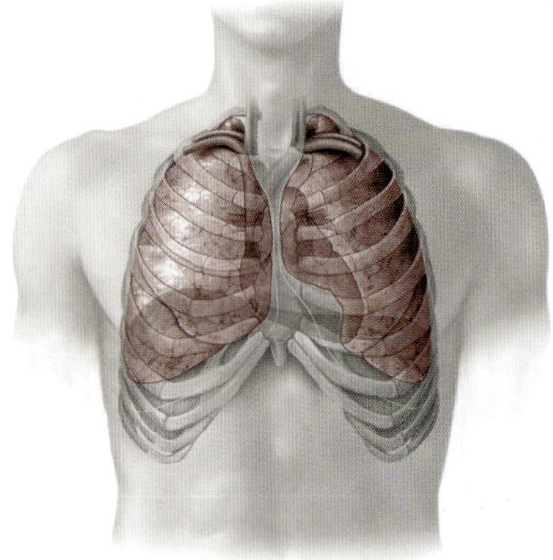

A Location of the lungs in the thorax: topographical relations

a Transverse section through the thorax, superior view. The lungs completely occupy the left and right pleural cavities flanking the mediastinum. Anteriorly, they approach each other in front of the pericardium and posteriorly they are located close to the spinal column. Due to the asymmetrical position of the heart, the left lung is slightly smaller than the right lung (see **D**).

b Projections of the lungs onto the thoracic skeleton, anterior view. Superiorly, both lungs extend above the superior thoracic aperture; inferiorly, the undersurface of the lungs arches over the domes of the diaphragm. The distinct notch at the inferior medial border of the left lung is due to the heart, which is partially overlapped by the medial border of the lungs.

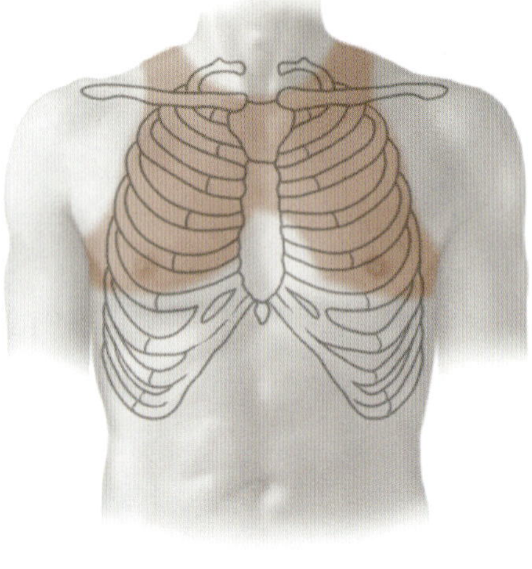

B Percussion field of the lungs

Anterior view. The air-filled lungs constitute a resonant cavity that produces a *sonorous lung sound* on percussion of the chest. The sonorous lung field extends cranially, with attenuation, to the apices of the lungs at the thoracic inlet. It also extends to the front of the chest, again with attenuation, and closely approaches the anterior midline (costomediastinal recess with anterior lung margin on deep inspiration, see pp. 140 and 143). The fluid-filled heart dampens the lung sounds, producing an area of cardiac dullness (see p. 97). A sharp transition from lung sound to liver sound is clearly audible at the inferior border of the right lung, since the liver is a solid organ with less resonance (medium-pitched, nonsonorous percussion sound).

Note: The lung percussion field does not precisely match the anatomical extent of the lungs because only well-aerated portions of the lung are sonorous to percussion. The anatomical extent of the lungs is greater than the percussion field.

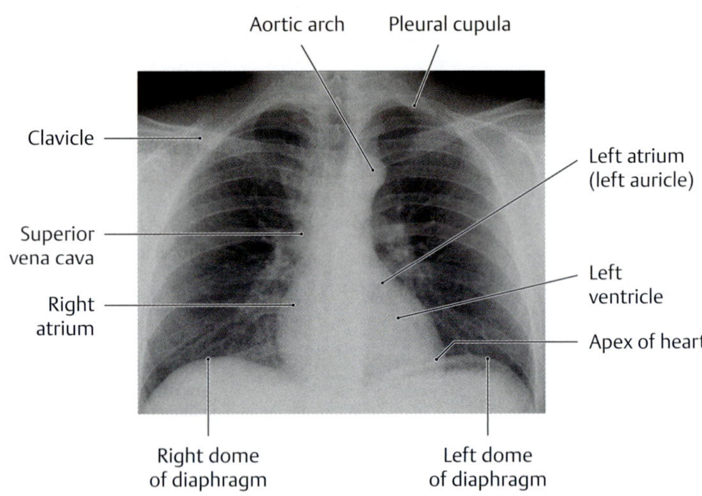

C Radiographic appearance of the normal lungs

Anterior view. Different regions of the lungs show different degrees of lucency in the chest radiograph. The perihilar region of the lung (where the main bronchi enter the lung and vessels enter and leave the lung) is less radiolucent than the peripheral region, which contains small-caliber vascular branches and segmental bronchi. Additionally, the perihilar lung region is partly covered by the heart. These "shadows" appear as white or bright areas on the radiograph. The same effect is observed in diseased lung areas, which appear more opaque as a result of fluid infiltration (inflammation) or tissue proliferation (neoplasia). These opacities are easier to detect in the peripheral part of the lung, which is inherently more radiolucent than the perihilar lung (from: Reiser M, Kuhn F, Debus J, eds. *Duale Reihe Radiologie*. 4th ed. Stuttgart: Thieme; 2017).

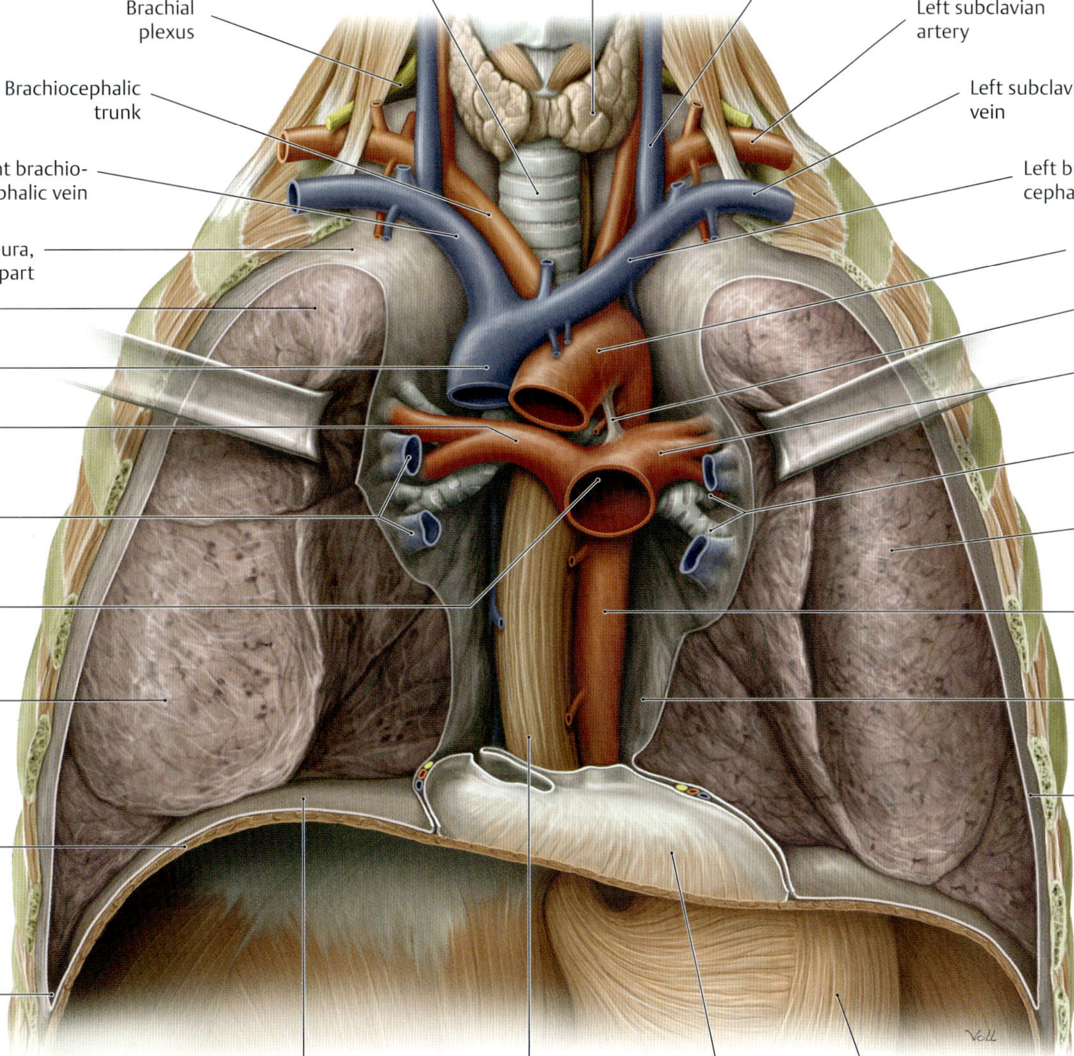

D The lungs in situ

Anterior view of the opened thorax (depiction simplified). The heart and pericardium have been removed. The vessels surrounding the heart have been transected, and all mediastinal connective tissues have been removed. The lungs have been retracted laterally to stretch and expose the main bronchi. The abdominal cavity has been opened and eviscerated, leaving only the stomach in place. The cervical part of the trachea is still visible below the cricoid cartilage. Shortly below its entry into the chest through the thoracic inlet, the trachea is almost completely obscured by the great vessels. The thoracic part of the esophagus can be seen below the tracheal bifurcation, which lies directly behind the ascending aorta. The lungs in the pleural cavities closely approach the vertebral column *posteriorly*, while *anteriorly* they extend in front of the pericardium and narrow the anterior mediastinum. Percussion of the chest yields a "sonorous" lung sound (see **B**) which is dulled by the heart and pericardium. The extent of the lungs depends on the phase of respiration (see p. 161), but the apices of the lungs always extend into the thoracic inlet, which is closed by a condensation of loose connective tissue—the suprapleural membrane. The apical lung tissue is pictured here as soft and pliant, corresponding to its natural consistency. It should be noted that when the pleural cavities are opned at operation, the lungs tend to collapse toward the hilum owing to their elastic recoil; they do not completely fill the pleural cavity as shown here. (For clarity, the lungs are portrayed in an expanded state.)

4.2 Pleural Cavities

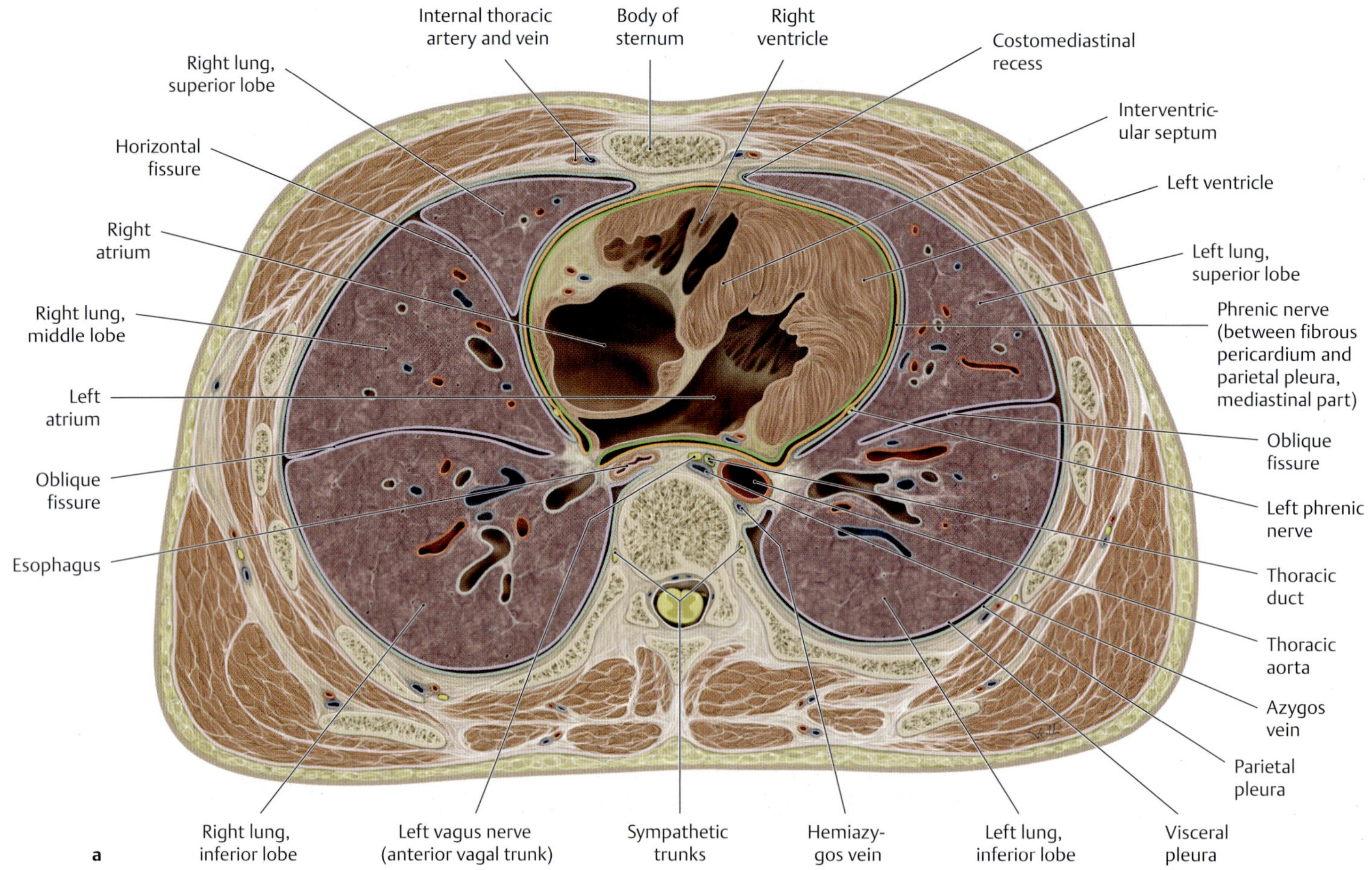

a

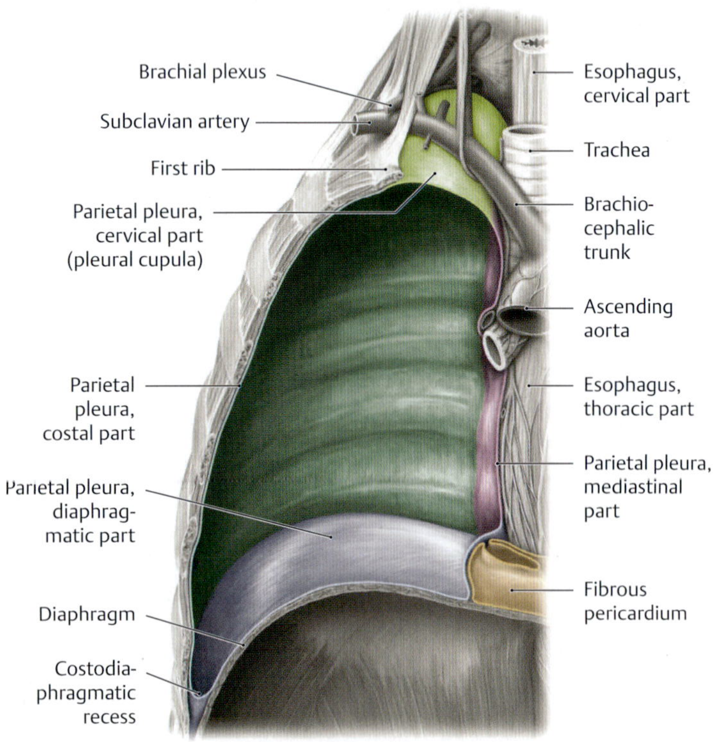

b

A Pleura and pleural cavities: structure and topography

a Transverse section through the thorax, inferior view; **b** Anterior view of the right pleural cavity, which has been opened.

The pleural cavities are paired like the lungs they enclose, which is one reason they have a greater extent than the lungs:

- anteriorly, they extend past the pericardium to just behind the sternum, and in the dorsomedial direction up to the spinal column (**a**);
- due to the arching of the dome of the diaphragm, the inferior margin of the pleural cavities extends downward and overlaps with the abdominal cavity (**b**);
- due to the asymmetrical position of the heart in the mediastinum, the left pleural cavity is slightly smaller than the right pleural cavity (**a**);
- because the pleural cavities have a greater extent than the lungs, recesses develop in them (see also p. 143).

Completely analogous to the peritoneal and pericardial cavities, each pleural cavity is composed of two serous layers: the visceral pleura (pulmonary pleura attached to the surface of the lung) and the parietal pleura (attached to the endothoracic fascia). As a result of the attachment to the thorax, the pleura and thus the lungs (which adhere to the walls of the pleural cavities through capillary forces) automatically follow the movements of the chest wall. The line of junction between the visceral and parietal layers occurs along at the medial surface of the lungs (see p. 36). The capillary fissure-like space between the visceral and parietal pleura contains a small amount of clear serous fluid. This fluid layer allows both layers of the pleura to glide past each other and at the same time serves to hold the pleural layers together by capillary forces. For more about the topographical parts of the pleural layers see **C**.

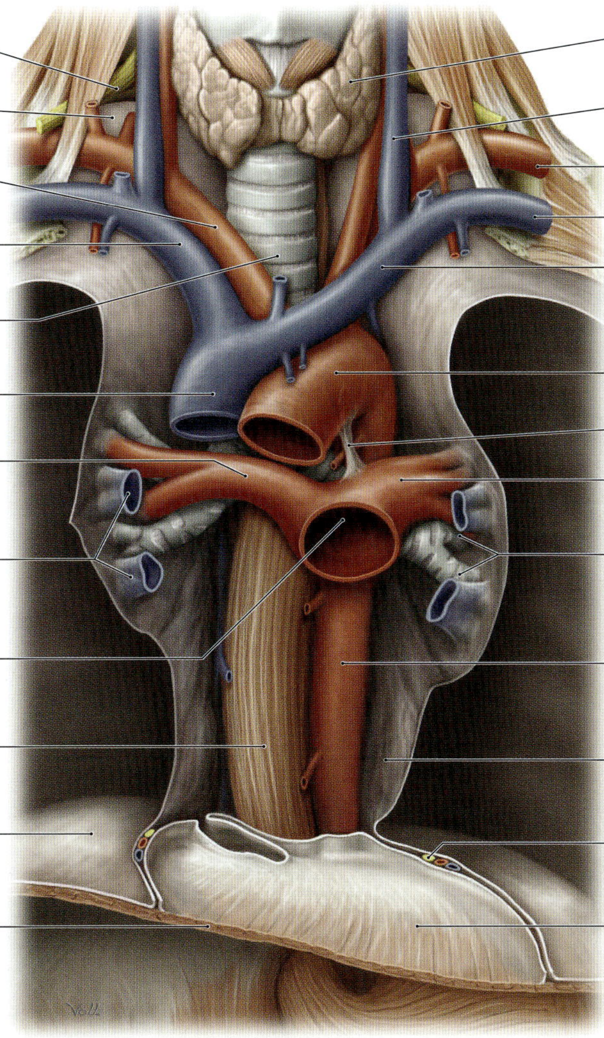

B Mediastinal part of the pleura and the mediastinum
The mediastinum is bounded on either side by the pleural cavities from which it is separated by the mediastinal part of the parietal pleura. The mediastinal pleura is in direct contact with the mediastinal connective tissue. All neurovascular structures running between mediastinum and lungs (e.g., bronchi, pulmonary arteries, pulmonary veins) are wrapped in mediastinal pleura, which fuses with the outer layer of the connective tissues of these neurovascular structures. The phrenic nerves and pericardiacophrenic vessels, which are only just visible at the bottom of the diagram, pass between the mediastinal pleura and pericardium.

C Portions of the parietal pleura

Portion	Location	Adjacent layer of connective tissue
Costal portion	Inner chest wall	Endothoracic fascia
Diaphragmatic portion	Surface of the diaphragm	Phrenicopleural fascia
Mediastinal portion	Lateral to mediastinum	Unnamed, direct transition to the connective tissue of the mediastinum
Cervical portion (Pleural cupula)	Apical, above the superior thoracic aperture	Suprapleural membrane (Sibson's fascia)

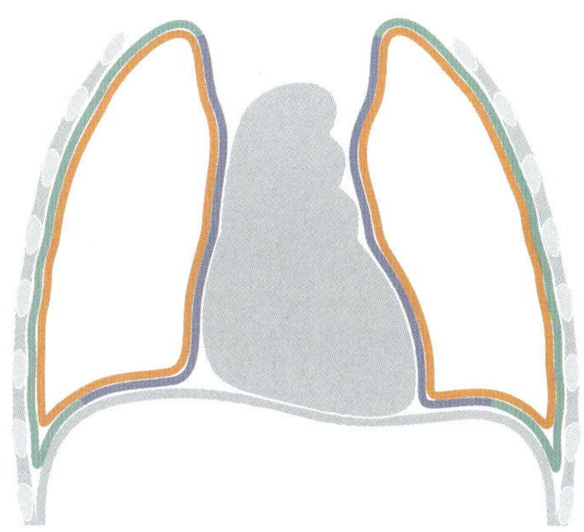

D Innervation of the pleura
The *parietal pleura*, as part of the trunk wall, is innervated by somatic sensory nerves: The mediastinal portion and the largest part of the diaphragmatic portion are supplied by the phrenic nerves. A small part of the diaphragmatic portion located close to the ribs is also supplied by intercostal nerves. The costal portion is innervated by intercostal nerves. The *visceral pleura* is the organ-related layer and as such receives a sparse innervation by visceral sensory fibers, probably from the sympathetic nervous system. The corresponding neuronal perikarya are located in spinal ganglia—their branching axons pass through the sympathetic ganglion without terminating.

4.3 Boundaries of the Lungs and Parietal Pleura

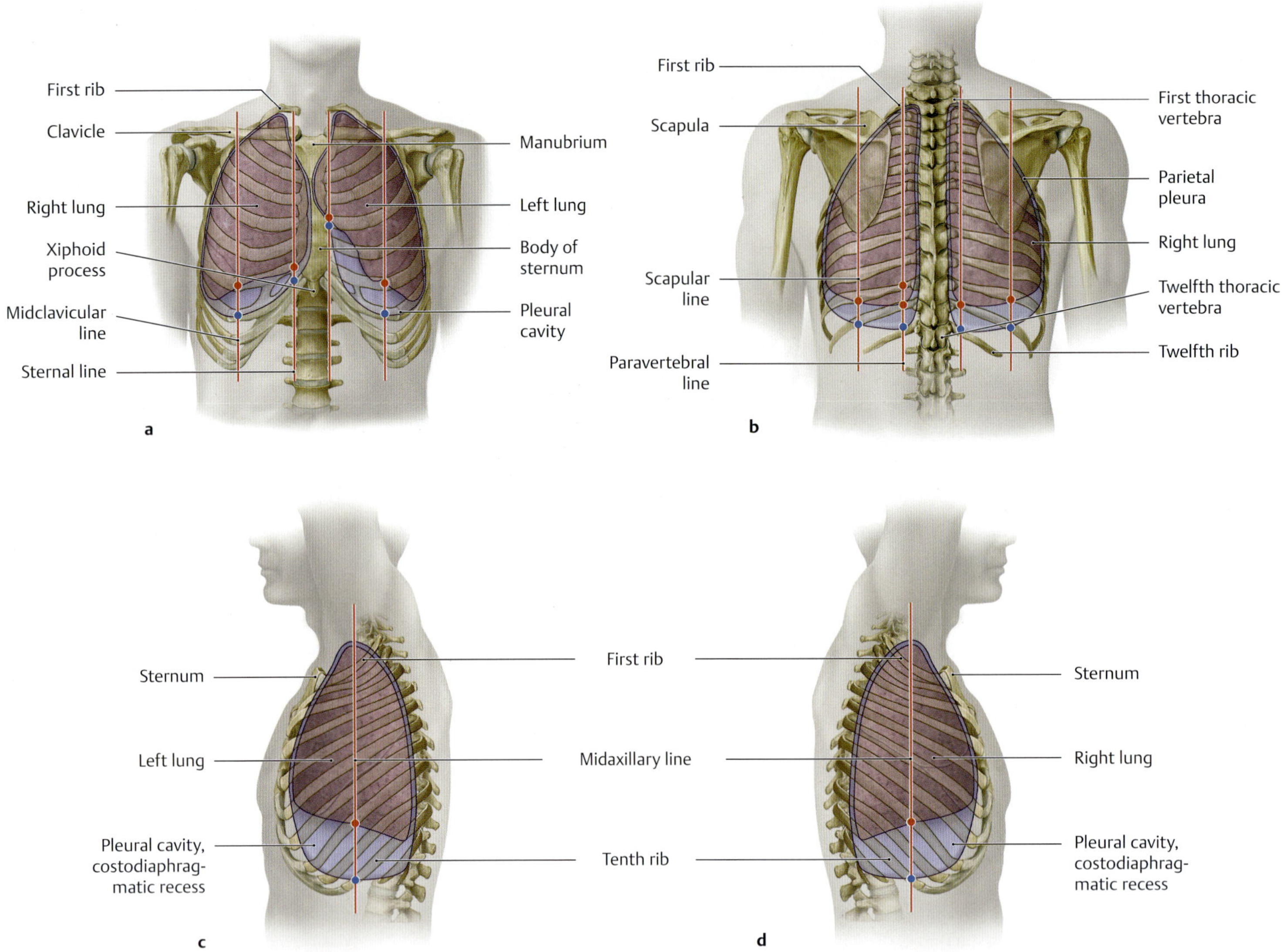

A Projections of the boundaries of the lungs and parietal pleura onto the thoracic skeleton

Anterior view (**a**), posterior view (**b**), view from the left and right sides (**c** and **d**). The diagrams show the boundaries of the parietal pleura and lungs. The table (see **B**) summarizes some of the projection sites of the pleura and lungs onto the anterior, posterior and lateral thoracic wall. The parietal pleura lines the inner surface of the thoracic skeleton and projects itself onto palpable or visible bony landmarks. The connection between these landmarks forms the boundaries of the parietal pleura (important in cases of pleural inflammations with effusion—visible on radiographs).

Note: The asymmetrical position of the heart makes the pleural cavity slightly smaller on the left side than on the right side. This causes the boundaries of the parietal pleura on the left side at the level of the heart to shift more laterally than on the right side.

B Relations of the lungs and pleural boundaries to landmarks on the thoracic skeleton

Reference line	Right lung	Right parietal pleura	Left lung	Left parietal pleura
Sternal line	Intersects the 6th rib	Between cartilage of 6th and 7th ribs	Intersects the 4th rib	Margin of cartilage of 4th rib
Mid-clavicular line	Runs parallel to the 6th rib	Intersects the 7th rib	Intersects the 6th rib	Intersects the 7th rib
Mid-axillary line	Intersects the 8th rib	Intersects the 10th rib	Same as right lung	Same as right side
Scapular line	Intersects the 10th rib	Intersects the 11th rib	Same as right lung	Same as right side
Paravertebral line	Intersects the 11th rib	Extends to the T12 vertebra	Same as right lung	Same as right side

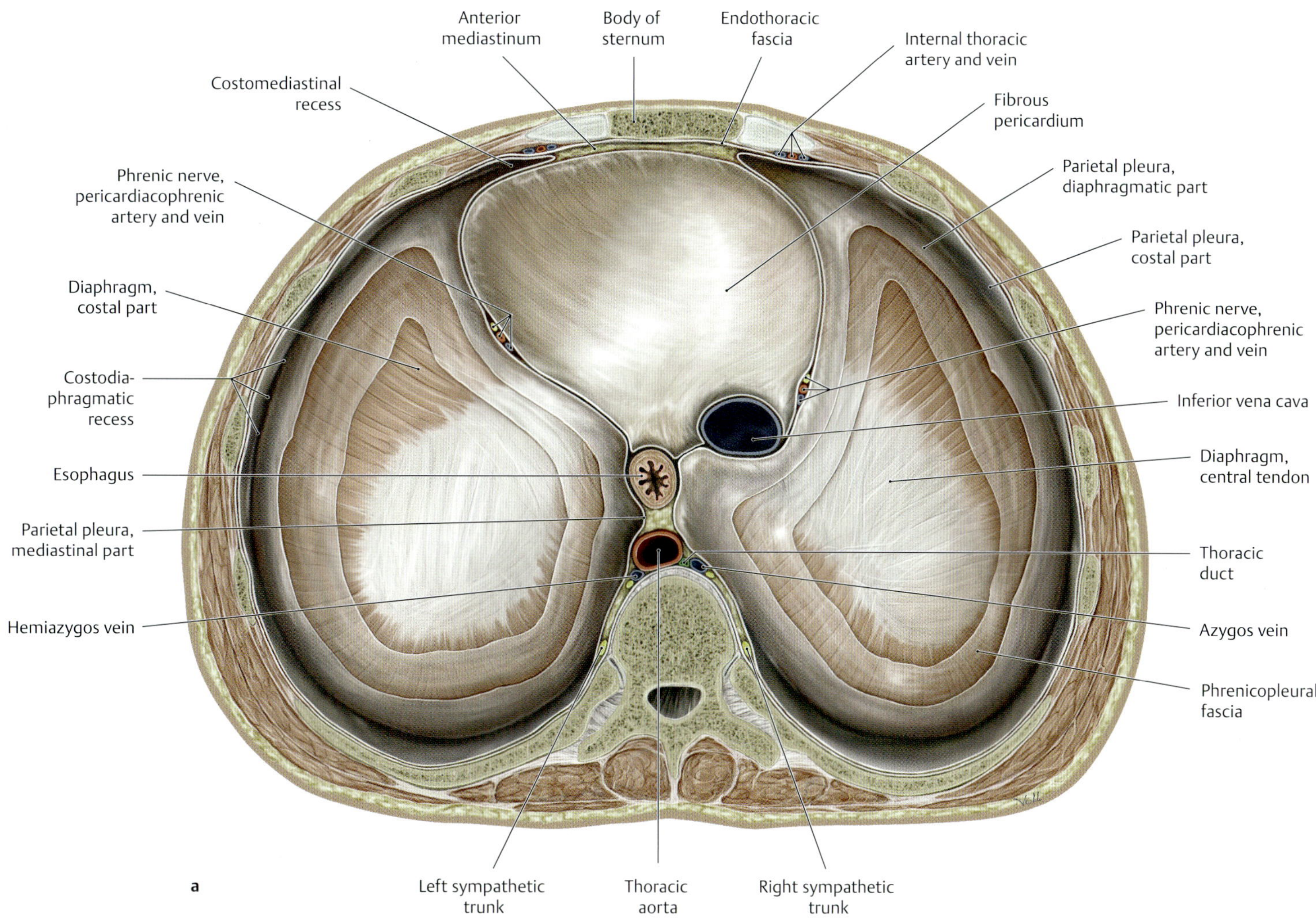

a

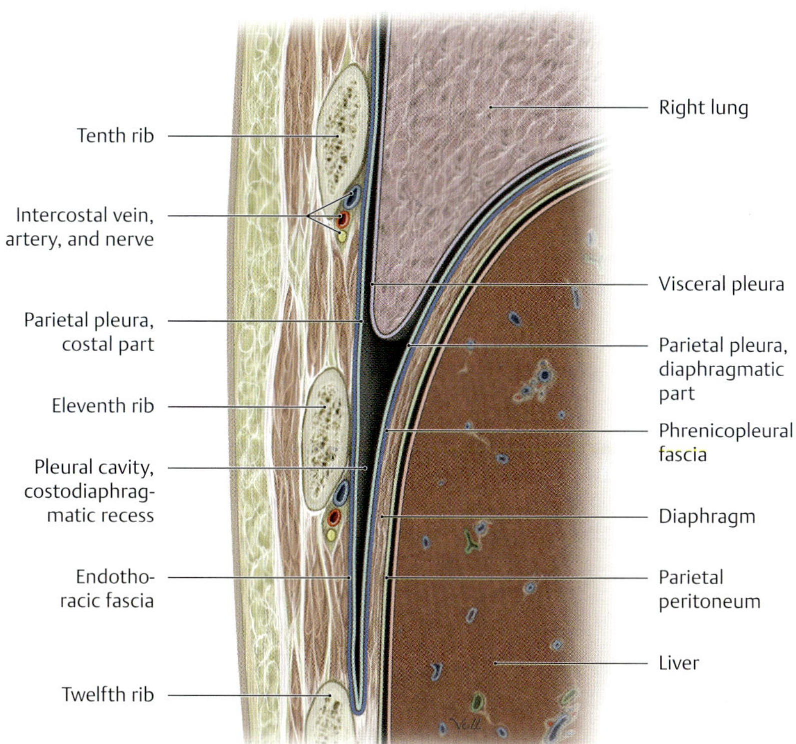

b

C Recesses of the parietal pleura

a Superior view, the heart and lungs have been removed, the parietal pleura has been removed over a large area of the diaphragm; **b** Detail from a parasagittal section through the right side of the thorax and abdomen, viewed from the lateral side.

The extent of the *visceral* pleura, which directly invests the lung, is identical to that of the lung. However, the *parietal* pleura, which completely lines the inner surface of the chest wall, has a greater extent than the lungs. This arrangement creates two major recesses within the pleural cavity:

- The *costodiaphragmatic recess*, located on each side of the domes of the diaphragm, facing the ribs (**b**), which is lined by the costal and diaphragmatic parts of the parietal pleura, and
- The *costomediastinal recess*, located anterior to the pericardium, on the left and right sides of the anterior mediastinum (**a**), which is lined by the costal and mediastinal parts of the parietal pleura.

For more about the function of the pleural recesses, see p. 161.

4.4 Trachea

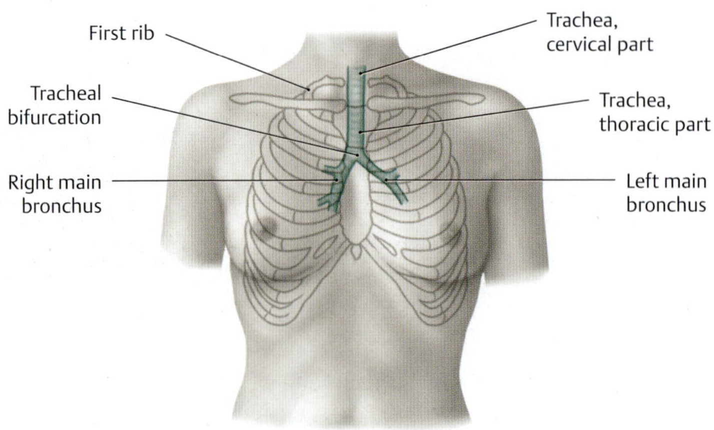

A The trachea projected onto the neck and thorax
The trachea is located in the mediastinum and lies precisely in the median plane. The initial, cervical part of the trachea begins just below the larynx, and its thoracic part ends at the tracheal bifurcation. The trachea expands during inspiration and contracts during expiration. The projection in the figure shows the appearance of the trachea at functional residual capacity (relaxed end-expiration).

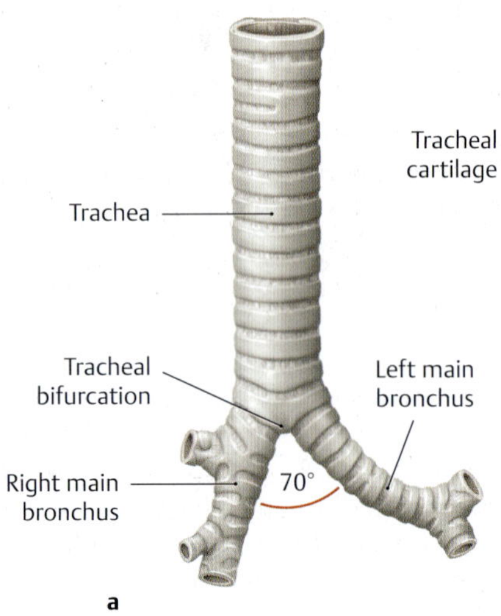

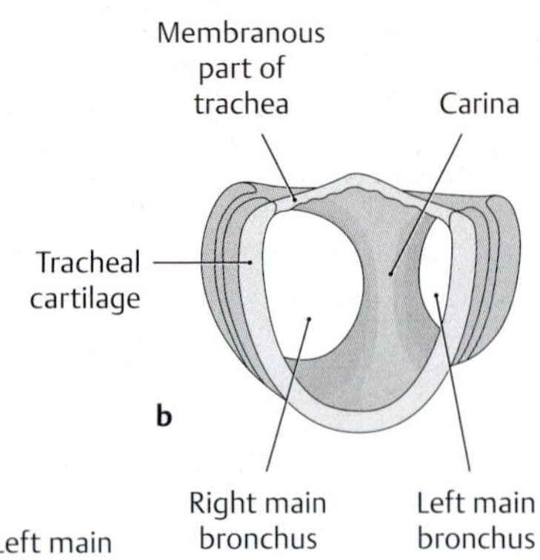

B Shape of the trachea
a Anterior view; **b** Superior view of the tracheal bifurcation.
The trachea is a flexible air-conducting tube 10 to 12 cm long. At the approximate level of the T3–T4 vertebral bodies, it bifurcates into the left and right main (principal) bronchi, which form an angle of approximately 55–70°. Viewed from the anterior side, the tracheal bifurcation lies just below the junction of the manubrium and body of the sternum. *Note:* The right main bronchus is more vertical than the left main bronchus, and therefore it is more common for aspirated foreign bodies to enter the right main bronchus than the left. This also makes it easier to view the interior of the right main bronchus with an endoscope. Owing to the asymmetry of the heart and the associated asymmetrical position of the lungs, the left main bronchus is slightly longer than the right.

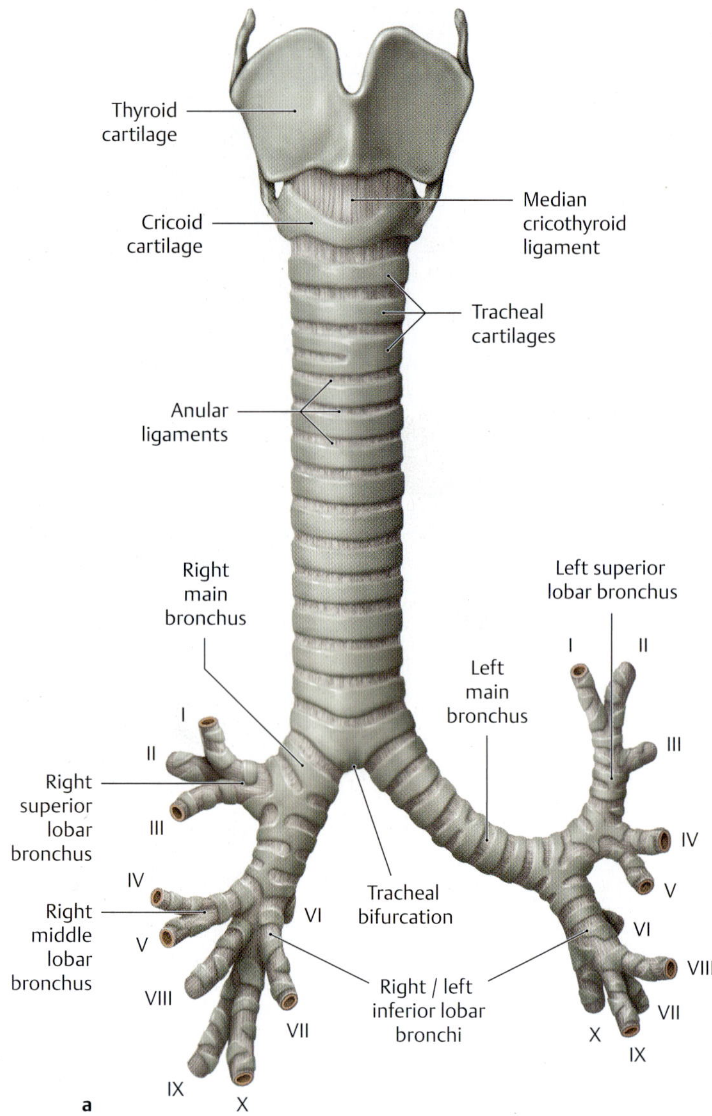

C Structure of the trachea and bronchial tree
a Anterior view; **b** Posterior view with opened posterior wall.
The trachea consists of 16–20 horseshoe-shaped rings composed of hyaline cartilage (the tracheal cartilages) and a membranous posterior wall composed of connective tissue and tracheal muscle (not shown here). The tracheal cartilages are interconnected longitudinally by collagenous connective tissue (anular ligaments). The two parts of the trachea are clearly distinguishable:

- Cervical part: extends from the first tracheal cartilage below the cricoid cartilage of the larynx at the level of the C 6/C 7 vertebrae to the thoracic inlet (see **A**);
- Thoracic part: extends from the thoracic inlet to the tracheal bifurcation, where the trachea divides into the right and left main bronchi at the level of the T4 vertebra. A cartilaginous spur (carina, see **Bb**) at the tracheal bifurcation (the carina, see **Bb**) projects upward into the tracheal lumen.

The left and right main bronchi divide into two or three lobar bronchi, respectively, which subsequently branch into segmental bronchi (see **D**).

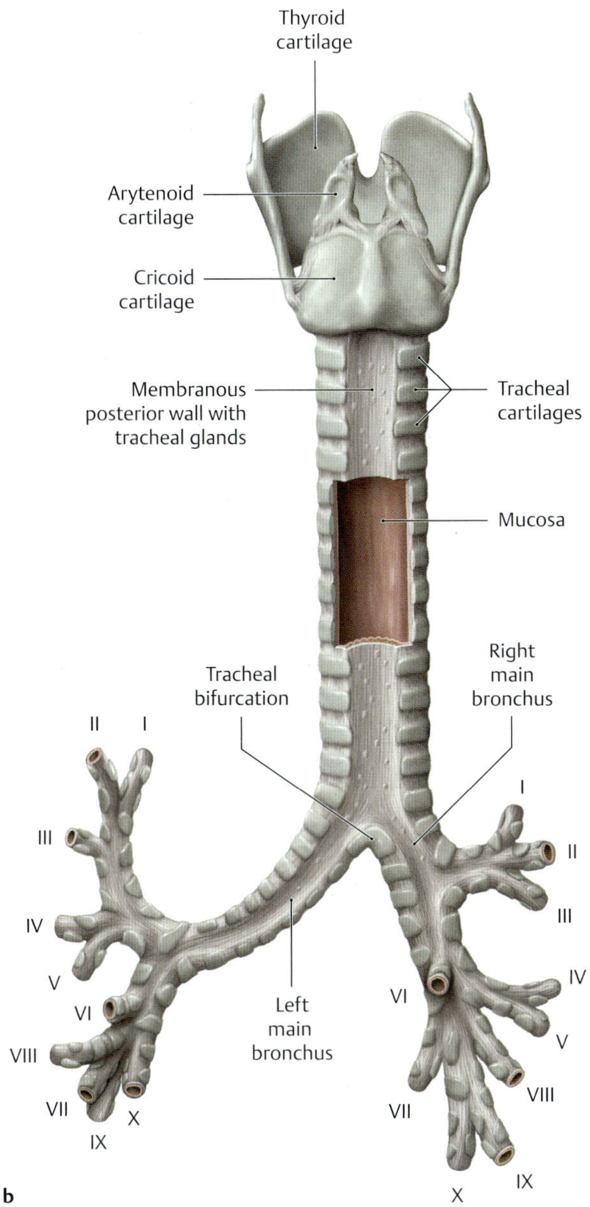

b

D Divisions of the trachea and bronchial tree

Right main bronchus	Left main bronchus
Right superior lobar bronchus Apical segmental bronchus (I) Posterior segmental bronchus (II) Anterior segmental bronchus (III)	*Left superior lobar bronchus* Apicoposterior segmental bronchus (I, II) Anterior segmental bronchus (III)
Right middle lobar bronchus Lateral segmental bronchus (IV) Medial segmental bronchus (V)	 Superior lingular bronchus (IV) Inferior lingular bronchus (V)
Right inferior lobar bronchus Superior segmental bronchus (VI) Medial basal segmental bronchus (VII) Anterior basal segmental bronchus (VIII) Lateral basal segmental bronchus (IX) Posterior basal segmental bronchus (X)	*Left inferior lobar bronchus* Superior segmental bronchus (VI) Medial basal segmental bronchus (VII) Anterior basal segmental bronchus (VIII) Lateral basal segmental bronchus (IX) Posterior basal segmental bronchus (X)

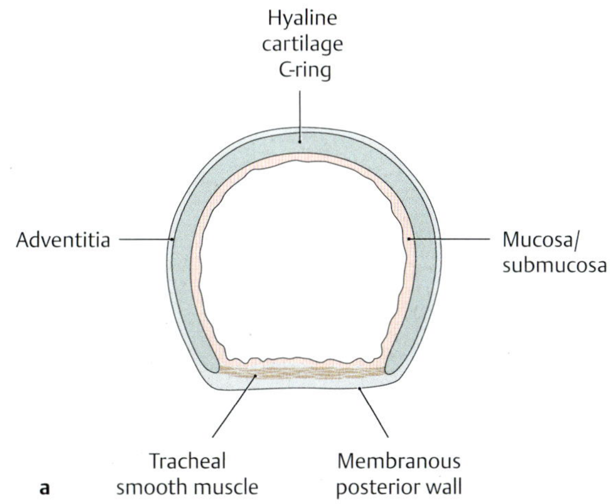

a

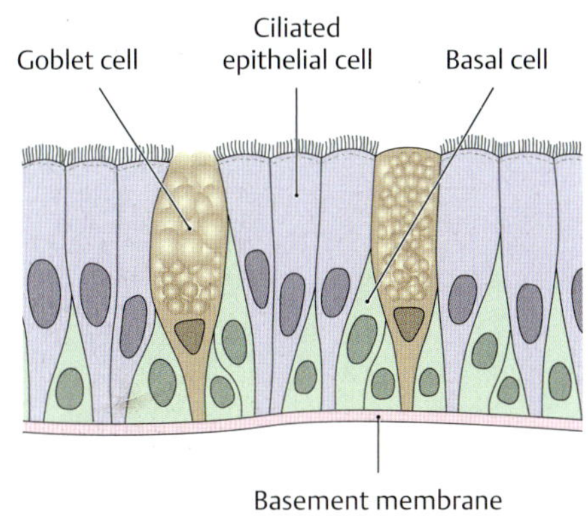

b

E Wall structure of the trachea and main bronchi

a Wall structure (for the ultrastructure of the bronchial tree see p. 150f and 156f):

- Tracheal mucosa with an epithelial layer and a lamina propria: The lamina propria contains seromucous glands (tracheal glands) which secrete a mucous film on the surface (for the epithelium see below).
- Fibromuscular-cartilaginous coat: This contains the C-shaped rings of hyaline cartilage and, on the posterior tracheal wall, the smooth muscle of the trachealis and abundant connective tissue.
- Adventitial sheath of connective tissue: This integrates the trachea into the adjacent connective tissue of the neck and mediastinum and allows mobility.

Note: The epithelium of the carina, unlike that of the rest of the trachea, consists of nonkeratinized squamous epithelium.

b Structure of the epithelium: The mucosa of the trachea and bronchi contains a pseudostratified columnar respiratory epithelium. All cells contact the basement membrane, but not all cells extend to the surface of the lumen. The cells in contact with the surface are ciliated. These hairlike structures propel small foreign bodies that have been inhaled toward the larynx. Smoking tobacco decreases the flow of secretions, compromising airway clearance. Mucus secreting goblet cells without cilia are interspersed among the epithelial cells.

4.5 Lungs: Shape and Structure

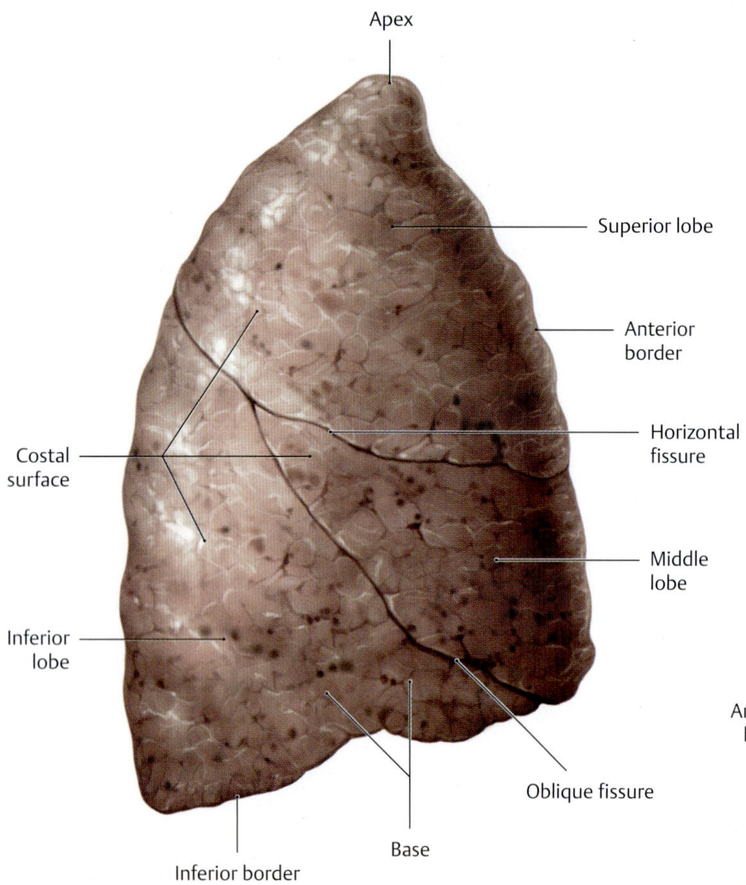

a Right lung, lateral view

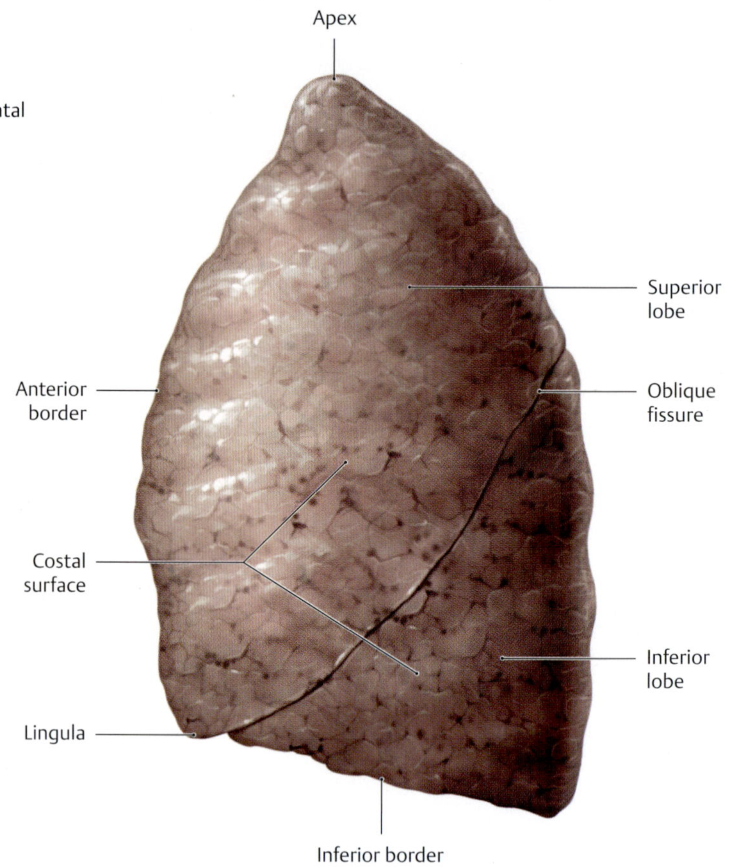

b Left lung, lateral view

A Gross anatomy of the left and right lungs
a, **b** Lateral view. **c**, **d** Medial view.
The color of the healthy lung ranges from gray to bluish-pink. Grayish-black particles are often visible beneath the pleural surface (as shown here) and are found even in nonsmokers. They do not necessarily have pathological significance, consisting of dust or carbonaceous particles that have been inhaled and deposited in the lung. A lung that has not been chemically fixed has a soft, spongy texture and collapses when taken from the chest. The shape shown above is the in vivo shape of the dynamically expanded lung (see p. 159). The right lung, with a volume of approximately 1500 cm, is slightly larger than the left lung, which has a volume of approximately 1400 cm (due to the inclination of the heart to the left side.) Each of the lungs is divided into *lobes* by one or more interlobar *fissures:*

- The left lung is divided into two lobes (superior and inferior) by one oblique fissure.
- The right lung consists of three lobes (superior, middle, and inferior) separated by one *oblique* fissure and one *horizontal* fissure. The pulmonary fissures are completely lined by visceral pleura.

Note: Owing to the steep angle of the oblique fissure in the left lung, the lingula of the upper lobe forms part of the base of the left lung. The smallest morphologically distinct and autonomous structural unit of the lung is the *lobule*, which is aerated by a bronchiole. The pulmonary lobules are separated from one another by (often incomplete) fibrous interlobular septa, demarcating numerous polyhedral areas that may be visible on the lung surface.
Aside from the differences noted above, both lungs have the same basic parts:

- The apex, which extends into the thoracic inlet
- The base, which rests on the diaphragm

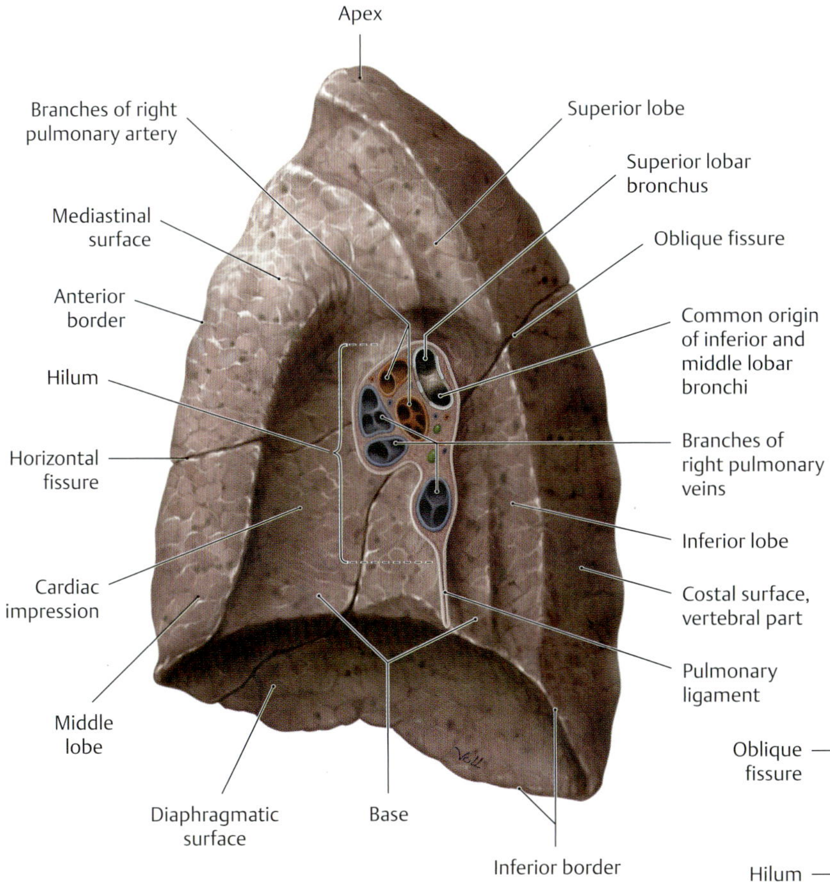

c Right lung, medial view

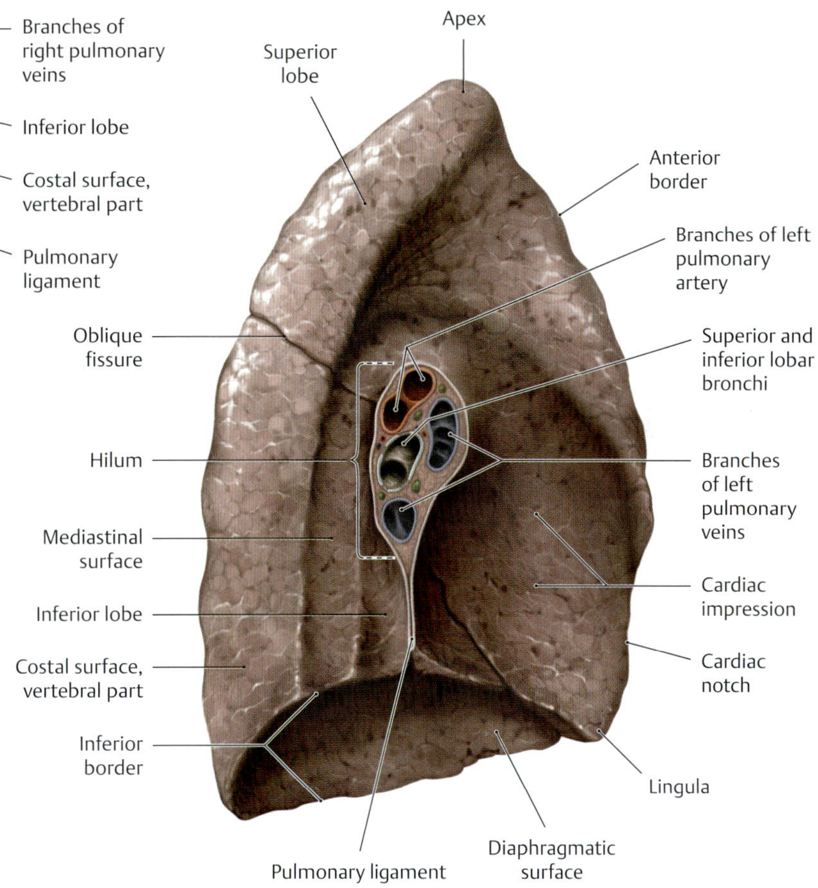

d Left lung, medial view

- Surfaces of the lung:
  - Costal surface: relates laterally and posteriorly to the ribs. The vertebral part of the costal surface faces the vertebral column (see **c**, **d**);
  - Mediastinal surface: relates medially to the mediastinum.
  - Diaphragmatic surface (see **c**, **d**): relates inferiorly to the diaphragm.
  - Interlobar (fissural) surfaces. In the chemically fixed specimen, impressions from the ribs are visible on the costal surface, a cardiac impression on the mediastinal surface, and an impression from the diaphragm leaflet on the diaphragmatic surface. The left lung additionally has a distinct cardiac *notch* in its anterior border.
- Borders of the lung:
  - Anterior border: sharp, thin border located at the junction of the costal and mediastinal surfaces (inserts into the costomediastinal recess).
  - Inferior border: located at the junction of the diaphragmatic and costal or mediastinal surfaces, sharp at the costal surface (inserts into the costodiaphragmatic recess) and blunt at the mediastinal surface.
- Hilum: area where bronchi and neurovascular structures enter and leave the mediastinal surface. The *root* of the lung comprises all of the blood vessels, lymphatics, bronchi, and nerves that enter and emerge at the hilum. Elements of the bronchial tree are generally located in the posterior part of the hilum. Pulmonary venous branches are anterior and inferior, and pulmonary arterial branches are found mainly in the upper part of the hilum. A simple mnemonic to help remember the relative positions is this: bronchi are posterior, veins are ventral, arteries are apical. The main difference between the left and right hilum is that the most superior structure on the right is a bronchus (eparterial bronchus) whereas on the left it is the artery (hyparterial bronchus).

Both lungs are invested by a serous membrane, the *visceral pleura* (pulmonary pleura), which is reflected at the mediastinal surface to continue as the parietal pleura. This pleural fold is ruptured when the lung is removed, appearing as the *pulmonary ligament*.

4.6 Lungs: Segmentation

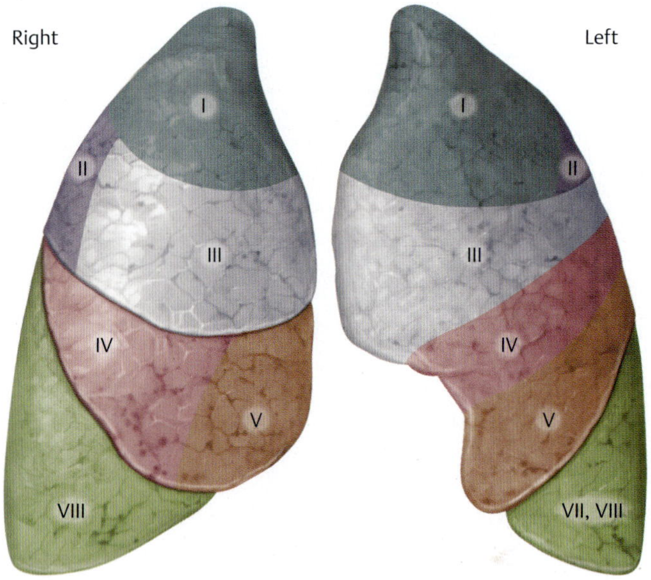

a Lungs, anterior view

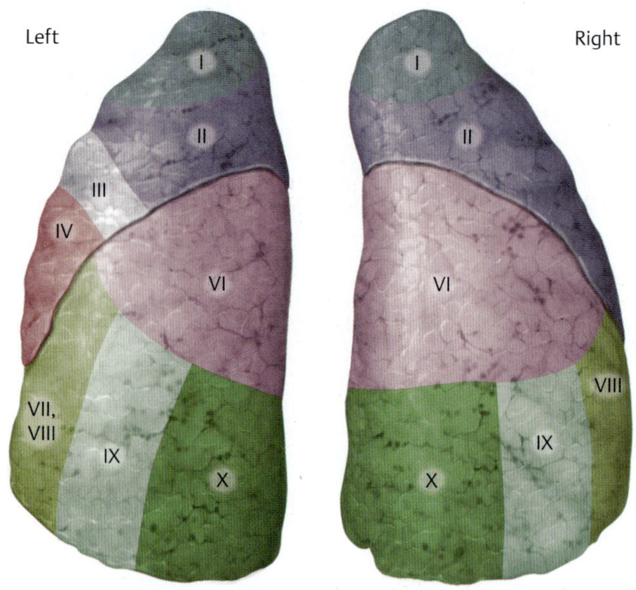

b Lungs, posterior view

A Segmental architecture of the lungs
Anterior view (**a**) and posterior view (**b**) of the right and left lungs (lateral and medial views are shown in **C**).
The segmental architecture of the lung relates directly to the branching pattern of the bronchial tree (see p. 145). The basic structural unit of the lung is the *lobe*, whose boundaries are clearly defined on the surface of the lung by the interlobar fissures. Each lobe is further subdivided into *segments*—wedge-shaped functional units whose apex points toward the pulmonary hilum. The pulmonary segments are incompletely separated from one another by thin connective tissue and are not discernible as separate units on the lung surface. Passing to the center of each segment are a *segmental bronchus* and a *segmental branch of the pulmonary artery* (segmental artery), constituting the "bronchopulmonary segment" or "bronchoarterial segment." The segments, in turn, consist of subsegments defined by the further branching pattern of the segmental bronchi. Each lung consists basically of ten segments. Due to the presence of the cardiac notch in the *left* lung (see p. 149, **Da**), however, segment VII of that lung is often so small that it is not considered a separate segment but part of segment VIII. As noted above, the segmental boundaries are not visible on the surface of the lung. For partial resections of the lung (see **D**), the targeted segments are identified by clamping off the segmental artery. As the devascularized segment blanches, it contrasts sharply with the surrounding tissues that are still perfused. Intrasegmental blood flow can also be demonstrated by ultrasound scanning. The pulmonary segments are named and numbered as shown in table **B**.

B Segmental architecture of the lungs

Right lung	Left lung
Superior lobe	*Superior lobe*
Apical segment (I)	Apicoposterior segment (I + II)
Posterior segment (II)	
Anterior segment (III)	Anterior segment (III)
Middle lobe	
Lateral segment (IV)	Superior lingular segment (IV)
Medial segment (V)	Inferior lingular segment (V)
Inferior lobe	*Inferior lobe*
Superior segment (VI)	Superior segment (VI)
Medial basal segment (VII)	Medial basal segment (VII)
Anterior basal segment (VIII)	Anterior basal segment (VIII)
Lateral basal segment (IX)	Lateral basal segment (IX)
Posterior basal segment (X)	Posterior basal segment (X)

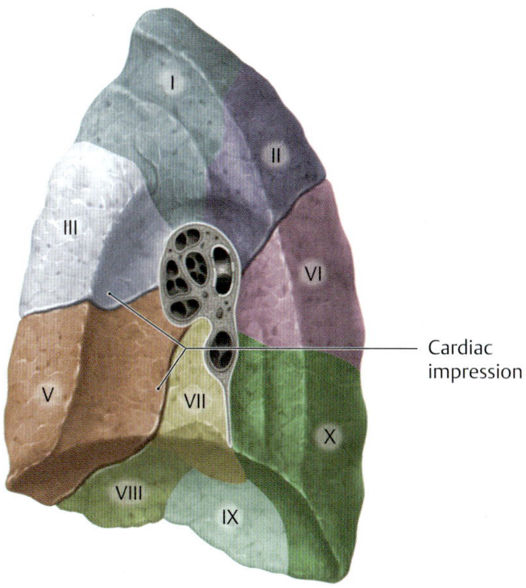

a Right lung, medial view

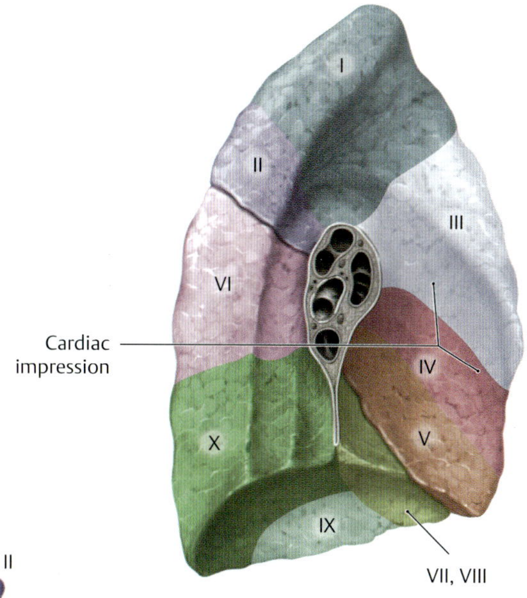

b Left lung, medial view

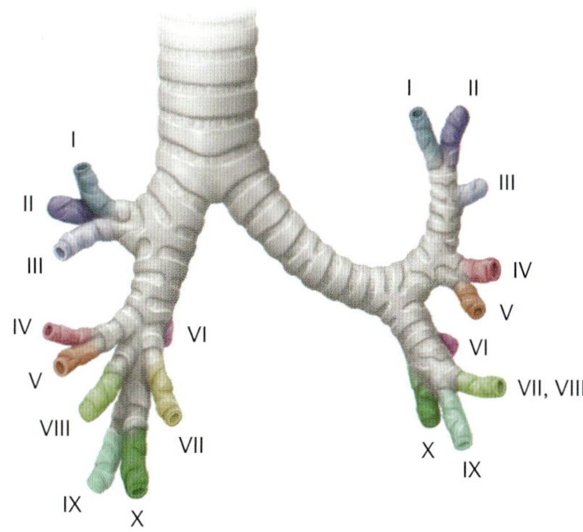

e

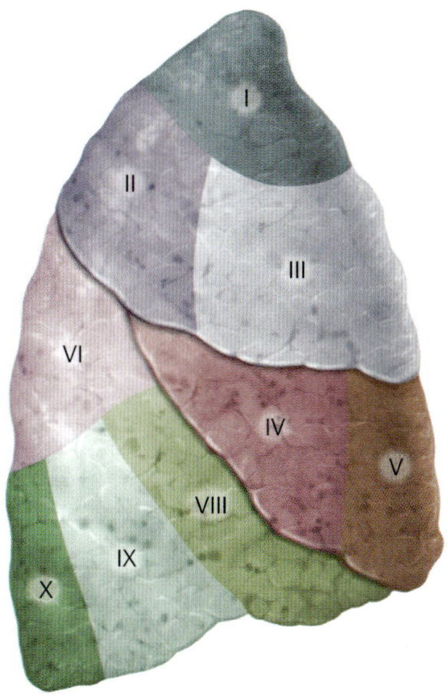

c Right lung, lateral view

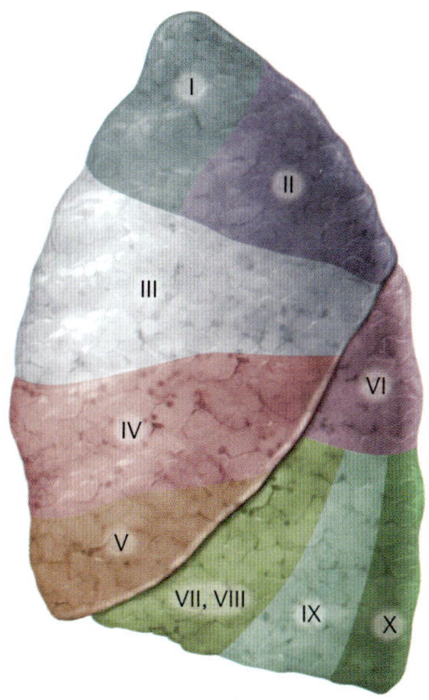

d Left lung, lateral view

C Segmental architecture of the lungs: bronchopulmonary segments
Lateral and medial views of the right (**a**, **c**) and left lung (**b**, **d**).

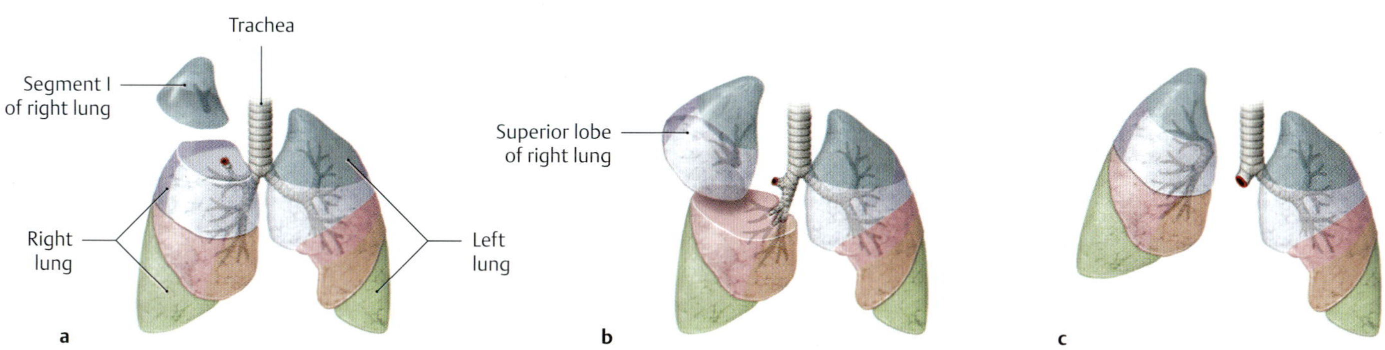

D Partial lung resections
The anatomical subdivision of the lungs into lobes and segments (see **B**) is exploited in partial lung resections:

- Segmentectomy (wedge resection): (**a**) removal of one or more segments
- Lobectomy: (**b**) removal of an entire lobe or (**c**) the complete resection of a lung (pneumonectomy).

4.7 Functional Structure of the Bronchial Tree

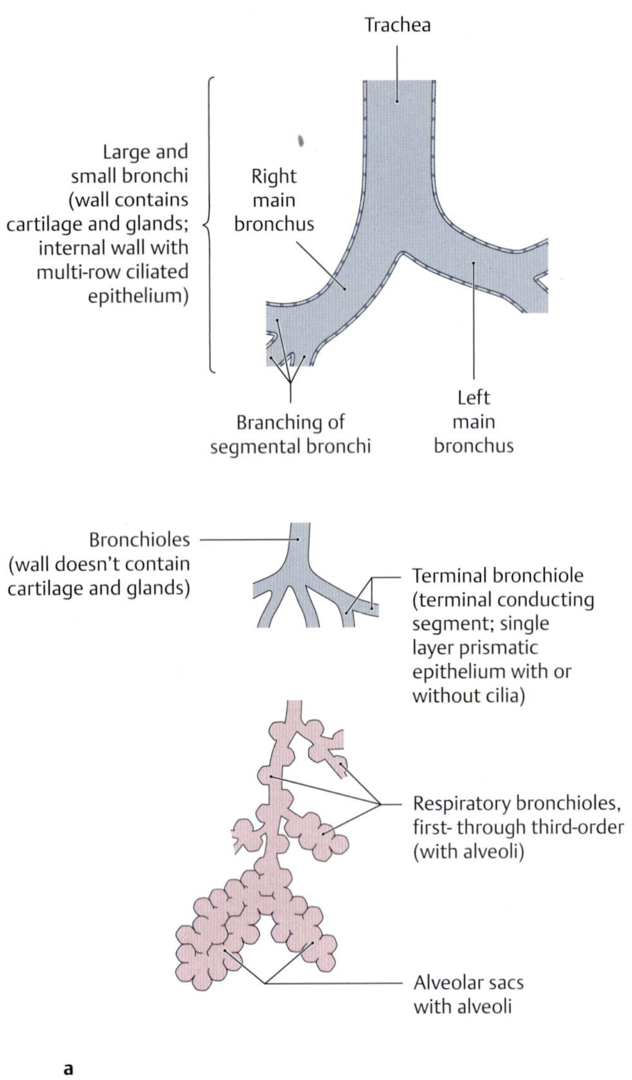

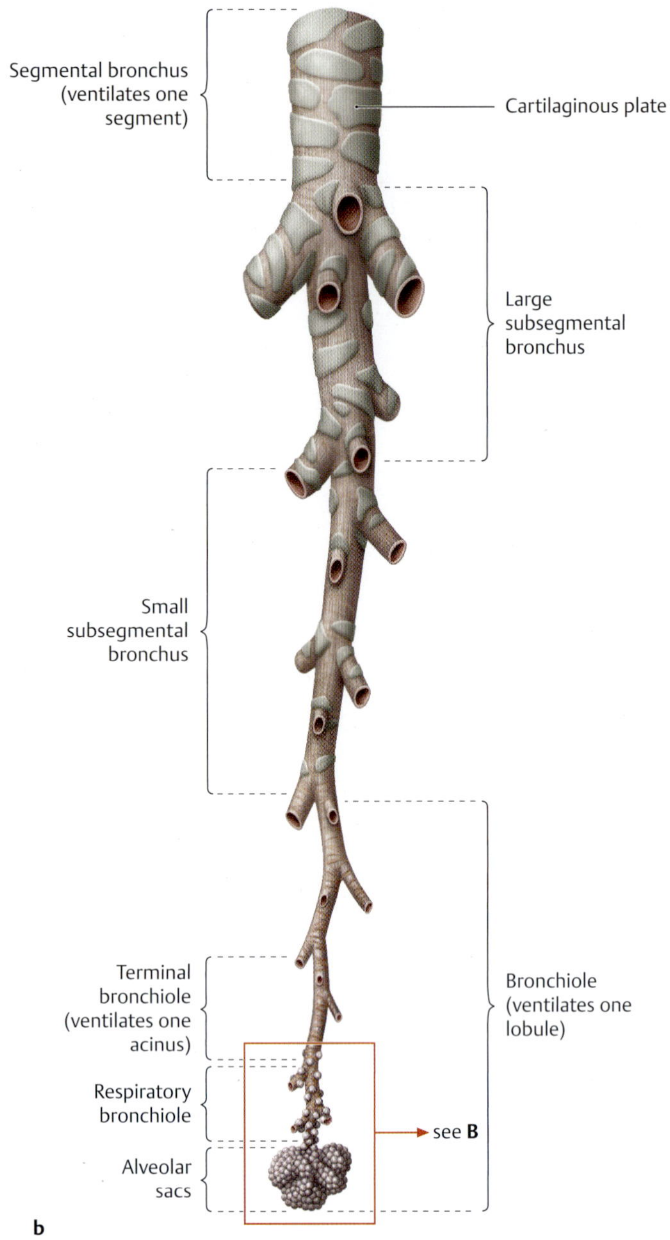

A Conducting and respiratory parts of the bronchial tree

The structure of the lung is organized to maximize the surface area available for gas exchange, and the bronchial tree is arranged to deliver the gases, in warmed and humidified (saturated with water vapor) air, to that specialized surface area. The exchange takes place mostly in *pulmonary alveoli*, microscopic pouches approximately 200–250 µm in diameter. The adult lungs contain about 300 million alveoli with a total surface area of nearly 150 m2. From the trachea, the bronchial tree branches into successively finer divisions (22 "dichotomous" divisions, in which each passage divides into two smaller passages). The parts of the bronchial tree are classified functionally as *conducting* or *respiratory*:

- Conducting part (blue): main bronchi, lobar bronchi, segmental and subsegmental bronchi, bronchioles, and terminal bronchioles
- Respiratory part (red): respiratory bronchioles, alveolar duct (not visible), and alveolar sacs.

The bronchial tree presents a uniform structure of a specialized air-conduction tube out to the level of the segmental bronchi. The bronchial wall is reinforced by cartilage rings or plates and is lined internally by a pseudostratified columnar, ciliated epithelium (with goblet cells; see p. 145). The walls of the *smaller* bronchi do not have cartilage reinforcement. The concentric musculature of these bronchi acquires a lattice-like structure (see **B**), and the pseudostratified epithelium is replaced by a single layer of prismatic epithelial cells, some of which are ciliated. Goblet cells become less numerous and are no longer present past the level of the terminal bronchiole. The terminal bronchiole is the final segment of the air-conducting portion of the bronchial tree. Each terminal bronchiole aerates one *acinus*. A group of three to five acini whose terminal bronchioles arise near one another on the bronchial tree forms a lobule, which is the smallest morphologically distinct structural unit of the lung.

Note: Although the vascular and bronchial trees are closely related functionally, the vascular tree (see p. 156) is discussed following the sections about the pulmonary and bronchial vessels. Since the vascular tree is composed of the terminal branches of the pulmonary and bronchial vessels, knowledge of these vessels is essential for understanding the structure of the vascular tree.

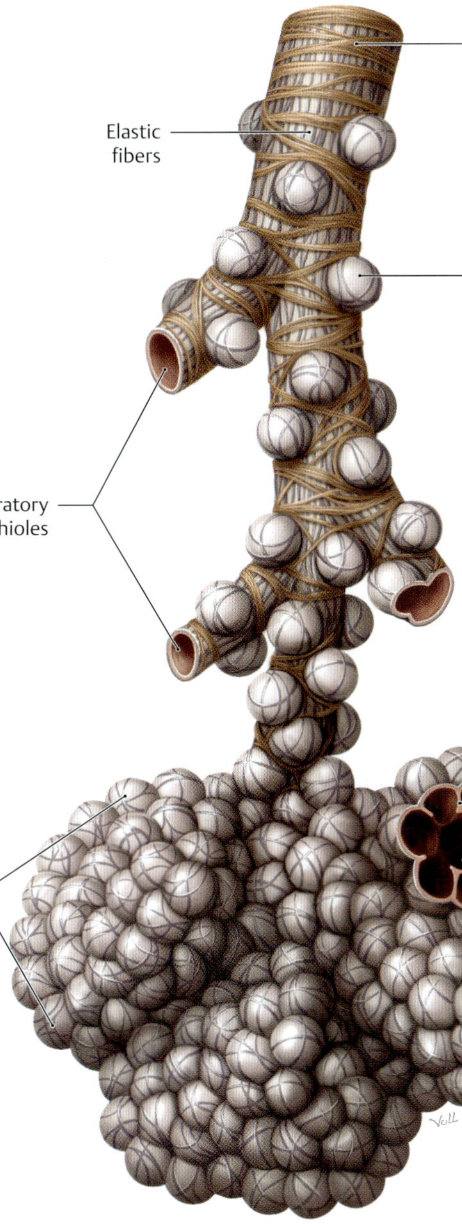

B Structure of a respiratory bronchiole

The respiratory bronchioles dichotomously divide into first- through third-order respiratory bronchioles, the thinnest of which is less than 0.5 mm in diameter. Alveoli begin to appear on the first-order respiratory bronchioles, marking the start of the respiratory portion of the lung. The alveoli are isolated initially, then become more numerous and are collected into sacs. Each sac has a central open space, an alveolar duct, that is continuous with the lumen of its respiratory bronchiole. The alveolar walls are composed of thin squamous epithelium and are in direct contact with the capillaries to allow for gas exchange. Adjacent alveoli are separated from one another by a porous interalveolar septum. Connective tissue with abundant elastic fibers is interposed between the branches of the bronchial tree and the alveoli. When these elastic fibers are stretched during inspiration, they store energy and provide the mechanism for the elastic recoil of the lung during expiration.

In patients with bronchial asthma the bronchioles are hypersensitive, and constriction of the smooth muscle in the bronchiolar walls can be triggered by allergens (e.g., pollen) or by stimuli like cold that are trivial to non-asthmatics. Since these walls are not cartilage-reinforced, the bronchioles narrow and restrict the passage of air to the alveoli (obstructive ventilatory impairment), causing dyspnea (respiratory distress).

4.8 Pulmonary Arteries and Veins

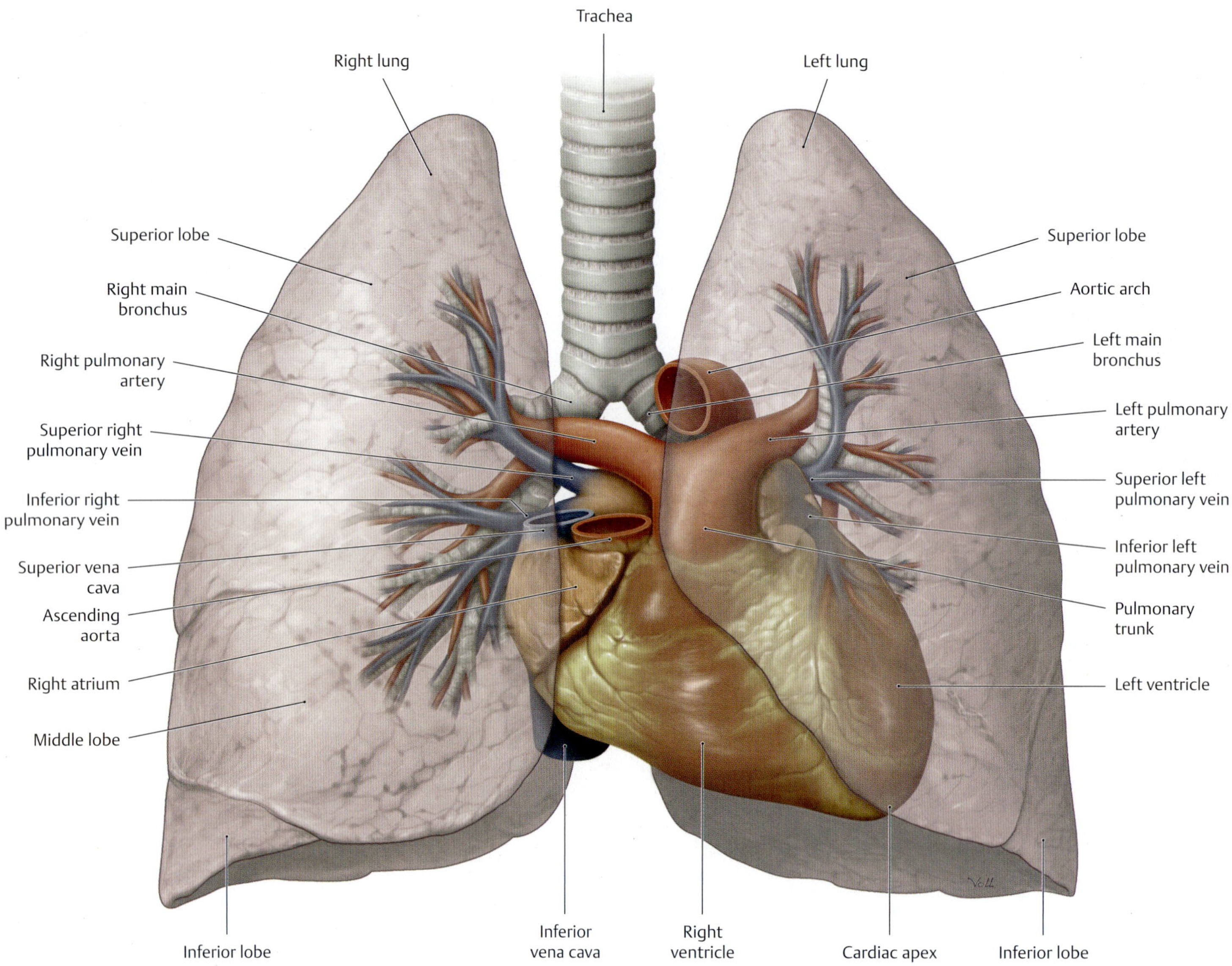

A Overview of the pulmonary vessels
Anterior view of a "heart-lung preparation."
The venae cavae have been cut close to the heart, and a segment has been removed from the ascending aorta and arch to display the division of the pulmonary trunk, which is inferior to the aortic arch, and the origin of the right pulmonary artery. The lungs and heart are shown partially transparent. The arteries and veins that pass to the lung are divided into two groups:

- *Pulmonary arteries and veins*, which carry blood to the lungs and back for *gas exchange* (O_2, CO_2)
- *Bronchial arteries and veins* (not shown here), which *supply blood* to parts of the lungs themselves (see p. 154)

The **divisions of the pulmonary arteries** basically follow the branching pattern of the bronchial tree (see p. 144). Two or three arterial branches, called lobar arteries, accompany the two (left) or three (right) lobar bronchi into the lung. (The lobar arteries are larger than the lobar bronchi.) As the bronchial tree branches into *segmental bronchi*, the arteries similarly divide into *segmental arteries*. The artery and its associated bronchus are always placed at the center of the structural lung unit, first occupying the center of a lobe, then the center of a *bronchopulmonary segment* (see p. 148).

The **divisions of the pulmonary veins** do not follow the branching pattern of the bronchial tree, instead coursing between pulmonary segments to collect blood from within (*intrasegmental* veins) and among (*intersegmental* veins) adjacent segments. Thus pulmonary veins are named differently than pulmonary arteries (see **C** and **D**). In cases of left ventricular insufficiency, blood backs up in the pulmonary veins. As a result, the boundaries of the pulmonary segments become visible on radiographs.

Note: The pulmonary arteries carry deoxygenated blood to the lungs, and the pulmonary veins carry oxygenated blood from the lungs to the heart. In order to ensure a consistent presentation throughout this atlas, the arteries are still colored red and the veins are colored blue.

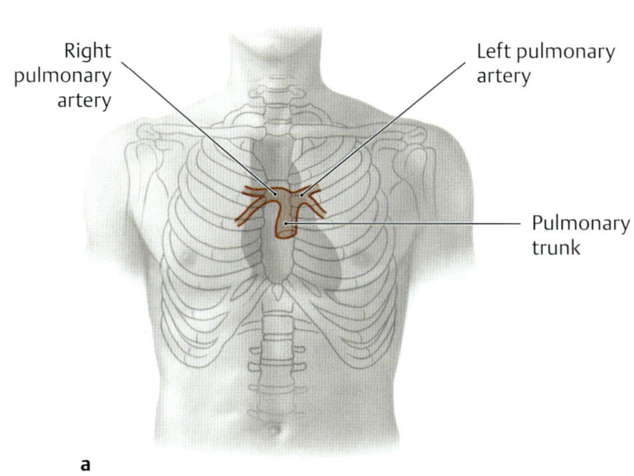

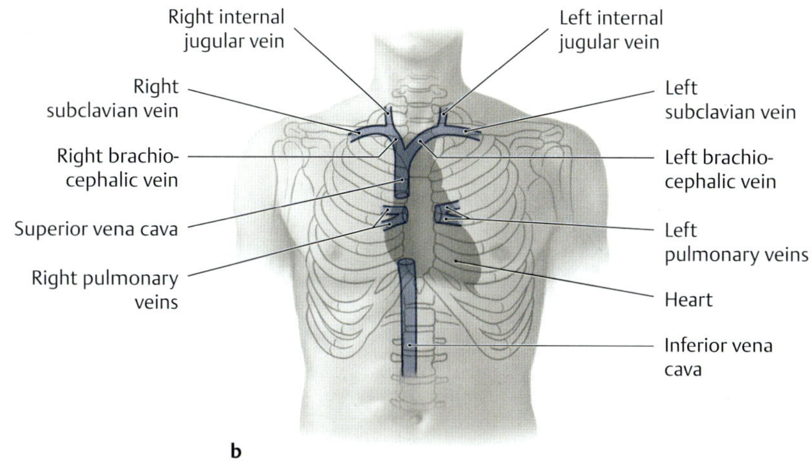

B Projection of the pulmonary arteries and veins onto the chest wall

Anterior view.

a Projection of the pulmonary arteries onto the chest wall. The pulmonary trunk arises from the right ventricle, which is anterior owing to the slightly rotated position of the heart, and divides into a left and right pulmonary artery for each lung. The pulmonary trunk appears on chest radiographs as a knob-like shadow on the left cardiac border above the ventricles.

Note: The pulmonary trunk lies to the left of the midline in the chest. As a result, the right pulmonary artery (length approximately 2–3 cm) is longer than the left pulmonary artery.

b Projection of the pulmonary veins onto the chest wall: Normally, a pair of pulmonary veins open into the left atrium on each side. Taken together, the right and left pulmonary veins and both venae cavae form an asymmetrical cruciform pattern on the chest radiograph.

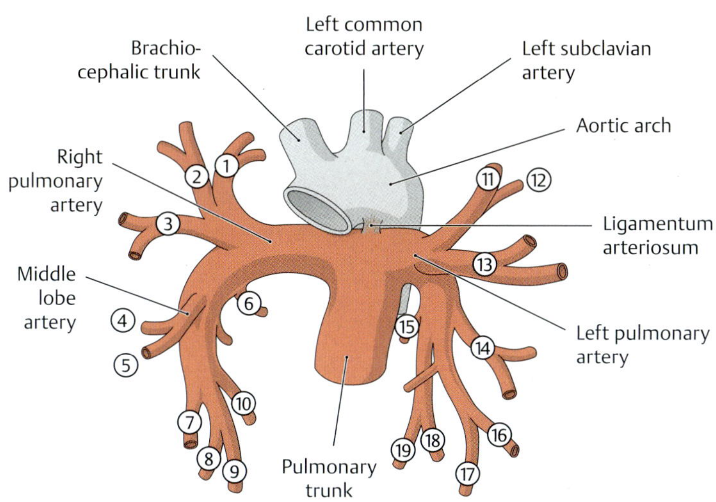

C The pulmonary arteries and their branches

Right lung Right pulmonary artery	Left lung Left pulmonary artery
Superior lobe arteries ① Apical segmental artery ② Posterior segmental artery ③ Anterior segmental artery	*Superior lobe arteries* ⑪ Apical segmental artery ⑫ Posterior segmental artery ⑬ Anterior segmental artery
Middle lobe artery ④ Lateral segmental artery ⑤ Medial segmental artery	⑭ Lingular artery
Inferior lobe arteries ⑥ Superior segmental artery ⑦ Anterior basal segmental artery ⑧ Lateral basal segmental artery ⑨ Posterior basal segmental artery ⑩ Medial basal segmental artery	*Inferior lobe arteries* ⑮ Superior segmental artery ⑯ Anterior basal segmental artery ⑰ Lateral basal segmental artery ⑱ Posterior basal segmental artery ⑲ Medial basal segmental artery

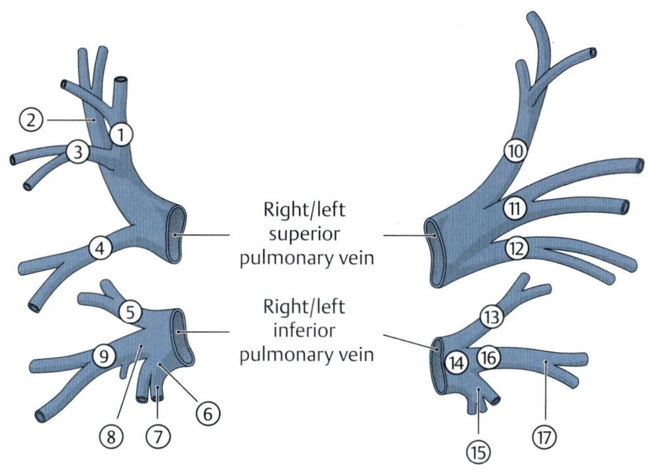

D The pulmonary veins and their tributaries

Right lung Right pulmonary veins	Left lung Left pulmonary veins
Right superior pulmonary vein ① Apical vein ② Posterior vein ③ Anterior vein ④ Middle lobe vein	*Left superior pulmonary vein* ⑩ Apicoposterior vein ⑪ Anterior vein ⑫ Lingular vein
Right inferior pulmonary vein ⑤ Superior vein ⑥ Common basal vein ⑦ Inferior basal vein ⑧ Superior basal vein ⑨ Anterior basal vein	*Left inferior pulmonary vein* ⑬ Superior vein ⑭ Common basal vein ⑮ Inferior basal vein ⑯ Superior basal vein ⑰ Anterior basal vein

4.9 Bronchial Arteries and Veins

A Bronchial arteries and veins
Anterior view. The trachea and bronchi are shown partially transparent.

a Arterial supply of the bronchi: The bronchi derive their blood supply from the thoracic aorta via bronchial arterial branches that follow the divisions of the main bronchi. It is not uncommon for one of the bronchial arteries to arise from a posterior intercostal artery (usually on the right side), rather than directly from the aorta. Given the relationship of the bronchi to the thoracic aorta, the bronchial arteries usually enter the bronchi from the posterior side. The blood pressure within these arteries is equal to the systemic pressure, not the pulmonary pressure (as is the case in the pulmonary arteries).
Note: The trachea is supplied with arterial blood by small tracheal branches (not shown here) that may arise from the thoracic aorta, the internal thoracic artery, or the thyrocervical trunk, depending on the level of the trachea that is supplied.

b Venous drainage of the bronchi: The bronchi are drained by bronchial veins, which usually open into the accessory hemiazygos vein on the left side. On the right side, the veins may drain via collaterals into the azygos vein, but may also empty into the pulmonary veins, causing a small amount of deoxygenated bronchial blood to be mixed with the much larger outflow of pulmonary blood on its way to the left atrium. Small tracheal veins (not shown here) empty into the superior vena cava, left brachiocephalic vein, or internal thoracic vein at different levels of the trachea.

Note: A pulmonary embolism occurs when a blood clot forms in a vein (usually a leg or pelvic vein) and is carried into one of the pulmonary arteries. Depending on its size, the clot blocks one of the branches of the pulmonary artery and in extreme cases the entire artery. The mechanical blockage of a large artery to the lungs leads to acute increased pressure in the right ventricle of the heart, which can result in acute right-sided heart failure. Large pulmonary emboli are often fatal. If, however, a pulmonary embolism occludes a small-caliber vessel, the mechanical blockage and increased pressure on the heart are considerably less severe and the heart compensates for it without any significant problems. Arterial occlusion usually does not result in necrosis of lung tissue as the bronchial arteries ensure delivery of nutrients and oxygen to the tissues of the lungs.

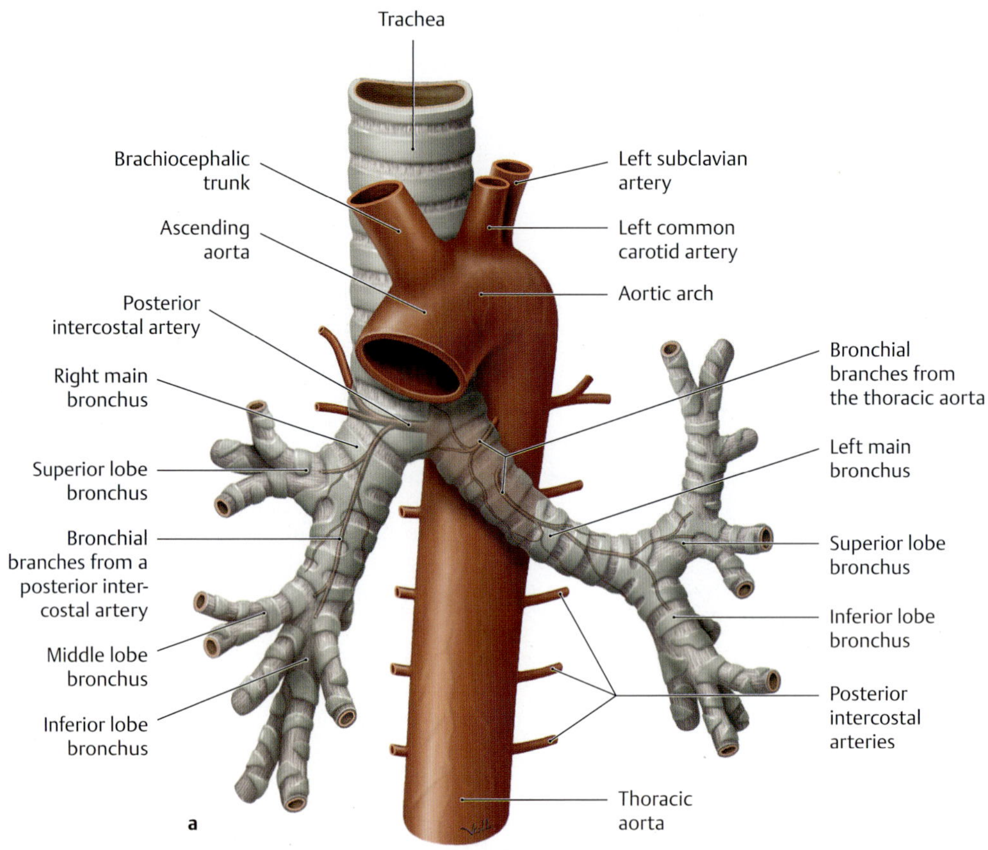

a

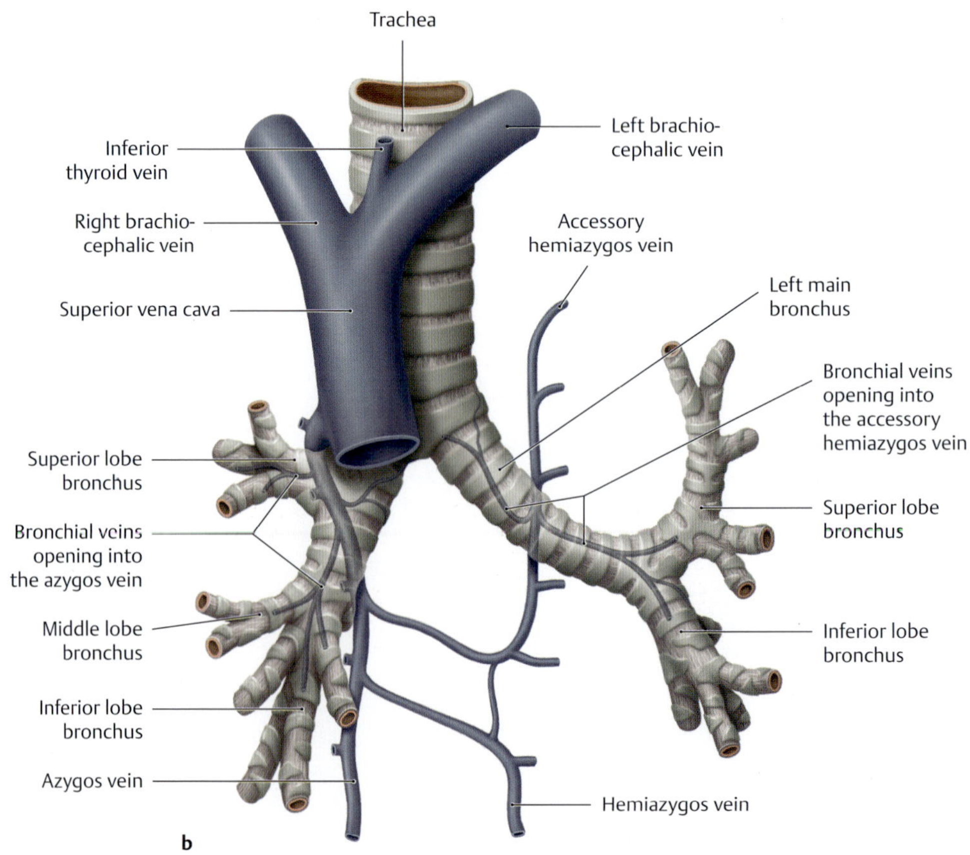

b

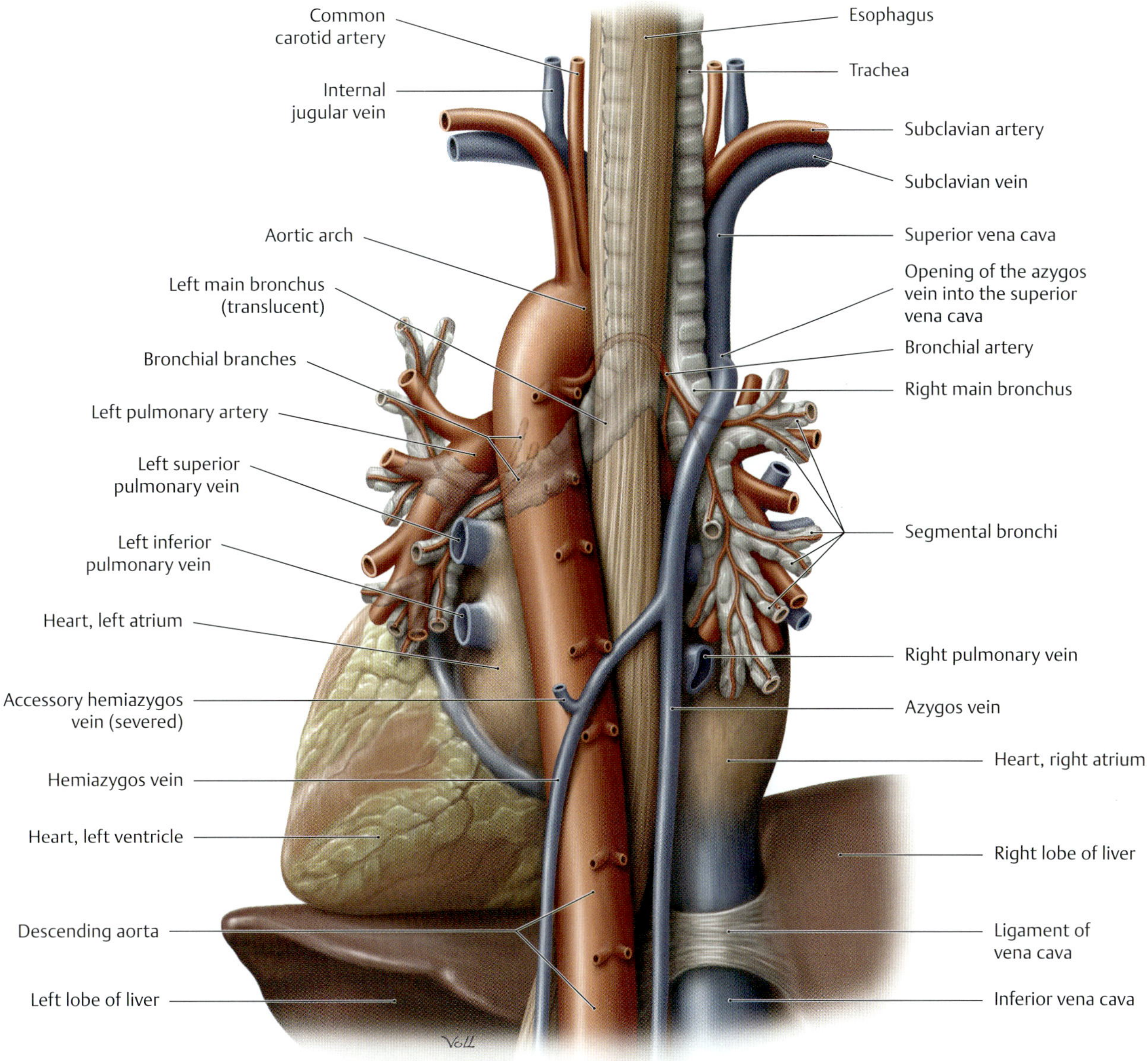

B Bronchial arteries and their topographical relation to the pulmonary arteries

Isolated organ group composed of heart, major vessels, trachea, esophagus and liver, posterior view.

Note: The bronchial arteries originate from the proximal portion of the descending aorta.

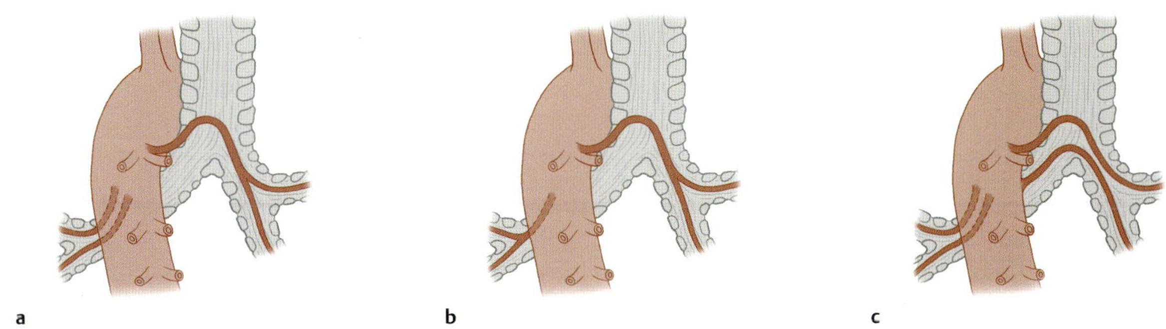

C Origin of the bronchial arteries from the aorta: normal anatomy and variations (after Platzer)

Posterior view.

a Normal anatomical case (40% of cases): on the right side of the aorta arise a bronchial artery and a posterior intercostal artery, on the left side arise two bronchial arteries;

b Variation 1 (15–30 % of cases): only *one* bronchial artery arises from the left and the right sides of the aorta;

c Variation 2 (12–23 %): *two* bronchial arteries arise from the left and the right sides of the aorta.

4.10 Functional Structure of the Vascular Tree

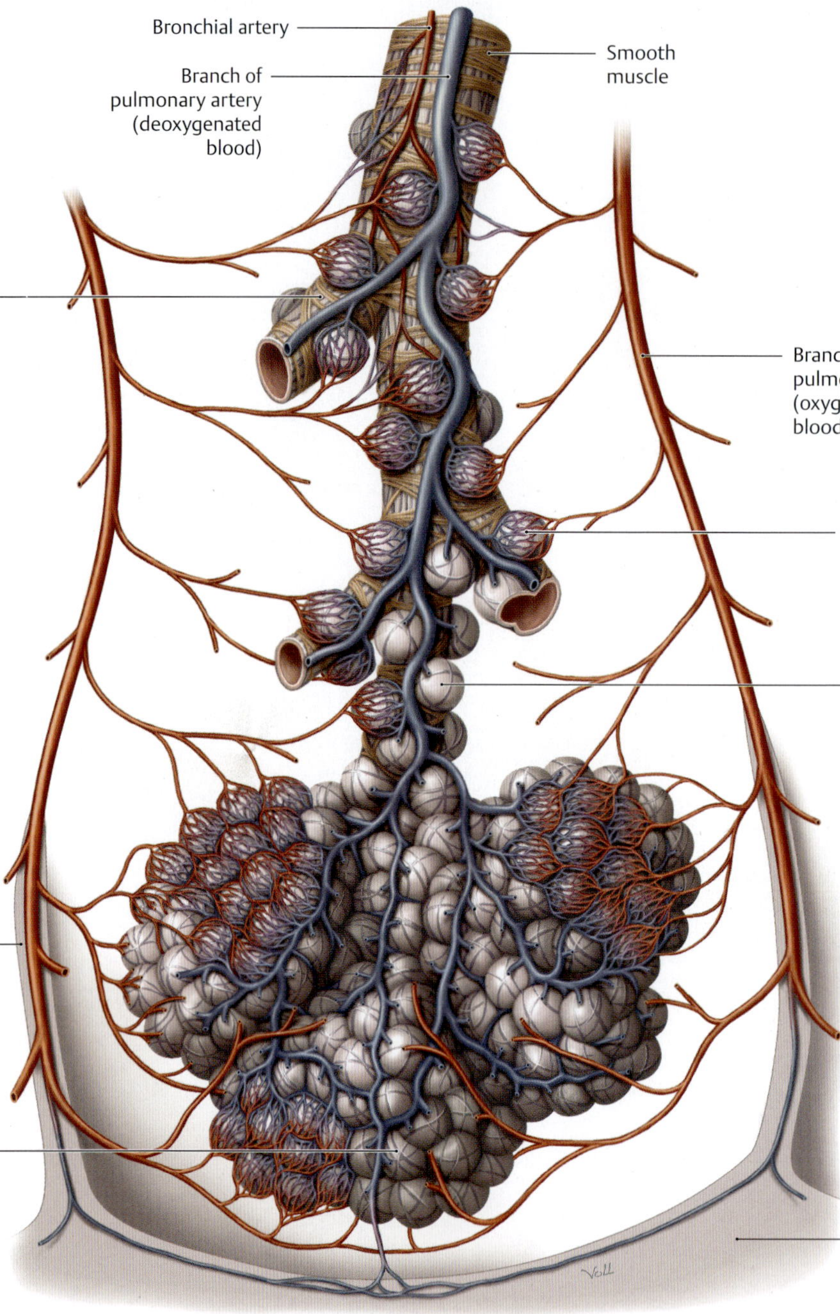

A Overview of vascular tree structure

Note: In previous sections, arteries have been colored in red and veins have been colored in blue. However, since this paragraph discusses in particular the functional structure of the vascular tree, this standard convention of coloring is not followed here. Instead, branches of the pulmonary artery (arterial side of circulation) are colored in blue, because of low oxygen levels, and branches of the pulmonary veins (venous side of circulation) are colored in red because of high oxygen levels.

The vascular tree is made up of the finest terminal branches of the pulmonary arteries and veins as well as the bronchial arteries and veins. These branches of the vasa publica (pulmonary arteries and veins) and vasa privata (bronchial arteries and veins) are analogous to those of the bronchial tree (see p. 154). Because of this arrangement, gas exchange can occur between air in the alveoli (in the finest branches of the bronchial tree) and blood (in the finest branches of the pulmonary vessels).

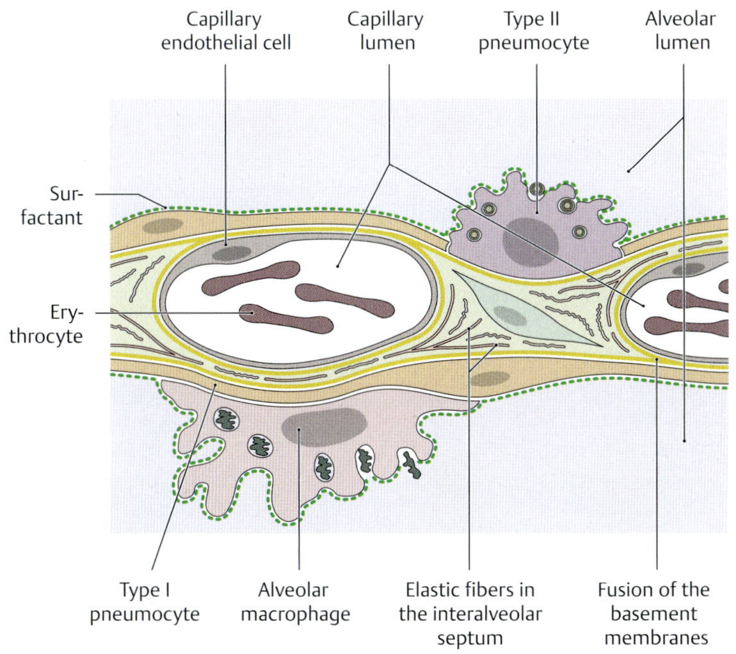

B Epithelial lining of the alveoli
The alveoli are lined by two types of alveolar epithelial cells (pneumocytes):

- Type I pneumocytes: They cover approximately 90 % of the alveolar surface, are spread out flat and form a continuous layer (cap cells). They are closely interconnected by tight junctions.
- Type II pneumocytes: Relative to total number, they are as common as type I pneumocytes. However, because of their rounded shape they are thicker than type I pneumocytes but not as expansive as them. They cover only about 10% of the alveolar surface. They are found among type I pneumocytes, often at alveolar-septal junctions, and thus they are also referred to as niche cells. They produce and secrete a protein-phospholipid film called surfactant, which is distributed over the entire alveolar surface and lowers the surface tension of the alveoli, making it easier for the lung to expand. The immature lung of the preterm infant often fails to produce sufficient surfactant. Thus, preterm infants often suffer from respiratory problems. Type II pneumocytes continuously produce and reabsorb surfactant so that a large amount of surfactant is reused. Only a fraction is cleared by alveolar macrophages.

At the sites where type I alveolar epithelial cells come into contact with the capillary endothelial cells, their basement membranes are fused together. The anatomical distance from the alveolar lumen to the capillary lumen, over which gaseous diffusion takes place, measures only 0.5 μm at that location.
Note: All diseases which

- increase the diffusion distance between the alveolar lumen and capillary lumen (edematous fluid collection or inflammation),
- decrease the aeration of the lung (alveolar destruction due to emphysema, for example) or decrease lung perfusion (capillary obliteration), or
- cause fluid infiltration of the alveoli (pneumonia)
- will decrease the efficiency of alveola–capillary gas exchange, leading to respiratory compromise.

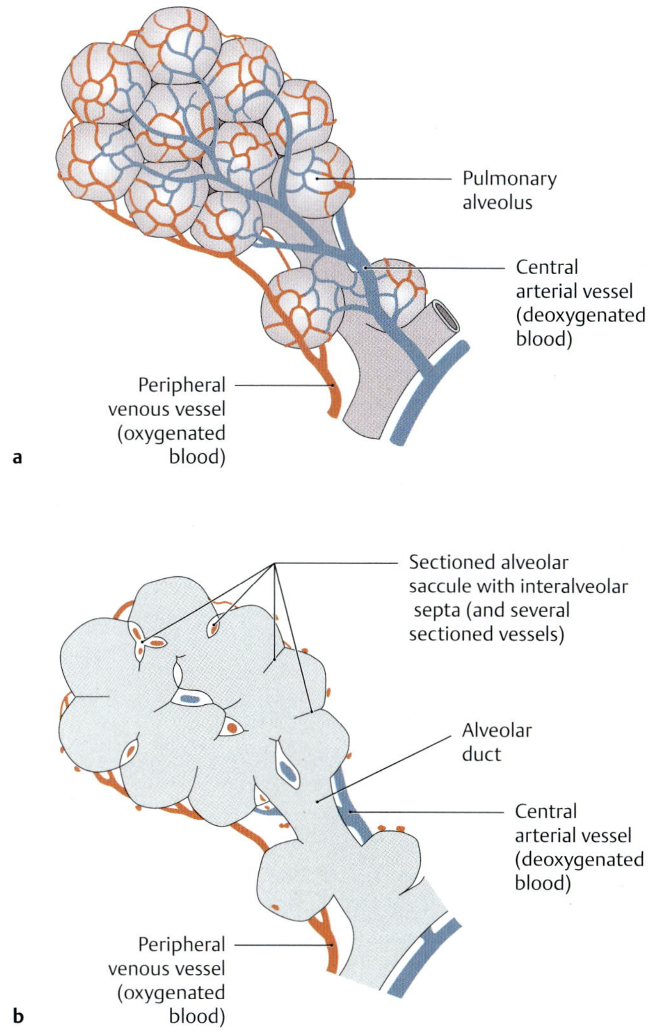

C Relationship between the alveolar sac and pulmonary vessels
In **a**, a branch of the pulmonary artery carrying oxygen-depleted blood from the right ventricle is depicted in blue. A corresponding branch of the pulmonary venous system is shown in red, carrying oxygen-enriched blood back to the left heart. Pulmonary arterial branches are intimately apposed to, and follow closely the course of, the respiratory bronchiole branches, sending capillaries over the alveolar sacs and invading the alveolar septa. The sectioned alveolar sac (**b**) clearly shows that the vessels not only surround the alveoli on the outer surface of the sac but also penetrate the interalveolar septa, enabling the capillaries to undergo gas exchange with multiple adjacent alveoli.
Note: In most of the circulatory system, small arterial and corresponding venous branches tend to follow parallel courses, but this is not true in the pulmonary circulation. While pulmonary arterial branches follow the same segmental and lobular branching pattern as the bronchial tree, the pulmonary veins have a more independent course, not closely apposed to the bronchioles, remaining on the periphery of lobules and segments, and often crossing lobular boundaries. This difference in conformation between pulmonary arteries and veins is demonstrated dramatically in **A**.

4.11 Innervation and Lymphatic Drainage of the Trachea, Bronchial Tree, and Lungs

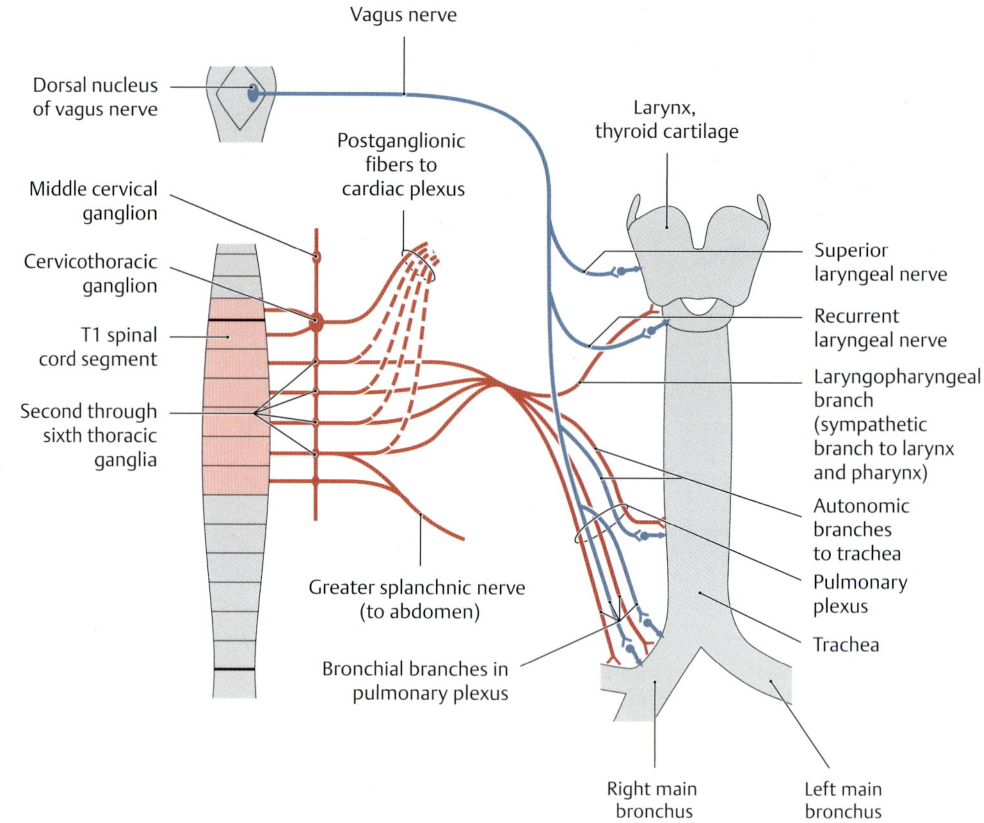

A Autonomic innervation of the trachea and bronchial tree

Parasympathetic: Branches from both vagus nerves are distributed to the cervical part of the trachea, mostly via the recurrent laryngeal nerves. At the thoracic level they form tracheal branches that continue as bronchial branches and enter the pulmonary plexus, which is heavily branched at the pulmonary hilum.

Sympathetic: Few postsynaptic fibers are distributed to the trachea; numerous thoracic pulmonary branches (postsynaptic branches of the thoracic ganglia) pass into the pulmonary plexus.

The pulmonary plexus regulates the caliber and secretory activity of the bronchi and influences the caliber of the pulmonary vessels. Activation of the parasympathetic nervous system causes the bronchi to constrict (as in bronchial asthma), while activation of the sympathetic nervous system causes bronchial dilation. Thus, drugs that activate the sympathetic nervous system cause bronchial dilation and may be useful in the treatment of acute bronchial asthma. The autonomic effects on the pulmonary vessels provide a means of varying the perfusion to different areas of the lung by controlling vascular calibers. For example, the autonomic system can greatly reduce the blood flow to poorly ventilated lung areas during shallow respiration.

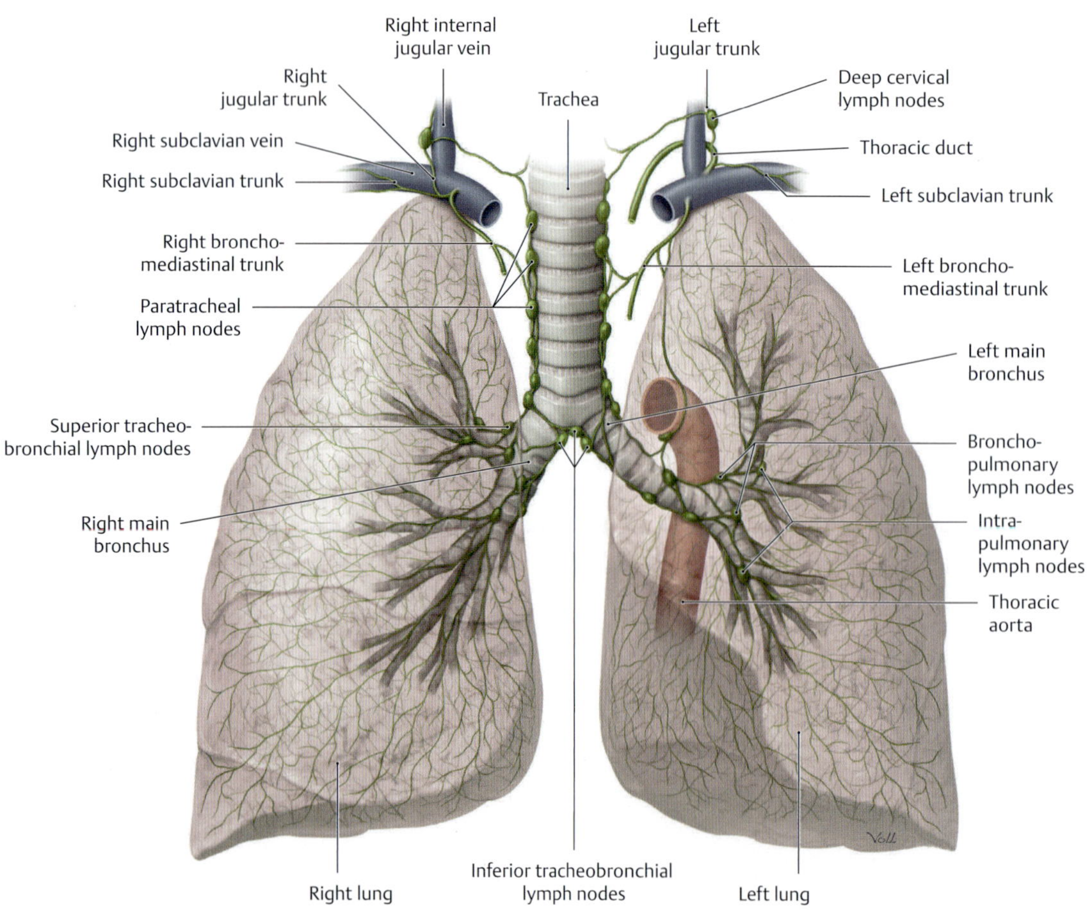

B Lymph nodes of the trachea, bronchi, and lungs

Anterior view. The following lymph nodes can be distinguished inside and outside the lungs, listed in order from deep to superficial:

- Inside the lung: intrapulmonary lymph nodes in the lung tissue and at the divisions of the segmental bronchi; bronchopulmonary lymph nodes at the division of the lobar bronchi.
- Outside the lung: inferior and superior tracheobronchial lymph nodes at the tracheal bifurcation and on both main bronchi; paratracheal lymph nodes along both sides of the trachea.

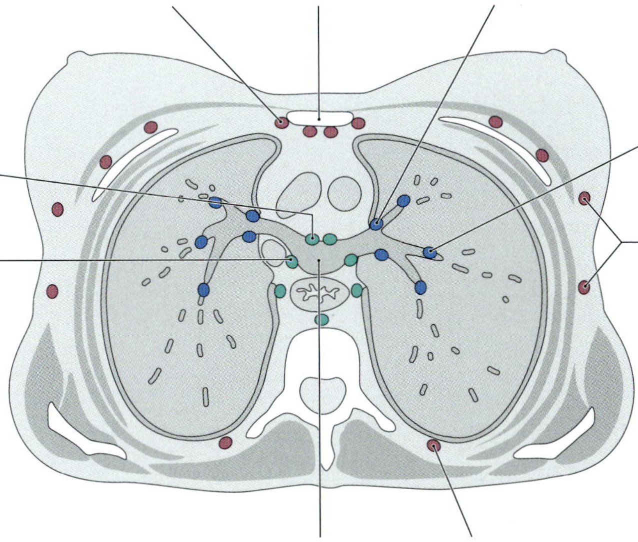

a

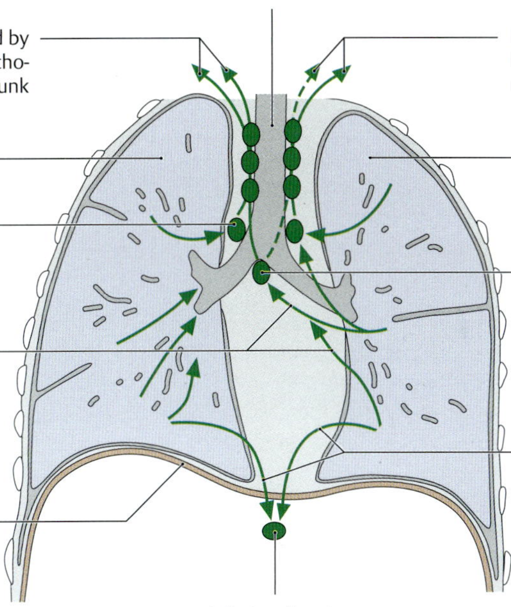

b

C Lymphatic drainage of the lungs, bronchial tree, and trachea

a, **b** Transverse and coronal sections viewed from above (**a**) and from the front (**b**). The lymphatic drainage of the *lungs and bronchi* is handled by two separate networks of delicate lymphatic vessels (see **b**):

- The *peribronchial network* follows the branching pattern of the bronchial tree (see p. 145) and collects lymph from the bronchi and most of the lungs.
- The *subpleural network* (smaller) bordering the lungs collects lymph from peripheral lung areas and from the *visceral* pleura. The parietal pleura (part of the chest wall) is drained by the intercostal and parasternal lymph nodes of the chest wall.

These two networks communicate at the pulmonary hilum and convey lymph *cranially*, ultimately to the tracheobronchial lymph nodes (deep tissue areas may drain to the intrapulmonary or bronchopulmonary nodes, but the lung as a whole is drained by the tracheobronchial nodes). Lymph flows from the tracheobronchial lymph nodes to the paratracheal nodes and bronchomediastinal trunks, which terminate at the junction of the subclavian and internal jugular veins independently or after joining the thoracic duct or right lymphatic duct.

Note: Lymph from the *left* inferior lobe may also drain to the right bronchomediastinal trunk via (inferior) tracheobronchial lymph nodes. The inferior lobes of *both* lungs may drain cranially, but they may also drain inferiorly to the superior phrenic lymph nodes or may drain through the diaphragm to the inferior phrenic nodes.

The **trachea** drains to the paratracheal lymph nodes, which may empty directly into the jugular trunk or indirectly via the bronchomediastinal lymph nodes.

Note: Tracheobronchial lymph nodes that lie very close to the pulmonary hilum are known in clinical parlance as the “hilar lymph nodes.” Their enlargement in response to pathological processes may be detectable by imaging studies.

4.12 Respiratory Mechanics

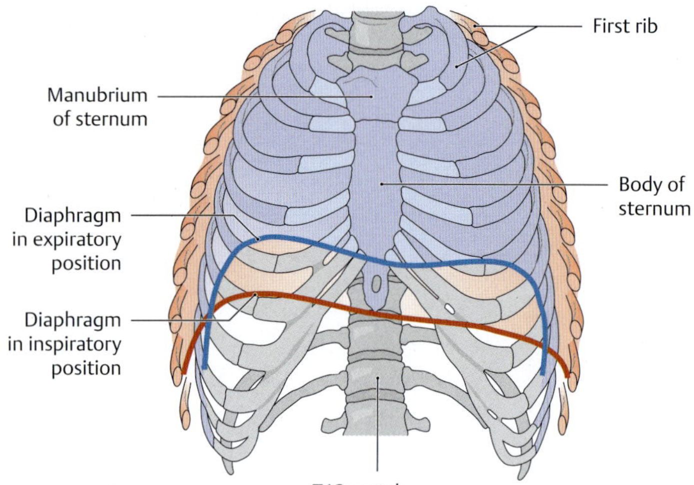

a

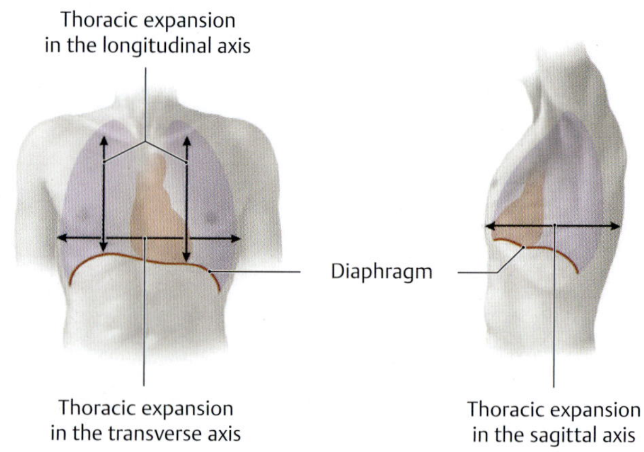

b

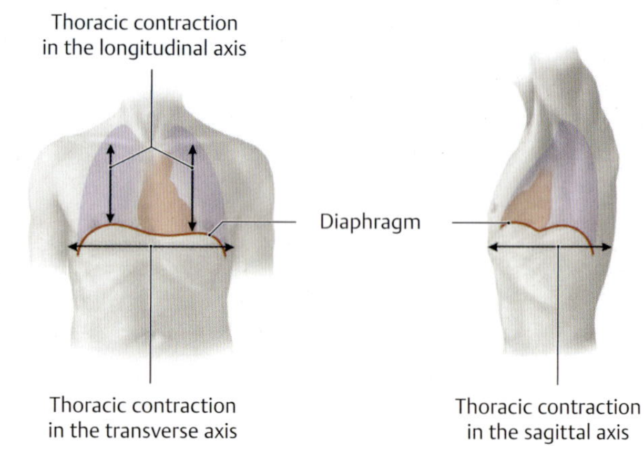

c

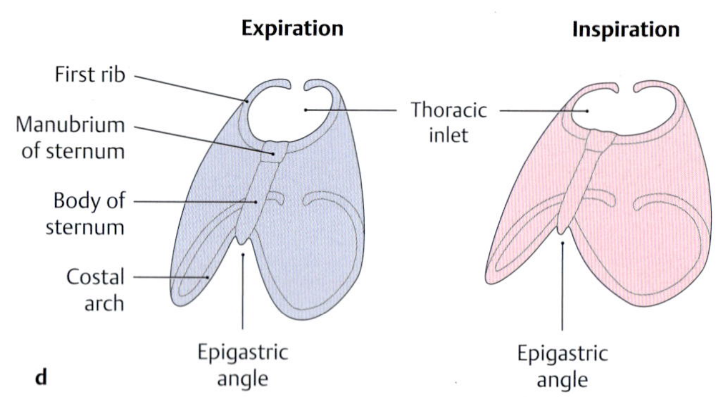

d

A Basic principles of respiratory mechanics

The mechanics of external respiration (as opposed to the internal respiration of cells and tissues) are based on a rhythmical increase and decrease in the thoracic volume, with an associated expansion and contraction of the lungs. As the lung expands, the pressure within the lung falls and air is drawn into the lung (inspiration). As the lung contracts, the pulmonary pressure rises and air is expelled from the lung (expiration). Thus, contrary to a common misconception, air is not pumped into the lungs during respiration but is sucked into the lungs by the "bellows effect," a negative intrapulmonary pressure. The ribs, the thoracic muscles (especially the intercostal muscles), and the elastic fibers in the lung interact as follows during respiration:

- When the diaphragm moves to the **inspiratory position** (red), the ribs are elevated by the intercostal muscles (chiefly the external intercostals) and the scalene muscles. Because the ribs are curved and are directed obliquely downward, elevation of the ribs expands the chest transversely (toward the flanks) and anteriorly. Meanwhile the diaphragm leaflets are lowered by muscular contraction (red outline in **a**), causing the chest to expand inferiorly. The epigastric angle is also increased (see **d**). These processes result in an overall expansion of the thoracic volume.
- When the diaphragm moves to the **expiratory position** (blue), the chest becomes smaller in all dimensions and the thoracic volume is decreased. This process does not require additional muscular energy. The muscles that are active during inspiration are relaxed, and the lung contracts as the myriad elastic fibers in the lung tissue that were stretched on inspiration release their stored energy, causing an elastic recoil. For forcible expiration, however, the muscles that assist expiration (mainly the internal intercostal muscles) can actively lower the rib cage more rapidly and to a greater extent than is possible by passive elastic recoil alone.

B Respiratory muscles

Active during inspiration	Active during expiration
Scalene muscles	Internal intercostal muscles
External intercostal muscles	Transversus thoracis
Intercartilaginous muscles	Subcostal muscles
Serratus posterior superior and inferior	
Diaphragm	

When the upper limb is fixed (e.g., by bracing the arm on a table), the muscles of the shoulder girdle, whose primary action is to move the shoulder girdle, can elevate and expand the thorax, to which they are attached. They can also function as auxiliary respiratory muscles during forced respiration, when breathing is made difficult (dyspnea) by disease.

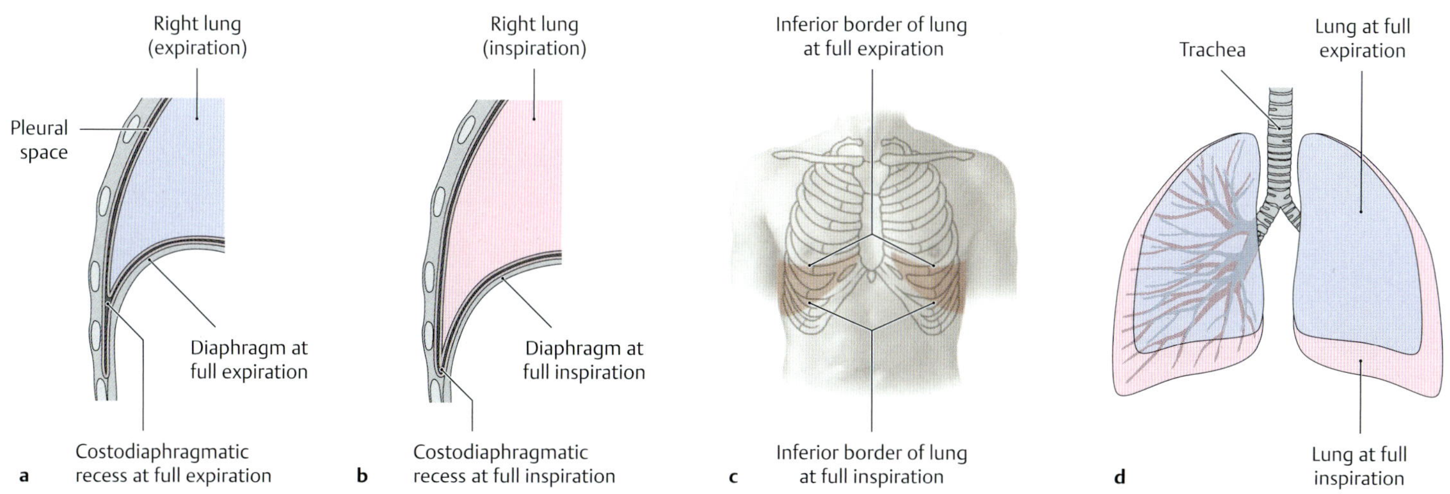

C Respiratory changes in lung volume

a–c Respiratory contraction and expansion of the lung. Capillary forces in the pleural space cause the lung to "stick" to the wall of the pleural cavity, forcing the lung to follow changes in the thoracic volume. This is particularly evident in the pleural recesses—sites where the lung does not fully occupy the pleural cavity at functional residual capacity (the resting position between inspiration and expiration, see p. 143). As the dome of the diaphragm flattens during inspiration (see **A**), the costodiaphragmatic recess expands and the lung is "sucked" into the resulting space, though it does not fill it completely. During expiration, the lung retracts from the recess somewhat. The respiratory changes in the volume of the costodiaphragmatic recess lead to considerable displacement of the inferior lung borders (**c**).

d Respiratory movements of the bronchial tree. As the thoracic volume changes during respiration, the entire bronchial tree moves within the lung. These structural movements are more pronounced in portions of the bronchial tree that are more distant from the pulmonary hilum.

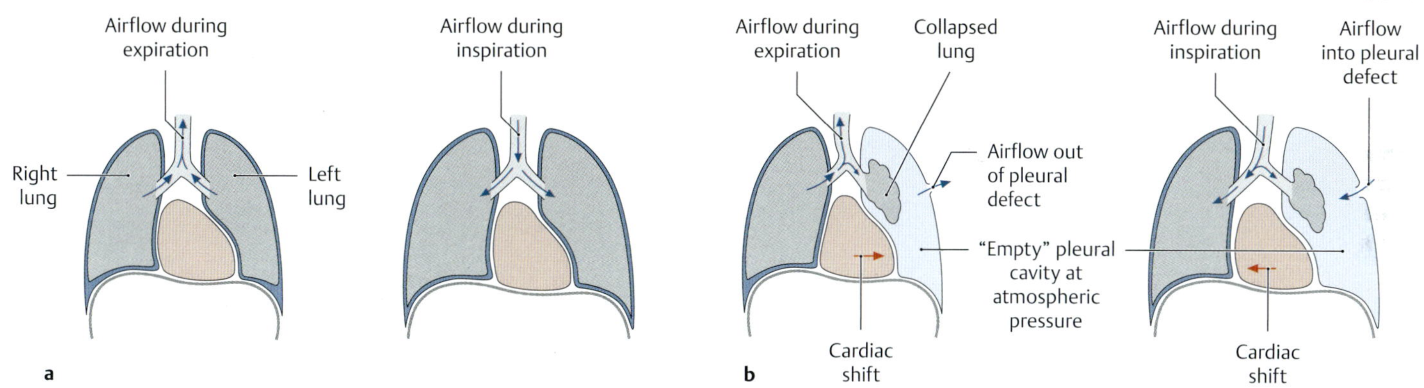

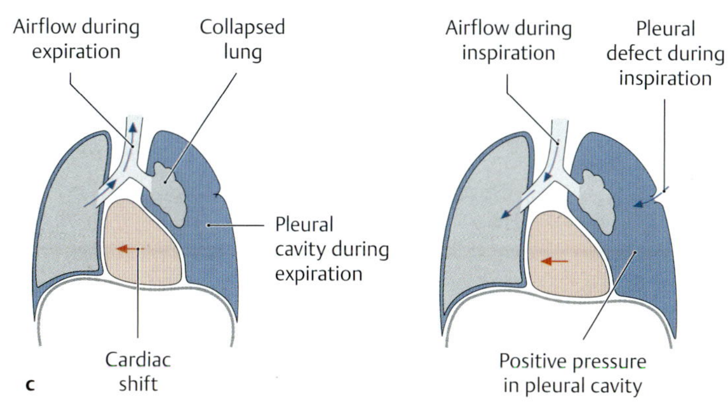

D Change in respiratory mechanics due to pneumothorax

a Normal respiratory mechanics: The pleural space is hermetically sealed on all sides.

b Pneumothorax: With injury to the left parietal pleura, outside air can enter the pleural space. The mechanical effect of the capillary pleural space (see **C**) is lost, and the left lung collapses from the inherent elasticity of its connective tissue. It no longer participates in respiration. The right pleural cavity is intact and can function independently. Air is sucked into the opened pleural cavity during inspiration and is expelled during expiration. Because normal respiratory pressure variations still prevail in the right pleural cavity but are absent on the left side due to the pleural defect, the mediastinum shifts toward the normal side during expiration and returns toward the midline during inspiration ("mediastinal flutter").

c Tension pneumothorax (valve pneumothorax): Tissue that has been traumatically detached and displaced covers the defect in the pleural cavity from the inside like a mobile flap, preventing the expulsion of air. Air passes through the defect in one direction only: from outside to inside. Because of this check-valve mechanism, a small amount of air enters the pleural cavity with each breath but cannot escape, similar to air being pumped into a bicycle tire. The mediastinum is gradually shifted toward the normal side (mediastinal shift), which may cause kinking of the vessels around the heart. Without treatment, tension pneumothorax is invariably fatal.

4.13 Radiological Anatomy of the Lungs and Vascular System

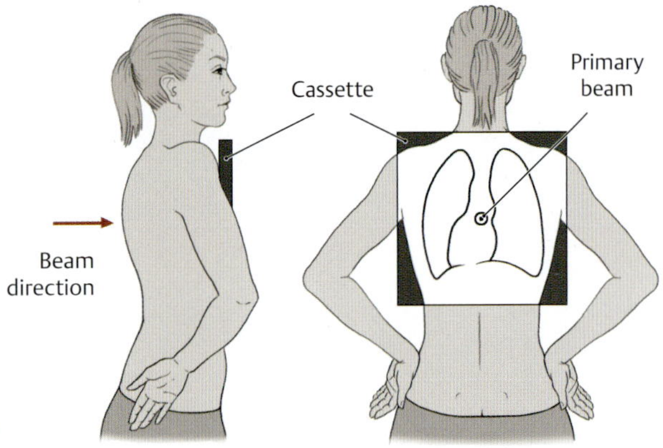

a

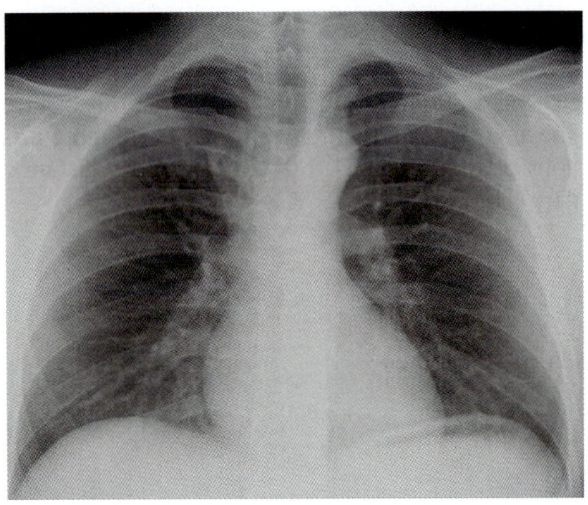

b

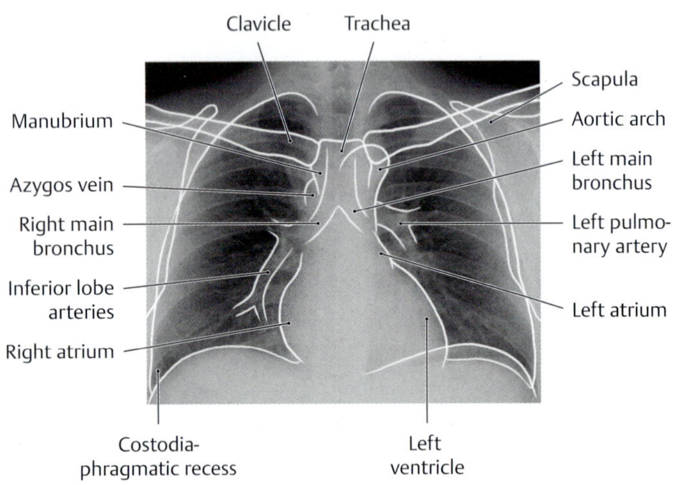

c

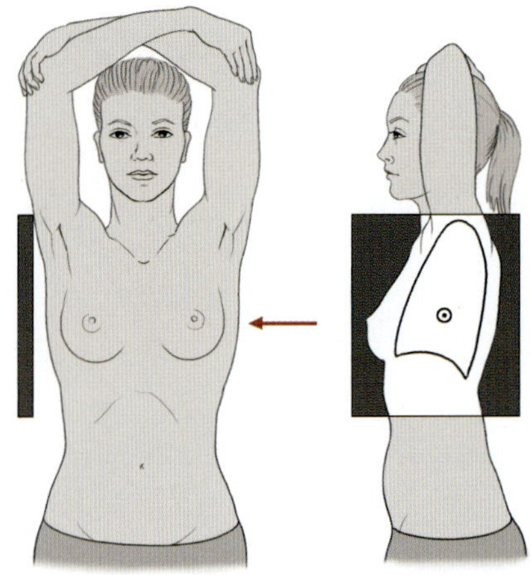

a

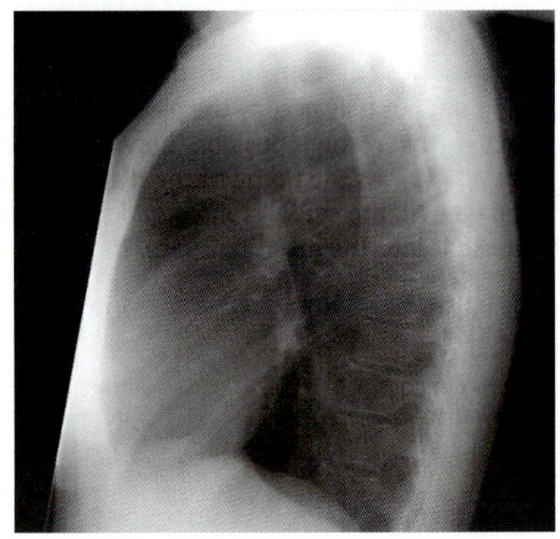

b

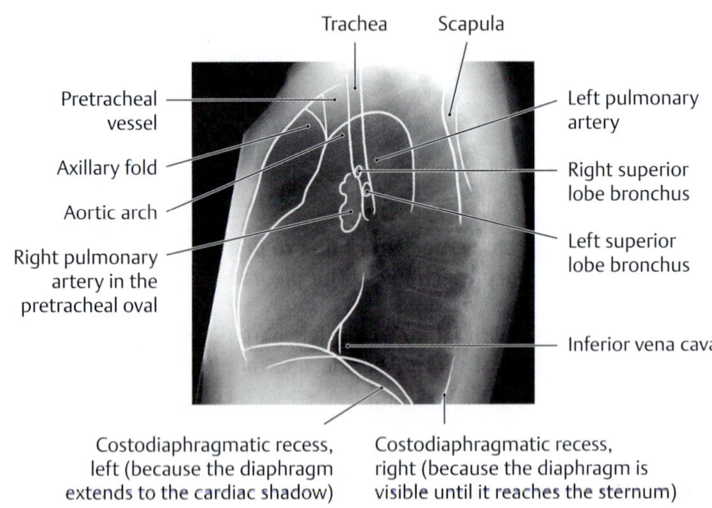

c

A Posterior-anterior (PA) chest radiograph

a The patient stands with the anterior chest wall on the cassette (the beam "passes" through the patient in a posterior-to-anterior direction with the central beam targeted at the level of the 6th thoracic vertebra). The radiographs are taken with the patient keeping the mouth open, breathing in and holding the breath. The back of the hands are placed on the hips with the elbows turned forward;

b Posterior-anterior chest radiograph (PA radiograph; viewed from an anterior to posterior direction);

c Explanation of the visible structures.

B Lateral chest radiograph

a The patient is standing with the left or right side against the cassette, with both arms raised above the head. The central beam is targeted a hand's width below the left (right) armpit;

b Lateral chest radiograph;

c Explanation of the visible structures.

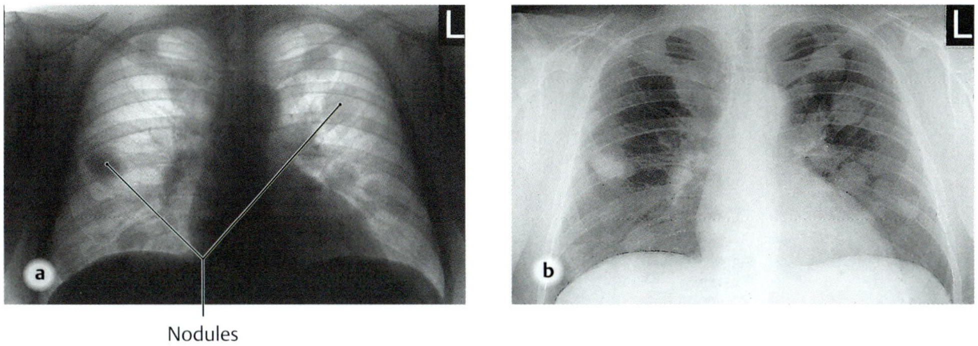

C Terminology to describe conventional radiographic findings

The terminology used to describe conventional radiographic findings dates back to the era of *photofluorography*. On the fluorescent screens that were used back then, radiopaque areas, such as the heart and bones, but also lung metastases (also known as nodules), appear as shadows because they show weaker *light emission* (**a**). Compared with the fluorescent screen, modern radiographs (**b**) produce inverted images (negative images): The *low absorption areas* (radiolucent areas) appear as dark areas and the *opacities* (radiopaque areas) as bright areas.

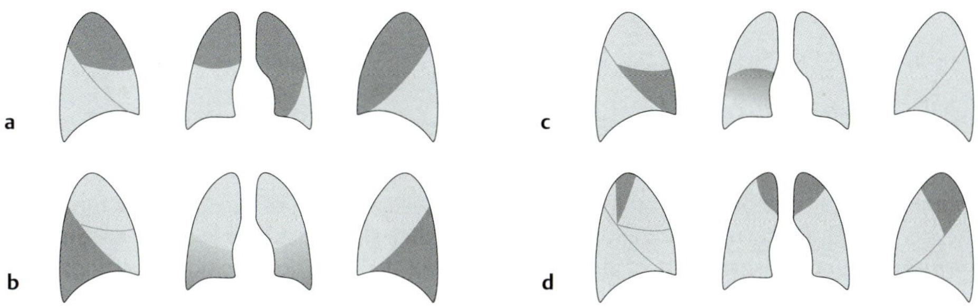

D Opacity in lung diseases

Lateral and anterior views of the right and left lungs.

a Opacity of both superior lobes; **b** Opacity of both inferior lobes; **c** Opacity of the middle lobe (right); **d** Opacity of apical segment on both sides.

In most cases, opacities that follow the lines of segmental lung boundaries are almost always due to inflammation of the lungs.

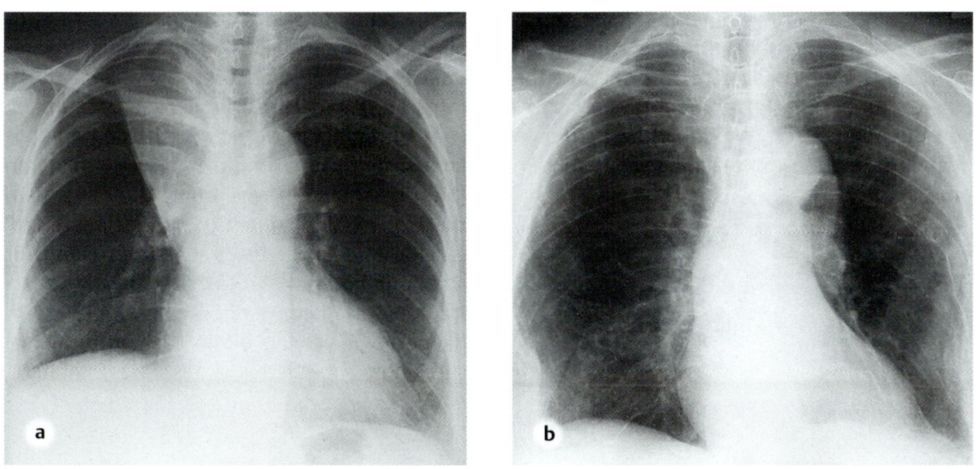

E Pulmonary opacities on an AP chest radiograph

a Right superior lobe atelectasis due to damage to the right superior lobe bronchus caused by a central carcinoma. This resulted in reduced ventilation of the affected superior lobe and subsequent collapse of lung tissue;

b Right basal pleural effusion causing complete opacification of the lateral costodiaphragmatic recess. Opacity is higher laterally, concave to the lung and does not follow lobar boundaries.

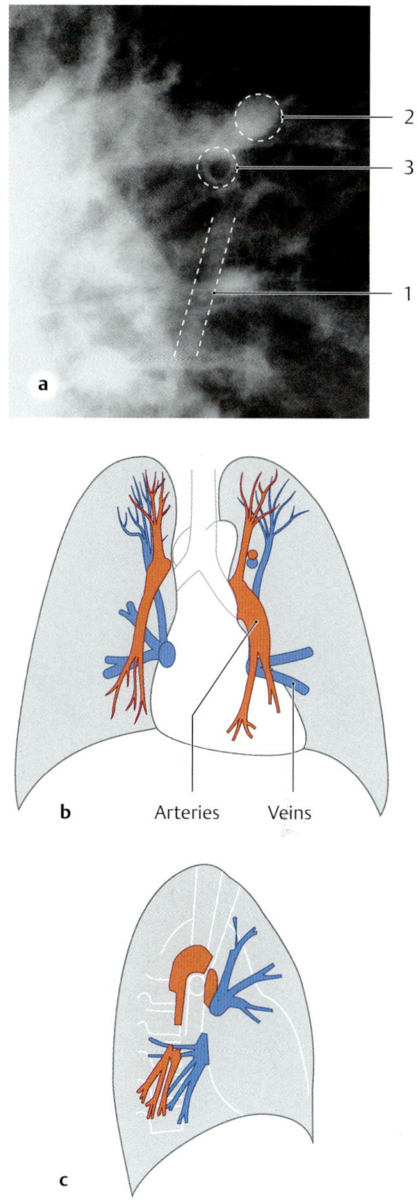

F Radiographic appearance of pulmonary vessels

a Detail from AP chest radiograph close to the pulmonary hilum: The image shows a longitudinal view of a vessel (1), an oblique view of a vessel (2) and an oblique view of a bronchus (3). Farther out in the periphery, opacities are usually not detectable.

b Schematic view of the vascular bundle in an AP projection.
Note: Arteries always run adjacent to the bronchi; arteries to the superior lobes run medial to the veins, and inferior lobe veins run horizontally and cross the inferior lobe arteries.

c Schematic view of the vascular bundle, lateral view.
Note: In the retrocardiac vascular bundle, the veins descend more anteriorly than the arteries.

(All photos in this learning unit from: Reiser M, Kuhn F, Debus J, eds. *Duale Reihe Radiologie*. 4th ed. Stuttgart: Thieme; 2017.)

4.14 Computed Tomography of the Lung and Mediastinum (Thorax CT)

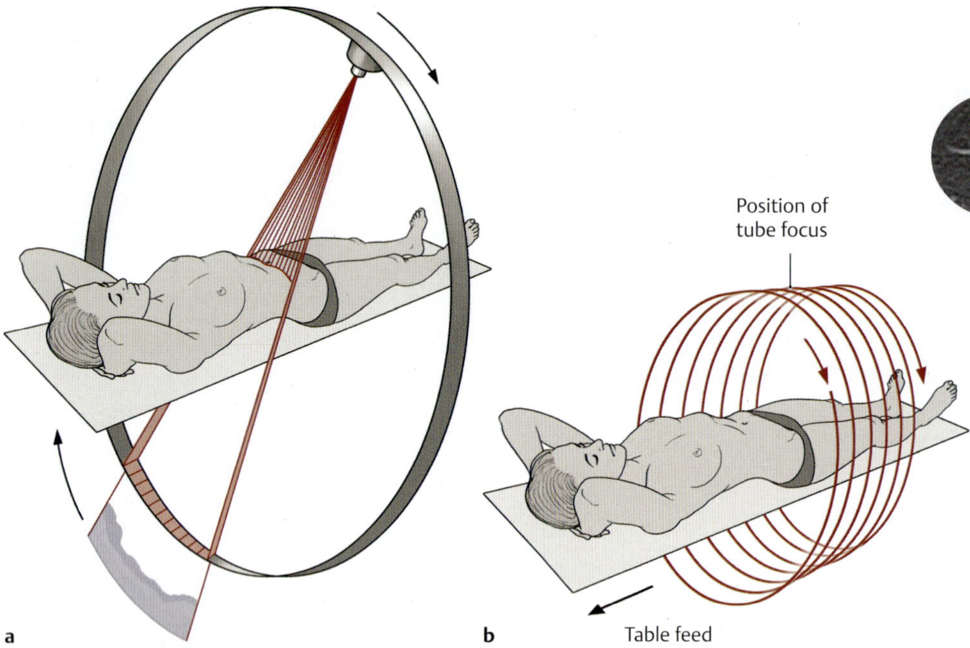

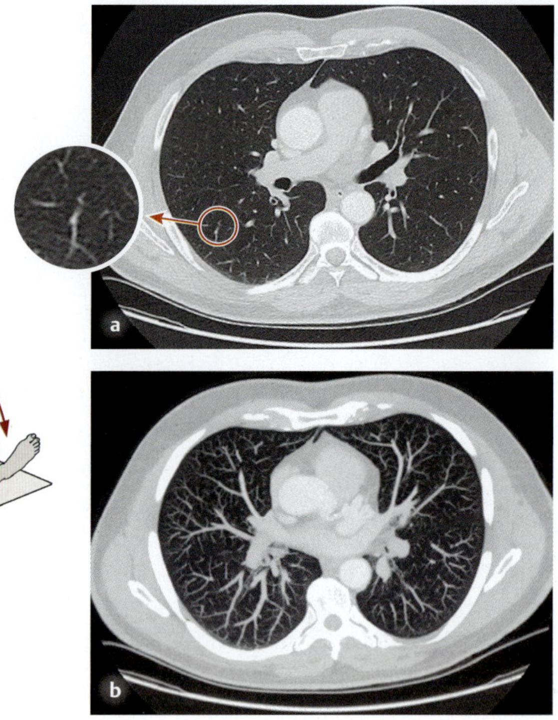

A Principle of computed tomography

a Principle of image acquisition in computed tomography: **b** diagram of spiral path of X-ray tube around the body (helical CT). Tube rotation and the table feed are continuous motions in CT. The measurements are acquired as a volume data set from which slices of any desired thickness and at variable distance can be calculated.

Computed tomography is a radiographic process that creates transverse (axial) slices through the body (Greek *tomos*, slice). The technique was developed in the 1960s by Hounsfield and Cormack. The decisive difference to conventional radiography is that the images are not obtained directly but are calculated by a computer. Depending on which and how much image data are acquired in the radiographic process, two-dimensional images or three-dimensional reconstructions can be obtained in any spatial plane (sagittal, coronary, etc. see **D**). Computed tomography also allows unobstructed visualization of structures (no radiographic shadows of superimposed organs or tissues). A computed tomography system essentially consists of a gantry with an X-ray tube and detector (see **a**), an examining table for the patient, a control console, and a computer. Depending on the density of the tissue through which it passes, the X-ray beam is attenuated to varying degrees. Soft tissue is significantly more absorbent than tissue containing air; that is, the different tissue densities are essentially what provides the image contrast. The electronic detectors measure the differences in intensity of the X-rays and convert them into electronic signals that are then digitalized and fed into the image construction process.

B Visualization of the lung as a function of slice thickness and window settings

a Axial CT on lung window settings; **b** MIP (= maximum intensity projection) on the lung window (for window settings, see **C**).

How structures are visualized on CT depends on the selected slice thickness as well as other factors. Normally the examined slices are 1.25–2.5 mm thick. At this slice thickness and with corresponding magnification, interlobar structures in the lung and secondary pulmonary lobules, the smallest building blocks of the pulmonary parenchyma, are well visualized (see **a**). Visualizing larger structures requires slightly thicker slices (approximately 10 mm thick) and also a higher contrast image (see **b**). This can be achieved using what is known as the maximum intensity projection (MIP) technique in which only the pixels with the highest signal intensity are included. MIP is used in such cases as when searching for focal pulmonary lesions; that is, nearly spherical areas of circumscribed density 1–3 cm in diameter of varying origin such as bronchial carcinoma, metastases, abscesses, infarcts, etc.

C Typical densities of various types of tissue in Hounsfield units

The densities of tissues in computed tomography are specified in Hounsfield units (HU). They express the absorption values (attenuation values) of the imaged tissue in relation to the absorption values of air and water: Air is assigned the absorption value –1000 and water the absorption value 0. In this context, ventilated lung tissue has a value of –500 HU and the dense cortex of bone a value of 1000 to 2000 HU.

Tissue or finding	Hounsfield units (HU)
Air	–1000
Lung tissue	–500
Fatty tissue	–50 to –100
Water	0
Cerebrospinal fluid	+15
Liver tissue	+40 to +60
Liver tissue with contrast agent	+150
Acute bleeding	+70 to +90
Cortex	+1000 to +2000

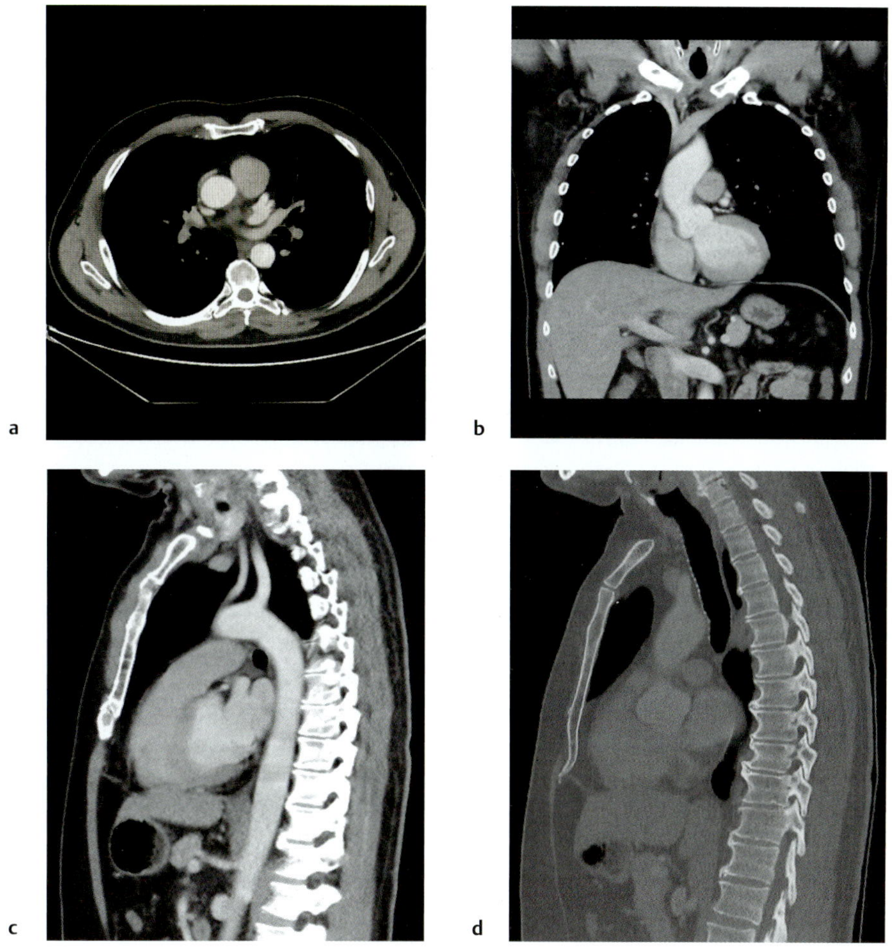

D Visualization of structures as a function of window settings

a–c Soft tissue window on **a** axial, **b** coronal, and **c** sagittal slices; **d** bone window on a sagittal slice.

In addition to slice thickness, see **B**, the window setting plays an important role in computed tomography. CT images are able to depict significantly more shades of gray than the human eye can detect. For this reason the detected gray scales must be limited according to which structures one wishes to examine. This is achieved by selecting the appropriate *window setting*. One selects a certain density value (HU value) as the center (or level) of the gray scale image or window and magnifies this center to a certain degree (window width). Small windows have higher contrast, wider windows have less. The respective window then optimally shows only those gray scales that one wants to evaluate. Here, with respect to the thorax:

- The **soft tissue or mediastinal window** shows the mediastinal structures, especially on axial (**a**), coronal (**b**), and sagittal (**c**) slices.
- The **bone window** shows bony structures, especially on sagittal slices (**d**).
- The **lung window** shows pulmonary structures, especially in axial slices (see Fig. **Ba** and **b**).

Example: For the lung one selects a center of −650 HU and a window width of 1500 HU. This value of −650 HU is selected because the lung has −500 HU (see Table **C**) and the center is chosen to match the HU density value of the tissue to be examined as closely as possible. Instead of only −500 HU, one selects −650 HU in order to visualize air, vascular structures, and connective tissue as well. A lung window with these values then extends from −1400 HU to +100 HU. All structures whose density range lies above or below this HU value are shown as either completely black or completely white. Intravenous administration of iodinated contrast agents improves the demarcation of mediastinal structures and pulmonary vessels and provides information about the blood supply to pathologic structures.

(CT images on this page from: Prof. S. Müller-Hülsbeck, M.D., Institut für Diagnostische und Interventionelle Radiologie/Neuroradiologie, DIAKO Krankenhaus gGmbH Flensburg.)

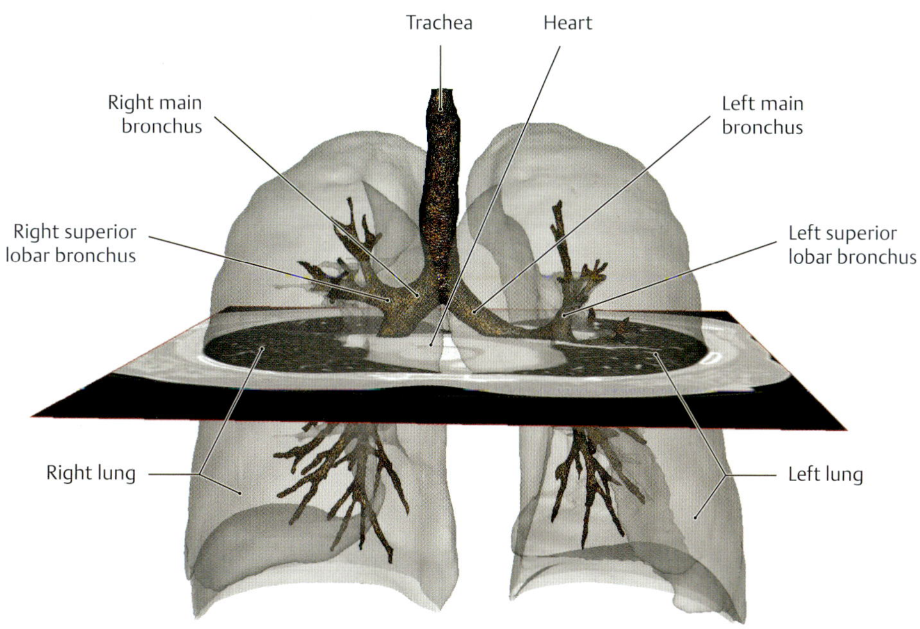

E Reconstruction of the bronchial tree from cross-sectional images

Anterior view; three-dimensional reconstruction of the bronchial tree from individual CT scans. The result is a high resolution, three-dimensional display. For orientation purposes, a CT section displaying the thorax with part of the heart and lungs is shown. Unlike the older technique of bronchography (radiographic contrast examination of the bronchi), this procedure is less debilitating for patients. Because of the high resolution of the scan, even small changes in the bronchial tree can be detected and accurately localized. Using this technique, a bronchial carcinoma, an often malignant tumor that is particularly common in smokers, can be precisely localized.

5.1 Esophagus: Location and Divisions

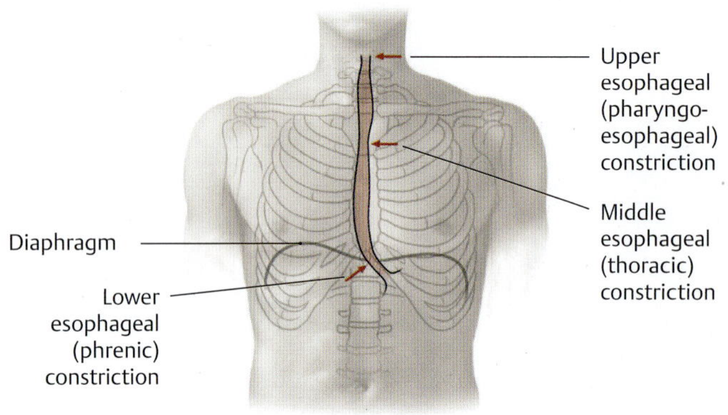

A Projection onto the thoracic skeleton
Anterior view. The esophagus is located slightly to the right of the midline, especially in its course through the thorax, where it descends along the right side of the aorta. It pierces the diaphragm just below the xiphoid process of the sternum. The arrows mark the sites of the three normal anatomical constrictions of the esophagus (see **C**).

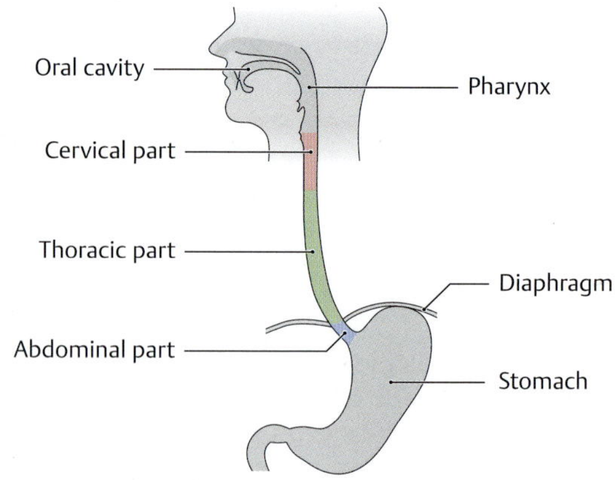

B Divisions of the esophagus
Anterior view with the head turned to the right. The esophagus is approximately 23–27 cm long, 1–2 cm in diameter, and is divided into three parts:

- Cervical part: just anterior to the vertebral column in the neck, extends from C 6 to T 1.
- Thoracic part: the longest part, located in the superior and posterior mediastinum, extends from T 1 to the esophageal hiatus of the diaphragm (at approximately T 11).
- Abdominal part: the shortest part, located in the peritoneal cavity, extends from the diaphragm to the cardiac orifice of the stomach.

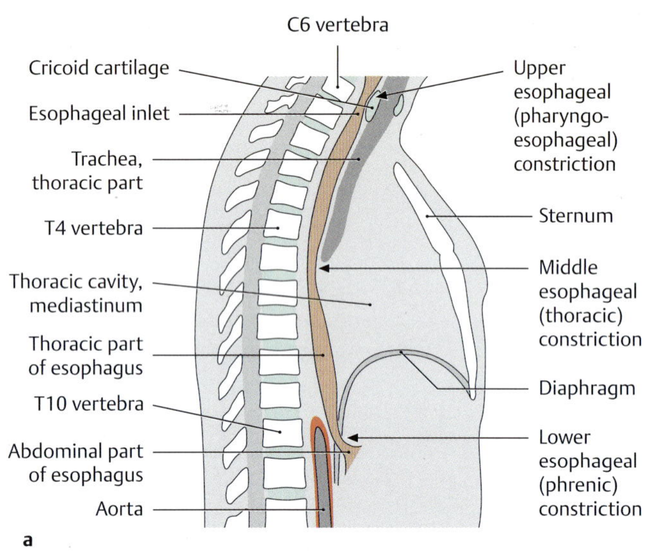

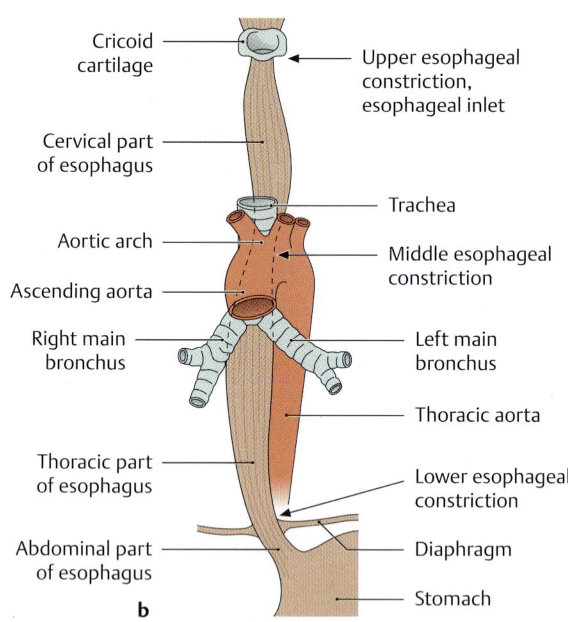

C Constrictions and curves of the esophagus
Right lateral view (**a**), anterior view (**b**).
The esophagus has three normal anatomical *constrictions*, which are projected at the levels of specific vertebrae (**a**). The constrictions are caused by adjacent structures that indent the esophagus and by functional closure mechanisms (lower constriction, see p. 169). These constrictions are visible during gastroscopy, and the scope must be carefully maneuvered past them (normal width of the esophagus is approximately 20 mm):

- Upper constriction (pharyngoesophageal constriction, 14–16 cm from the incisor teeth), corresponds to the esophageal inlet in the cervical part of the esophagus (see p. 168). It is located where the esophagus passes behind the cricoid cartilage (C 6) and has a maximum width of approximately 14 mm.
- Middle constriction (thoracic constriction, 25–27 cm from the incisors), located where the esophagus passes to the right of the aortic arch and thoracic aorta (at T 4/T 5). Maximum width is 14 mm.
- Lower constriction (phrenic constriction, 36–38 cm from the incisors), located at the start of the abdominal part of the esophagus, where it pierces the diaphragm (T 10/T 11). Functional closure of the esophagus by muscles and veins of the esophageal wall. The abdominal part is normally occluded except during swallowing (see p. 169). Maximum width is 14 mm.

Besides its constrictions, the esophagus also presents characteristic **curves** (**b**): an upper curve to the left (in the cervical part), a mid-level curve to the right (in the thoracic part, caused by the adjacent thoracic aorta), and a lower curve to the left (in the abdominal part). Additionally, the esophagus is slightly concave anteriorly in the sagittal plane, following the curvature of the vertebral column (thoracic kyphosis, **a**).

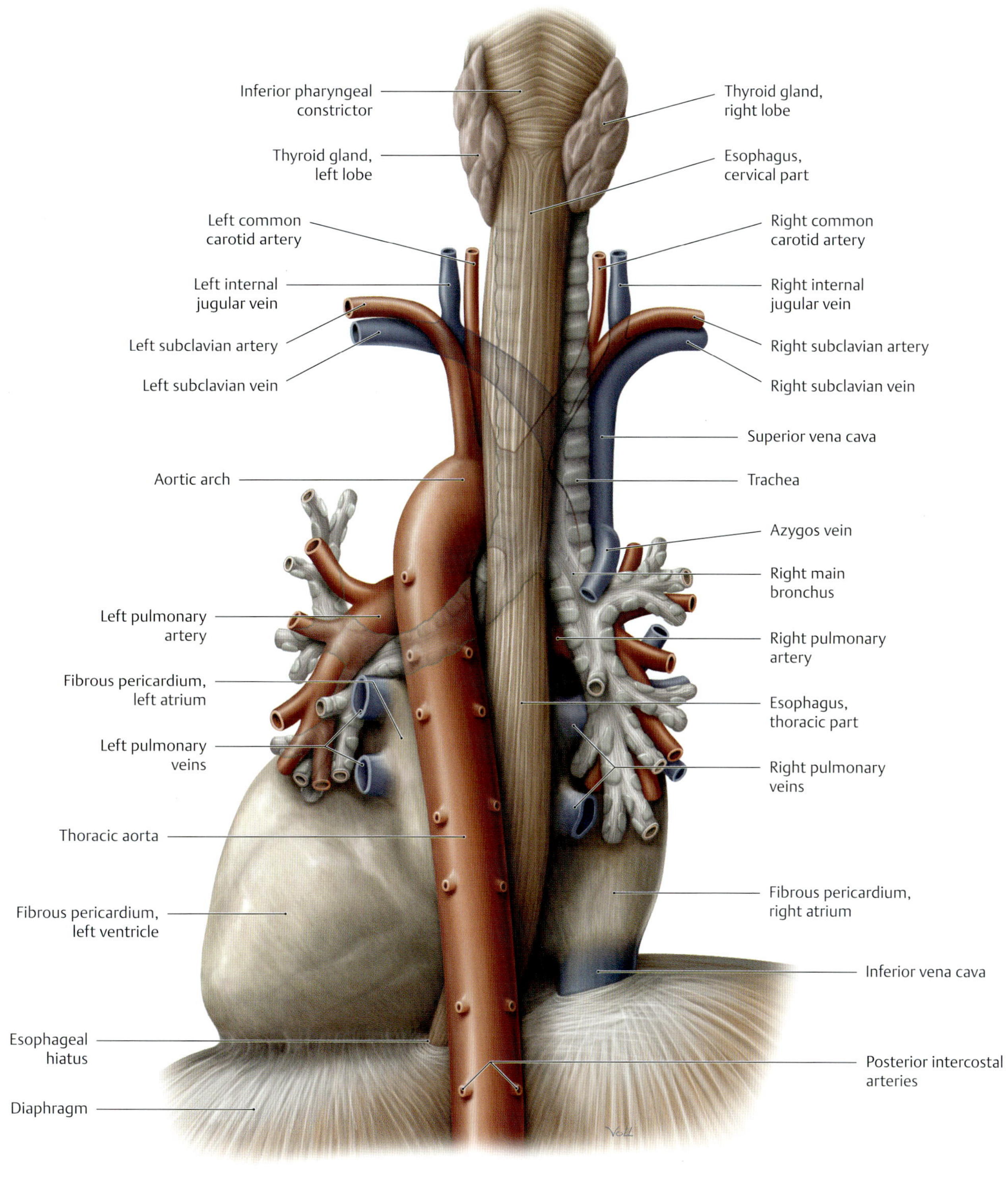

D Topographical relations of the esophagus, posterior view
The relations of the esophagus to the pericardium, great vessels, and trachea are depicted here. The close proximity of the esophagus to the left atrium and thoracic aorta can be seen. Due to the asymmetrical position of the heart in the thorax, the right pulmonary veins are closer to the esophagus than the left pulmonary veins. The esophagus initially descends to the right of the aorta, but just above the diaphragm it crosses in front of the aorta before piercing the diaphragm to enter the abdominal cavity (see **C**). The esophagus is loosely attached by its own connective tissue (adventitia) to the connective tissue of the mediastinum (important for swallowing). It is stabilized somewhat by the attachment of its anterior wall to the back of the trachea, again by numerous slips of connective tissue.
Note: The trachea develops as an outgrowth from the esophagus during early embryonic development, at which time a communication exists between the two structures. Normally this communication closes, but its persistence results in a tracheoesophageal fistula, which may allow food to enter the trachea and reach the lung, causing recurrent episodes of pneumonia.

5.2 Esophagus: Inlet and Outlet, Opening and Closure

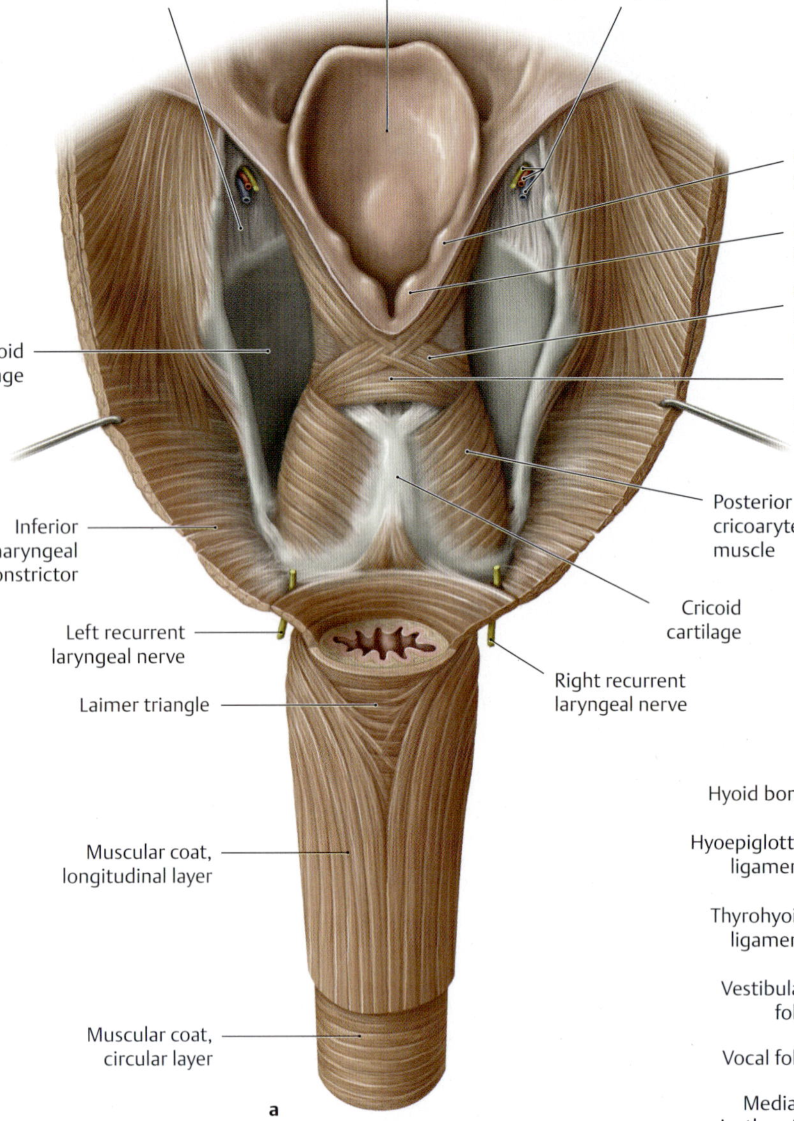

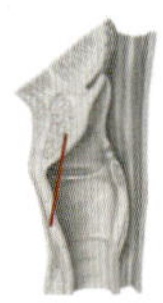

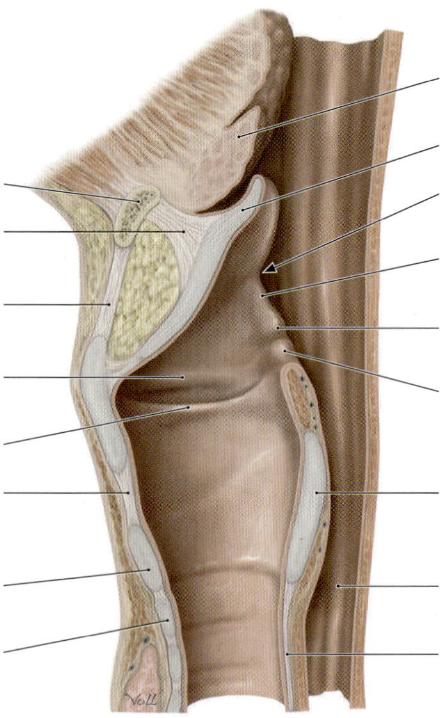

A Esophageal inlet (upper esophageal sphincter)

a Posterior view. The muscular posterior wall of the pharynx has been divided and reflected laterally, and the uppermost esophageal segment has been opened posteriorly. At the posterior junction of the longitudinal esophageal musculature with the pharyngeal musculature, the longitudinal muscles are thin and do not span the full circumference of the esophagus. This area of muscular weakness ("Laimer triangle") is a site of vulnerability for the development of diverticula (see p. 171). This diagram shows the esophagus with an expanded, stellate lumen near the esophageal inlet, as it would appear during swallowing. While in the resting state, the esophageal inlet usually has the form of a transverse slit. The musculature of the upper esophagus is a continuation of the (skeletal) pharyngeal muscles and consists of striated fibers that give way distally to smooth muscle (not shown here).

b Midsagittal section, viewed from the left side. In the lateral view, both the esophageal muscle and mucosa are visible. Additionally, the diagram shows the posterior dilation of the esophagus, and thus the size of the esophagus relative to the larynx. The upper esophageal constriction, located behind the cricoid cartilage, is also clearly visible.

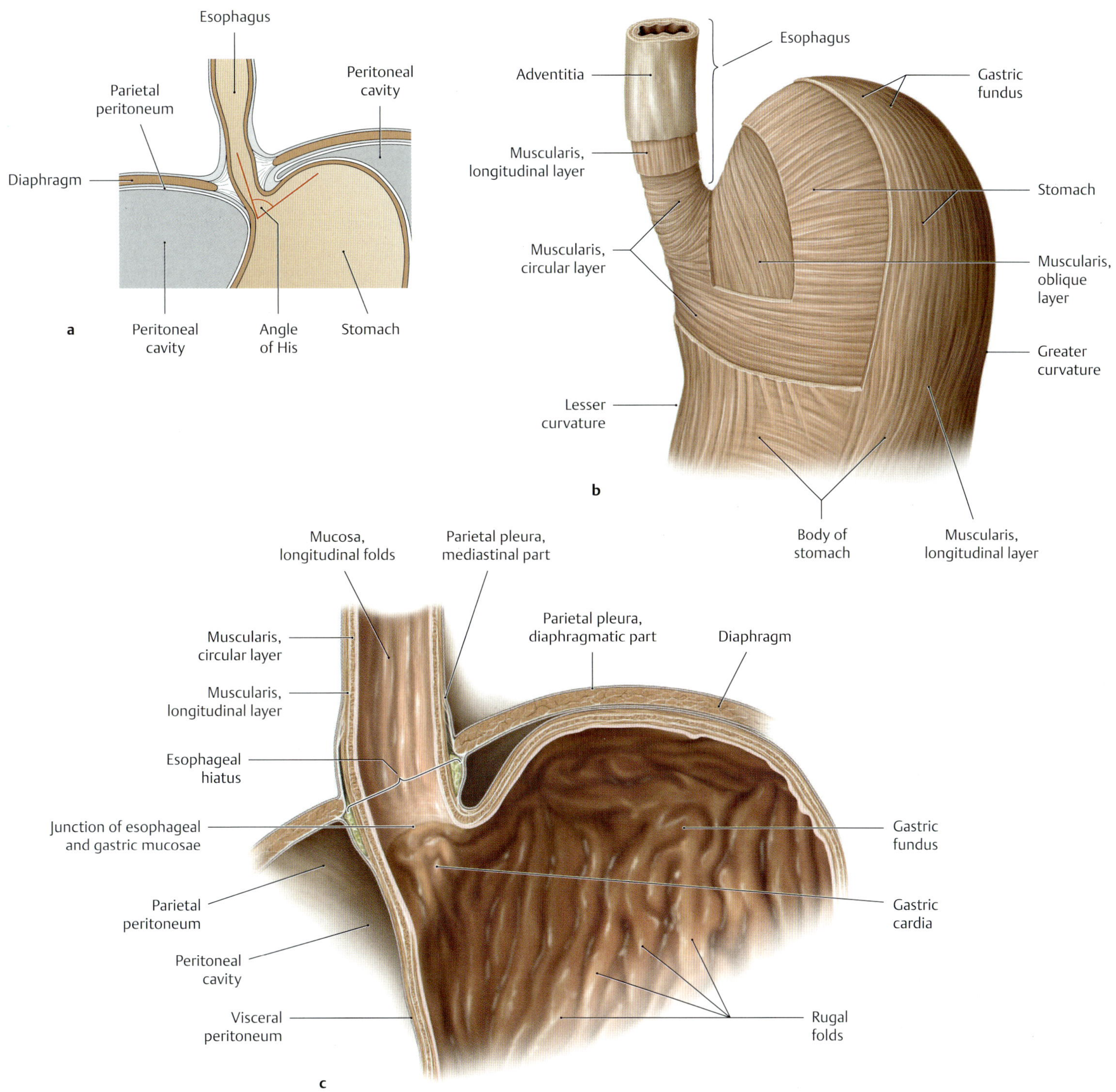

B Esophageal outlet and esophageal closure

Functional closure of the esophageal outlet is an important mechanism for preventing the backflow of gastric contents, especially hydrochloric acid, into the distal esophagus (gastroesophageal reflux). This mechanism is essential because the esophageal mucosa, unlike the gastric mucosa, is vulnerable to corrosive injury by stomach acid. As a result, repeated exposure to hydrochloric acid can cause esophageal inflammation (reflux esophagitis). Early, relatively mild forms of this reflux ("heartburn") are often manifested by a burning retrosternal pain that is most pronounced in the supine position (at night). Effective closure of the esophagus is based on several factors:

- Narrowing of the esophageal outlet by
  - the circular muscles of the esophagus (see **b**) and
  - submucous venous plexuses, which raise longitudinal folds in the esophageal mucosa (see **c**). These prominent veins function as portosystemic collaterals in response to an obstruction of portal venous blood flow (see p. 173). Together, the esophageal circular muscles and venous plexuses provide "angiomuscular closure" at the esophagogastric junction;
- The structurally narrow muscular esophageal hiatus in the diaphragm (see **c**);
- Connective tissue and fat surrounding the esophagogastric junction (**c**);
- Continuity of the esophageal and gastric musculature (**b**), and the oblique angle at which the esophagus joins the stomach just below the diaphragm (the angle of His, see **a**).

5.3 Esophagus: Wall Structure and Weaknesses

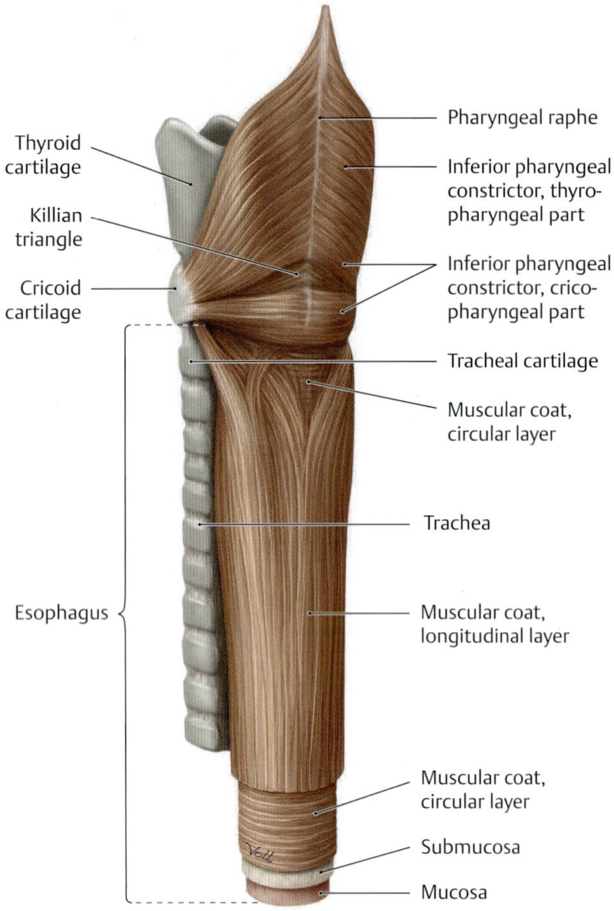

A Structure of the esophageal wall

Posterior view. Portions of the pharynx, larynx, and trachea are also shown; and the outermost layer (adventitia, see **B**) has been removed. The esophageal wall has been telescoped to display both layers of the muscular coat (the circular and longitudinal layers). They are connected to the pharyngeal muscles at the esophageal inlet (hidden here by the pharynx). The muscles of the esophagus can generate powerful peristaltic movements directed toward the stomach (actively propelling a food bolus to the stomach in 5–8 seconds), and they can reverse the direction of these movements during vomiting (antiperistalsis).

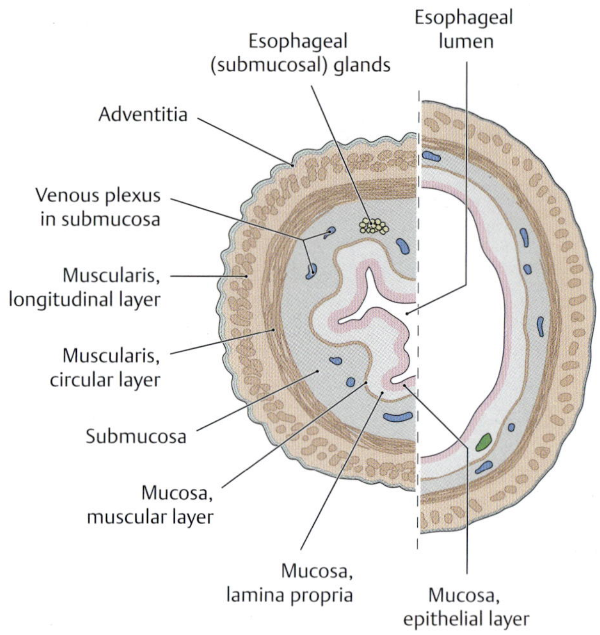

B Microscopic structure of the esophageal wall

Transverse section through an esophagus in the contracted (left) and relaxed state (right). The layers of the esophageal wall are typical of a hollow viscus in the digestive tract:

- The *mucosa*, which consists of an epithelial layer, lamina propria, and muscular layer. The epithelial layer is composed of stratified, nonkeratinized squamous epithelium (for mechanical resistance to food passage).
- The *submucosa*, a loose layer of connective tissue that contains numerous glands (esophageal glands) whose secretions lubricate the mucosa to facilitate food passage. Particularly in the lower esophagus, the submucosa contains numerous veins that participate in the closure of the esophageal outlet (see p. 169).
- The *muscularis*, consisting of an inner layer of circular muscle and an outer layer of longitudinal muscle. Smooth-muscle contractions aid in the peristaltic propulsion of food.
- The *adventitia*, a layer of loose connective tissue that tethers the esophagus to the mediastinal connective tissue and is firmly attached to the connective tissue of the posterior tracheal wall.

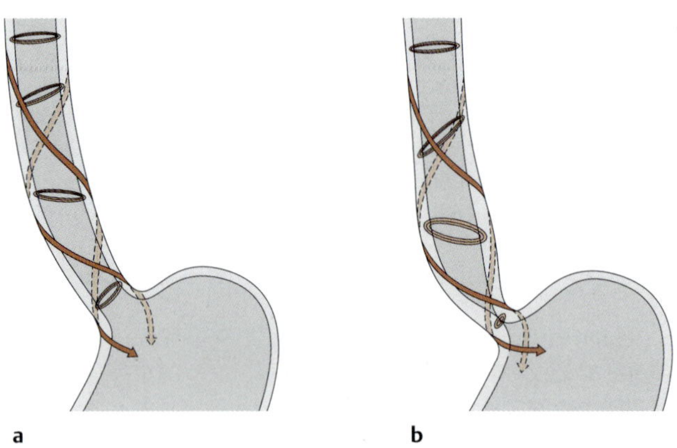

C Functional architecture of the esophageal muscles

During the act of swallowing, the esophageal outlet at the cardiac end of the stomach opens (**a**) and then immediately closes (**b**). The longitudinal and circular layers of the muscular wall of the esophagus (see **A**) contain numerous fibers that wind *obliquely* around the organ (see the circles in the figure). The musculature is additionally "twisted" due to the embryonic rotation of the gut (see p. 43). Owing to the presence of longitudinal, circular, and oblique fibers, the esophagus can be narrowed and closed as needed (by the action of the circular fibers) at its inlet and outlet (see p. 169), but it can also be simultaneously narrowed and shortened by the combined action of the longitudinal, circular and oblique fibers to generate peristaltic motion toward the stomach during swallowing.

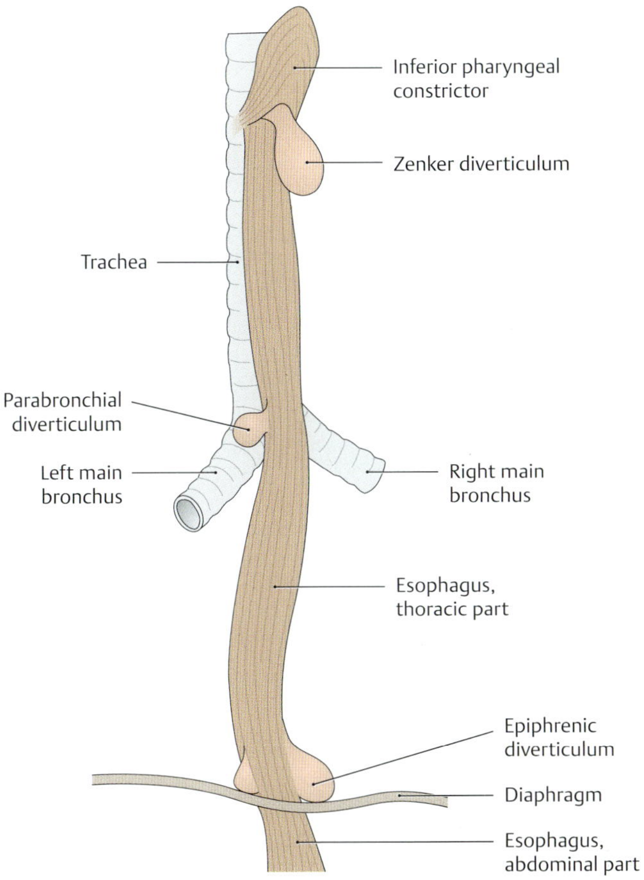

D Development of esophageal diverticula
Esophageal *diverticula* (abnormal outpouchings or sacs) most commonly develop at a weak spot like that located above the esophageal hiatus of the diaphragm (parahiatal or epiphrenic diverticulum, 10% of cases). These are "false" *pulsion diverticula* in which the mucosa and submucosa herniate through weak spots in the muscular coat due to a rise of pressure in the esophagus (e.g., during normal swallowing). A Zenker diverticulum, often described as the most common esophageal diverticulum (70% of cases), is actually a *hypopharyngeal* diverticulum occurring at the junction of the pharynx and esophagus (the "Killian triangle"). This wall protrusion is also called a pharyngoesophageal diverticulum. The remaining 20% of esophageal diverticula do not occur at typical weak spots and are characterized by the protrusion of all wall layers ("true" diverticula, *traction diverticula*). They usually result from an inflammatory process such as lymphangitis, in which case they occur at the site where the esophagus closely approaches the bronchi and bronchial lymph nodes (thoracic or parabronchial diverticulum).

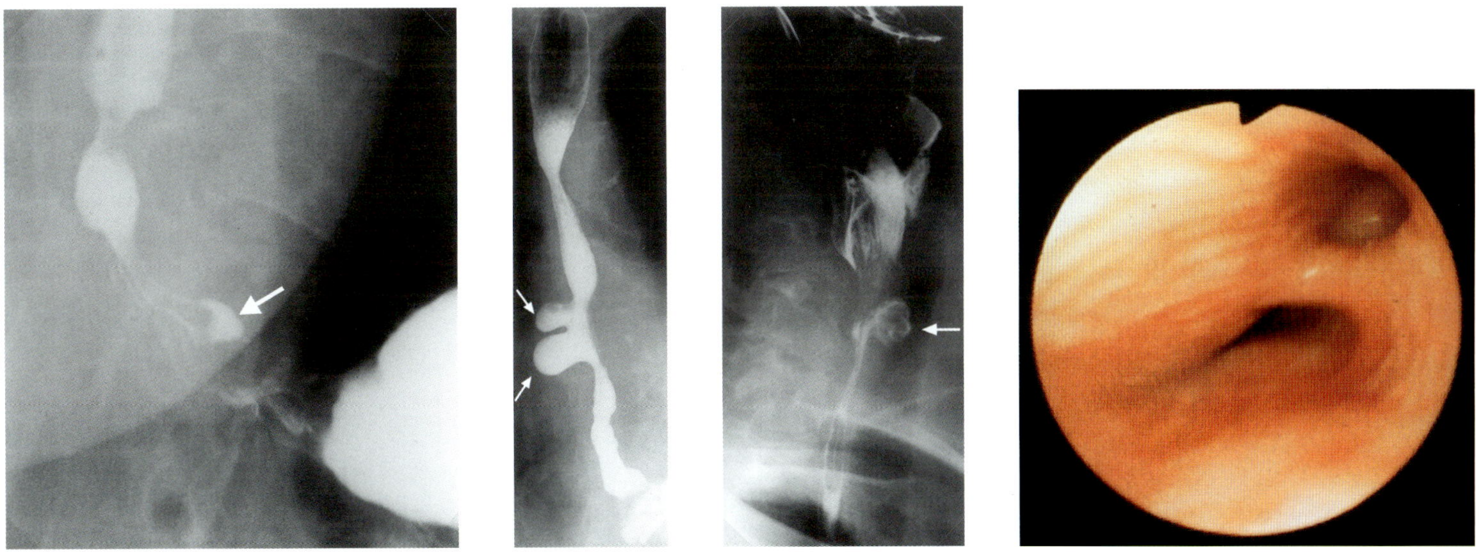

a b c d

E Barium swallow (a–c) and endoscopy (d) used to diagnose diverticula (from: Reiser M, Kuhn F, Debus J, eds. *Duale Reihe Radiologie*. 4th ed. Stuttgart: Thieme; 2017).

a Epiphrenic diverticulum with small pooling of contrast medium (arrow) directly above the diaphragm;

b Traction diverticulum (double-contrast view, arrows) at the level of the tracheal bifurcation;

c Zenker diverticulum directly below the cricoid cartilage, pooling of contrast material detected (arrow);

d Endoscopic view, the esophageal diverticulum is recognizable through an additional orifice in the esophageal wall.

5.4 Arteries and Veins of the Esophagus

A Blood vessels of the esophagus
a Arteries, **b** veins.
Posterior wall of the thorax and upper abdomen, viewed from the anterior aspect. All of the thoracic organs have been removed except for the esophagus and part of the trachea. The proximal portion of the stomach has been left in the abdomen.
Note: The esophagus is supplied by three groups of arteries, consistent with its division into three parts (see p. 166), and it is likewise drained by three venous groups (see **B**).

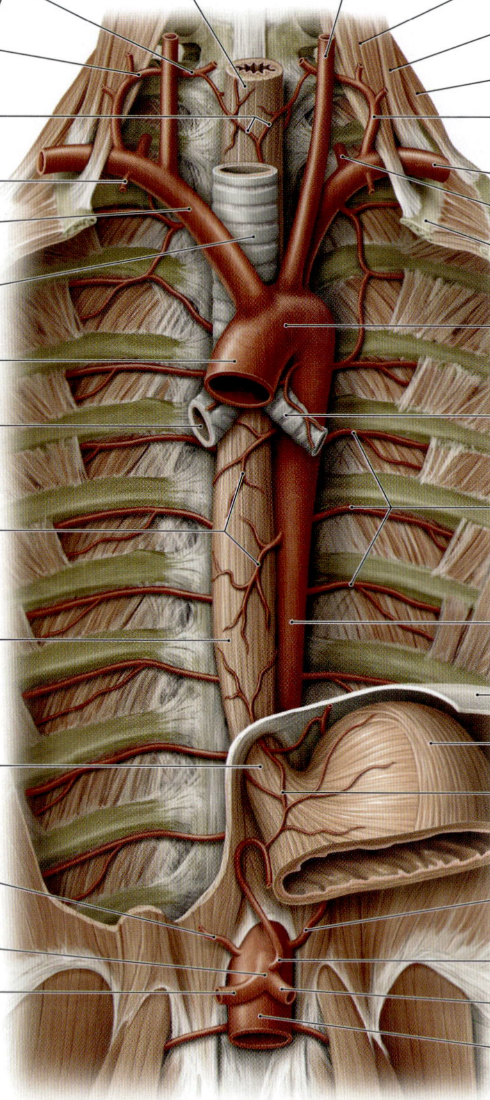

B Arterial supply and venous drainage of the esophagus

Part of esophagus	Arterial supply	Venous drainage (see **Ab**)
• Cervical part	• Esophageal branches – Usually from the inferior thyroid artery or – Direct branches (rare, not shown here) from the thyrocervical trunk or common carotid artery	• Esophageal veins – Drain to inferior thyroid vein or – Left brachiocephalic vein
• Thoracic part (largest arteries and veins serving the esophagus)	• Esophageal branches from the thoracic aorta, distributed to the anterior and posterior sides of the esophagus	• Esophageal veins – Drain at upper left into the accessory hemiazygos vein or left brachiocephalic vein – Drain at lower left into the hemiazygos vein – Drain into the azygos vein on the right side
• Abdominal part (smallest arteries and veins serving the esophagus)	• Esophageal branch of the left gastric artery	• Esophageal veins draining into the left gastric vein

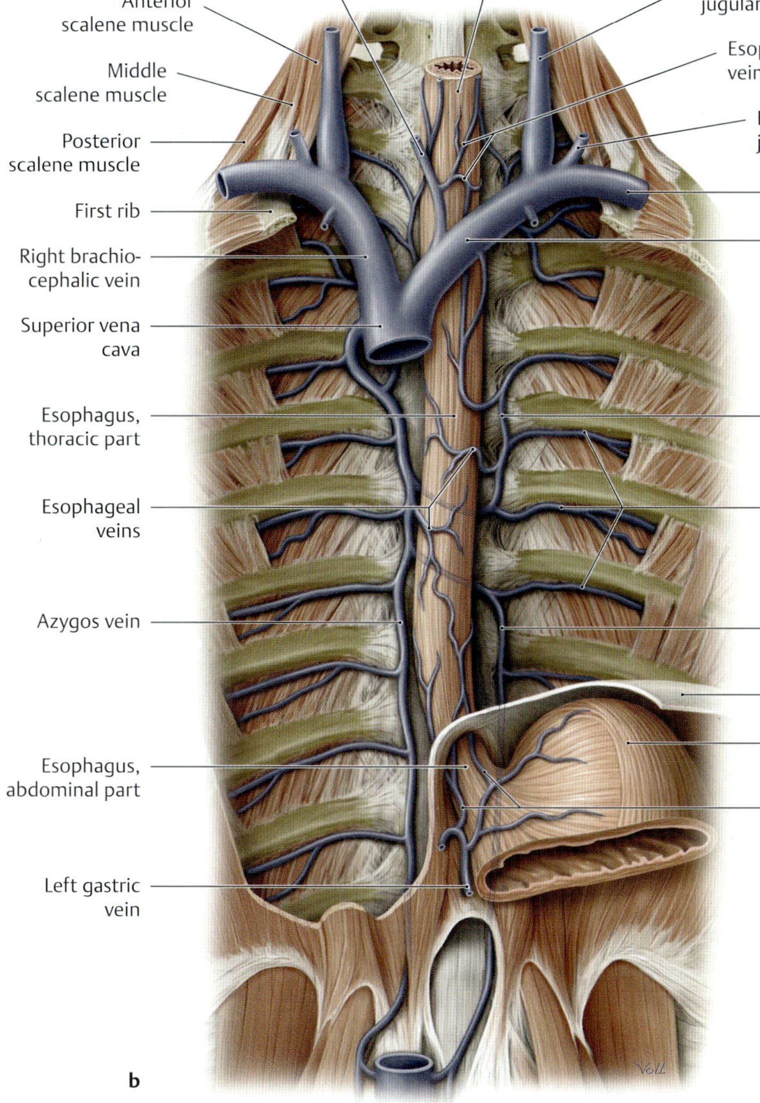

b Veins of the esophagus (legend on previous page).

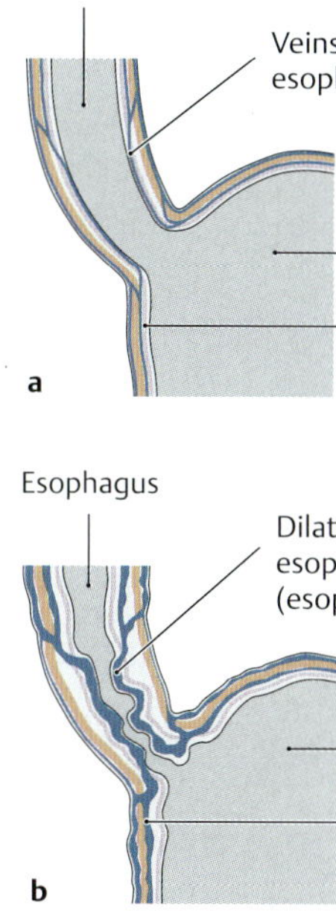

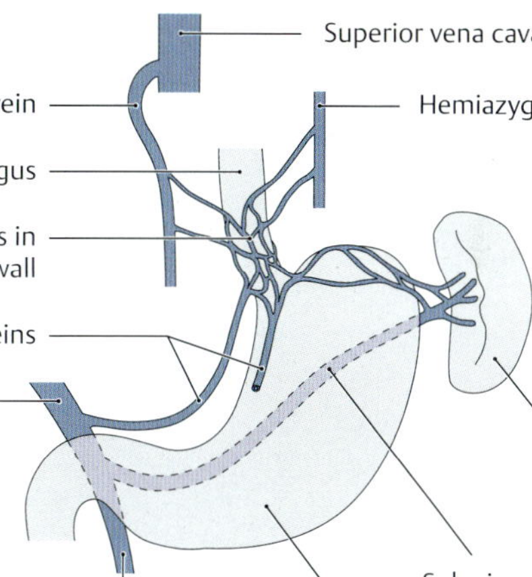

C Submucous venous plexuses and venous collaterals

a, b Submucous venous plexuses and varices in the esophagus: The smallest tributaries of the esophageal veins pass through all layers of the esophageal wall, accompanied by arterial branches, to the lamina propria of the mucosa. In the adjacent, thicker submucosa they form an extensive plexus that contributes to functional closure of the esophagus at the junction of its thoracic and abdominal parts (see p. 169). This venous plexus is continuous with an analogous plexus at the gastric inlet. With any obstruction of portal venous flow to the liver (as in cirrhosis associated with chronic alcoholism), these anastomoses provide a collateral pathway by which the venous blood flow may be diverted into the submucous venous plexuses of the esophagus, causing them to undergo varicose dilation (esophageal varices, see **b**). There may be associated abnormal dilation of the gastric veins.

c Esophageal venous collaterals: Venous anastomoses provide two routes for draining the veins at the junction of the thoracic and abdominal parts of the esophagus:

1. Via the azygos or hemiazygos vein to the superior vena cava (thoracic route)
2. Via the left gastric vein to the portal vein (abdominal route)

Thus, when portal venous flow becomes obstructed in the liver (cirrhosis), blood may be diverted through the esophageal veins to the superior vena cava (portosystemic collaterals, see p. 235). The esophageal veins are fed through the venous plexus of the esophageal wall.

5.5 Lymphatic Drainage of the Esophagus

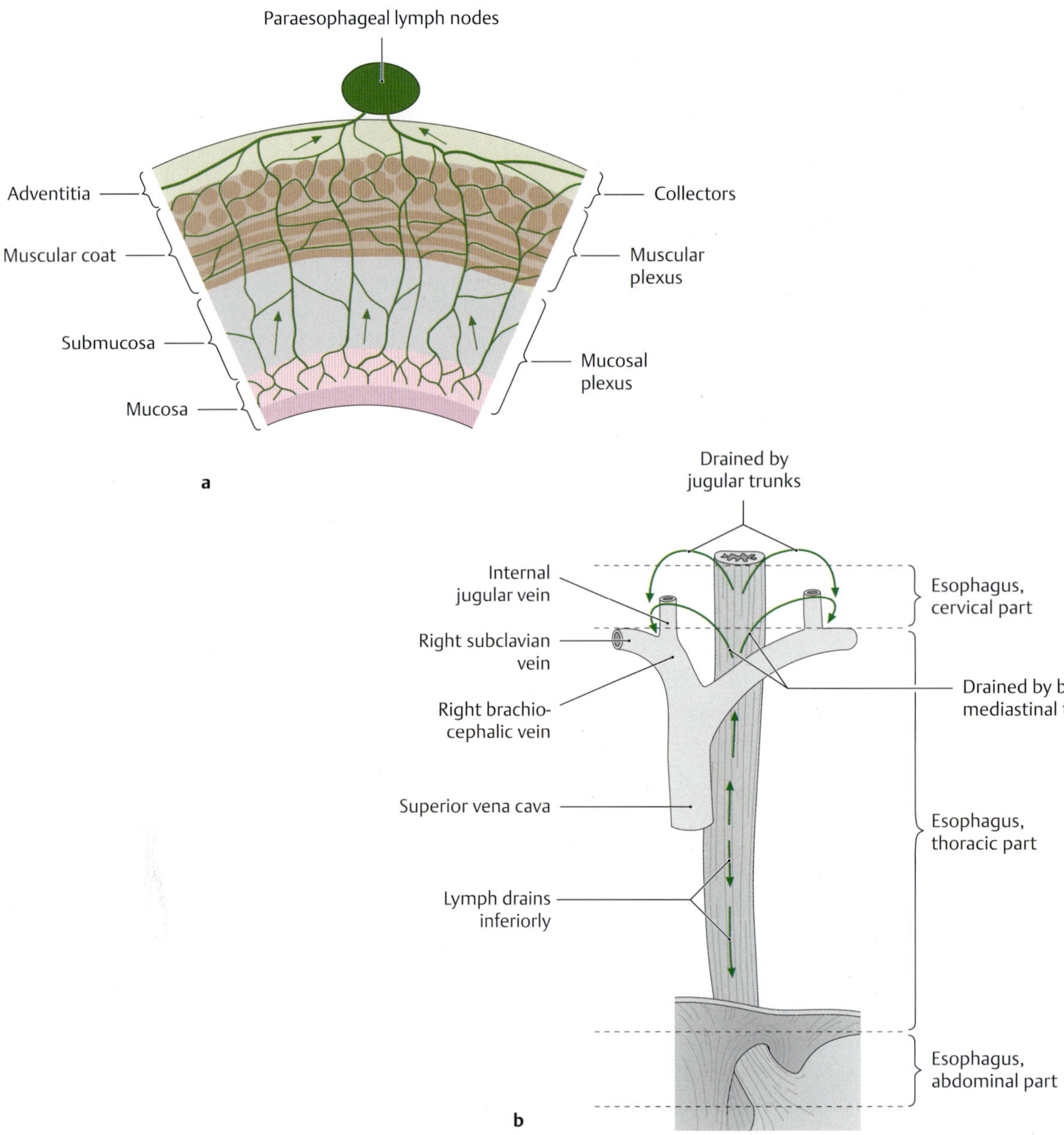

A Lymphatic drainage of the esophagus

a Lymphatic drainage of the esophageal wall, **b** lymphatic drainage at different levels of the esophagus.

Lymph from the esophagus flows from inside to outside through the various wall layers (**a**), draining initially to the lymph nodes that are distributed along the esophageal wall (paraesophageal lymph nodes, see **B**). There are three principal directions of lymphatic drainage, which correspond roughly to the three divisions of the esophagus (**b**):

- The *cervical part* of the esophagus drains cranially, mainly to the deep cervical lymph nodes and then to the jugular trunk.
- The *thoracic part* of the esophagus drains in two principal directions:
  - Cranially to the bronchomediastinal trunks (upper half).
  - Inferiorly (partly via the superior phrenic lymph nodes) to the bronchomediastinal trunks (lower half). Fine lymphatic vessels may convey a small amount of lymph through the esophageal hiatus into the upper abdomen to the abdominal part of the esophagus (lymph may drain to the *inferior* phrenic lymph nodes as well as the celiac nodes). The "watershed" area for these two flow directions lies at the approximate midpoint of the thoracic esophagus, whose upper part may also drain to tracheal lymph nodes.
- The *abdominal part* of the esophaqus, like the stomach, drains to the celiac lymph nodes (not shown here). Thus, when the flow direction in these lowest esophageal lymph nodes is reversed (a simple change of body posture or intracavitary pressure change due to breathing or bearing down can alter the direction of lymph flow), lymph from the stomach (which may bear malignant cells from gastric carcinoma) can reflux across the diaphragm and enter the thoracic nodes.

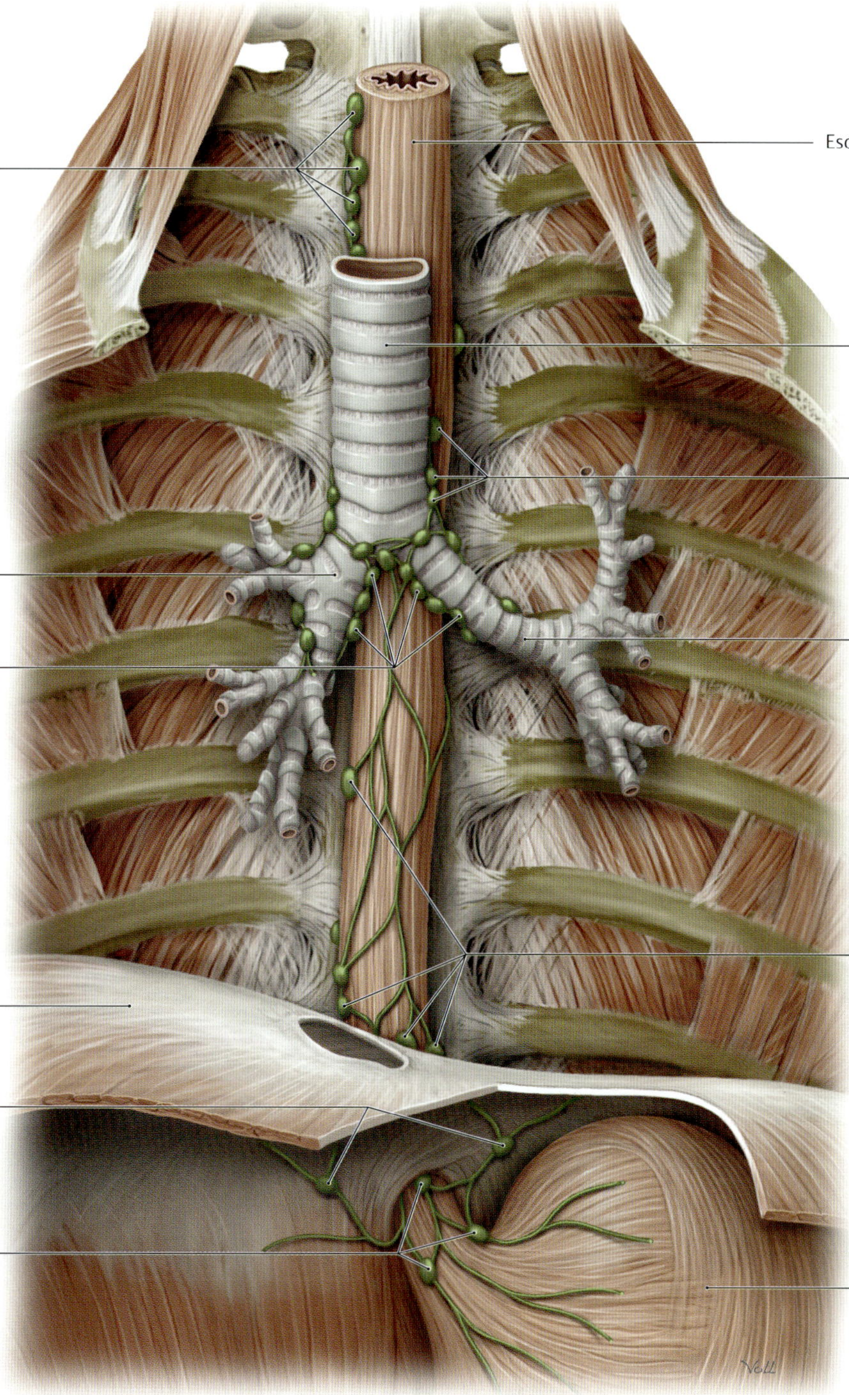

B Lymph nodes of the esophagus

Anterior view of the opened thorax. All thoracic organs, with the exception of a portion of the trachea, the main bronchi, and the esophagus have been removed. Part of the abdomen is shown, and the stomach has been retracted slightly downward. A portion of the diaphragm has been excised to display the esophageal hiatus. The esophagus is covered by a network of fine lymphatic vessels that carry lymph to the paraesophageal lymph nodes. Lymph from the paraesophageal nodes drains to collecting nodes or directly into the jugular trunk or the right and left bronchomediastinal trunks (see **A**). Esophageal lymphatics near the tracheal bifurcation also communicate with the (inferior) tracheobronchial lymph nodes. Lymphatic vessels descend with the esophagus through the esophageal hiatus, and they may connect at the abdominal level with the inconstant cardiac lymphatic ring that surrounds the cardiac orifice of the stomach (drains to the celiac lymph nodes). The esophageal lymph nodes at this level may also connect with the lymph nodes on the inferior surface of the diaphragm (inferior *phrenic* lymph nodes).

Note: The paraesophageal lymph nodes are classified as a subgroup of the mediastinal lymph nodes (see also p. 91).

5.6 Innervation of the Esophagus

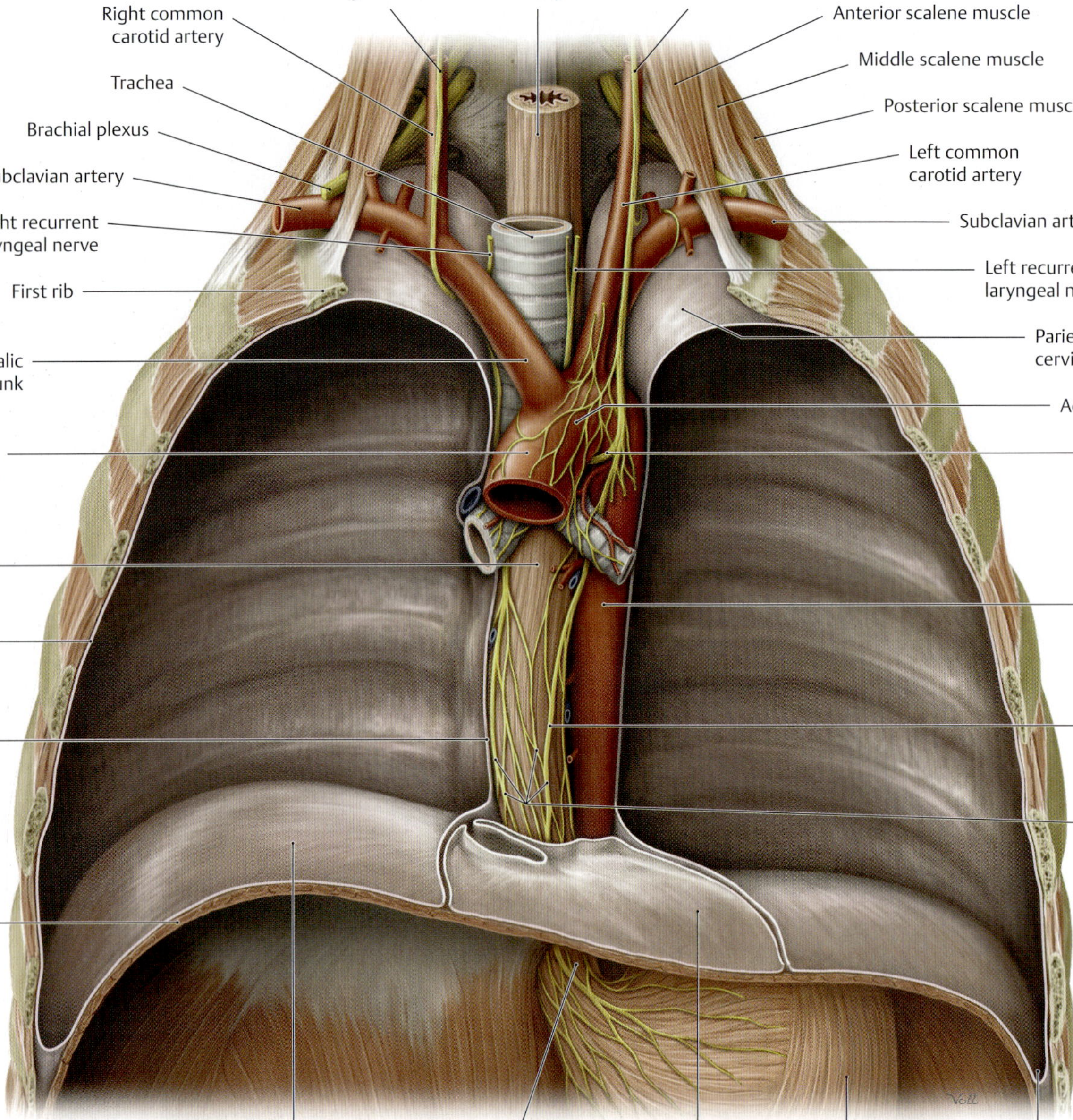

A Innervation of the esophagus: Overview
Anterior view with the thorax opened. All organs except for the trachea and esophagus have been removed. The left and right vagus nerves give off branches to the esophagus. These branches form the esophageal plexus. The plexus, located on the anterior and posterior esophageal walls, further descends and enters the abdomen as the anterior and posterior vagal trunks. The esophageal plexus also receives fibers from the sympathetic chain.

B Effects of the sympathetic and parasympathetic nervous systems on the esophagus

Sympathetic nervous system	Parasympathetic nervous system
• Decreases peristalsis	• Increases peristalsis
• Decreases esophageal gland secretions	• Increases esophageal gland secretions

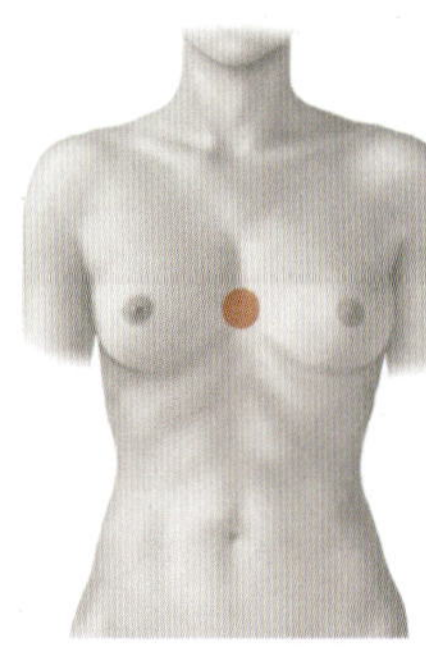

C Referred pain from the esophagus
Anterior view. As with other visceral structures, pain in the esophagus may not be localized to the organ itself, but may instead seem to originate elsewhere. Esophageal pain may be referred to cutaneous areas over the sternum. The phenomenon is called "referred pain."

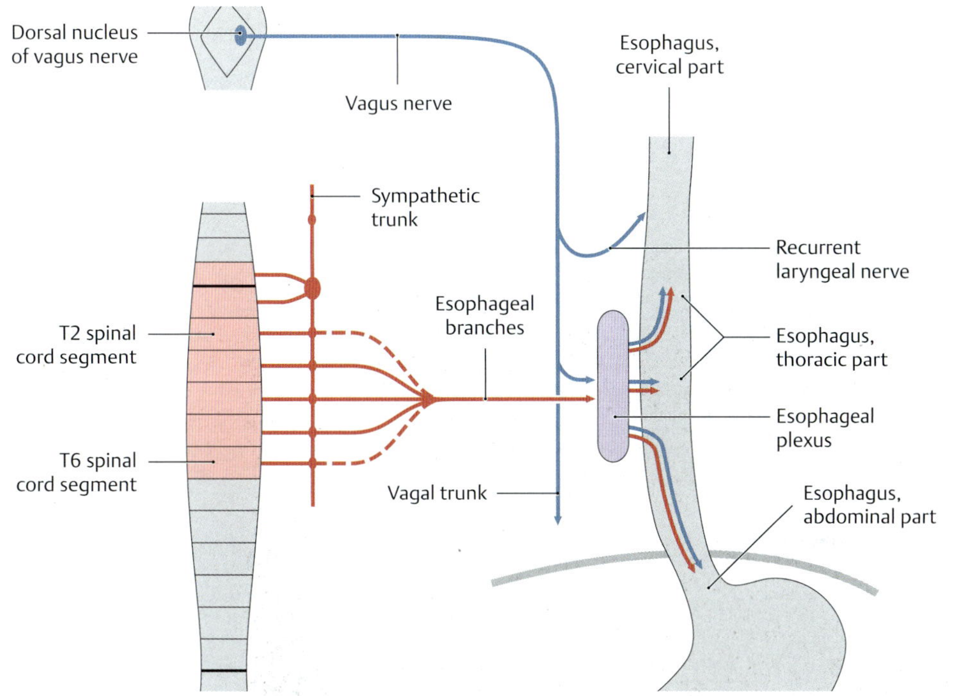

D Autonomic innervation of the esophagus

Parasympathetic fibers arise from the dorsal vagal nuclei and enter the vagus nerves. The vagus gives off parasympathetic motor fibers to the cervical part of the esophagus via the recurrent laryngeal nerve. Other vagal axons form an extensive esophageal plexus, which extends to abdominal levels of the esophagus. These presynaptic fibers synapse on scattered parasympathetic ganglion cells (not depicted here) in the esophageal wall. The embedded ganglion cells in turn innervate esophageal smooth muscle and glands.

Note: The vagus nerve also conveys direct motor innervation, without an intervening local synapse, from the nucleus ambiguus in the brainstem (not shown here) to striated muscle in the cervical esophagus via the recurrent laryngeal nerve.

Sympathetic fibers are contributed mostly by the second through sixth thoracic paravertebral ganglia. These postsynaptic axons enter the esophageal plexus but directly innervate the esophagus. The middle cervical sympathetic ganglion contributes innervation to the cervical part of the esophagus. On the whole, sympathetic innervation is much less extensive than the parasympathetic supply to the esophagus.

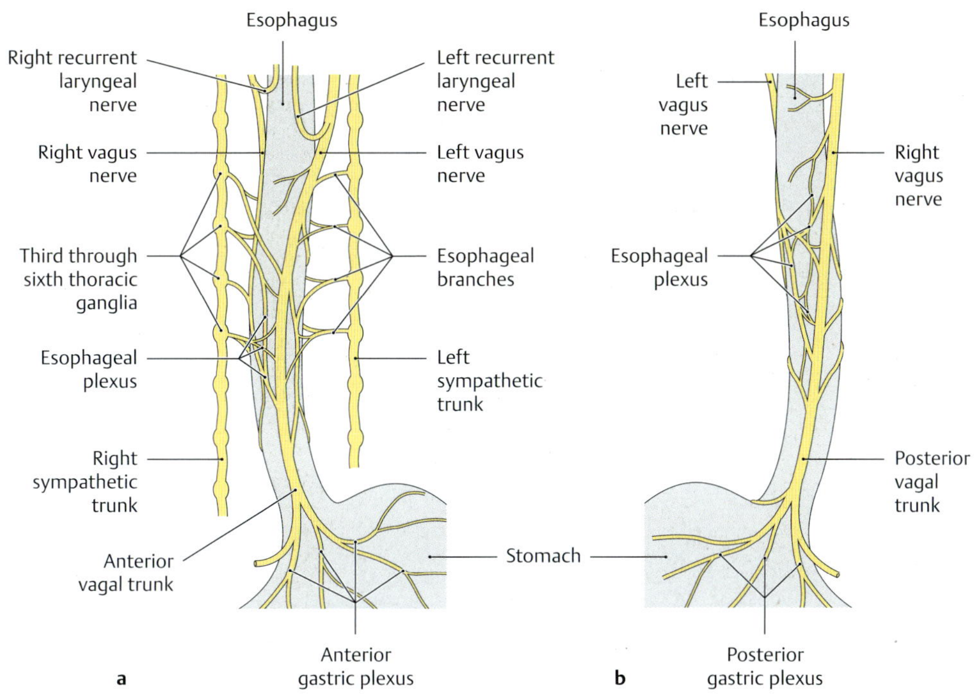

E Formation of the esophageal plexus

The esophagus and part of the stomach, viewed from the anterior side (**a**) and posterior side (**b**).

Initially the vagus nerves descend a short distance on the left and right sides of the esophagus as the left and right vagus nerves, but then they turn anteriorly and posteriorly owing to the 90° clockwise rotation of the esophagus (viewed from above) that occurs during embryonic development. The left vagus nerve now becomes the anterior vagal trunk, and the right vagus nerve becomes the posterior vagal trunk. Both trunks exchange a considerable number of fibers, however, so that the anterior vagal trunk (actually a derivative of the left vagus nerve) also contains fibers from the right vagus nerve, and vice versa. Both vagus nerves and both vagal trunks distribute numerous fibers to the esophagus, which form the anterior and posterior esophageal plexuses. The esophageal plexus is continuous inferiorly with the gastric plexus. The cervical part of the esophagus is supplied by the recurrent laryngeal nerves, which arise from the vagus nerves. The postganglionic sympathetic fibers enter the esophageal plexus, which thus contains both parasympathetic and sympathetic fibers. On the whole, however, the parasympathetic innervation of the esophagus is greater than its sympathetic innervation.

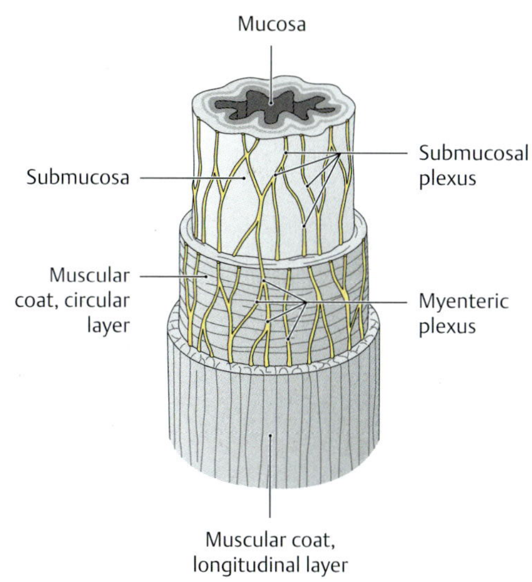

F Autonomic nerve plexuses in the esophageal wall

Oblique view of the esophagus, dissected to show the different wall layers. Like all hollow organs in the gastrointestinal tract, the esophagus has its own autonomous intramural nervous system. This system consists mainly of two plexuses, which are located in the submucosa (submucosal plexus) and in the muscular coat (myenteric plexus). These plexuses are composed of intramural ganglion cells that are interconnected by an extensive network and control the muscular functions of the esophagus (e.g., peristalsis). The activity of this autonomous network is modulated by the sympathetic and parasympathetic nervous systems (see **B**).

5.7 Thymus

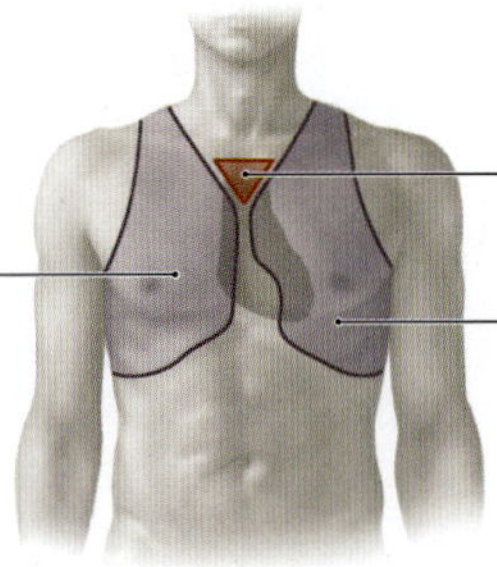

A Projection of the thymus onto the chest wall
For clarity, the pleural cavities have also been projected onto the chest wall. The thymus lies in the superior mediastinum and extends down into the anterior mediastinum, where it is anterior to the heart and great vessels and posterior to the sternum. The area in which the thymus projects onto the chest wall is sometimes called the "thymic triangle." On the chest radiograph of a very small child, the large thymus may appear to broaden the silhouette of the cardiac base.

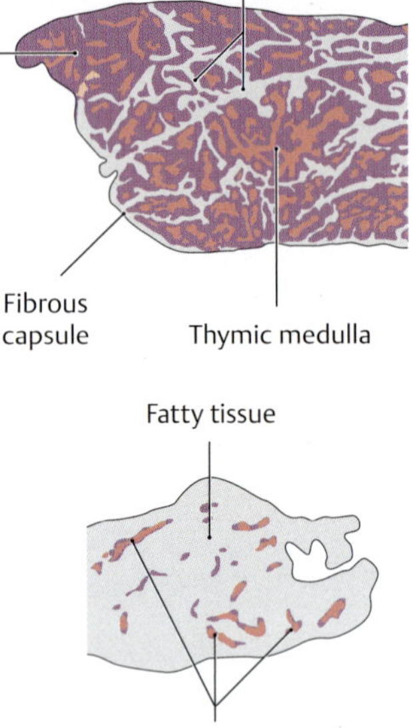

a

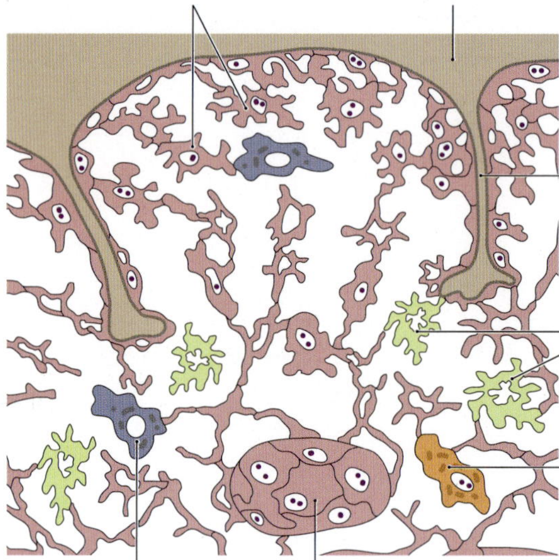

b

B Histological structure of the thymus

a Structure of the thymus in adolescence (above) and old age (below). The thymus is a primary lymphatic (lymphoepithelial) organ that has a predominantly endodermal origin (third pharyngeal pouch) but also contains ectodermal elements. It plays a central role in the maturation of T (*thymus*) lymphocytes and their differentiation into immunologically competent cells. Additionally, immunemodulating hormones (thymosin, thymopoietin, thymulin) are produced in the thymus. Congenital absence of the thymus results in severe immunodeficiency. The thymus consists of a cortex and medulla. The cortex appears much darker-staining due to the predominance of thymocytes (precursors to T-lymphocytes). The inner medullary region appears lighter-staining as a result of fewer thymocytes and an increase in the number of epithelial cells. Fine, vascularized trabeculae extend from the delicate fibrous capsule of the thymus into the parenchyma, subdividing the organ into numerous lobules.

b Functional architecture (as described by Lüllmann-Rauch). The thymus consists of a basic epithelial framework (lymphoepithelial organ). During embryonic development, the precursors of T-lymphocytes migrate into the thymus and mature (under the control of the epithelial cells) into immunocompetent T-lymphocytes. The epithelial cells form a densely packed, subcapsular layer that creates a boundary between the interior of the thymus and the cortical capillaries in the fibrous trabeculae (the "blood–thymus barrier," not shown here). Epithelial (epithelial reticular) cells with long processes join together in the cortex and medulla to form a three-dimensional network that encloses the thymocytes. (Thymocytes are not shown here in order to display other cell types clearly.) Epithelial cells in the medulla aggregate to form the thymic (Hassall's) corpuscles. The innermost cells in large thymic corpuscles often degenerate into a homogeneous mass. The function of the thymic corpuscles is not yet fully understood. The thymus contains several other cell types as well:

- Macrophages (phagocytosis of thymocytes)
- Dendritic cells (antigen presentation)
- Myoid cells (function unclear)

Maturation of the thymocytes occurs during their migration from the cortex to the medulla. A mature T-lymphocyte can recognize foreign antigens and differentiate them from endogenous cells ("autotolerance").

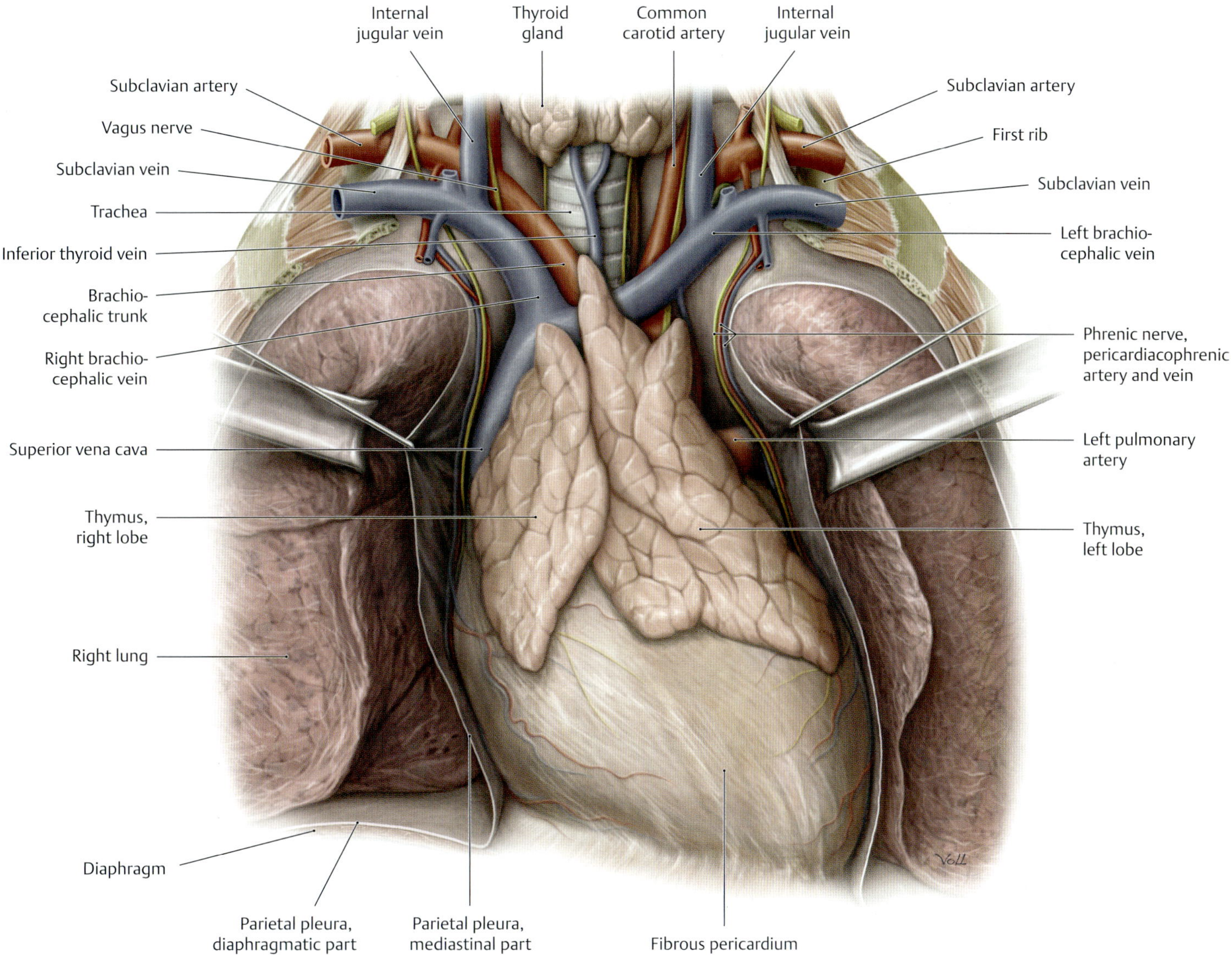

C Size and shape of the thymus
Anterior view into the superior mediastinum of a 2-year-old child. The thymus is still well developed at this age, consisting of two prominent lobes (right and left) that are subdivided by fibrous septa into numerous lobules. Usually the thymus is apposed to the anterior surface of the pericardium and lies anterior to the superior vena cava, brachiocephalic veins, and aorta. In a small child, the thymus may extend up into the neck almost to the level of the thyroid gland, lying posterior to the pretracheal lamina of the cervical fascia. When the thymus reaches its greatest size during puberty, it has a maximum weight of 20–50 g.

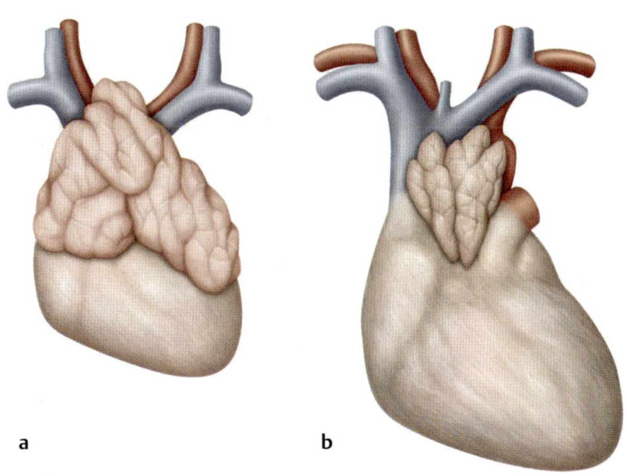

D Size of the thymus in newborns (a) and in adults (b)
In adults, the thymus is smaller than in newborns and lies in the superior mediastinum. In newborns, the thymus extends down into the inferior mediastinum.

6.1 Surface Anatomy, Topographical Regions, and Palpable Bony Landmarks

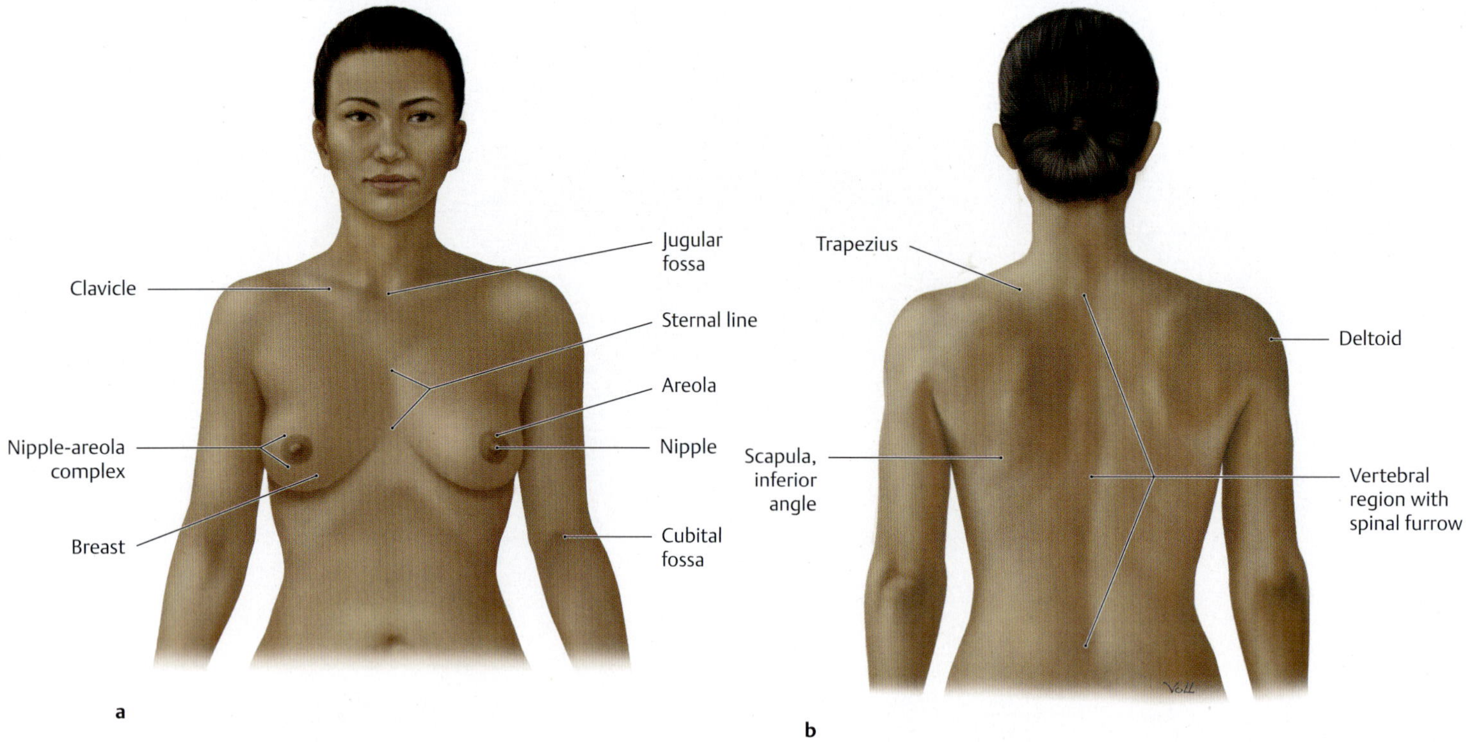

A Surface of the female thorax
a Anterior view; **b** Posterior view.

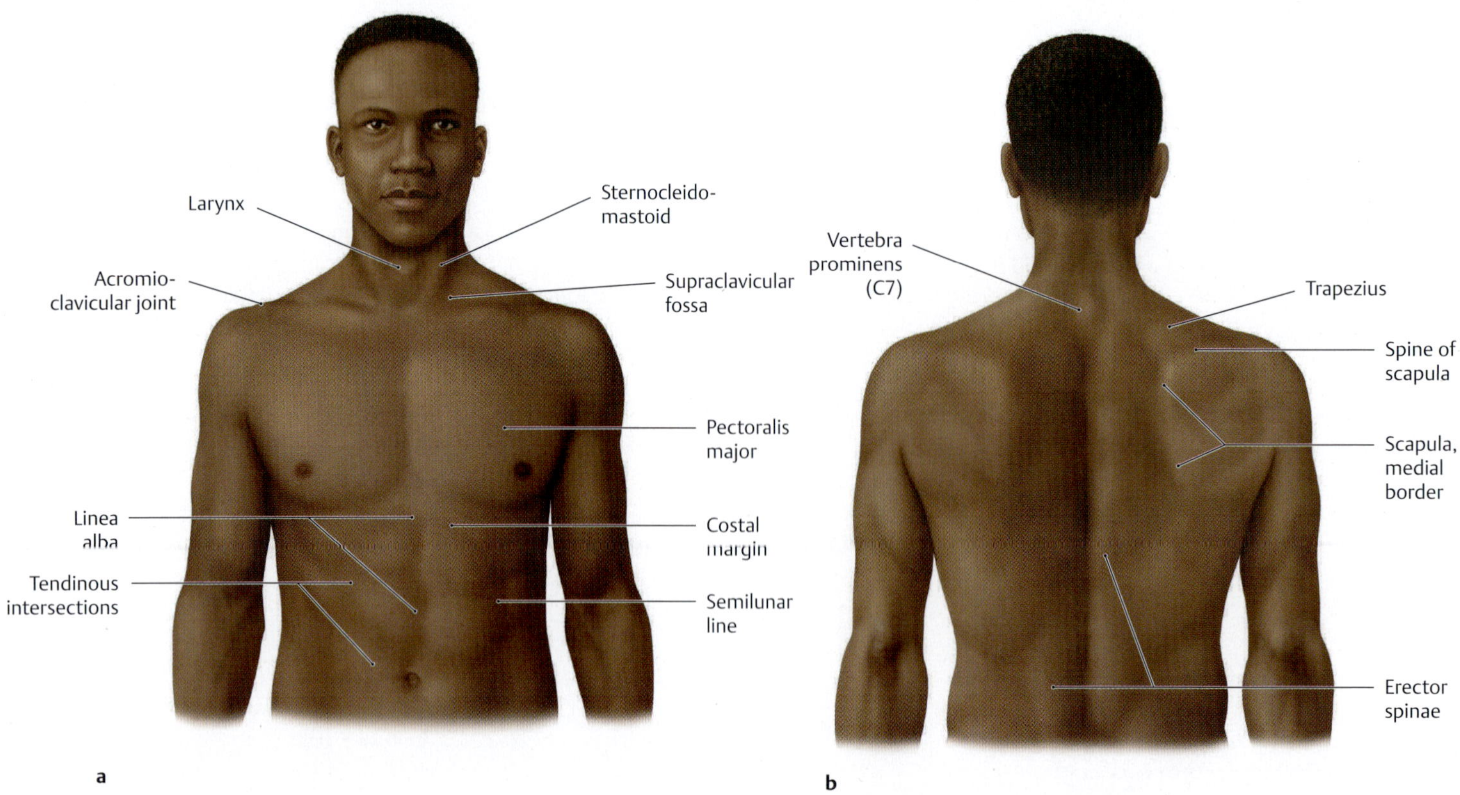

B Surface of the male thorax
a Anterior view; **b** Posterior view.

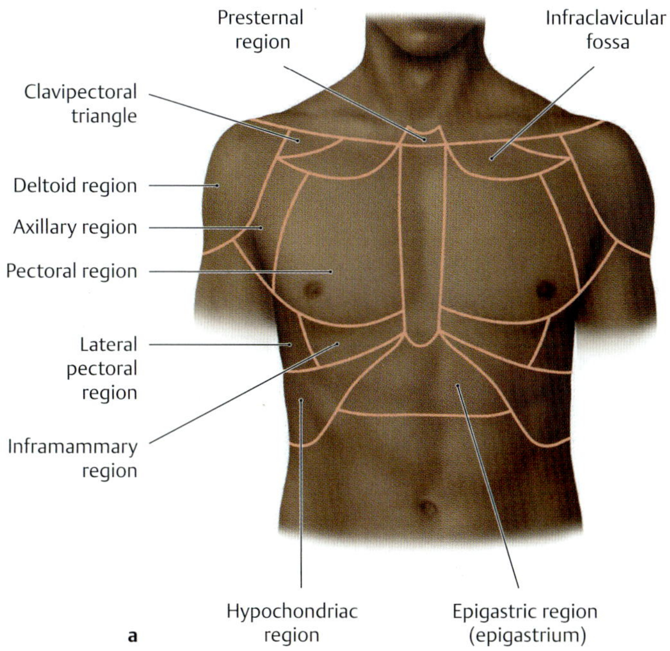

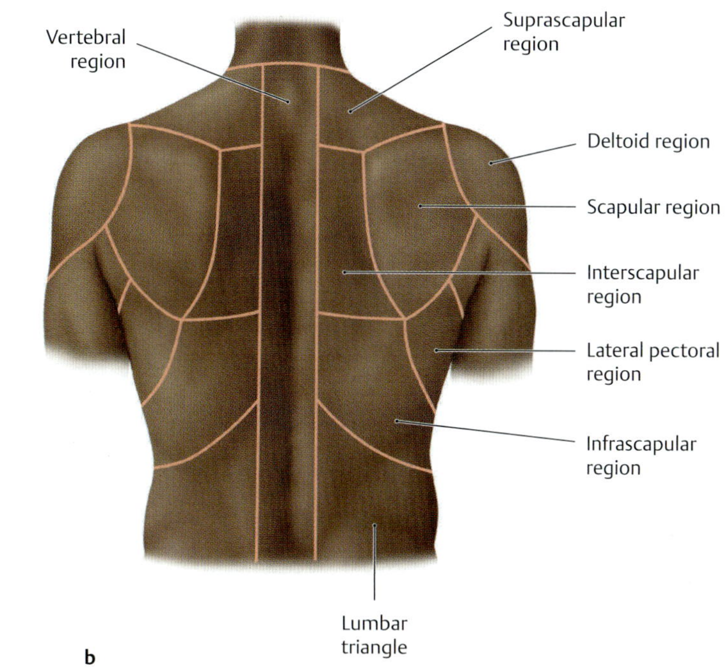

C Topographical anatomy of the male thorax
a Anterior view; **b** Posterior view.

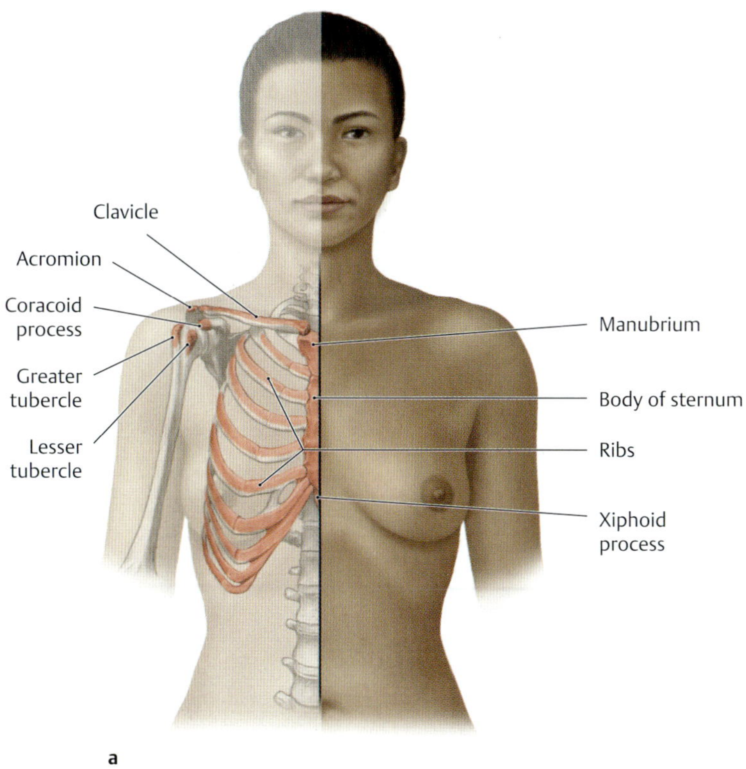

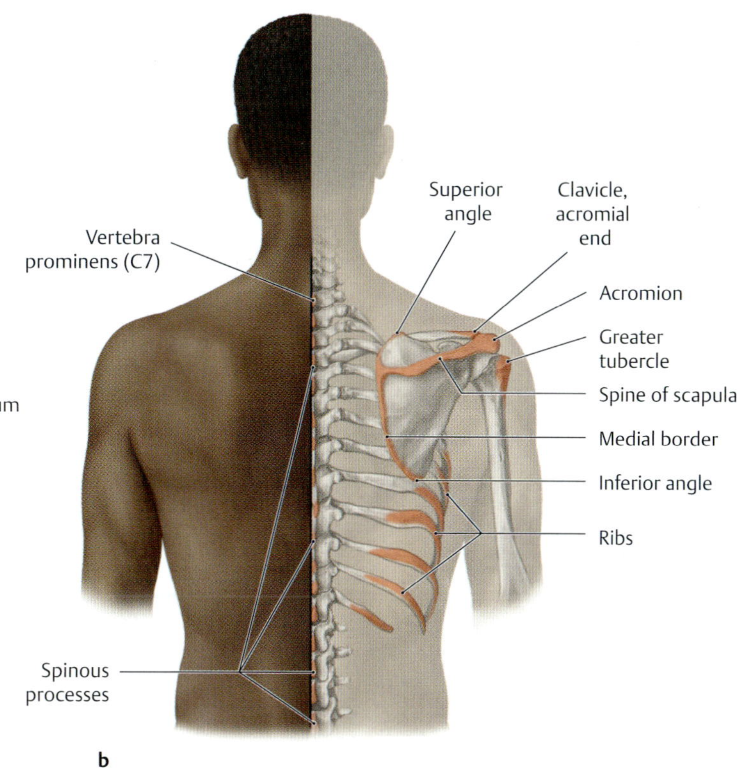

D Surface anatomy and palpable bony landmarks in the thoracic region
a Anterior view; **b** Posterior view.

6.2 Anatomical Landmarks of the Thoracic Skeleton (Projection of Organs)

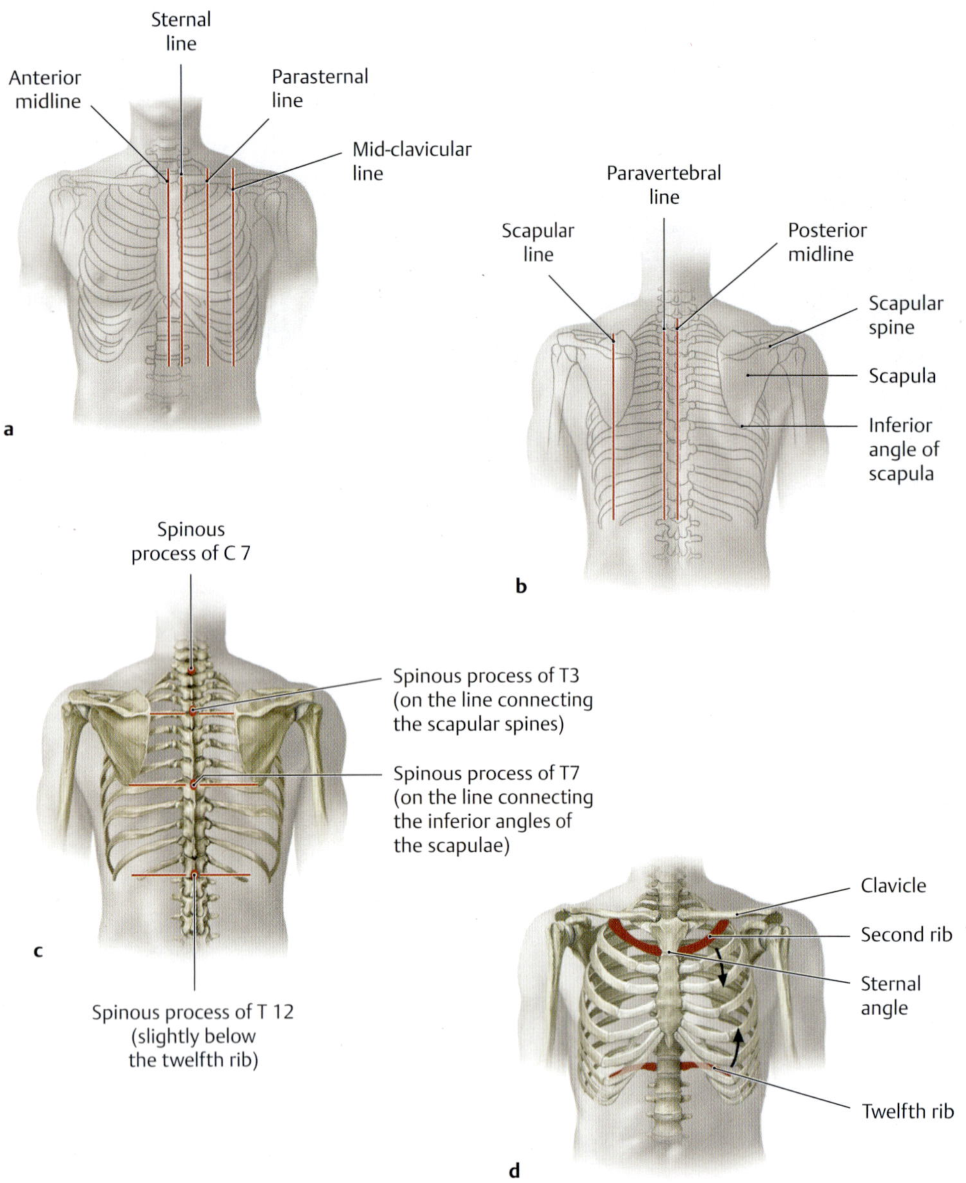

A Anatomical landmarks of the thoracic skeleton

The thoracic skeleton presents a number of visible and palpable landmarks that are accessible to physical and radiographic examination (see **B**). These landmarks can be used to define reference lines for describing and evaluating the location and extent of organs based on their relationship to the lines:

- Longitudinal reference lines (**a**, **b**) are defined by visible or palpable anterior (**a**) and posterior (**b**) bony structures and provide information on the location and extent of specific thoracic organs (e.g., the apical heartbeat is palpable in the left mid-clavicular line).
- Most horizontal reference lines (**c**) are defined by the position of specific thoracic vertebrae. The seventh cervical vertebra (C 7) is easily identified by palpating its very prominent spinous process. It provides a starting point from which the examiner can locate all 12 thoracic vertebrae (T 1–T 12). The levels of the T 3 and T 7 vertebrae correspond respectively to the medial end of the scapular spine and the inferior angle of the scapula.
- The ribs as anatomical landmarks (**d**). The levels of intrathoracic organs also correlate with specific ribs and intercostal spaces, particularly on the anterior side. The first rib is usually difficult to palpate because it is behind the clavicle. The second, however, is attached to the palpable sternal angle (where the body and manubrium of the sternum join). Past the second rib, the examiner should have no difficulty counting down the remaining ribs.

B Projection of anatomical structures onto the thoracic vertebrae

Level	Structure
T 1	Superior border of the scapula
T 2/3	Jugular notch of the sternum
T 3	• Medial border of the scapular spine • Posterior end of the pulmonary oblique fissure
T 3/4	• Tracheal bifurcation • Root of the aortic arch
T 3–4	Manubrium of sternum
T 4	End of the aortic arch
T 4/5	Sternal angle
T 5	Thoracic duct crosses the midline
T 5–8	Sternum
T 7	• Inferior scapular angle • Accessory hemiazygos vein crosses the midline to the right and opens into the azygos vein
T 8	• Caval opening of the diaphragm – Inferior vena cava – Right phrenic nerve • Left phrenic nerve pierces the diaphragm to the left of the central tendon • Hemiazygos vein crosses the midline to the right and opens into the azygos vein
T 8/9	• Xiphisternal synchondrosis • Superior epigastric vessels pass through the diaphragm • Xiphoid process
T 8–10	Superior border of the liver (moves with respiration)
T 10	• Esophageal hiatus of the diaphragm: – Esophagus – Anterior vagal trunk – Posterior vagal trunk
T 12	• Aortic hiatus of the diaphragm: – Aorta – Azygos and hemiazygos veins – Thoracic duct • Origin of the celiac trunk (inferior border of T 12) • Splanchnic nerves pass through the crura of the diaphragm • Sympathetic trunk passes below the medial arcuate ligament: transpyloric plane (line in abdomen, see p. 160)

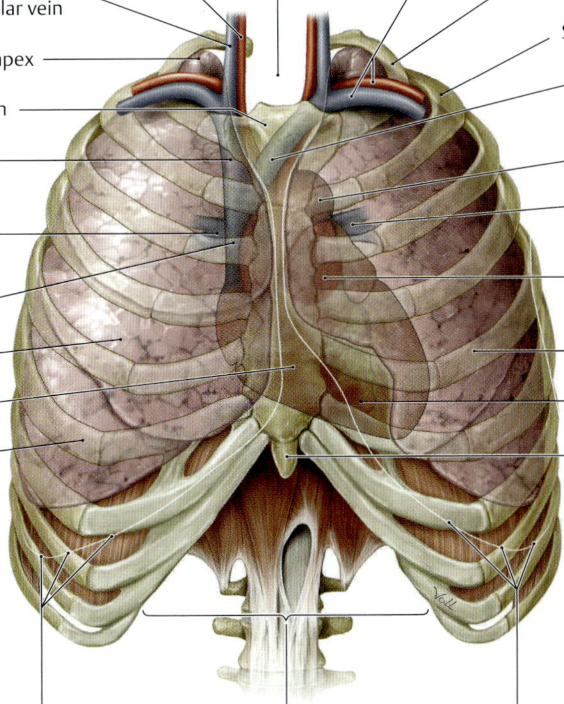

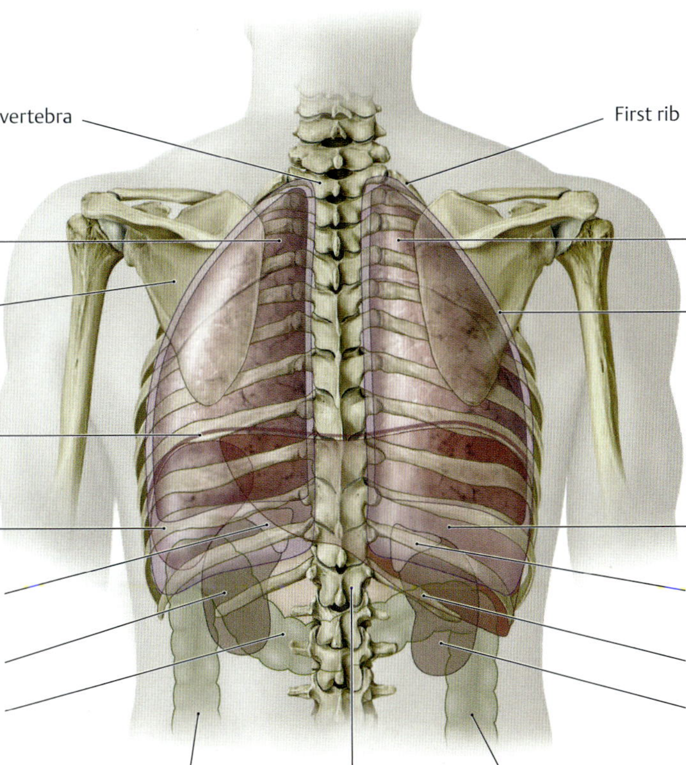

C Overview of the thorax

a Anterior view. The intercostal muscles, fasciae, and abdominal organs have been removed. **b** Simplified schematic view from the posterior side. The scapulae and several abdominal organs have been outlined for clarity.

The thoracic cavity is one of the three main body cavities, along with the abdominal and pelvic cavities. The wall surrounding the thoracic cavity consists of

- bones: 12 thoracic vertebrae, 12 pairs of ribs, and the sternum
- connective tissue: internal fasciae of the thorax, muscle fasciae
- muscles: chiefly the intercostal muscles, internal muscles, and diaphragm

The thoracic cavity is divided into the centrally located unpaired mediastinum, which contains the mediastinal organs, and the paired pleural cavities. The *mediastinum* contains the central motor of the circulatory system, the heart, and the thoracic part of the digestive system, the esophagus. The *pleural cavities* enclose the major organs of respiration, the lungs. Also, a number of neurovascular structures pass through or terminate within the thorax.

The bony thoracic cage is open at its apex at the superior thoracic aperture (thoracic inlet), which is closely bounded and protected by muscles and connective tissue but communicates structures from the neck. The inferior aperture of the thoracic cage (thoracic outlet) is almost completely sealed from the abdominal cavity by the diaphragm and its fasciae (shown most clearly in **a**).

Note: The diaphragm is normally in the shape of a high dome, with a substantial superior convexity that places part of the abdominal cavity above the thoracic outlet (see the abdominal organs shadowed in **b**). A perforating injury perpendicular to the trunk wall, as from a gunshot or stab wound, may thus simultaneously breach both the abdominal and thoracic cavities ("multicavity injury").

6.3 Structure of the Anterior Thoracic Wall and its Neurovascular Structures

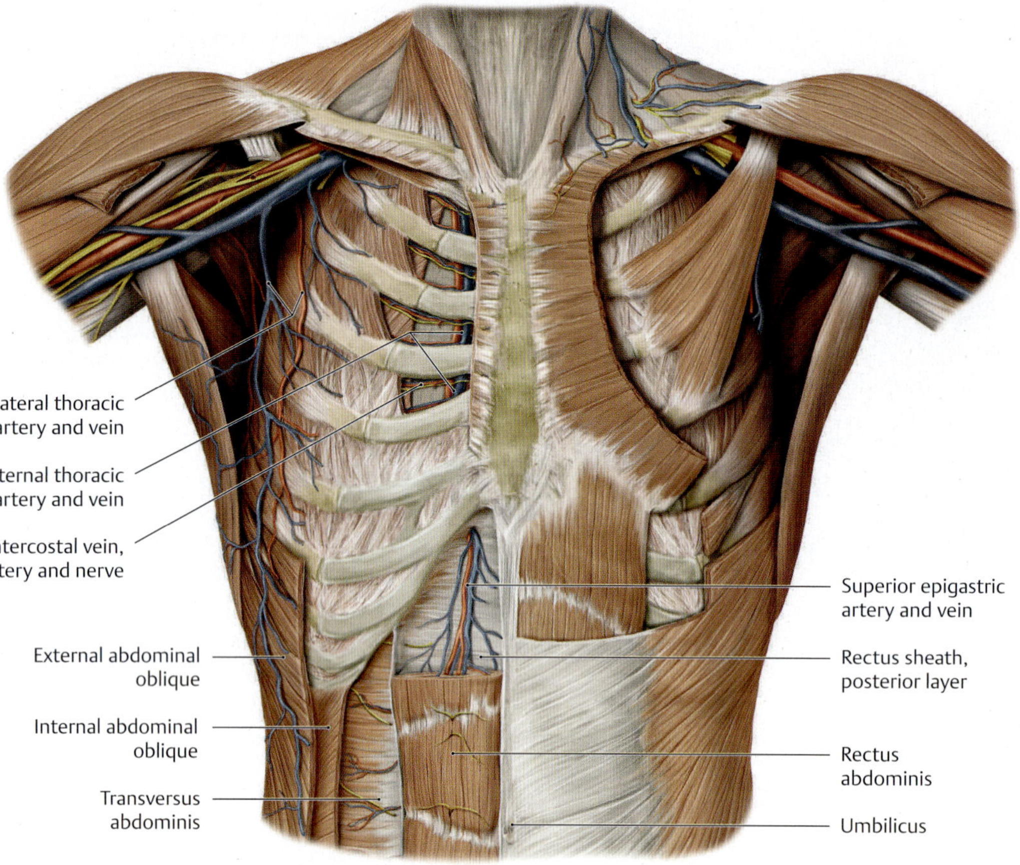

A Neurovascular structures of the anterior trunk wall
Anterior view. On the right side of the trunk, the pectoralis major and minor have been completely removed and the external and internal abdominal obliques have been partially removed to display both epifascial (subcutaneous) and deep (subfascial) neurovascular structures. For the depiction of the superior epigastric vessels the superior part of the right rectus abdominis has been removed or rendered transparent. In order to illustrate the course of the intercostal vessels, the intercostal spaces have been exposed.

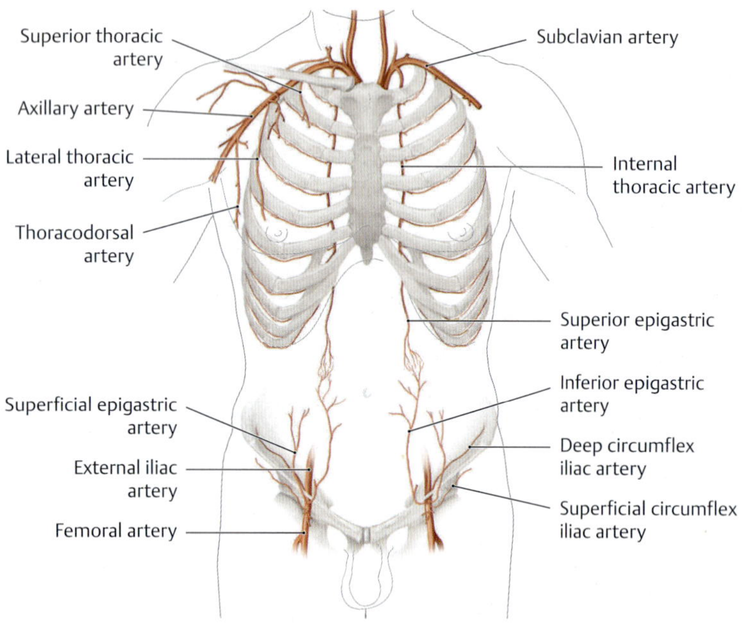

B The arterial supply of the anterior trunk wall
Anterior view. The anterior trunk wall receives its blood supply from two main sources: the internal thoracic artery, which arises from the subclavian artery, and the inferior epigastric artery, which arises from the external iliac artery. It is also supplied by smaller vessels arising from the axillary artery (superior thoracic artery, thoracodorsal artery, and lateral thoracic artery) and from the femoral artery (superficial epigastric artery and superficial circumflex iliac artery).

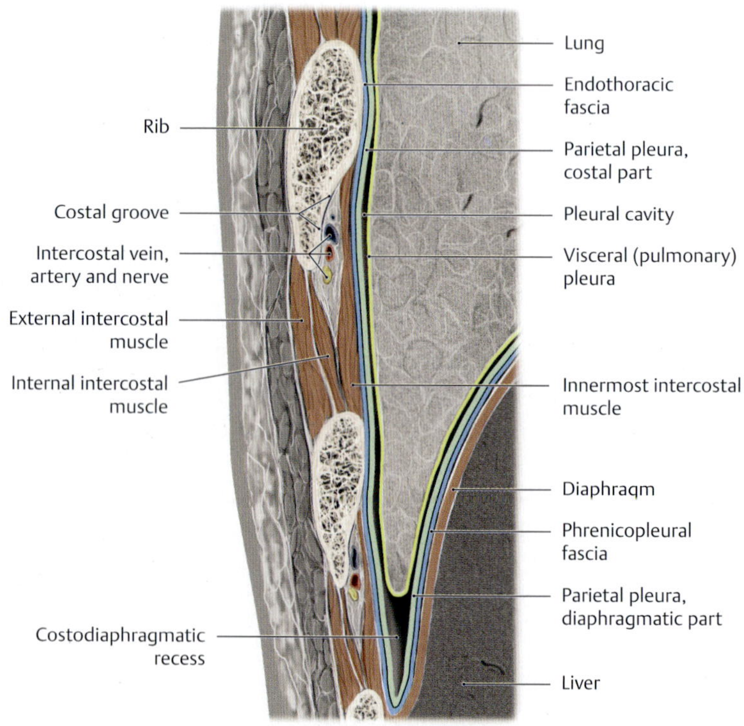

C Structure of the lateral thoracic wall
Coronal section through the lateral thoracic wall and costodiaphragmatic recess.

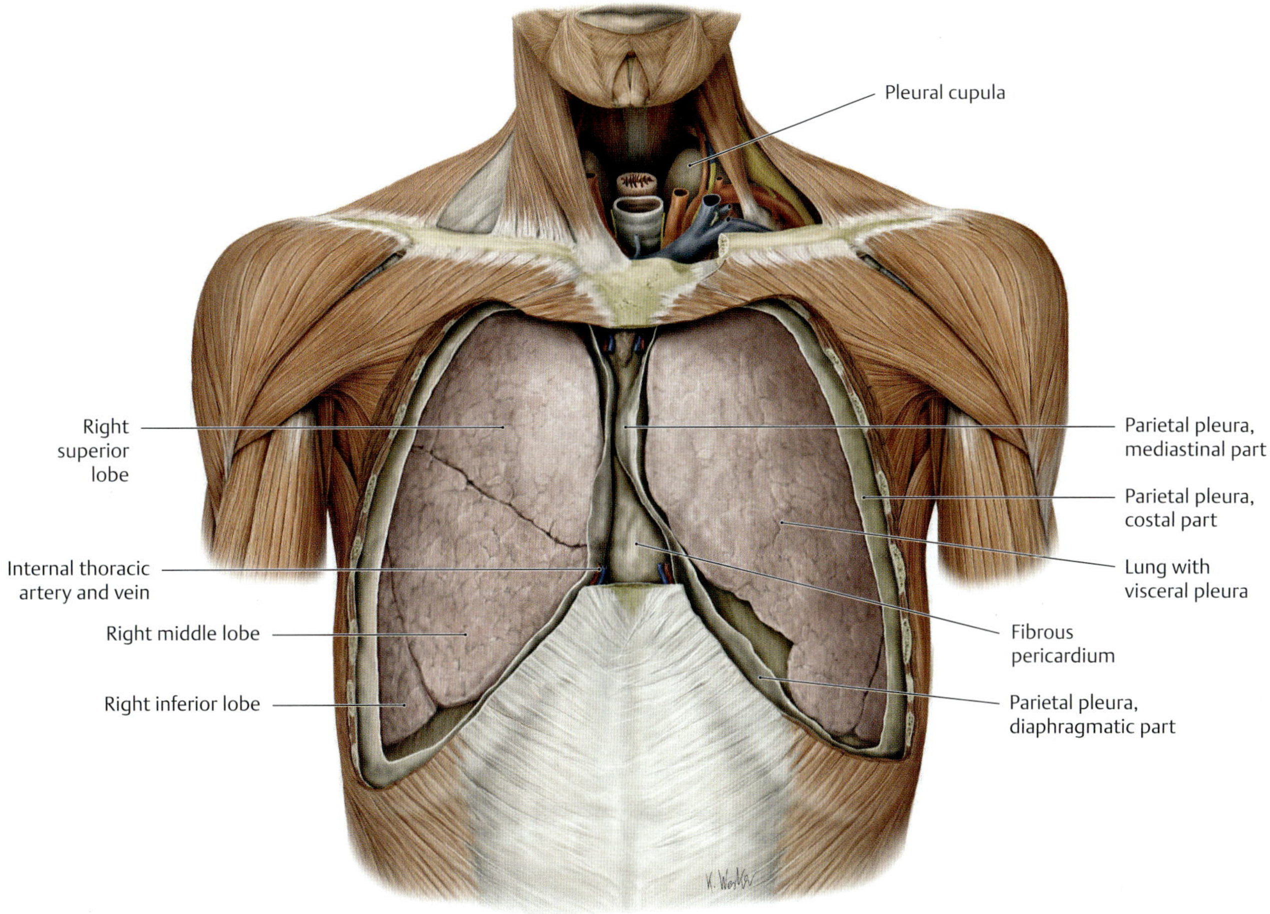

D Thorax, pleural cavities have been opened
Anterior view.

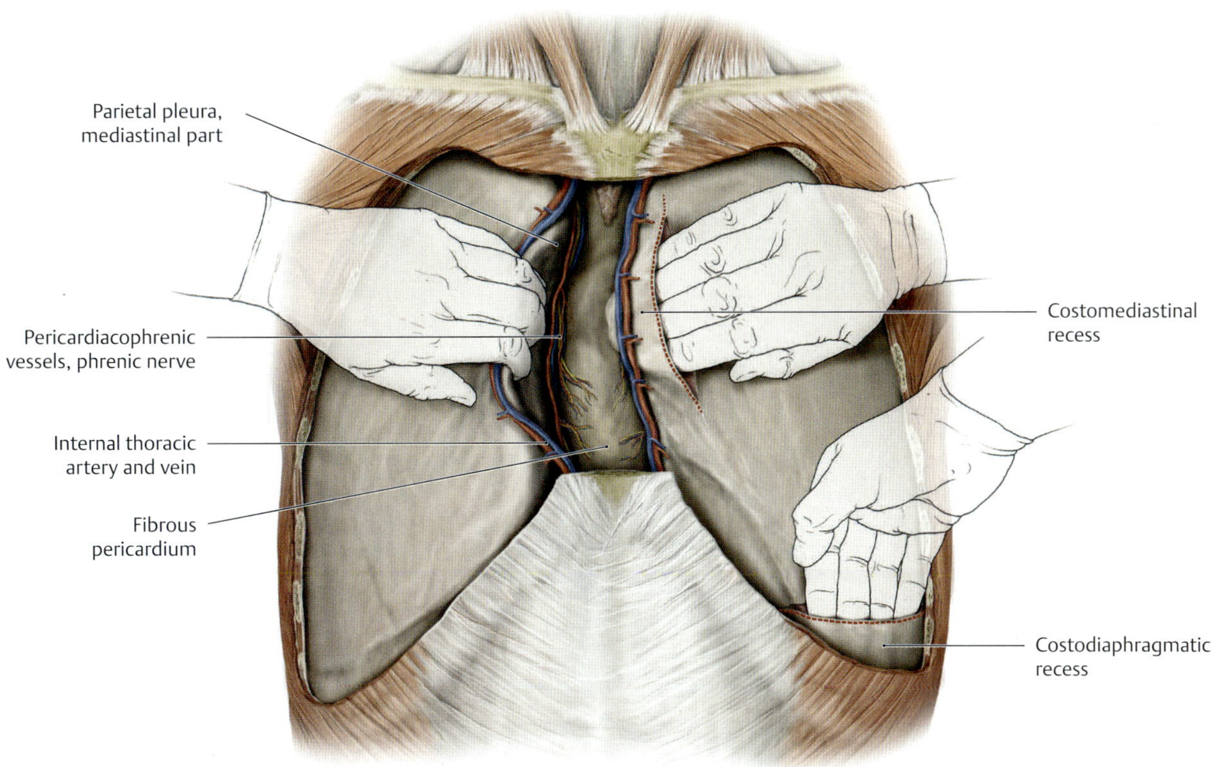

E Costomediastinal and costodiaphragmatic recesses
On the left side, the parietal pleura has been slit open parasternally and above the 9th rib so that the costomediastinal and costodiaphragmatic recesses can be located with the fingertips. On the right side, the lung together with its mediastinal pleura has been carefully loosened from the pericardium in order to display the pericardiacophrenic vessels and phrenic nerve.

6.4 Thoracic Organs in situ: Anterior, Lateral, and Inferior Views

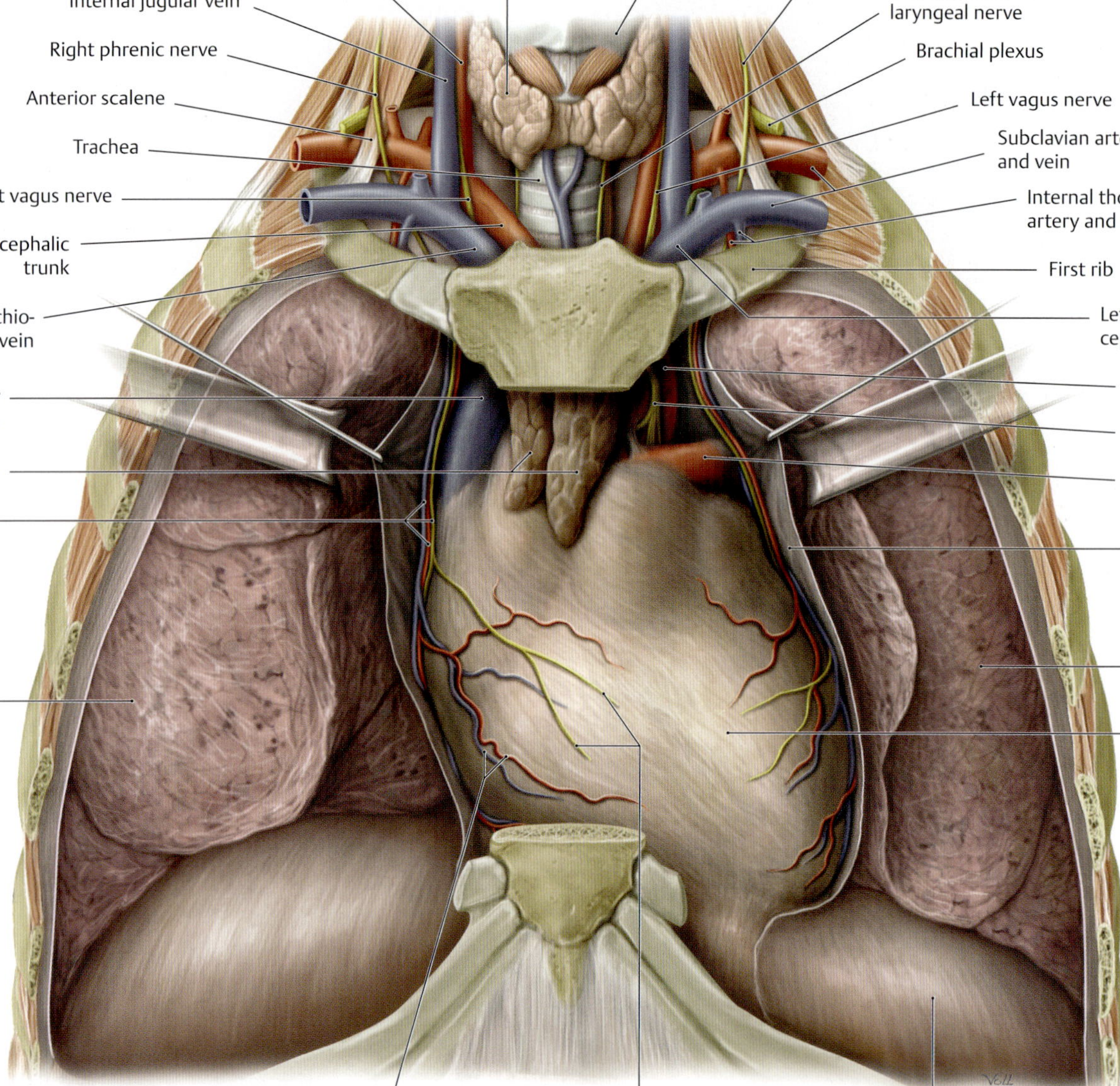

A Mediastinum, anterior view with the anterior thoracic wall removed

Coronal section through the thorax. All connective tissue has been removed from the *anterior mediastinum*.

This dissection displays a prominent thymus, occupying the *superior mediastinum* and extending inferiorly into the anterior mediastinum. Visible structures that are continued from the superior mediastinum into the neck or upper limb include branches of the aortic arch, the superior vena cava, and the trachea, although the latter is mostly obscured by the vessels surrounding the heart. The *middle mediastinum*, visible in this coronal section, is dominated by the heart and pericardium (fused to the diaphragm) and the associated neurovascular structures—the phrenic nerve and pericardiacophrenic vessels. These vessels descend along the pericardium toward the diaphragm while giving off pericardial branches.

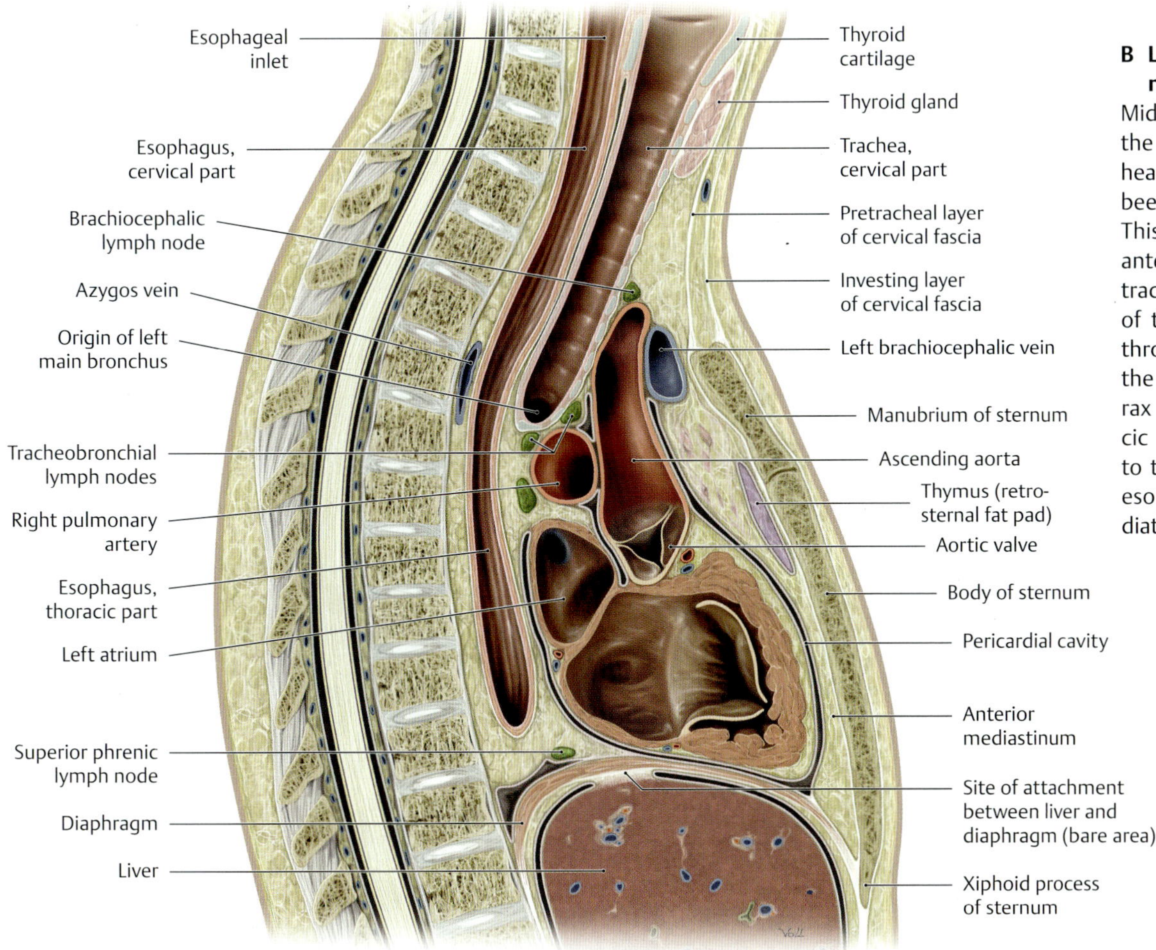

B Lateral view of the mediastinum

Midsagittal section; viewed from the right side. The pericardium, heart, trachea and esophagus have been cut open, simplified drawing. This lateral view demonstrates the anterior-to-posterior shift of the trachea, located directly in front of the esophagus, as it descends through the neck and extends into the thorax. After entering the thorax through the superior thoracic aperture, it passes *posteriorly* to the vessels near the heart. The esophagus is located in the immediate vicinity of the left atrium.

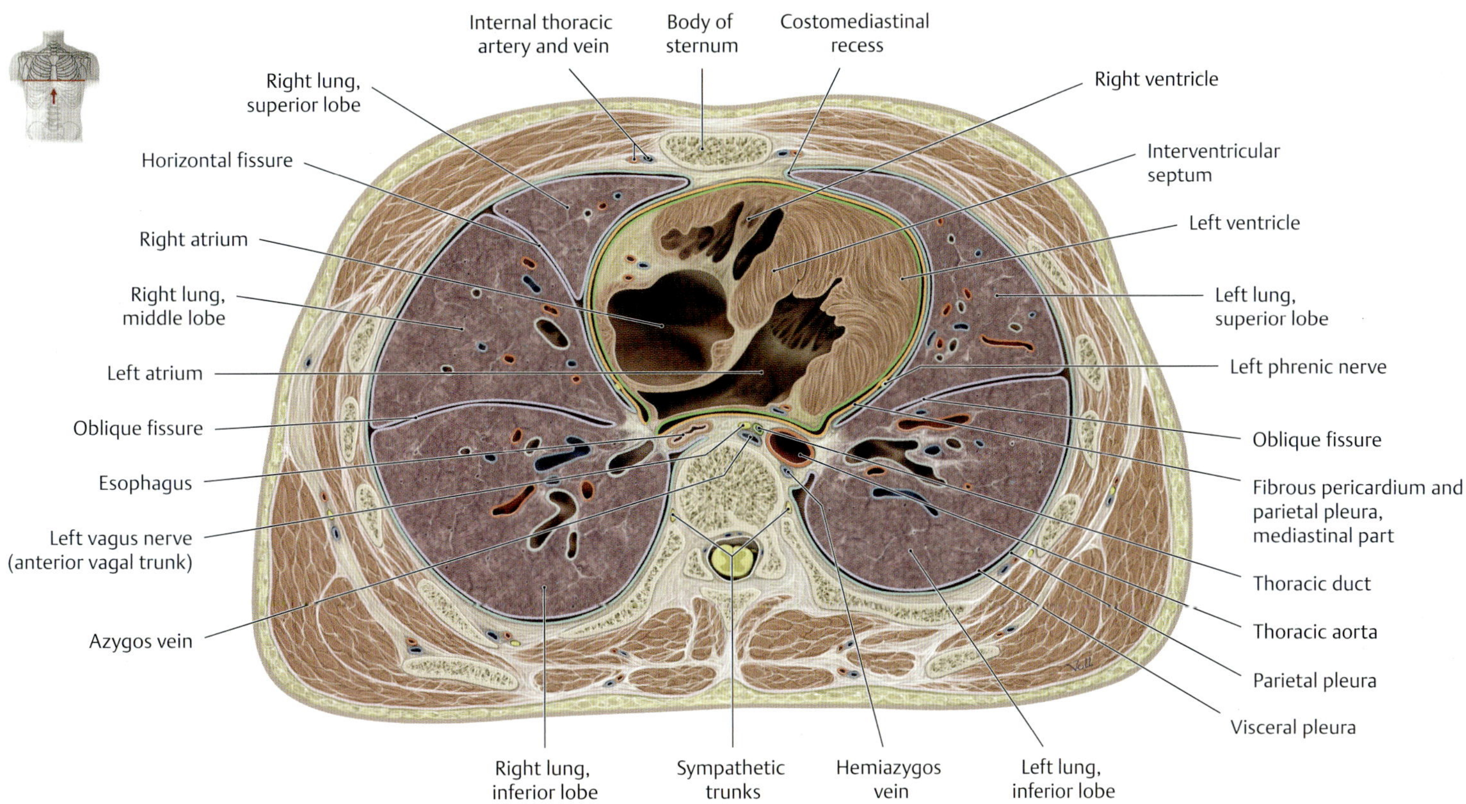

C Inferior view of the mediastinum

Transverse section at the level of the 8th thoracic vertebra.

This diagram clearly shows the asymmetrical position of the heart in the thorax (see also p. 97). From both sides, the costomediastinal recesses extend between the heart and sternum (see p. 185).

6.5 Thoracic Organs in situ: Posterior Views

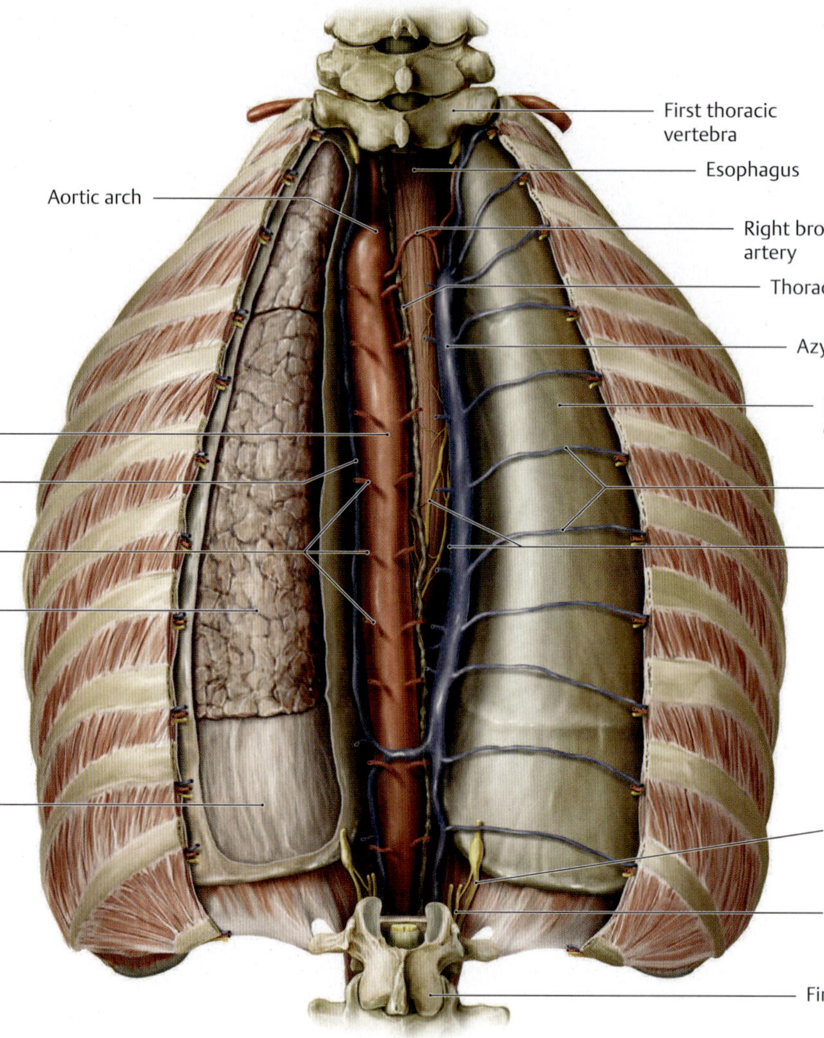

A Posterior view of the mediastinum
The thoracic spine has been removed, and parts of the posterior thoracic wall and left parietal pleura have been removed, in order to display the lungs.
Note the course of the thoracic duct between the thoracic aorta and esophagus.

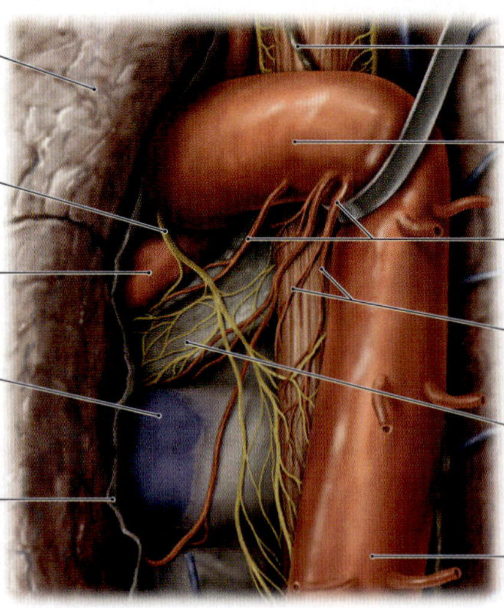

a

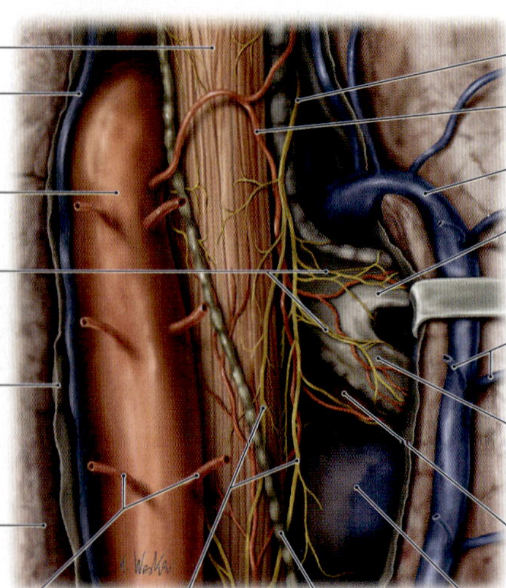

b

B Hilum of the left (a) and right (b) lung, posterior view
In order to show the left hilum, the aorta at the junction of the aortic arch and thoracic aorta has been retracted laterally in (**a**). In (**b**), the azygos vein has been retracted laterally to display the right hilum.

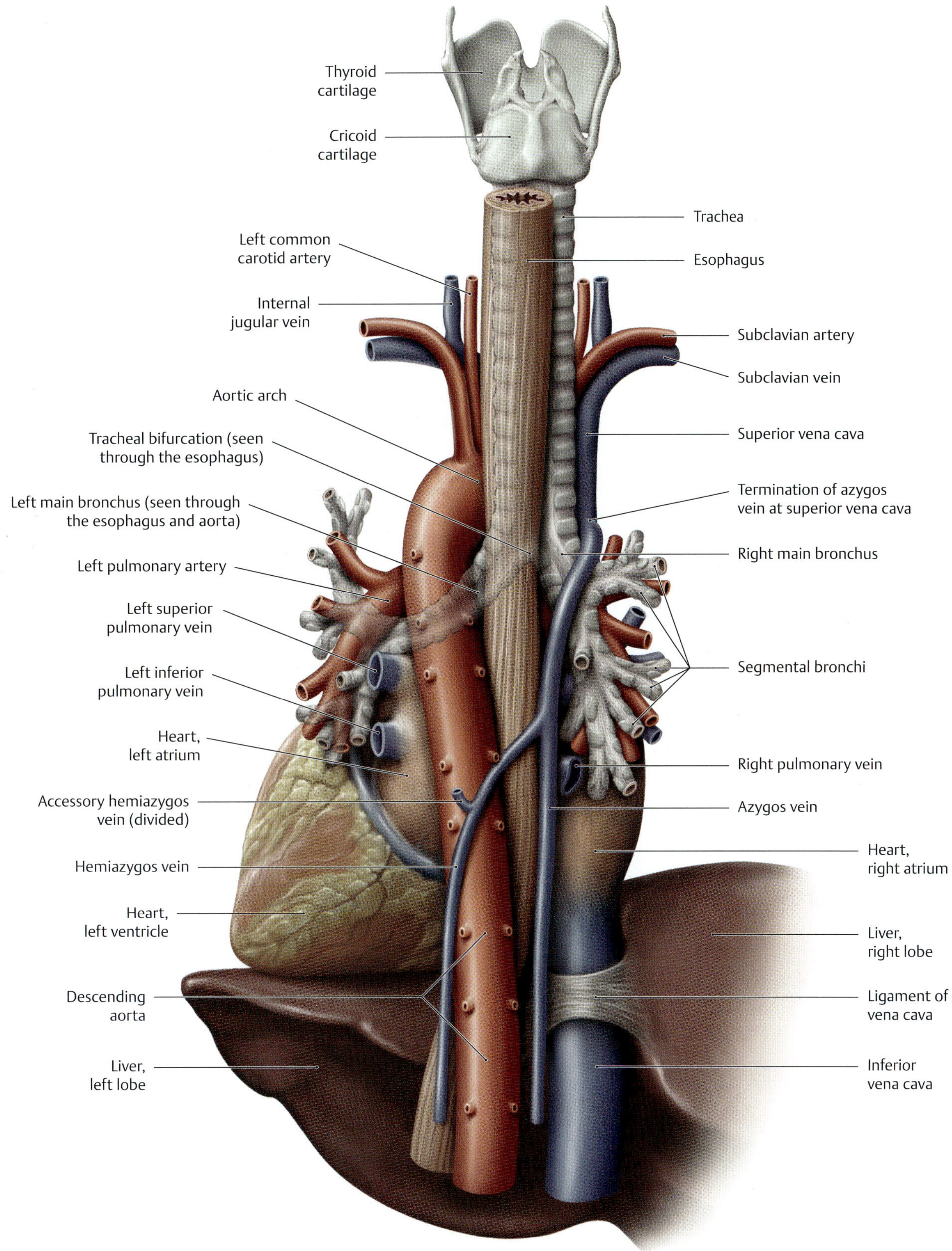

C Contents of the mediastinum, posterior view
The structures in the *posterior mediastinum* are depicted in this view. Note particularly the course of the descending aorta, the azygos and hemiazygos veins, and the esophagus, which is posterior to the trachea and partially obscures it. (An anterior view of the posterior mediastinum is shown on p. 194.) The topographical relations of the aorta change several times along its course. The proximal part of the aorta ascends in the middle mediastinum, which is a subdivision of the inferior mediastinum. At that level the aorta lies anterior to the trachea and esophagus. It then ascends into the superior mediastinum, where it curves posteriorly and to the left to form the aortic arch. This curve lies to the left of the esophagus and trachea, and it arches over the left main bronchus (the aorta "rides" upon that bronchus). In its further course the aorta turns back slightly medially and posteriorly and descends behind the esophagus in the posterior mediastinum, where it is closely related to the azygos and hemiazygos veins. Note also the very close proximity of the liver to the right side of the heart.

6.6 Heart: Pericardial Cavity

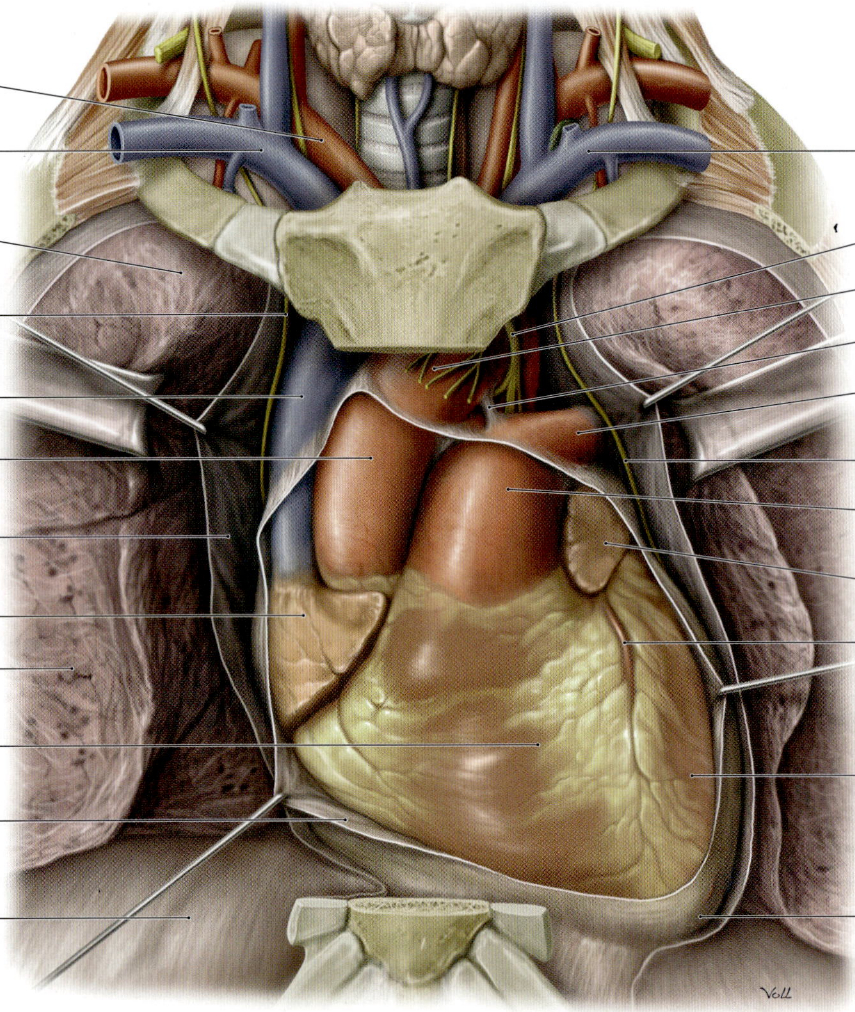

A The pericardial cavity has been opened to display the sternocostal surface of the heart

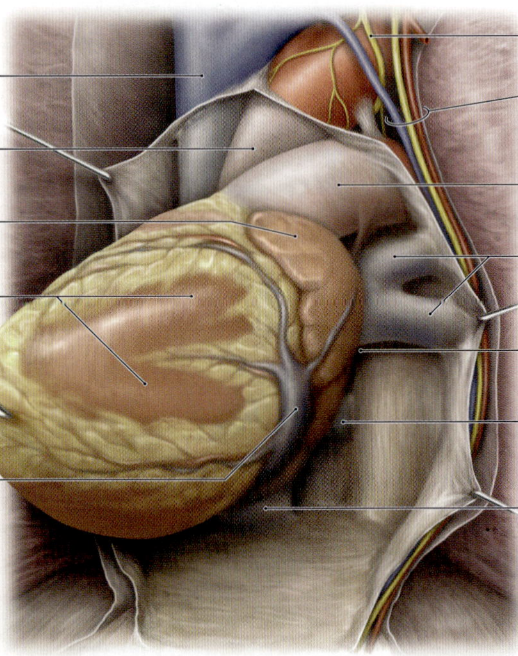

B Diaphragmatic surface of the heart (also known as posterior wall of the heart)
After lifting the heart, the diaphragmatic surface of the heart and the oblique pericardial sinus become visible.

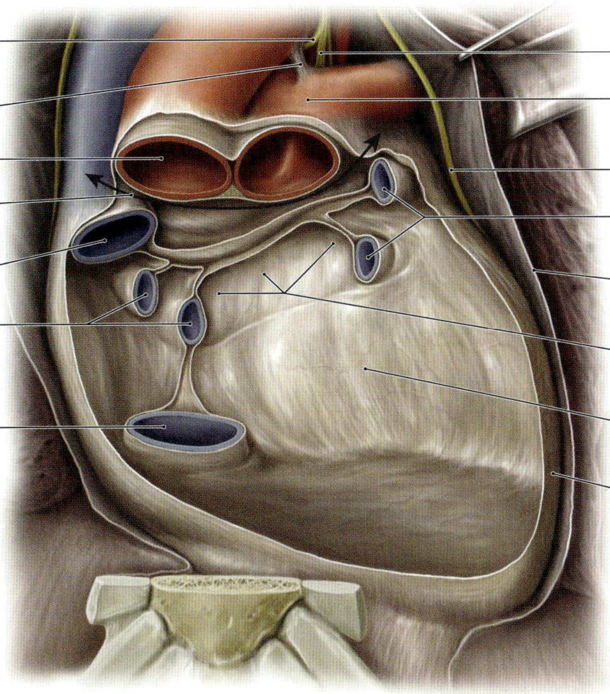

C Pericardial cavity after the heart has been removed

Note the location where the parietal layer is folded back onto the visceral layer, and the attachment between the pericardium and diaphragm.

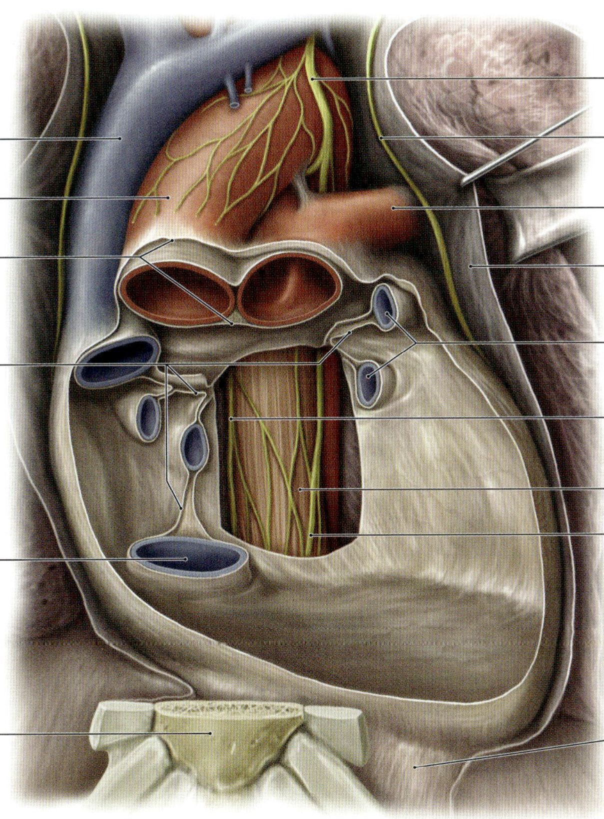

D Course of the esophagus along the posterior aspect of the left atrium

After a window is cut in the pericardium in the area of the oblique pericardial sinus, the esophagus, which courses in the immediate vicinity, and the anterior vagal trunk become visible.

6.7 Overview of the Mediastinum

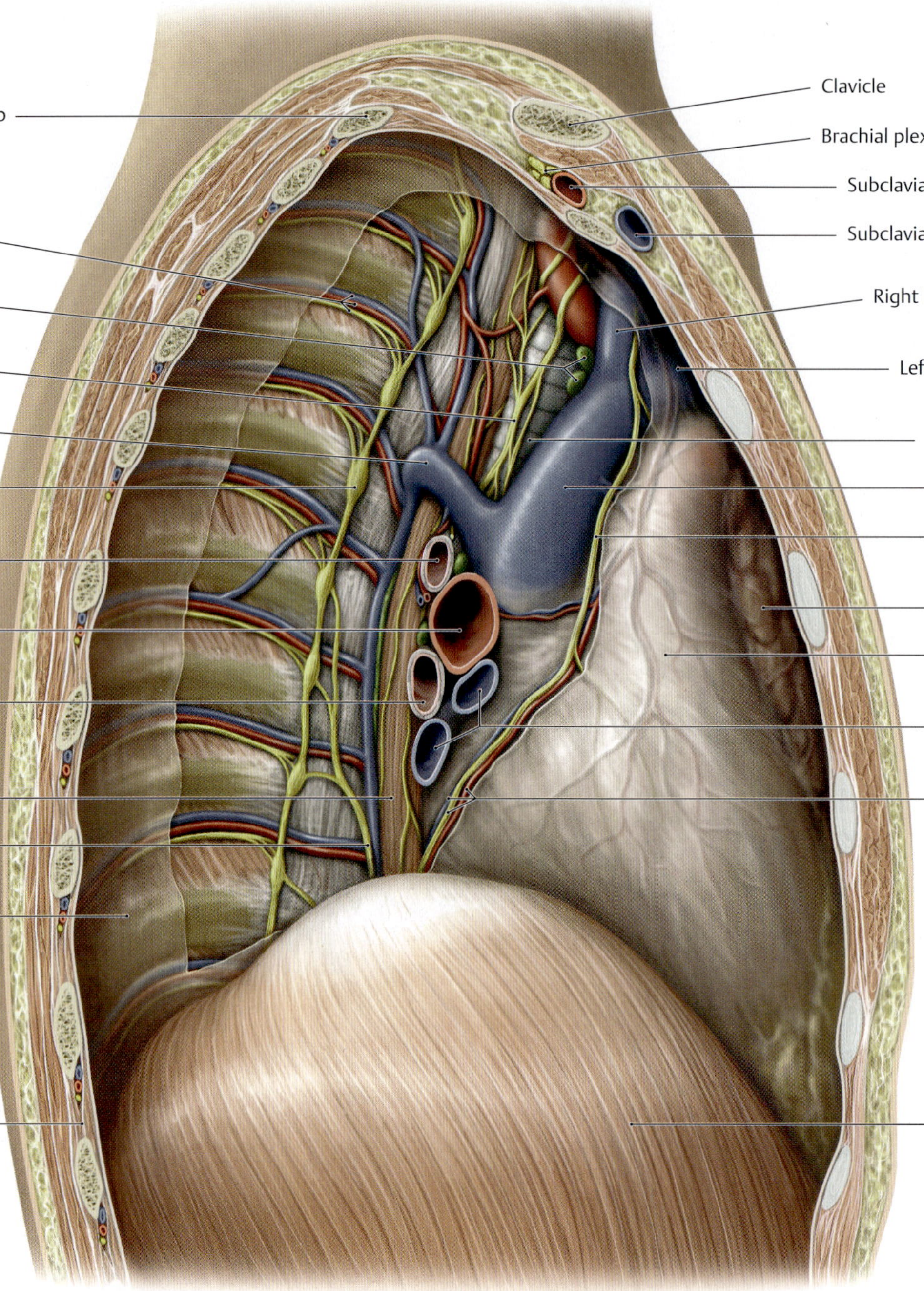

A Mediastinum viewed from the right side

Parasagittal section. The entire right lung and most of the wall of the pleural cavity have been removed (parietal pleura, see p. 194) to display the structures of the *posterior mediastinum* adjacent to the vertebrae, most notably the sympathetic trunk, and the azygos vein opening into the superior vena cava. In the *middle mediastinum*, the (right) phrenic nerve and the (right) pericardiacophrenic artery and vein are visible on the pericardium. The (right) vagus nerve is directly visible on the lateral wall of the esophagus. The trachea, which lies on the median plane, is partially obscured by other structures (vagus nerve, azygos vein, lymph nodes). The transected superior lobar bronchus and common trunk of the middle and inferior lobar bronchi are clearly visible. Coming from the mediastinum, these bronchi lie superior and inferior to the pulmonary artery and extend into the right lung. The thymus, relatively prominent here, is large in early postnatal life, but regresses in adulthood, eventually replaced in old age by a small retrosternal fat pad (involuted thymus).

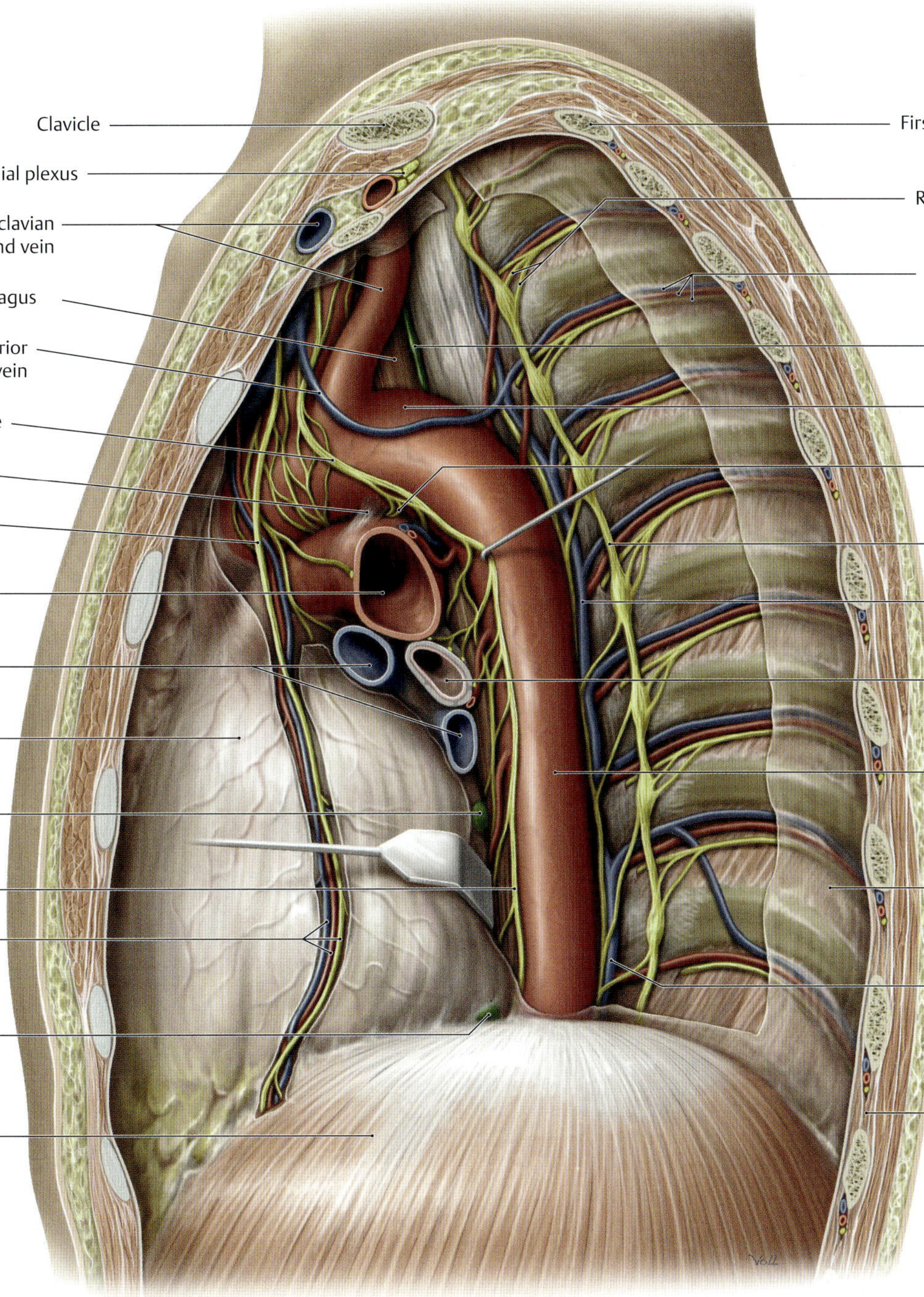

B Mediastinum viewed from the left side
Parasagittal section. The entire left lung and most of the parietal pleura of the left pleural cavity have been removed, but the pericardium remains intact. The left-sided elements of paired mediastinal structures (sympathetic trunk, vagus nerve, phrenic nerve, pericardiacophrenic vessels) can be identified. Visible unpaired structures include the hemiazygos vein and the (inconstant) accessory hemiazygos vein. The dominant vessel in this field is the aorta, of which the aortic arch and descending aorta can be seen anterior and lateral to the esophagus. Both left pulmonary veins have been transected near their terminations in the left atrium of the heart, again demonstrating the close topographical relationship between the left atrium and esophagus. The trachea is almost entirely obscured in a left paramedian section. Only the transected left main bronchus is clearly visible between the left pulmonary veins.

6.8 Posterior Mediastinum

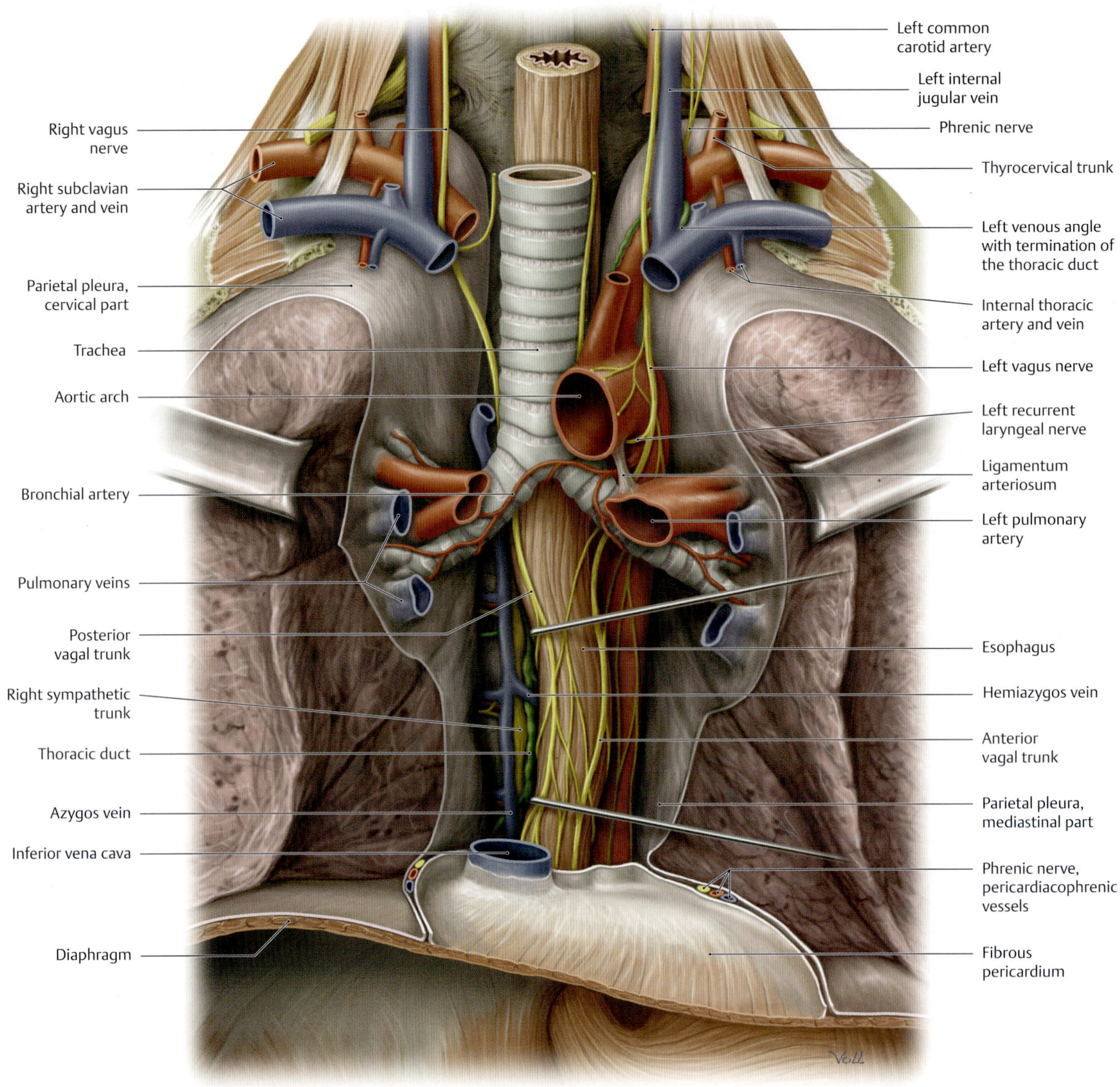

A Posterior mediastinum, anterior view

The heart has been removed, and the esophagus has been slightly retracted laterally. The major structures of the posterior mediastinum are visible: esophagus, vagus nerves, thoracic aorta, intercostal vessels, azygos and hemiazygos veins and sympathetic trunk.

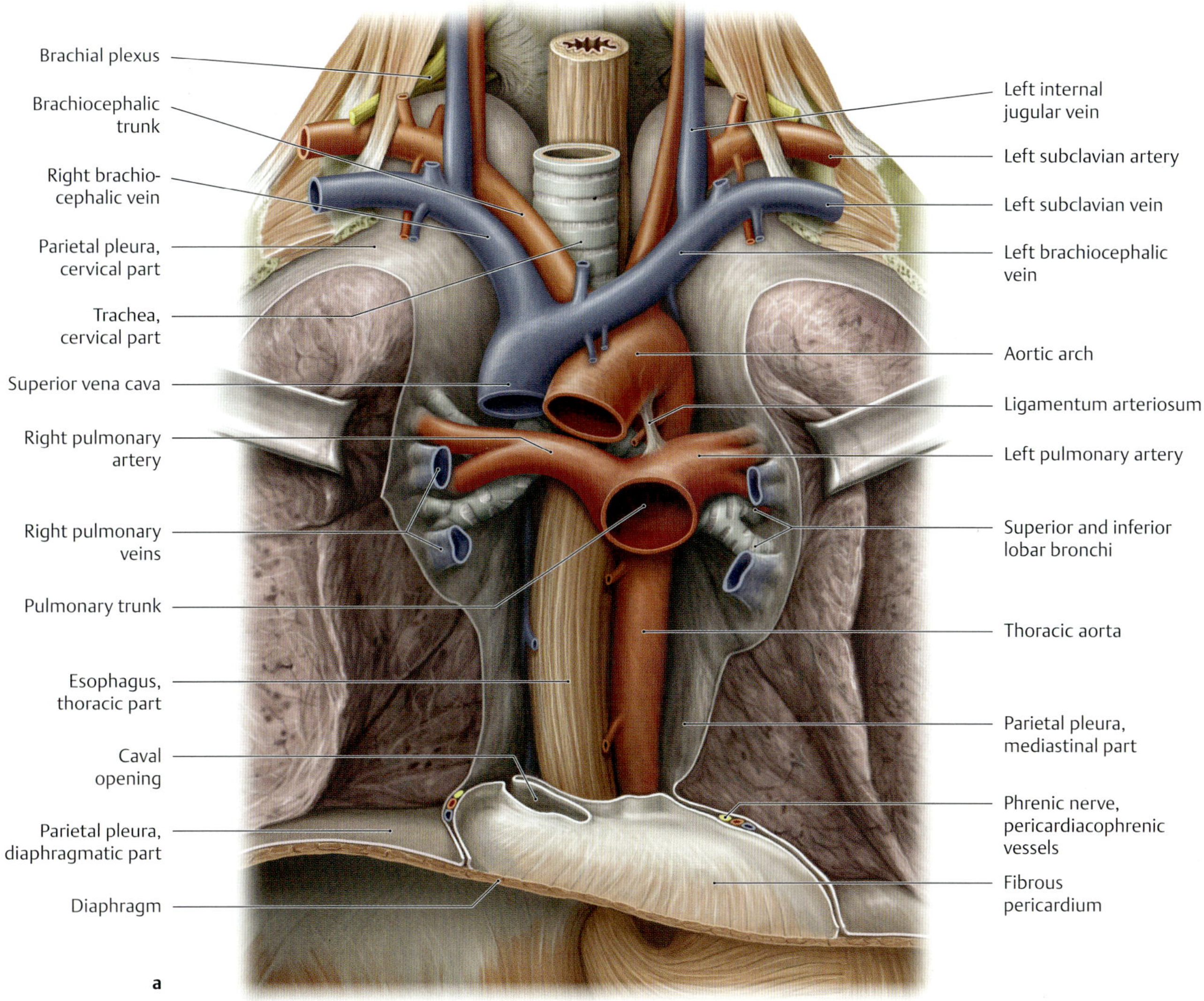

a

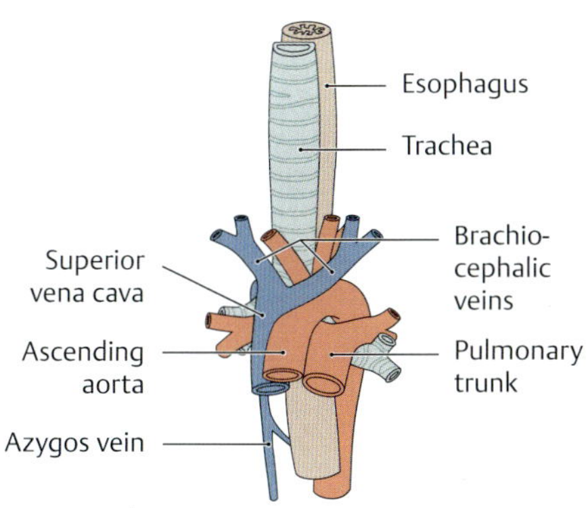

b

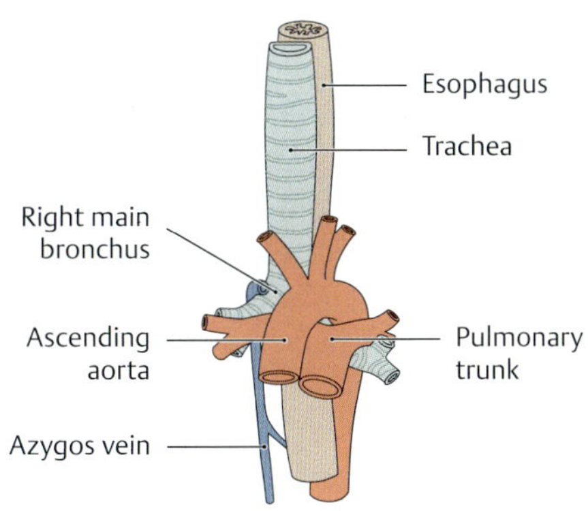

c

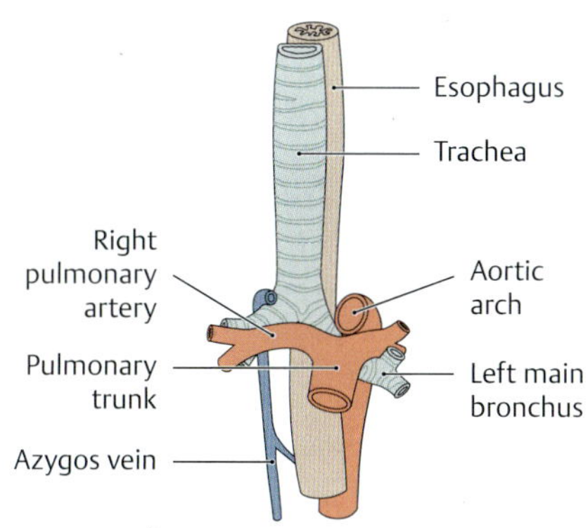

d

B Topographical relations

a Anterior view; the heart has been removed; **b–e** In the drawings above, structures are progressively removed to obtain greater exposure of the trachea and bronchi:

b situs similar to **a**. With all structures intact, the trachea can be seen anterior to the esophagus. The tracheal bifurcation is covered by the aortic arch and pulmonary artery;

c with the superior vena cava and brachiocephalic veins removed, the right main bronchus is just visible and the azygos vein is seen "riding" on the right upper lobar bronchus;

d the ascending aorta and much of the aortic arch have been removed, exposing the tracheal bifurcation and pulmonary arteries;

e with the pulmonary trunk removed, the aorta "rides" upon the left main bronchus.

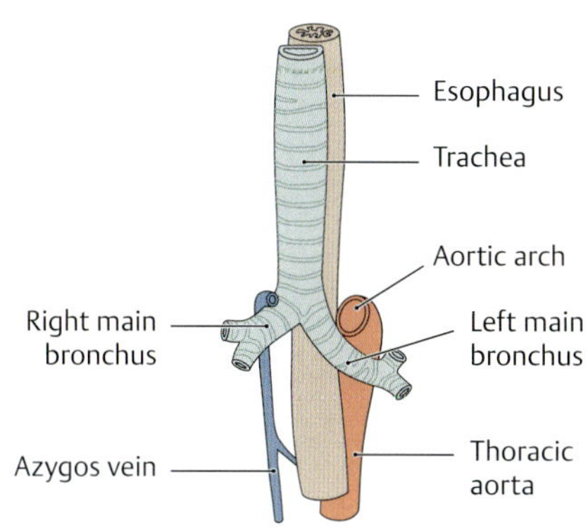

e

6.9 Superior Mediastinum

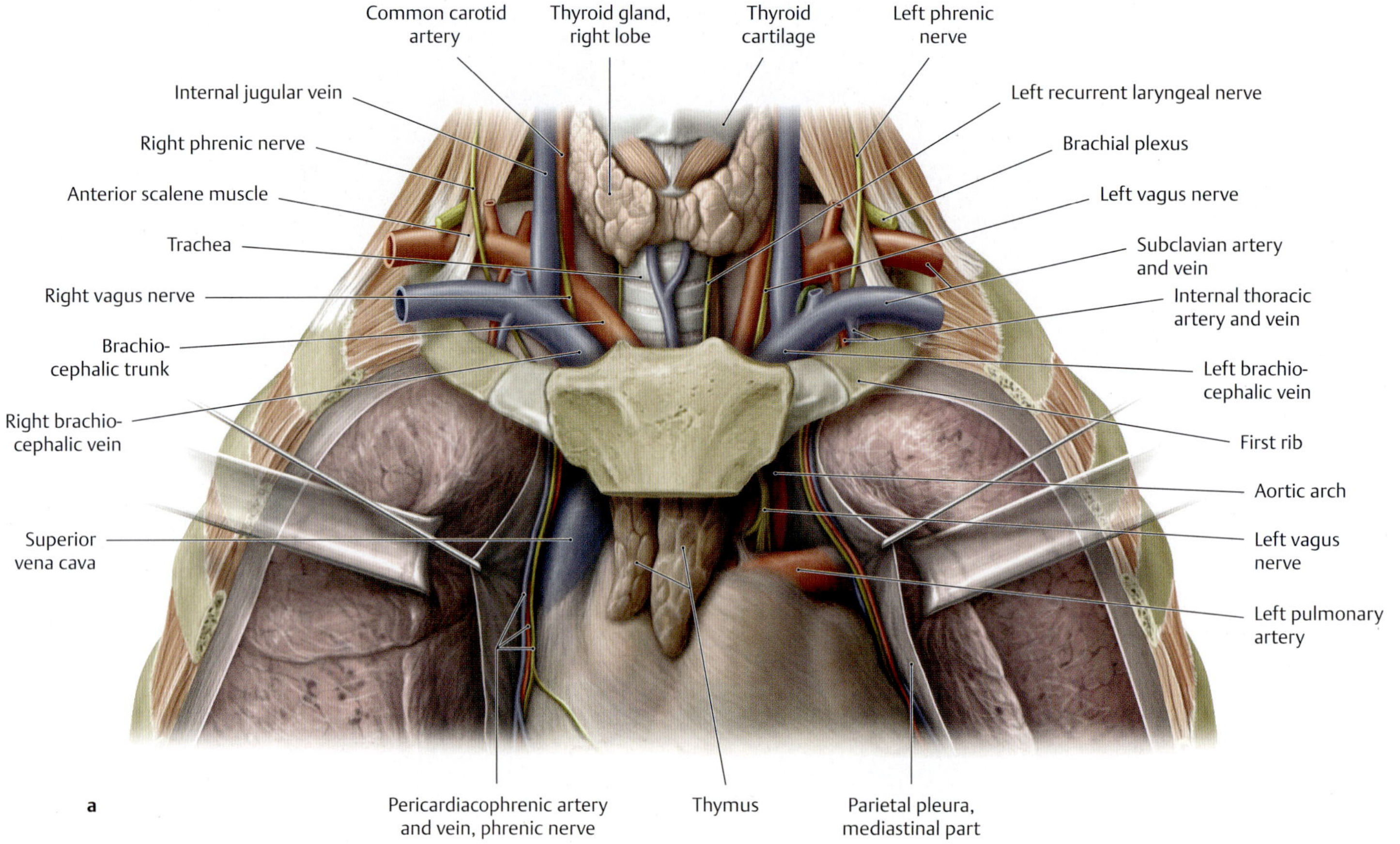

a

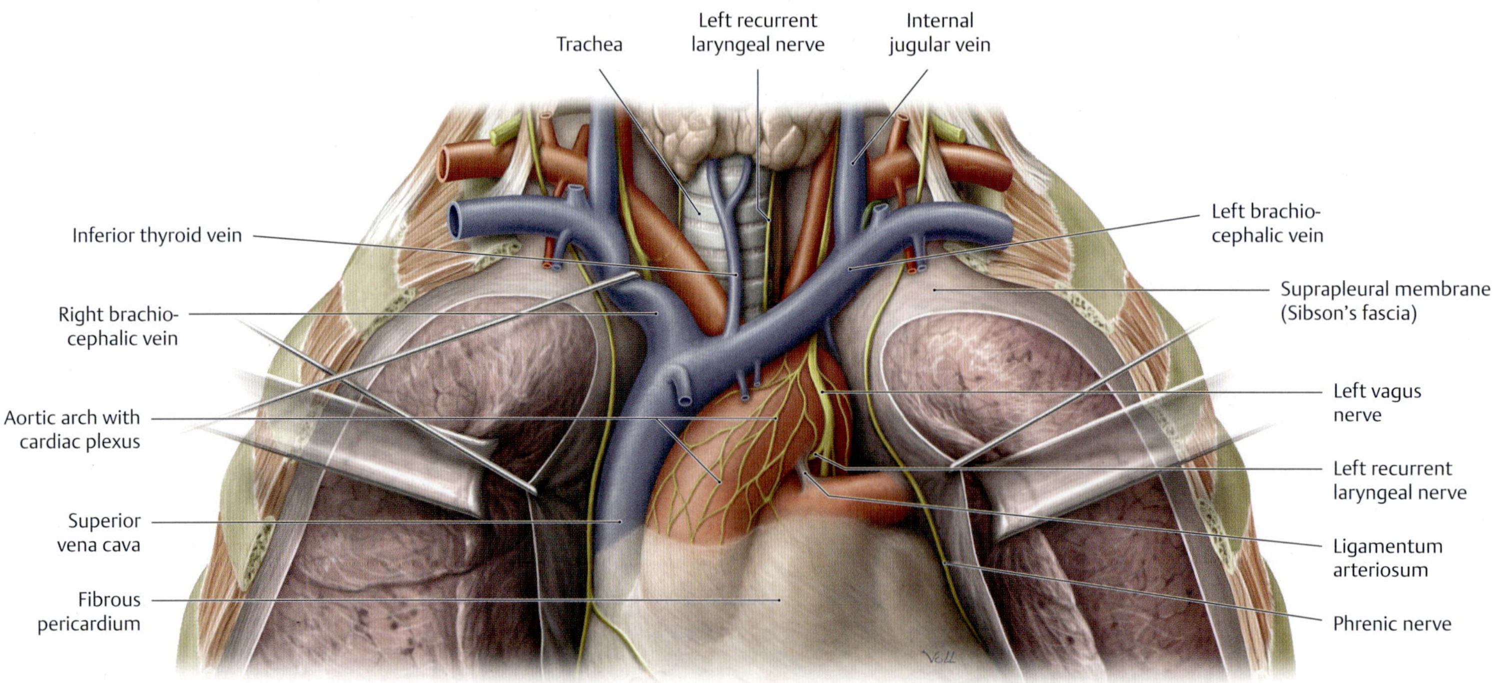

b

A View of the superior thoracic aperture and the superior mediastinum

a The body of sternum and adjacent ribs have been removed; at the level of the superior thoracic aperture, the superior mediastinum borders the neck; the actual structures of the superior mediastinum become visible only after removal of the manubrium of the sternum (see **b**);

b The superior mediastinum is exposed: the manubrium of the sternum, and the thymus or thymus remnants (retrosternal fat pad) have been removed.

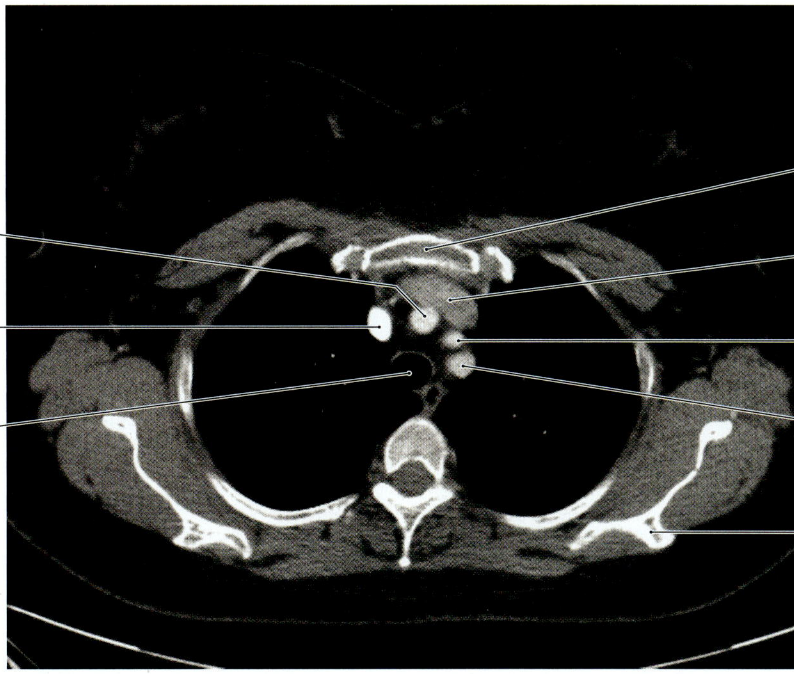

B Cross-sectional anatomy of the superior thoracic aperture
Transverse (axial) CT scan (soft-tissue window) at the level of the superior thoracic aperture (manubrium of sternum or T 3), inferior view.

(Original image from: Prof. S. Müller-Hülsbeck, M.D., Institut für Diagnostische und Interventionelle Radiologie/Neuroradiologie, DIAKO Krankenhaus gGmbH Flensburg.)

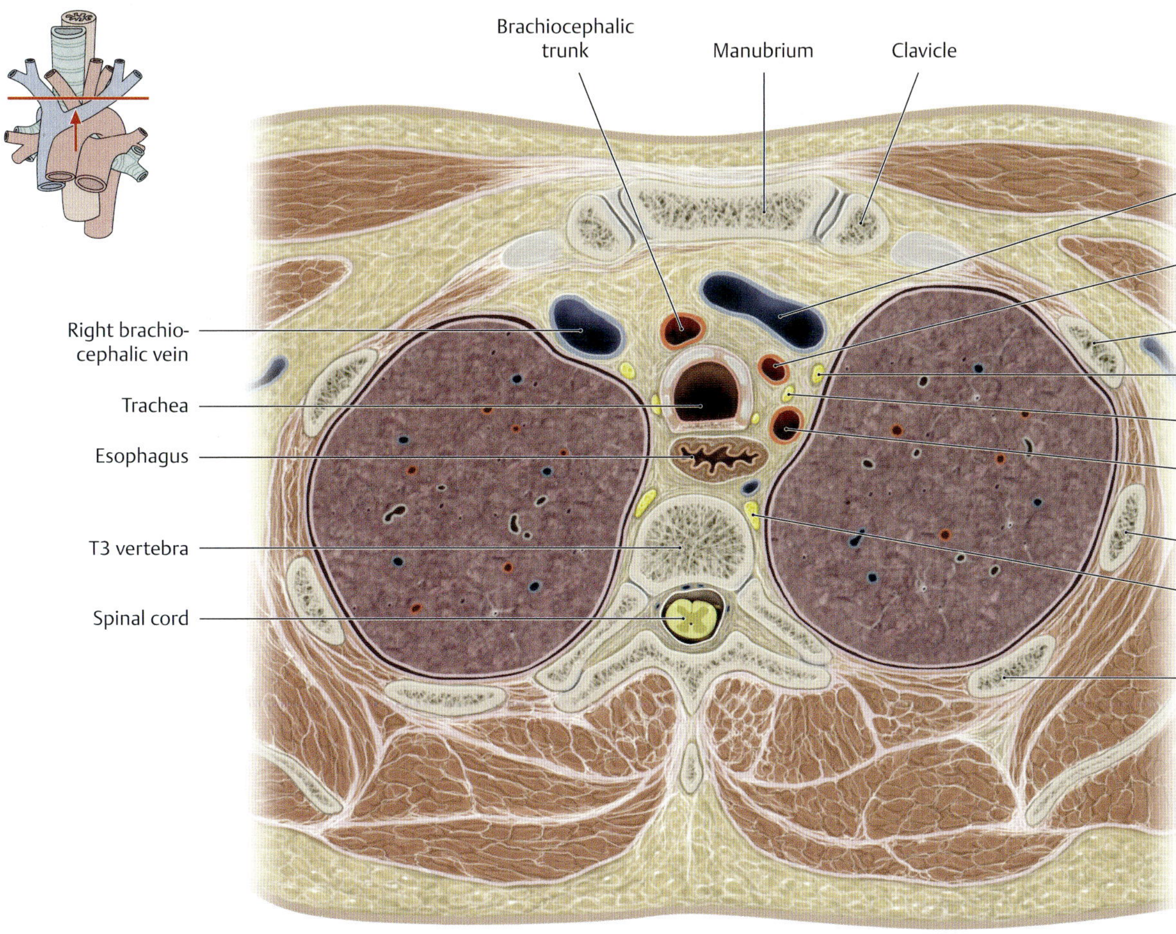

C Transverse section at the level of the superior thoracic aperture
Inferior view.

6.10 Aortic Arch and Superior Thoracic Aperture

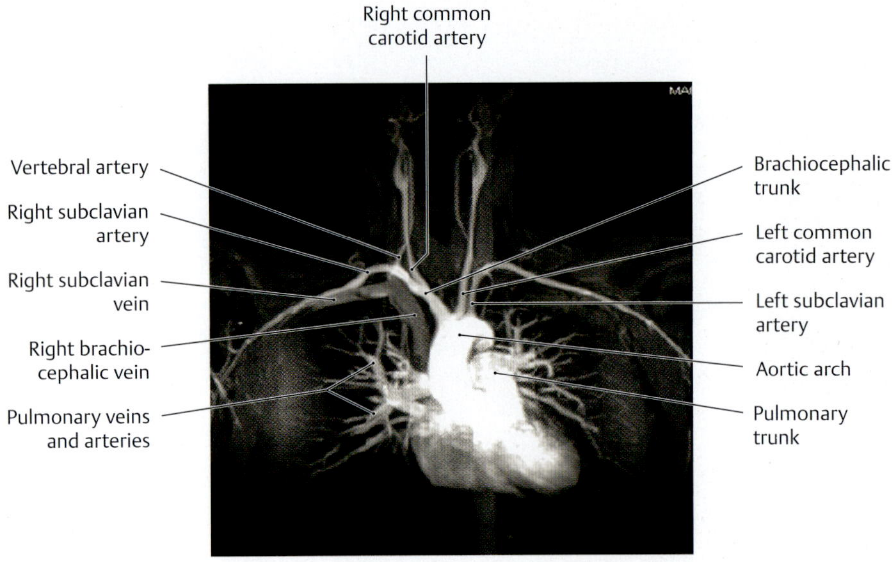

A Contrast-enhanced MR angiography of the vessels near the heart

The image shows an MR angiogram of the normal anatomy of the vessels near the heart (contrast agent administered intravenously via the cubital fossa). The image was generated using the MIP (maximum intensity projection) technique. It uses 3D fast gradient echo sequences, measured at the identical location before and after administration of contrast agent. The subsequent subtraction of images generates 3D data, which includes only vessel information. Using this technique, images from a dynamic series (e.g., pulmonary circulation) can be obtained within a few seconds. (Original image from: Prof. S. Müller-Hülsbeck, M.D., Institut für Diagnostische und Interventionelle Radiologie/Neuroradiologie, DIAKO Krankenhaus gGmbH Flensburg.)

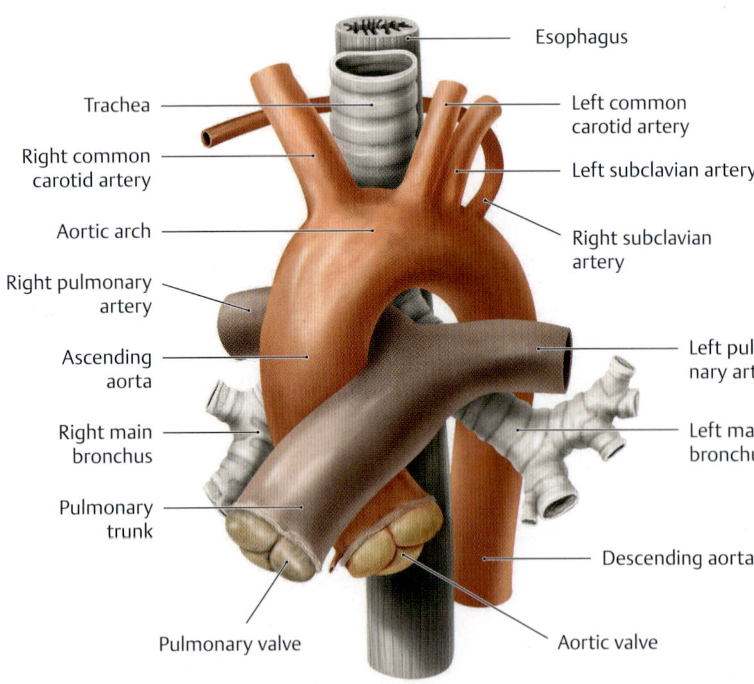

B Congenital anomalies of the aortic arch: Aberrant subclavian artery (arteria lusoria)

If the right subclavian artery arises as the last vessel from the aortic arch distal to the left subclavian artery and then courses behind the trachea and esophagus it may produce a condition called aberrant subclavian artery (arteria lusoria) (see also **C**). Indications for surgery exist only if the patient presents with clinical symptoms (dysphagia, dyspnea, and stridor).

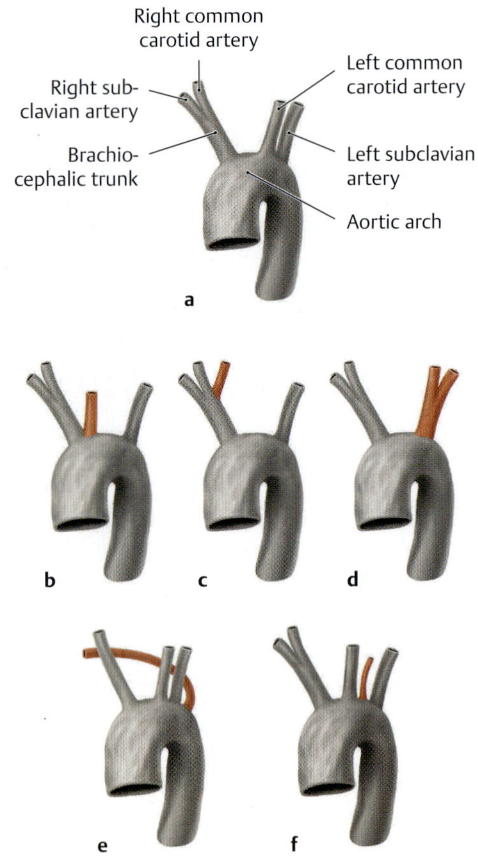

C Origin of the branches of the aortic arch: common pattern and variations (after Lippert and Pabst)

Anterior view.

- **a** Common pattern (70% of cases): The right subclavian artery and right common carotid artery arise together from the brachiocephalic trunk, which arises from the aortic arch; however, the left common carotid artery and left subclavian artery arise directly from the aortic arch.
- **b** Variation 1 (13% of cases): The brachiocephalic trunk (with its two branches, the right subclavian artery and the right common carotid artery) and left common carotid artery arise together from the aortic arch.
- **c** Variation 2 (9% of cases): In addition to the right subclavian artery and right common carotid artery, the *left* common carotid artery also arises from the brachiocephalic trunk.
- **d** Variation 3 (1% of cases): There are two brachiocephalic trunks: one divides into the right subclavian artery and right common carotid artery, the other divides into the left subclavian artery and left common carotid artery.
- **e** Variation 4 (1% of cases): The right subclavian artery is the last branch to arise from the aortic arch. This is called arteria lusoria (from Lat. *lusorius* = play).
- **f** Variation 5 (1% of cases): The left vertebral artery arises directly from the aortic arch.

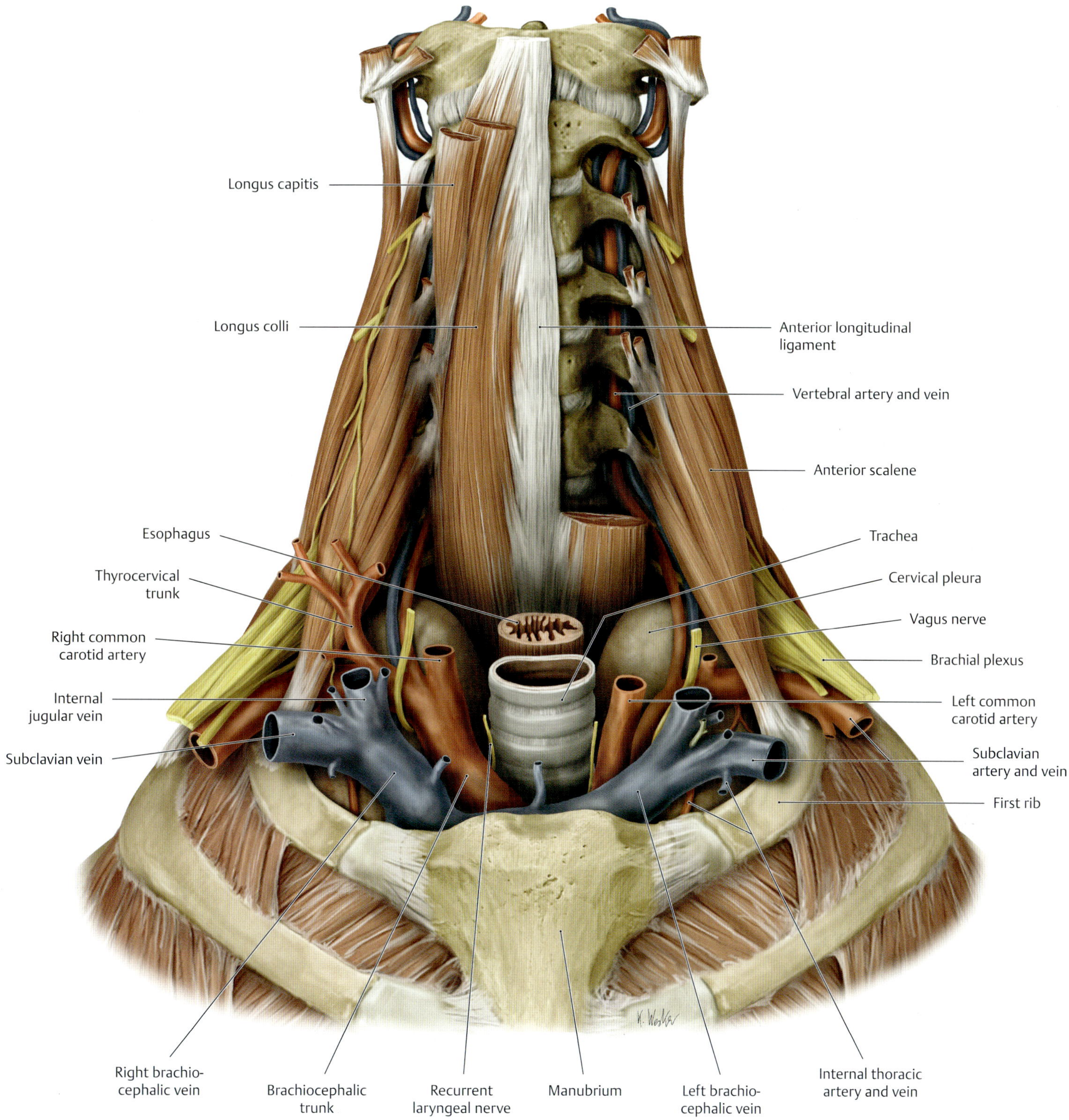

D Topography of the branches of the aortic arch in the superior thoracic aperture

Anterior view after the cervical viscera have been removed. Parts of the prevertebral muscles (longus capitis and longus colli) have also been removed to display the course of the left vertebral artery.

6.11 Clinical Aspects: Coarctation of the Aorta

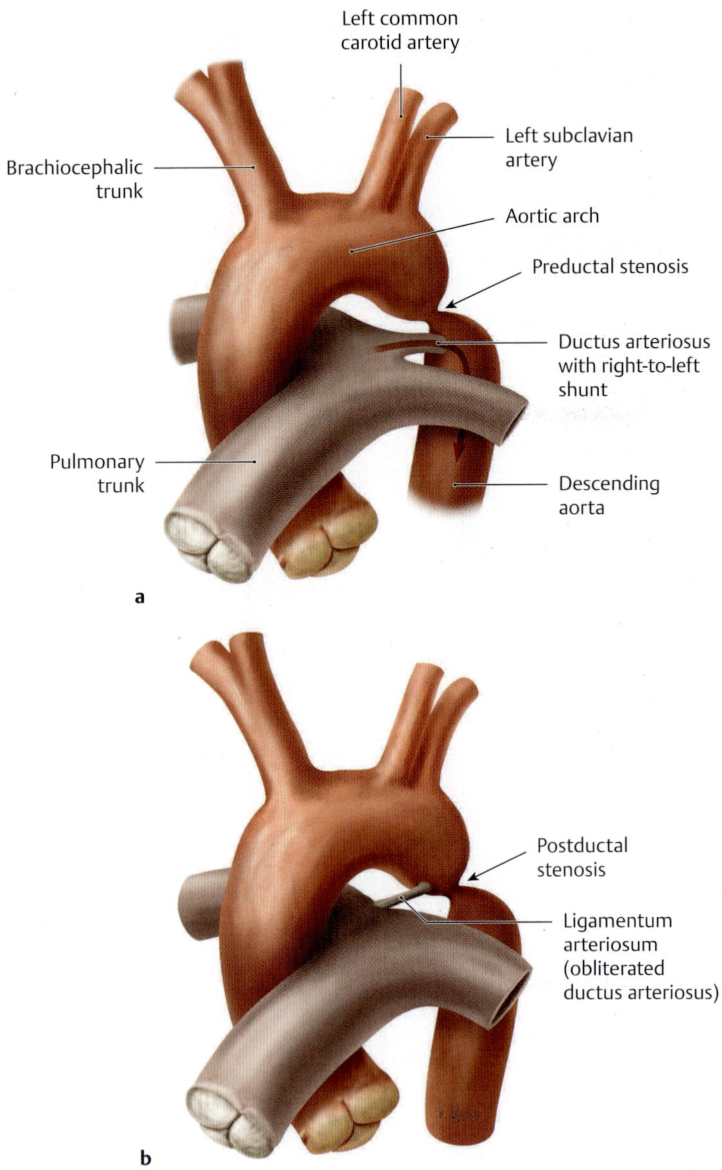

A Definition, organization and epidemiology
a Preductal aortic isthmus stenosis; **b** Postductal aortic isthmus stenosis.

Aortic isthmus stenosis (coarctation of the aorta) is characterized by a localized narrowing between the aortic arch and the descending aorta (the aortic isthmus). Thus, it is distal to the origin of the left subclavian artery, approximately at the level of the ligamentum arteriosum (the obliterated ductus arteriosus). Corresponding with the topographical relation to the ligamentum arteriosum, the two types are classified as preductal and postductal forms:

- preductal form: the narrowing is proximal to the patent ductus arteriosus, and
- postductal form: the narrowing is distal to the obliterated ductus arteriosus (ligamentum arteriosum).

Because preductal coarctation leads to symptoms in the first few years of life, it is also called the "infantile form." The postductal form, which usually develops after the child has reached adolescence, is also known as the "adult form." A narrowing of the aortic arch in the aortic isthmus is a relatively common anomaly (5–7 % of all congenital cardiac and vascular malformations; boy:girl ratio is 3:1). Because clinical symptoms don't always occur (see **B**), the clinical presentation is rare.

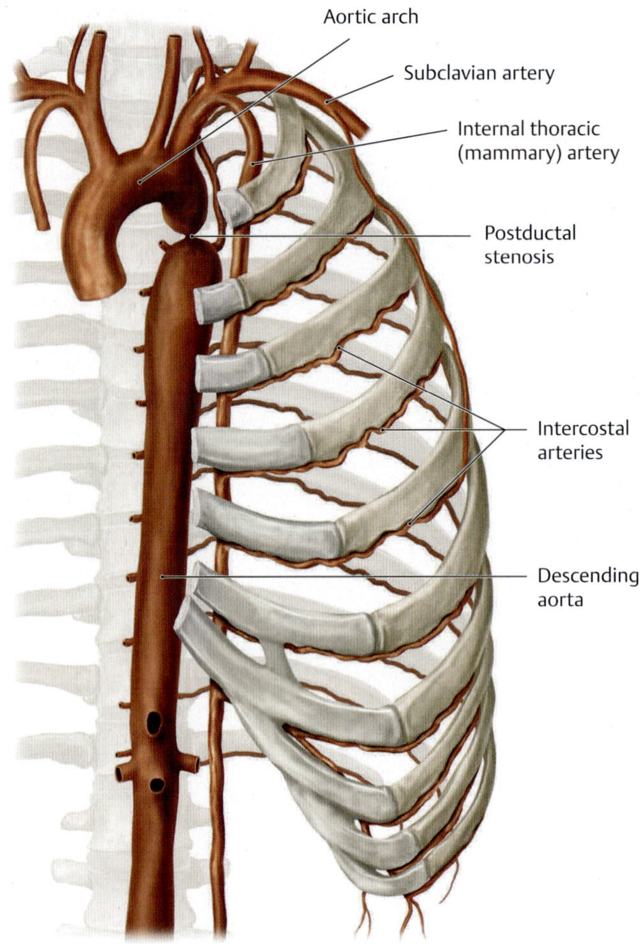

B Pathophysiology and clinical symptoms
Coarctation of the aorta leads to a characteristic increase in blood pressure (hypertension) in the upper systemic circulation while at the same time blood pressure in the lower half of the body drops (hypotension). Cardinal signs include the difference in arterial pressure between upper and lower limbs (weak or absent femoral pulses) as well as cold feet and intermittent claudication caused by insufficient supply of blood.

- Low blood pressure in the lower body caused by **preductal stenosis** with a patent ductus arteriosus results in a *right-to-left shunt* accompanied by cyanosis of the lower body and right ventricular loading (dyspnea, tachypnea). This condition can lead to a life-threatening emergency in infants that requires surgery to correct (resection of the stenotic segment and end-to-end anastomosis).
- **Postductal stenosis** with an obliterated ductus arteriosus (shown here) results in the development of collateral circulation between the thoracic aorta and abdominal aorta (via the subclavian artery, internal thoracic artery and/or intercostal arteries). Depending on how well-functioning the collateral circulation is, patients may experience few or no symptoms at all. If patients do suffer from symptoms, the cardinal sign is often treatment-resistant hypertension, which early in life is often accompanied by headaches, ringing in the ear, dizziness, and nosebleeds. Complications of chronic hypertension in the upper body (left ventricular hypertrophy, coronary heart disease, cerebral hemorrhage) develop only later in life.

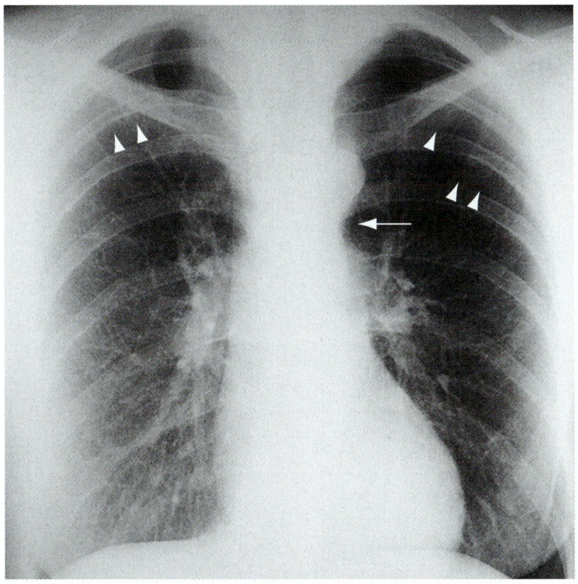

a

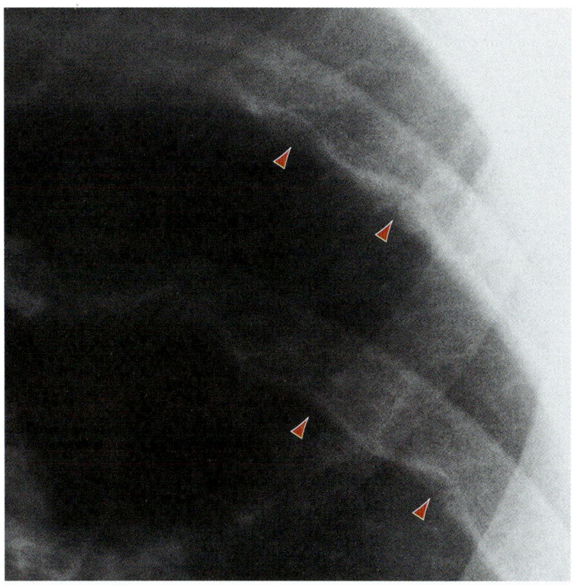

b

C Conventional diagnostic radiology

a and **b** Postductal aortic isthmus stenosis in an anterior-posterior projection (from: Reiser M, Kuhn F, Debus J, eds. *Duale Reihe Radiologie*. 4th ed. Stuttgart: Thieme; 2017).

The thoracic aorta shows mild changes in aortic contour. The post-stenotic descending aorta is dilated, the aortic arch is narrowed and the outer outline of the aorta shows a visible indentation at the level of the stenotic segment (arrow). Rib notching (enlarged detail in **b**, red arrowheads) refers to bone changes around the costal groove caused by dilation and elongation of the enlarged intercostal arteries. It is typically visible at the inferior edges of the ribs.

The extent and localization of the stenosis is best displayed in an angiographic projection using either MRI or spiral CT including three-dimensional reconstruction (see p. 165).

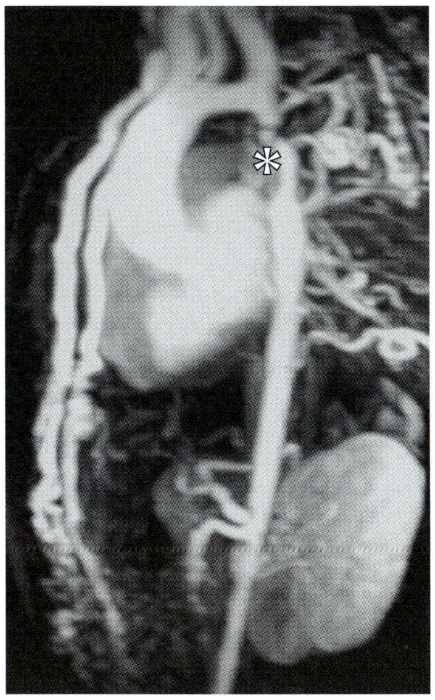

a

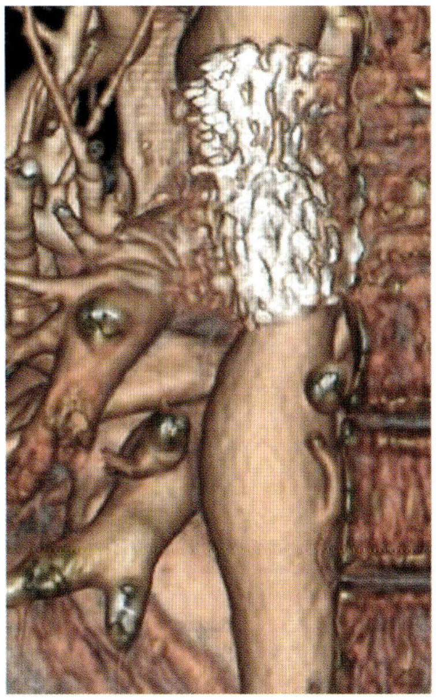

b

D Interventional therapy of aortic isthmus stenosis

Unlike surgical treatment of aortic isthmus stenosis in infants, over the past few years aortic isthmus stenosis in adults has been increasingly treated with minimally invasive, interventional techniques (balloon dilatation and/or stent placement).

a 3D MIP reconstruction of contrast MR angiography of aortic isthmus stenosis in an adult, with severe stenosis (*) and pronounced collaterals prior to implantation; **b** 3D volume rendering of a CT angiogram after stent placement (from: Gutberlet M. *Bildgebende Diagnostik angeborener Herzfehler*. Stuttgart: Thieme; 2017).

6.12 Clinical Aspects: Aortic Aneurysm

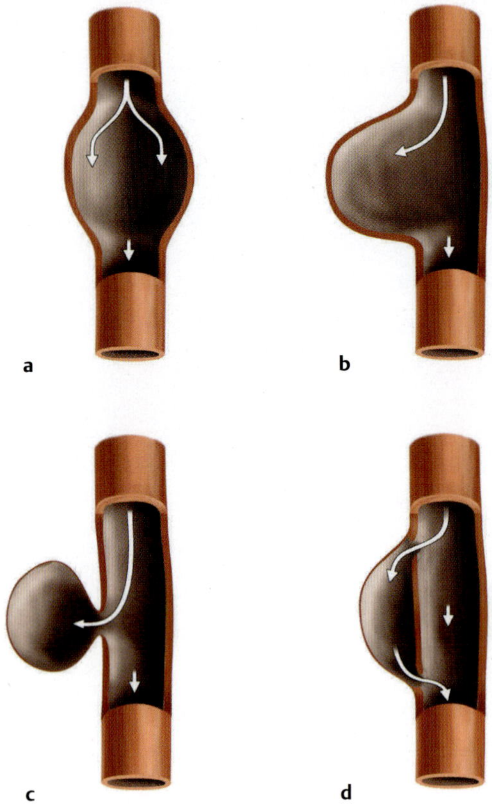

A Definition and classification

An aneurysm is an abnormal enlargement of an artery, usually caused by atherosclerosis. An aneurysm can develop in any artery but usually occurs in the infrarenal abdominal aorta (90% of cases); peripheral aneurysms are predominantly found in the popliteal arteries. Aneurysms are classified as follows:

- **True aneurysms (a, b):** enlargement of the vascular lumen involving all layers of the arterial wall with the vascular wall remaining intact. A morphologic distinction exists between spindle-shaped (*fusiform*) aneurysms involving the entire circumference of the vascular wall and saccular (*sacciform*) aneurysms, which involve only part of the circumference.
- **False aneurysms (pseudoaneurysms) (c):** a perivascular hematoma, which often develops following perforation of the vascular wall (e.g., arterial puncture) or at anastomotic sites after vascular surgery. If the vessel fails to occlude, blood escapes into the perivascular connective tissue leading to the formation of an aneurysmal cavity lined with thrombotic material.
- **Dissecting aneurysms (d):** a tear of the intima/media and subsequent dilatation of the media/adventitia leads to the formation of a second "false" lumen in the vascular wall. This leads to development of a vessel with two channels, one non-perfused and the other perfused. Depending on the location of the intimal tear, also known as the entry site, the entire aorta or only the abdominal aorta can be affected. As the disease progresses, external perforation (rupture with subsequent bleeding) or perforation of the dissected membrane back into the perfused lumen (called re-entry) can occur, see **C**.

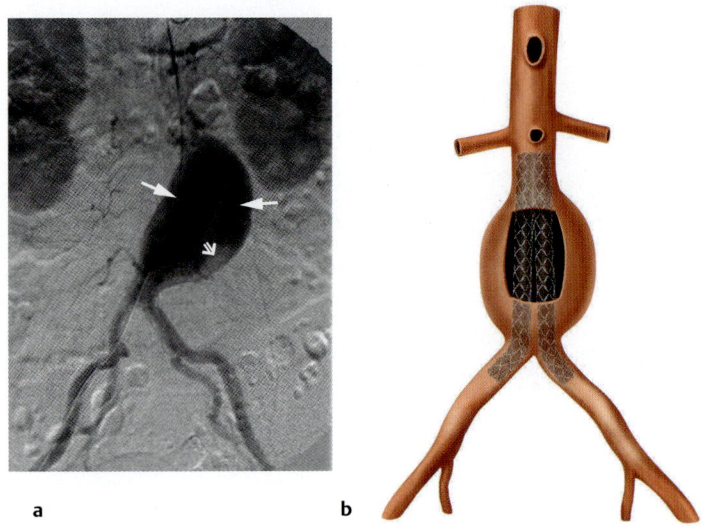

B Infrarenal aortic aneurysm: symptoms, diagnosis and treatment

a Evidence of a saccular infrarenal aortic aneurysm without involvement of the renal or pelvic arteries, obtained from digital subtraction angiography (DSA). Thrombotic deposits on the wall of the aneurysm are visible (from: Reiser M, Kuhn F, Debus J, eds. *Duale Reihe Radiologie*. 4th ed. Stuttgart: Thieme; 2017);

b Schematic representation of a vascular prosthesis for bypassing infrarenal aortic aneurysms (an aortoiliac bifurcation prosthesis).

Symptoms: abdominal aneurysms cause symptoms when the enlarged vessel compresses other structures (neighboring vertebrae) or organs (ureter, nerves, etc.) (Symptoms are typically thoracic or abdominal pain as well as back pain radiating in a belt-like fashion). Parietal thromboses can lead to embolisms with acute peripheral ischemia. However, a ruptured aneurysm manifests itself as constant severe pain (acute abdominal) and signs of shock.

Note: A ruptured aortic aneurysm is a severe and acute life-threatening emergency. Only immediate surgery can save the patient's life (surgical death rate between 30 and 50%).

Diagnosis: Most aortic aneurysms are diagnosed with the help of ultrasound examinations. This least invasive technique usually ensures a reliable assessment regarding localization and extent of the aneurysm. CT examination with contrast media is the preferred technique when assessing the size (relative to the perfused lumen and wall thrombosis) and relative anatomical positions of thoracic and abdominal aneurysms. Transarterial digital subtraction angiography (usually DSA) provides information about the vascular branches, particularly the renal arteries.

Treatment: The indication for treatment is based on the risk of rupture. Characteristic symptoms, distinct patterns of asymmetry (as shown here) as well as a diameter of more than 5 cm and rapid growth (more than 1 cm per year), are considered an absolute indication for surgery. The surgical procedure consists of resection of the aortic aneurysm and graft replacement. Nowadays, interventional therapy is often used to treat infrarenal aortic aneurysms. Using a femoral approach a catheter is placed into the aorta. With the help of the catheter a covered, fixed plastic prosthetic stent is positioned (endoluminal stent placement).

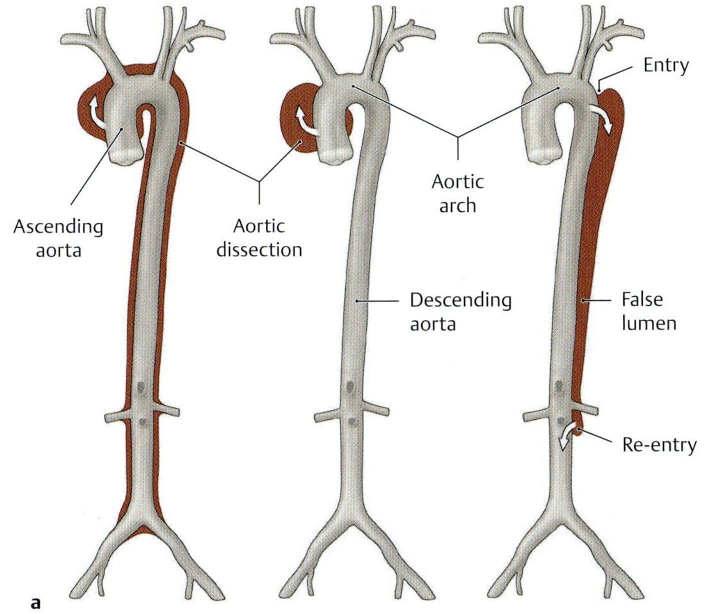

DeBakey:	I	II	III
Stanford:	Type A		Type B

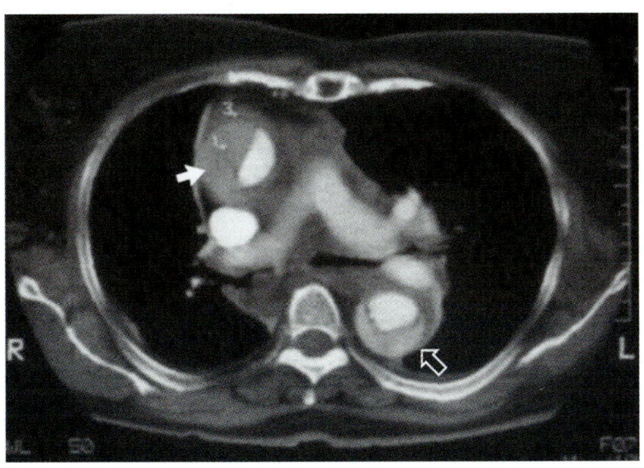

b

C Aortic dissection: Classification based on anatomical location

a Aortic dissections can be classified according to anatomical location in the Stanford or DeBakey systems. The most common is the **Stanford classification**, which is based on the location of the entry site of the dissection:

- Dissections involving the ascending aorta (Stanford type A, approximately 80% of cases)
- Dissections involving the descending aorta (Stanford type B, approximately 20% of cases).

The **DeBakey classification** further differentiates Stanford type A:

- DeBakey type I (involves the whole aorta) and
- DeBakey type II (involves the ascending aorta);
- DeBakey type III equals Stanford type B (dissection involves the descending aorta).

b Axial computed tomography (inferior view) of an aortic dissection type I according to DeBakey (Stanford type A) demonstrating the ascending (white arrow) and descending (open arrow) aortas: Delayed filling of the false lumen shows up as a lower density than the true lumen (from: Reiser M, Kuhn F, Debus J, eds. *Duale Reihe Radiologie*. 4th ed. Stuttgart: Thieme; 2017).

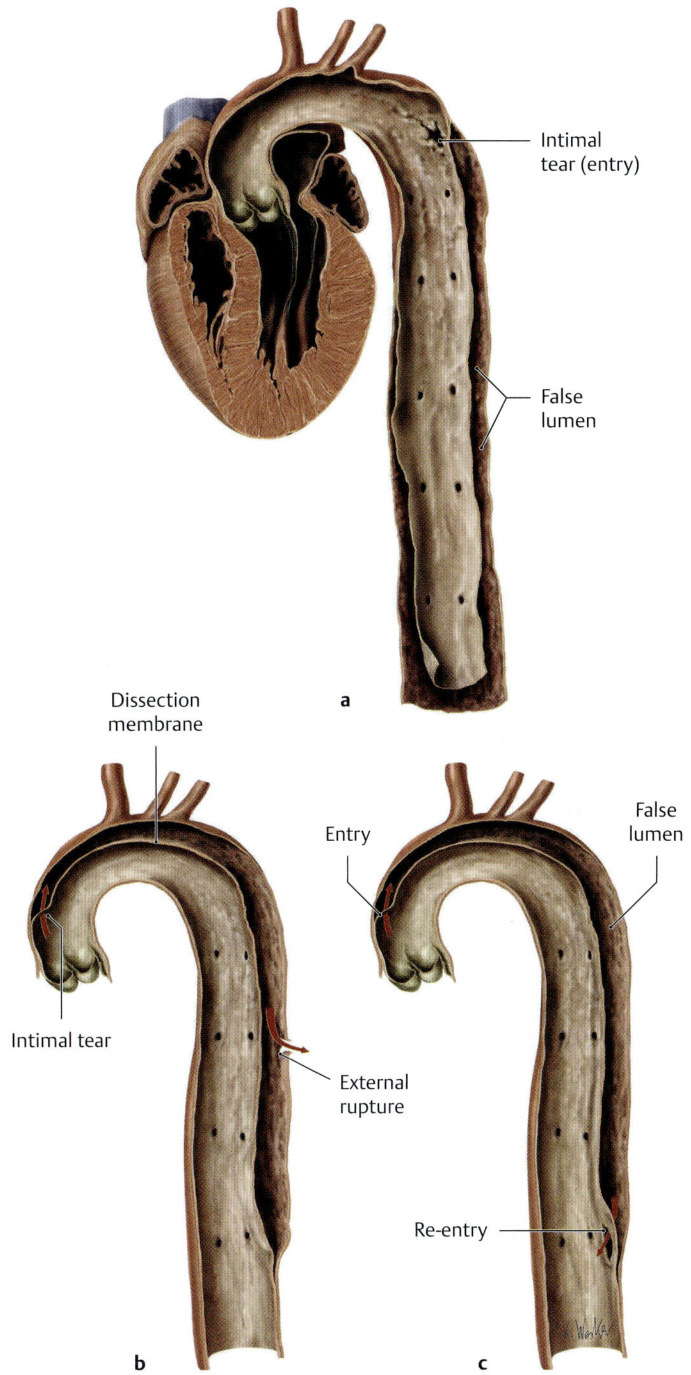

D Pathophysiology of aortic dissection

a Aortic dissection with intimal tear and false lumen; **b** Aortic dissection with intimal tear and rupture through outside wall; **c** Aortic dissection with intimal tear (entry) and re-entry tear.

In a classic aortic dissection (incidence of 2.6–3.5/100,000 population), arterial hypertension initially leads to degenerative changes in the layers of the aortic wall, which results in an intimal tear and a partial media tear. The aortic wall splits producing false and true lumens, which are separated by the dissection membrane. Depending on the location of the initial intimal tear, the whole aorta (intimal tear at the level of the thoracic aorta) or only the abdominal aorta is involved. Protrusion of the dissection membrane may lead to secondary occlusion of visceral branches resulting in ischemic syndromes. As the disease progresses, a perforation through the outside wall of the aorta (rupture and hemorrhage) or back into the true lumen (prognostically beneficial re-entry) may occur.

7.1 Cross Sections through the Thorax at the Level of Vertebrae T1–T2

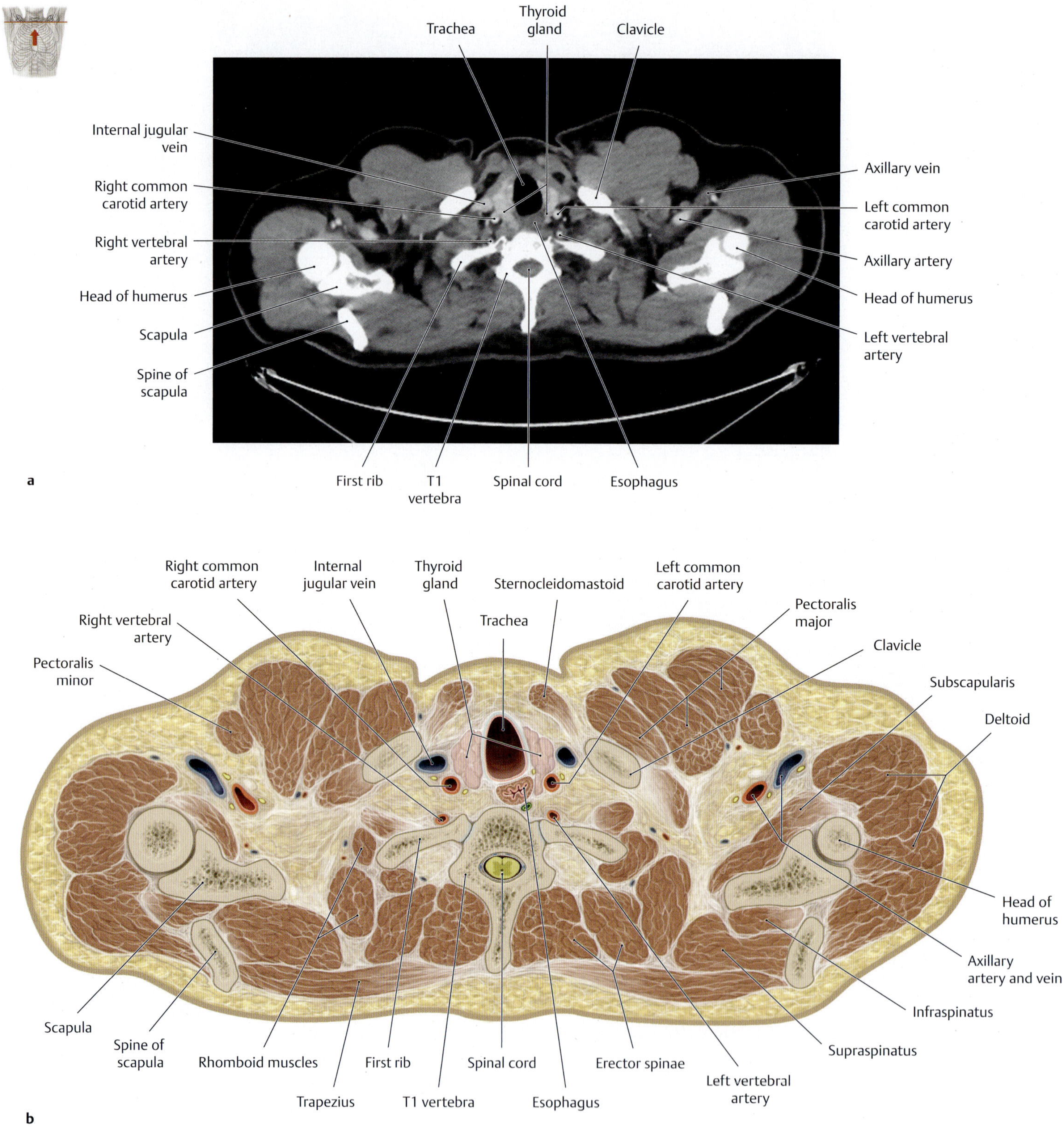

A Cross section through the thorax at the level of vertebra T1
a Axial (horizontal) CT image (soft tissue window); **b** horizontal section. Both are caudal views. In this plane the humeral head and scapula are sectioned. As the connection between the spine of the scapula and the rest of the scapula lies below the selected imaging plane, the spine of the scapula appears here as a separate bone. Anterior cervical viscera visualized here include the two lobes of the thyroid gland that lie adjacent to the trachea. Posterior structures include the common carotid arteries extending superiorly on each side. The esophagus courses posterior to the trachea. This visceral space is demarcated anteriorly by the two sternocleidomastoid muscles.

We thank Prof. S. Müller-Hülsbeck, M.D., Institut für Diagnostische und Interventionelle Radiologie/Neuroradiologie, DIAKO Krankenhaus gGmbH Flensburg, for kindly providing the CT images in Chapter 7.

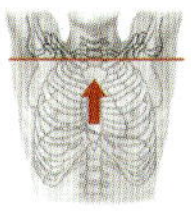

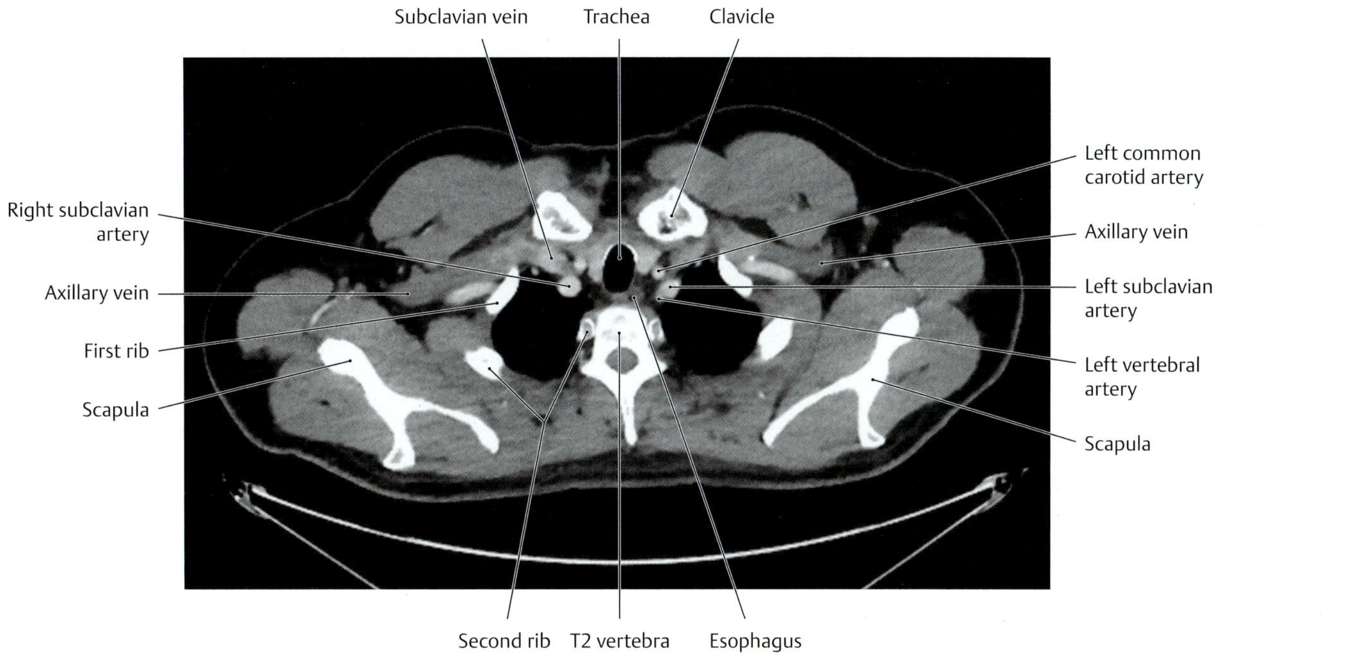

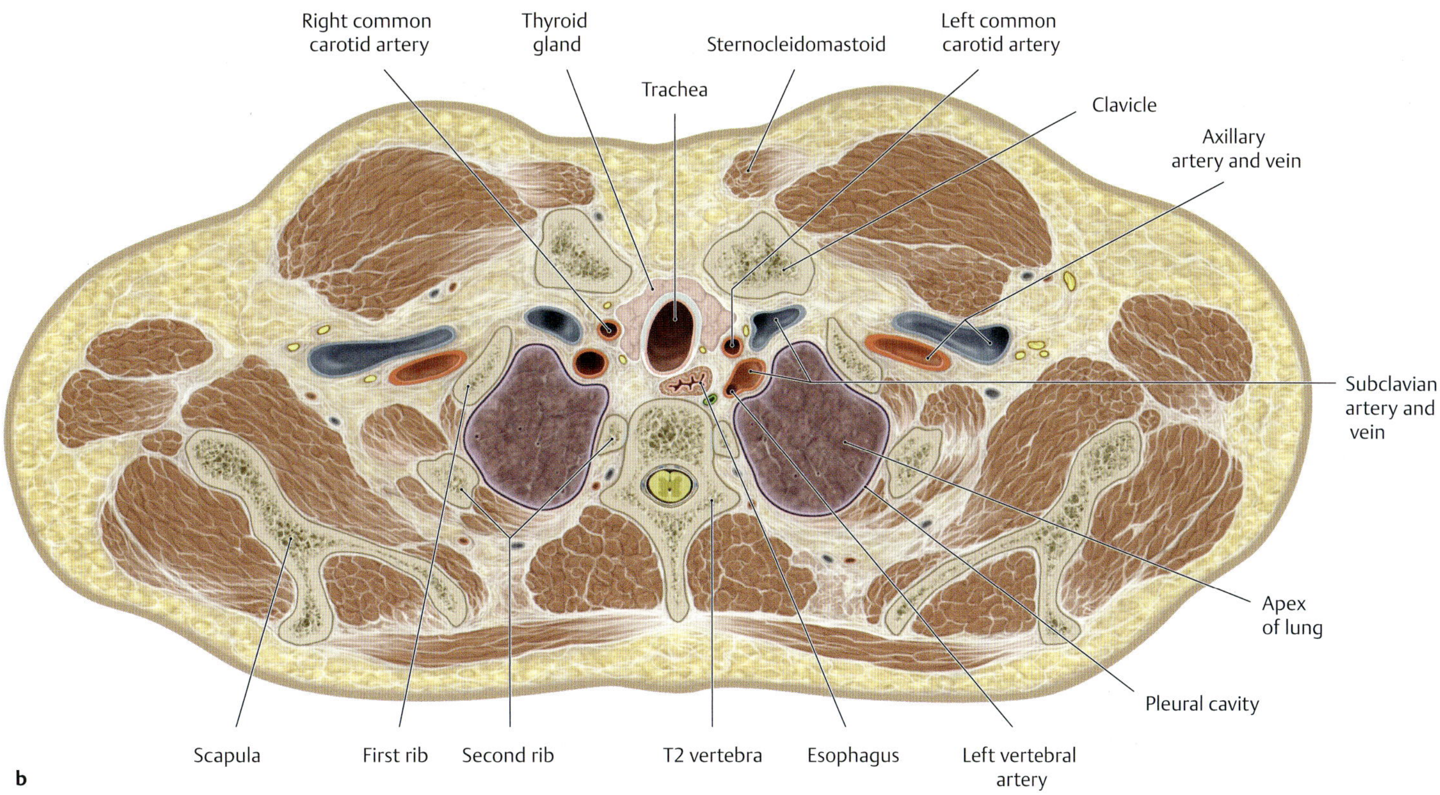

B Cross section through the thorax at the level of vertebra T2

a Axial (horizontal) CT image (soft tissue window); **b** horizontal section. Both are caudal views. The clavicle as well as the first and second ribs are sectioned due to the thoracic kyphosis, whereas the sternum is not. We are in the superior portion of the oblique plane of the superior thoracic aperture. The inferior pole of the two lobes of the thyroid gland are covered on each side anteriorly by the sternocleidomastoid muscles. The apexes of both lungs are sectioned; both extend past the superior thoracic aperture. The subclavian artery and vein course from medial to lateral. Slightly superior to this level the subclavian vein courses directly over the apexes of the lungs, which at that location are separated from the subclavian vein only by the fascia of Sibson. Due to this close topographical proximity approximately every tenth puncture of the subclavian vein results in pneumothorax (therefore proper placement of a subclavian vein catheter should be verified by fluoroscopy).

7.2 Cross Sections through the Thorax at the Level of Vertebrae T3–T4

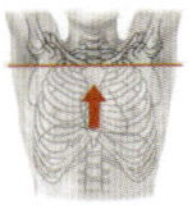

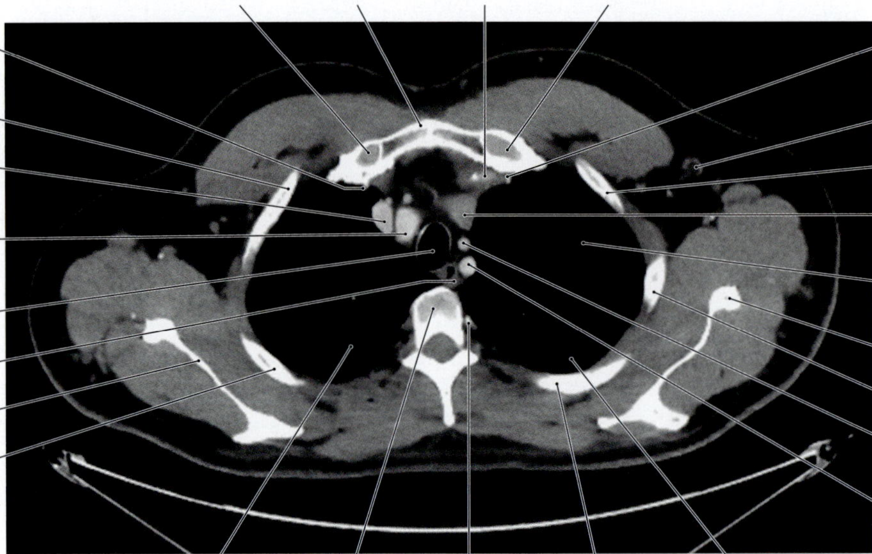

a

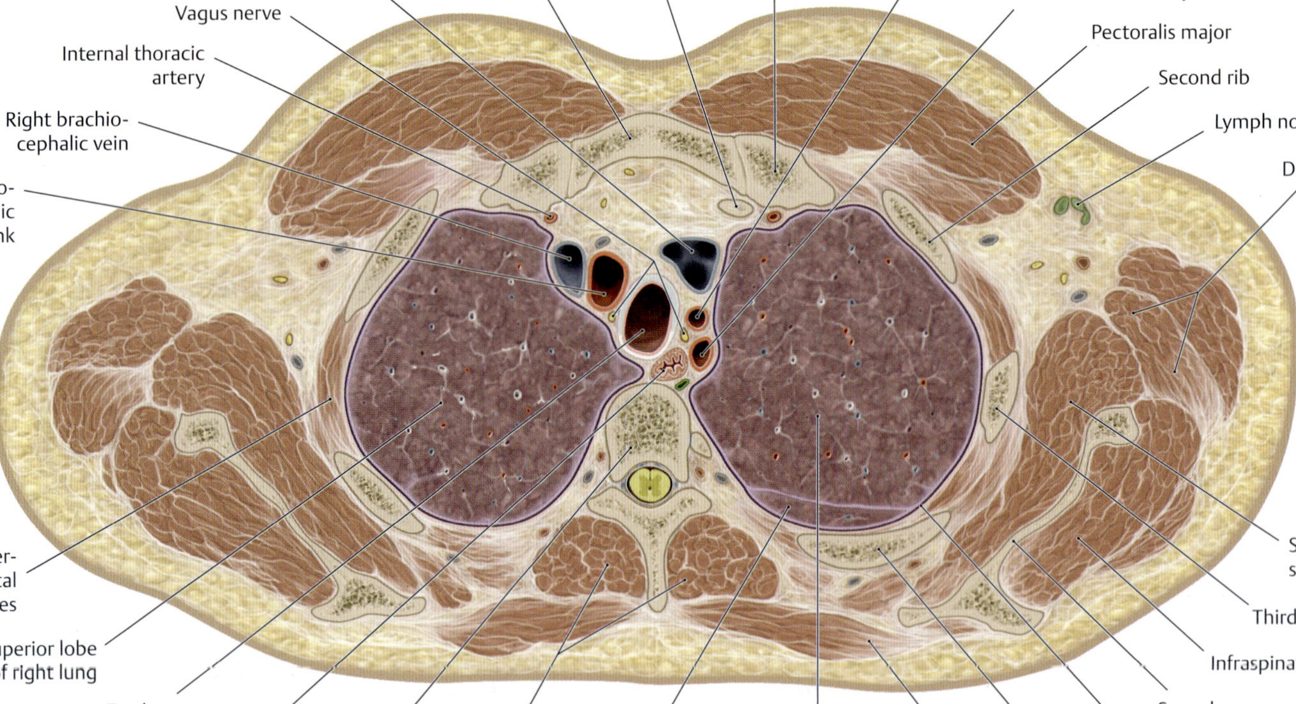

b

A Cross section through the thorax at the level of vertebra T3

a Axial (horizontal) CT image (soft tissue window); **b** horizontal section. Both are caudal views. Sectioned skeletal structures include the scapula, vertebra T3, the first through fourth ribs, and the sternum. We are in the plane of the inferior portion of the superior thoracic aperture. The intercostal musculature is found between the sectioned ribs. Major neurovascular structures visualized here include the brachiocephalic trunk, the common carotid artery on the left, and the subclavian artery. As the subclavian artery is sectioned tangentially here, it appears larger than the common carotid artery. The vagus nerve is found on either side of the trachea (not visualized on the CT image).

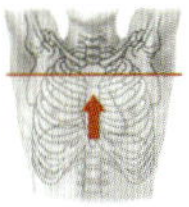

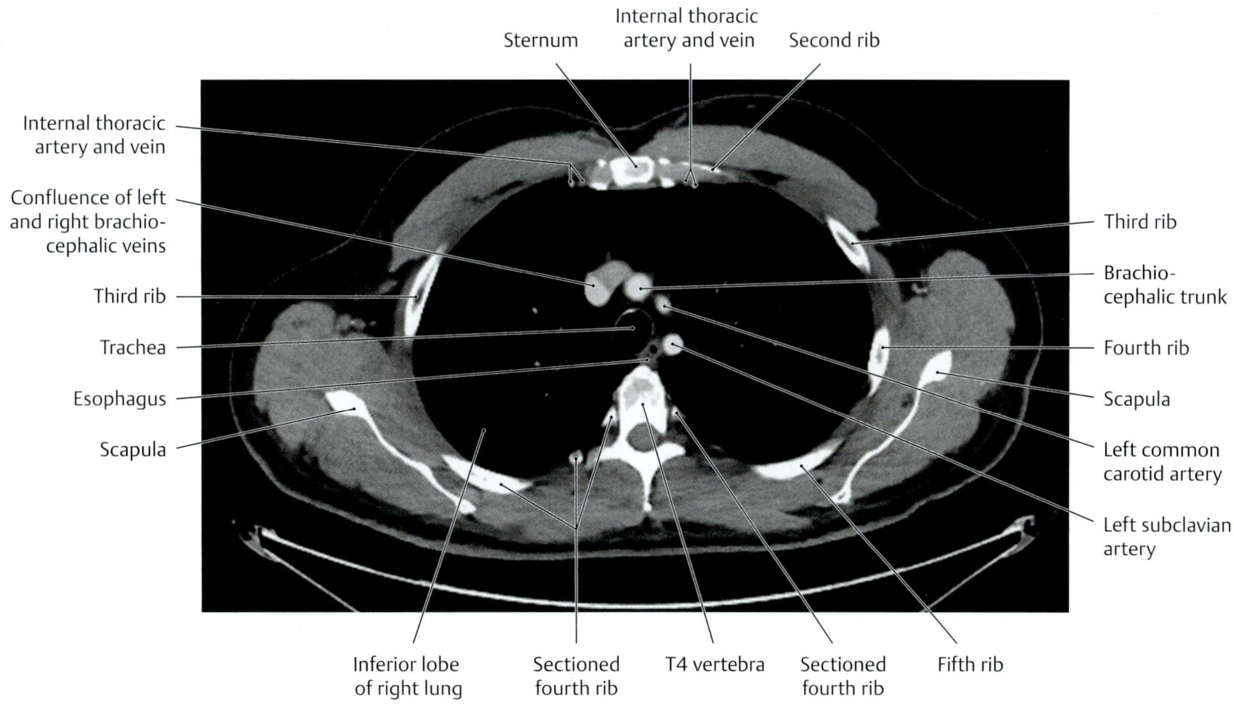

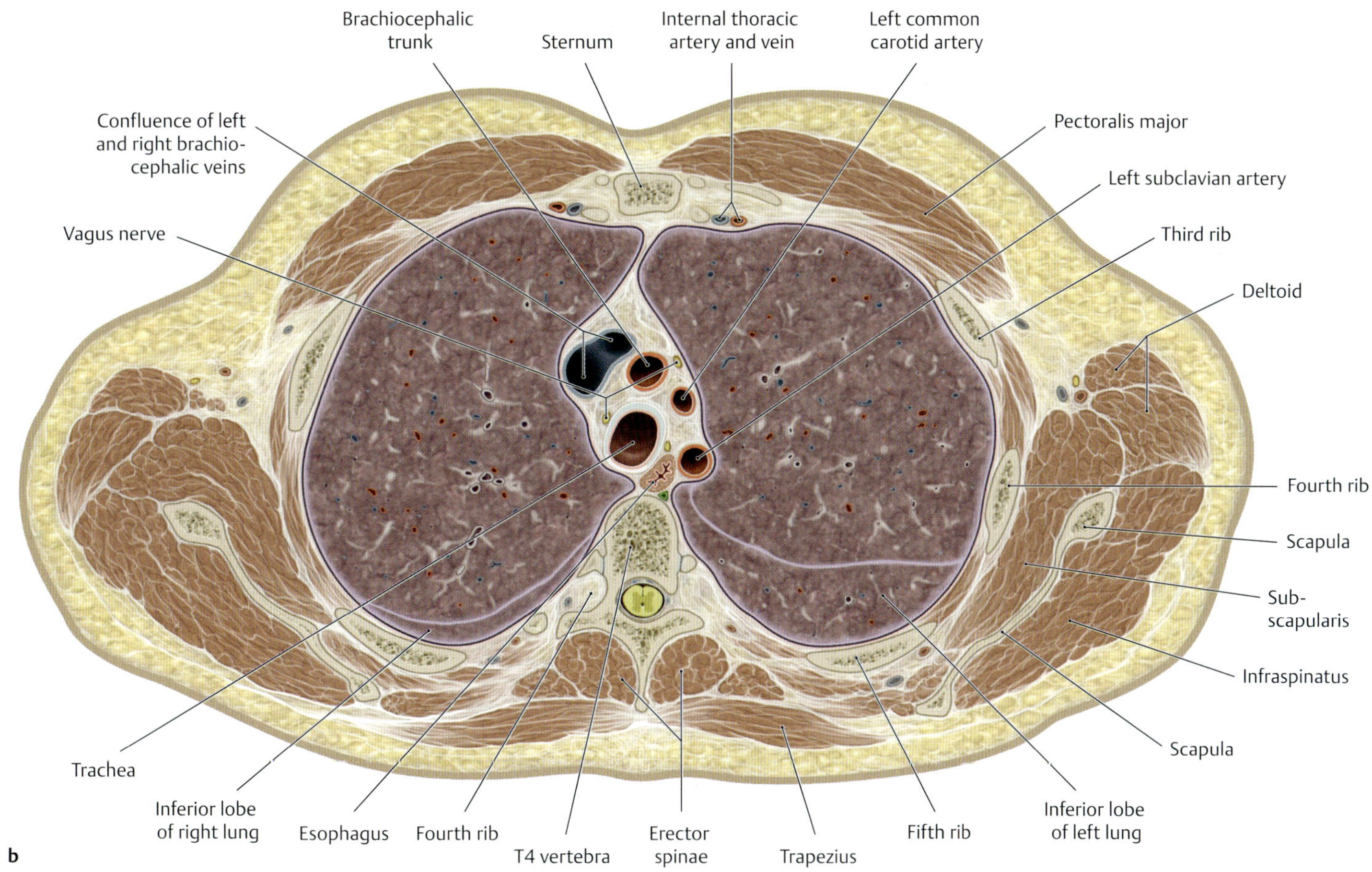

B Cross section through the thorax at the level of vertebra T4

a Axial (horizontal) CT image (soft tissue window); **b** horizontal section. Both are caudal views. The sternum, fourth rib, and vertebra T4 are sectioned. The following structures in the superior mediastinum are of particular interest: The esophagus is directly adjacent to the vertebra; anterior to it lies the trachea, accompanied on both sides by the vagus nerve. The vessels anterior and adjacent to the trachea are important: the confluence of the left and right brachiocephalic veins, the brachiocephalic trunk, and the left common carotid artery behind it as well as the subclavian artery which has just arisen from that artery.

7.3 Cross Sections through the Thorax at the Level of Vertebrae T5–T6

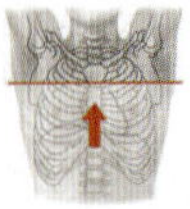

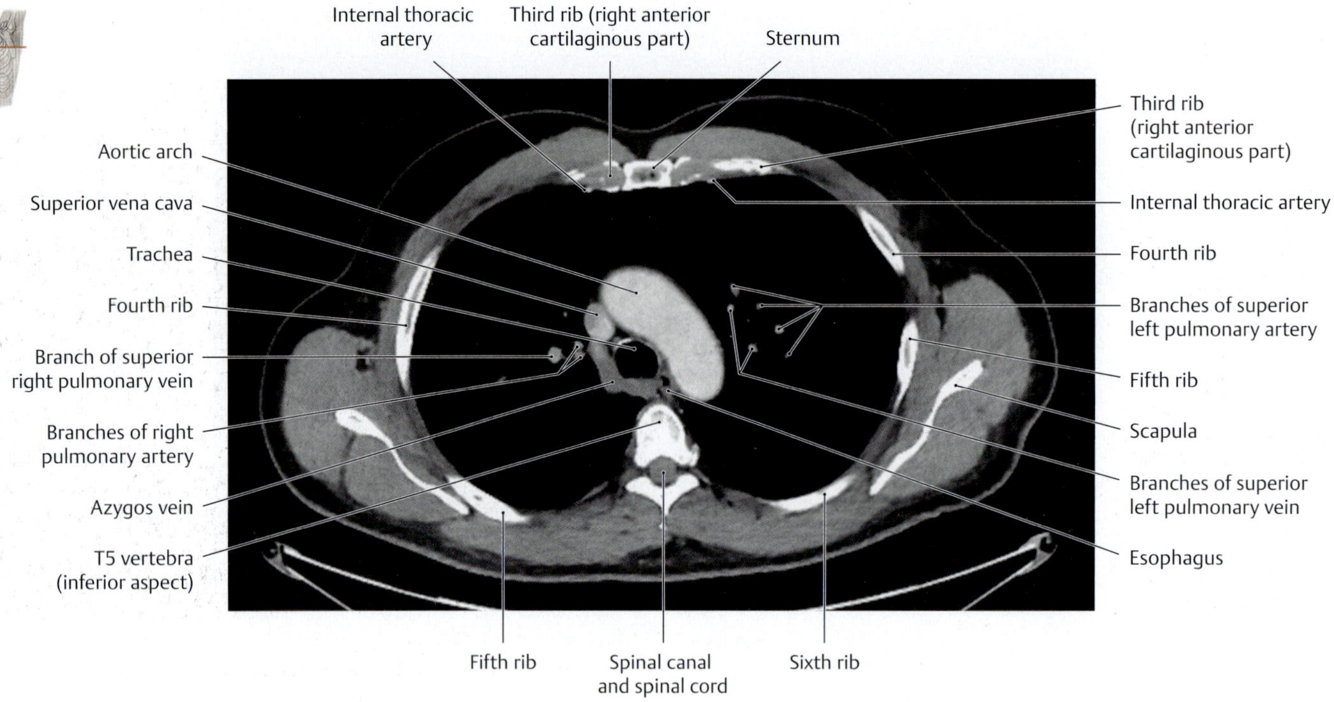

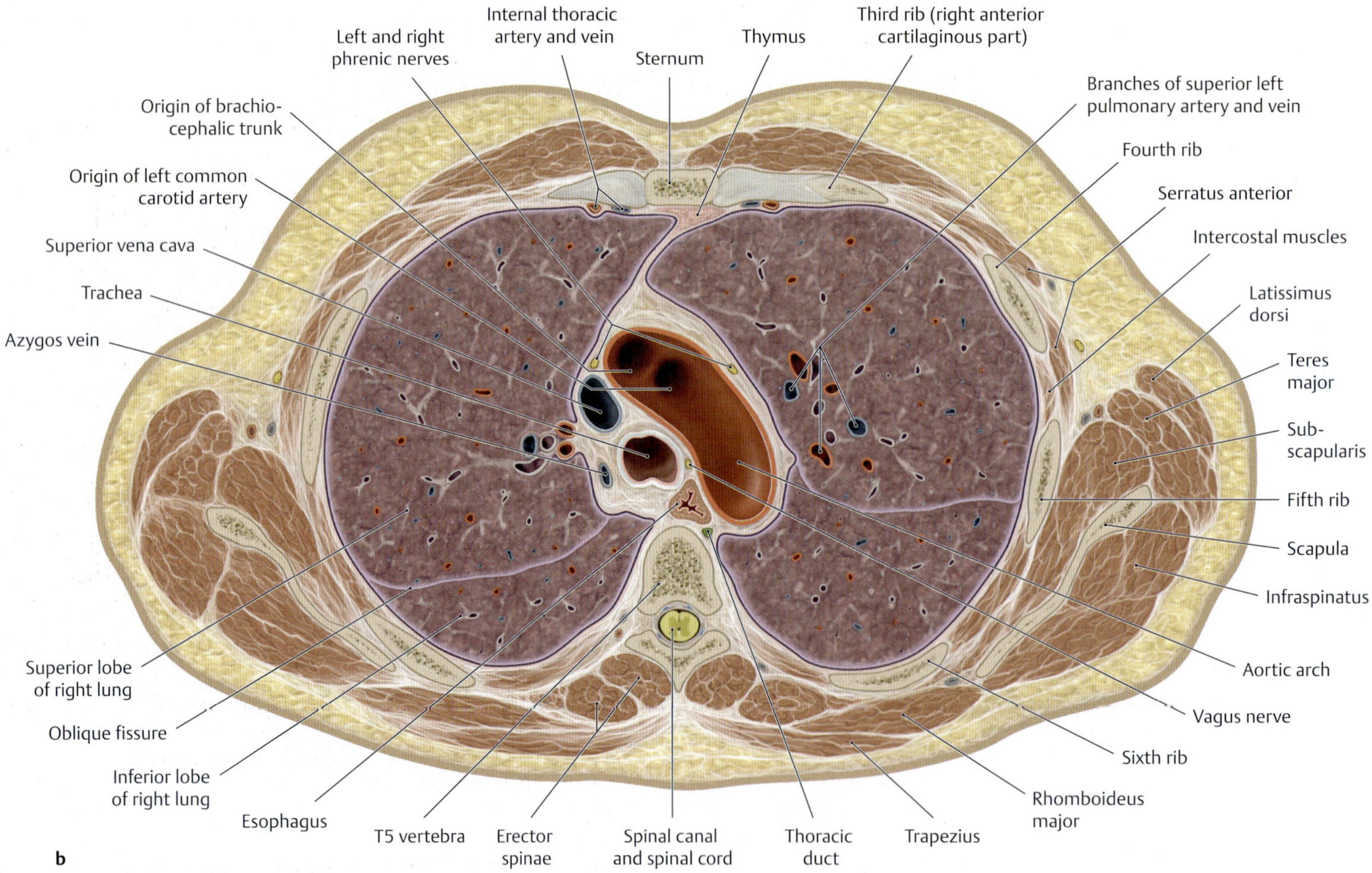

A Cross section through the thorax at the level of vertebra T5
a Axial (horizontal) CT image (soft tissue window); **b** horizontal section. Both are caudal views. The superior vena cava, aortic arch, esophagus, and thymus all lie in the superior mediastinum (for the contents of the superior mediastinum, see p. 196).

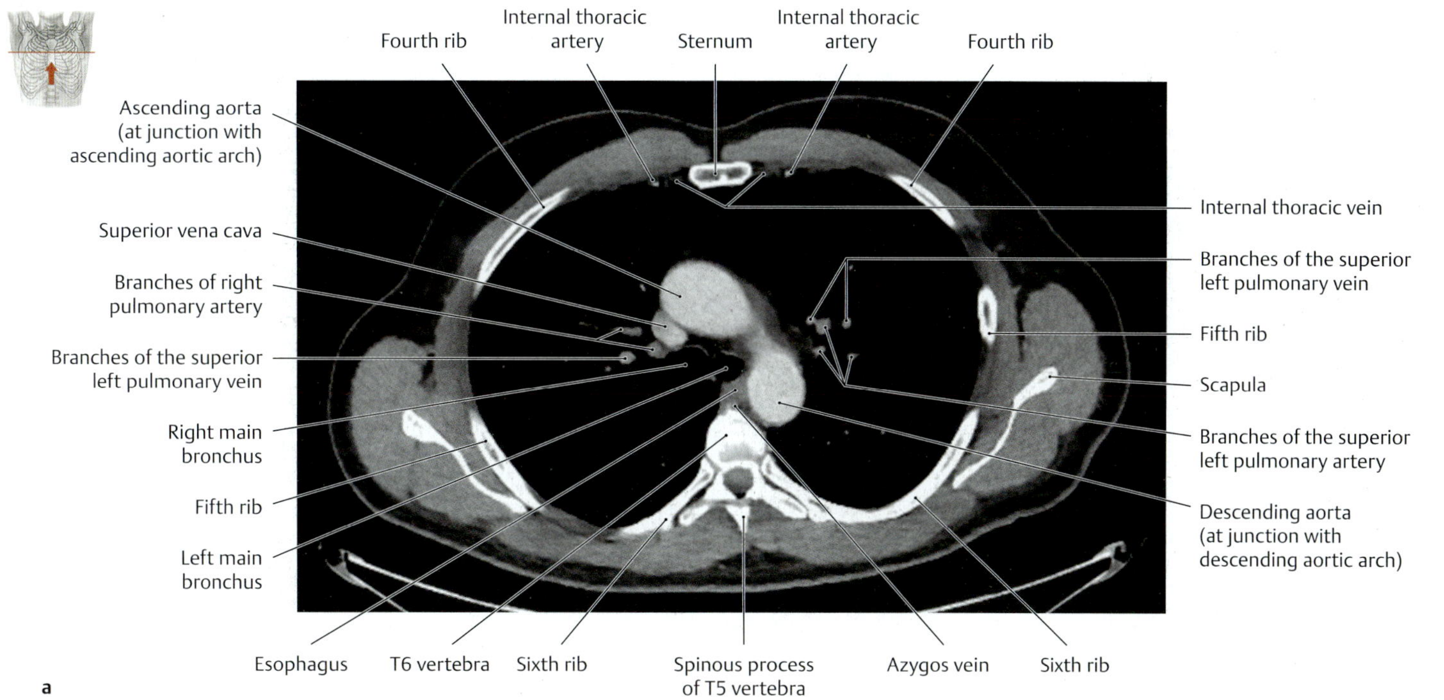

a

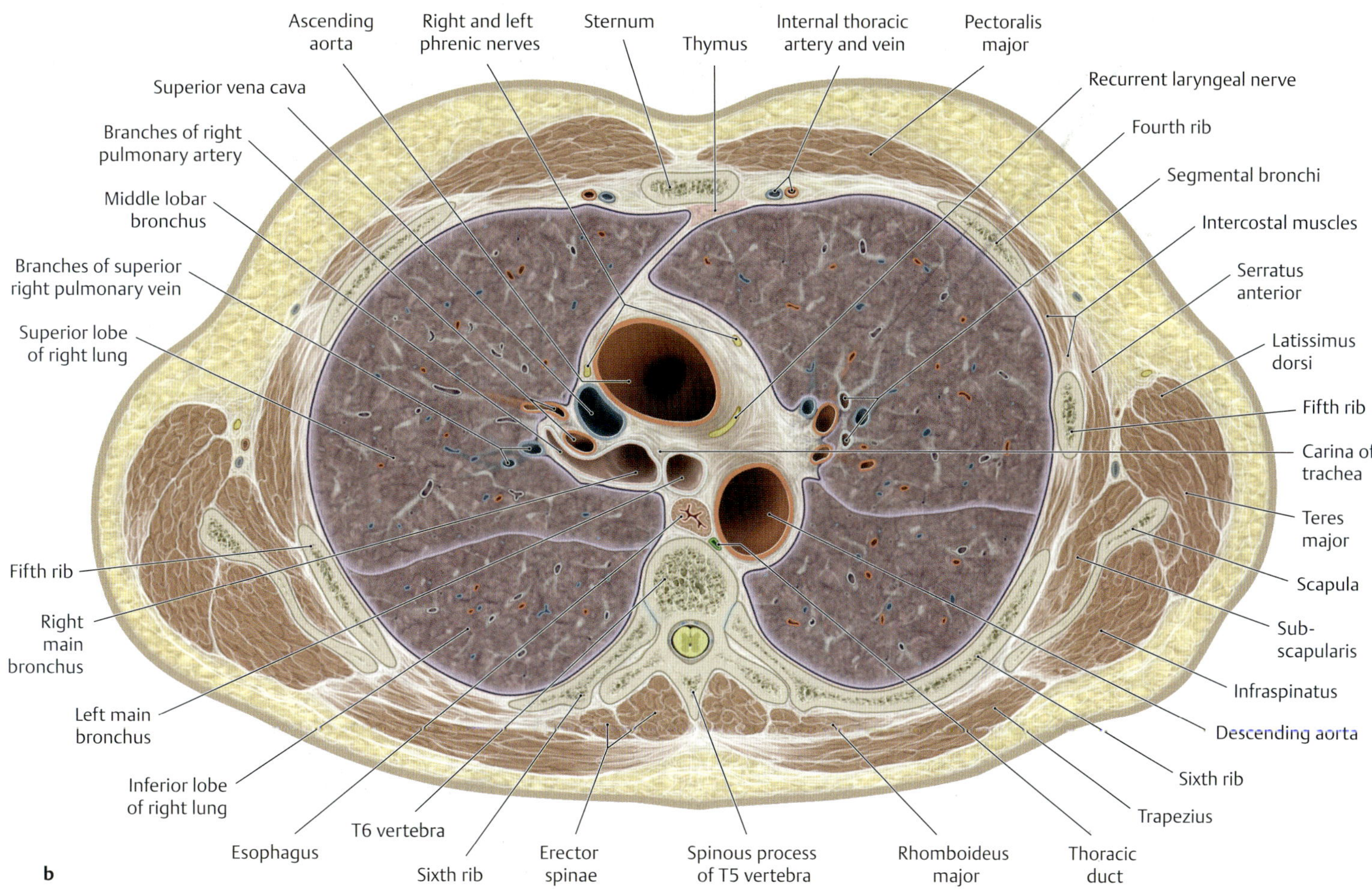

b

B Cross section through the thorax at the level of vertebra T6
a Axial (horizontal) CT image (soft tissue window); **b** horizontal section. Both are caudal views. The thoracic artery and vein (mammary artery and vein) are located in the anterior thorax, directly posterior to the sternum. The superior vena cava right lies anterior to the main bronchus, and the aortic arch lies anterior to the vein. The esophagus and thoracic duct are located posterior to the left main bronchus, and posterior and lateral to them lies the descending aorta.

7.4 Cross Sections through the Thorax at the Level of Vertebrae T6–T7

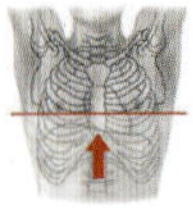

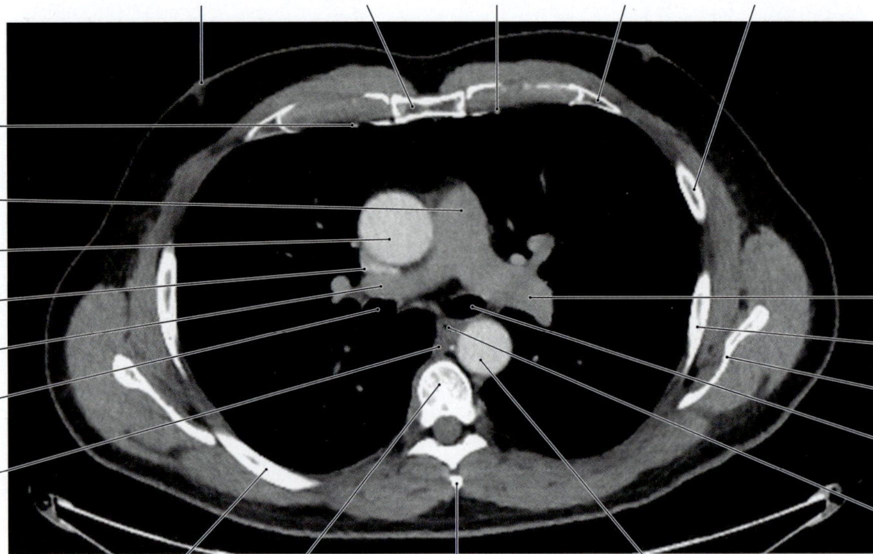

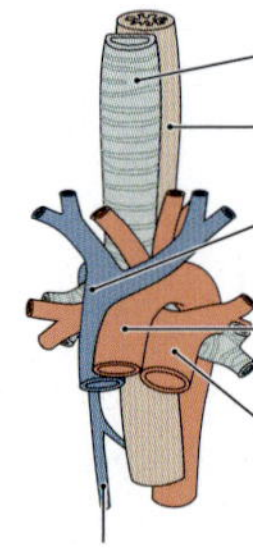

a

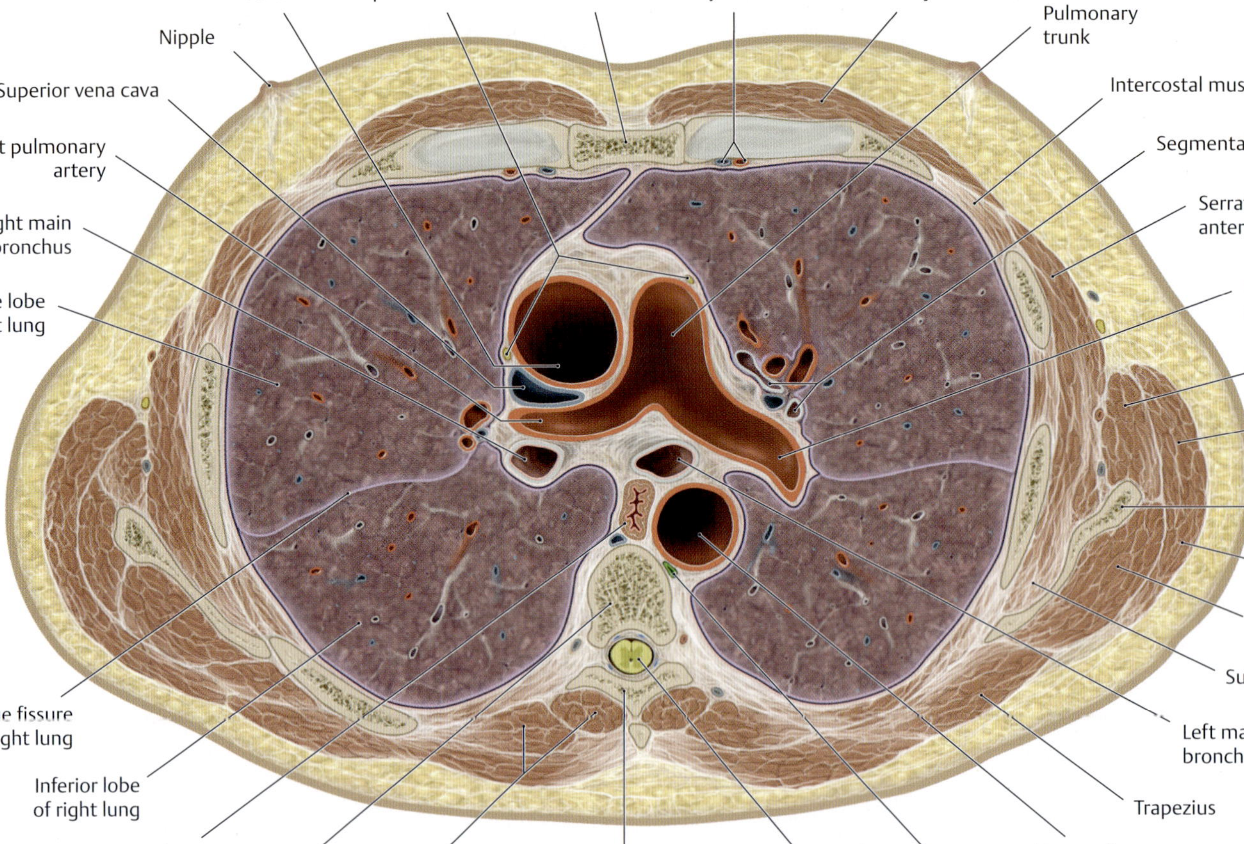

b

A Cross section through the thorax at the level of vertebra T6
a Axial (horizontal) CT image (soft tissue window); **b** horizontal section. Both are caudal views. The pulmonary trunk splits into the right and left pulmonary arteries. The superior vena cava lies anterior to the right pulmonary artery, followed by the ascending aorta. The phrenic nerves lie lateral to the aorta; the esophagus and descending aorta lie posterior to the left main bronchus.

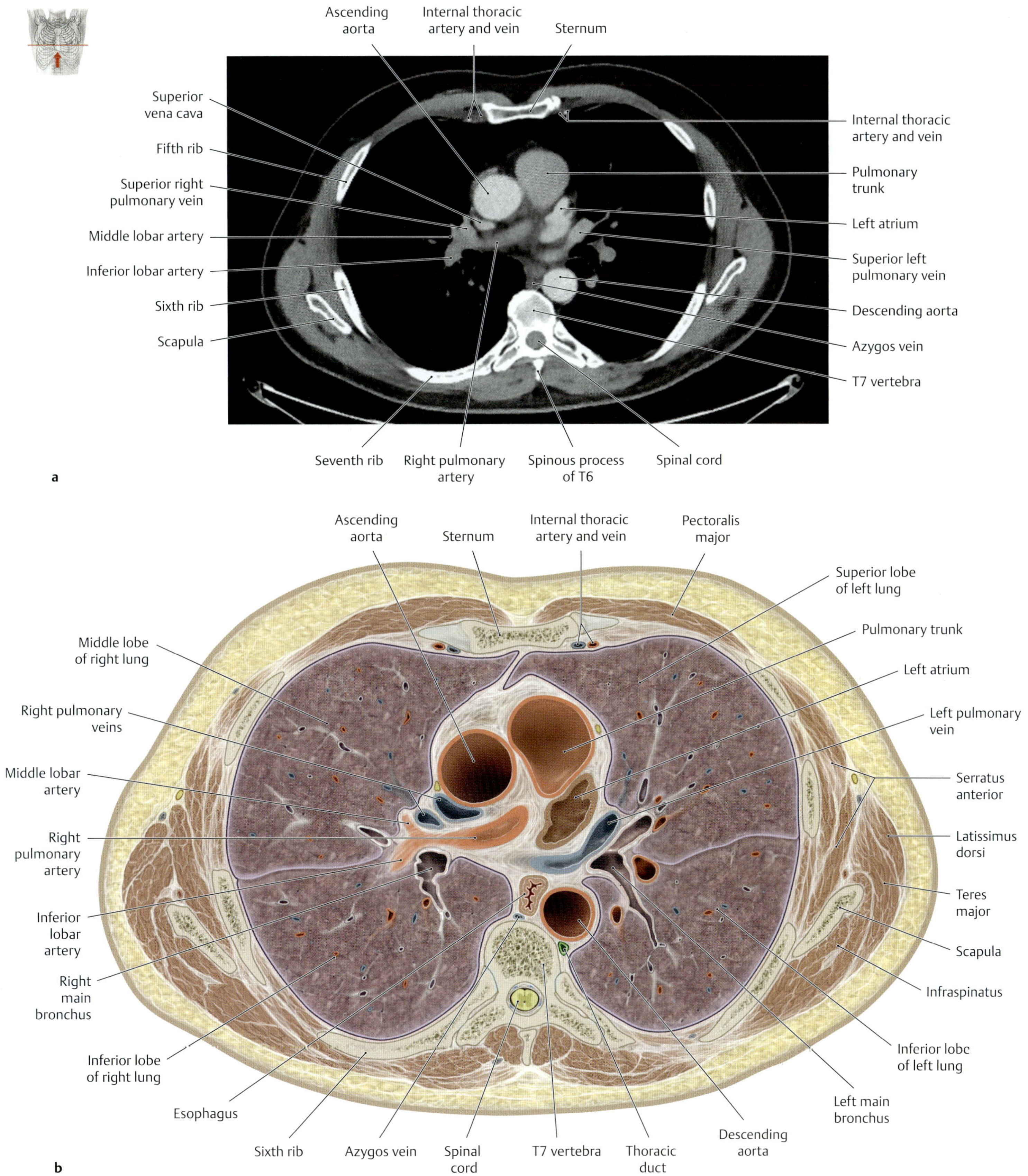

B Cross section through the thorax at the level of vertebra T7

a Axial (horizontal) CT image (soft tissue window); **b** horizontal section. Both are caudal views. The two main bronchi and their branches are sectioned. The pulmonary trunk and right pulmonary artery should be used as anatomic landmarks. Between the two structures lies the ascending aorta; the left pulmonary vein and left atrium lie posterior to it. The left pulmonary vein is immediately posterior to the left atrium, followed by the esophagus and descending aorta. Medial to it lies the azygos vein, and posterior to it lies the thoracic duct, which is not visualized on the CT image.

7.5 Cross Sections through the Thorax at the Level of Vertebra T8

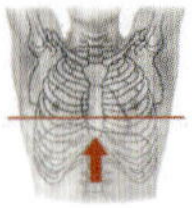

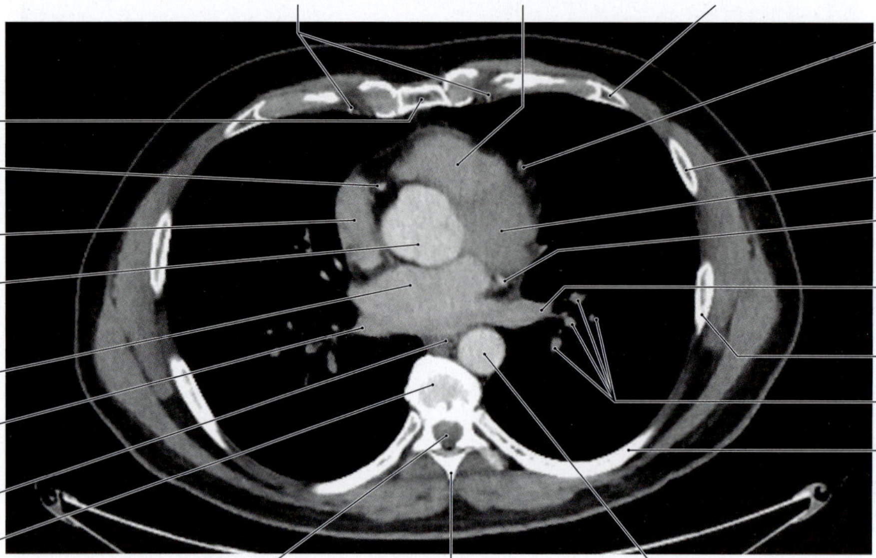

a

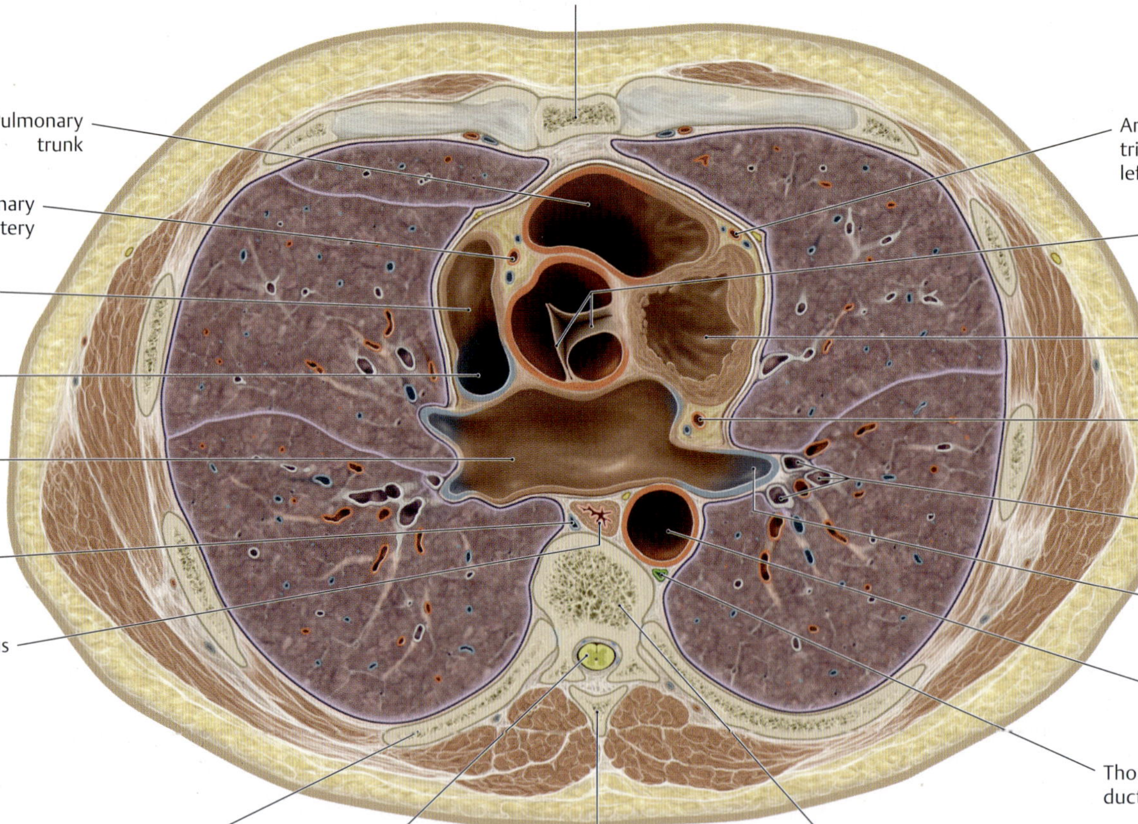

b

A Cross section through the thorax at the level of vertebra T8
a Axial (horizontal) CT image (soft tissue window); **b** horizontal section. Both are caudal views. The right coronary artery is sectioned in the connective tissue space adjacent to the heart between the right atrium and the pulmonary trunk. Posterior to the right atrium lies the left atrium, and the esophagus and descending aorta are located posterior to it. The thoracic duct lies posterior to the descending aorta but is not visualized on the CT image.

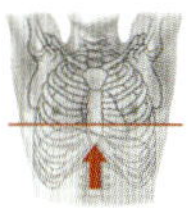

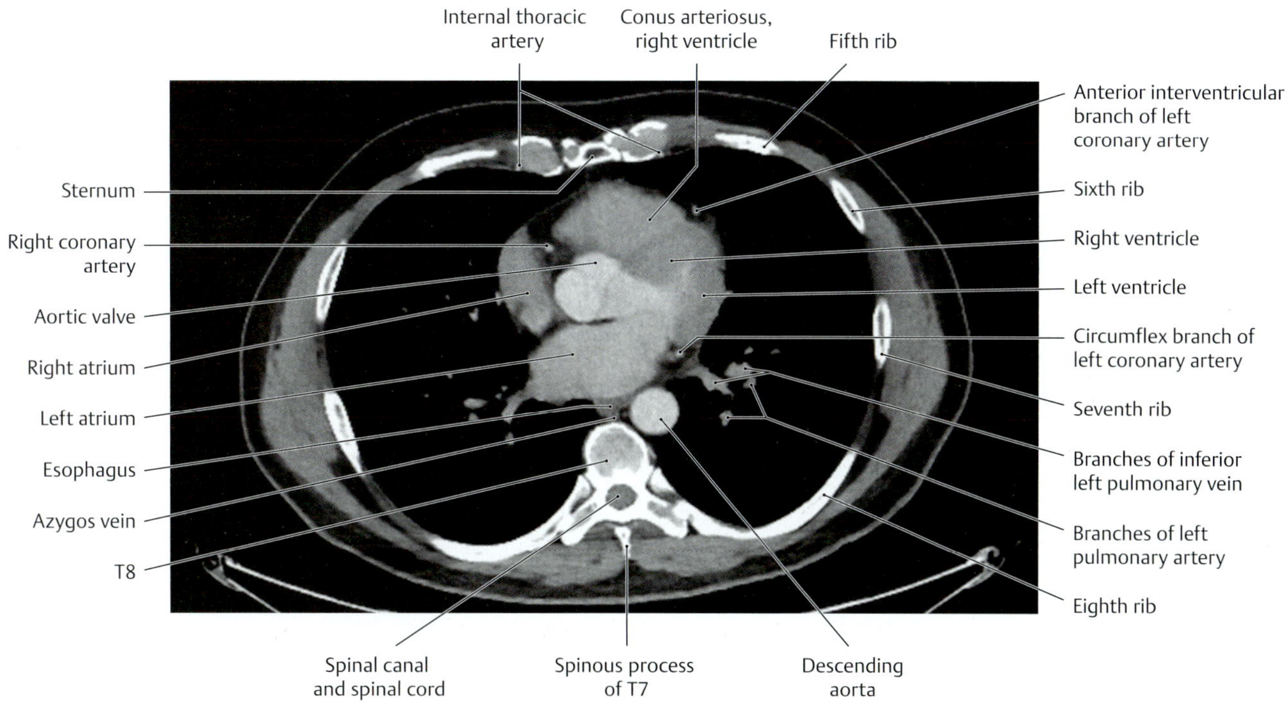

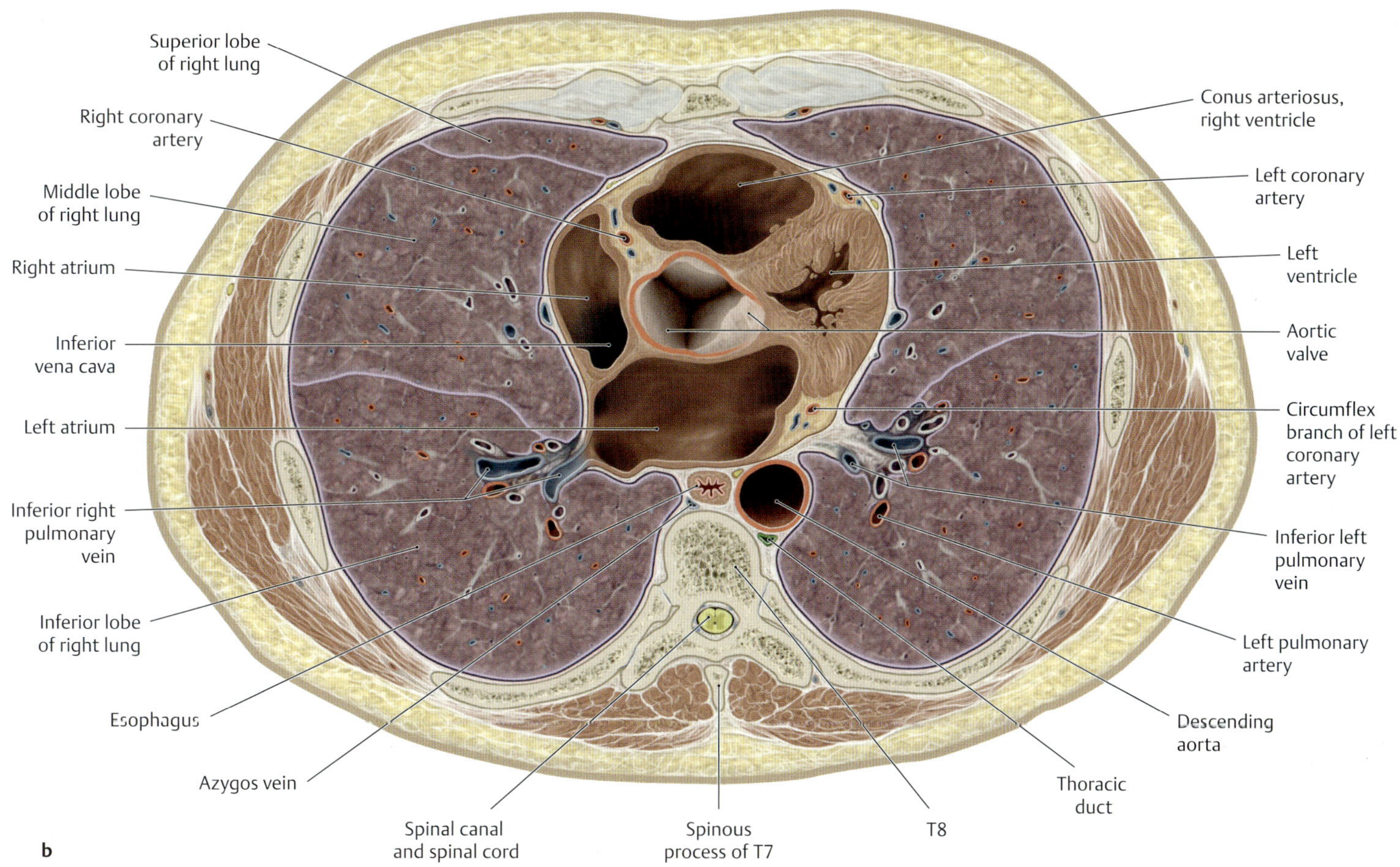

B Cross section through the thorax at the level of vertebra T8

a Axial (horizontal) CT image (soft tissue window); **b** horizontal section. Both are caudal views. Sectioned midline structures from anterior to posterior include the conus arteriosus of the right ventricle, the aortic valve of the left ventricle, and the left atrium. The right atrium is located to the right lateral to these midline structures. The superior and inferior pulmonary veins enter the left atrium on both sides, whereby the opening of the left pulmonary veins is not visualized here. The azygos vein, esophagus, and descending aorta lie posterior to the left atrium. The right coronary artery is sectioned at the posterior margin of the conus arteriosus. The superior lobe of the right lung is barely sectioned in this view.

7.6 Cross Sections through the Thorax at the Level of Vertebrae T9–T10

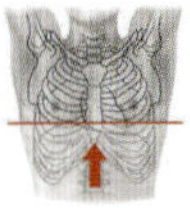

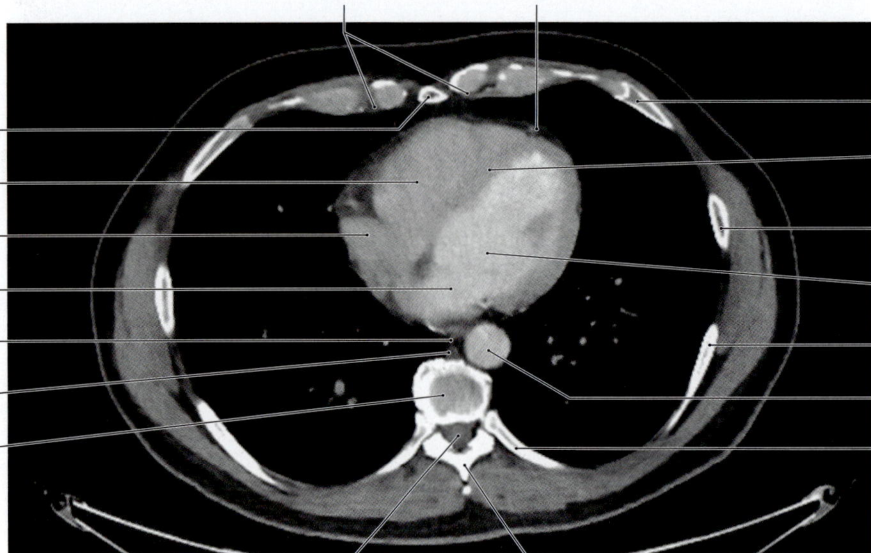

a

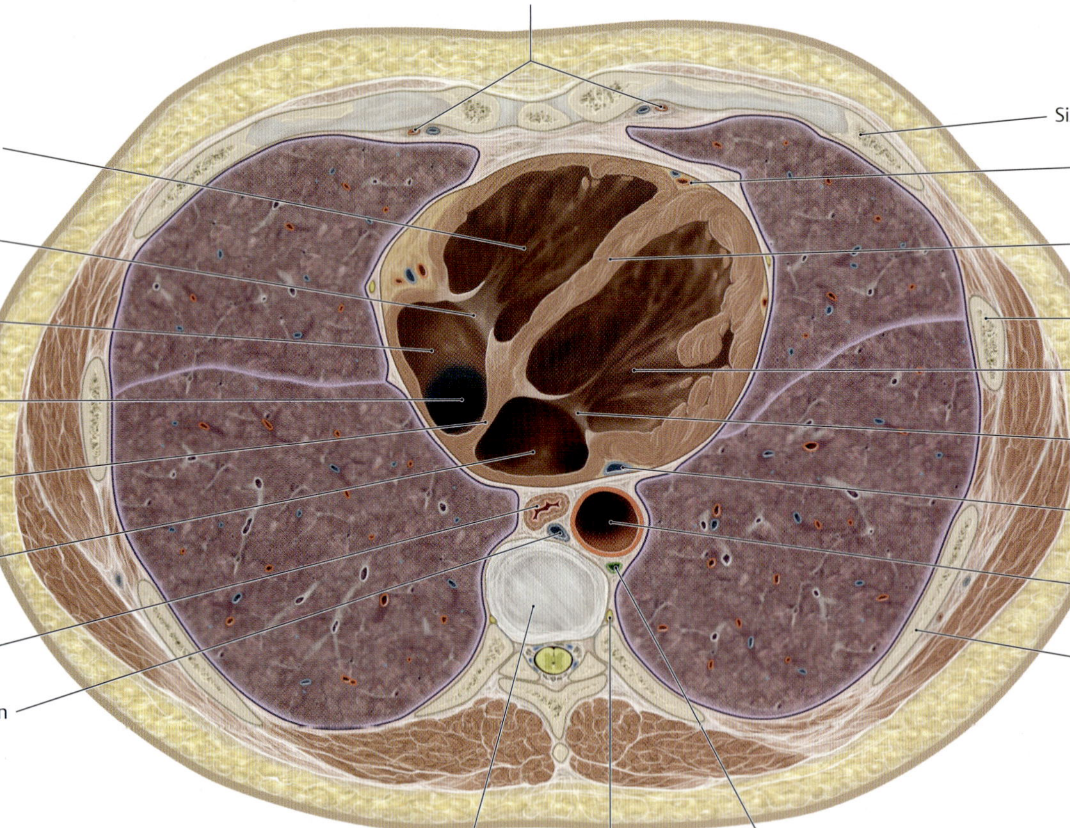

b

A Cross section through the thorax at the level of vertebra T9
a Axial (horizontal) CT image (soft tissue window); **b** horizontal section. Both are caudal views. The right ventricle with its sectioned tricuspid valve is directly adjacent to the sternum and ribs. The right atrium is located posterolateral to it on the right. Left of and lateral to right ventricle and separated by the interventricular septum lies the left ventricle with the bicuspid valve separating it from the left atrium, which lies posterior. The descending aorta, azygos vein, thoracic duct, and sympathetic trunk lie posterior to the heart.

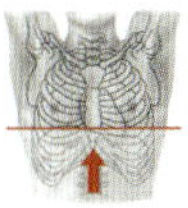

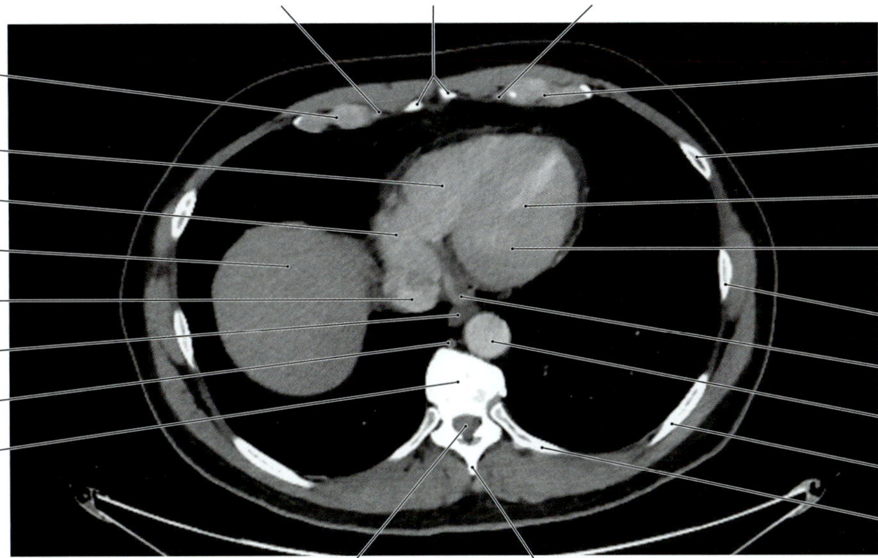

a

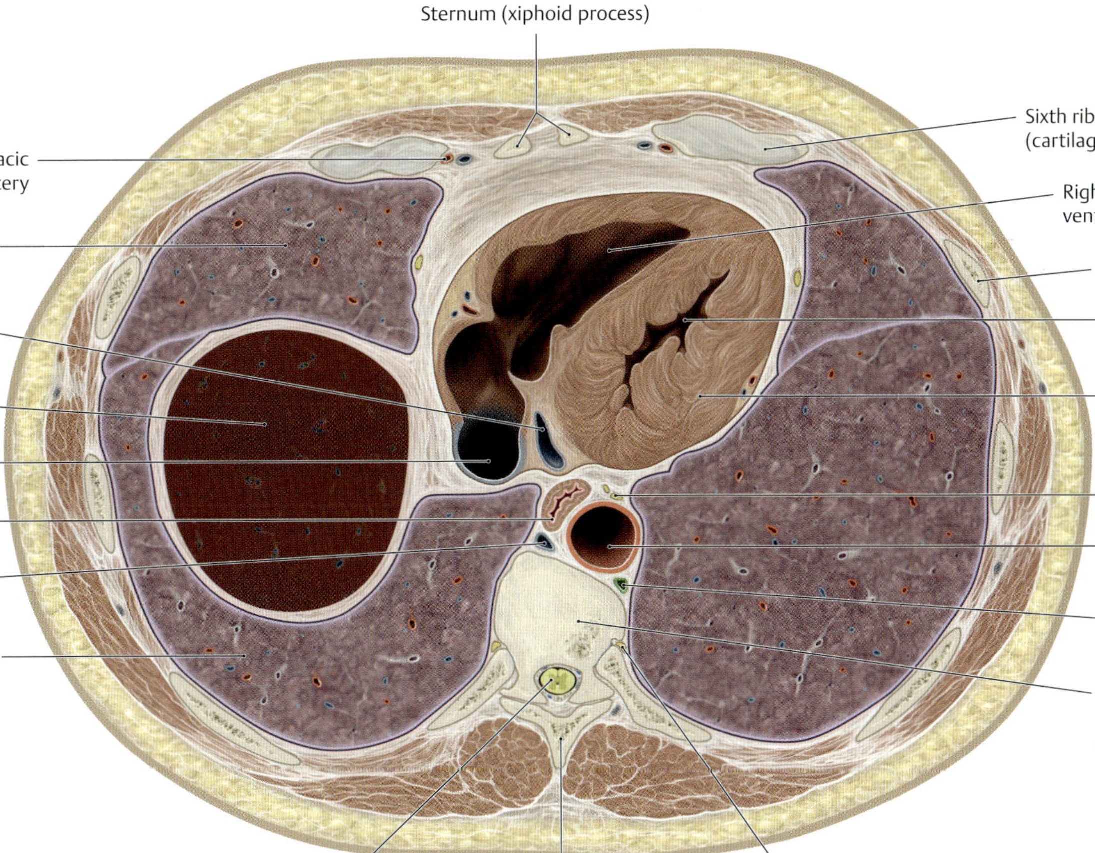

b

B Cross section through the thorax at the level of vertebra T10

a Axial (horizontal) CT image (soft tissue window); **b** horizontal section. Both are caudal views. At this level the inferior vena cava is sectioned again; it lies posterior to the right atrium. The coronary sinus lying medial to it is also sectioned, and a large portion of the left ventricular myocardial musculature is also sectioned tangentially. A section of the liver is also visualized for the first time in this view.

7.7 Cross Sections through the Thorax at the Level of Vertebrae T10–T11

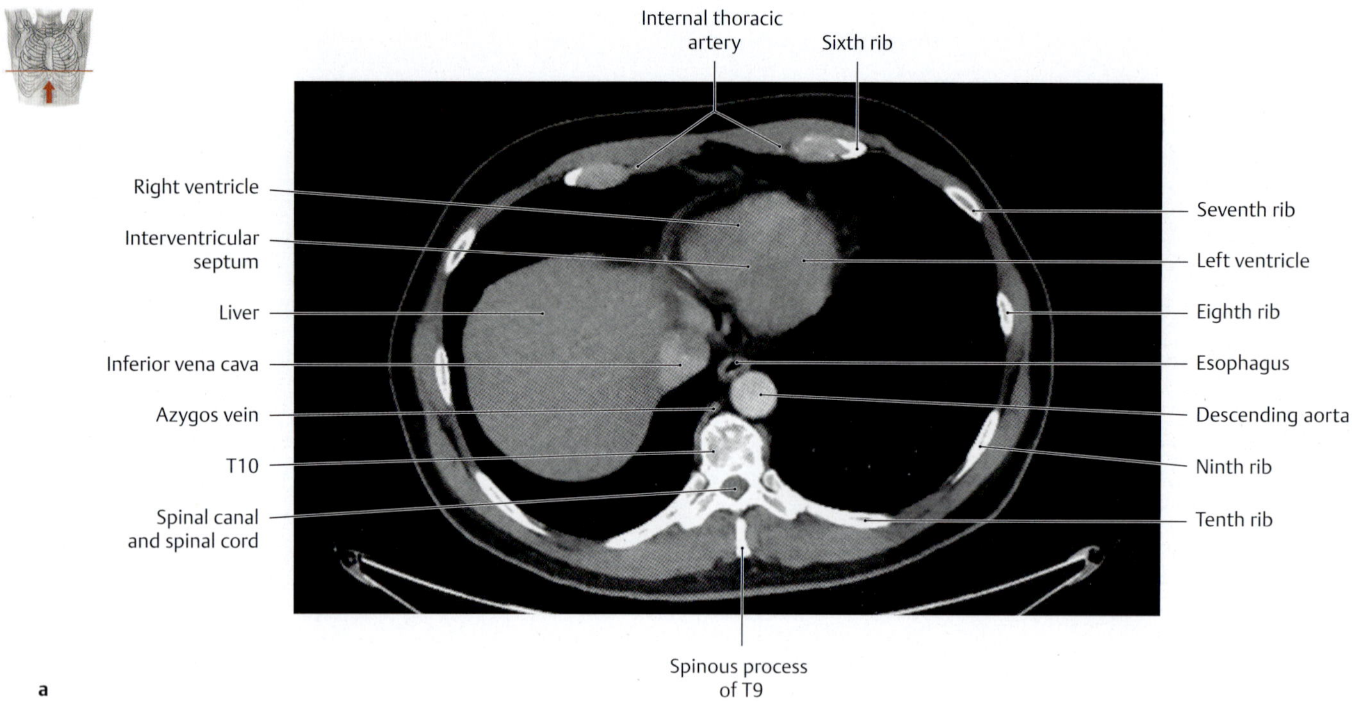

a

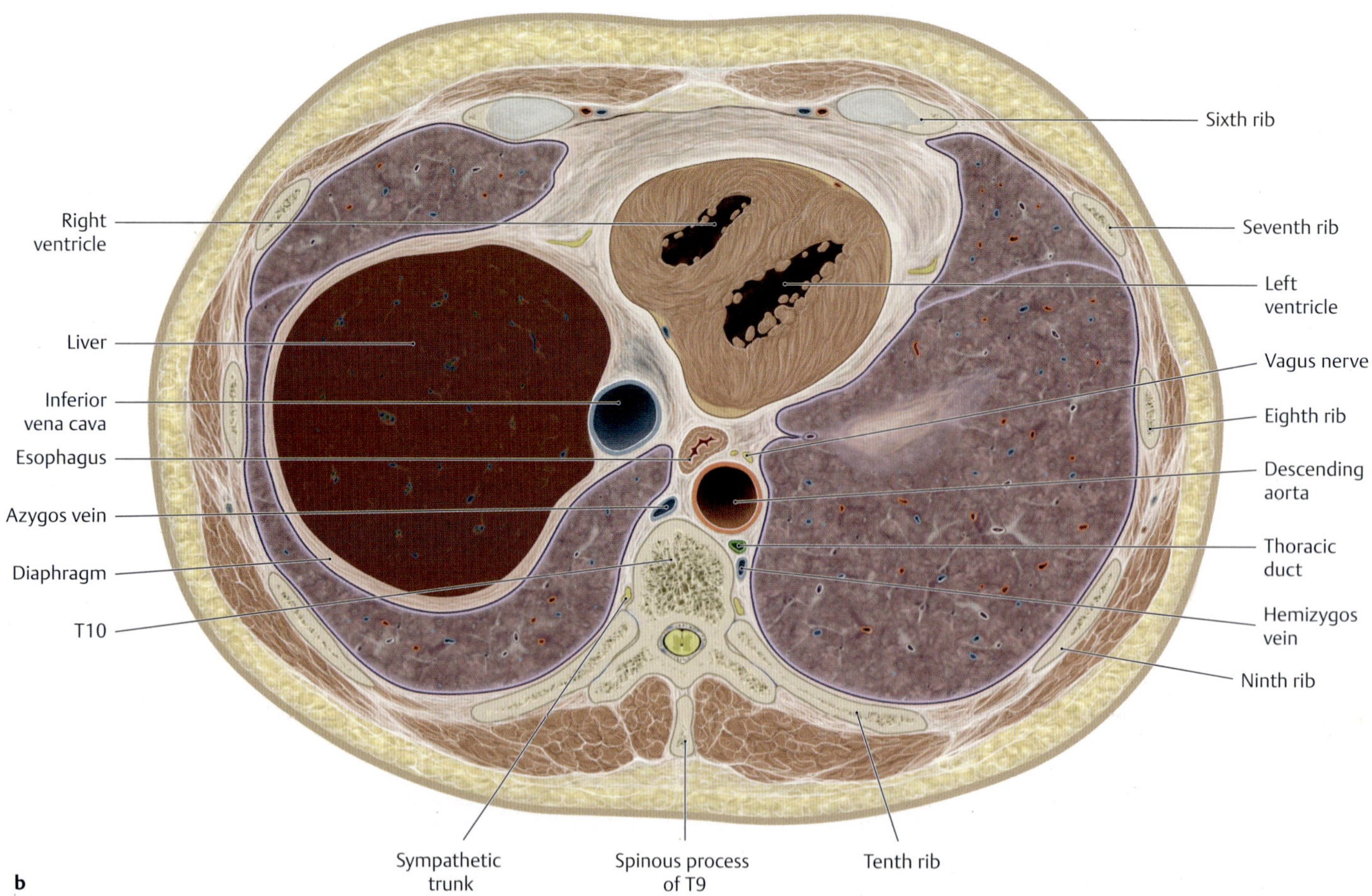

b

A Cross section through the thorax at the level of vertebra T10
a Axial (horizontal) CT image (soft tissue window); **b** horizontal section. Both are caudal views. In this plane the dome of the diaphragm extends into the thoracic cavity on the right. The liver is located beneath it and adjacent to the inferior vena cava. As the spleen does not push the dome of the diaphragm as far superiorly as the liver does on the right, the myocardium of both ventricles is sectioned in this view.

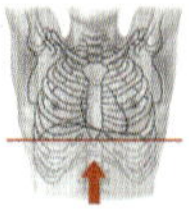

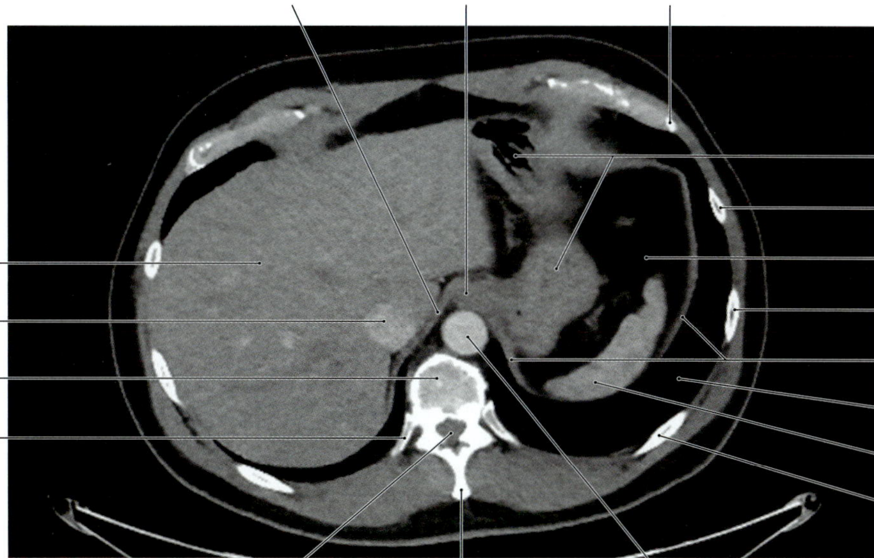

a

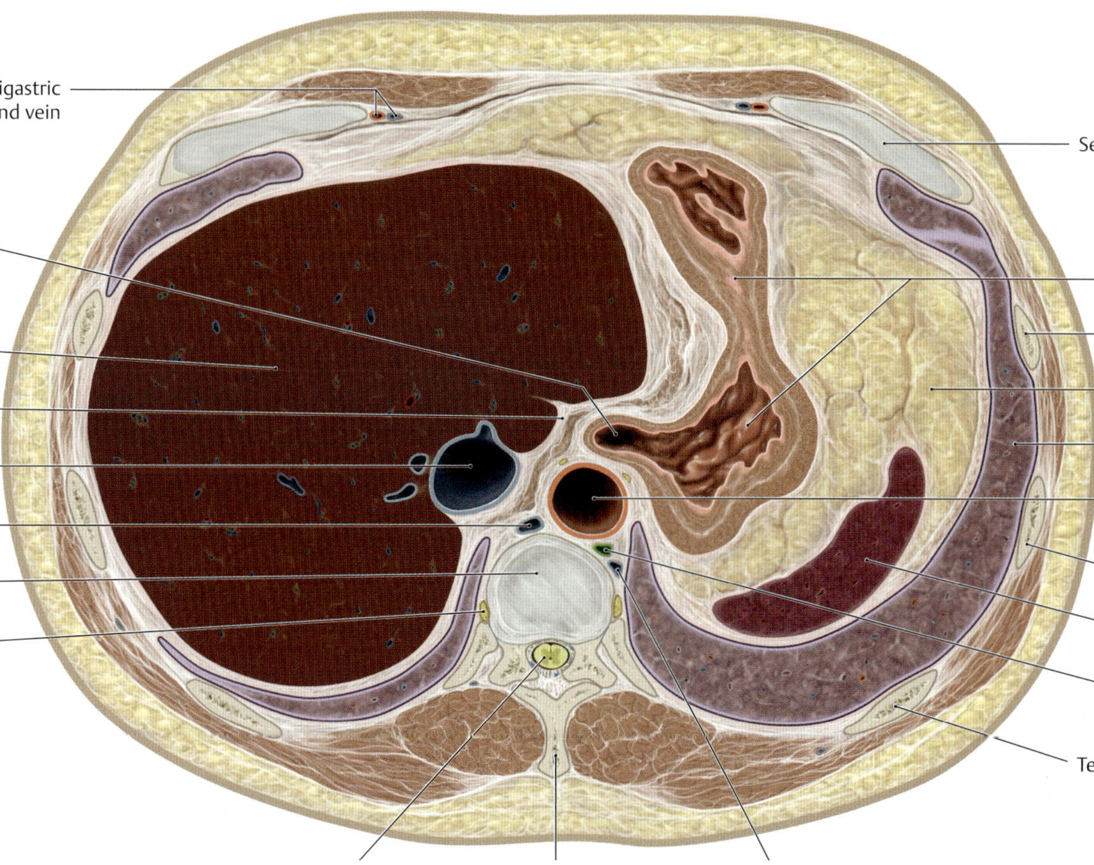

b

B Cross section through the thorax at the level of vertebra T11

a Axial (horizontal) CT image (soft tissue window); **b** horizontal section. Both are caudal views. Here we are in the region of the attachments of the diaphragm to the wall of the thorax. The only thoracic structures visible are the neurovascular structures along the spinal column and the two lungs. The predominant abdominal structures are the liver, stomach, and spleen.

C Abdomen and Pelvis

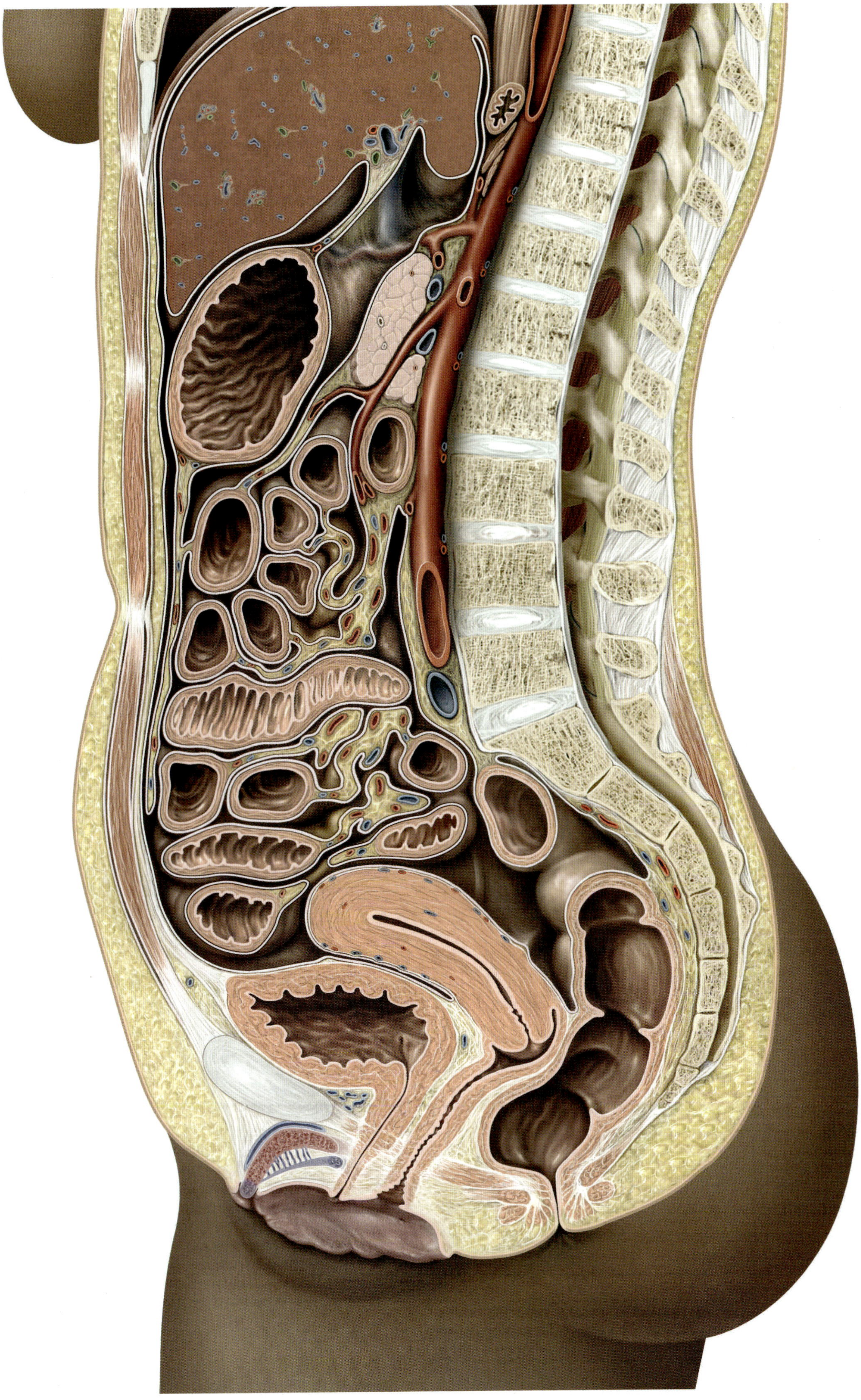

1.1 Architecture, Wall Structure, and Functional Aspects

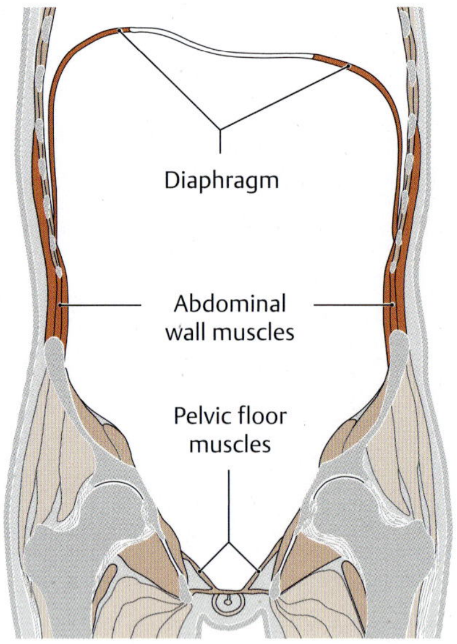

A Architecture and wall structure of the abdominal and pelvic cavities

Whereas the thoracic and abdominal cavities are separated by the diaphragm, the abdominal and pelvic cavities are continuous with each other. They are divided topographically by the linea terminalis. Thus, they form a single functional unit (see p. 2). Bones (vertebral column, thorax, and pelvis) as well as muscles (diaphragm, abdominal, and pelvic floor muscles) along with their fasciae and aponeuroses form the walls of this space. It is bounded by the following structures:

- Superiorly (see **Ca**): diaphragm with right and left domes and central tendon
- Inferiorly (see **Cb**): bony pelvis, muscles of the pelvic wall (iliacus, obturator internus, piriformis, and coccygeus) and pelvic floor muscles (mainly the levator ani forming most of the pelvic diaphragm)
- Posteriorly (see **Cc**): lumbar vertebral column, deep muscles of the abdominal wall (quadratus lumborum and psoas major), and intrinsic back muscles
- Anteriorly and laterally (see **Cd**): anterior and lateral muscles of the abdominal wall together with their aponeuroses (rectus abdominis and transversus abdominis as well as internal and external abdominal obliques)

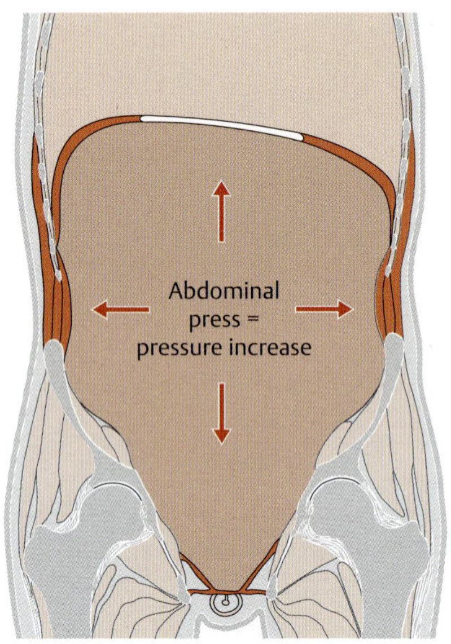

a

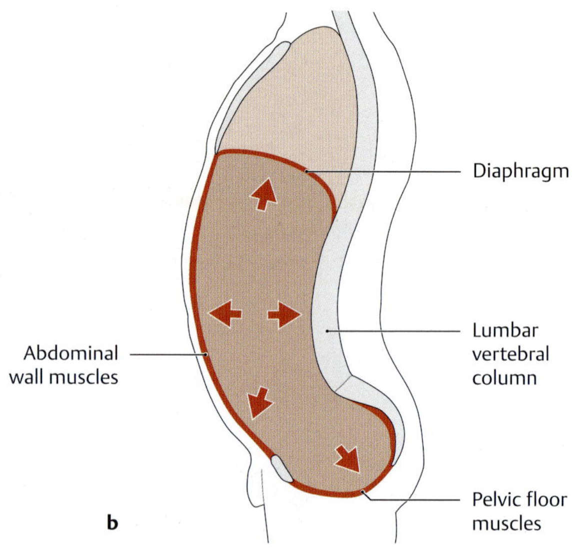

b

B Functional aspects of abdominal and pelvic wall structure: abdominal press

Abdominal press is made possible by the structure of the abdominal and pelvic walls, which plays an important role in their elastic properties. "Abdominal press" describes the voluntary contraction of the diaphragm, and abdominal and pelvic muscles. When the muscles contract they reduce the volume of the abdominal cavity thereby significantly raising the intra-abdominal pressure: pressure in the standing position is approximately 1.7 kPa (12.75 mmHg), when lying down it is approximately 0.2 kPa (1.5 mmHg), and under strain including coughing or squeezing it is 10–20 kPa (75–150 mmHg).
Abdominal press is important in

- Emptying of the rectum (defecation), of the bladder (micturition), and of the stomach (vomiting),
- Uterine contractions during the expulsive phase of labor ("expulsive pains"),
- Stabilizing the spinal column (mainly the lumbar spine) and the trunk (the wall stiffens like the wall of an inflated ball), for example when lifting heavy loads, but also in the standing posture (hydrostatic effect of abdominal press).

Hernias occur when the pressure load is greater than the strength of the complex myofascial network. They develop either in the anterior abdominal wall or more commonly in the groin region because the weight of the pelvic and abdominal organs puts increasing strain on the wall structures, which increases from superior to inferior. Additionally, the pelvic floor muscles in particular are much less able to withstand the increased abdominal pressure than the abdominal wall muscles or the diaphragm. During abdominal press, closure of the glottis and the retaining of air in the lungs gives support to the diaphragm; there is no such compensatory mechanism in the pelvic floor muscles making it a characteristic weak spot. After excessive stretching (e.g., caused by vaginal delivery) the pelvic floor is unable to maintain the pelvic organs in their normal position (pelvic floor descent) and provides inadequate support for the abdominal press. The results are urinary and fecal incontinence.

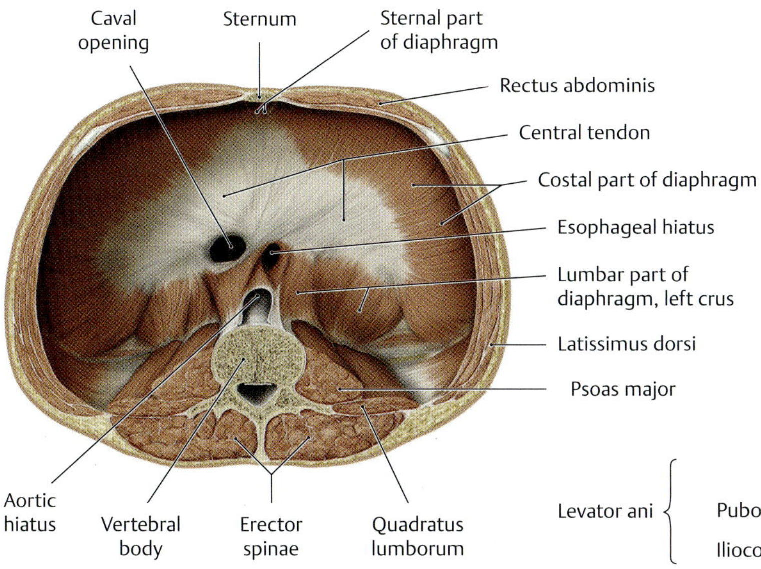

a Superior boundary.

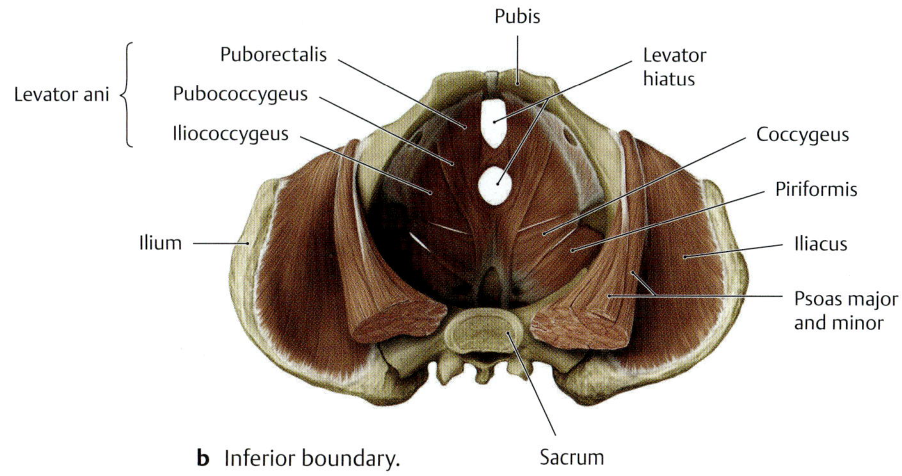

b Inferior boundary.

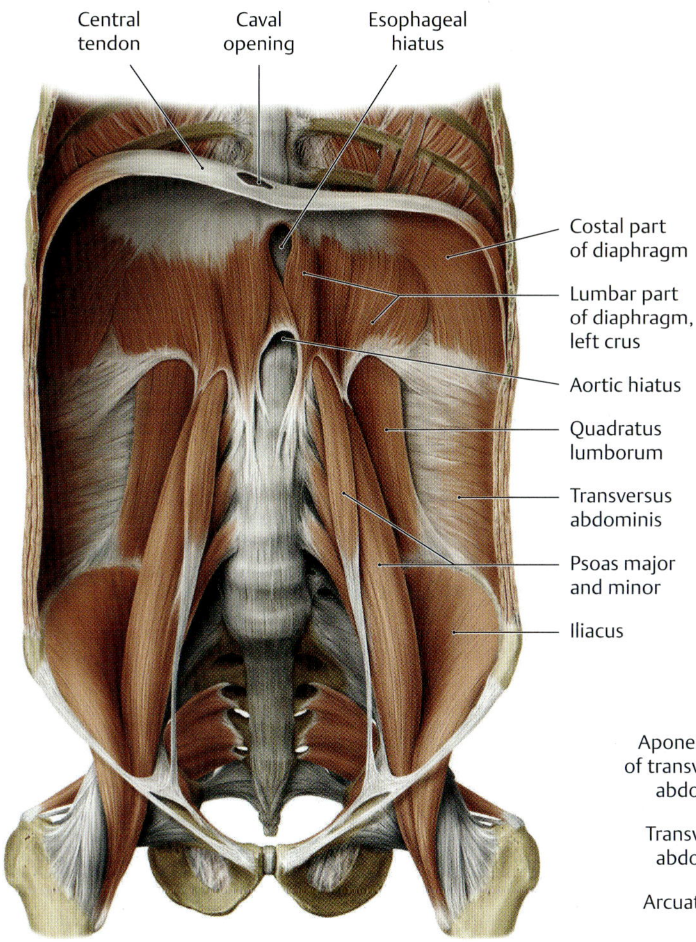

c Posterior boundary.

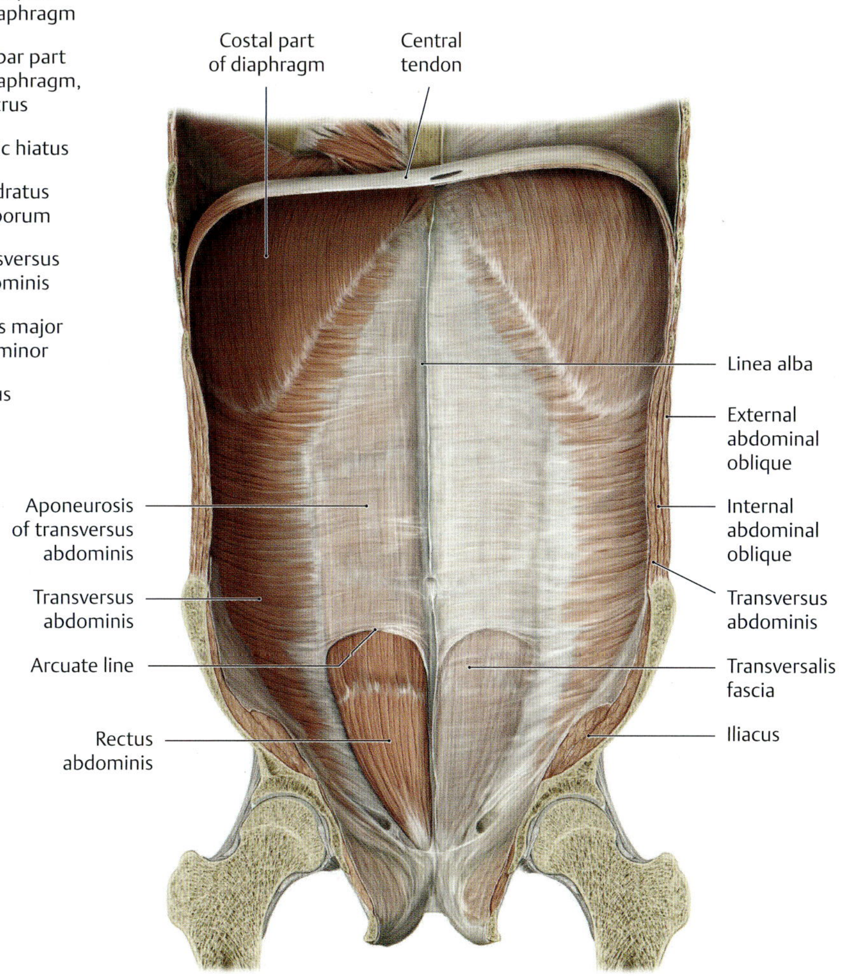

d Anterior and lateral boundaries.

C Boundaries of the abdominal and pelvic cavities

a Diaphragm, inferior view; **b** Pelvic floor, superior view; **c** **(d)** Anterior (posterior) view of the posterior (anterior) trunk wall.

1.2 Divisions of the Abdominal and Pelvic Cavities

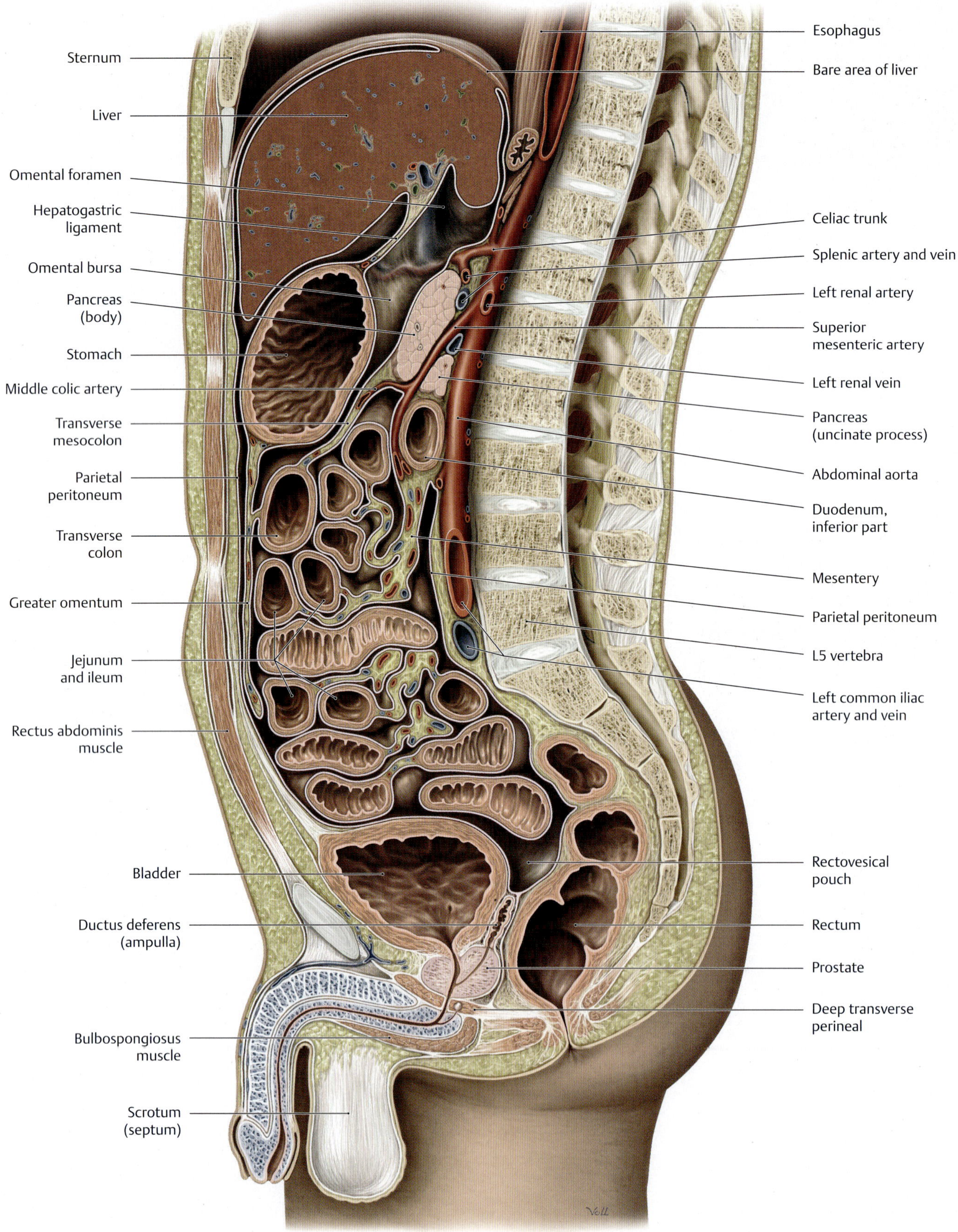

A **Midsagittal section through the abdomen and pelvis, viewed from the left side**

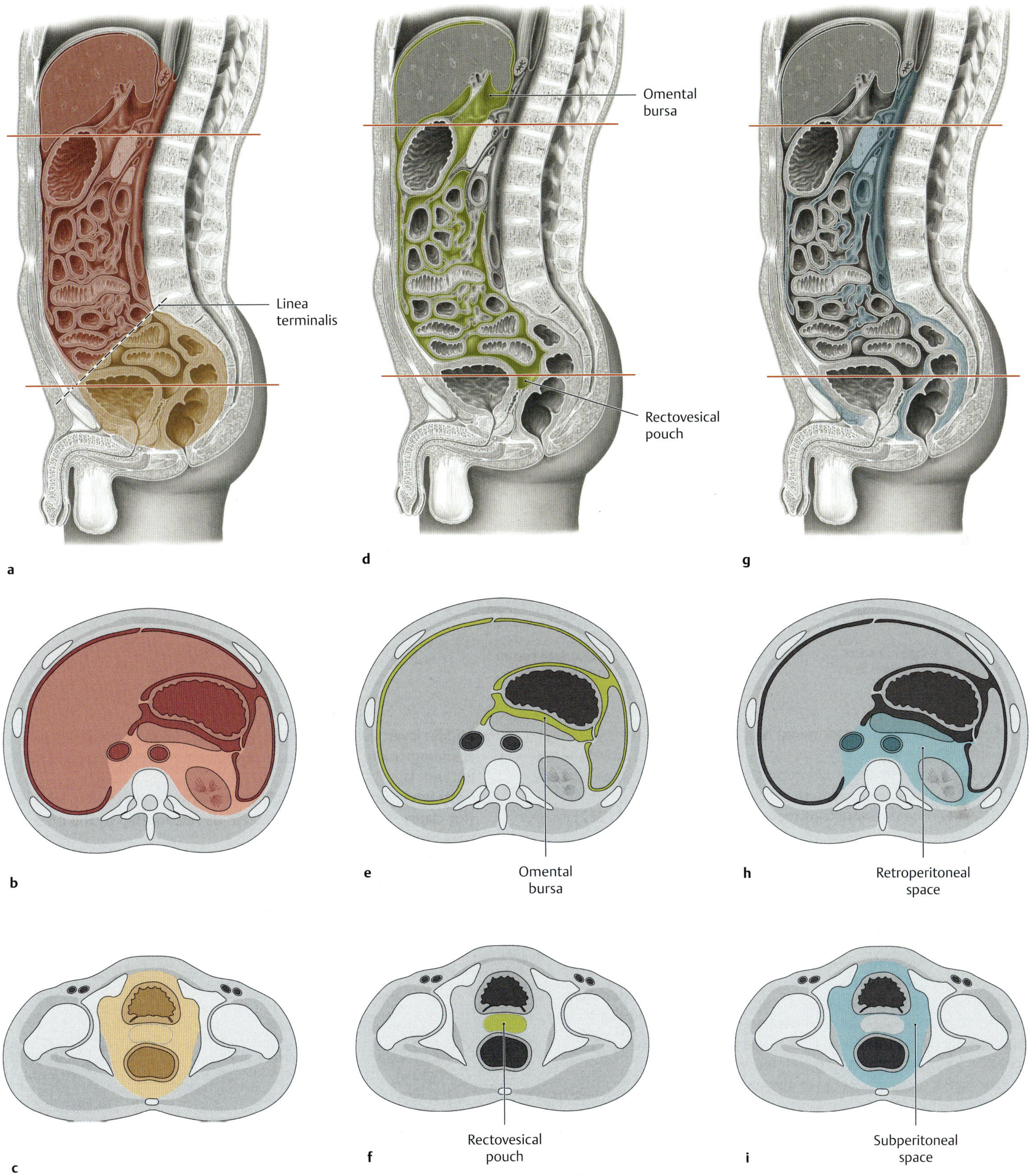

B Divisions of the pelvic and abdominal cavities
Each column of diagrams shows a midsagittal section viewed from the left side, as well as two axial sections, one at the L1 level and the other at the lower part of the sacrum, both viewed from below.

a–c Topography of body cavities: abdominal cavity and pelvic cavity (imaginary line separating the two cavities is the linea terminalis);

d–f Serous cavities (peritoneal spaces): abdominal peritoneal cavity and pelvic peritoneal cavity;

g–i Connective tissue spaces (extraperitoneal spaces): retroperitoneal space and subperitoneal space; serous cavities and extraperitoneal spaces are separated by peritoneum (see p. 225).

1.3 Classification of Internal Organs Based on their Relationship to the Abdominal and Pelvic Cavities

The organs of the abdomen and pelvis can be classified according to various topographical criteria:

- By layers in the anteroposterior direction (**A**)
- By levels in the craniocaudal direction (**B**)
- As intra- or extraperitoneal based on their peritoneal investment (**C**, **D**)

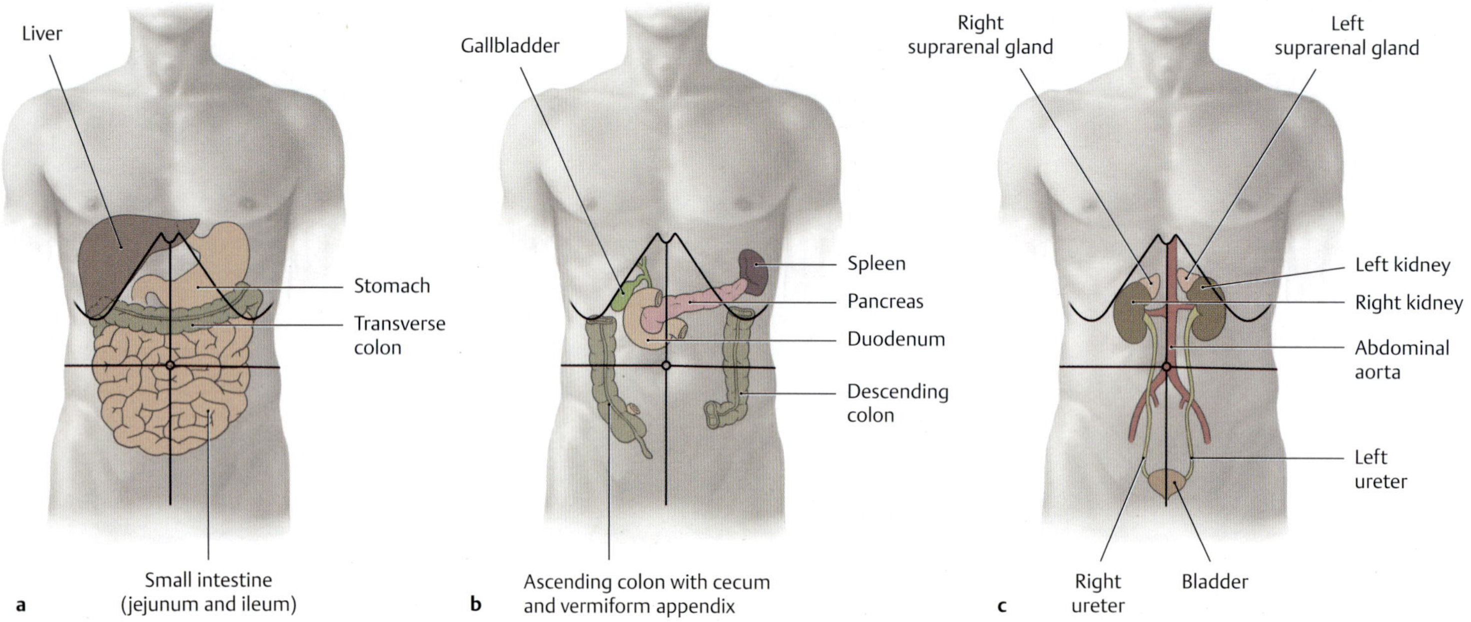

A Classification of the abdominal and pelvic organs by layers
The abdominal and pelvic organs can be roughly divided into three layers in the anteroposterior direction. This classification is particularly useful from a surgical standpoint.
Note: Larger organs may occupy more than one layer (see p. 222).

a Anterior layer: liver, stomach, transverse colon, jejunum, ileum, and bladder (for clarity not shown here, but shown with the other urinary organs in **c**);
b Middle layer: liver, duodenum, pancreas, spleen, ascending and descending colon, and uterus (not shown for clarity, extends into the anterior layer);
c Posterior layer: great vessels, kidneys, ureters, and suprarenal glands (for clarity, the bladder is shown in its relationship to the other urinary organs, see **a**).

B Classification of the abdominal and pelvic organs by levels
In this classification the organs are roughly assigned to craniocaudal levels based on their relationship to the transverse mesocolon (upper and lower abdominal organs) and lesser pelvis (pelvic organs). Because the kidneys and suprarenal glands are retroperitoneal, they are not listed in the table. When the kidney is projected onto the abdominal wall, its inferior pole extends into the lower abdomen.

Level	Organs located there
• **Upper abdomen** (above the transverse mesocolon)	• Stomach • Duodenum • Liver • Gallbladder and biliary tract • Spleen • Pancreas
• **Lower abdomen** (between the transverse mesocolon and pelvic inlet plane)	• Jejunum and ileum • Cecum and parts of the colon *Note:* The transverse colon, while located in the upper abdomen, is classified functionally as part of the lower abdomen.
• **Lesser pelvis**	• Bladder • Terminal portion of ureter • Rectum • Uterus, uterine tube, ovary, and vagina • Portions of the ductus deferens, prostate, and seminal vesicle (the testis and epididymis are outside the pelvic cavity)

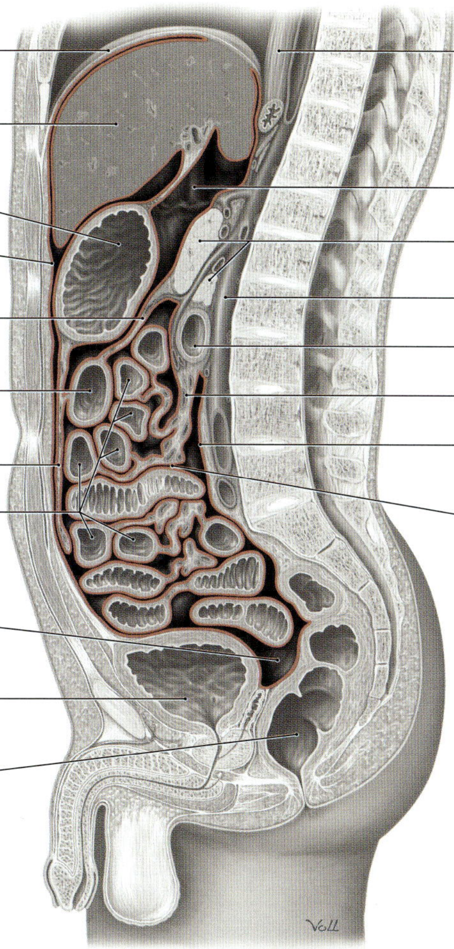

C Location of intraperitoneal and extraperitoneal organs in the abdomen and pelvis

Midsagittal section (kidneys outside the sectional plane) viewed from the left side.

The peritoneal cavity is a closed cavity that is lined by **peritoneum** and surrounded on all sides by the extraperitoneal cavity. Laterally, anteriorly and superiorly, the extraperitoneal cavity appears like a very narrow slit (see p. 223). Only its posterior portion (retroperitoneal space) and inferior portion (extraperitoneal space of the pelvis) are true spaces that contain organs. Because peritoneum covers the organs (*visceral peritoneum*) and walls (*parietal peritoneum*), the intraperitoneal organs can easily glide upon one another. The extraperitoneal organs, such as the bladder or rectum are not, or are only partially, covered by peritoneum. The bladder is covered by peritoneum only on one side (on its superior surface), which enables it to expand upward as it becomes distended with urine. This part of the peritoneum, which in females also covers large parts of the uterus, is known as *urogenital peritoneum*.

The **mesentery** is a band of connective tissue (a suspensory ligament also referred to as "meso"), which is also covered by peritoneum—by parietal peritoneum near where the mesentery is attached to the body wall and by visceral peritoneum near where it is attached to the organs. The mesentery contains the neurovascular structures of the intraperitoneal organs that are "suspended" from it. This suspensory ligament allows the intraperitoneal organs to have greater mobility than extraperitoneal organs, which are embedded in the connective tissue of the wall of the peritoneal cavity, either primarily because they were retroperitoneal when they formed or secondarily because they "migrated" behind the peritoneum during the course of embryonic development (see **D** and p. 47).

D Intra- and extraperitoneal organs of the abdomen and pelvis

Location in relation to the peritoneum	Organs
Intraperitoneal (Organs are completely covered by peritoneum and are suspended by mesentery)	
• In the abdominal peritoneal cavity	• Stomach, spleen, liver and gallbladder, small intestine (parts of the superior and ascending duodenum plus jejunum and ileum), transverse and sigmoid colon, cecum (portions of variable size may be extraperitoneal, see below)
• In the pelvic peritoneal cavity	• Fundus and body of the uterus, the ovaries, and the uterine tubes and possibly the superior portion of the rectum
Extraperitoneal (Organs without a mesentery; their neurovascular structures are located in the extraperitoneal connective tissue)	
Primarily extraperitoneal (extraperitoneal from the outset)	
• Behind the abdominal or pelvic peritoneal cavity, thus retroperitoneal	• Kidneys, suprarenal glands, ureters
• Below the pelvic peritoneal cavity, thus infra- or subperitoneal	• Urinary bladder, prostate, seminal vesicle, uterine cervix, vagina, and rectum past the sacral flexure (the urinary bladder is covered by peritoneum superiorly [urogenital peritoneum])
Secondarily extraperitoneal (become extraperitoneal during the course of embryonic development; the organs are covered by peritoneum anteriorly)	
• Behind the abdominal or pelvic peritoneal cavities, thus retroperitoneal	• Small intestine (duodenum: descending, horizontal, and part of the ascending portions), pancreas, ascending and descending colons, parts of the cecum (see above), rectum up to the sacral flexure

2.1 Branches of the Abdominal Aorta: Overview and Paired Branches

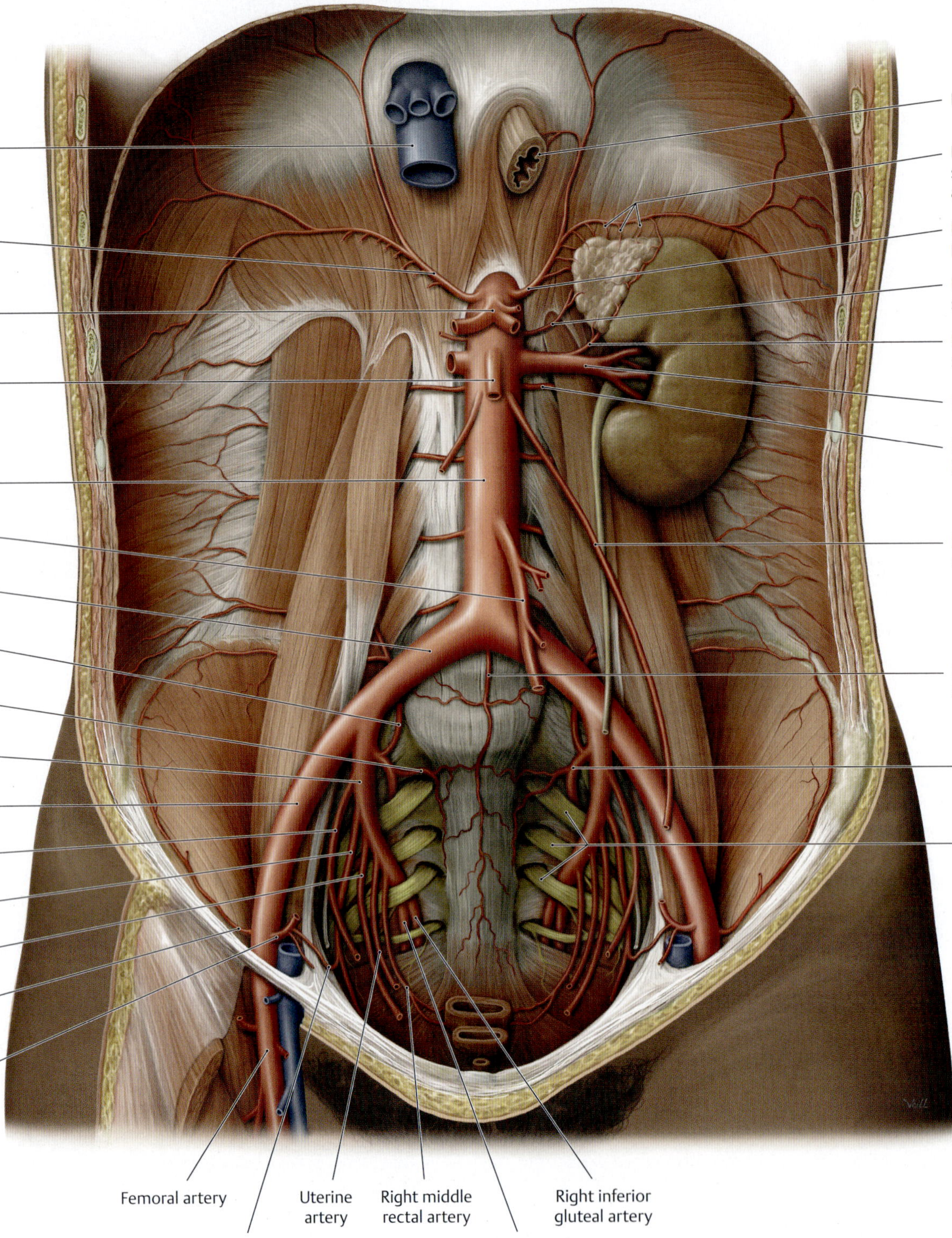

A Overview of the abdominal aorta and pelvic arteries (abdominal organs removed)

Anterior view (female pelvis). The esophagus has been pulled slightly inferiorly, and the peritoneum has been completely removed.

The abdominal aorta is the distal continuation of the thoracic aorta. It descends slightly to the left of the midline to approximately the level of the L 4 vertebra, as shown in **B** (or possibly to the L 5 vertebra in older individuals). There it divides into the paired common iliac arteries (aortic bifurcation). The common iliac arteries divide further into the internal and external iliac arteries. The abdominal aorta (see **C**) and its major branches give origin to various "subbranches" that supply the abdomen and pelvis (see **D**, p. 229).

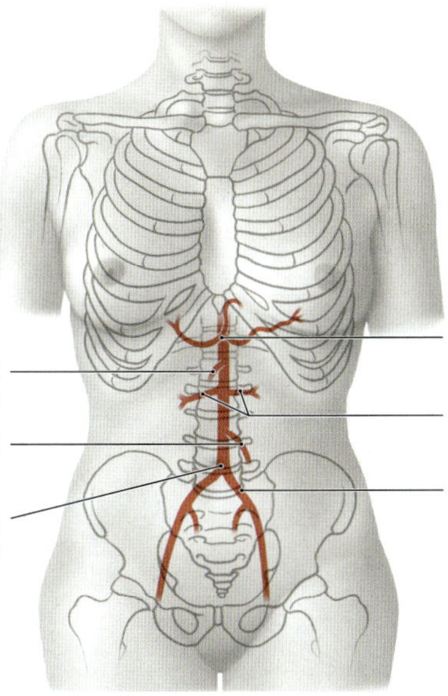

B Projection of the abdominal aorta and its major branches onto the vertebral column and pelvis

Anterior view of the five major arterial trunks. The major branches of the abdominal aorta can be identified in imaging studies based on their relationship to the vertebrae.

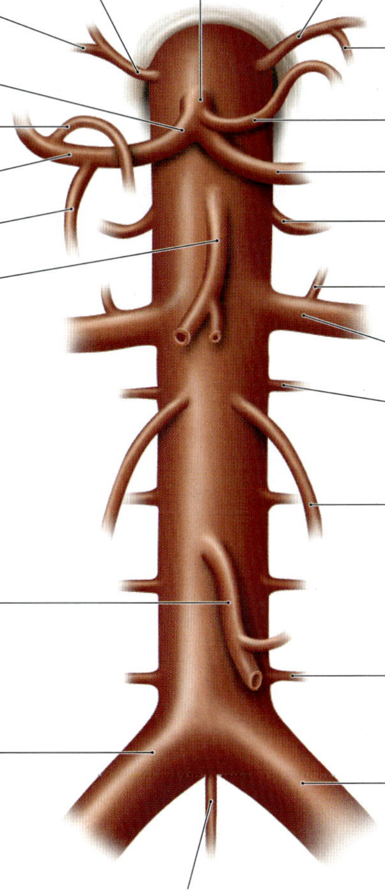

C Sequence of branches from the abdominal aorta

D Functional groups of arteries that supply the abdomen and pelvis

The branches of the abdominal aorta and pelvic arteries can be divided into five broad functional groups (→ = give rise to). For details about the areas supplied by the unpaired branches see p. 229.

Paired branches (and one unpaired branch) that supply the diaphragm, kidneys, suprarenal glands, posterior abdominal wall, spinal cord, and gonads (see **C**)
• Right and left inferior phrenic arteries → Right and left superior suprarenal arteries • Right and left middle suprarenal arteries • Right and left renal arteries → Right and left inferior suprarenal arteries • Right and left testicular (ovarian) arteries • Right and left lumbar arteries (first through fourth) • Median sacral artery (with lowest lumbar arteries)
One unpaired trunk that supplies the liver, gallbladder, pancreas, spleen, stomach, and duodenum (see **C**, pp. 229 and 283)
• Celiac trunk with – Left gastric artery – Splenic artery – Common hepatic artery
One unpaired trunk that supplies the small intestine and large intestine as far as the left colic flexure (see **C**, pp. 229 and 287)
• Superior mesenteric artery
One unpaired trunk that supplies the large intestine from the left colic flexure (see **C**, p. 229)
• Inferior mesenteric artery
One indirect (see below) paired trunk that supplies the pelvis (see **A**, p. 229)
• Internal iliac artery (from the common iliac artery, not directly from the aorta, hence an "indirect paired trunk")

2.2 Branches of the Abdominal Aorta: Unpaired and Indirect Paired Branches

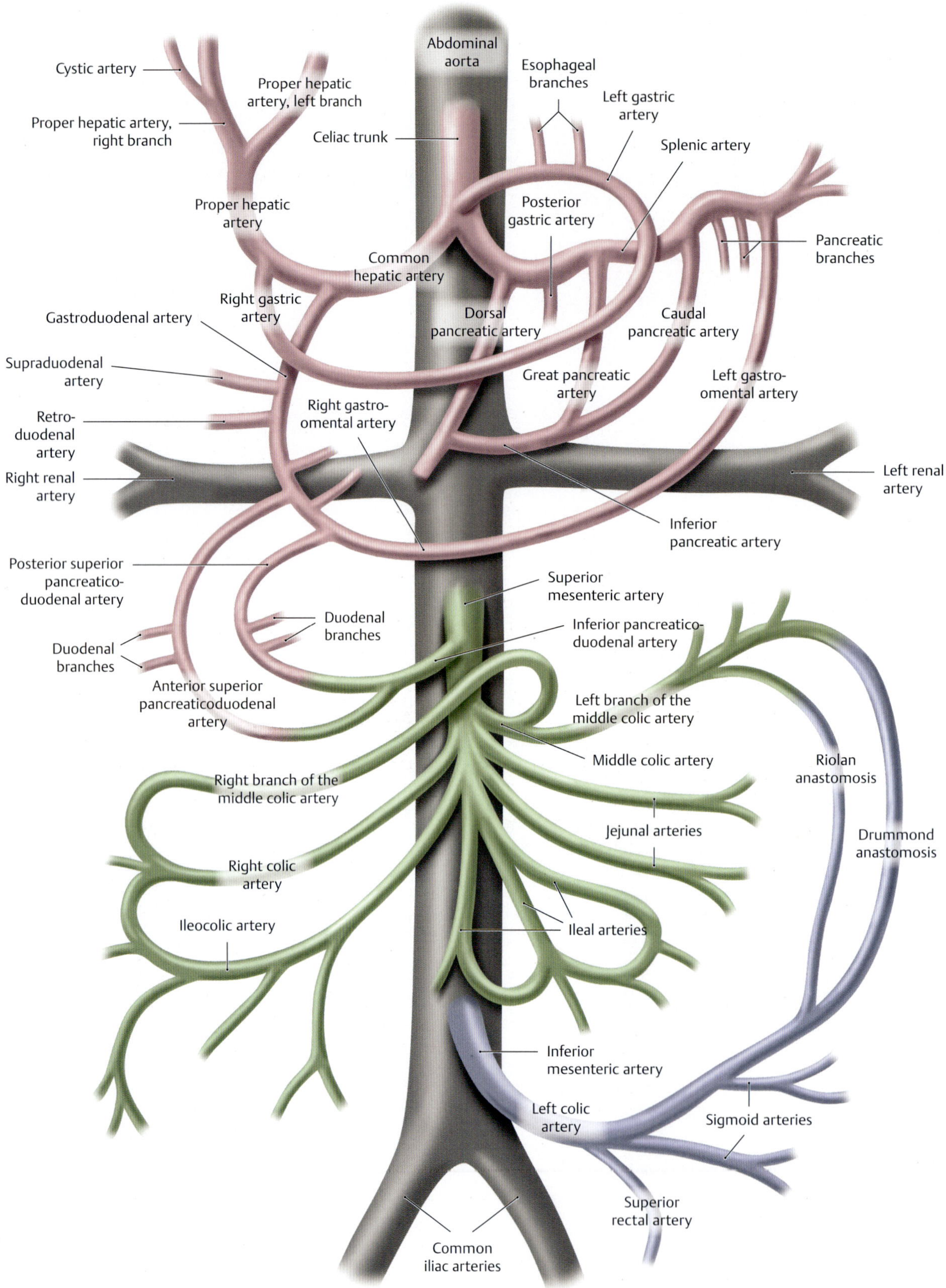

A Classification of arteries supplying the abdomen and pelvis

Red: Branches of the celiac trunk. These supply the proximal bowel segments from the abdominal esophagus to the pancreas and duodenum.

Green: Branches of the superior mesenteric artery. These supply the middle bowel segments from the pancreas and duodenum to the left colic flexure.

Blue: Branches of the inferior mesenteric artery. These supply the distal bowel segments from the left colic flexure to the rectum.

Note: For the sake of a systematic overview, the origin of the superior mesenteric artery has been drawn a little further caudally in this schematic illustration, deliberately foregoing topographical precision.

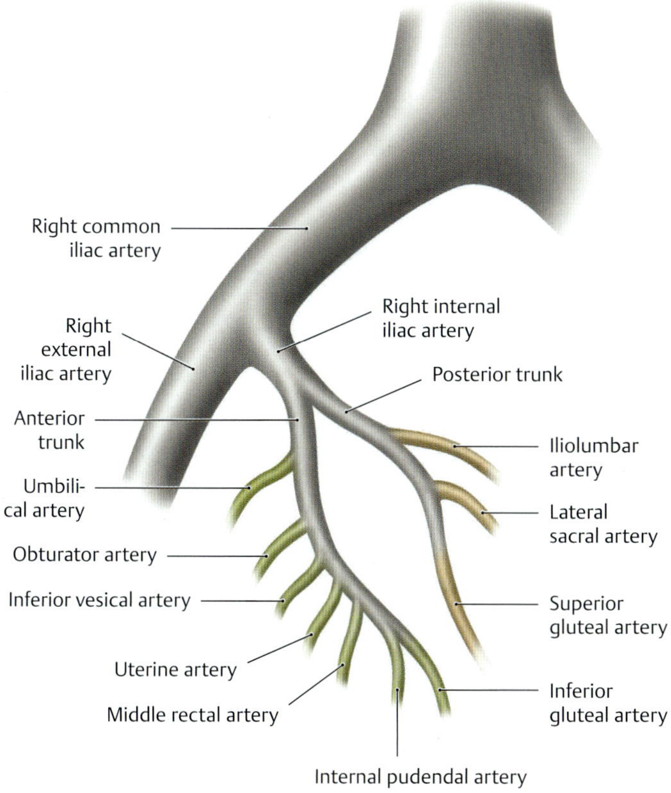

B Right common iliac artery with subbranches

The aortic bifurcation is the point where the abdominal aorta bifurcates into the two common iliac arteries, which give off multiple subbranches that supply the viscera and pelvic walls (see **D**).

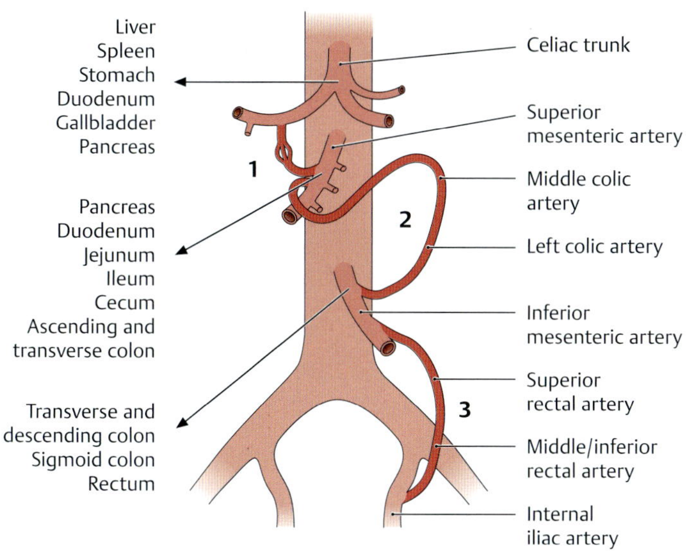

C Abdominal arterial anastomoses

1 Between the celiac trunk and superior mesenteric artery via the pancreaticoduodenal arteries
2 Between the superior and inferior mesenteric arteries (middle and left colic arteries; Riolan and Drummond anastomoses, see **A**)
3 Between the inferior mesenteric artery and internal iliac artery (superior rectal artery and middle or inferior rectal artery)

These anastomoses are important in that they can function as collaterals, delivering blood to intestinal areas that have been deprived of their normal blood supply.

D Classification of the arteries supplying the abdomen and pelvis

For the area supplied by the paired branches see p. 227 (→ = is continuous with).

Note the anastomoses particularly between the unpaired trunks (see Fig. **A** and **C**).

One unpaired trunk that supplies the liver, gallbladder, pancreas, spleen, stomach, and duodenum (see **A**)

- Celiac trunk with
  - Splenic artery
    - → Left gastro-omental artery
    - → Posterior gastric artery (and short gastric arteries)
    - → Pancreatic branches
    - → Caudal pancreatic artery
    - → Great pancreatic artery
    - → Dorsal pancreatic artery
    - → Inferior pancreatic artery
    - → Transverse pancreatic artery
  - Left gastric artery
    - → Esophageal branches
  - Common hepatic artery
    - → Gastroduodenal artery
      - → Supraduodenal artery (inconstant branch of the gastroduodenal artery)
      - → Retroduodenal artery
      - → Right gastro-omental artery
      - → Anterior or posterior superior pancreaticoduodenal artery
      - → Duodenal branches
    - → Right gastric artery
    - → Proper hepatic artery
      - → Cystic artery

One unpaired trunk that supplies the small intestine and large intestine as far as the left colic flexure (see **A**)

- Superior mesenteric artery
  - → Inferior pancreaticoduodenal artery
  - → Jejunal and Ileal arteries
  - → Ileocolic artery
  - → Right colic artery
  - → Middle colic artery

One unpaired trunk that supplies the large intestine from the left colic flexure (see **A**)

- Inferior mesenteric artery
  - → Left colic artery
  - → Sigmoid arteries
  - → Superior rectal artery

One indirect (see below) paired trunk that supplies the pelvis (see **B**)

- Internal iliac artery (from the common iliac artery, not directly from the aorta, hence an "indirect paired trunk") with branches that supply
  - → Umbilical artery
    - → Superior vesical artery
    - → Artery of ductus deferens ♂
  - → Inferior vesical artery
  - → Uterine artery
  - → Middle rectal artery
  - → Internal pudendal artery

  The pelvic walls (parietal branches)
  - → Iliolumbar artery
  - → Lateral sacral artery
  - → Obturator artery
  - → Superior and inferior gluteal arteries

2.3 Inferior Vena Caval System

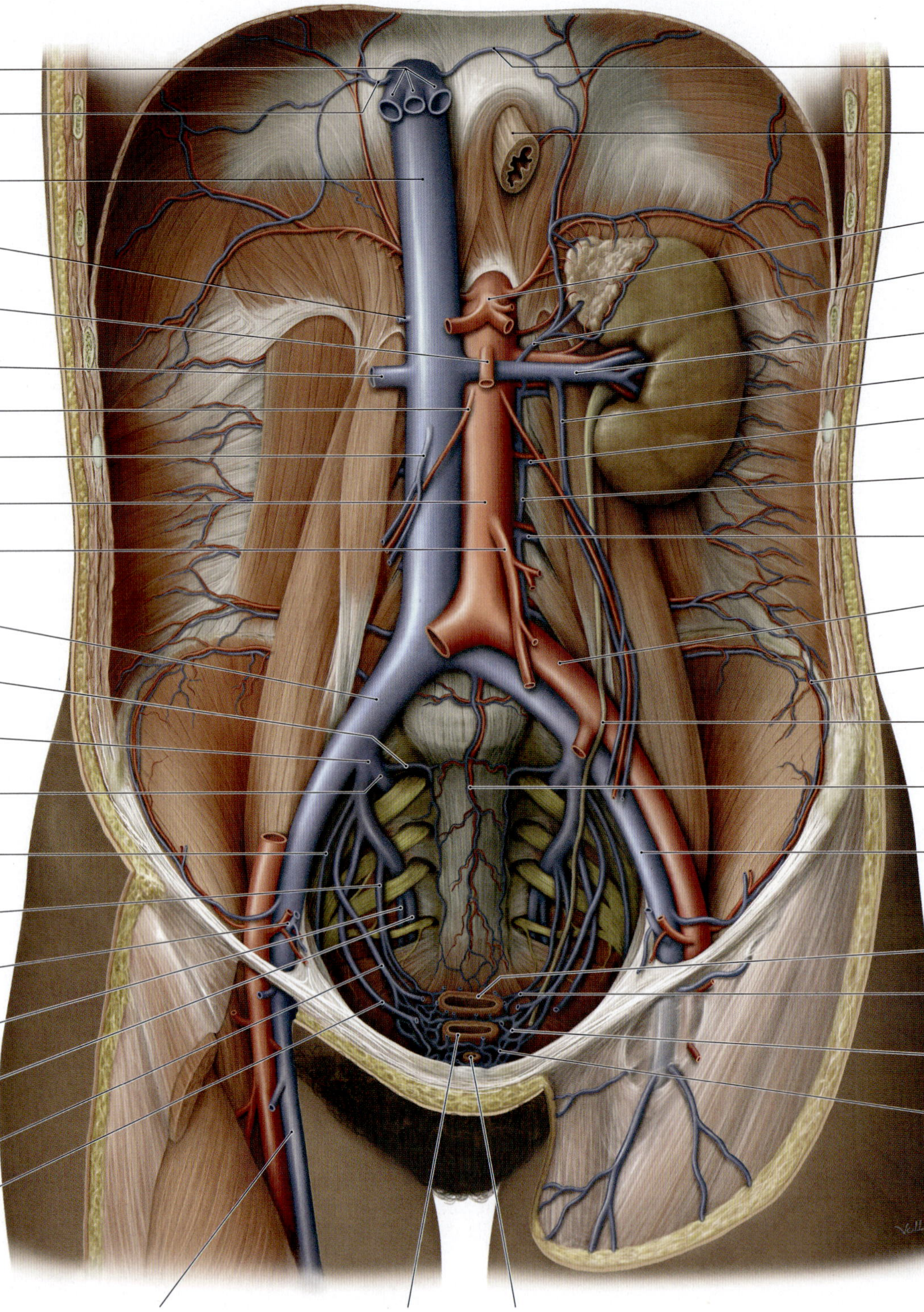

A Tributaries of the inferior vena cava in the posterior abdomen and pelvis

Anterior view of an opened female abdomen. All organs but the left kidney and suprarenal gland have been removed, and the esophagus has been pulled slightly inferiorly.

The inferior vena cava receives numerous tributaries that return venous blood from the abdomen and pelvis (and, of course, from the lower limbs), analogous to the distribution of the paired abdominal aortic branches in this region. The inferior vena cava is formed by the union of the two common iliac veins at the approximate level of the L 5 vertebra (see **C**), behind and slightly inferior to the aortic bifurcation.

Note the special location of the left renal vein and its risk of compression by the superior mesenteric artery (see p. 287): The left renal vein passes in front of the abdominal aorta but behind the superior mesenteric artery. Veins in the male pelvis are described on p. 365.

The veins in the pelvis have numerous variants. For example, the tributaries of the internal iliac vein are frequently multiple (unlike those shown above) but unite to form a single trunk before entering the iliac vein (see also p. 367).

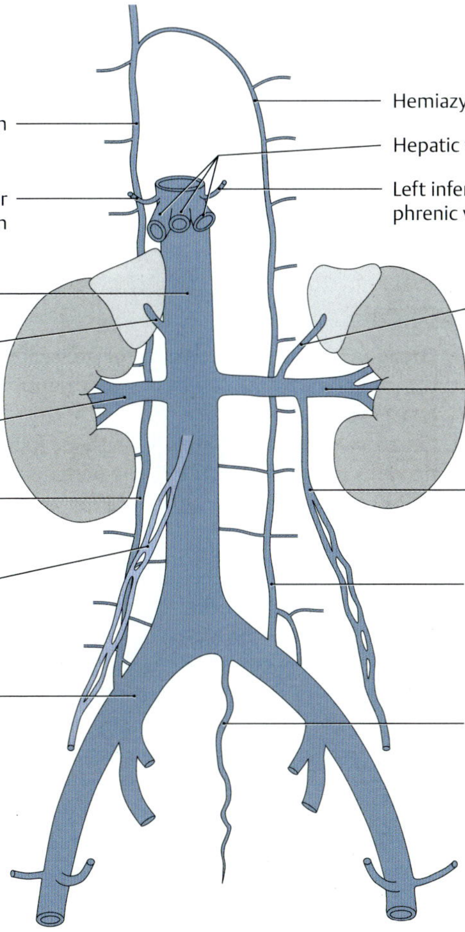

B Tributaries of the inferior vena cava

The difference in the venous drainage of the right and left kidneys is displayed more clearly here than in **A**. The continuity of the right ascending lumbar vein with the azygos vein is also shown.

Direct tributaries return venous blood directly to the inferior vena cava without passing through an intervening capillary bed. Direct tributaries drain the following organs:

- The diaphragm, abdominal wall, kidneys, suprarenal glands, testes/ ovaries, and liver
- For the *pelvis* (via the common iliac vein) from the pelvic wall and floor, uterus, uterine tubes, bladder, ureters, accessory sex glands, lower rectum, and lower limb.

Indirect tributaries return blood that has passed through the capillary bed of the liver via the hepatic portal system (see p. 233). The following organs have indirect tributaries:

- The spleen
- The organs of the digestive tract: pancreas, duodenum, jejunum, ileum, cecum, colon, and upper rectum

Note: Venous blood from the inferior vena cava may drain through the ascending lumbar veins into the azygos or hemiazygos vein and thence to the *superior* vena cava. Thus a connection between the two venae cavae exists on the posterior wall of the abdomen and thorax: a cavo-caval or intercaval anastomosis. The location and significance of cavo-caval anastomoses are discussed on p. 234. Frequently an anastomosis exists between the suprarenal vein and inferior phrenic vein (not shown here, see **A**) on the left side of the body.

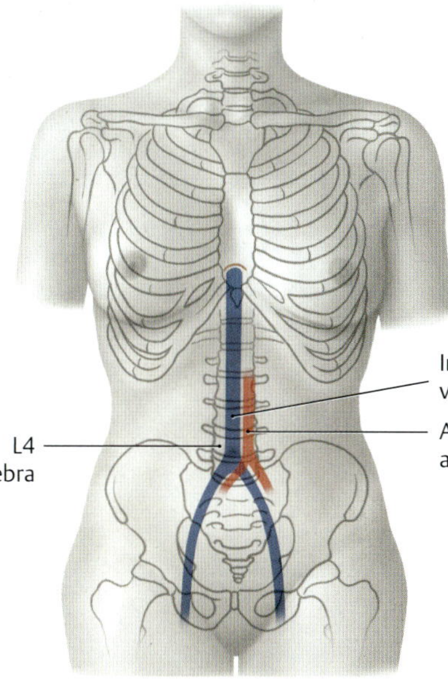

C Projection of the inferior vena cava onto the vertebral column

The inferior vena cava ascends on the right side of the abdominal aorta and pierces the diaphragm at the caval opening located at the T 8 level. The common iliac veins unite at the L 5 level to form the inferior vena cava (see also **A**).

D Direct tributaries of the inferior vena cava

- Right and left inferior phrenic veins
- Hepatic veins
- Right suprarenal vein
- Right and left renal veins at the L 1/L 2 level (the left testicular/ ovarian vein and left suprarenal vein terminate in the left renal vein)
- Lumbar veins
- Right testicular/ovarian vein
- Common iliac veins (L 5 level)
- Median sacral vein (often terminates in the left common iliac vein)

2.4 Portal Venous System (Hepatic Portal Vein)

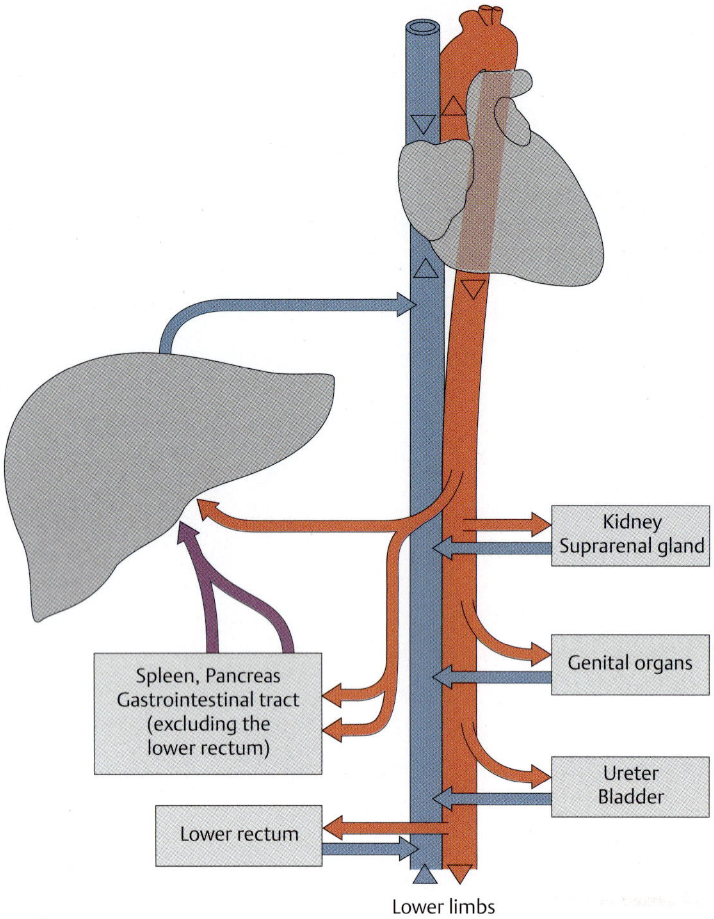

A The portal venous system in the abdomen

The arterial blood supply and venous drainage of the abdominal and pelvic organs differ in their functional organization: While they derive their arterial blood supply entirely from the abdominal aorta or one of its major branches, *venous drainage* is accomplished by one of two *different venous systems*:

1. Organ veins that drain directly or indirectly (via the iliac veins) into the inferior vena cava, which then returns the blood to the right heart (see also p. 230);
2. Organ veins that first drain directly or indirectly (via the mesenteric veins or splenic vein) *into the portal vein*—and thus to the liver—before the blood enters the inferior vena cava and returns to the right heart.

The *first pathway* serves the urinary organs, suprarenal glands, genital organs, and the walls of the abdomen and pelvis. The *second pathway* serves the organs of the digestive system (hollow organs of the gastrointestinal tract, pancreas, gallbladder) and the spleen (see **D**). Only the lower portions of the rectum are exempt from this pathway and drain directly through the iliac veins to the inferior vena cava. This (re)routing of venous blood through the hepatic portal system ensures that the organs of the digestive tract deliver their nutrient-rich blood to the liver for metabolic processing before it is returned to the heart. It also provides a route by which elements of degenerated red blood cells can be conveyed from the spleen to the liver. Thus, the portal vein functions to deliver blood to the liver to support metabolism. This contrasts with the proper hepatic artery, which supplies the liver with oxygen and other nutrients. Anastomoses may develop between the portal venous system and vena caval system (*portacaval anastomosis*) and function as collateral pathways in certain diseases (see p. 234).

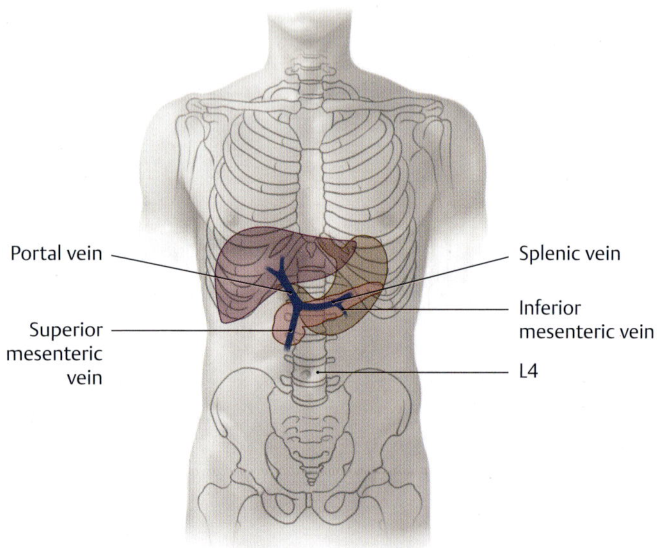

B Projection of the portal vein and its two major tributaries onto the vertebral column

The portal vein of the liver is formed by the union of the *superior* mesenteric vein and splenic vein to the right of the midline at the L 1 level. The *inferior* mesenteric vein typically opens into the splenic vein, also conveying its blood to the portal vein via this route.

Note the relationship of the portal vein to the liver, stomach, and pancreas.

C Tributaries of the portal vein

- **Superior mesenteric vein** (see p. 294) with its tributaries:
  - Pancreaticoduodenal veins
  - Pancreatic veins
  - Right gastro-omental vein
  - Jejunal veins
  - Ileal veins
  - Ileocolic vein
  - Right colic vein
  - Middle colic vein
- **Inferior mesenteric vein** (see p. 295) with its tributaries:
  - Left colic vein
  - Sigmoid veins
  - Superior rectal vein
- **Splenic vein** (see p. 293) with its tributaries:
  - Left gastro-omental vein
  - Pancreatic veins
  - Short gastric veins
- **Direct tributaries** (see p. 293)
  - Cystic vein
  - Left gastric vein with esophageal veins
  - Right gastric vein
  - Posterior superior pancreaticoduodenal vein
  - Prepyloric vein
  - Paraumbilical veins

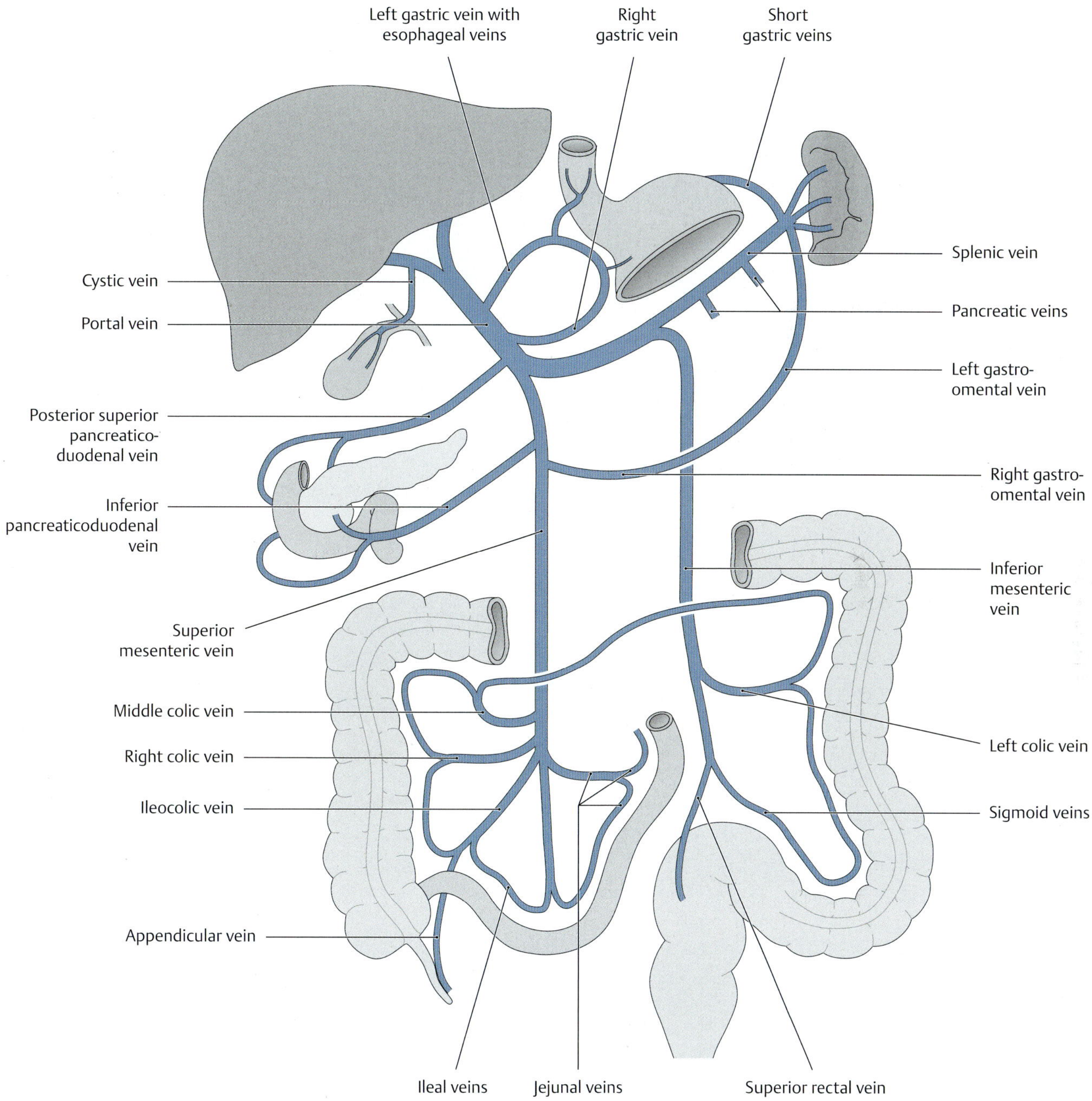

D Distribution of the portal vein (see also **C**)

The portal vein of the liver is a short vessel (total length 6–12 cm) with a large caliber. On entering the liver, it divides into two main branches, one for each of the hepatic lobes. The region drained by the portal vein corresponds to the region supplied by the celiac trunk and the superior and inferior mesenteric arteries. The portal vein receives venous blood from the hollow organs of the gastrointestinal tract (excluding the lower rectum) and from the pancreas, gallbladder, and spleen. Some of this blood flows directly to the portal vein through the corresponding organ veins, and the rest reaches the portal vein indirectly by way of the mesenteric veins or splenic vein.

2.5 Venous Anastomoses in the Abdomen and Pelvis

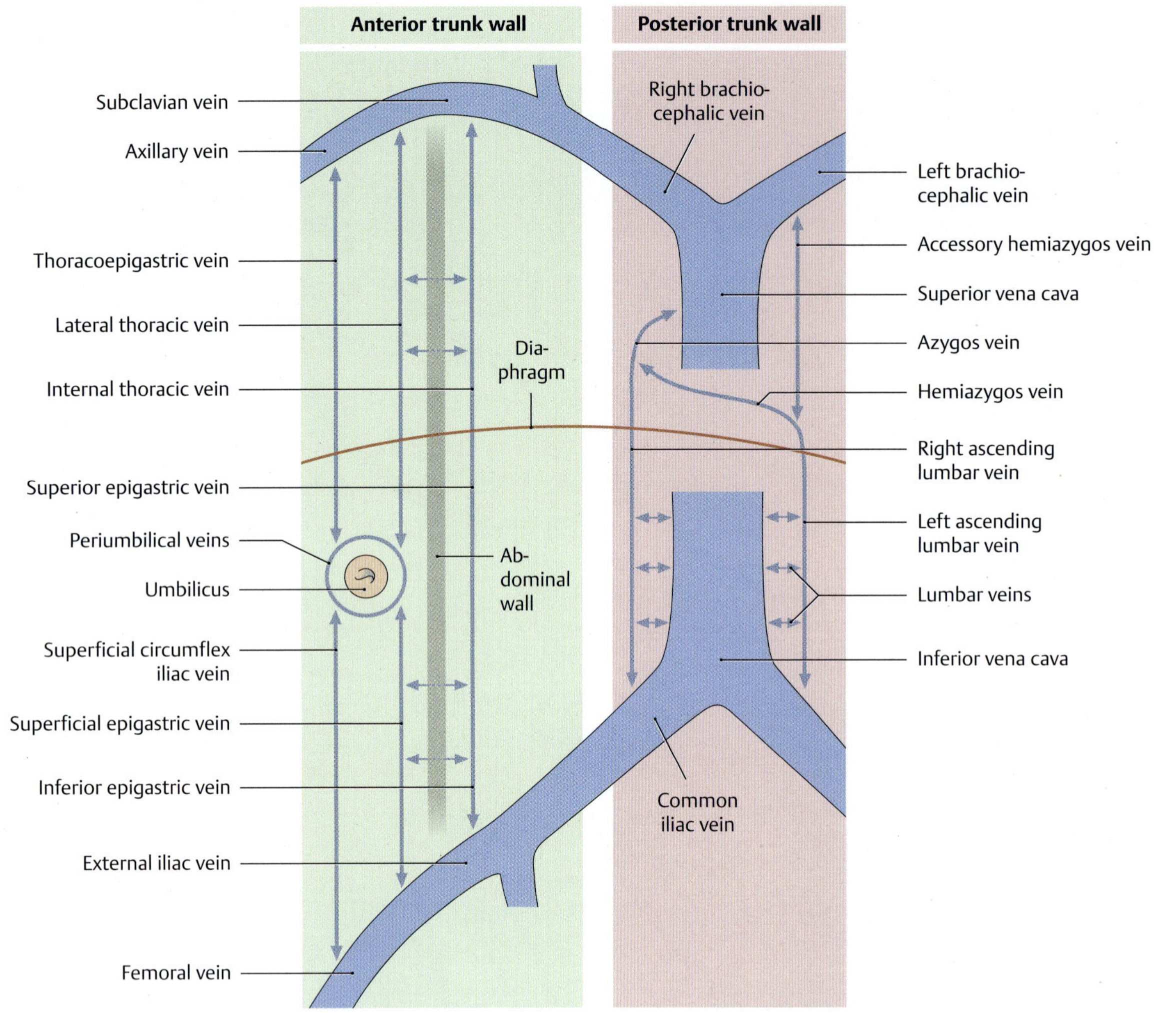

A Cavocaval (intercaval) anastomoses

Large venous anastomoses are present between the inferior and superior vena cava on the anterior and posterior trunk walls. Known as *cavocaval* or *intercaval anastomoses*, they provide collateral pathways for returning venous blood to the *superior* vena cava and right heart in patients with outflow obstructions affecting the *inferior* vena cava in the abdomen or the common iliac veins in the pelvis. Veins of the chest wall form the cranial portion of this collateral network. The veins of the *anterior* abdominal wall provide both a *superficial* pathway (anterior to the rectus abdominis) and a *deep* pathway (posterior to the rectus abdominis). (In the chest, these pathways lie outside or inside the thoracic skeleton.)

Note: On the *anterior* trunk wall, the paraumbilical veins (see **B**) establish a collateral pathway between the portal vein and drainage to the venae cavae. This portosystemic (portacaval) pathway is important in patients with obstructed portal venous flow and may affect the superficial and deep anterior pathways.

- Anastomoses on the *posterior wall* of the abdomen. They utilize the connection between the ascending lumbar vein and the azygos/hemiazygos vein. Two pathways are available:
  1. A *direct* pathway between the ascending lumbar vein and azygos/hemiazygos vein:
     Inferior vena cava → (possibly via the common iliac vein) ascending lumbar vein → azygos/hemiazygos vein → **superior vena cava**.
  2. An *indirect* pathway between the ascending lumbar vein and azygos/hemiazygos vein by way of horizontal trunk wall veins (intercostal and lumbar veins, mediated by venous plexuses on the spinal column; for clarity, not shown here):
     Inferior vena cava → (possibly via the common iliac vein) ascending lumbar vein → lumbar veins → vertebral venous plexus → posterior intercostal veins → azygos/hemiazygos vein → **superior vena cava**.
- Anastomoses on the *anterior* wall of the abdomen. They utilize superficial and deep cutaneous veins, which may exchange blood between them. Two pathways are available:
  1. Deep pathway (posterior to the rectus abdominis):
     Inferior vena cava → common iliac vein → external iliac vein → inferior epigastric vein → superior epigastric vein → internal thoracic vein → subclavian vein → brachiocephalic vein → **superior vena cava**.
  2. Superficial pathway (anterior to the rectus abdominis):
     Inferior vena cava → common iliac vein → external iliac vein → femoral vein → superficial epigastric vein/superficial circumflex iliac vein → thoracoepigastric vein/lateral thoracic vein → axillary vein → subclavian vein → brachiocephalic vein → **superior vena cava**.

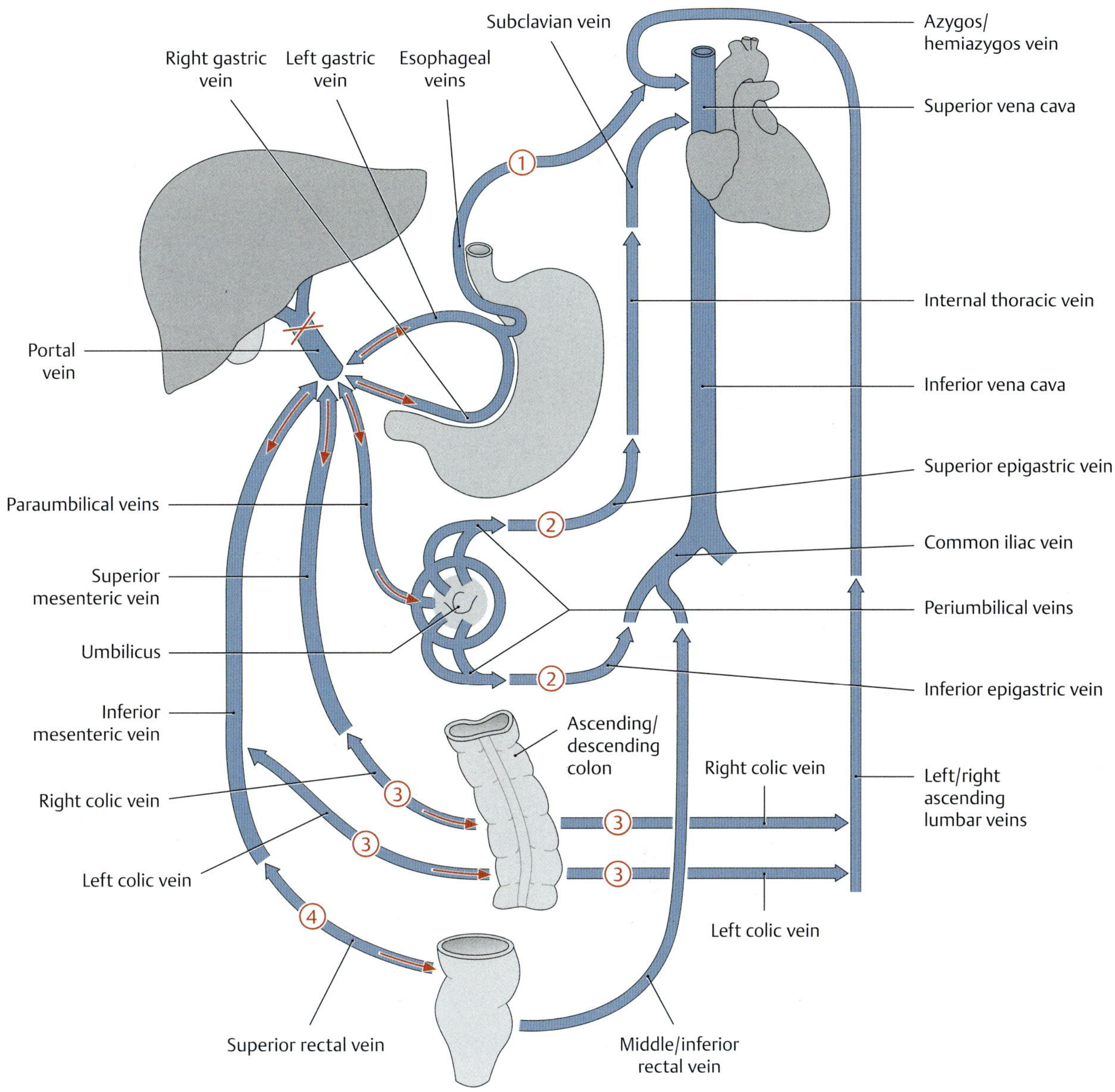

B Schematic of collateral pathways for the portal vein (porto-systemic collaterals)

Venous collateral pathways are also available between the portal venous system and the inferior and superior venae cavae. These *porto-systemic* collaterals are physiological pathways that can develop in response to (1) overlapping venous territories in organs (venous plexuses in the esophagus, colon, rectum) or (2) the persistence of patent blood vessels that are normally obliterated after birth (umbilical vein, paraumbilical veins). These collateral pathways become clinically significant when the portal system is compromised (as in hepatic cirrhosis, for example). As venous pressure increases, the portal vein can divert blood away from the liver and return it to the supplying vessels. Thus, veins that are normally *afferent* vessels for the liver undergo a *flow reversal* (see red arrows) and transport blood back through the inferior or superior vena cava and back to the heart. Portosystemic shunts can be lifesaving, but nevertheless cause significant additional problems, because some of the vessels in the shunt pathways (in the esophagus and rectum, specifically) are barely capable of handling the significant redirected blood flow, with consequent rise of pressure in the system, and are thus liable to rupture. The following four **collateral pathways** are of key importance:

① Through veins of the stomach and distal esophagus (dilation of these veins may lead to esophageal varices, with risk of life-threatening hemorrhage):
Portal vein ← gastric veins ← *esophageal veins* → azygos/hemiazygos vein → **superior vena cava.**

② Through veins of the anterior abdominal wall:
Portal vein ← umbilical vein (patent part) ← *paraumbilical veins* → periumbilical veins →superior epigastric vein → internal thoracic vein → subclavian vein → **superior vena cava** or
Portal vein ← umbilical vein (patent part) → *paraumbilical veins* → periumbilical veins →inferior epigastric vein → external iliac vein → **inferior vena cava**.
Note: Drainage from paraumbilical veins into the superficial veins (rare) of the anterior abdominal wall (thoracoepigastric vein, lateral thoracic vein, superficial epigastric vein, see **A**) leads to dilation of these tortuous veins (Medusa head, caput medusae).

③ Through veins of the posterior abdominal wall:
Portal vein ← superior and inferior mesenteric vein ← left and right *colic veins* → left and right ascending lumbar veins → azygos/hemiazygos vein → **superior vena cava**. The ascending lumbar veins may also divert blood to the inferior vena cava.

④ Through the rectal venous plexus (with dilation):
Portal vein ← inferior mesenteric vein ← superior rectal vein ← middle/*inferior rectal veins* → internal iliac vein → **inferior vena cava**.

2.6 Lymphatic Trunks and Lymph Nodes

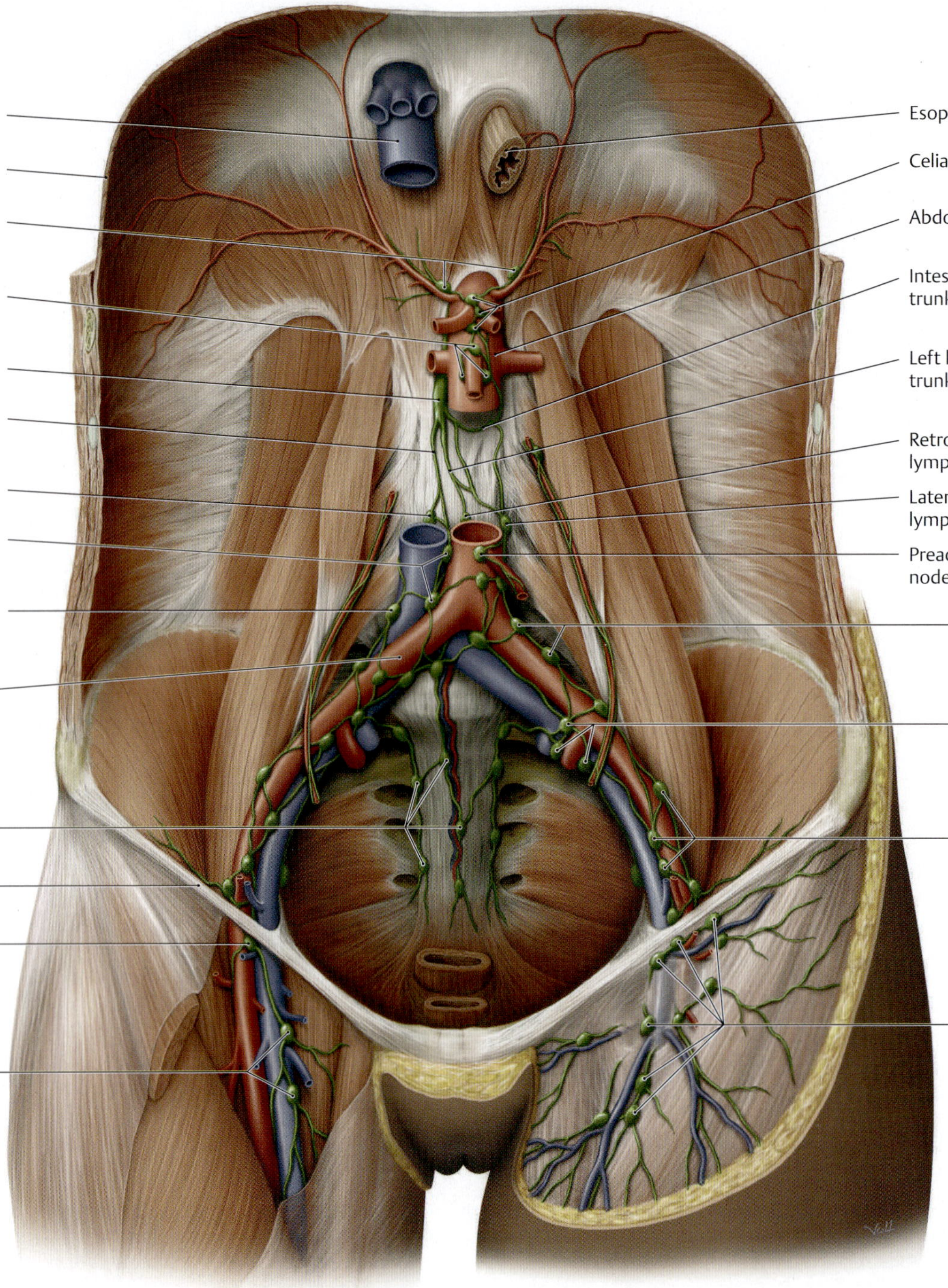

A Overview of parietal lymph nodes in the abdomen and pelvis
Anterior view of an opened female abdomen. All visceral structures have been removed except for major vessels, and the lymphatic vessels are shown larger for clarity. Size disparities between the lymph nodes (1 mm to over 1 cm) and actual numbers (several hundred) are ignored. Regional lymph nodes (see **C**) may be arranged so densely that individual groups can scarcely be identified. Lymph nodes in the abdomen and pelvis are classified by their location as *parietal* or *visceral*. Parietal lymph nodes are located *near* the *trunk wall* (often distributed along blood vessels), while visceral lymph nodes are located *near organs* in the connective tissue of the extraperitoneal space or in the mesentery attached to an organ. A large percentage of parietal lymph nodes are located on the posterior wall of the abdomen and pelvis: they are clustered around the large vessels that course on the posterior abdominal and pelvic walls, such as the abdominal aorta and inferior vena cava in the abdomen and the iliac arteries and veins and their branches in the pelvis. Only a few lymph nodes are located on the anterior wall, such as the inguinal lymph nodes and the nodes around the external iliac artery (iliac lymph nodes). The lymph nodes and lymphatic vessels are arranged in an intricate network in the abdomen and pelvis, as they generally are elsewhere in the body. As a result, lymphatic drainage tends to follow multiple regional patterns of flow rather than a single well-defined pathway (see p. 238). Potential drainage routes are particularly numerous for the organs of the pelvis, where several organs may share lymphatic pathways. For example, certain lymph nodes are utilized (with varying degrees of preference) by the bladder, genital organs, and rectum.

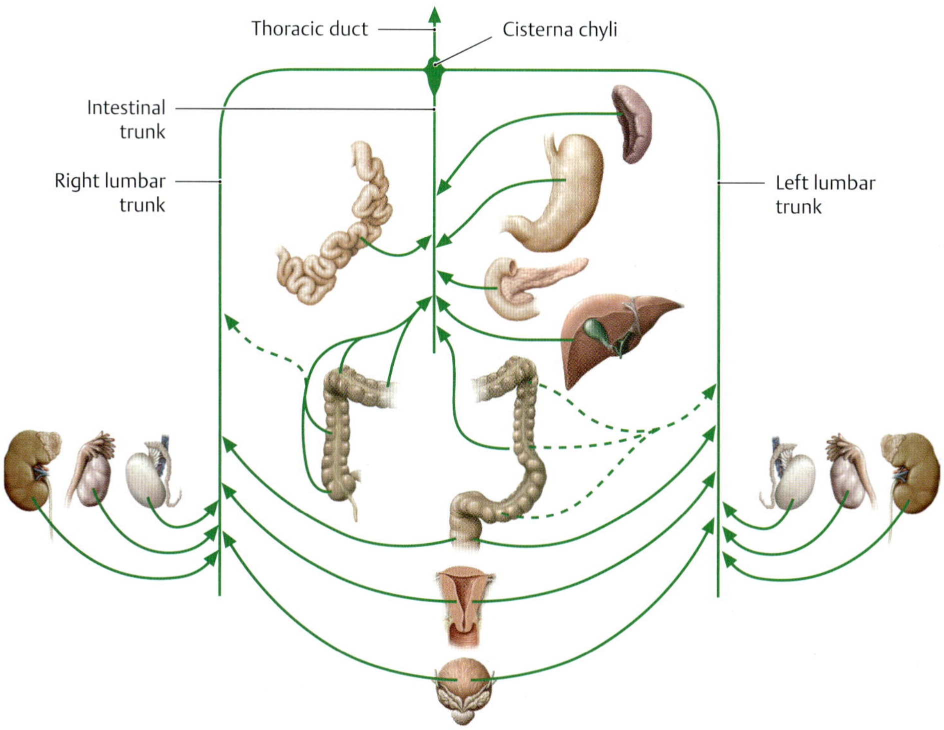

B Lymphatic trunks in the abdomen and pelvis

Lymph from the abdominal and pelvic organs drains to the lumbar and intestinal trunks (see p. 238) after first passing through one or more lymph node groups (see **C**). An expansion, the cisterna chyli, is frequently present at the union of these trunks. Lymph from the cisterna chyli drains through the thoracic duct to the junction of the left subclavian and internal jugular veins. The thoracic duct is the principal lymphatic trunk that returns lymph to the venous system.

Solid arrows: main drainage pathways; dashed arrows: secondary drainage pathways via secondary retroperitoneal flow from the ascending and descending colon.

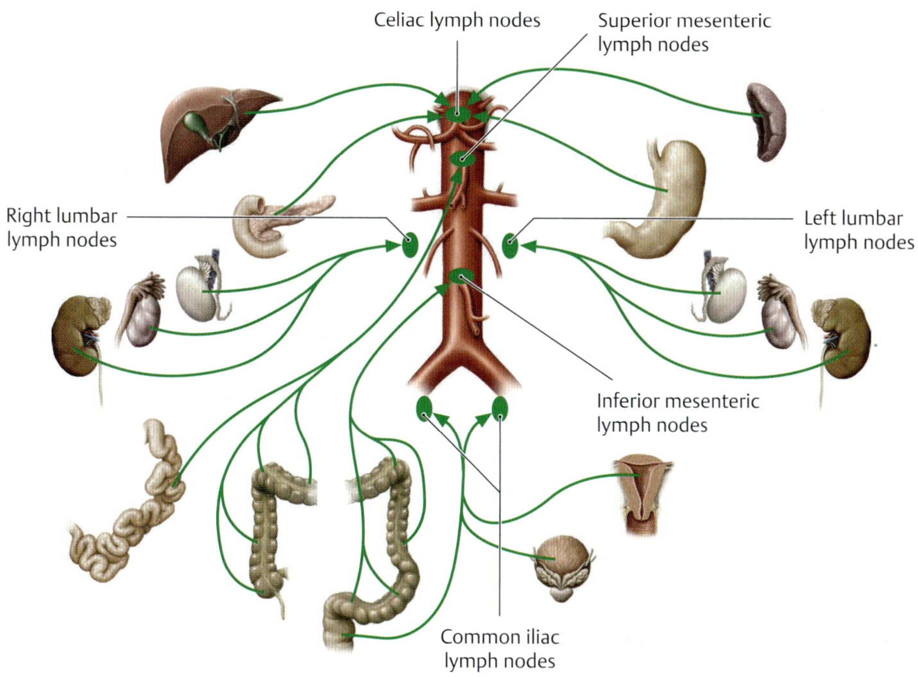

C Lymph node groups in the abdomen and pelvis

Before lymph from the organs of the abdomen and pelvis enters the lymphatic trunks, it is filtered by **lymph nodes** that collect the lymph from a particular organ (or region). After leaving the regional nodes, the lymph drains to **collecting lymph nodes**. These are the nodes that collect lymph from several lymph node groups and carry it to the lymphatic trunks. In the abdomen and pelvis, these are the lumbar and intestinal trunks.

Note: One lymph node may function as a *regional lymph node* for *various* organs, but at the same time it may collect lymph from several regional nodes, functioning also as a *collecting lymph node*. This principle is illustrated in the abdomen and pelvis by the lumbar lymph nodes: They function as regional lymph nodes for the kidneys, suprarenal glands, gonads, and adnexa (see p. 332) and as collecting lymph nodes for the iliac nodes.

D Lymph node groups and tributary regions

Lymph node groups and collecting lymph nodes	Location (see **C**)	Organs or organ segments that drain to these lymph node groups (tributary regions)
Celiac lymph nodes	Around the celiac trunk	Distal third of esophagus, stomach, greater omentum, duodenum (superior and descending parts), pancreas, spleen, liver, and gallbladder
Superior mesenteric lymph nodes	At the origin of the superior mesenteric artery	Second through fourth parts of duodenum, jejunum and ileum, cecum with vermiform appendix, ascending colon, transverse colon (proximal two-thirds)
Inferior mesenteric lymph nodes	At the origin of the inferior mesenteric artery	Transverse colon (distal third), descending colon, sigmoid colon, rectum (proximal part)
Lumbar lymph nodes (right, intermediate, left)	Around the abdominal aorta and inferior vena cava	Diaphragm (abdominal side), kidneys, suprarenal glands, testis and epididymis, ovary, uterine tube, uterine fundus, ureters, retroperitoneum
Iliac lymph nodes	Around the iliac vessels	Rectum (anal end), bladder and urethra, uterus (body and cervix), ductus deferens, seminal vesicle, prostate, external genitalia (via inguinal lymph nodes)

2.7 Overview of the Lymphatic Drainage of Abdominal and Pelvic Organs

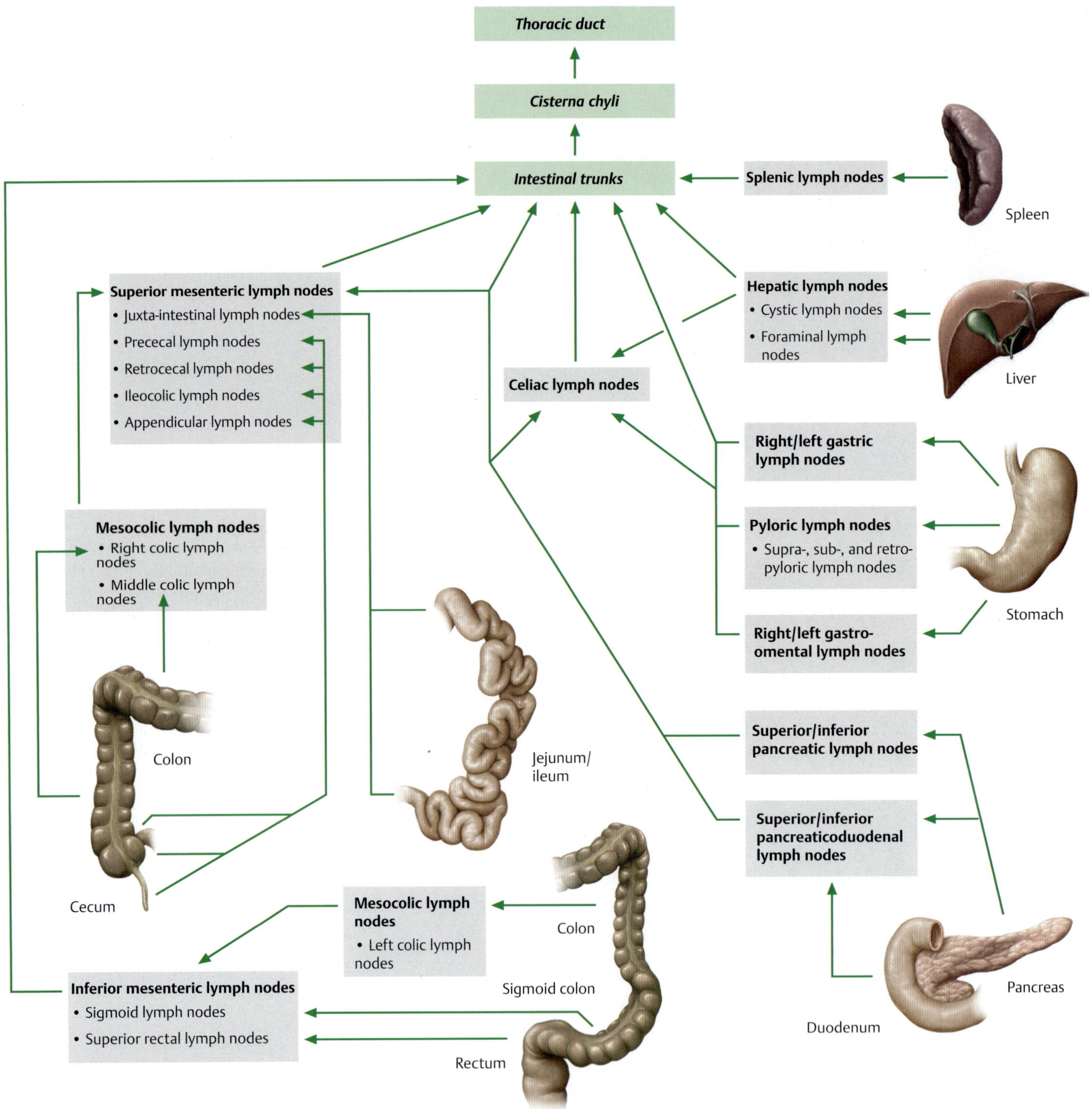

A Principal lymphatic pathways draining the digestive organs and spleen

Lymph from the spleen and most of the digestive organs drains directly from regional lymph nodes or through intervening collecting lymph nodes to the *intestinal trunks*. Exceptions are the descending colon, sigmoid colon, and the upper part of the rectum, which are drained by the *left lumbar trunk*. The organs and visceral lymph nodes in the above schematic are served mainly by three large collecting stations (individual lymph nodes see p. 298 ff):

- Celiac lymph nodes: collect lymph from the stomach, duodenum, pancreas, spleen, and liver. Topographically and at dissection, they are often indistinguishable from the regional lymph nodes of nearby upper abdominal organs.
- Superior mesenteric lymph nodes: collect lymph from the jejunum, ileum, ascending colon, and transverse colon.
- Inferior mesenteric lymph nodes: collect lymph from the descending colon, sigmoid colon, and rectum.

These collecting lymph nodes drain *principally* through the intestinal trunks to the cisterna chyli. There is also an *accessory* drainage route to the cisterna chyli by way of the left lumbar lymph nodes.
The lymphatic drainage of the rectum is described on p. 301.

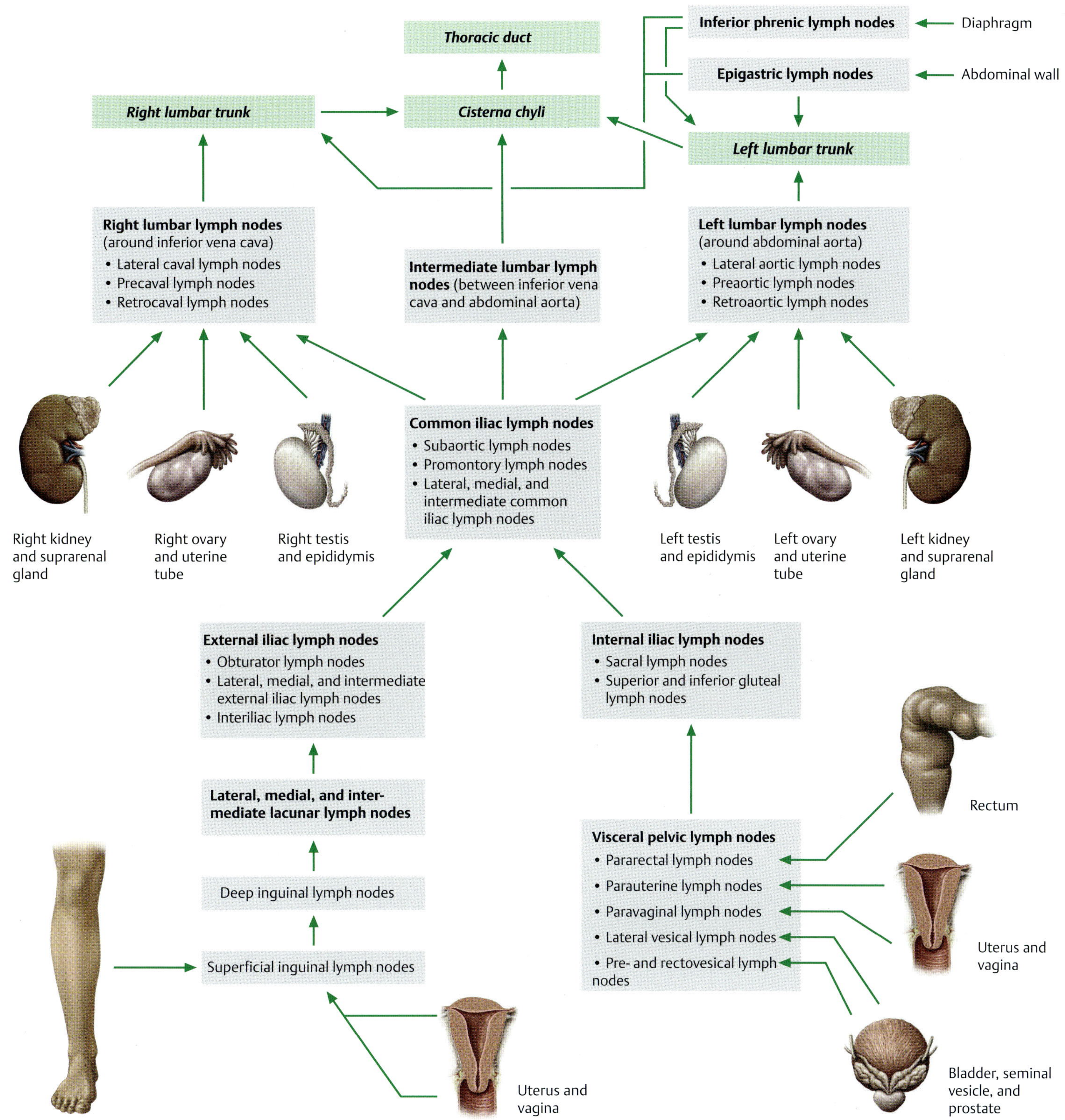

B Principal lymphatic pathways draining the organs of the retroperitoneum and pelvis (and lower limb)

Lymph from these organs drains principally to the right and left lumbar trunks. The following are important lymph node groups for the organs of the retroperitoneum and pelvis (and lower limb):

- Common iliac lymph nodes: collect lymph from the pelvic organs and lower limb.
- Right and left lumbar lymph nodes: collecting lymph nodes for the common iliac nodes, also regional lymph nodes for the organs of the retroperitoneum *and* the gonads, although the latter are located in the pelvis or scrotum. As the gonads undergo their developmental descent, they maintain their lymphatic connection to the lumbar lymph nodes (analogous to their blood supply, see p. 368). As a result, when tumors of the testis (or ovary), for example, undergo lymphogenous spread, they tend to metastasize directly to the abdomen rather than to the pelvis.

Both the iliac lymph nodes and the lumbar lymph nodes are classified as *parietal* nodes, a category that includes the phrenic and epigastric nodes. Lymph nodes such as the pararectal and parauterine lymph nodes are classified as *visceral* nodes.

2.8 Autonomic Ganglia and Plexuses

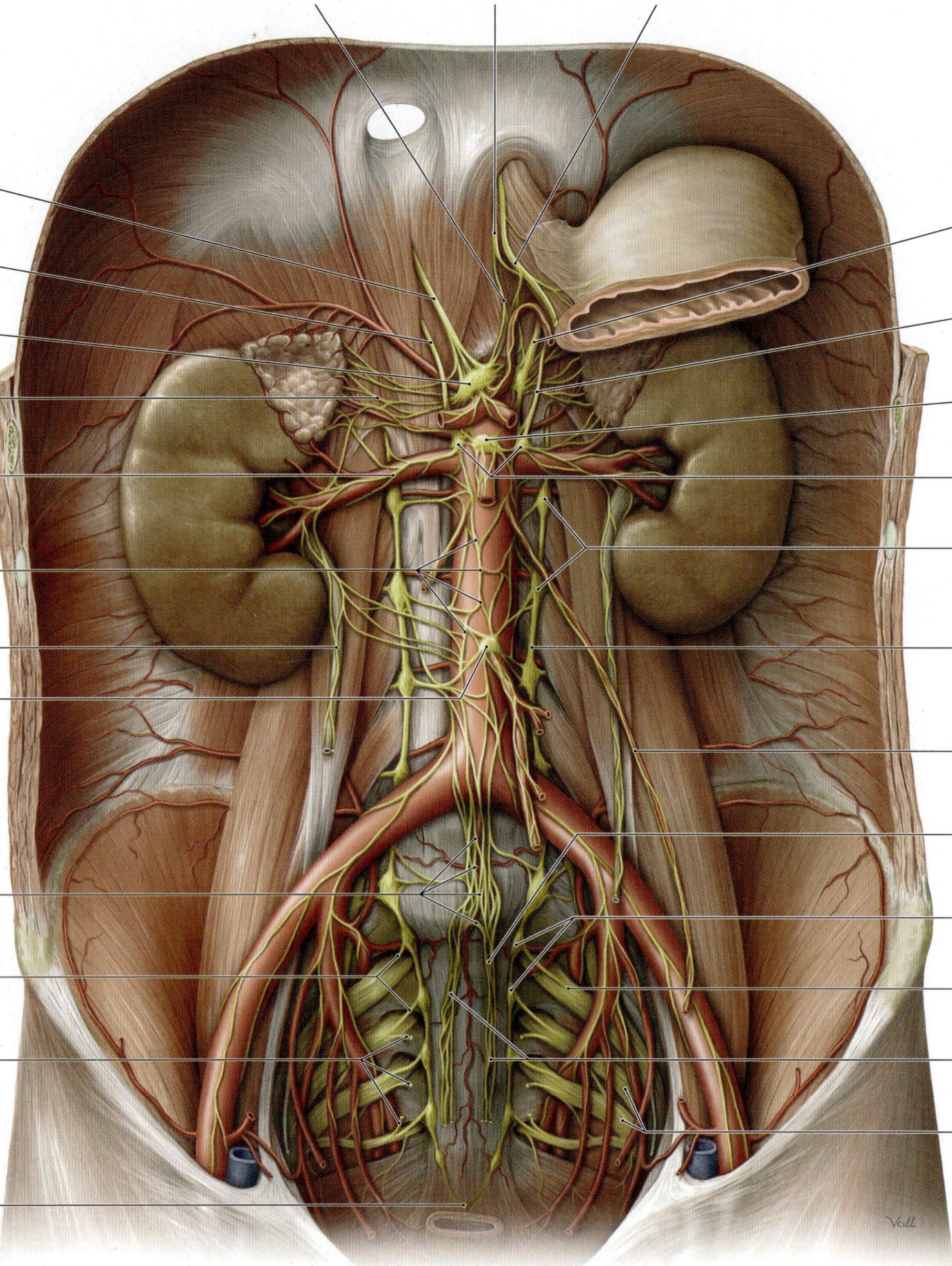

A Overview of autonomic ganglia and plexuses in the abdomen and pelvis

Anterior view of an opened male abdomen and pelvis with all of the peritoneum removed. Almost all of the stomach has been removed, and the gastric stump and esophagus have been pulled slightly inferior. The pelvic organs have been removed except for a rectal stump. The autonomic nervous system forms extensive *plexuses* and a number of *ganglia* around the abdominal aorta and within the pelvis, the ganglia marking the sites where the first presynaptic neuron synapses with the second postsynaptic neuron. All of the autonomic plexuses in front of and alongside the abdominal aorta are collectively termed the *abdominal aortic plexus*. This structure also includes the individual plexuses located at the origins of the paired and unpaired branches of the abdominal aorta (see **B**). As a general rule, sympathetic and parasympathetic nerve fibers come together in the plexuses on their way to the target organ.

Note: The left and right vagus nerves are organized around the esophagus to form the anterior and posterior vagal trunks. Both trunks contain fibers from both vagus nerves, the *anterior* vagal trunk containing more fibers from the left vagus nerve, the *posterior* trunk containing more fibers from the right vagus nerve. While the anterior vagal trunk generally terminates at the stomach, the posterior vagal trunk goes on to supply the entire small intestine and the large intestine approximately to the junction of the middle and distal thirds of the transverse colon.

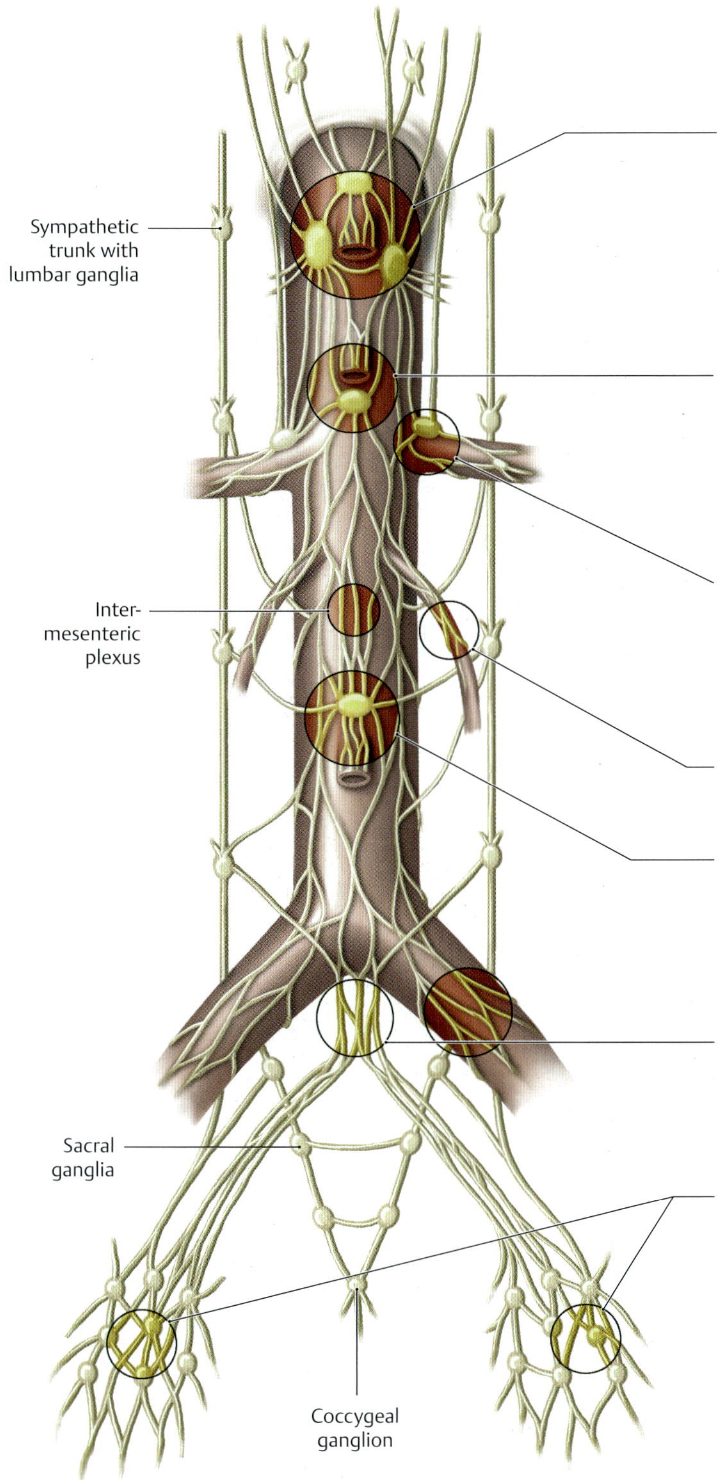

Celiac plexus
with celiac ganglia

- Hepatic plexus → Liver, gallbladder
- Gastric plexus → Stomach
- Splenic plexus → Spleen
- Pancreatic plexus → Pancreas, duodenum

Superior mesenteric plexus
with superior mesenteric ganglion

- No subplexuses → Pancreas (head only), duodenum, jejunum, ileum, cecum, colon to left colic flexure, ovary

Suprarenal and renal plexus
with aorticorenal ganglio

- Ureteral plexus → Suprarenal gland, kidney, proximal ureter

Ovarian/testicular plexus → Ovary, testis

Inferior mesenteric plexus

- Superior rectal plexus → Left colic flexure, descending and sigmoid colon, upper rectum

Superior hypogastric plexus

- Branches to ureter and genital organs → Ureter, epididymis, testis, ovary

Inferior hypogastric plexus
with pelvic ganglia

- Middle and inferior rectal plexus → Middle and lower rectum
- Prostatic plexus → Prostate, seminal vesicle, bulbourethral gland, ejaculatory duct, penis, urethra
- Deferential plexus → Ductus deferens, epididymis
- Uterovaginal plexus → Uterus, uterine tube, vagina, ovary
- Vesical plexus → Bladder
- Ureteral plexus → Ureter, ascending from pelvis

B Organization of autonomic ganglia and plexuses in the abdomen and pelvis

The ganglia and plexuses of the autonomic nervous system are named for the arteries that they accompany or around which they are distributed (e.g., the celiac ganglion and mesenteric plexus). In the *sympathetic* system, the presynaptic neuron synapses with the postsynaptic neuron in ganglia *distant* from the organs (or ganglion cells in a plexus distant from the organs); in the *parasympathetic* system, this synapse occurs in ganglia *near* the organs (or ganglion cells in a plexus near the organs). Thus, the parasympathetic ganglia are usually located on the target organ or in its wall, where they receive branches from the vagal trunks or pelvic splanchnic nerves.

Note: Even plexuses may contain aggregations of ganglion cells, sometimes very small. An example is the renal plexus, which contains the renal ganglia (too small to be shown in the drawing).

The autonomic plexuses contain efferent (visceromotor) fibers as well as numerous afferent (viscerosensory) fibers for both their sympathetic and parasympathetic components.

2.9 Organization of the Sympathetic and Parasympathetic Nervous Systems

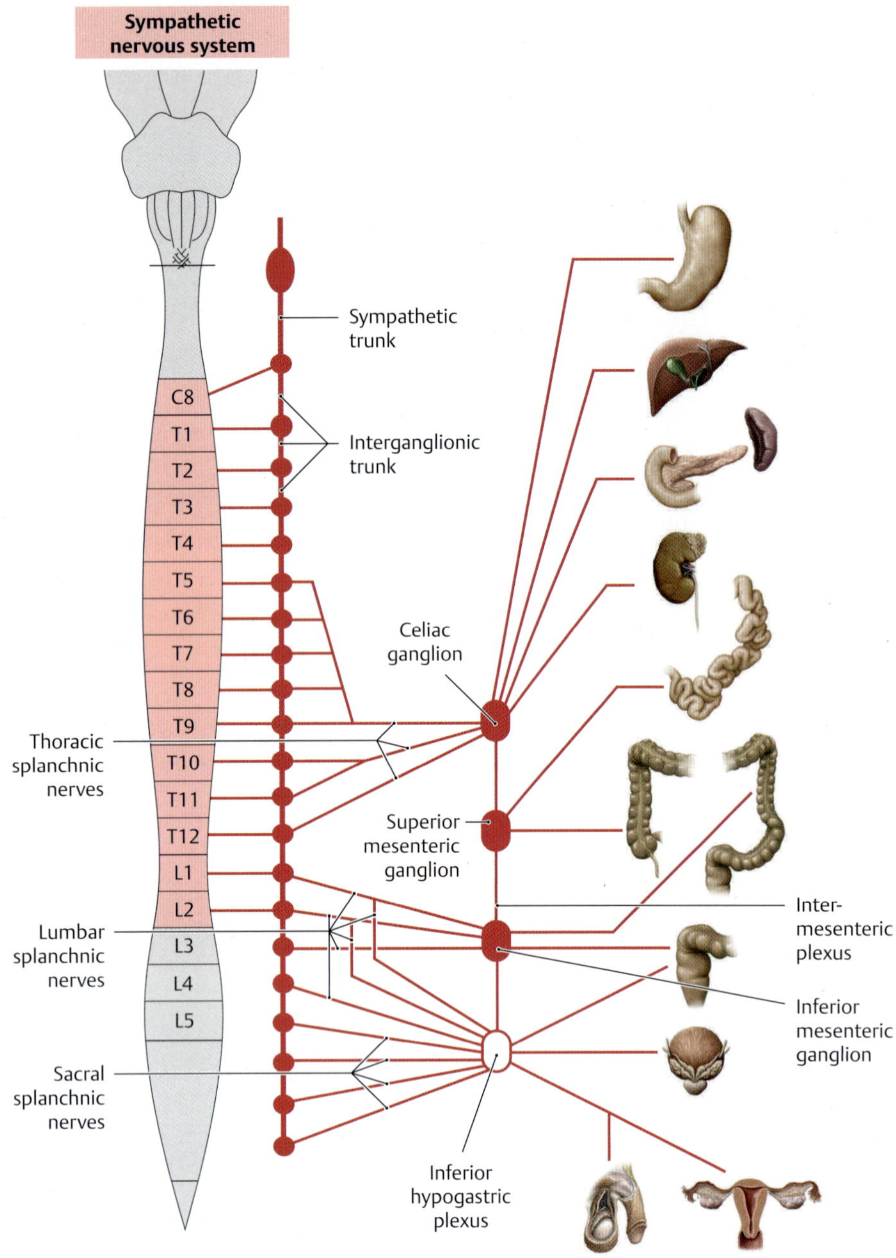

B Effects of the sympathetic nervous system on organs in the abdomen and pelvis

Organ, organ system	Sympathetic nervous system effects
• Gastrointestinal tract	
– *Longitudinal and circular muscle fibers*	Decreased motility
– *Sphincter muscles*	Contraction
– *Glands*	Decreased secretions
• Splenic capsule	Contraction
• Liver	Increased glycogenolysis/ gluconeogenesis
• Pancreas	
– *Endocrine pancreas*	Decreased insulin secretion
– *Exocrine pancreas*	Decreased secretion
• Bladder	
– *Detrusor vesicae*	Relaxation
– *Functional bladder sphincter*	Contraction
• Seminal vesicle	Contraction (ejaculation)
• Ductus deferens	Contraction (ejaculation)
• Uterus	Contraction or relaxation, depending on hormonal status
• Arteries	Vasoconstriction

A Organization of the sympathetic nervous system in the abdomen and pelvis

The **first**, or presynaptic, neurons of the sympathetic system that supply the **organs of the abdomen** are located in the lateral horns of spinal cord segments T 5–T 12. Their presynaptic axons pass *without synapsing* through the ganglia of the sympathetic trunk and form the thoracic splanchnic nerves (greater and lesser thoracic splanchnic nerves, and occasionally a least thoracic splanchnic nerve from T 12). The *synapse with the second, or postsynaptic, neuron* is located in the celiac ganglion, the superior (or inferior) mesenteric ganglion, or the aorticorenal ganglion (see p. 305).

The **first**, or presynaptic, neurons of the sympathetic system that supply the **organs of the pelvis** are located in the lateral horns of spinal cord segments L 1 and L 2. Their presynaptic axons pass through the lumbar ganglia of the sympathetic trunk and form the lumbar splanchnic nerves. The *synapse with the second, or postsynaptic, neuron* may be located in the lumbar ganglia, inferior mesenteric ganglion, or inferior hypogastric plexus. Beyond that point the postsynaptic fibers of the postsynaptic neuron generally pass to the target organ with its artery, usually accompanied by parasympathetic fibers of the autonomic nervous system.

Note: The peripheral ganglia of the sympathetic nervous system are distributed along the sides of the vertebral column (paravertebral). Peripheral ganglia in the abdomen and pelvis are also placed anterior to the vertebral column (prevertebral) and sacrum.

The paravertebral ganglia are interconnected by interganglionic connections to form the sympathetic trunk—two long pathways extending along each side of the vertebral column. The ganglia are named for the corresponding levels of the spine (thoracic ganglia, lumbar ganglia, etc.) and are variable in number. The prevertebral ganglia are located at the origins of the major arteries from the abdominal aorta and are named accordingly (celiac ganglion, superior and inferior mesenteric ganglia, etc.).

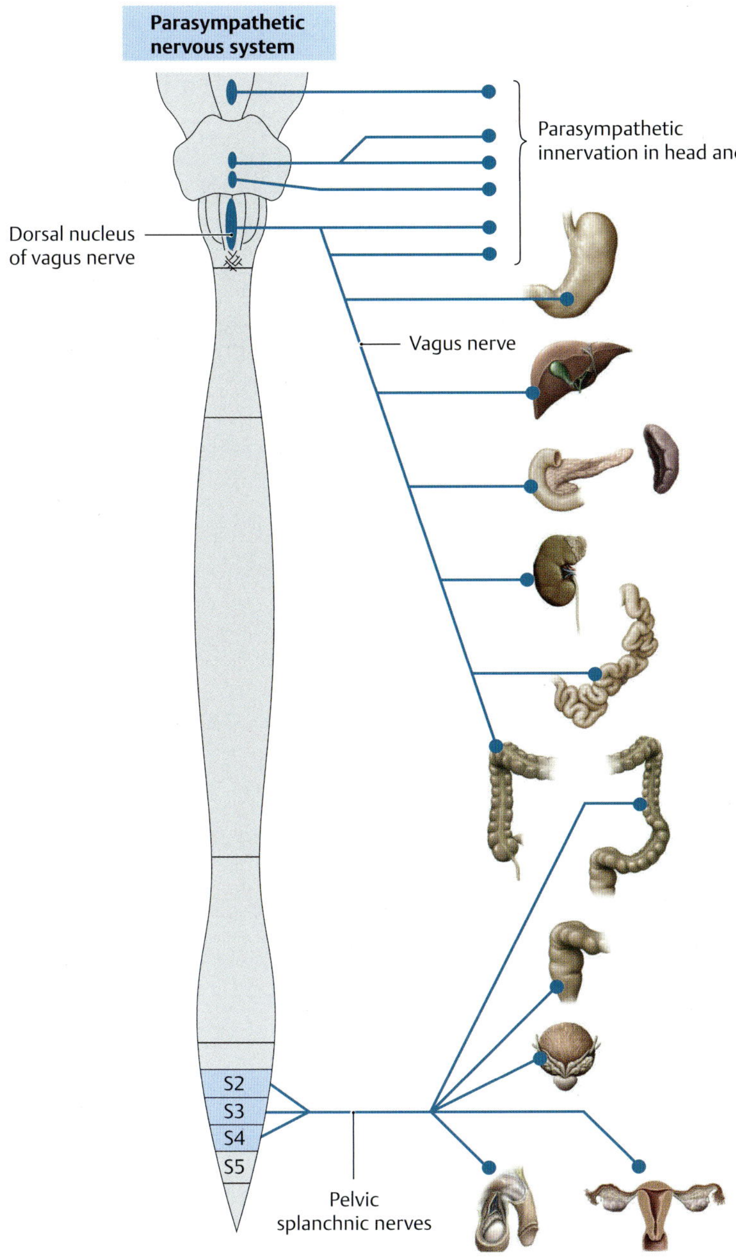

D Effects of the parasympathetic nervous system on organs in the abdomen and pelvis

Organ, organ system	Parasympathetic nervous system effects
• Gastrointestinal tract	
– *Longitudinal and circular muscle fibers*	Increased motility
– *Sphincter muscles*	Relaxation
– *Glands*	Increased secretions
• Splenic capsule	–
• Liver	–
• Pancreas	
– *Endocrine pancreas*	–
– *Exocrine pancreas*	Increased secretion
• Bladder	
– *Detrusor vesicae*	Contraction
– *Functional bladder sphincter*	–
• Seminal vesicle	–
• Ductus deferens	–
• Uterus	–
• Arteries	Vasodilation of the arteries in the penis or clitoris (erection)

Note the special role played by the suprarenal medulla and kidneys: the suprarenal medulla is phylogenetically and functionally analogous to a "sympathetic ganglion." It is thus part of the sympathetic nervous system and is therefore not listed in this table. The renal vessels are not regulated by the sympathetic or parasympathetic nervous systems, but by autoregulation (occurs only for renal blood flow). For functional reasons, the kidneys self-regulate renal blood pressure.

C Organization of the parasympathetic nervous system in the abdomen and pelvis

Contrasting with the thoracolumbar organization of the sympathetic nervous system, the parasympathetic nervous system in the abdomen and pelvis consists of *two topographically distinct systems*: a cranial part and a sacral part. This system also differs from the sympathetic nervous system in that the synapse of the first, or presynaptic, neuron with the second or postsynaptic neuron is located in the intramural ganglia of the organ walls.

- **Cranial part of the parasympathetic nervous system in the abdomen and pelvis:** The presynaptic neuron is located in the dorsal nucleus of the vagus nerve (i.e., the nucleus of cranial nerve X in the medulla oblongata). The axons (presynaptic nerve fibers) course with the vagus nerve to visceral or intramural ganglia, where they synapse with the postsynaptic neuron. The *distribution* of the cranial part includes the stomach, liver, gallbladder, pancreas, duodenum, kidney, suprarenal gland, small intestine, and the large intestine from the ascending colon to near the left colic flexure.
- **Sacral part of the parasympathetic nervous system in the abdomen and pelvis:** Its origin is located in the lateral horns of spinal cord segments S2–S4 (sacral intermediolateral nucleus). The axons (presynaptic nerve fibers) run a very short distance with spinal nerves S2–S4, then separate from them and course as the pelvic splanchnic nerves to ganglion cells in the inferior hypogastric plexus or organ wall, where they synapse with the postsynaptic neuron. The *distribution* of the sacral part of the parasympathetic nervous system in the abdomen and pelvis includes left colic flexure, the descending and sigmoid colon, rectum, anus, bladder, urethra, and the internal and external genitalia.

3.1 Stomach: Location, Shape, Divisions, and Interior View

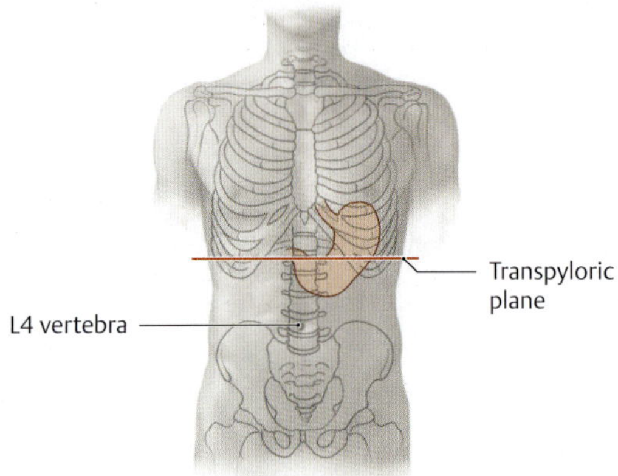

A Projection onto the trunk
Anterior view. The stomach is intraperitoneal and located in the left upper quadrant (epigastrium).
Note the transpyloric plane (halfway between the superior border of the pubic symphysis and superior border of the manubrium, see p. 378). It serves as an important anatomical landmark: the pylorus is located at or slightly below the transpyloric plane. Unlike other parts of the stomach, the pylorus hardly moves at all since it is connected to the duodenum, which is retroperitoneal (and thus relatively immobile).

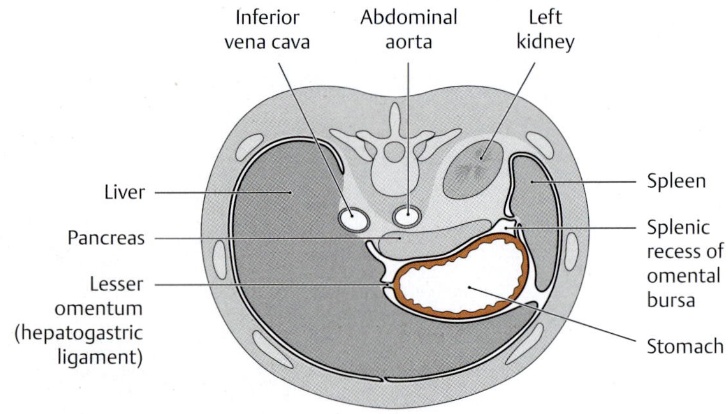

B Topographical relationships
Transverse section at approximately the T 12/L 1 level. Viewed from above.
Note the relationship of the stomach to the spleen, pancreas, liver, and omental bursa: The greater curvature extends to the spleen; the left lobe of the liver extends in front of the stomach and into the left upper quadrant. When the abdomen is opened, very little of the stomach is visible as most of it is obscured by the liver. Posterior to the stomach lies a narrow peritoneal space called the omental bursa. Its posterior wall is largely formed by the pancreas. Due to its peritoneal covering, the stomach is very mobile relative to the neighboring organs. This is important for facilitating the stomach's peristaltic movements. Due to its embryonic placement in the ventral and dorsal mesogastrium (see p. 42), the stomach has direct peritoneal attachments to the spleen and liver.

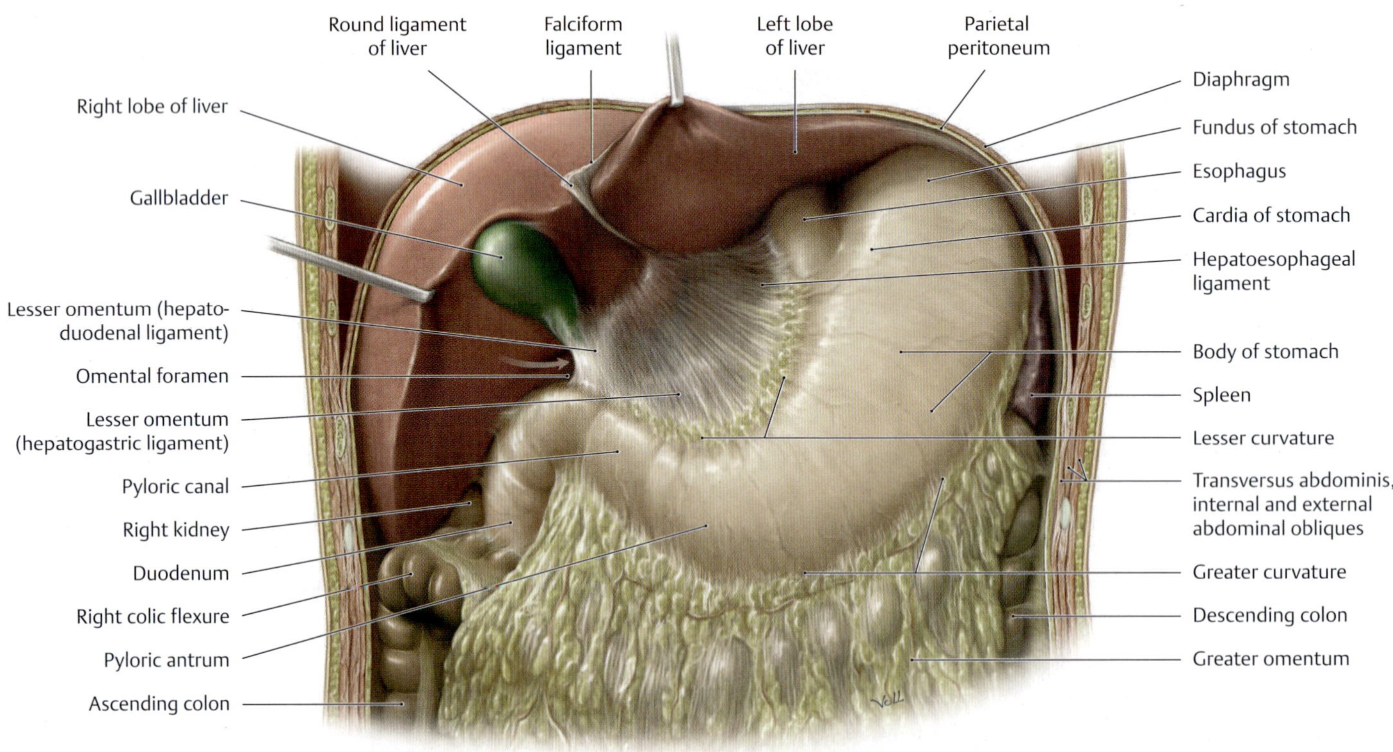

C The stomach in situ
Anterior view of the opened upper abdomen. The liver has been retracted superolaterally, and the esophagus has been pulled slightly downward for better exposure. The arrow points to the omental foramen, the opening in the omental bursa behind the lesser omentum. Peritoneal adhesions are visible between the liver and the descending part of the duodenum. The lesser omentum is visibly subdivided into a relatively thick hepatoduodenal ligament (transmitting neurovascular structures to the porta hepatis) and a thinner hepatogastric ligament, which is attached to the lesser curvature of the stomach. A hepatoesophageal ligament can also be identified. The greater curvature of the stomach is closely related to the spleen in the left upper quadrant (LUQ). The greater omentum is a duplication of peritoneum that covers the transverse colon and drapes over the loops of small intestine (not visible here).

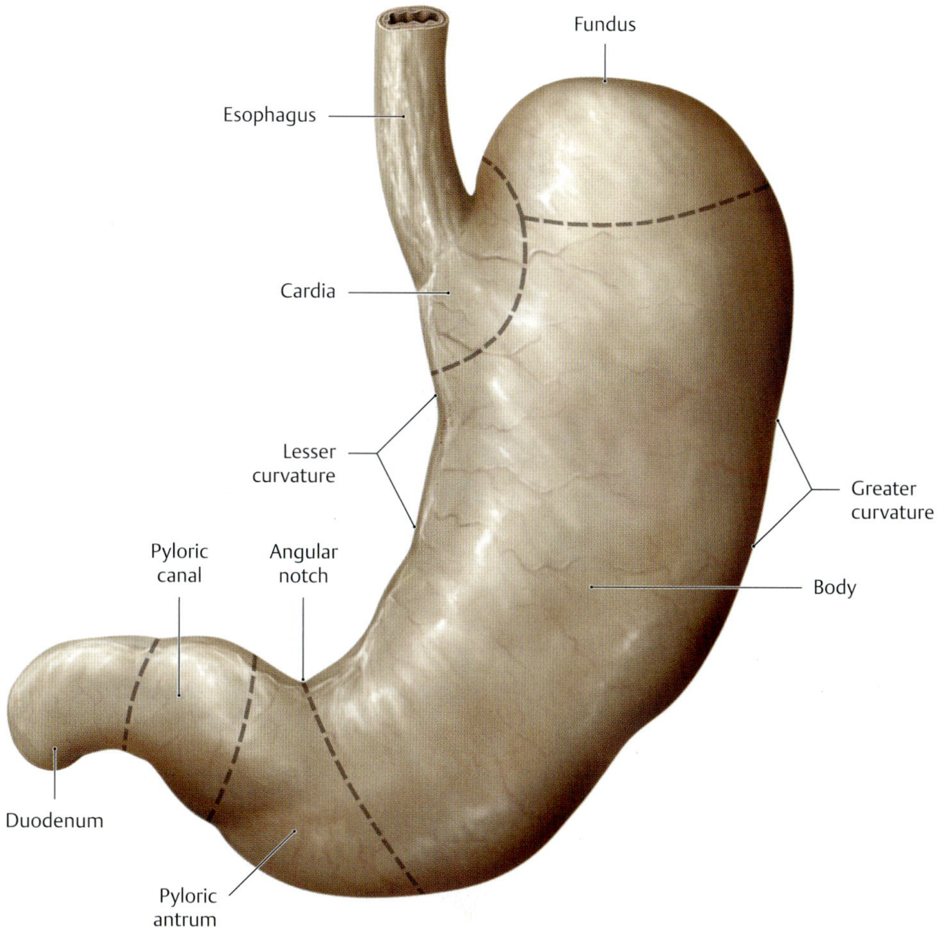

D Shape and anatomical divisions
Anterior view of the anterior wall. The body (corpus) of the stomach is the largest part of the stomach. It terminates blindly at the gastric fundus, which in the standing patient is the highest part of the stomach and is usually filled with air (visible on radiographs as the "gastric bubble").
Note: The cardia is the area of the gastric inlet where the esophagus opens into the stomach (at the cardiac orifice). While the esophagus is invested by adventitial connective tissue, the stomach has a visceral peritoneal covering or serosa. The transition from adventitia to serosa is sharply defined, and occasionally the serosa continues a short distance onto the lower end of the esophagus.
The part of the stomach that opens into the duodenum, the pyloric part, consists of a broad pyloric antrum, a narrow pyloric canal, and the pylorus itself (pyloric orifice). The circular muscle layer of the stomach is markedly thickened at the end of the pyloric canal to form the pyloric sphincter (see **E**), which produces a visible external constriction of the pyloric canal.

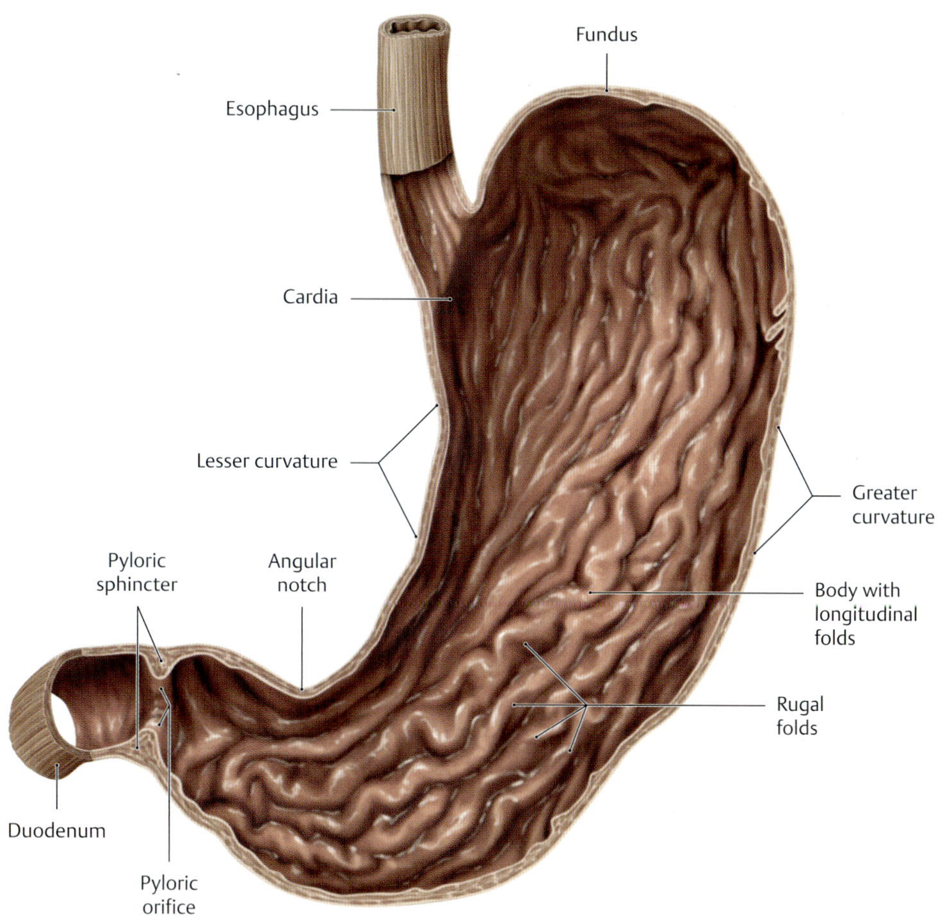

E Interior of the stomach
Anterior view of the stomach with the anterior wall removed. For clarity, small portions of the esophagus and duodenum are also shown. The gastric mucosa forms prominent folds (rugal folds) that serve to increase its surface area. These folds are directed longitudinally toward the pylorus, forming "gastric canals." The rugal folds are most prominent in the body of the stomach and along the greater curvature and diminish in size toward the pyloric end. The mucosa imparts a glossy sheen to the stomach lining.
Note: The pyloric orifice is quite large in this dissection. Normally, the orifice usually opens to a luminal diameter of only 2–3 mm.

3.2 Stomach: Wall Structure and Histology

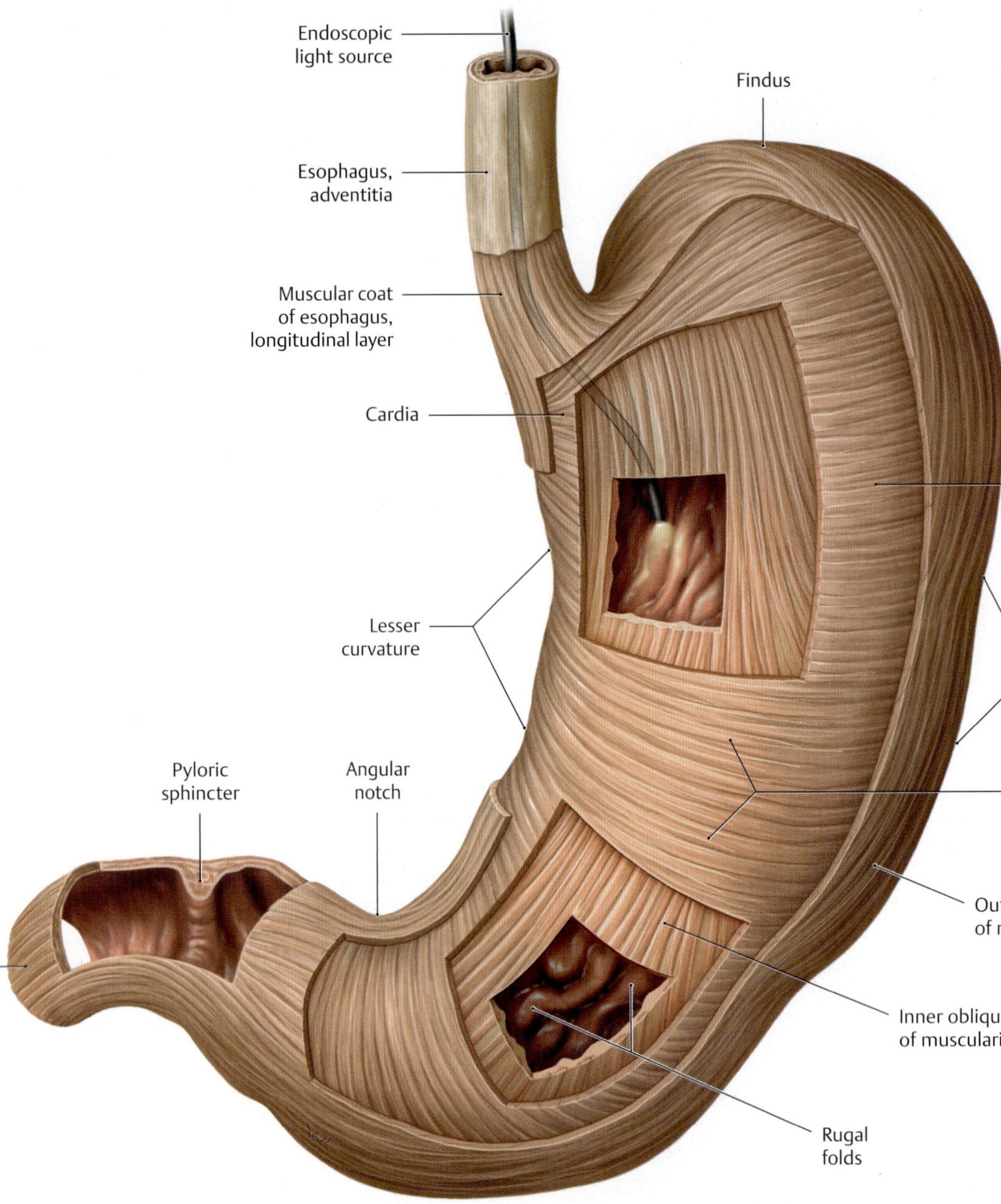

A Muscular layers
Anterior view of the anterior stomach wall with the serosa and subserosa removed. The muscular coat of the stomach has been windowed at several sites. The *entire stomach wall* ranges from 3 mm to approximately 10 mm in thickness (see **B** for individual layers). Most of its muscular coat consists not of two layers (as in other hollow organs of the gastrointestinal tract) but of *three* muscular layers:

- An outer longitudinal layer, which is most pronounced along the greater curvature (greatest longitudinal expansion)
- A middle circular layer, which is well developed in the body of the stomach and most strongly developed in the pyloric canal (anular sphincter, see p. 245)
- An innermost layer of oblique fibers, which is derived from the circular muscle layer and is clearly visible in the body of the stomach.

The three-layered structure of its muscular wall enables the stomach to undergo powerful churning movements. The muscles can forcefully propel solid food components against the stomach wall in the acidic gastric juice, breaking the material up into particles approximately 1 mm in size that can pass easily through the pylorus. The longitudinally oriented rugal folds (reserve folds that disappear when the stomach is distended) form channels, called gastric canals, that rapidly convey liquids from the gastric inlet to the pylorus.

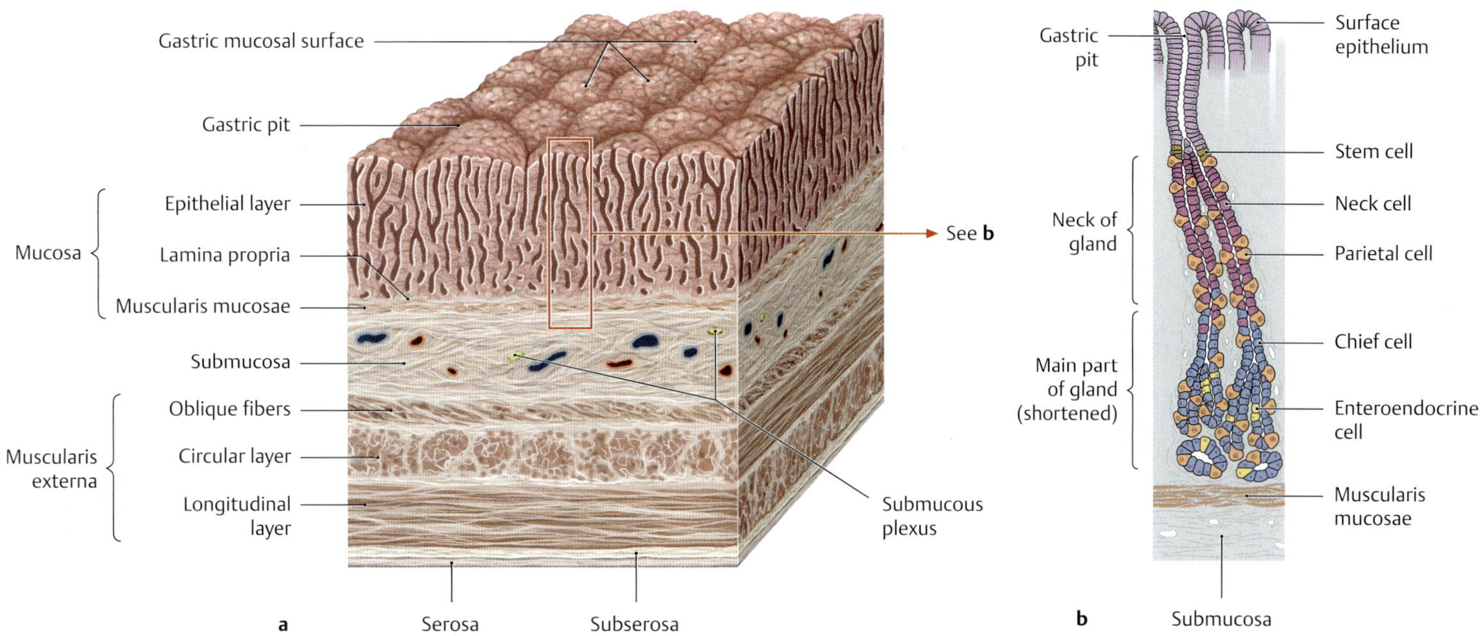

B Structure of the stomach wall and gastric glands

a The **structure of the stomach wall** illustrates the layered wall structure that is typical of the hollow organs throughout the gastrointestinal tract. The stomach is unique, however, in that its muscular coat consists of three rather than two layers (see **A**).

Note: The serosa (visceral layer of the peritoneum) and subserosa (connective-tissue layer giving attachment to the serosa and transmitting neurovascular structures for the muscular coat) are present only in areas where the organ in question is covered by visceral peritoneum. In wall areas that lack a peritoneal covering (e.g., large portions of the duodenum and colon), the serosa and subserosa are replaced by a fibrous adventitia, which connects the wall of the organ to the connective tissue of surrounding structures.

The *mucosa* contains specialized cells that are aggregated into *glands* (visible microscopically). The glandular *orifices* open at the base of the gastric pits (see **b**). In the body and pylorus of the stomach these glands extend down to the muscular layer of the mucosa, the muscularis mucosae (deeper glands = more cells = higher secretory output). The submucosa (layer of connective tissue transmitting neurovascular structures for the muscular coat) contains the *submucous plexus* for visceromotor and viscerosensory control of the hollow organs in the gastrointestinal tract. This plexus, like the *myenteric plexus* (located in the muscular coat for visceromotor control of the visceral muscle, not shown here), is part of the *enteric* nervous system, which contains, in total, millions of scattered ganglion cells.

b Structure of the gastric glands (after Lüllmann-Rauch) (simplified schematic of a gland from the body of the stomach). Several types of cells are distinguished in the fundus and body of the stomach:

- Surface epithelial cells: cover the surface of the mucosa and secrete a mucous film.
- Neck cells: produce mucin to strengthen the mucous film (make it more anionic).
- Parietal cells: produce HCl and intrinsic factor, which is necessary for vitamin B_{12} absorption in the ileum.
- Chief cells: produce pepsinogen, which is converted to pepsin (for protein breakdown) in the stomach.
- Enteroendocrine cells: different subtypes producing gastrin (G cells), somatostatin (D cells), or other factors controlling motility and secretion
- Stem cells: reservoir for replenishing the surface epithelial cells and gland cells

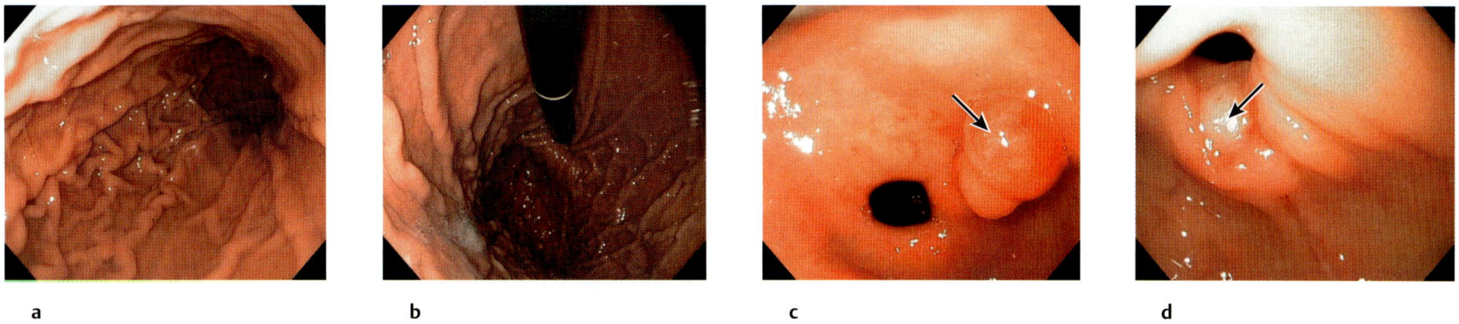

C Endoscopic appearance of the gastric mucosa

a and **b** Healthy gastric mucosa with a glistening surface; **c** and **d** Pathologic changes in the gastric mucosa.

a View upward into the body and fundus (inverted): The mucosa is raised into prominent folds due to the tortuous gastric rugae of the submucosa;

b Inspection of a normal pyloric antrum shows significantly less prominent folds than in the body of the stomach;

c Polyp (arrow) in the pyloric antrum;

d Gastric ulcer (arrow) in the pyloric antrum. A gastric ulcer is defined as a tissue defect that extends at least into the muscularis mucosae, but many ulcers extend into deeper layers of the stomach wall. Most gastric ulcers are caused by infection by *Helicobacter pylori*, a bacterium resistant to stomach acid (original images from: Johannes-Martin Hahn, M.D., Tübingen).

3.3 Small Intestine: Duodenum

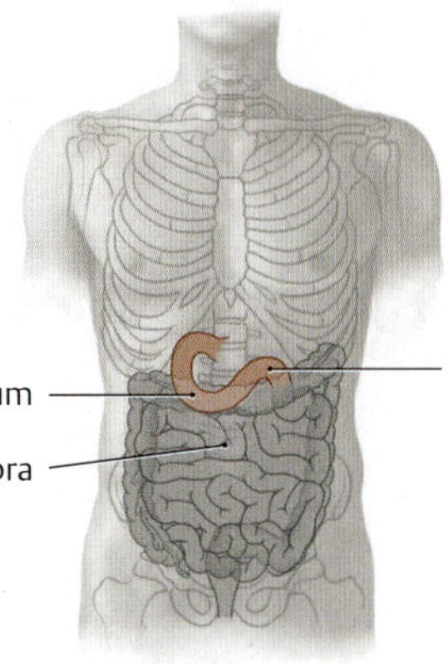

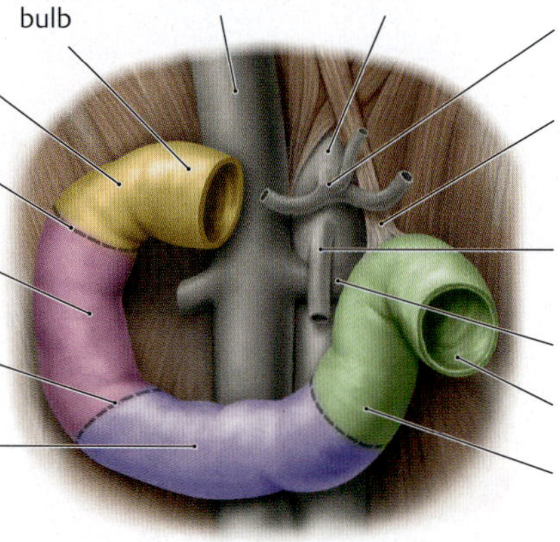

A Projected onto the vertebral column
The duodenum is a C-shaped loop of small intestine lying predominantly on the right side of the vertebral column in the right upper quadrant (RUQ) and encompassing the L 1 through L 3 vertebrae and occasionally extending to L 4. The concavity of the duodenum normally encloses the head of the pancreas at the L 2 level (see **D**).

B Parts of the duodenum
Anterior view. The anatomical parts of the duodenum (superior, descending, horizontal, and ascending parts with intervening flexures) have a total length of approximately 12 fingerwidths (L. *duodeni* = "twelve at a time").
Note the suspensory ligament of the duodenum (called also the ligament of Treitz), which often contains smooth-muscle fibers. Mobile loops of small intestine may wrap around this ligament and become entrapped between the ligament and the vessels behind it (most notably the abdominal aorta). This "Treitz hernia" may cause mechanical obstruction of the affected bowel loop and strangulate its blood supply.

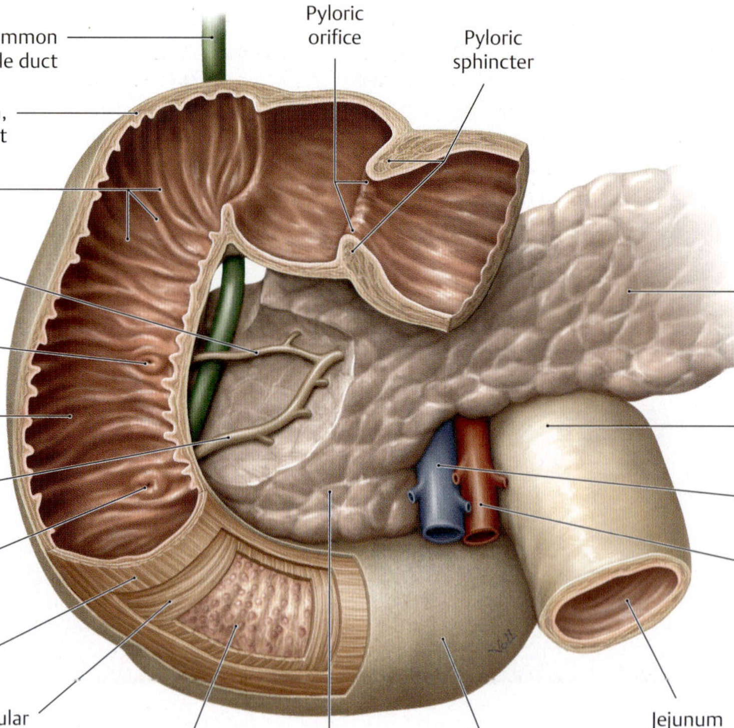

C Wall structure and duct orifices
Anterior view. Most of the duodenum has been opened. The pyloric orifice (here greatly dilated) opens to a luminal diameter of only about 2–3 mm for the passage of chyme. The duodenum has basically the same wall structure as the other hollow organs of the gastrointestinal tract (see **B**, p. 247). The structure of the mucosa is shown in **F**. The descending part of the duodenum has two small elevations along its inner curve: the minor duodenal papilla, which bears the orifice of the accessory pancreatic duct, and the major duodenal papilla (called also the *papilla of Vater*), which has a common orifice for the pancreatic duct and common bile duct. Thus, the release of bile and pancreatic juice to aid digestion takes place in the upper part of the duodenum.

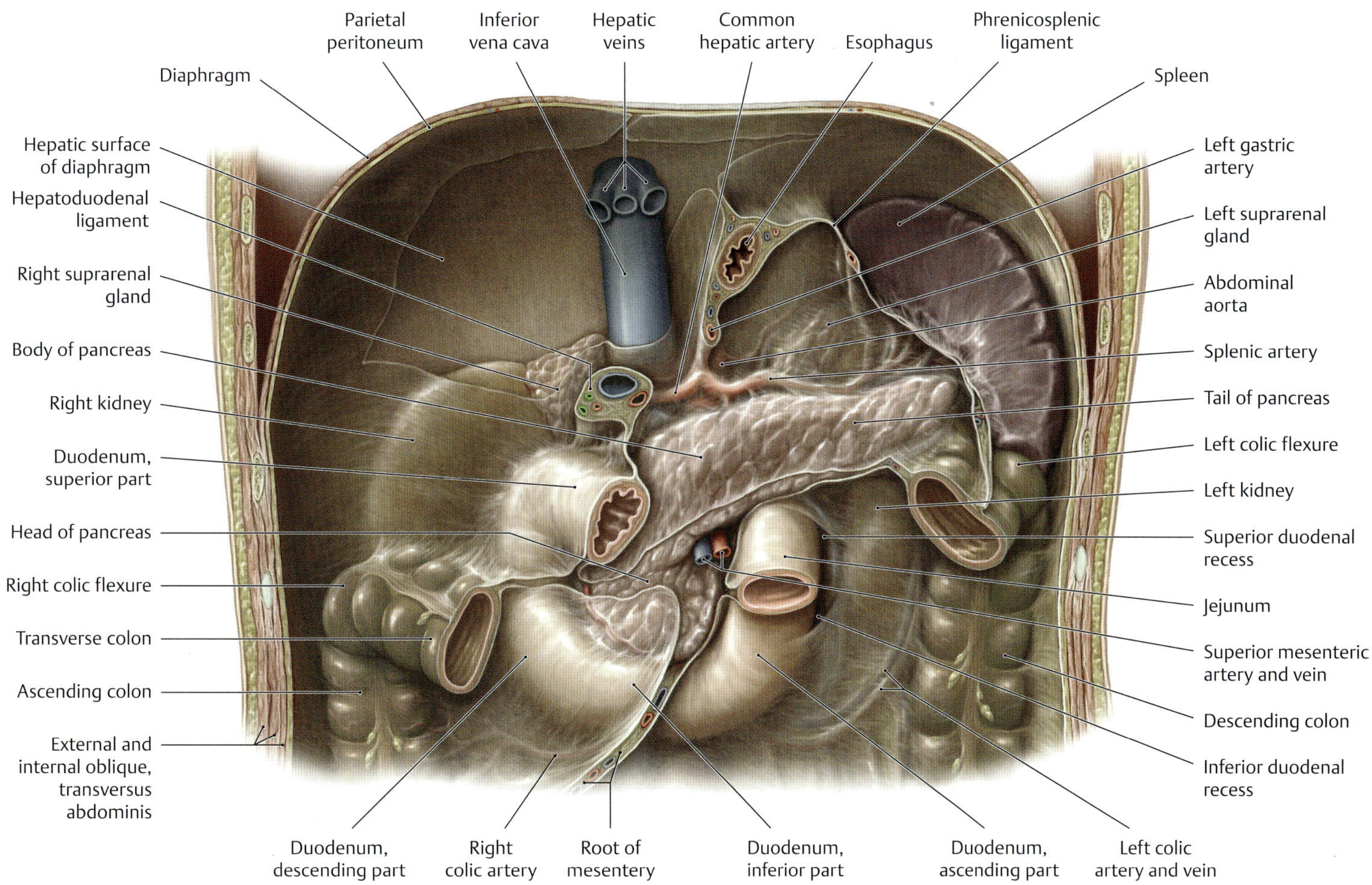

D The duodenum in situ
Anterior view. The stomach, liver, small intestine, and large portions of the transverse colon have been removed. The retroperitoneal fat and connective tissue, including the perirenal fat capsule, have been substantially thinned. The head of the pancreas lies in the concavity of the C-shaped loop of the duodenum. The first 2 cm of the superior part of the duodenum is still intraperitoneal (attached to the liver by the hepatoduodenal ligament), but most of the duodenum is retroperitoneal.

Owing largely to the proximity of the duodenum and the head of the pancreas, lesions of the pancreas (tumors) or malformations (anular pancreas) may cause duodenal obstruction. The peritoneum at the duodenojejunal junction forms the superior and inferior duodenal recesses. Mobile loops of small intestine may enter these peritoneal recesses and become entrapped there (*internal hernia*), causing a potentially life-threatening bowel obstruction.

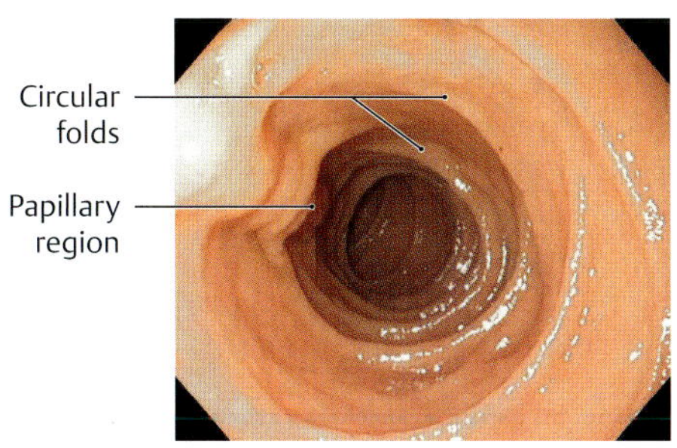

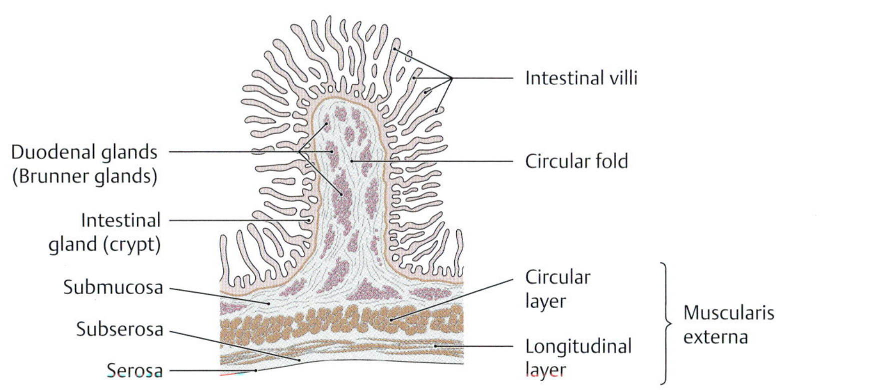

E Endoscopic view
The endoscope is pointing down into the descending part of the duodenum. The papillary region where the bile duct and pancreatic duct open into the duodenum is visible on the left side of the image at approximately the 10 o'clock position. The circular folds (valves of Kerckring) are typical of those found in the small intestine, diminishing in size in the proximal to distal direction (original image from: Johannes-Martin Hahn, M.D., Tübingen).

F Histological structure
Longitudinal section through the duodenal wall. The duodenum has basically the same histological structure as the other hollow organs of the gastrointestinal tract (see **B**, p. 247), with some notable differences such as the presence of duodenal (Brunner) glands (secrete mucins and bicarbonate to neutralize the acidic gastric juice) and valves of Kerckring (specialized circular folds). Other features that distinguish the duodenum from the jejunum and ileum are its more prominent mucosal folds, which diminish in size toward the end of the small intestine.
Note: The muscularis externa of *all* portions of the intestine, unlike that of the stomach, consists of only two layers: an inner layer of circular muscle fibers and an outer layer of longitudinal muscle fibers.

3.4 Small Intestine: Jejunum and Ileum

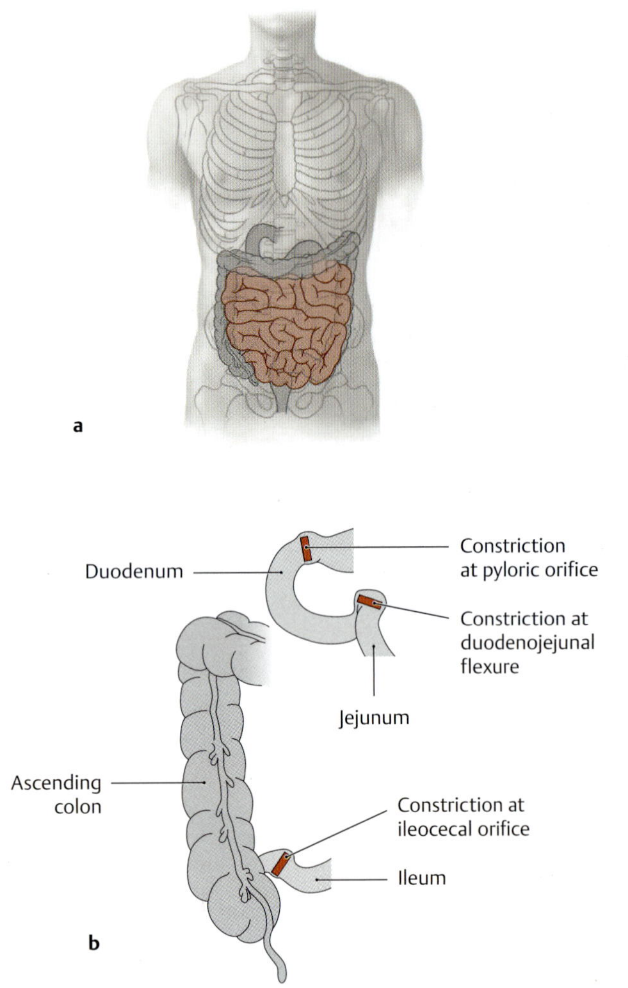

A Parts of the small intestine: overview (a) and anatomical constrictions (b)

Anterior view. The large intestine surrounds the loops of small intestine like a frame. Because the small bowel loops are intraperitoneal and therefore very mobile, it is not possible to define their location by reference to skeletal landmarks. If the intestinal loop rotates normally during embryonic development (see p. 46), the duodenum lies *behind* the transverse colon. If the intestinal loop rotates in the wrong direction, the duodenum will come to lie *in front* of the transverse colon.
Note the following normal anatomical constrictions:

- Junction of the pylorus and duodenum (luminal diameter of the pyloric orifice is only about 2–3 mm)
- Duodenojejunal flexure
- Ileocecal orifice

Swallowed foreign bodies may become lodged at these sites, obstructing intestinal transit and causing mechanical intestinal paralysis (*mechanical ileus*, a life-threatening condition that is an absolute indication for surgical treatment).

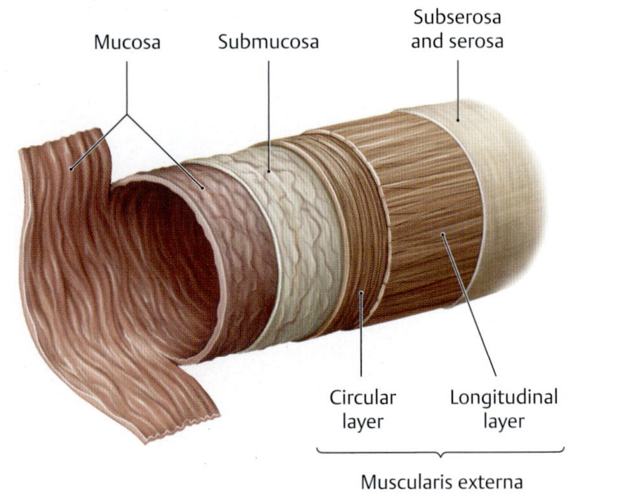

B Wall structure of the jejunum and ileum

The wall layers of the small intestine are displayed in a "telescoped" cross-section. The mucosal layer has been incised longitudinally and opened. The jejunum and ileum have basically the same wall structure as the other hollow organs of the gastrointestinal tract (see **B**, p. 247), but local differences are observed in the circular folds (see **C**) and vascular supply (see p. 286).

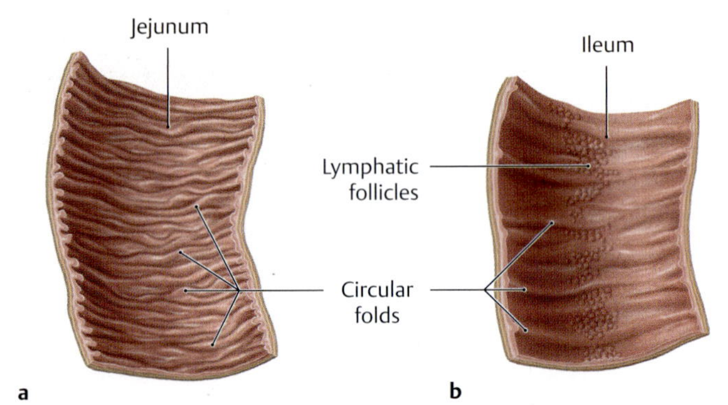

C Differences in the wall structure of the jejunum and ileum

Macroscopic views of the jejunum (**a**) and ileum (**b**), which have been opened longitudinally to display their mucosal surface anatomy.
Note: The transversely oriented circular folds in the jejunum are spaced much closer together than in the ileum. Lymphatic follicles are particularly abundant in the wall of the ileum (from the lamina propria to the submucosa) for mounting an immune response to antigens in the intestinal contents ("aggregated lymph nodules," Peyer's patches).

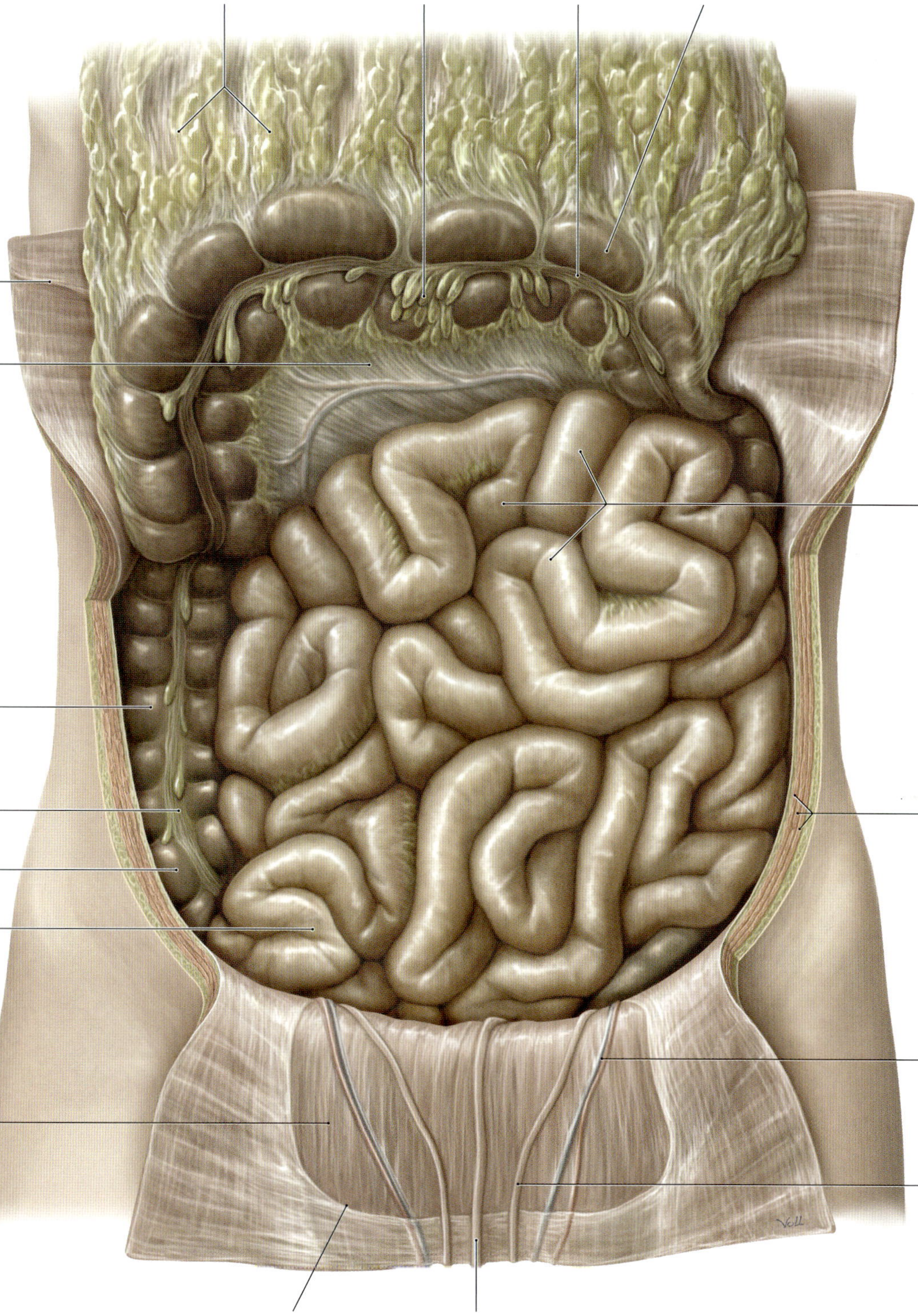

D The jejunum and ileum in situ

Anterior view. The abdominal wall has been opened and the transverse colon has been reflected upward. Coils of jejunum and ileum completely fill the four quadrants of the peritoneal cavity below the transverse mesocolon and are framed by the colon segments. In this dissection the loops of small intestine have been displaced slightly to the left in front of the descending colon, hiding it from view. The ascending colon and cecum are visible along the right flank of the abdomen.

3.5 Large Intestine: Colon Segments

A Anatomical divisions of the large intestine

The large intestine consists of the following divisions in the proximal-to-distal direction:

- Cecum with the vermiform appendix
- Colon, consisting of four parts:
  - Ascending colon
  - Transverse colon
  - Descending colon
  - Sigmoid colon
- Rectum

Note: For various reasons, some authors consider the rectum to be a separate section of the intestine, and not a part of the large intestine. However, according to the Terminologia Anatomica, which serves as the international standard on human anatomic terminology, the rectum is a segment of the large intestine.

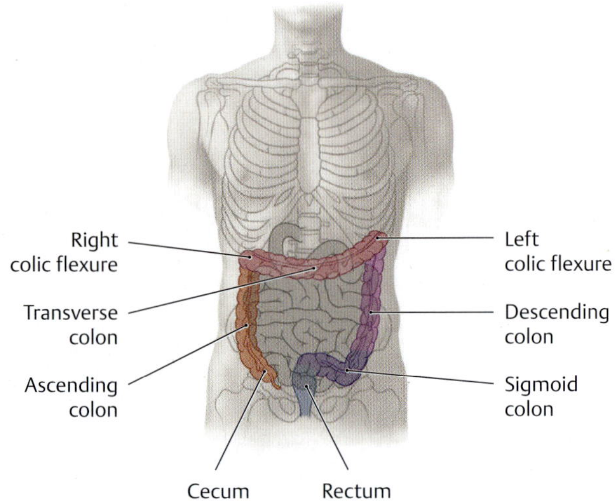

B Projection of the large intestine onto the skeleton

Because of the embryonic rotation of the primary intestinal (midgut) loop, the large intestine typically forms a frame encompassing the small intestine. The position and length of the colon segments may vary, however, depending on the course of intestinal rotation. For example, when the intestinal loop rotates normally, the ascending colon acquires a "normal" length (as shown here). If intestinal rotation is incomplete, the ascending colon is shortened. The transverse colon is particularly mobile owing to its mesocolon, while the ascending and descending colon are less mobile because they are fixed to the posterior wall of the peritoneal cavity. The left colic flexure usually occupies a somewhat higher level than the right colic flexure due to the space occupied by the large right lobe of the liver. Also, the descending colon is usually more posterior than the ascending colon.

C Distinctive morphological features of the large intestine

There are four morphological features—three visible externally and one internally—that distinguish the large intestine from the small intestine. It should be noted that these features do not occur equally in all parts of the large intestine and are absent in the cecum, vermiform appendix, and rectum.

Taeniae coli	In most portions of the large intestine, the longitudinal muscle fibers do not form a continuous layer around the intestinal wall but are concentrated to form three longitudinal bands, the taeniae (see **D**). Taeniae are not present in the rectum or vermiform appendix. The three taeniae converge to form the muscularis externa of the appendix.
Epiploic appendices	Fat-filled protrusions of the serosa, scattered over the surface of the large intestine except on the cecum (absent or sparse) and rectum (absent).
Haustra (haustrations)	Saccular wall protrusions between the transverse folds of the large intestine (see p. 254), absent in the rectum.
Semilunar folds	Visible only *internally*, in contrast to the external features above. They are functional features caused by contraction of the muscular coat. The internal folds correspond to external constrictions that separate the haustra.

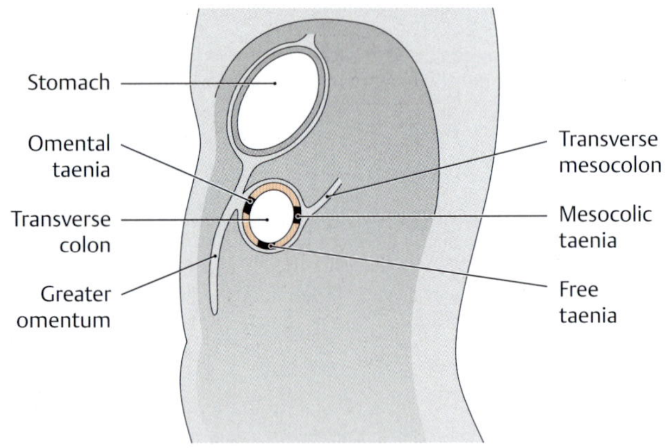

D The three taeniae of the colon

Sagittal section, viewed from the left side. The three taeniae are named for their position on the colon:

- Free taenia (Taenia libera)
- Omental taenia (the taenia at the attachment of the greater omentum)
- Mesocolic taenia (the taenia at the attachment of the mesocolon)

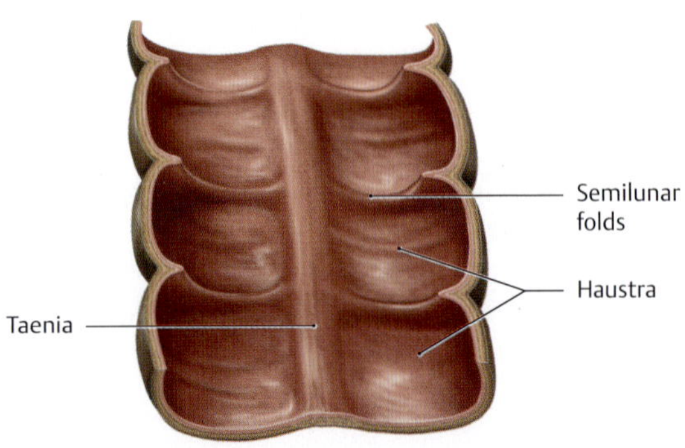

E Interior of the colon

The image shows the transversely oriented semilunar folds and the sacculations between the folds, the haustra. The semilunar folds are created by contraction of the muscularis of the wall of the colon and thus appear or disappear depending on the muscular tension in the muscular layer of the wall. The folds and haustra move slowly down the colon with waves of peristaltic activity.

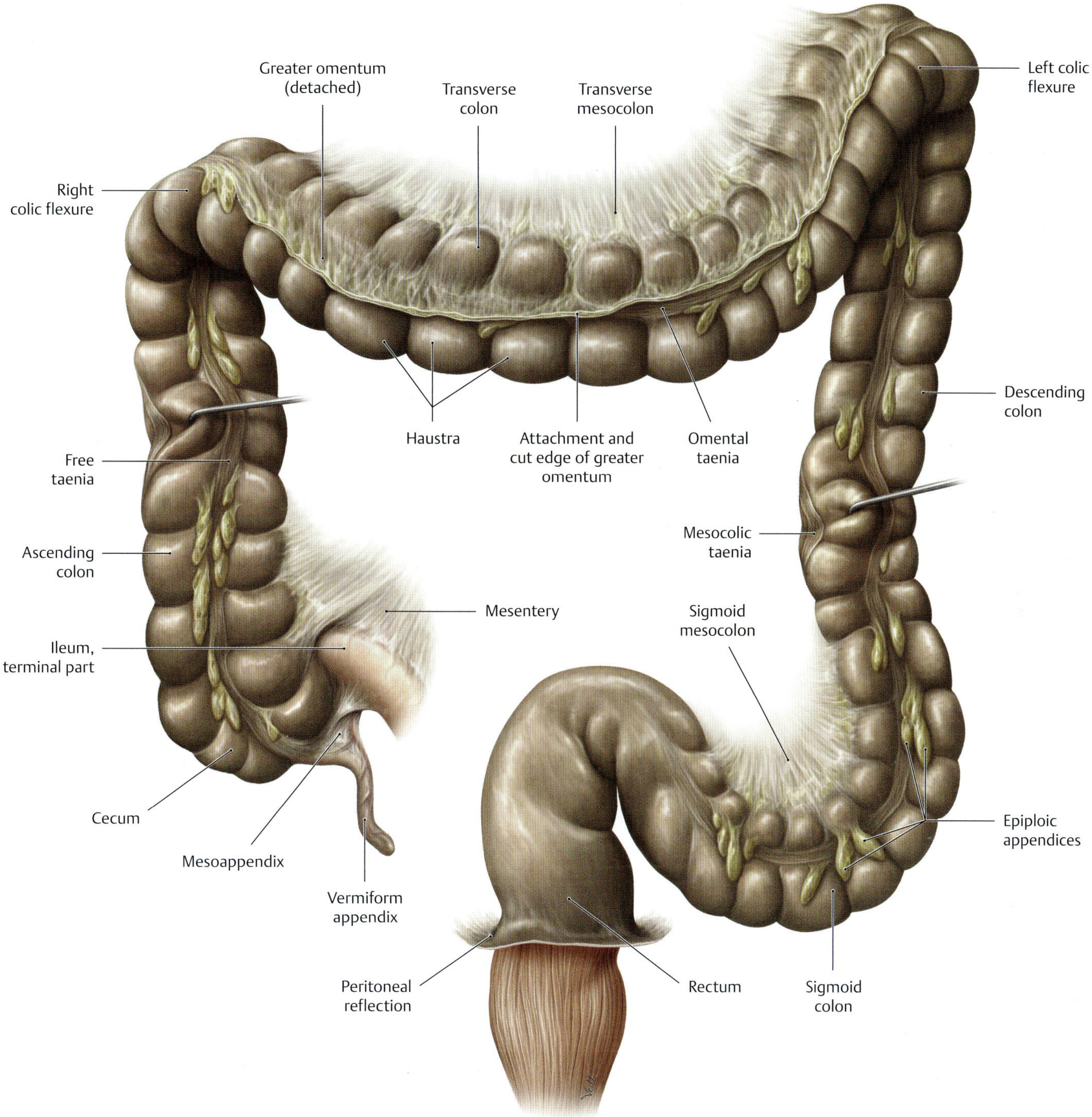

F Large intestine: segments, shape, and distinctive features
Anterior view, large intestine. The terminal part of the ileum and portions of the transverse and sigmoid mesocolon are shown. The ascending and descending colon have been rotated to display their taeniae.
Note: Colorectal cancer, which has become one of the most common cancers in industrialized countries, has a special predilection for the rectosigmoid junction and the rectum itself (i.e., sites distal to the left colic flexure see p. 264).
The various colon segments possess all the morphological characteristics of the large intestine (haustra, taeniae, epiploic appendices, see **C**). Typically these features disappear past the rectosigmoid junction. As the taeniae disappear, they are replaced on the rectum by a continuous layer of longitudinal muscle fibers. Instead of haustra, the rectum has three permanent constrictions that are produced by internal transverse folds (see p. 257). The peritoneal reflection on the anterior rectal wall represents the site where the peritoneum is reflected onto the posterior wall of the uterus (in the female) or onto the upper surface of the bladder (in the male).
Note: The ascending and descending colon are (secondarily) retroperitoneal and therefore, unlike the sigmoid and transverse colon, they do not have a mesocolon and are covered only anteriorly by peritoneum. The rectum is extraperitoneal in the lesser pelvis, lacks a “suspensory ligament,” and bears other unique features.

3.6 Large Intestine: Wall Structure, Cecum, and Vermiform Appendix

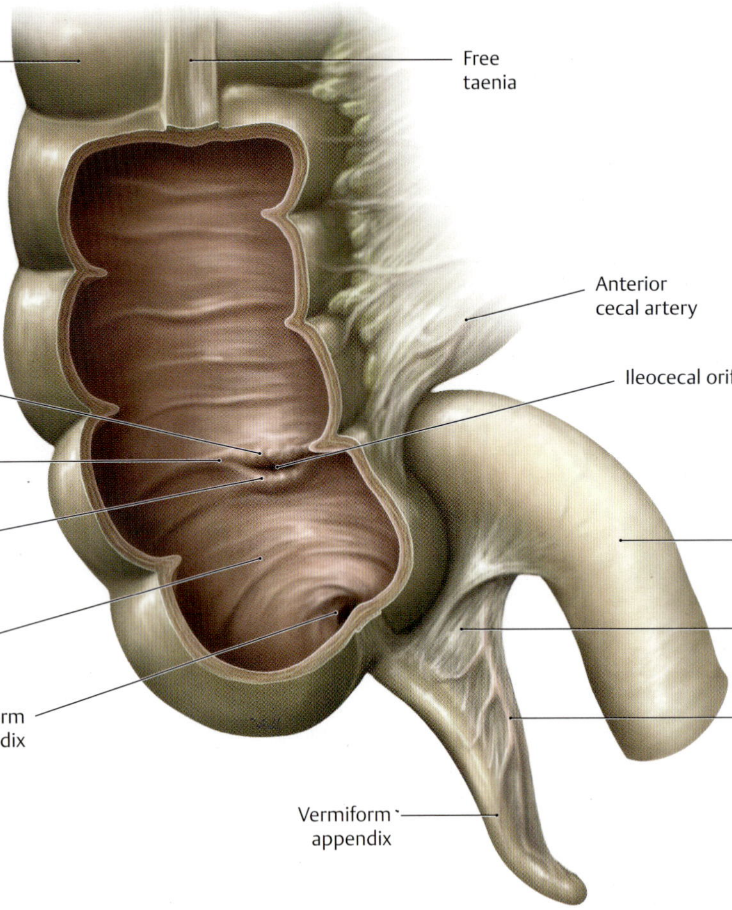

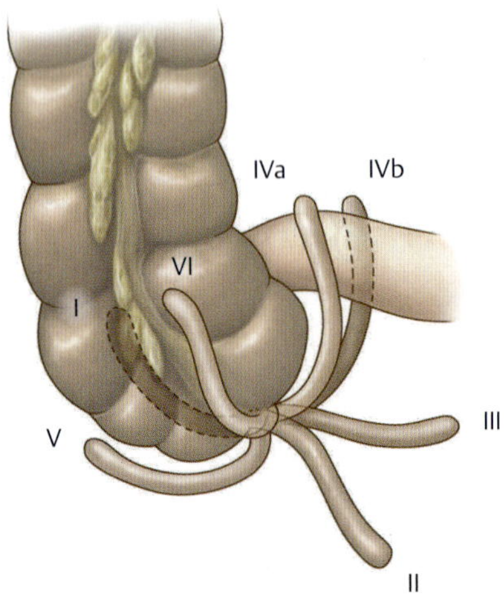

Variants (rounded to whole numbers)

I	= retrocecal	approx. 30 %
II	= pelvic	approx. 27 %
III	= subcecal	approx. 13 %
IV	= ileal	approx. 14 %
	IV a = preileal	approx. 9 %
	IV b = postileal	approx. 5 %
V	= paracecal	approx. 7 %
VI	= anterocecal	approx. 4 %
VII	= other (not shown)	approx. 5 %

A Cecum and terminal ileum

a Anterior view; **b** Positional variants of the vermiform appendix (data from Kacprzyk A, Droś J, Stefura T et al.). The cecum is unique in its end-to-side connection with the terminal part of the small intestine (ileum) and the presence of its vermiform appendix (average length approximately 8–10 cm, average diameter: 0.5–1.0 cm). As a result, it has two openings: a superior one, the ileocecal orifice on a small papilla (ileal papilla) and an inferior one, the orifice of the vermiform appendix leading into the lumen of the appendix. The ileocecal orifice is approximately round in the living individual but is often slit-like in the postmortem colon, bounded by superior and inferior flaps or "lips," the ileocolic labrum (superior lip) and the ileocecal labrum (inferior lip). Both are continued as a narrow band of mucosa, the frenulum of the ileocecal orifice.

Note: Acute inflammation of the vermiform appendix (appendicitis) is one of the most common surgically treated diseases of the gastrointestinal tract. Untreated acute appendicitis can lead to the spread of bacteria from the intestinal lumen into the peritoneal cavity (a "ruptured appendix" in popular jargon). The bacteria can in turn gain access to the large peritoneal surface, quickly inciting a life-threatening inflammation of the peritoneum (peritonitis).

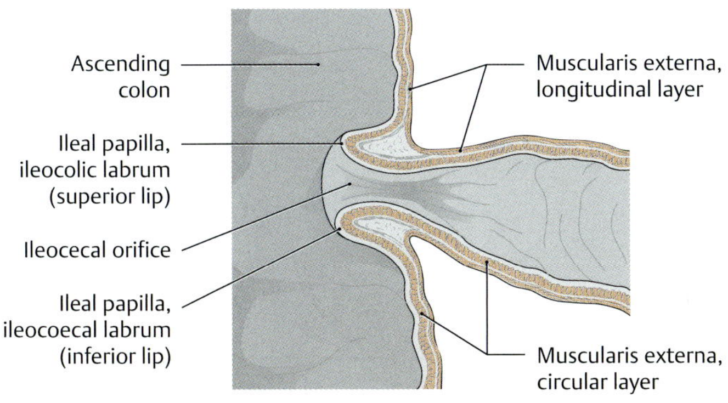

B Ileocecal Orifice

Anterior view of a longitudinal coronal section of the cecum and ileum. The ileocecal orifice hermetically seals the terminal ileum from the cecum and prevents the reflux of contents from the large intestine (structural constriction, see **A**, p. 254). At the ileocecal orifice, the end of the ileum evaginates the circular muscle layer of the large intestine into the cecal lumen. All layers of the ileal wall except the longitudinal muscle and peritoneum contribute to the structure of the ileocecal orifice. The circular muscle layers of the ileum and cecum function as a sphincter, which periodically opens the orifice. This allows the contents of the small intestine to enter the large intestine while effectively preventing reflux. The function of the sphincter is similar to that of the pylorus.

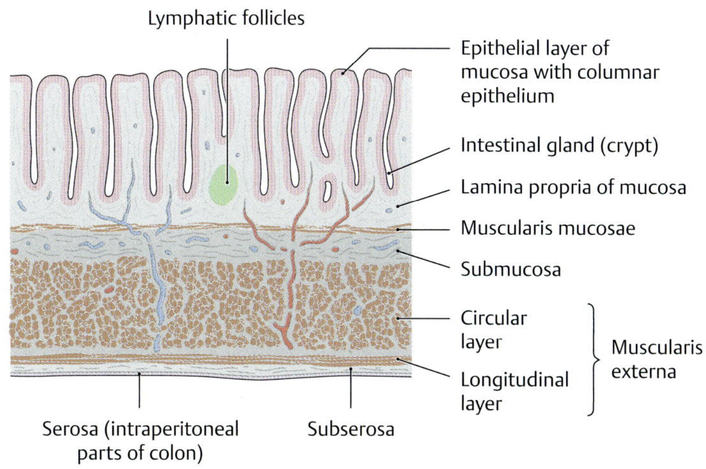

C Wall structure of the colon and cecum

Longitudinal section through the bowel wall. All the typical wall layers of the gastrointestinal canal are present: the mucosa, submucosa, muscularis externa, and serosa (or adventitia in the retroperitoneal parts of the colon, see **B**, p. 247). There are several features, however, that distinguish the wall structure of the colon and cecum from that of the stomach and small intestine:

- The mucosa is *devoid* of villi (i.e., the total surface area is not enlarged as much as in the small intestine). Instead of villi, there are large numbers of deep *crypts* (Lieberkühn crypts), more numerous than in the small intestine.
- The epithelial layer of the mucosa contains large numbers of goblet cells (for clarity, not shown here).
- The colonic mucosal surface undulates in large-scale, crescent-shaped, semilunar folds (see **E**, p. 252).
- The muscularis externa consists of an inner circular layer and an outer longitudinal layer, which is concentrated in three longitudinal bands, the taeniae (see p. 252).

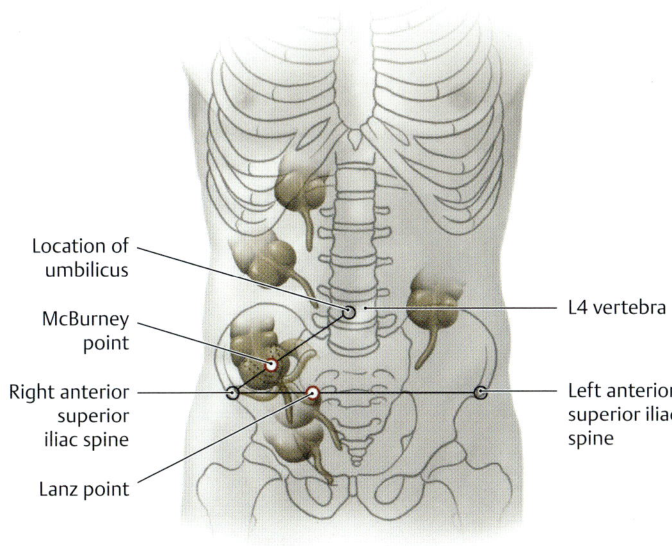

D Variants in the position of the vermiform appendix

Disturbances in the rotation of the embryonic gut can result in numerous positional variants of the cecum and vermiform appendix. The appendix may even come to lie in the left side of the abdomen. The inflammation of an appendix in the *typical position* is characterized by tenderness at two points:

- McBurney point: Position on a line connecting the umbilicus and the right anterior superior iliac spine. The McBurney point is one-third of the distance along this line from the iliac spine.
- Lanz point: Position on a line connecting the anterior superior iliac spines. The Lanz point is one third of the distance along this line from the right spine.

Although very useful, these are not definitive clinical signs. Tenderness may be felt at other abdominal sites, especially if the appendix is in an atypical position.

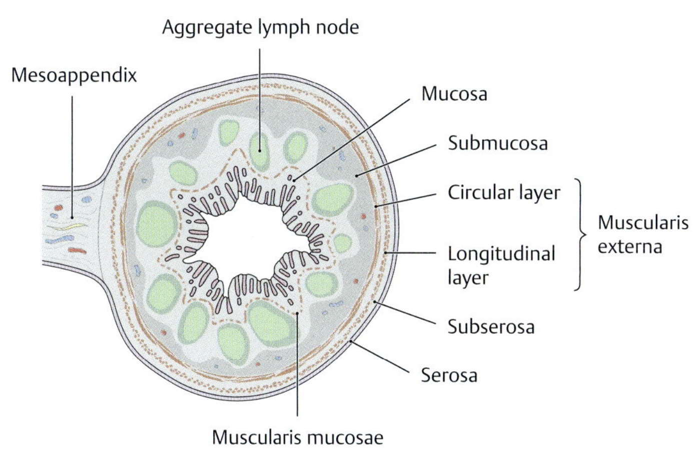

F Wall structure of the vermiform appendix

The vermiform appendix has the typical wall structure of an intraperitoneal intestinal tube. One striking feature is the abundance of lymphatic follicles in the submucosa (also present in the colon and cecum, but in much smaller numbers). With its high degree of immunological activity, the appendix has been characterized as the "intestinal tonsil." The mucosa has numerous deep crypts that are in intimate contact with the lymphatic follicles in the lamina propria and the submucosa (crypts and lymphatic follicles are not visible here). Since the vermiform appendix is intraperitoneal, it possesses a small mesentery, the mesoappendix, which transmits neurovascular structures.

3.7 Large Intestine: Location, Shape, and Interior View of Rectum

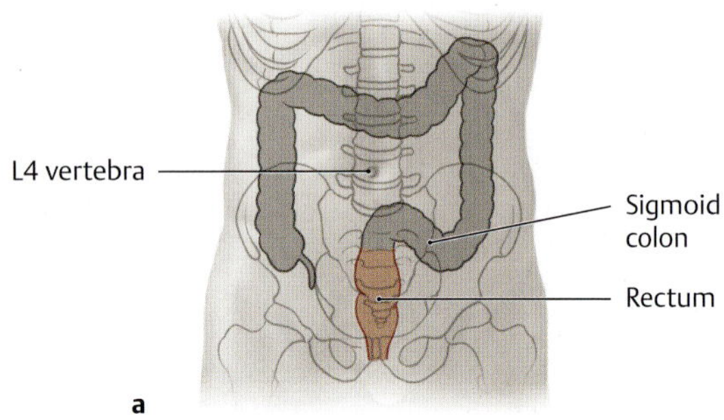

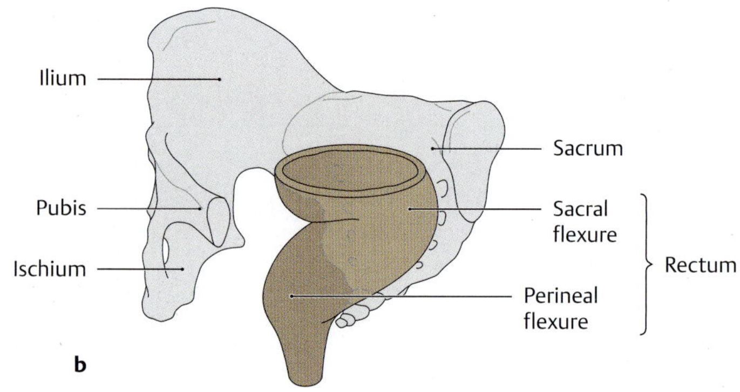

A Location and curves of the rectum
Anterior view (**a**) and left anterior view (**b**). The rectum is 15–16 cm long and extends approximately from the superior border of the third sacral vertebra to the perineum. It is "straight" only in the frontal projection (as shown in **a**); it presents two flexures in the sagittal projection (see **b**): the sacral flexure (retroperitoneal) and the perineal flexure (extraperitoneal), which represents the start of the anal canal and is already extraperitoneal. The sacral flexure—conforming to the shape of the os sacrum—is concave anteriorly. The perineal flexure is an important functional component of rectal continence (see p. 258f).

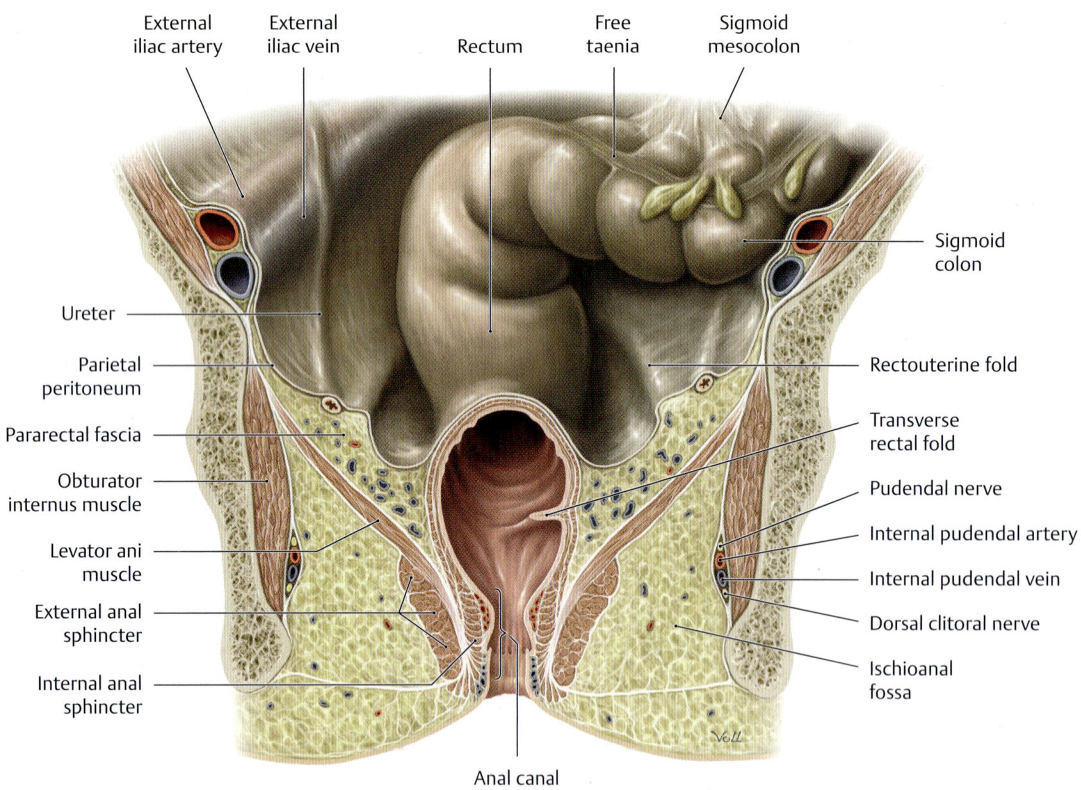

B The rectum in situ
Coronal section of the female pelvis, anterior view, with the rectum opened from about the level of the middle transverse inferior rectal fold. The taeniae of the sigmoid colon are not continued onto the rectum. The constrictions in the outer wall of the rectum correspond to the transverse folds on the inner wall. The rectum (which would appear in this form only if the ampulla were full) is shown in a slightly raised position. Below the levator ani muscle is the powerful external anal sphincter, the muscular component of the rectal continence organ. The pararectal connective tissue below the peritoneal cavity contains numerous vessels that supply the rectum.
This drawing was made from the dissection of a female cadaver. Thus, the peritoneum would be reflected from the anterior wall of the rectum onto the posterior wall of the uterus. Although both the anterior rectal wall and uterus are not visible here (anterior to this plane of section), parts of the rectouterine folds are still visible.

C Distinct morphological features of the rectum

The mucosa and wall structure of the rectum does not differ from the large intestine, including the colon and cecum. Nevertheless, it lacks several colonic characteristics:

- no taeniae, the rectum has a continuous longitudinal muscle layer;
- no omental appendices;
- no haustra;
- no semilunar folds, the rectum has transverse rectal folds;
- the wall of rectum is devoid of ganglion cells;
- embryonic development: The part above the anorectal line, like the colon, is derived from endoderm, the anal canal is derived from ectoderm (which is why some authors don't consider it part of the rectum).

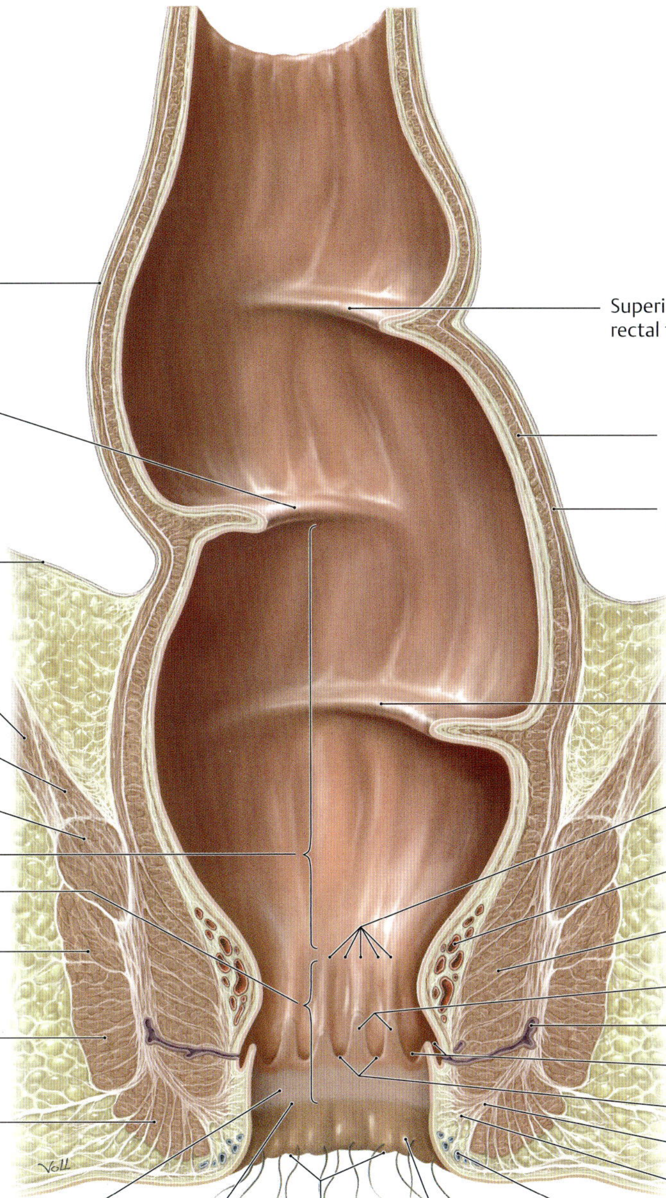

D Rectum and anal canal: divisions, internal surface and wall structure

Anterior view of the rectum in coronal section with the anterior wall removed. Instead of semilunar folds, the rectum contains three permanent transverse folds. The distal portion of the rectum, also known as the *anorectum*, is recognizable by a palpable protrusion (puborectalis sling or anorectal junction) which is visible on the mucosal surface. The anorectum is divided into two segments, the *rectal ampulla* and the *anal canal*.

- **Rectal ampulla:** the lowest portion of the rectum between the middle transverse rectal fold (Kohlrausch fold) and the anorectal junction. The rectal ampulla is the most distensible part of the rectum. It is normally empty. Once a certain volume of stool accumulates there, a specific mechanism triggers defecation (see p. 261). The middle transverse fold, which projects into the rectum from its right posterior wall, is approximately 6–7 cm from the anus and can just be reached with the palpating finger. Rectal tumors located below the Kohlrausch fold may therefore be palpable (see p. 264).
- **Anal canal:** located below the anorectal junction at the distal perineal flexure (see **A**). It is approximately 4 cm long and normally kept closed by the anal sphincter muscles. The clinically important "*surgical anal canal*" begins at the level of the anorectal junction and extends to the anocutaneous line, which is also palpable. It is a groove located between the margins of the internal and external anal sphincters (intersphincteric groove) at the junction of the anoderm (white zone), a region with very dense somatic innervation, and the pigmented perianal skin (see p. 258, **B**). Above the anoderm are located 8–10 longitudinal mucosal folds (anal columns), produced by the arterial cavernous body of the rectum (hemorrhoidal plexus), located in the submucosa (see p. 258). The distal ends of the mucosal folds are connected by valve-like transverse folds (anal valves). All anal valves together form the *dentate line*, which is an important landmark because it is visible. Behind the anal valves are pocket-like depressions (anal sinuses or pouches of Morgagni), into which empty 6–8 outflow ducts of the rudimentary mucus-secreting anal glands (proctodeal glands). The most common site of these glands is the posterior commissure (approximately at 6 o'clock in the lithotomy position), either in the submucosa or intersphincteric (between the internal and external anal sphincter) space, so that the outflow ducts partially transverse the internal anal sphincter.

Note: Bacterial infections of the glands may cause perianal abscesses and anal fistulas, which are difficult to treat (see p. 263).

3.8 Continence Organ: Structure and Components

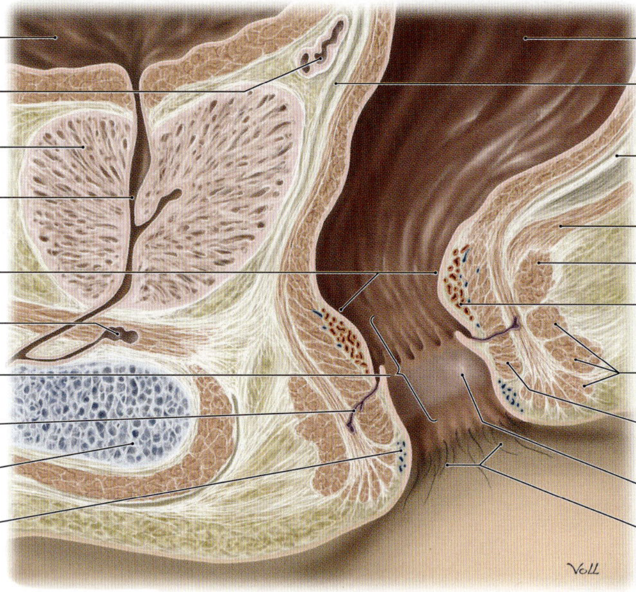

A Components of the continence apparatus
Midsagittal section at the level of the anal canal in the male, viewed from the left side.
The continence apparatus, or continence *organ*, controls the closing (continence) and opening (defecation) of the rectum and provides a tight closure before and after evacuation of solid, liquid and gas bowel contents.
It consists of a distensible hollow organ as well as vascular and muscular continence mechanisms, including their neural control. These angiomuscular continence mechanisms are integrated into a structurally narrow segment, which begins at the level of the perineal flexure and continues along the anal canal:

- Distensible hollow organ:
  - rectum with stretch receptors, mainly in the rectal ampulla (viscerosensory innervation)
  - anus with distensible skin in the anal canal (somatosensory innervation);
- Muscular continence:
  - internal anal sphincter (visceromotor innervation)
  - external anal sphincter (somatomotor innervation)
  - levator ani, especially the puborectalis muscle (somatomotor innervation);
- Vascular continence:
  - hemorrhoidal plexus (permanently distended cavernous tissue that subsides only during defecation;
- Neural control:
  - visceral and somatic nervous system (mainly from S2–S4) with the pelvic splanchnic nerves, pudendal nerve and rectal plexus.

Functionally, both continence and defecation are the result of a fine-tuned feedback loop between receptors and effectors of the continence apparatus with involvement of the central nervous system (see p. 260f).

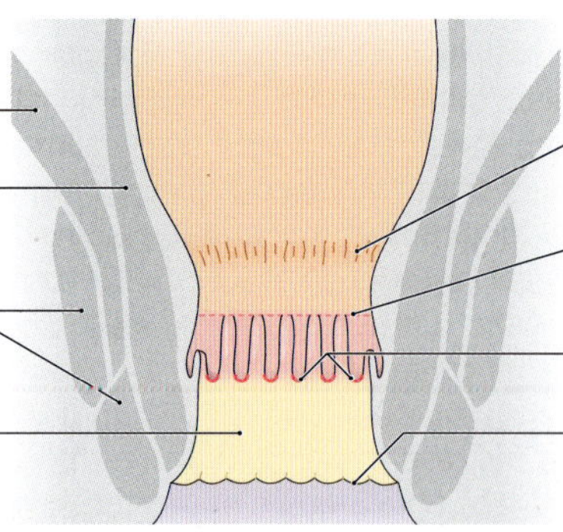

B Epithelial regions of the anal canal (after Lüllmann-Rauch)
In the anal canal, the unilayered columnar epithelium of the colorectal mucosa at the level of the transition zone is continuous with the stratified squamous epithelium of the anoderm and perianal skin. The transition occurs near characteristic landmarks. The anal canal can be divided into the following epithelial regions:

- **Colorectal zone** between anorectal junction and supratransitional line; homogeneous colorectal mucosa with crypts;
- **Transition zone** at the level of the anal columns (between supratransitional line and dentate line) mosaic patterns of colorectal mucosa, unilayered columnar epithelium and stratified squamous epithelium;
- **Squamous zone** between dentate line and anocutaneous line: evenly covered by stratified, nonkeratinized squamous epithelium, which is intimately attached to the underlying internal anal sphincter, hence its whitish appearance (white zone). Deep sensory innervation with touch, pressure, temperature and mainly pain receptors (clinically: anoderm);
- **Perianal skin** below the anocutaneous line: start of the stratified squamous epithelium of the outer layer of the skin (heavy pigmentation, eccrine and apocrine sweat glands and hair follicles).

Note: Knowledge about the epithelial regions of the anal canal is important mainly for the differentiation between rectal (usually adenocarcinoma) and anal carcinoma (of keratinizing or non-keratinizing squamous epithelium).

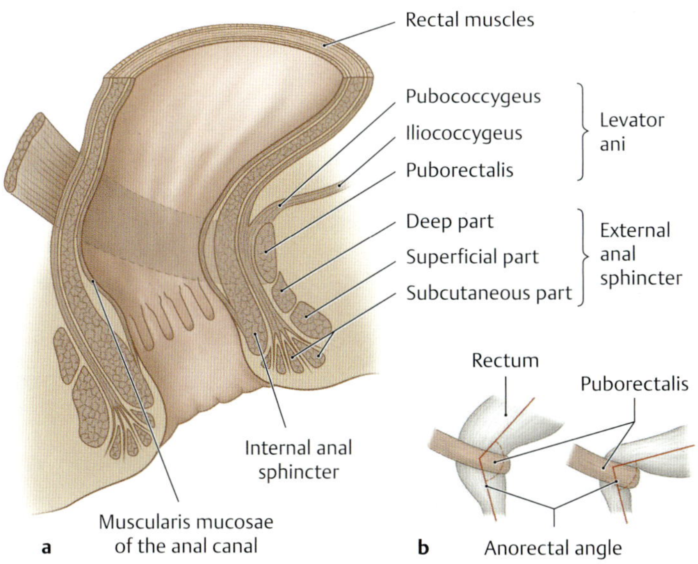

C Structure of the muscular continence mechanism

a Midsagittal section, viewed from the left side; **b** Puborectalis sling and anorectal angle: relaxed muscle (left) and contracted muscle (right). The complex system of anal sphincters involves both smooth and striated muscles. Whereas the smooth muscles represent the direct continuation of the muscles of the rectal wall, the striated muscles are formed by specialized areas of the pelvic floor muscles. Thus, these muscular continence mechanisms are maintained under both somatic-voluntary and visceral-involuntary control.

Involuntarily innervated smooth muscles:

- *Internal anal sphincter*: most significant smooth muscle; as the continuation of the circular muscle layer of the rectum, it forms a strong circular ring. Sympathetic nerve fibers and a significantly reduced number of enteric ganglion cells (hypoganglionosis) allow it to maintain constant tonic activity to help constrict the anal canal (the internal sphincter is responsible for 70% of fecal continence);
- *Muscularis mucosae of the anal canal*: as the continuation of the muscular layer of the mucosa, it extends beyond the hemorrhoidal plexus and ends at the dentate line; stabilizes the hemorrhoidal plexus and holds it in place;
- *Corrugator ani*: as the continuation of the longitudinal muscle layer of the rectum, the muscle fibers extend beyond the anal canal, permeate through the subcutaneous part of the external anal sphincter and insert into the perianal skin. Corrugator ani owes its name to the fact that muscle contraction produces radial wrinkles on the perianal skin.

Voluntarily innervated striated muscles:

- *External anal sphincter*: cylindrical muscle that encircles the outside wall of the anal canal, made up of three recognizable parts: deep, superficial, and subcutaneous. Whereas the deep and subcutaneous parts are arranged in circular layers, the superficial part extends between the anteriorly located perineal body and the posterior anococcygeal ligament and surrounds the anal canal and serves as a clamp. It is largely composed of type I fibers, which are slow, durable, and fatigue resistant.
- *Puborectalis muscle*: as the innermost portion of the levator ani muscle, it forms a strong sling of muscle, which loops around the rectum at the level of the anorectal junction and is closely aligned to the deep part of the external anal sphincter. It arises from the fixed end of the pubic bone, so when the puborectalis muscle contracts it creates a "kink" between anal canal and rectum at the anorectal angle.

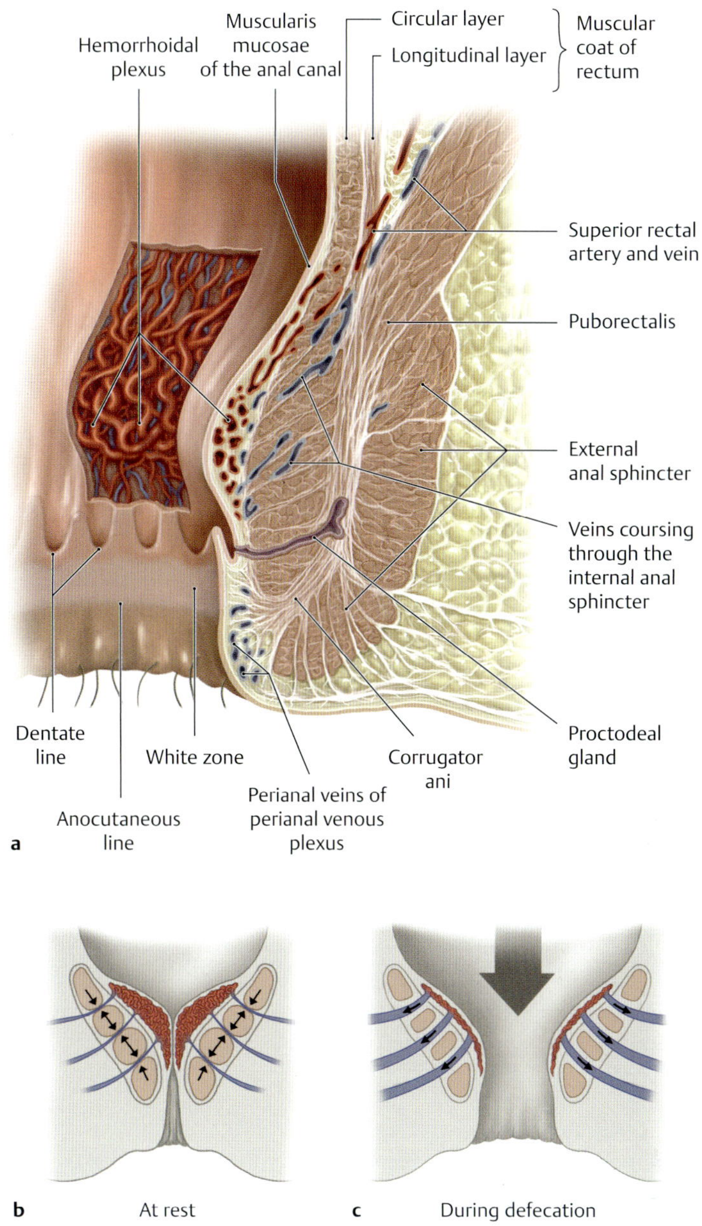

D Structure of the vascular continence mechanism

a Longitudinal section of the anal canal with the hemorrhoidal plexus windowed; **b** and **c** Hemorrhoidal plexus at rest and during defecation. Above the dentate line at the level of the anal columns in the submucosa lies a cavernous body, the hemorrhoidal plexus. Its elasticity largely ensures liquid-and gas-tight closure of the rectum. The circular configuration of the hemorrhoidal plexus is similar in structure to the cavernous body of the penis but differs in that it is permanently distended. The hemorrhoidal plexus is a network of cavernous tissue and is almost exclusively supplied by three branches of the superior rectal artery (at 3, 7, and 11 o'clock in the lithotomy position), which further divide near the anal columns (see p. 291). Blood reaches the venous drainage system via arteriovenous anastomoses through transsphincteric veins—largely along the internal anal sphincter—and reaches the drainage area of the inferior mesenteric vein (and is carried to the portal vein) but also partially through the middle and inferior rectal veins to the perianal veins of the external venous plexus. When the sphincter apparatus relaxes during defecation, it allows blood to drain from the hemorrhoidal plexus.

Note: Abnormal dilation (hyperplasia) of the hemorrhoidal plexus beyond the physiological range leads to hemorrhoidal disease, one of the most common proctological disorders (see p. 262f).

3.9 Continence Organ: Function

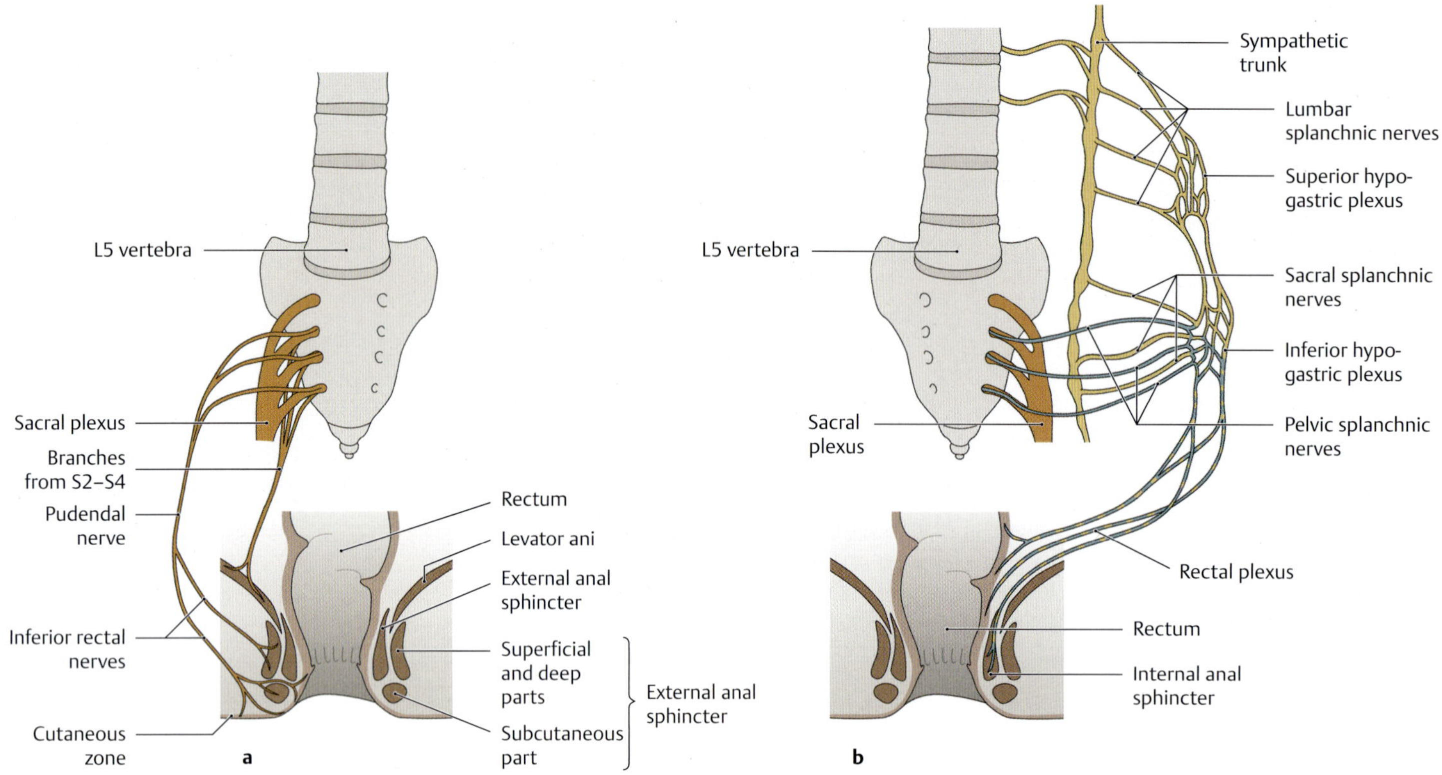

A Innervation (after Stelzner)
a Somatomotor and somatosensory innervation; **b** Visceromotor and viscerosensory innervation.

- Somatomotor: pudendal nerve for the external anal sphincter, levator nerves for the levator ani muscle (especially the puborectalis). They provide active, partially voluntary innervation of the external anal sphincter and levator ani.
- Somatosensory: inferior rectal nerves for the anus and perianal skin. Arising from the pudendal nerve, they transmit touch and especially pain sensation. The skin of the anus is extremely sensitive to pain. Even small tears in the anal skin, which often show inflammatory changes, tend to be extremely painful.
- Visceromotor: pelvic splanchnic nerves (S2–S4) for the internal anal sphincter. The resting tone of the internal sphincter (lumbar and sacral splanchnic nerves) helps to maintain closure of the anal canal and inhibits venous drainage from the hemorrhoidal plexus; the cavernous body remains distended, contributing to fecal continence and flatus control. Topographically, the pelvic splanchnic nerves are closely related to the rectal plexuses.
- Viscerosensory: pelvic splanchnic nerves (S2–S4) supply the wall of the rectum, particularly the stretch receptors in the rectal ampulla. Stretching of the ampulla by the fecal column triggers a subjective awareness of the need to defecate.

B Mechanism of defecation (after Wedel; see right page)
a Filling of the rectal ampulla; **b** Relaxation of the voluntarily controlled sphincters and propulsion of fecal column.
Both defecation and continence are under central nervous system control involving different anatomical structures ranging from the cerebral cortex to the perianal skin, with the anorectum being one of multiple effectors. Directly involved are the pelvic floor, muscles used during squatting, the abdominal press as well as autonomic and sensory nerves along with their higher nerve centers.

Filling of the rectal ampulla and stimulation of local stretch receptors in the ampullary wall: when the fecal bolus is propelled into the rectal ampulla by anterogradely propagating waves, mechanoreceptors detect distension and transmit the information via visceral afferents in the posterior funiculus to the sensory cortex, which perceives the urge to defecate. Olfactory, visual, or acoustic stimuli can either accelerate or decelerate the perception and subsequent voluntary action, which results in defecation.

Rectoanal inhibitory reflex and relaxation of the voluntarily innervated sphincters: When the ampulla fills with feces, the intrarectal pressure increases and the internal anal sphincter relaxes, followed by voluntary relaxation of the puborectalis sling and the external anal sphincter. As a result, the anorectal angle straightens and the anal canal widens.
Propulsion of fecal column: Rectal evacuation is assisted by a direct involuntary increase in pressure in the rectal area and by simultaneous increase in pressure by the contraction of voluntarily innervated muscles: abdominal (abdominal press), perineal (pelvic floor lift), diaphragmatic (diaphragm contraction) and glottic (glottis closure) muscles. The squatting position further increases abdominal pressure (flexor reflex). With the propulsion of the fecal column, the hemorrhoidal cushions are drained and pushed out.
Completion of defecation: After the sphincter apparatus allowed the fecal column to pass through, it comes in contact with the highly sensitive anoderm, which perceives the volume, consistency, and location of the stool. This perception initiates the voluntary process of completing defecation. Defecation is completed once the sphincter apparatus contracts and the hemorrhoidal plexus fills up.

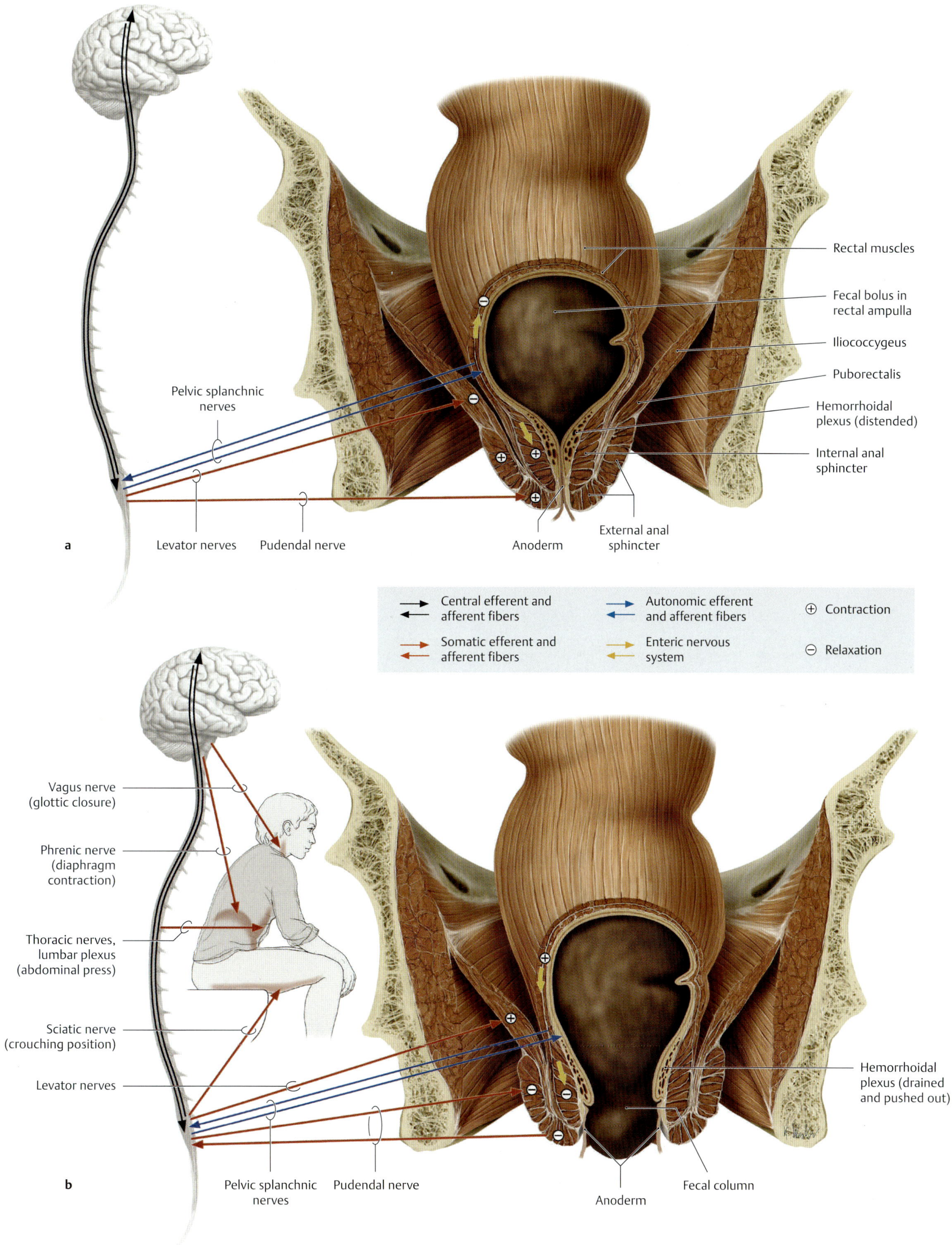
Rectal muscles
Fecal bolus in rectal ampulla
Iliococcygeus
Puborectalis
Hemorrhoidal plexus (distended)
Internal anal sphincter
Pelvic splanchnic nerves
Levator nerves
Pudendal nerve
Anoderm
External anal sphincter
a
Central efferent and afferent fibers
Autonomic efferent and afferent fibers
Contraction
Somatic efferent and afferent fibers
Enteric nervous system
Relaxation
Vagus nerve (glottic closure)
Phrenic nerve (diaphragm contraction)
Thoracic nerves, lumbar plexus (abdominal press)
Sciatic nerve (crouching position)
Levator nerves
Hemorrhoidal plexus (drained and pushed out)
b
Pelvic splanchnic nerves
Pudendal nerve
Anoderm
Fecal column

3.10 Disorders of the Anal Canal: Hemorrhoidal Disease, Anal Abscesses, and Anal Fistulas

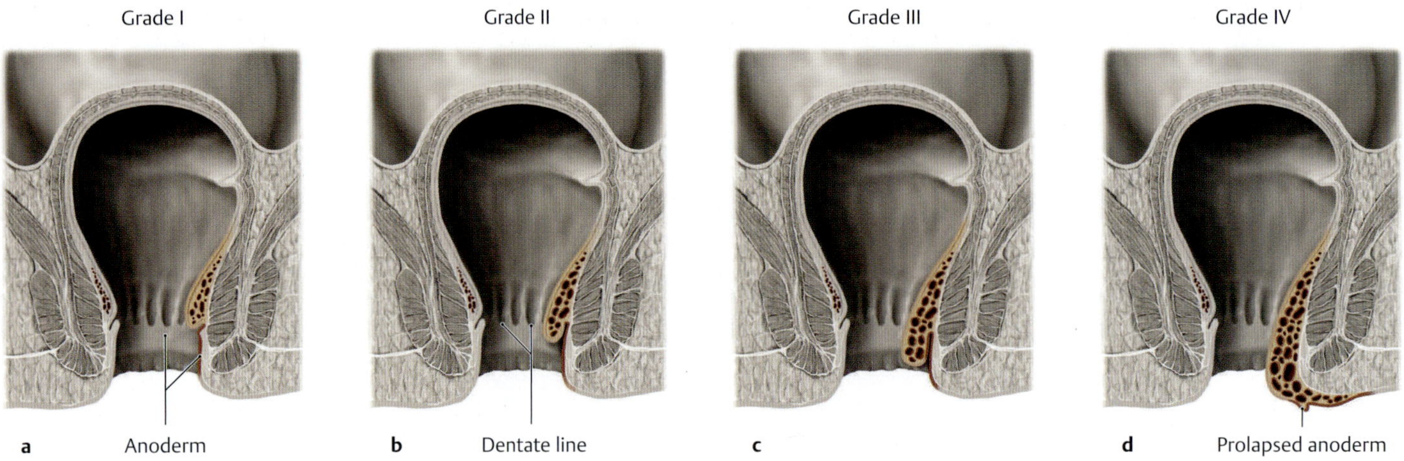

A Hemorrhoidal disease

Hemorrhoidal disease is one of the most common proctological disorders. The site of origin is the circular hemorrhoidal plexus of the cavernous body of the rectum located above the dentate line. It is largely responsible for the fine adjustment of anal continence. *Hemorrhoid* is a general term used to describe hyperplasia (enlargement) of a cavernous body with arterial blood supply, a condition which initially does not cause any symptoms. Hemorrhoids become pathological once they become symptomatic (bleeding is bright red from arterial blood, mucus discharge, itching, burning, fecal soiling, etc.) and when they require treatment (hemorrhoidal disease). Most commonly, hemorrhoids result from increased pressure on the anus during defecation, often caused by chronic constipation as a result of a lack of fiber and fluids in the diet. Another cause is impaired venous return due to increased anal sphincter tone as this may lead to the hemorrhoidal plexus taking on a gnarled appearance. Diagnosis and classification of hemorrhoids are based on examination, palpation, and proctoscopy of the anal canal. Depending on the severity of the hemorrhoids and their symptoms, they are divided into four grades:

- **Grad I (a):** swollen, elastic cushions of tissue that are visible only on proctoscopy (located above the dentate line) and may cause painless bright red bleeding (painless because the swollen cushions are located above the anoderm);
- **Grade II (b):** visibly hyperplastic vascular cushions, which can prolapse inside or outside of the anal canal during defecation or while pressing but retract immediately after emptying the bowels. Dripping blood and mucus discharge may cause oozing or itching, a condition also known as perianal eczema;
- **Grad III (c):** during defecation or while the intra-abdominal pressure is increased, hemorrhoids prolapse spontaneously and require manual repositioning. Possible thrombosis or incarceration of the prolapsed knot may cause significant pain;
- **Grad IV (d):** at this stage, the nodular enlargements and large parts of the anal canal, including the highly pain-sensitive anoderm, are permanently prolapsed (irreducible) and attached to the anal margin (also known as an anal prolapse).

Note: Unlike in the German medical terminology, the Anglo-American and Swiss terminology distinguish between *internal* and *external hemorrhoids*. Internal hemorrhoids originate from the internal rectal venous plexus, external hemorrhoids are subcutaneous clots at the margin of the anus (e.g., perianal thromboses). In our assessment, however, external hemorrhoids are simply hyperplastic vascular cushions of the rectal cavernous body with their arterial blood supply that have prolapsed to the outside.

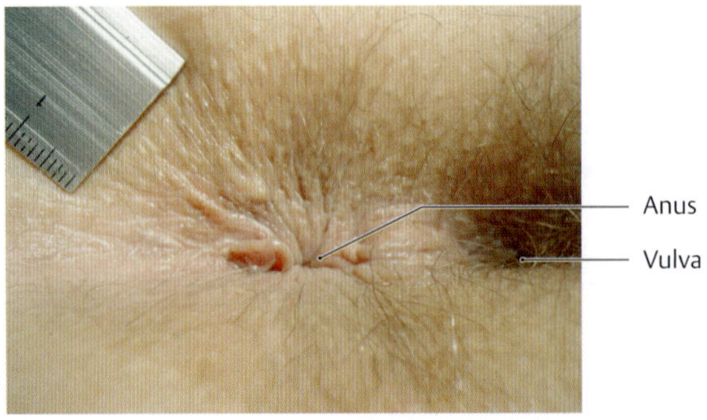

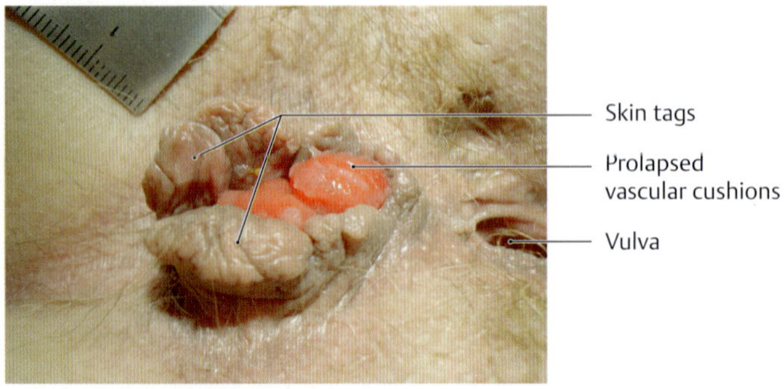

B Conditions of the perianal skin with and without hemorrhoidal disease

a Normal anatomy of the perianal area in a 38-year-old female patient;
b Grade IV hemorrhoids in a 54-year-old female patient: mucosal prolapse at the anterior commissure combined with right- and left-lateral anal skin tags (harmless, generally asymptomatic perianal skin folds) (from Rohde, H.,: Lehratlas der Proktologie. Thieme, Stuttgart 2007).

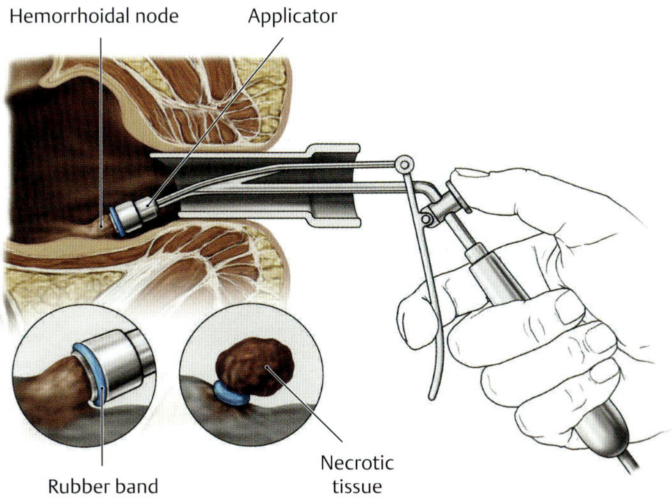

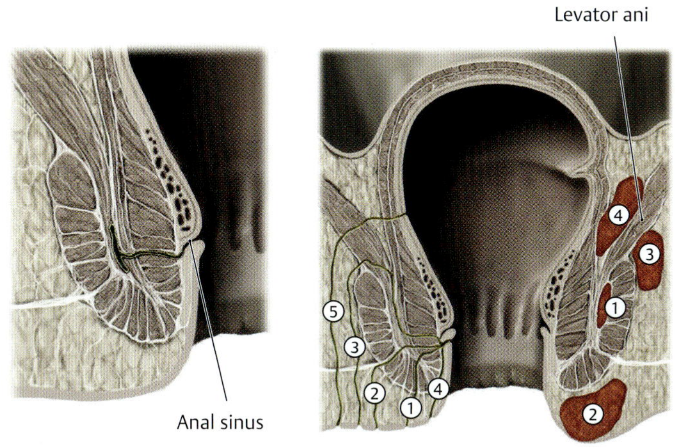

a Proctodeal gland **b** Anal fistulas Anal abscesses

C Therapeutic possibilities in hemorrhoidal disease

Treatment for hemorrhoidal disease is mainly aimed at prevention, removal of hemorrhoids, and restoration of the normal anatomy and physiology of the affected areas. Thus, the therapeutic possibilities can be divided into preventive measures and symptomatic (conservative, semi-invasive, surgical) treatment:

- **Preventive measures:** focus on informing patients about advisable nutritional habits (switching to a fiber-rich, low-fat diet with sufficient fluid intake, avoiding alcohol, tobacco, and hot spices) and improving bowel habits (defecating only when feeling the urge to have a bowel movement, avoid straining, no laxatives, proper but not excessive anal hygiene);
- **Conservative measures:** local treatment using ointments, suppositories, anal tampons, and sitz baths to alleviate symptoms;
- **Semi-invasive measures:** sclerotherapy (e.g., after Blond), rubber band ligation (after Barron), and Doppler ultrasound-guided hemorrhoidal arterial ligation have proven effective as treatments especially for grade I and grade II hemorrhoids. In sclerotherapy, 0.5–1.0 ml polidocanol is injected submucosally above the dentate line. Polidocanol is a sclerosing agent that damages the endothelium of the blood vessels, which are then replaced by fibrous tissue. This treatment is aimed at fixing the hemorrhoids. Rubber band ligation is the preferred method to treat grade II hemorrhoids (see **A**). Using a special applicator, excess hemorrhoidal tissue is tied off with a rubber band. The necrotic tissue falls off within one to two weeks. Hemorrhoidal artery ligation (HAL) helps to reduce the blood supply to the enlarged vascular cushions and makes them shrink.
- **Surgical measures:** grade III and grade IV hemorrhoids require surgical intervention. Common surgical procedures include hemorrhoidectomy after Millian-Morgan and a procedure known as stapled hemorrhoidopexy after Longo. Hemorrhoidectomy involves radial-segmental excision and ligation of the enlarged cushions. For stapled hemorrhoidopexy, a special device is inserted with which to reposition the prolapsed hemorrhoids and to resect a ring of mucosa from the proximal anal canal along with parts of the hemorrhoidal tissue. A circular stapler is used to fix the remaining tissue in place. This procedure offers a significant advantage in that it results in less postoperative pain because the staple line is placed in the area of the rectal mucosa that does not receive sensory innervation.

D Anal fistulas and anal abscesses

The symptoms of both of these conditions are closely related and are almost always caused by the same disorder: an infection of the rudimentary proctodeal glands (see p. 257). Usually, the anal abscess represents the acute and the anal fistula the chronic manifestation of the cryptoglandular infection. Based on the anatomy of the proctodeal glands—which most commonly are located within the intersphincteric space near the posterior commissure and open into the anal sinuses (**a**)—anal fistulas and anal abscesses (**b**) are classified according to their course or location relative to the sphincter apparatus:

- **Anal fistulas** (typical fistulas are complete, meaning they have an internal opening into the anal canal and an external opening in the skin; hence two openings—one in the anal sinus and one in the perianal skin):

  ① Intersphincteric fistula: 50–70% of all anal fistulas, pierces the internal anal sphincter;
  ② Transsphincteric fistula: 30–40% of all anal fistulas, pierces both the internal and the external sphincter;
  ③ Suprasphincteric fistula: approximately 5% of all anal fistulas, passes upward between the sphincters and crosses the puborectalis sling;
  ④ Subcutaneous or subanodermal fistula: 5–10% of all anal fistulas, does not pierce either sphincter but passes directly below the anal canal and opens in the perianal skin (synonym: marginal fistula);
  ⑤ Atypical fistula: approximately 5% of all anal fistulas, does not begin at the proctodeal glands but passes from the rectal ampulla through the levator ani and has an external opening on the skin (also known as extrasphincteric fistula), common symptom of Crohn's disease.

- **Anal abscesses** (result from fistulas that don't have an external opening and thus end blindly):

  ① Intersphincteric abscess: within the proctodeal glands;
  ② Subcutaneous or subanodermal abscess: perianal or around the anal canal;
  ③ Ischiorectal or infralevator abscess: below levator ani in the ischiorectal (-anal) fossa;
  ④ Pelvirectal or supralevator abscess: between the rectum and levator ani funnel in the pararectal fascia.

Note: Anal fistulas and anal abscesses always require adequate surgical therapy. Anal abscesses in particular are accompanied by severe pain, fever, and leukocytosis and are generally an indication for emergency treatment. The aim of surgical treatment of anal fistulas in addition to sealing the fistula channel is to treat the infection of the proctodeal glands to prevent relapse. Exact knowledge of the anatomical relationships is crucial for a successful treatment.

3.11 Colorectal Tumors: Frequency, Risk Factors, and Screening

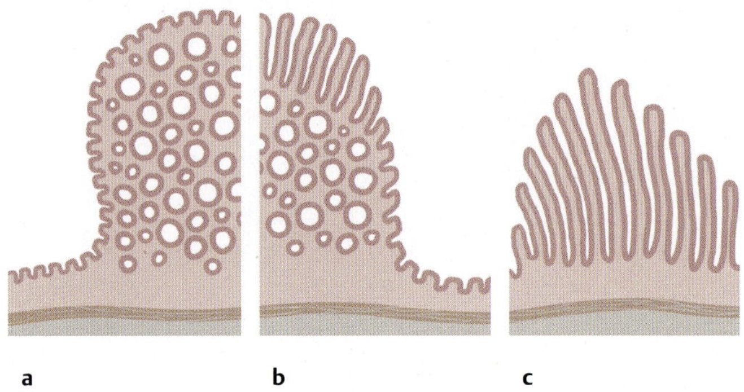

A Adenomatous polyps of the large intestine

a Tubular; **b** Tubulovillous; **c** Villous polyps.

Adenoma is a type of benign epithelial tumor (neoplasia) that originates in glandular tissue. When it originates in the large bowel mucosa, it often extends beyond the mucosa and grows in a polypous fashion (hence the term "large bowel polyps"). According to their morphological appearance, they are divided into

- Tubular adenomas (75% of all large bowel polyps): most commonly pedunculated and smaller than 2 cm;
- Tubulovillous adenomas (15% of all large bowel polyps): mixed, significantly higher risk of malignant transformation than tubular adenoma;
- Villous adenomas (10% of all large bowel polyps; high—30% risk of malignant transformation): hairy-appearing surface and overall flatter than tubular adenomas; because they are broad-based they are more difficult to remove endoscopically, hence there is a high risk of relapse.

Note: All adenomas can develop into cancer. The risk of malignant transformation correlates with the size of the polyp, its histological type, and the degree of dysplasia (e.g., degree of differentiation).

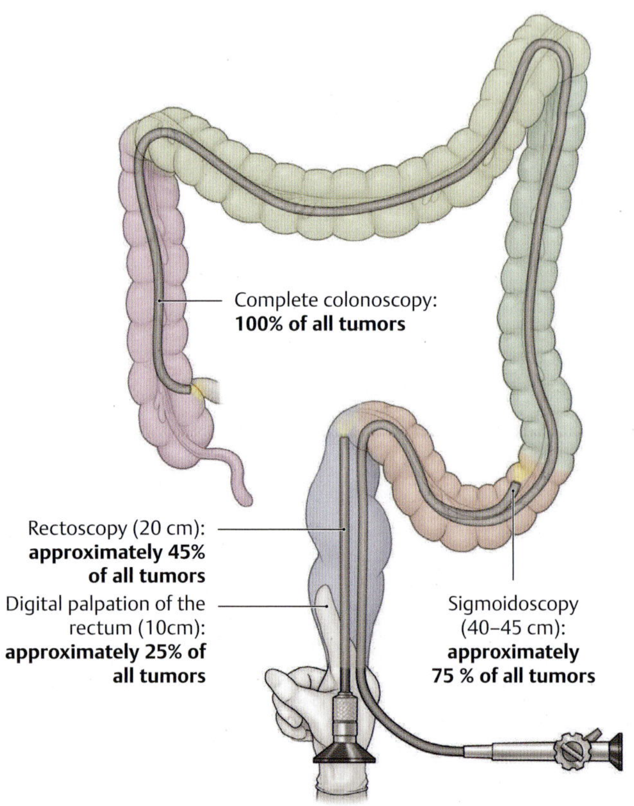

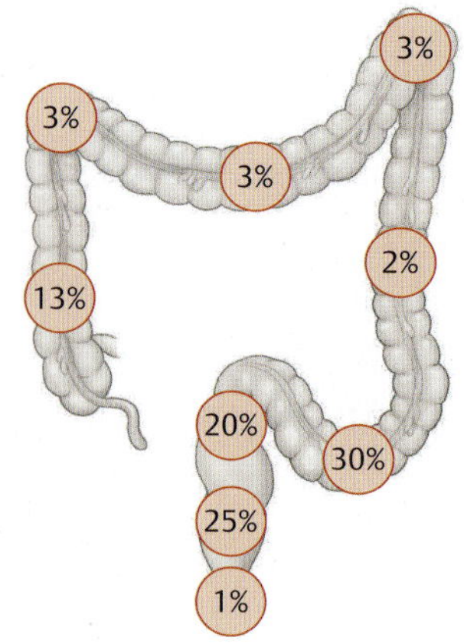

B Frequency and risk factors of colorectal carcinoma

Colorectal carcinoma is the most common cancer of the gastrointestinal tract in the Western world. In Europe and the United States, colorectal carcinoma accounts for 15% of all newly diagnosed cancers with increasing incidence rates. In Germany alone, with 60,000 new cases each year, colorectal adenocarcinoma is the second most common form of cancer regardless of gender (more than half of patients die from it). Almost 45% of these tumors develop in the rectum (see fig.). It is not clear what causes colorectal cancer but the following exogenous and endogenous risk factors appear to play a role:

- **Exogenous risk factors:**
  - high-meat, high-fat, low-fiber diet
  - insufficient intake of vitamins (folic acid, vitamins A, C, E) and trace elements (selenium)
  - alcohol consumption
  - asbestos exposure
  - low socioeconomic status (associated with malnutrition, see above)
  - physical inactivity;
- **Endogenous risk factors:**
  - denomatous polyps of the large intestine
  - frequent occurrence of colon cancer in families
  - inflammatory bowel diseases (e.g., ulcerative colitis, Crohn's disease).

Note: Colorectal cancer does not include anal canal tumors (1%).

C Cancer screening

Early detection of cancer through screening is particularly helpful in the case of colorectal carcinoma. This is due to the relatively long latency period of several years that it takes for the primarily benign adenoma to transform into cancer. Benign colorectal tumors predominantly begin as polypoid changes in the colorectal mucosa (tubular, villous, and tubulovillous adenomas that may be pedunculated or broad-based and occur as solitary or multiple lesions), with the greatest tendency for malignant change in villous adenomas (30%) (see **A**). Guideline-recommended colorectal cancer screenings include annual fecal occult blood testing (hemoccult testing to begin at age 40), digital rectal examination and a colonoscopy (to begin at age 55) with the option of direct primary intervention to remove neoplastic cells. CT colonography (virtual colonoscopy, p. 266) offers an additional, less invasive alternative to the conventional endoscopic examination. An extensive body of research shows that endoscopic diagnosis results in an impressive reduction of the incidence and mortality rate by 60–80%.

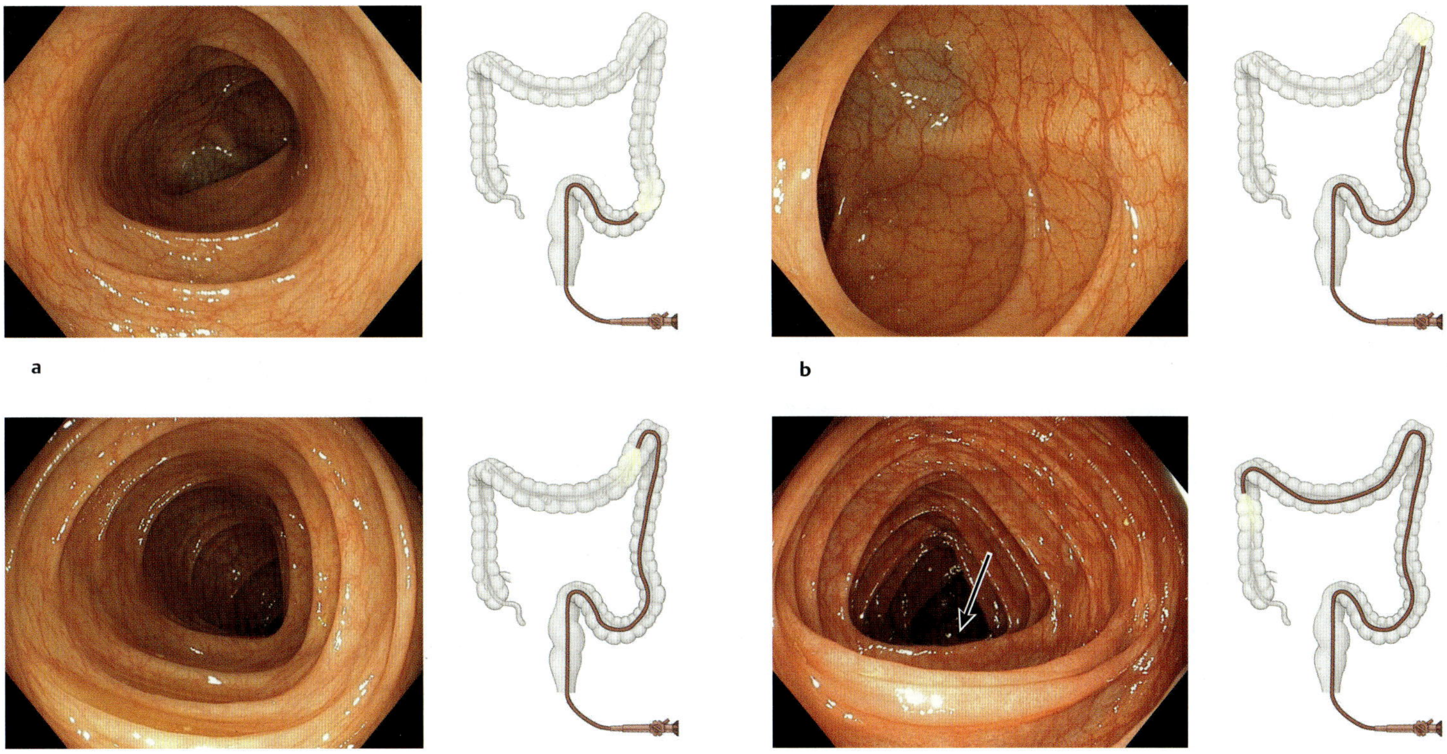

a b c d

D Colonoscopy and normal internal surface of various segments of the large intestine

a View of the descending colon (oval lumen and regular haustration); **b** Left colic flexure with adjacent impressing spleen: **c** View of the transverse colon with its typical triangular configuration; **d** View of the ascending colon with the ileocecal valve in the deep plane (arrow). The schematic diagram to the right of each image shows the respective position of the endoscope (photos from: Messmann H, editor. *Lehratlas der Koloskopie*. 2nd ed. Stuttgart: Thieme; 2014).

Note: The examiner's perspective in endoscopy is different from that in other imaging modalities: Here the examiner sees the internal surface of the intestine, which appears nearly triangular in cross section (see **c**). Coursing along the respective angles of this triangle are three cord-like bands in thickened areas of the longitudinal musculature (taeniae, see p. 252) along which crescent-shaped transverse folds (semilunar folds or plicae semilunares) alternate with sacculations (haustra).

Proper endoscopic inspection of the colon requires prior peroral bowel lavage to thoroughly clear the intestine (on the evening before the examination the patient drinks 4 liters of an inert electrolyte solution such as polyethylene glycol). Following analgesic preparation where indicated, the endoscopic examination begins with inspection and palpation of the perianal region. The intestinal lumen is expanded by means of CO_2 insufflation or with warm water (infusion technique) to minimize discomfort as the endoscope is advanced. After the cecum has been reached and the endoscope has been advanced into the terminal ileum, the phase of instrument withdrawal begins (starting with Fig. **d**) during which each of the individual segments of the colon are meticulously inspected. Therapeutic interventions (such as managing bleeding, resecting mucosal neoplasms, removing tumors, etc.) are generally performed while withdrawing the endoscope.

Note: The overall rate of complications of colonoscopy is about 0.3%.

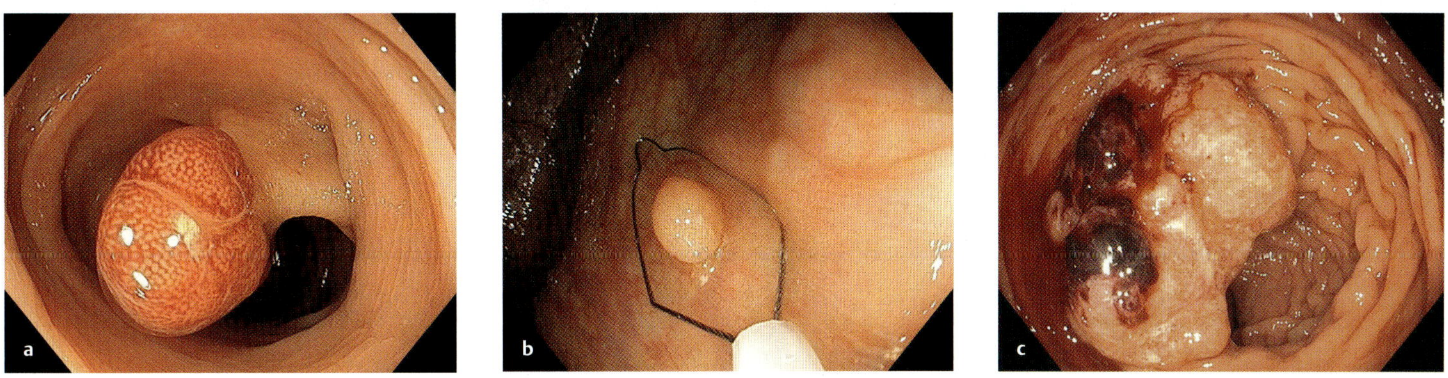

E Examples of benign (a and b) and malignant (c) colorectal tumors

a Pedunculated polyp; **b** Polyp in an open snare; **c** Exophytic carcinoma at the rectosigmoid junction with typical ulceration and bleeding (from: Messmann H, editor. *Lehratlas der Koloskopie*. 2nd ed. Stuttgart: Thieme; 2014). The vast majority of colorectal malignancies are adenocarcinomas that arise from the columnar epithelium of the colon or rectum. They are usually preceded by benign stages (adenomatous polyps). Characteristic symptoms of advanced carcinomas include destruction of the luminal surface, ulceration, bleeding (see **c**), and stenosis of the lumen of the colon.

3.12 Colorectal Tumors: Diagnostic Imaging and Surgical Treatment

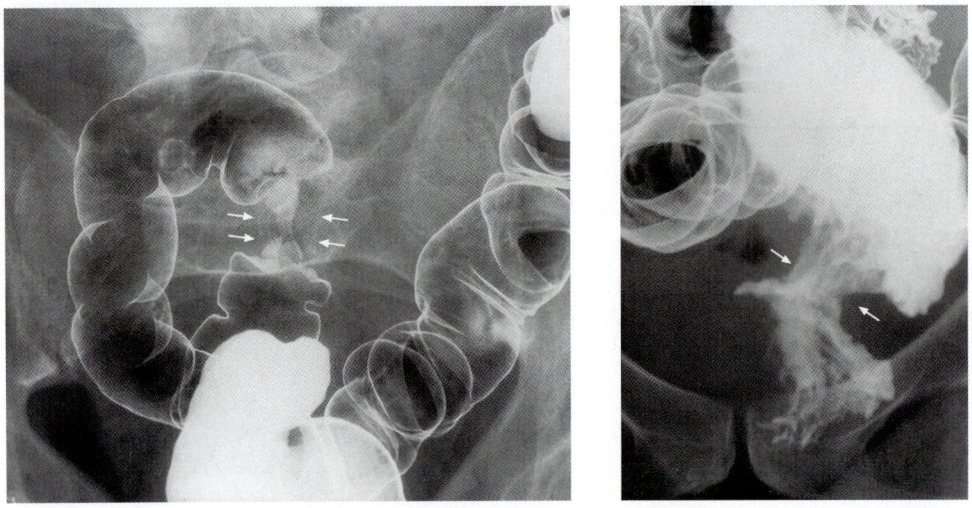

a b

A Double-contrast study of colon and rectum

a Carcinoma in the sigmoid colon with typical "apple bite" configuration (arrows) in the late phase of the tumor. A mural filling defect is visible and the interrupted wall contour indicates how the tumor projects into the lumen of the colon ("apple bite").

b The more the tumor advances, the more it constricts the lumen of the colon (arrows). Prestenotic dilation of the lumen is then observed, as in this example of a rectal carcinoma (from: Reiser M, Kuhn F, Debus J, eds. *Duale Reihe Radiologie*. 4th ed. Stuttgart: Thieme; 2017).

Note: CT and MRI (see **B** and **C**) have largely supplanted the double-contrast study as a standard radiologic procedure for diagnosing colorectal carcinomas. Both modalities are suitable primarily for tumor staging as well. Colonoscopy remains the most important procedure for the primary diagnosis of colorectal carcinomas (see p. 265).

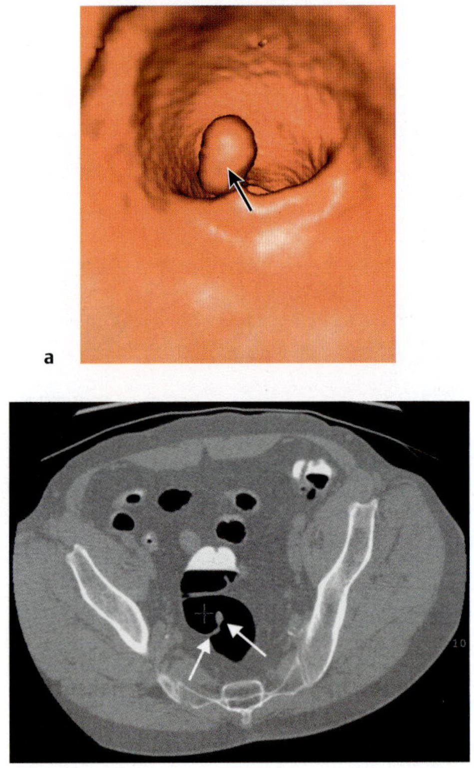

a b

B Virtual colonoscopy (CT colonography) of colon and rectum

a 3D reconstruction and CT image (**b**) of a pedunculated rectal polyp in virtual colonoscopy. Circumscribed intraluminal mass arising from the wall of the colon (**a** black arrow, **b** white arrow) (from: Henne-Bruns D, editor. *Duale Reihe Chirurgie*. 4th ed. Stuttgart: Thieme; 2012). Virtual colonography is not an invasive procedure like conventional colonoscopy. Rather it is based on cross-sectional CT scans of the abdomen from which a computer generates three-dimensional images that reconstruct the colon. Using a virtual endoscopic camera the radiologist can take a virtual trip through the colon. Studies indicate that polyps and neoplasms larger than 10 mm can be diagnosed with high sensitivity (> 90%) whereas smaller ones (less than 10 mm) are not be clearly identifiable. As the examination also involves not insignificant exposure to ionizing radiation, virtual colonoscopy has yet to become a standard procedure.

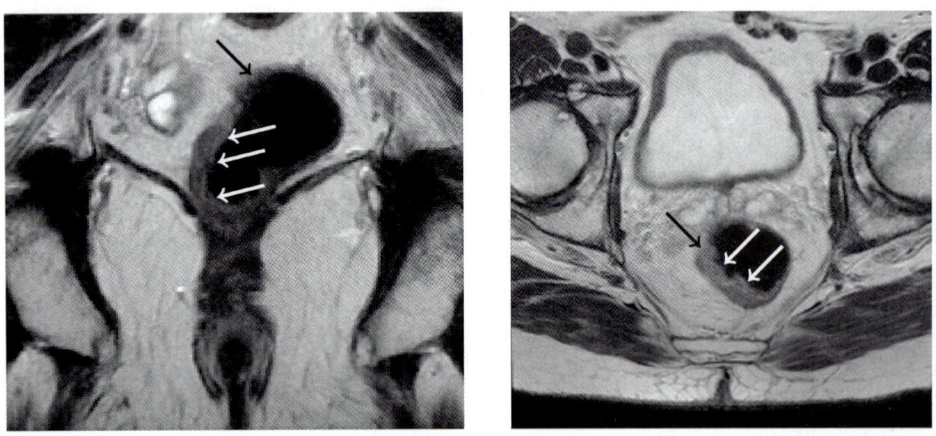

a b

C MRI of an infiltrating rectal carcinoma

Coronal (**a**) and axial (**b**) T2-weighted images of the small pelvis at the level of the hip (from: Reiser M, Kuhn F, Debus J, eds. *Duale Reihe Radiologie*. 4th ed. Stuttgart: Thieme; 2017). The images show a mural mass projecting into the rectal lumen (white arrows) which has infiltrated the mesorectal fatty tissue (see **E**; black arrow). Due to its high soft-tissue contrast MRI plays a decisive role in the diagnosis and staging of rectal carcinomas (depth of infiltration, etc.). This modality can also detect metastases to regional lymph nodes as well as remote metastases.

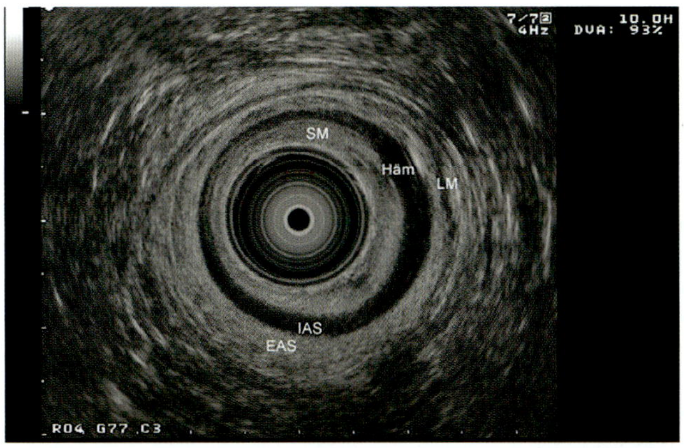

a

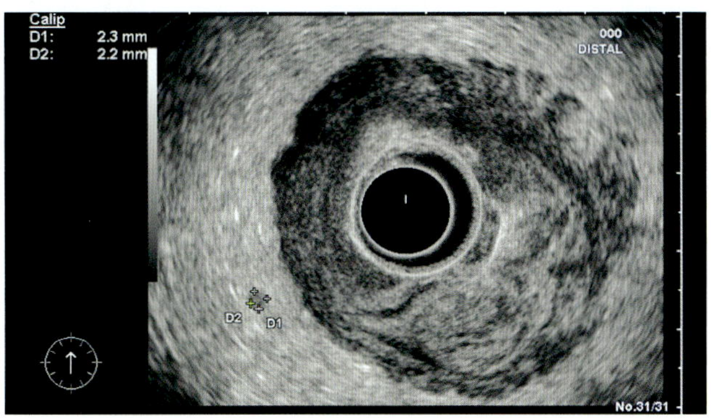

b

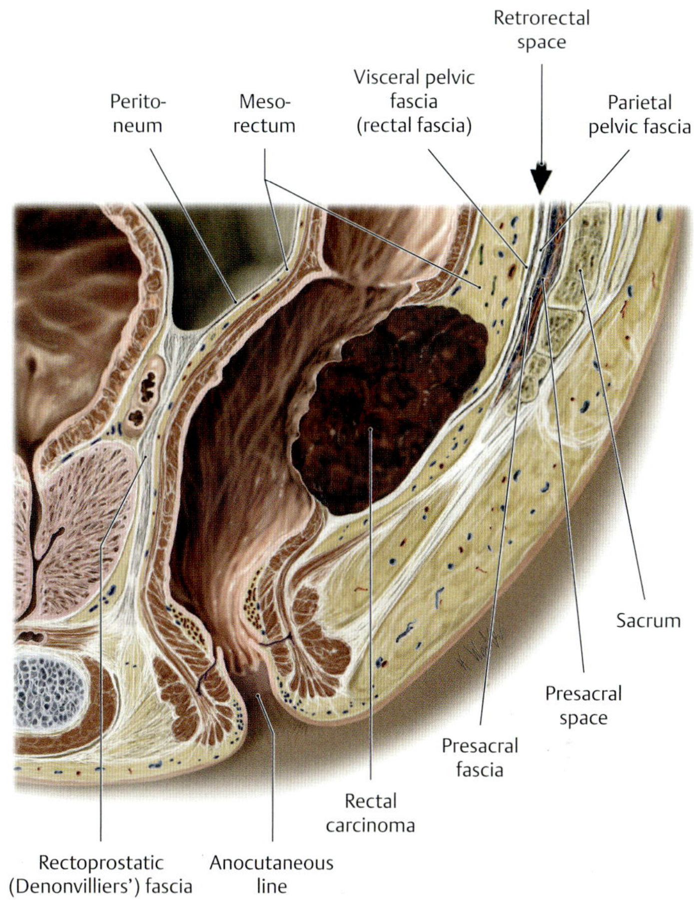

D Rectal and anal endosonography

In rectal and anal endosonography, the layers of the anorectal wall and surrounding structures are clearly displayed with high spatial resolution. Whereas endorectal ultrasound images display primarily the layers of the rectal wall, endoanal ultrasound allows the evaluation of the sphincters and the pelvic floor. In order to correctly assess results of endosonographic imaging, thorough knowledge of the anatomy is crucial. The transverse orientation with a 360-degree transducer is the most commonly used imaging plane employed in endosonography; it facilitates precise anatomical localization of the visualized structures.

- **a Anal endosonography:** technique to display the sphincter apparatus in the anal canal; the circular hypoechoic internal anal sphincter (IAS), which is continuous with the hyperechoic submucosa (SM) (parts of the hemorrhoidal plexus), serves as a landmark. Outside the internal sphincter lies the external anal sphincter (EAS), which exhibits a mixed pattern of echogenicity. As a continuation of the longitudinal muscles (LM), fibers of the corrugator ani are visible as a thin hypoechoic layer in the intersphincteric space.
- **b Rectal endosonography:** large circular rectal tumor that infiltrates the perirectal fat tissue. Rectal endosonography is used in the preoperative staging of rectal carcinoma to determine the depth of penetration into the rectal wall and the number of malignant regional lymph nodes. This information is essential with regard to the surgical approach: Must the rectum be completely removed (abdominoperineal excision), or can surgery preserve fecal continence (total mesorectal excision, see **E**), or is purely local treatment of the tumor possible? (From: Dietrich, Ch. editor. *Endosonography, Lehrbuch und Atlas des endoskopischen Ultraschalls*. Stuttgart: Thieme; 2007).

E Total mesorectal excision (TME)

Sphincter preservation can be achieved in 80% of surgeries for rectal cancer. One precondition for a sphincter sparing procedure is that the distal margin of the tumor is at least 6 cm above the anocutaneous line. Introduction of total mesorectal excision (TME) has significantly improved oncologic outcomes (reduction of local recurrence rates) especially for carcinomas situated in the middle or lower third of the rectum. TME takes into account the pattern of regional metastasis by removing not only the tumor, which may have infiltrated the perirectal fatty tissue (mesorectum), but also by radically resecting the regional lymphatic drainage area. Additionally, the surgical treatment is guided by the automatic nerve plexuses of the pelvis (inferior hypogastric plexus) mainly to prevent voiding and prostate dysfunction. Hence, the procedure is also referred to as nerve-oriented or nerve-guided mesorectal excision (see p. 401).

Operative approach: After preparing the lymphovascular pedicle of the superior rectal vessels, the inferior mesenteric artery and vein are ligated centrally (vascular ligation). The inferior mesenteric artery is ligated 2 cm distal to its origin so as not to damage the autonomic nerve plexus around the aorta. In the posterior direction, the actual TME includes the entire retrorectal pad of fat (i. e., the mesorectum is included in the mobilized segment) and occurs along the retrorectal space (black arrow; see also p. 401) between the visceral pelvic fascia (rectal fascia) and the parietal pelvic fascia. In the anterior direction the mobilization occurs in the prerectal space along the rectoprostatic (Denonvilliers') fascia. In the lateral direction the entire area extending to the pelvic wall (the pararectal fascia) is mobilized while protecting the hypogastric and pelvic splanchnic nerves. After mobilization of the rectum to the levator ani and after the puborectalis sling has been identified, the rectum is resected with a safety margin of 2 cm. A stapling device is used to attach the colon to the rectal stump, a procedure known as a coloanal anastomosis.

3.13 Liver: Position and Relationship to Adjacent Organs

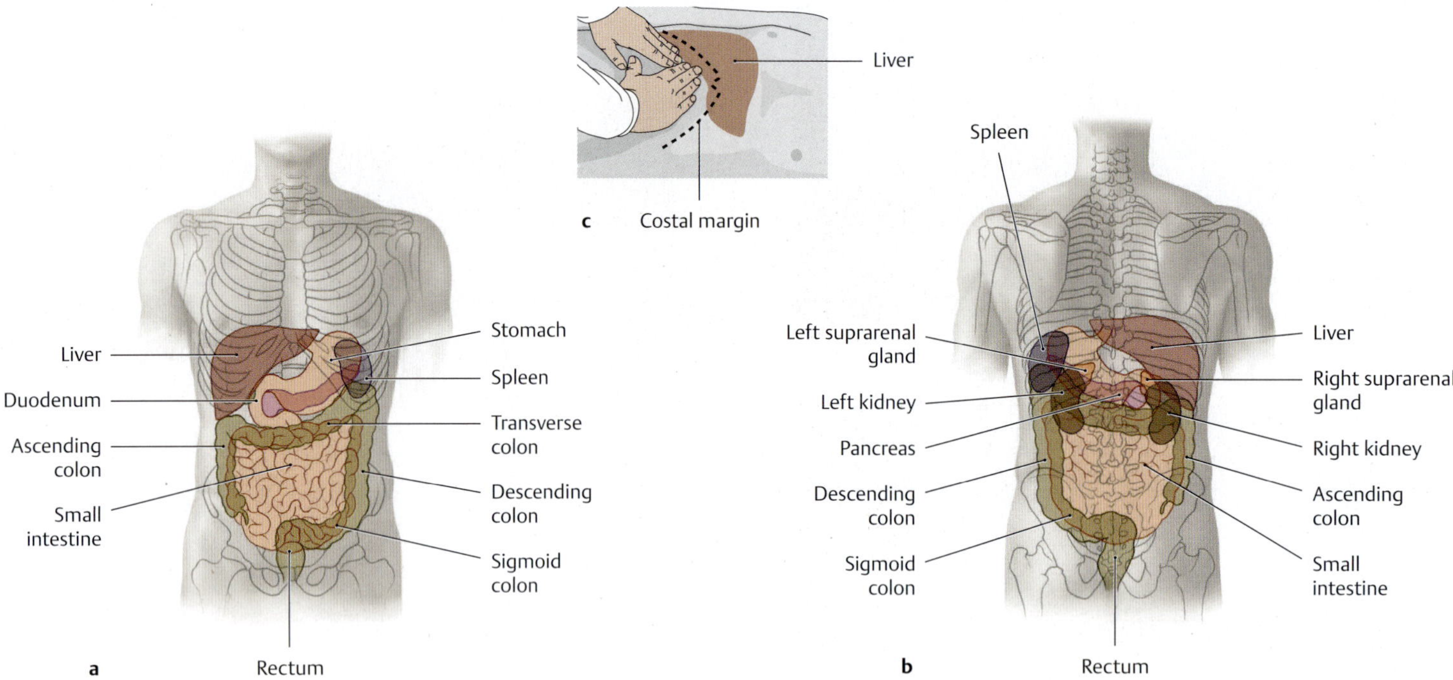

A Projection of the liver onto the trunk and adjacent organs; palpation of the liver

a Anterior view, **b** posterior view, **c** palpation of the liver.

The liver is situated mainly in the right upper quadrant but extends across the epigastrium into the left upper quadrant, lying anterior to the stomach. The right lobe of the liver is closely related to the right kidney and right colic flexure. Owing to the dome of the hemidiaphragm, the pleural cavity overlaps the anterior and posterior surfaces of the liver. Because the liver is attached to the inferior surface of the diaphragm, its position is significantly affected by respiratory excursions. It also depends on posture and age: The liver descends in the standing position, and it is also affected by the gradual settling of organs that occurs with aging. The liver is palpated (**c**) most easily by having the patient lie supine with the abdominal wall relaxed (legs drawn up) and exhale fully (the liver rises with the diaphragm), followed by a full inhalation. This causes the liver to fall, and its sharp inferior border (see **B**) can be palpated at the margin of the ribs. If the liver is abnormally enlarged (hepatomegaly), it may occasionally extend to the pelvic brim.

B Liver in situ: location of the liver in the abdominal cavity

Anterior view of the opened abdomen, the heart and lungs have been removed; the falciform ligament and round ligament of the liver have been transected anteriorly.

The liver occupies the right hypochondriac region and extends across the epigastric region and into the left upper quadrant. The stomach is visible at the inferior border of the left lobe of the liver, and the gallbladder is visible at the inferior border of the right lobe.

Note: Owing to the dome-shaped structure of the diaphragm, the liver and thoracic cavity lie on the same horizontal plane and they partially overlap. Thus, perforating injuries of the thoracic cavity containing the lungs may also involve the abdominal cavity containing the liver. This is known as a multicavity injury.

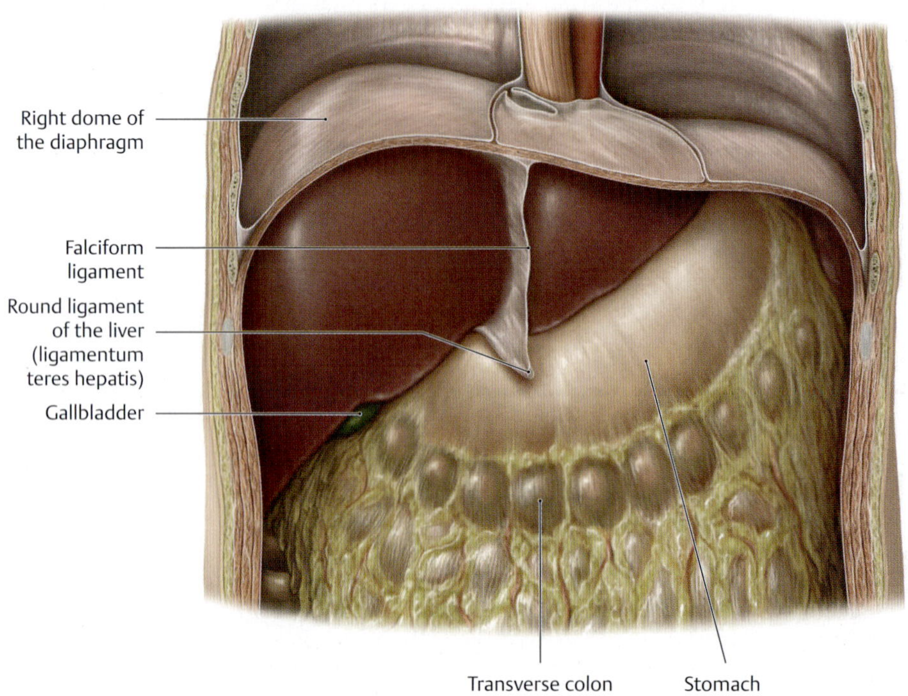

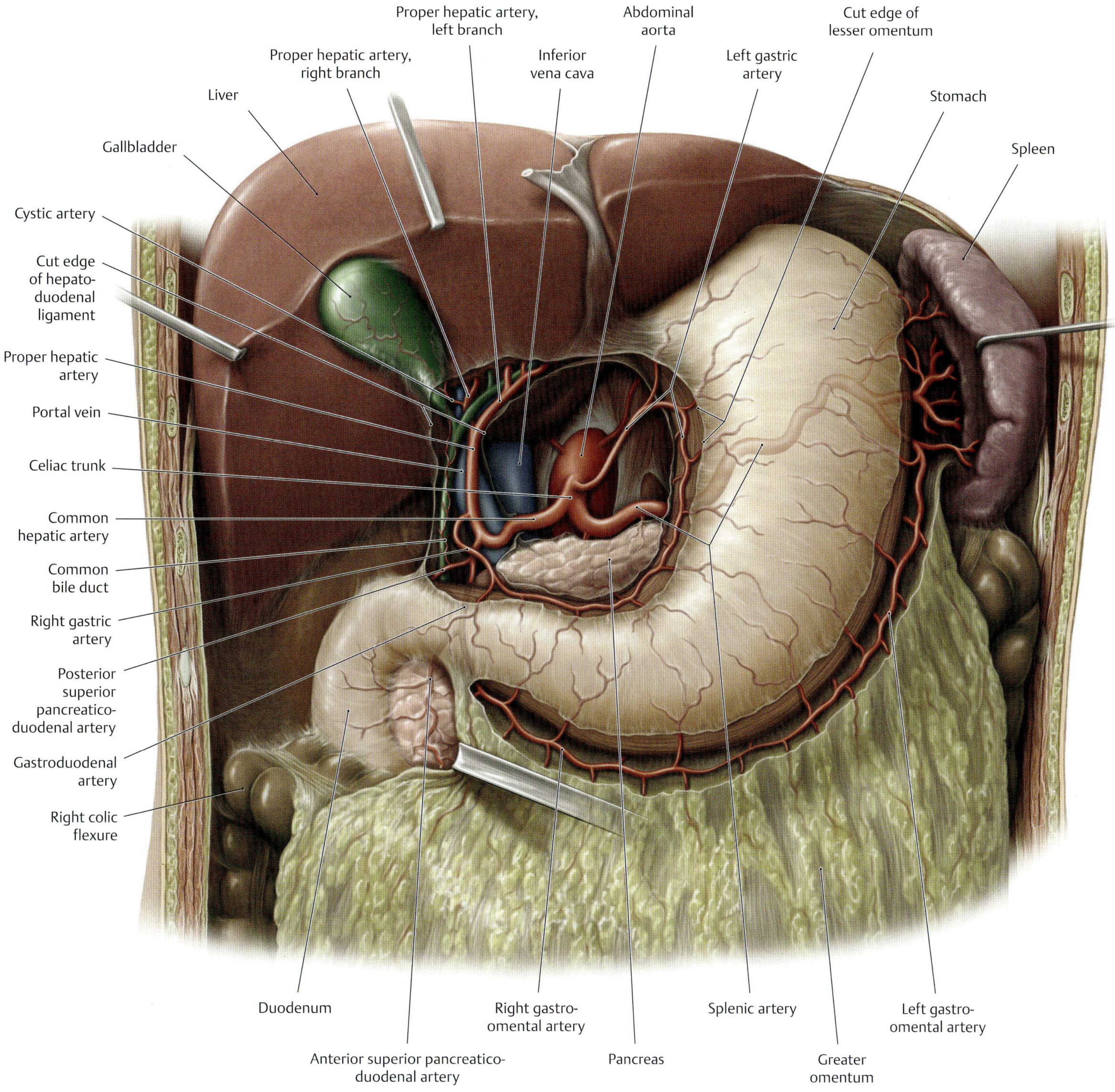

C The liver in situ after the lesser omentum has been opened
Anterior view of the opened upper abdomen, the liver and spleen have been lifted.

The lesser omentum has been opened allowing a direct view into the omental bursa. A small section of the pleural cavity is visible immediately to the right and slightly above the right lobe of the liver (see p. 271). The anterior border of the liver, which points downward in situ, has a sharp edge that is clearly palpable when the liver is enlarged. The inferior surface of the liver bears a fossa for the gallbladder (see p. 274), whose fundus is directed anteriorly toward the abdominal wall and extends slightly past the inferior hepatic border. The right portion of the lesser omentum, the hepatoduodenal ligament, transmits the blood vessels of the liver (proper hepatic artery and portal vein) and the common bile duct. The contour of the right kidney can be seen on the inferior surface of the right lobe of the liver.

Note: The opening of the hepatic veins into the inferior vena cava is located just below the diaphragm (see p. 275), just a few centimeters from the right atrium of the heart. Thus, in cases where the right side of the heart has lost pumping power (right-sided heart failure), blood may engorge the liver, causing palpable hepatic enlargement. When palpating the liver, the examiner should take into account the variable position of the organ (see **Ac**).

3.14 Liver: Peritoneal Relationships and Shape

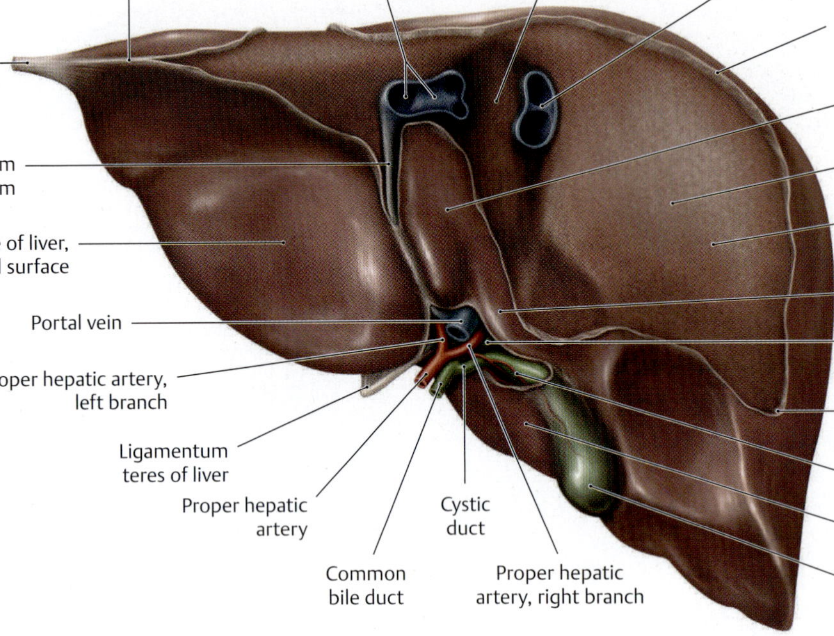

A Peritoneal covering of the liver
Posterior view of the upper part of the diaphragmatic surface of the liver. The liver is surrounded by a fibrous capsule with extensions that pass into the liver and transmit neurovascular structures. Most of the *surface* of the liver is covered by glistening visceral peritoneum, which is external to the fibrous capsule. Only the bare area, which is highly variable in extent, *lacks a peritoneal covering*; it has a rough appearance because the fibrous capsule forms its surface. The hepatic veins (usually three in number) leave the liver in the bare area, and thus *outside* the peritoneal covering. This is different from all other intraperitoneal organs, which have mesenteric structures for transmitting their veins and arteries. In the case of the liver, only the *afferent* artery, *afferent* portal vein, and common bile duct course in the hepatoduodenal ligament (see **Cb**), while the efferent veins do not. At sites where the visceral peritoneum is reflected into the parietal peritoneum on the inferior surface of the diaphragm, the delicate peritoneal epithelium is often backed by connective tissue to form a ligamentous band (coronary ligament, see **Ca**). This connective tissue is drawn out into a tapered band at the extremity of the left lobe (the fibrous appendix of the liver).

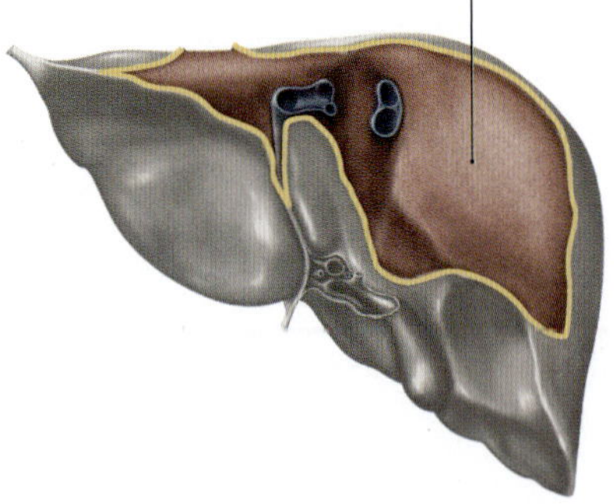

a

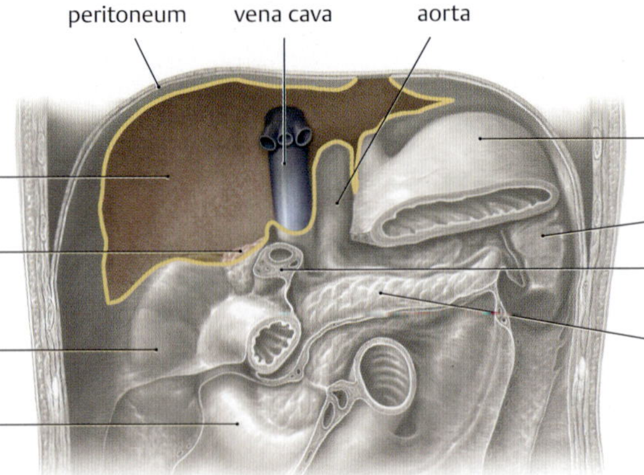

b

B Bare area of the liver and the hepatic surface of the diaphragm
Posterior view of the diaphragmatic surface of the liver (**a**) and the inferior surface of the diaphragm (**b**). The lines of peritoneal reflection on the liver and diaphragm demonstrate the mirror-image correspondence of the bare area with the hepatic surface of the diaphragm. The bare area is firmly attached to the inferior surface of the diaphragm by peritoneal reflection (coronary ligaments), rendering the liver immobile despite its intraperitoneal location.

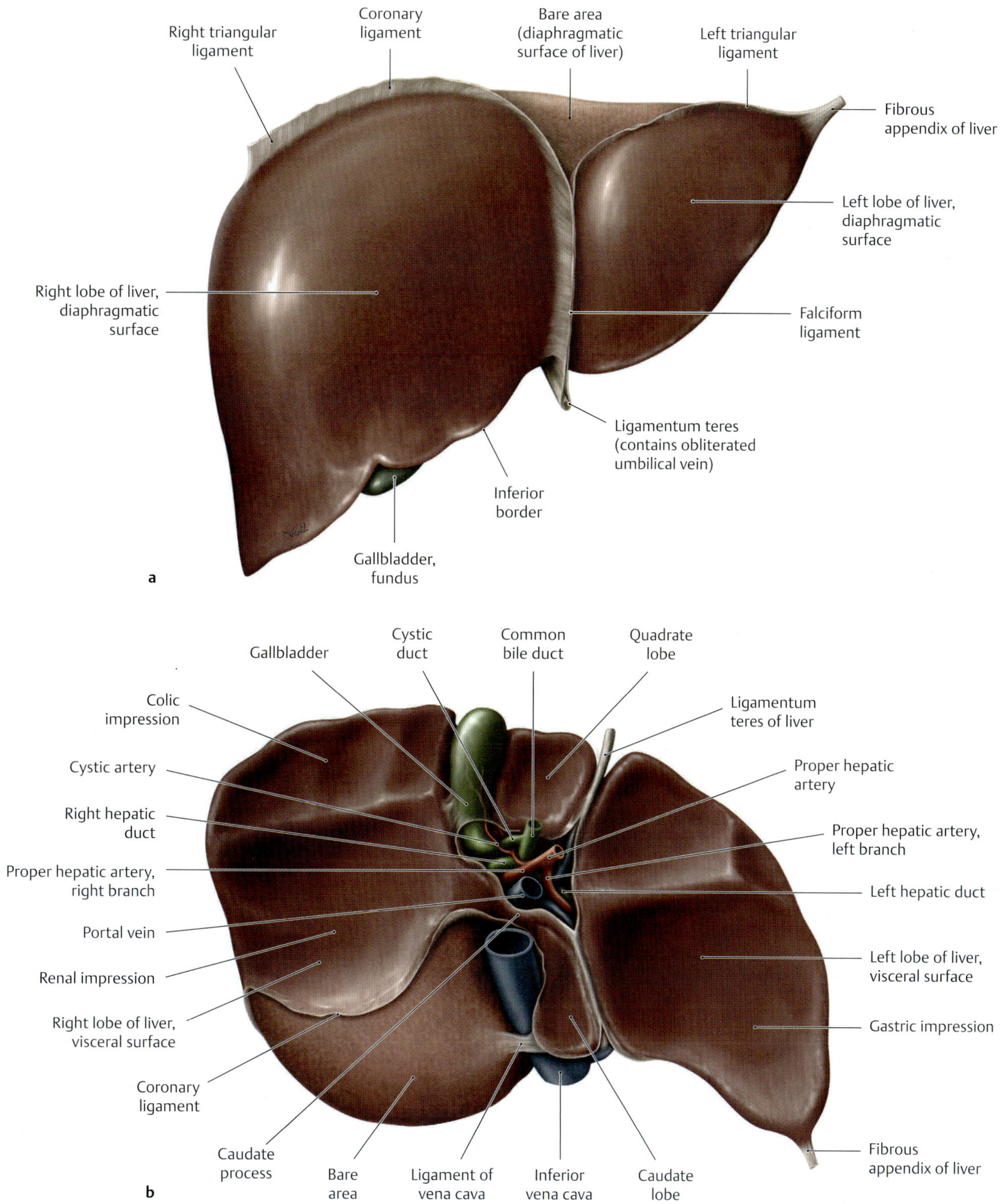

C Liver: diaphragmatic and visceral surfaces

a Anterior view of the diaphragmatic surface. Two lobes are visible in this view: the larger right lobe and the smaller left lobe. Between the two lobes is the falciform ligament of the liver, a "ventral mesentery" that extends to the anterior abdominal wall.

b Inferior view of the visceral surface. Two more of the four hepatic lobes are visible in this view: the caudate lobe and quadrate lobe. The visceral surface also contains the porta hepatis where neurovascular structures enter and leave the liver (common hepatic duct, proper hepatic artery, portal vein). Topographically, the hepatoduodenal ligament is a component of the lesser omentum. The extent of the hepatoduodenal ligament can be appreciated by noting the cut edge of visceral peritoneum surrounding the portal triad. Along with the hepatogastric ligament, it creates a "dorsal mesentery" for the liver. The numerous impressions from adjacent organs are seen this plainly only in a liver that has been chemically preserved. The gallbladder is closely applied to the visceral surface of the liver. Its fundus extends slightly past the inferior hepatic border, and its neck is directed toward the porta hepatis, where it comes into contact with the extrahepatic bile ducts.

3.15 Liver: Segmentation and Histology

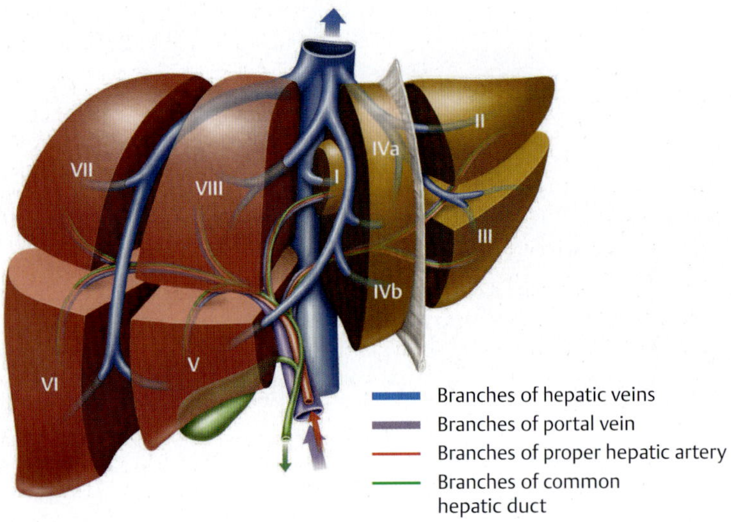

A Segmentation of the liver
Anterior view. *Note:* Three vascular structures enter or exit the liver at the porta hepatis:

- portal vein
- proper hepatic artery, and
- common hepatic duct

The central branch of the portal vein functionally subdivides the liver into a left part (yellow) and a right part (red). The boundary between the left and right parts of the liver is an imaginary line that roughly connects the gallbladder bed to the inferior vena cava (caval-gallbladder line, see **Cb**). Thus it is not identical to the externally visible boundary of the lobes formed by the falciform ligament (see p. 271). The portal triad subdivides within the two large parts, forming a total of eight segments that are more or less functionally independent of one another. This allows the surgeon to resect one or more hepatic segments without damaging the liver as a whole. Additionally, the remaining hepatic segments have a high regenerative potential. In the diagram above, the liver has been "exploded" at its virtual segmental boundaries to demonstrate the position and shape of its segments (numerical designations are shown in **B** and **C**).

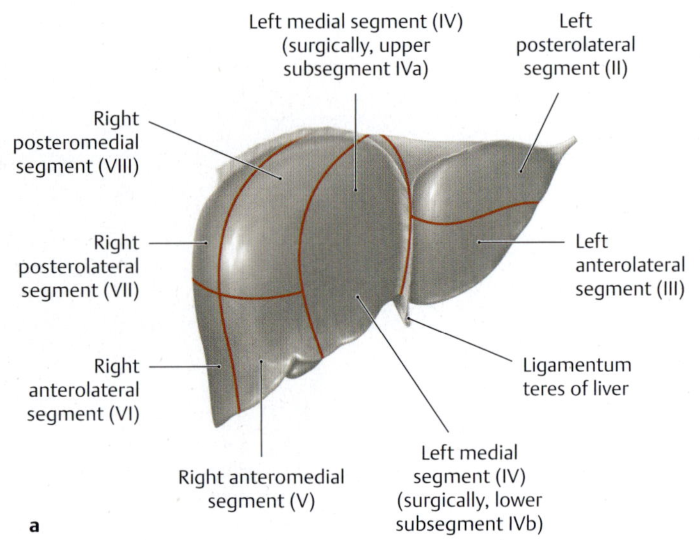

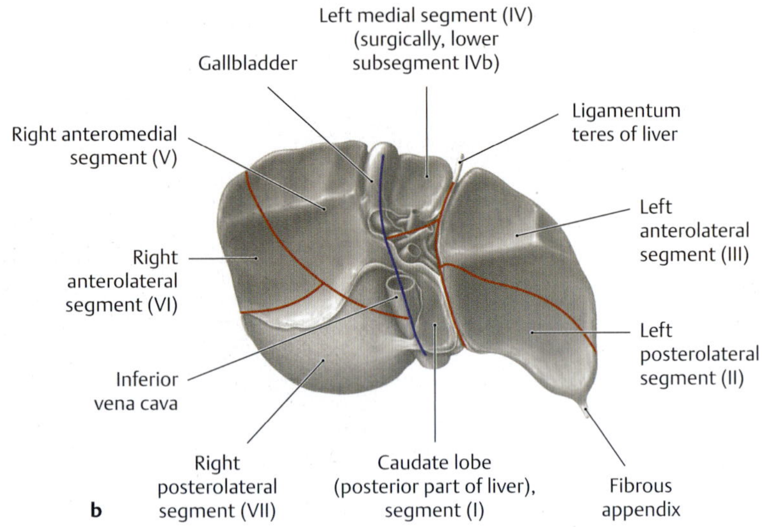

B Hepatic segments grouped by parts and divisions

Left part of the liver	• Posterior part, caudate lobe	• Segment I
	• Left lateral division	• Left posterolateral segment (segment II) • Left anterolateral segment (segment III)
	• Left medial division	• Left medial segment (segment IV), subdivided into subsegment IVa (above) and IVb (below)
Right part of the liver	• Right medial division	• Right anteromedial segment (segment V) • Right posteromedial segment (segment VIII)
	• Right lateral division	• Right anterolateral segment (segment VI) • Right posterolateral segment (segment VII)

C Projection of segmental boundaries onto the surface of the liver
Views of the diaphragmatic surface (**a**) and visceral surface of the liver (**b**).* The segments defined by the divisions of the portal vascular triad (see **A**) are projected onto the surface of the liver with their virtual boundaries. In this way the pattern of hepatic segmentation, which is based on vascular distribution, can be directly compared with the traditional division of the liver into four lobes based on external morphological criteria. For surgical purposes, it is useful to group the segments by parts and divisions (see **B**) because the portion of the liver selected for surgical resection may encompass not just one segment but two neighboring segments or the entire right or left part of the liver. Surgeons can positively identify the hepatic segments by ligating the feeding vessels until the segment or segments become discolored due to loss of blood supply.

* Blue line in **b**: caval-gallbladder line

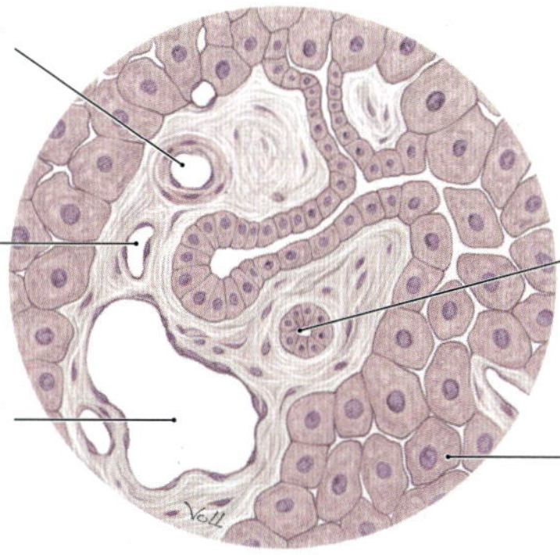

D Histologic appearance of a portal area

The portal triad (for the triad concept see also **E**) ramifies extensively and on the microscopic scale is referred to as the *peri*portal triad (*Glisson triad*) which lies in a *portal area* lined with connective tissue. The vascular structures of the portal triad at this level include the *interlobular artery and vein* and the *interlobular bile duct,* so named because they lie between the lobules (see **E**). The triad's vascular structures are easily distinguished from one another by differences in their calibers and wall structure:

- Interlobular artery: squamous epithelium, *thick* wall, *small* lumen
- Interlobular vein: squamous epithelium, *thin* wall, *large* lumen
- Interlobular bile duct: cuboidal epithelium and small lumen

Cirrhosis of the liver is characterized by a proliferation of connective tissue primarily in the portal area and about the central veins as necrotic hepatocytes are replaced by connective tissue. The capillary bed of the liver, the sinuses, are obliterated in the scarred areas, progressively diminishing the blood flow through the liver. Undiminished blood *inflow* into the liver through the proper hepatic artery and portal vein leads to engorgement of the portal vein (due to the greater *pressure* within the proper hepatic artery). This in turn causes an abnormal increase in blood pressure (portal hypertension). In many cases the blood is shunted into the vena cava system upstream of the liver via collateral veins (portocaval anastomoses, see p. 235).

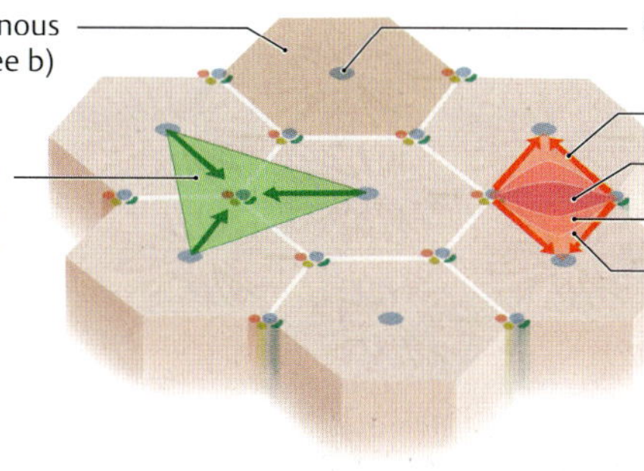

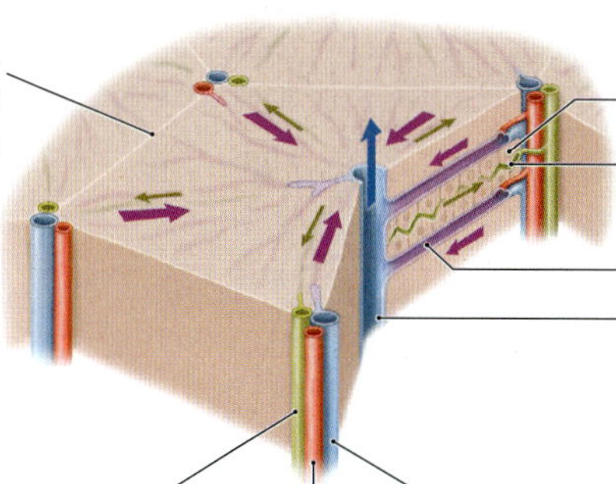

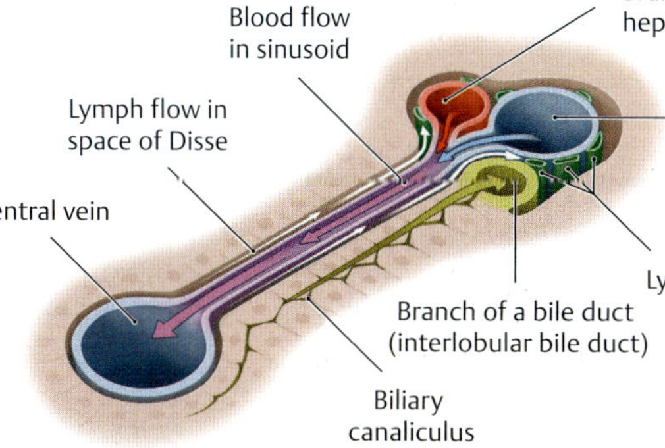

E Histologic architecture and flow of fluids in the liver

a Central venous lobule (brown); portal lobule (green), and hepatic acinus (red); **b** Three-dimensional structural model; **c** Flow of fluids in the liver.

a Functional histologic structure of the liver

- **Hexagonal central venous lobule:** Trabecular strands of hepatocytes are arrayed around a central vein in the center of the lobule. The hepatic sinusoids are blood conducting spaces that lie between the strands. The *periportal area* of connective tissue (see **b**) containing a vascular triad (portal or Glisson triad) is located at the edges, between neighboring lobules. Because of their position, the vascular structures are referred to as the *interlobular artery, vein, and bile duct* (see also **D**). For the triad concept see **c**. This classification reflects the histologic appearance and the *blood flow* from the portal area to the central vein.
- **Portal venous lobule:** Here the portal area is the center of a virtual triangle formed by three central veins of adjacent hepatic lobules. The green arrows indicate the *direction of bile flow* to the interlobular bile duct.
- **Hepatic acinus:** Blood flows from a line connecting two portal areas through the two adjacent lobules to the central vein (red arrows). The acinus describes the decreasing *oxygen and nutrient content* of the blood as it flows toward the central vein as areas of decreasing metabolic activity (I > II > III).

b and c Three-dimensional model of a hepatic lobule with flow of fluids: Blood in the hepatic lobule flows in the sinusoids away from the portal area and toward the central vein. Bile and lymph flow in the opposite direction. Glisson in his day did not yet describe periportal lymphatic vessels. Although there are actually **four** vascular structures in the portal area, one still refers to a "triad" in the traditional manner. The sinusoids are the common terminal capillary bed for the interlobular artery and vein. They thus contain mixed arterial and venous blood with a high level of nutrients from the gastrointestinal tract. Between the sinusoidal epithelium and the hepatocytes lies a narrow cleft, the perisinusoidal space of Disse. Pores in the discontinuous endothelium allow plasma components to pass into the space of Disse to be metabolized by the hepatocytes. The unabsorbed fluid is conducted as *hepatic lymph* through the space of Disse back to the portal area where it is removed via *lymphatic* vessels that empty into larger lymphatic vessels at the porta hepatis. The **bile** flows to the bile duct in *intercellular spaces lying between the hepatocytes* (biliary canaliculi, which have no walls of their own). If one looks at individual hepatocytes, the sinusoid and the space of Disse lie on one side whereas the canaliculus lies on the opposite side; the hepatocyte is functionally polarized whereby the biliary capillaries represent the apical pole of the cell. If biliary stasis develops, the resulting increase in pressure in the biliary canaliculus can cause loss of intercellular cohesion between the hepatocytes. The canaliculus develops leaks, allowing the bile to escape between the hepatocytes where it can enter the space of Disse and the sinusoid. When biliary components enter the bloodstream, one refers to jaundice.

3.16 Gallbladder and Bile Ducts: Location and Relationships to Adjacent Organs

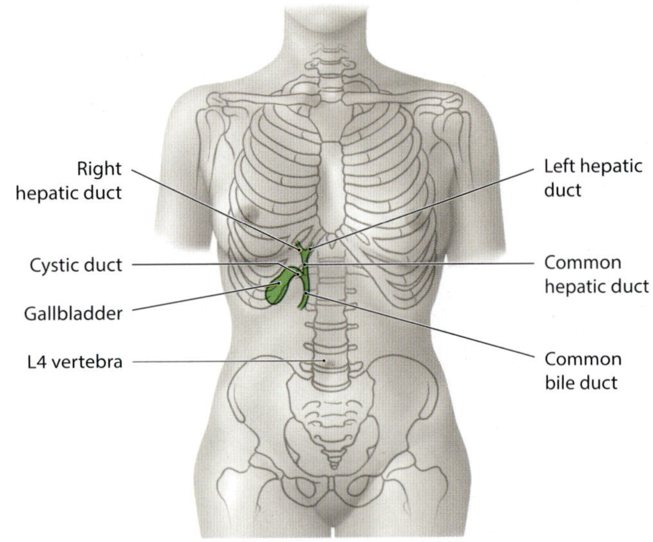

A Projection of the extrahepatic bile ducts onto the skeleton
Viewed from the front, the gallbladder is projected at a point where the mid-clavicular line intersects the inferior border of the ninth rib. The orifice of the common bile duct (which generally opens jointly with the pancreatic duct on the major duodenal papilla) lies approximately at the level of the L 2 vertebral body. The gallbladder emerges beneath the right costal arch at approximately the L 1/L 2 level. In certain diseases (e.g., cholecystitis), tenderness to pressure may be noted at this location.

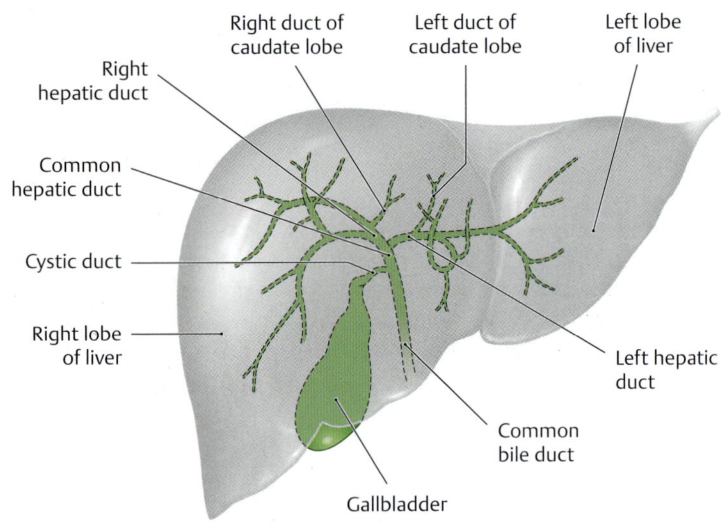

B Projection of the intra- and extrahepatic bile ducts onto the surface of the liver
Anterior view. Bile flows through the biliary canaliculi (microscopic) into the small interlobular bile ducts in the portal area (see p. 273). These ducts coalesce to form increasingly larger units that drain a hepatic segment. The bile from all the segments ultimately drains into two large collecting vessels, the left and right hepatic ducts, which receive the small left and right ducts of the caudate lobe, respectively, while still inside the liver. The right and left hepatic ducts unite to form the common hepatic duct. Almost immediately the excretory duct of the gallbladder, the cystic duct, enters the side of the common hepatic duct, which then becomes the common bile duct.

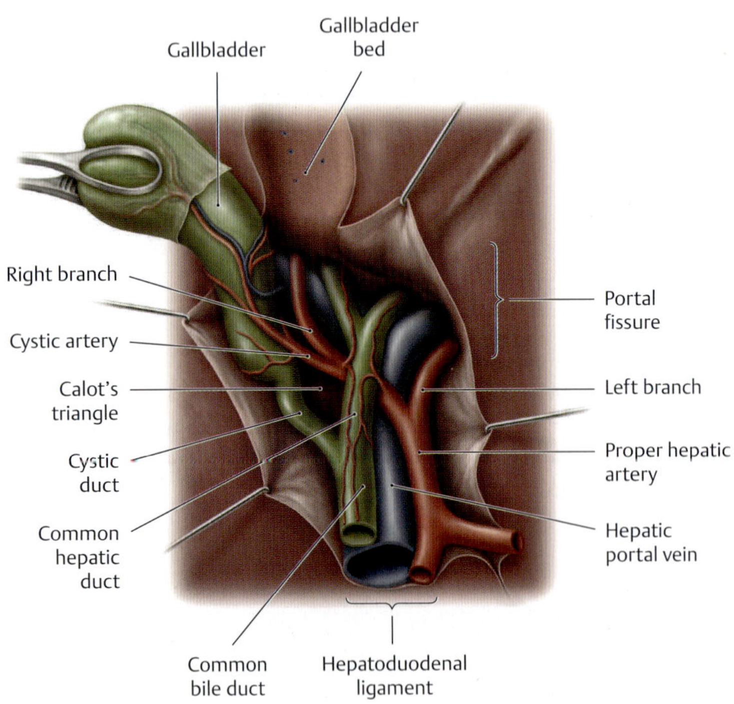

C Topography of Calot's triangle at the portal fissure
Inferoanterior view. The anterior margin of the right lobe has been pushed upward, the gallbladder has been lifted from its bed and retracted to the right. The peritoneum has been opened in the area of the portal fissure and the hepatoduodenal ligament. For better exposure, nerves, lymph nodes and their pathways have been removed. 95% of injuries to the extrahepatic bile ducts are sustained intraoperatively, most commonly during cholecystectomies. Particularly with the minimally invasive surgical method to remove the gallbladder (laproscopic cholecystectomy), the precise identification of anatomical structures is an essential aspect of this surgical procedure. Thus, before transecting the cystic artery and the cystic duct it is important to identify Calot's triangle, which is bordered by the cystic artery, cystic duct and common hepatic duct. The gallbladder fundus is grasped and retracted slightly superiorly to expose and open Calot's triangle. The structures that are to be transected are ligated with clips.

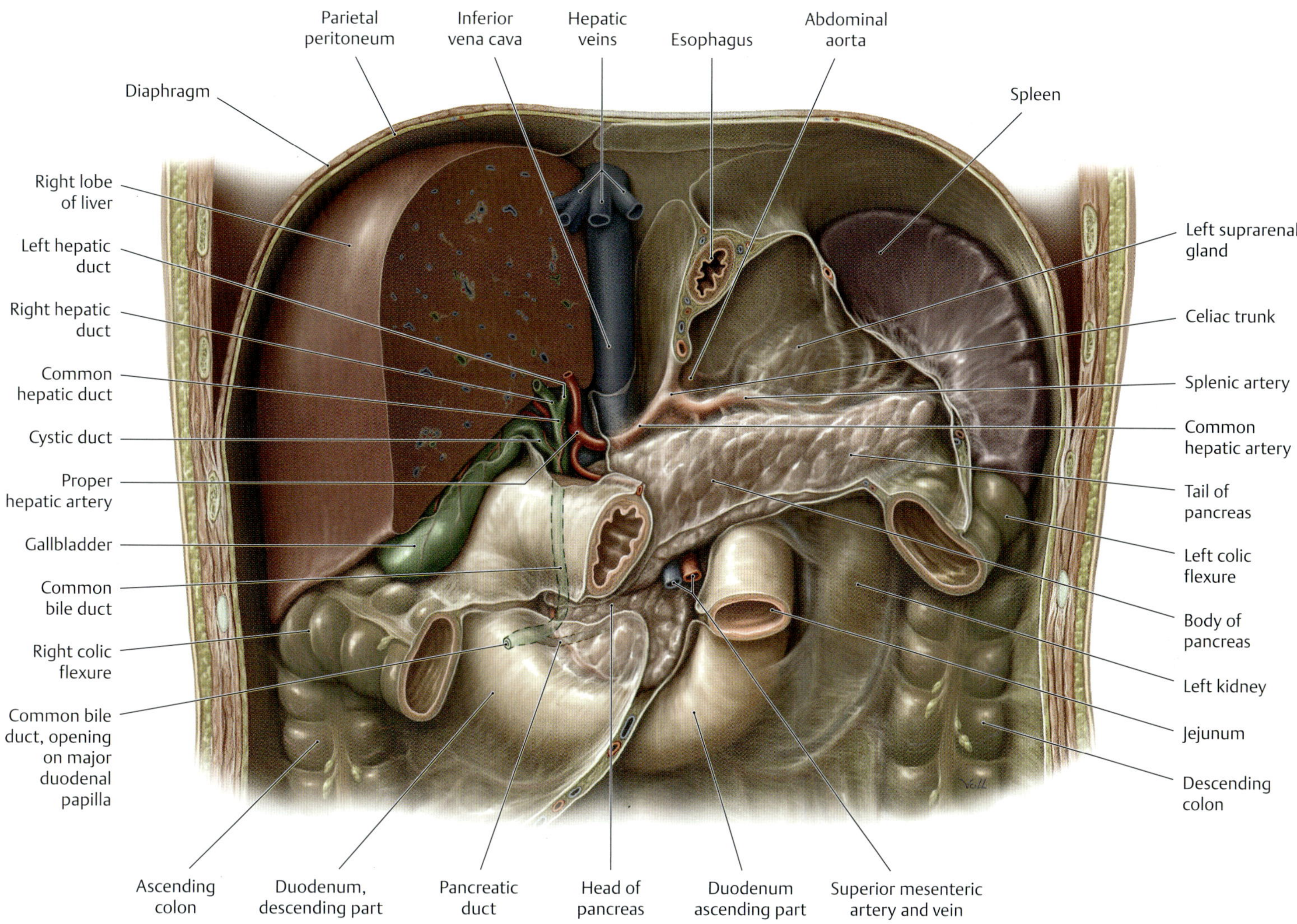

D Relationship of the biliary tract to adjacent organs

Anterior view of the opened abdomen. The stomach, small intestine, transverse colon, and large portions of the liver have been removed, and the peritoneum has been divided in the area of the hepatoduodenal ligament. The gallbladder is partially contained in a fossa on the visceral surface of the liver. The common bile duct passes behind the duodenum toward the head of the pancreas. After passing through the head of the pancreas, the bile duct frequently unites with the pancreatic duct, as shown here. Both ducts then open together at the major duodenal papilla in the descending part of the duodenum (see p. 276).

E Bile: secretion, composition and function

Secretion:
Bile is a thin secretion (up to1200ml/day) produced by the liver (hepatic bile). After water and salts have been removed, the bile is stored in the gallbladder (gallbladder bile) or runs into the duodenum via bile ducts. The major driving force for the secretion of bile is ATP-powered pumps, which transport mainly bile acids and other substances to the biliary canaliculi, and into which water follows by osmosis.

Composition:
Water, bile acids or their salts (e.g., cholate, deoxycholate), phospholipids (mainly lecithin), bile pigments (e.g., bilirubin), cholesterol, inorganic salts, etc.

Enterohepatic circulation:
98% of the bile salts secreted into the gallbladder are reabsorbed in the terminal ileum, returned to the liver via the portal vein, and secreted again from hepatocytes. In this way, bile salts are recycled up to 10 times per day before they are excreted in the feces.

Function:
Bile has essentially two major functions:

- Absorption of fat in the small intestine: together with phospholipids, the bile salts emulsify insoluble lipids (through formation of lipid micelles);
- Route for excretion of cholesterol and other waste products (e.g., bilirubin, a by-product of hemoglobin breakdown).

Gallstones:
Gallstones are caused by changes in gallbladder bile composition (cholesterol and pigment stones). The stones themselves usually do not produce any symptoms. Only the obstruction or inflammation of the bile ducts caused by the gallstones leads to symptoms (cholelithiasis, cholecystitis).

3.17 Extrahepatic Bile Ducts and Pancreatic Ducts

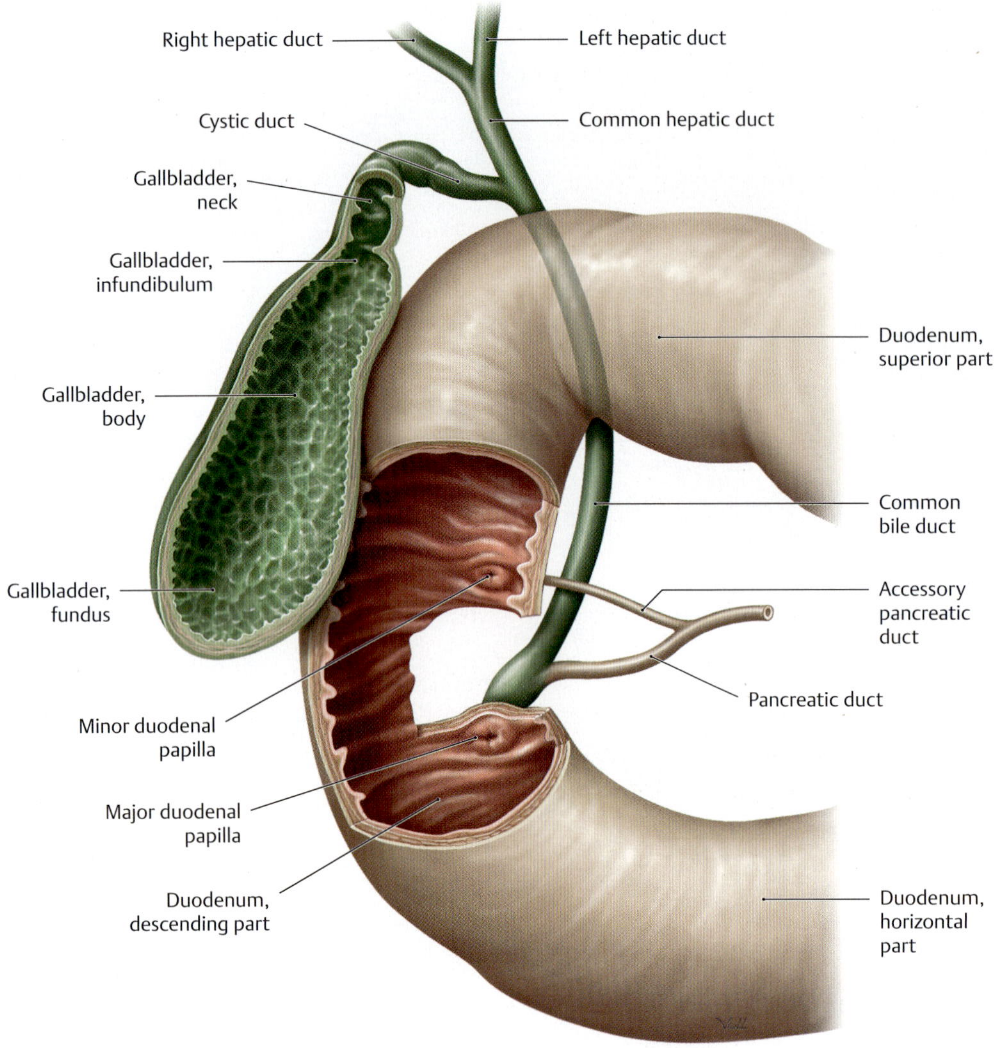

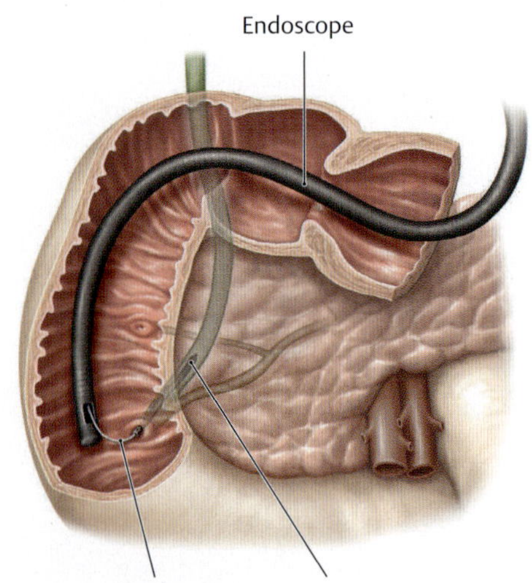

a

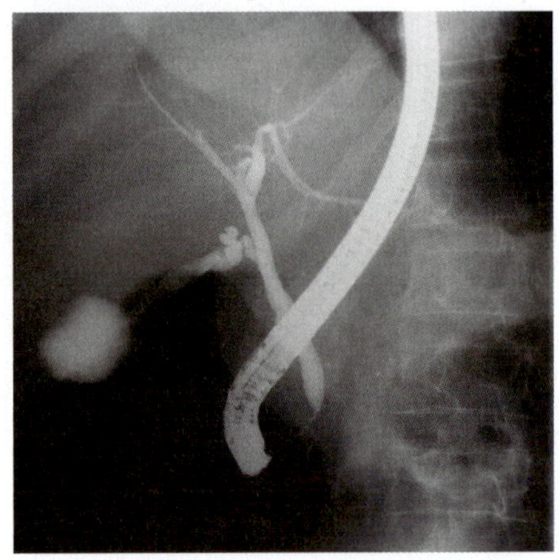

b

A Divisions of the extrahepatic bile ducts
Anterior view. The gallbladder has been opened, and the duodenum has been opened and windowed. The web-like pattern of folds in the gallbladder mucosa is plainly seen. The mucosa between the folds may be deepened to form crypts that can trap bacteria (with risk of cholecystitis). The largest part of the gallbladder is the *body*, which is joined to the neck by the funnel-shaped infundibulum. The neck leads to the cystic duct, which opens end-to-side into the common hepatic duct, formed by the union of the *right* and *left hepatic ducts*. The large duct formed by the union of the cystic duct and common hepatic duct is called the *common bile duct*. This duct often receives the pancreatic duct, both of which then discharge their secretions into the duodenum at the major duodenal papilla (of Vater). A short distance superior to the major papilla is the minor duodenal papilla, whose associated duct (accessory pancreatic duct) crosses in front of the common bile duct. The diagram illustrates a normal pattern of development in which the common hepatic and pancreatic ducts unite to form an ampulla (variants are shown in **D**).
Note: The combined termination of the common bile duct and pancreatic duct has two important implications: A tumor in the head of the pancreas may obstruct the common bile duct (causing biliary reflux into the liver with jaundice), and a gallstone that has migrated from the gallbladder into the common bile duct may obstruct the terminal part of the pancreatic duct. The obstruction of pancreatic secretions may incite a life-threatening pancreatitis.

B Endoscopic retrograde cholangiopancreatography (ERCP)
a Anterior view, duodenum opened anteriorly; **b** Image of the corresponding region using ERCP (b from: Möller, T.B,. E. Reif: Taschenatlas der Röntgenanatomie, 7th ed. Stuttgart: Thieme; 2021).
ERCP is a technique that uses radiographic contrast (see **b**) to display the bile ducts, gallbladder and pancreatic duct. An endoscope is used to locate the duodenal papilla (major or minor) and to inject contrast agent into the papillary orifice. A radiograph of the contrast-filled duct system can then be evaluated. ERCP can also be used to remove gallstones that have become impacted at the papilla (endoscopic papillotomy) with the help of a scissor-cutting device fitted to the tip of the endoscope. Thus, ERCP is used for diagnosis and treatment.

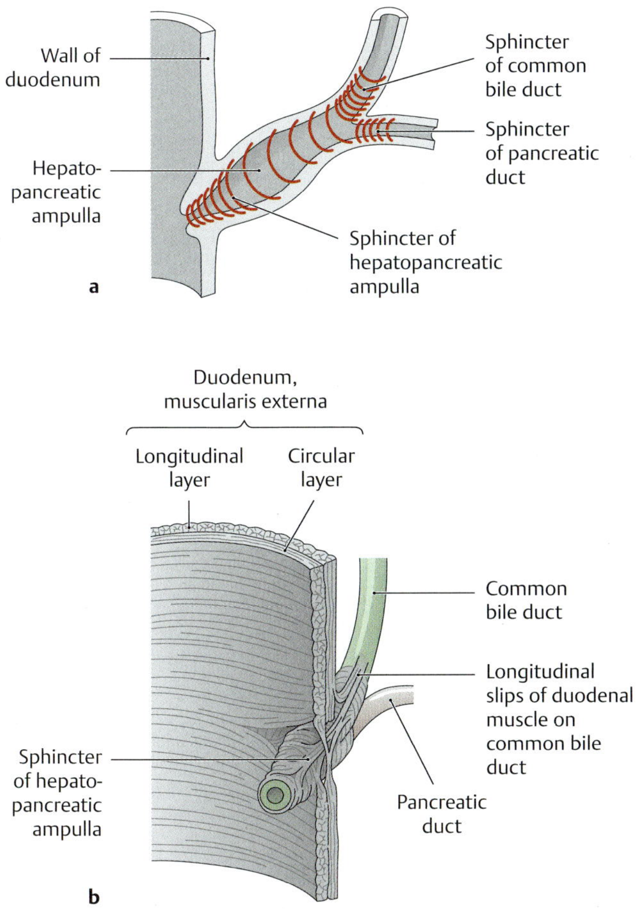

C Function and structure of the biliary sphincter system

a Sphincters of the common bile duct and pancreatic duct. Each duct has its own sphincter system. Typically both of the ducts unite to form a large ampulla, the hepatopancreatic ampulla, which also has its own sphincter. The sphincter mechanism is supported by adjacent venous pads (not shown here) in the walls of the ducts.

b Integration of the sphincter system in the duodenal wall. The muscles of both ducts blend with the sphincter muscle of the hepatopancreatic ampulla, which passes through the duodenal wall.

Note: The ampullary sphincter system works independently of the circular muscle layer of the duodenal wall, allowing the sphincters to function even during fasting when the duodenum is relaxed. In this state the ductal sphincters are contracted and bile is stored. When food is ingested, the sphincter system opens and allows bile to flow into the duodenum. The sphincter system forms a normal anatomical constriction where a gallstone may become lodged, obstructing the outflow of bile and pancreatic juice (pancreatitis, see **A**). The function of the sphincters, the discharge of bile by the gallbladder, and the production of bile by the liver are controlled partially by the autonomic nervous system (especially the parasympathetic system) and partially by gastrointestinal hormones (e.g., cholecystokinin and secretin).

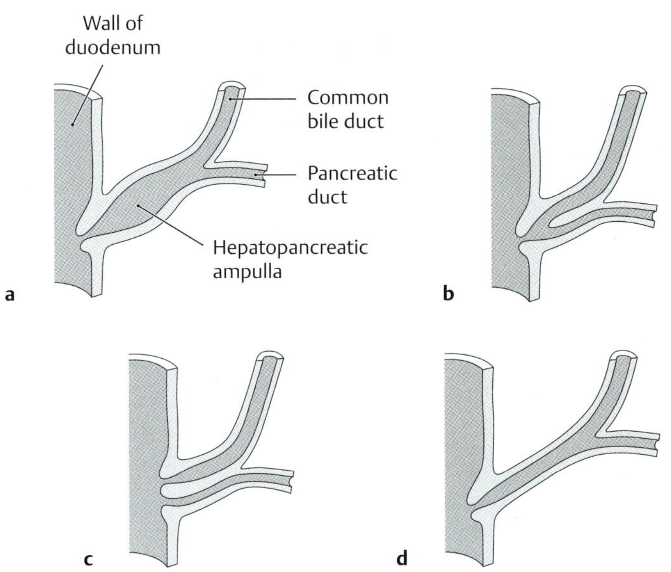

D Extrahepatic bile ducts: typical anatomy and variants
Variants in the termination of the common bile duct and pancreatic duct.

a Typical anatomy: Both ducts open at the major duodenal papilla by way of a common ampulla (the most common form).

b–d Variants:

b Varying degrees of septation of the common ampulla.

c Complete septation of the ampulla, with a separate opening for each duct.

d The ducts unite without forming a true ampulla.

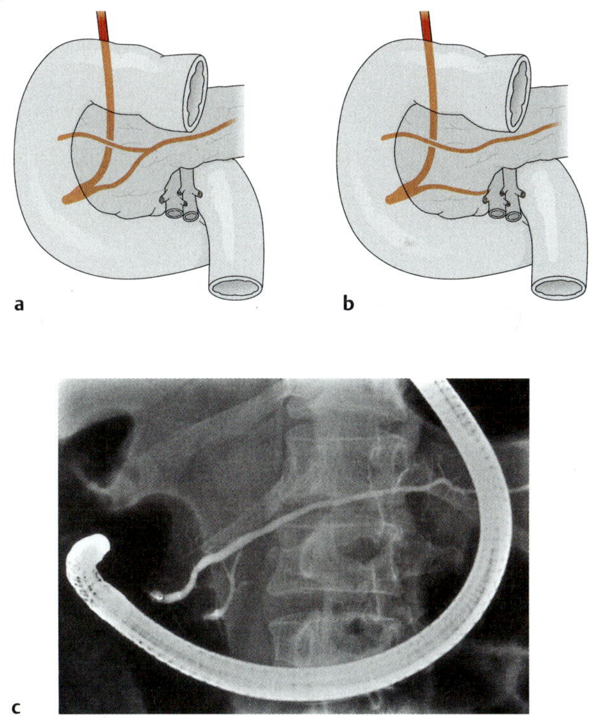

E Pancreas: normal anatomy and variants
a pancreatic buds have fused; **b** pancreas divisum (in up to 10% of examined patients); **c** pancreas divisum at ERCP (c from Brambs, H.-J.: Pareto Reihe Radiologie. Gastrointestinal system. Thieme, Stuttgart 2007). Failure of the dorsal pancreatic bud to fuse with the ventral bud (see p. 43) leads to a divided pancreas (pancreas divisum; no clinical disease, usually presents as an incidental finding). The ducts of both buds remain completely separate. The duct of the ventral pancreatic bud opens into the major duodenal papilla and the duct of the dorsal bud into the minor duodenal papilla. In ERCP (see **c**) both ducts were filled separately via the two papillae.

3.18 Pancreas

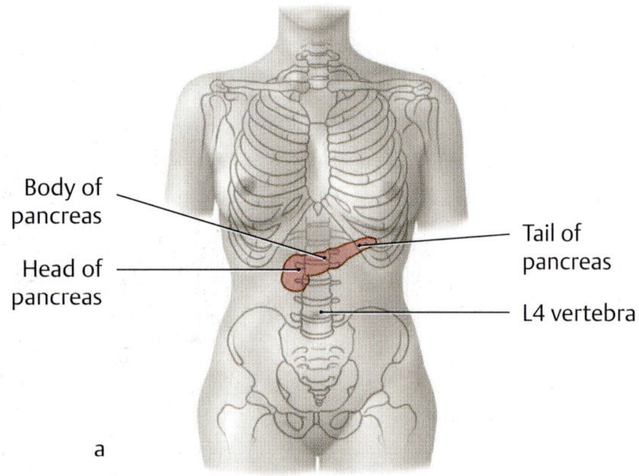

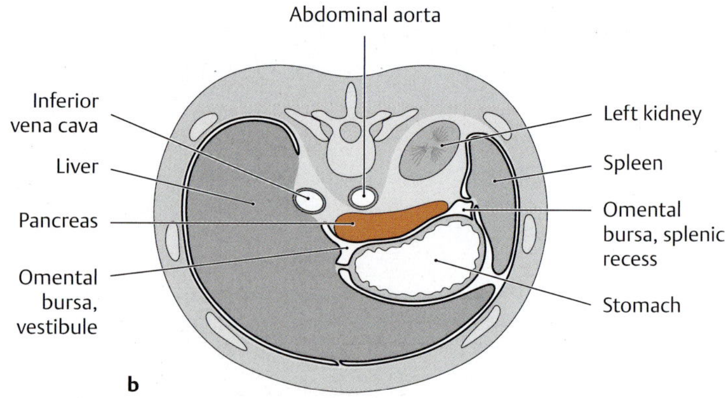

A Location of the pancreas

a Projection onto the vertebral column; **b** Transverse section through the abdomen at approximately the T 12/L 1 level, viewed from above. *Note*: The head of the pancreas is below the plane of section which is why the pancreas appears shortened at this level.

The pancreas is an elongated organ that is oriented transversely in the right and left upper quadrants, lying mainly in the epigastric region. Whereas most of the body of the pancreas crosses the midline at the L 1/L 2 level. The head of the pancreas is directed to the right and extends to the L 2/L 3 level. The tail of the pancreas may closely approach the spleen in the LUQ. The pain associated with diseases of the pancreas is often a "girdling pain" that encircles the upper abdomen and even the lower thorax (see p. 302).

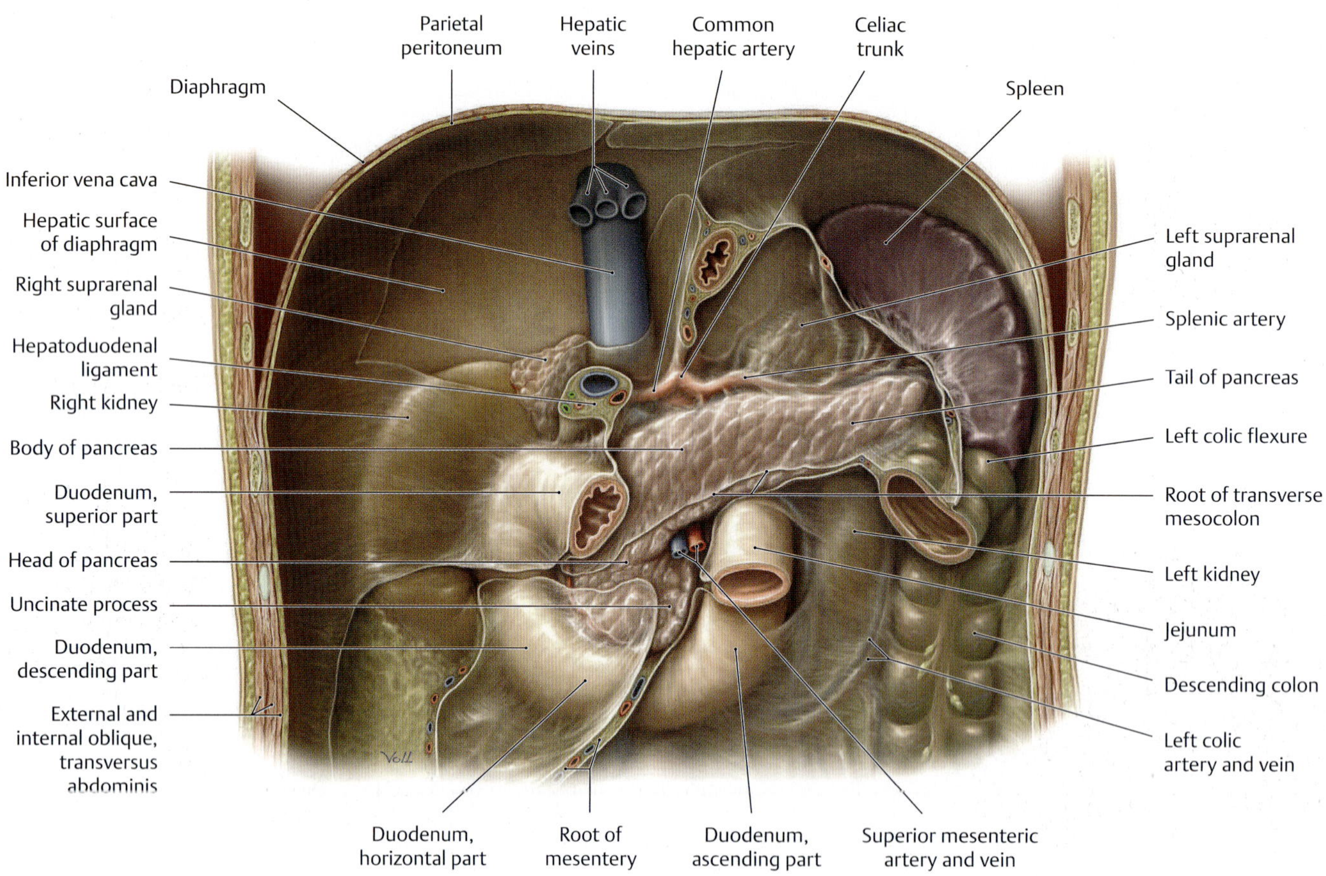

B The pancreas in situ

Anterior view. The liver, stomach, small intestine, and large intestine have been removed proximal to the left colic flexure. The retroperitoneal fat and connective tissue and the perirenal fat capsule have been greatly thinned to better demonstrate the structures in the retroperitoneum. The pancreas is a secondarily retroperitoneal organ located on the posterior wall of the omental bursa. Its head lies in the C-shaped loop of the duodenum. The transverse mesocolon is attached to the anterior surface of the pancreas. Because of its position posterior to or adjacent to other organs and large vessels, it is difficult to access surgically. At the same time, owing to its proximity, pancreatic tumors may invade and encase the superior mesenteric artery and vein (leading to impaired circulation of the organs they supply, such as the jejunum, ileum, and ascending colon). Inflammation of or tumors in the head of the pancreas may also lead to obstruction of the main bile duct (leading to obstructive jaundice).

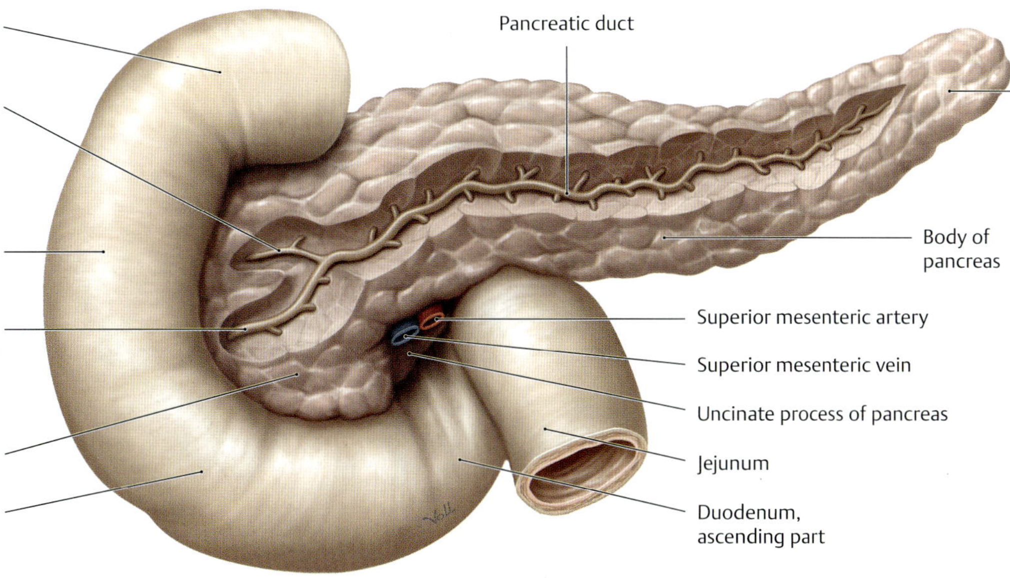

C Location and course of the pancreatic ducts

Anterior view. The anterior side has been partially dissected. The ducts of the former ventral and dorsal pancreatic buds have united to form a common duct, which is referred to as the main pancreatic duct (formed from the ventral pancreatic duct in the head of the pancreas and the distal portion of the dorsal pancreatic duct (most common case). It traverses the entire length of the pancreas and opens into the descending part of the duodenum, usually sharing an orifice with the common bile duct, on the major duodenal papilla. The small *accessory pancreatic duct* (the remaining proximal portion of the former dorsal pancreatic duct in the head of the pancreas) opens into the duodenum on the minor duodenal papilla (see p. 277). Several variants of ductal anatomy may exist:

- both ducts remain separate and open on two different papillae (pancreas divisum, see p. 277),
- both ducts unite to form a single duct that opens on one papilla,
- in both cases (though rarely), the common bile duct may open into the duodenum by a separate orifice.

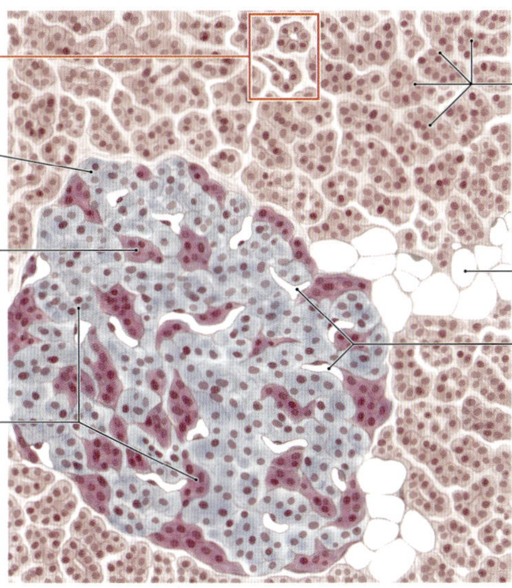

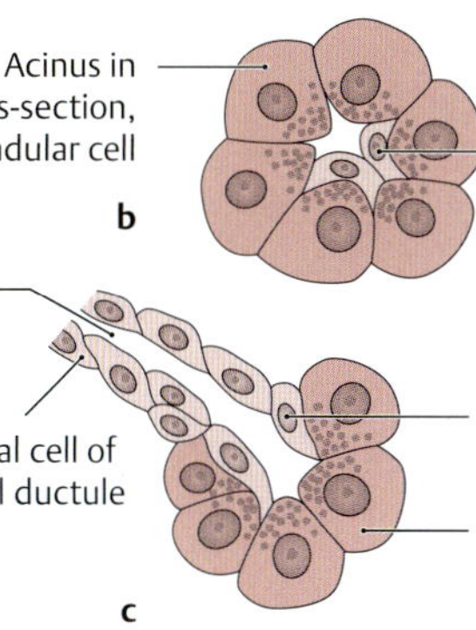

D Histological structure of the pancreas

a Pancreatic tissue; **b** and **c** detail from **a**: higher magnification views of acini shown in transverse and longitudinal sections.

a Histologically, the pancreas consists of two functionally distinct types of glandular tissue:

- The **exocrine pancreas** (98% of the organ mass, light pink in the upper part of the figure) consists of myriad berry-shaped glands (acini, see **b** and **c**), which secrete an enzyme-rich fluid through the pancreatic duct into the duodenum. Produced at a rate of approximately 2 liters/day, this fluid contains enzymes that assist numerous digestive processes in the bowel. Insufficiency of the exocrine pancreas leads to impaired digestive function.
- The **endocrine pancreas** (2% of the organ mass) also known as the islet apparatus: approximately 1 million epithelial cells (islets of Langerhans, pancreatic islets), which can be divided into alpha (A) cells (20% of islet cells) and beta (B) cells (80% of islet cells). The beta cells produce insulin, which lowers blood glucose levels, and the alpha cells produce the hormone glucagon. Other islet cell types include delta (D) and F cells, which produce somatostatin or pancreatic polypeptide. Special staining methods are used to make these cell types visible. The islet cells release hormones directly into the bloodstream (which is why there are many capillaries present in the pancreatic islets).

Note: A decrease in the number of beta-cells and deficient or defective production of insulin leads to the clinical picture of diabetes mellitus.

b The **acinar cells** produce approximately 2 liters of "pancreatic juice," an enzyme-rich secretion (containing numerous proteins) per day, which is passed into the duodenum via the pancreatic duct. This secretion is important for digestion. Thus, hypofunction of the exocrine pancreas leads to maldigestion.
Note: Acinar cells usually stain intensely with conventional techniques. Nonetheless, they don't appear equally dark in histological sections. The parts that transport secretions (the ductule cells) stain less intensely than the parts that produce secretions. Because the initial portion of the part that transports secretions is invaginated into the center of the acinus, which stains more intensely, they are conspicuous in histological sections. These cells that lie at the center of the acinus, but belong to the secretion-transporting part, are referred to as centroacinar cells. The pancreas is the only exocrine gland that contains centroacinar cells.

3.19 Spleen

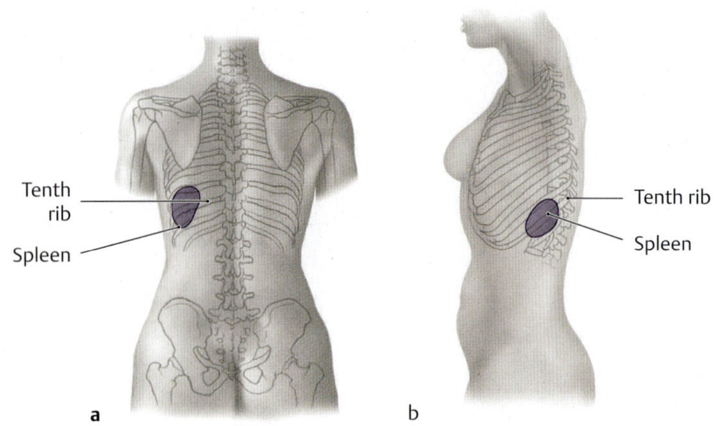

A Projection of the spleen onto the skeleton
Posterior view (**a**) and left lateral view (**b**). The spleen is located in the left upper quadrant. Its position varies considerably with respiration because it lies just below the diaphragm and is directly affected by its movements, even though (unlike the liver) it is not attached to the diaphragm. At functional residual capacity (the resting position between inspiration and expiration), the hilum of the spleen crosses the tenth rib on the left side. Generally a healthy, unenlarged spleen is not palpable on physical examination.

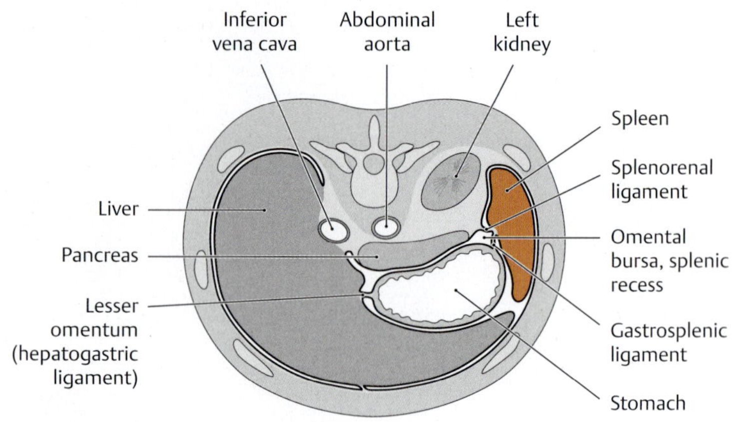

B Location of the spleen
Transverse section through the abdomen, viewed from above. This section demonstrates the relationship of the spleen to neighboring organs. The intraperitoneal spleen lies in its own compartment and is attached by folds of peritoneum to the posterior trunk wall (splenorenal ligament) and to the stomach (gastrosplenic ligament). A recess of the omental bursa (splenic recess) extends to the spleen.

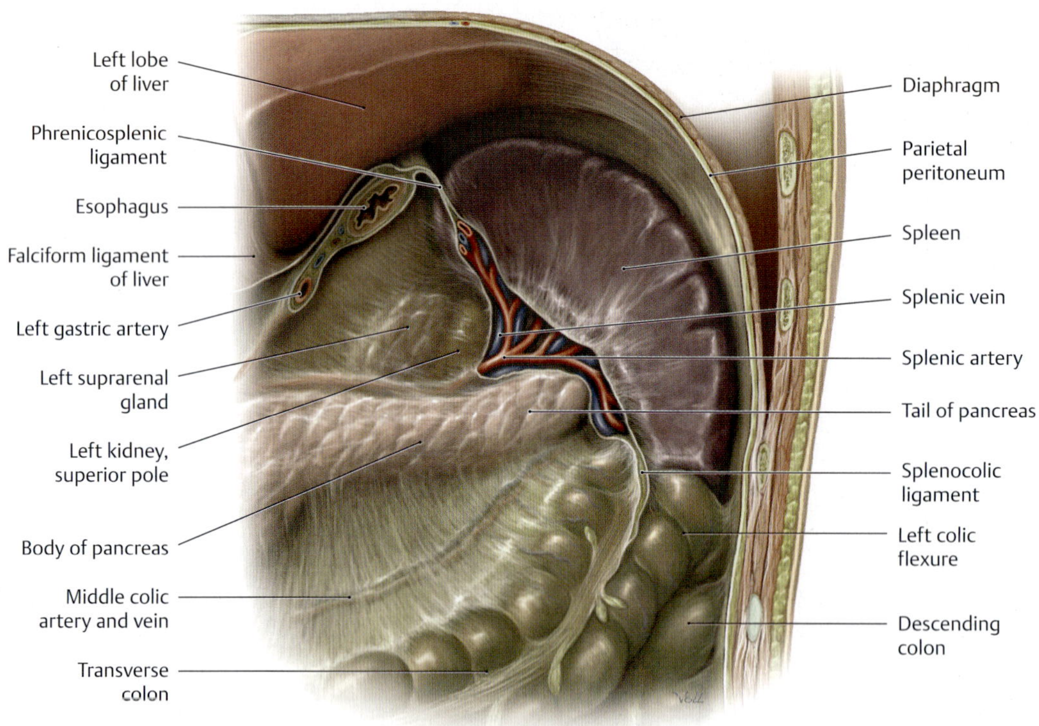

C The spleen in situ: peritoneal relationships
Anterior view into the LUQ with the stomach removed. When the spleen is abnormally enlarged, it may press heavily upon the stomach and colon, causing pain. The drawing illustrates the close proximity of the spleen to the tail of the pancreas and left colic flexure, which is also called the splenic flexure.
Note the peritoneal attachment between the spleen and transverse colon (splenocolic ligament, part of the greater omentum). Embryologically, the greater omentum is a dorsal mesentery in which the spleen develops. During rotation of the stomach in the embryo, the spleen moves from its original position posterior to the gut into the LUQ. A "side stitch" (piercing sensation felt below the rib cage during exercise) is believed to be caused by stretching of the peritoneal covering and splenocolic ligament due to swelling of the spleen during physical exercise.

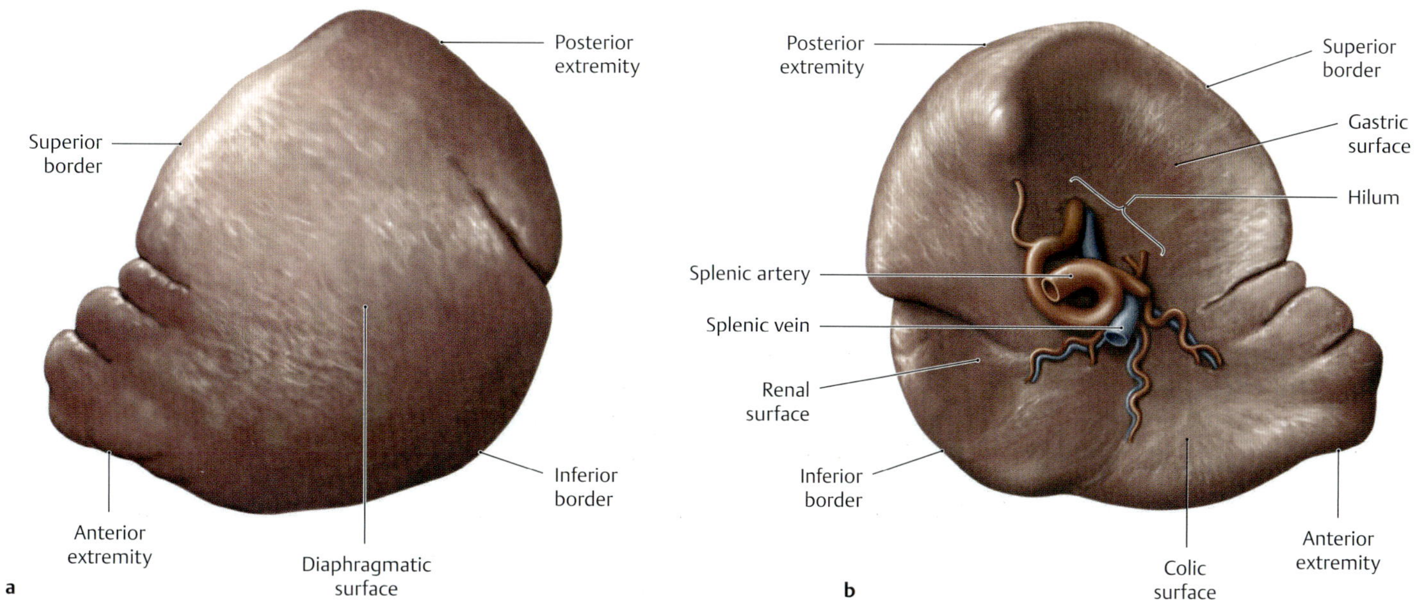

D Spleen: shape and surface anatomy
Views of the costal surface (**a**) and visceral surface (**b**) of the organ. The spleen is highly variable in its conformation in different people, but because this very soft organ is covered by a firm fibrous capsule, it maintains a relatively constant external shape ("coffee bean"). Since it is very difficult to suture the soft splenic tissue, it is not uncommon to treat splenic injuries by splenectomy, which eliminates a potential source of severe intraperitoneal bleeding. The blood vessels that enter and leave the organ at the splenic hilum are usually tortuous and form multiple coils.

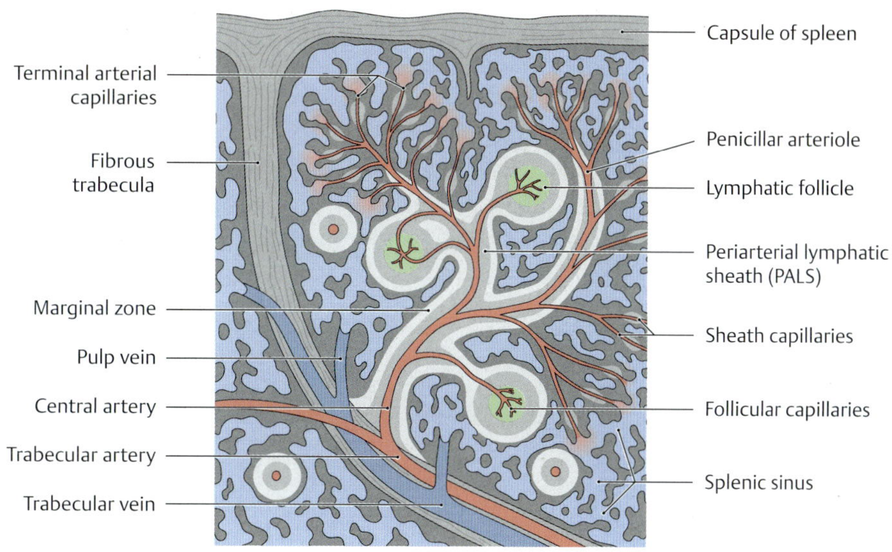

E Structure of the spleen
The spleen is the single largest lymphoid organ and the only lymphatic organ that is incorporated directly into the bloodstream (to screen out abnormal cells, see below). Strands of connective tissue called trabeculae extend from the firm fibrous capsule toward the hilum of the spleen, subdividing the splenic tissue into small chambers. The branches of the fibrous trabeculae and the vessels they transmit (*trabecular arteries and veins*) determine the architecture of the spleen. Between the fibrous trabeculae is a meshwork of fine reticular connective tissue, the splenic pulp. On entering the pulp, the blood vessels become known as the *pulp arteries* (central arteries) and *pulp veins*. The terminal arterial branches have the appearance of the mycelia of bread mold (*penicillium*), and are thus named "penicillar" arterioles. Two types of splenic pulp are distinguished: red pulp and white pulp:

- The red pulp consists of cavities (splenic sinuses) that are engorged with blood in the living organism (aggregation of large masses of red blood cells), accounting for its red color and its name (in the section shown here, the pulp is devoid of blood and is colorless). The function of the red pulp is to screen out aging and defective erythrocytes from the bloodstream. The numerous sinuses within the reticular meshwork give the spleen its soft, spongy consistency.
- The white pulp consists of splenic nodules (Malpighian bodies)—variable-sized aggregations of lymphocytes (periarterial lymphatic sheaths, lymphatic follicles) that consist of clones of beta cells that are proliferatory in response to antigens.

The lymphatic aggregations of the white pulp ensheath the central arteries in varying degrees to ensure close contact between the blood and lymphocytes. The central arteries ramify extensively before delivering their blood to the sinuses of the red pulp. From there the blood is conveyed by pulp veins to the trabecular veins, which in turn empty into the splenic vein.

3.20 Branches of the Celiac Trunk: Arteries Supplying the Stomach, Liver, and Gallbladder

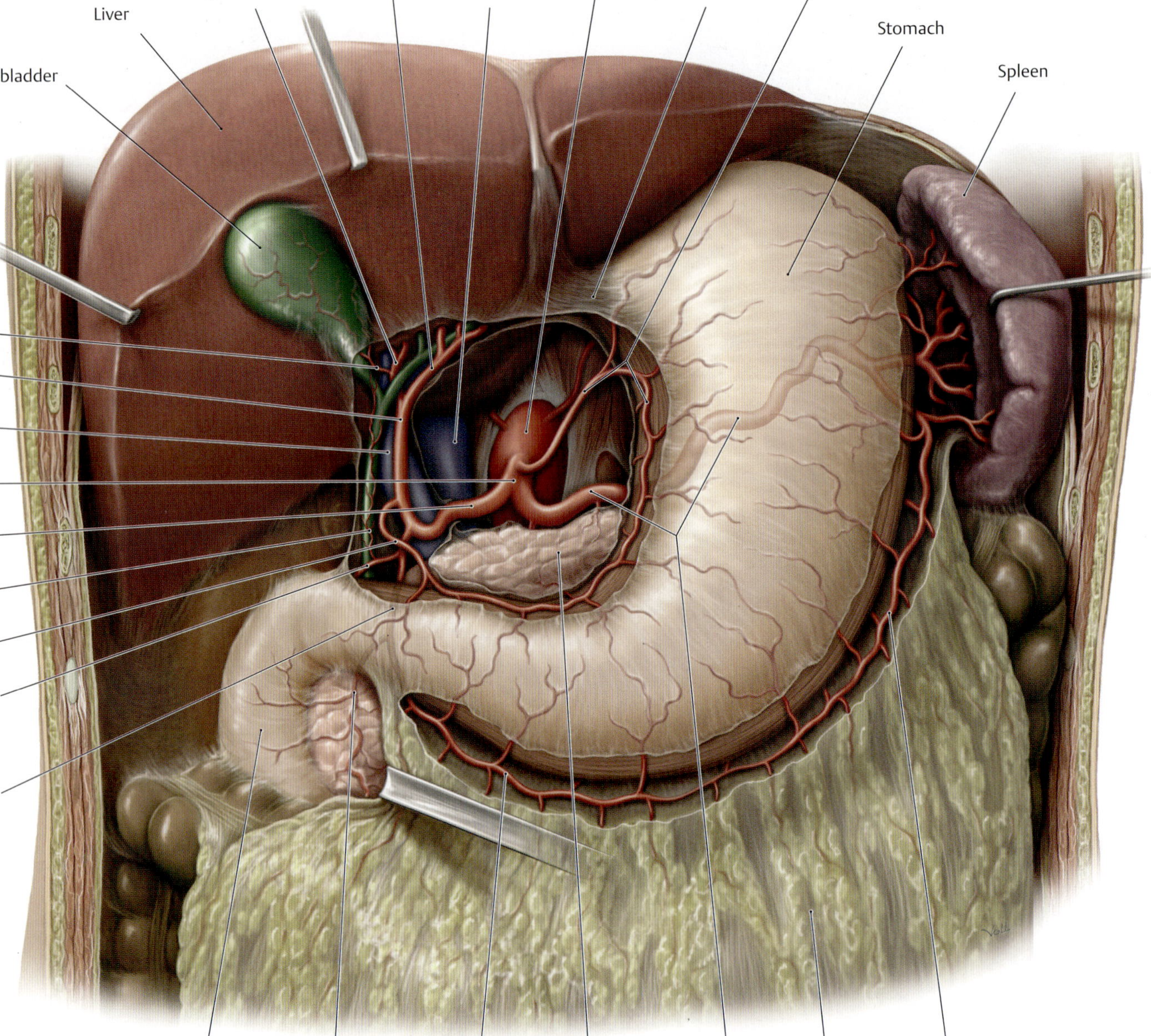

A Celiac trunk and arteries to the stomach, liver, and gallbladder
Anterior view. The lesser omentum has been opened to display the celiac trunk. The greater omentum has been incised to demonstrate the gastro-omental arteries.

The celiac trunk is the first anterior visceral branch of the abdominal aorta (see p. 227). It is only about 1 cm long. In 25% of cases it divides into three arterial branches in a tripod-like configuration, as illustrated here. The principal variants of the celiac trunk are shown in **C**.

Note that the proper hepatic artery, portal vein, and common bile duct reach the liver by passing through the hepatoduodenal ligament, which is part of the lesser omentum. These vessels must be protected in surgical operations on the gallbladder and bile duct.

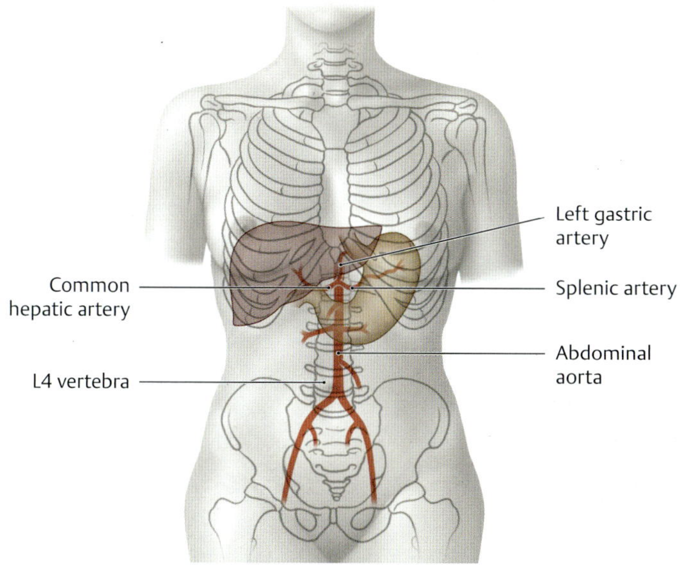

B Projection of the celiac trunk onto the vertebral column (T 12) and its relationship to the liver and stomach

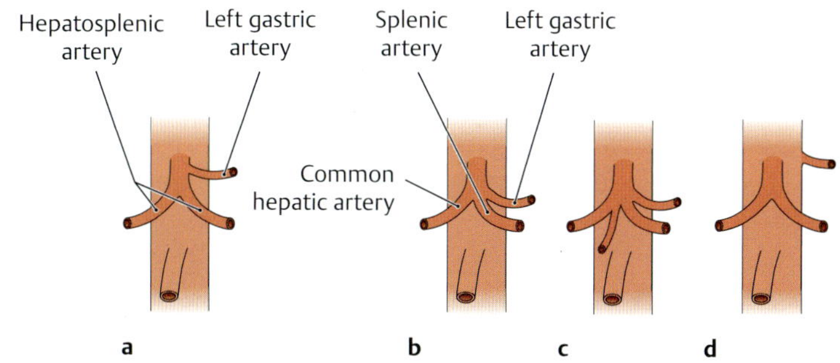

C Variants of the celiac trunk (after Lippert and Pabst)

a The celiac trunk divides into the left gastric artery and hepatosplenic artery (approximately 50% of cases).

b The common hepatic artery, left gastric artery, and splenic artery have a common origin (approximately 25% of cases).

c The celiac trunk gives off a fourth branch to the pancreas (approximately 10% of cases).

d The left gastric artery branches directly from the abdominal aorta (approximately 5% of cases). All other variants have an incidence of less than 5%.

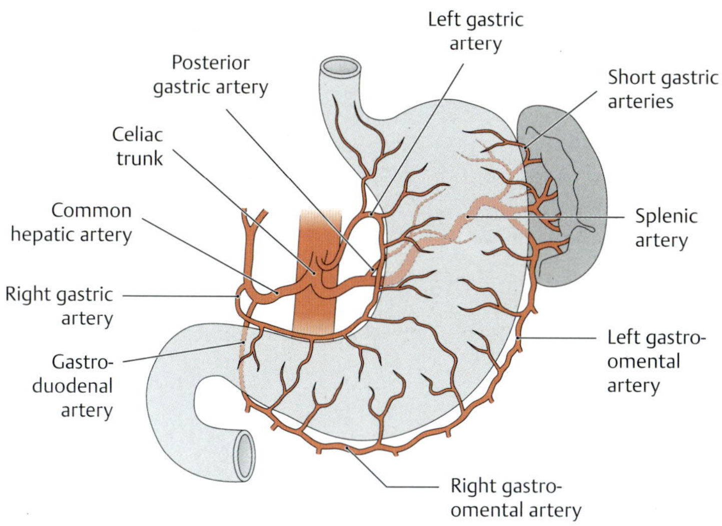

D Arteries of the stomach

Note that the *posterior wall* of the stomach is supplied by the posterior gastric artery, which arises from the splenic artery in 60% of cases. Variants of the gastric arteries do occur, but for simplicity they are not illustrated here.

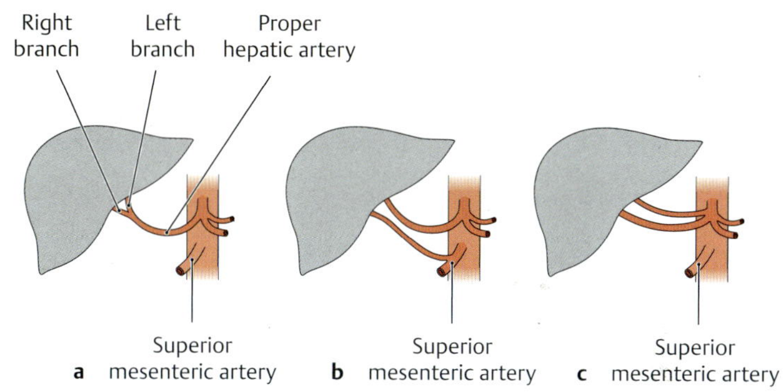

E Variants in the arterial supply to the liver (after Lippert and Pabst)

a The celiac trunk divides into the left gastric artery and hepatosplenic artery (approximately 50% of cases).

b The common hepatic artery, left gastric artery, and splenic artery have a common origin (approximately 25% of cases).

c Both branches arise separately from the celiac trunk (less than 5%).

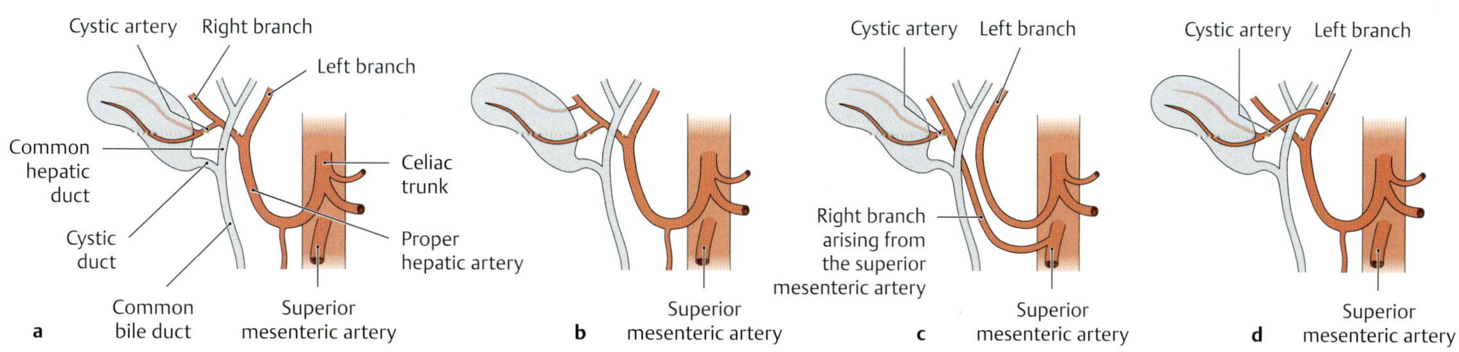

F Common variants of the cystic artery (after Lippert and Pabst)

a Cystic artery divides and passes to the anterior and posterior aspect of the gallbladder (46% of cases).

b Two cystic arteries supply the gallbladder (13% of cases).

c Cystic artery arising from the right branch of the superior mesenteric artery (12% of cases).

d Cystic artery arising from the left branch of the proper hepatic artery (5% of cases).

3.21 Branches of the Celiac Trunk: Arteries Supplying the Pancreas, Duodenum, and Spleen

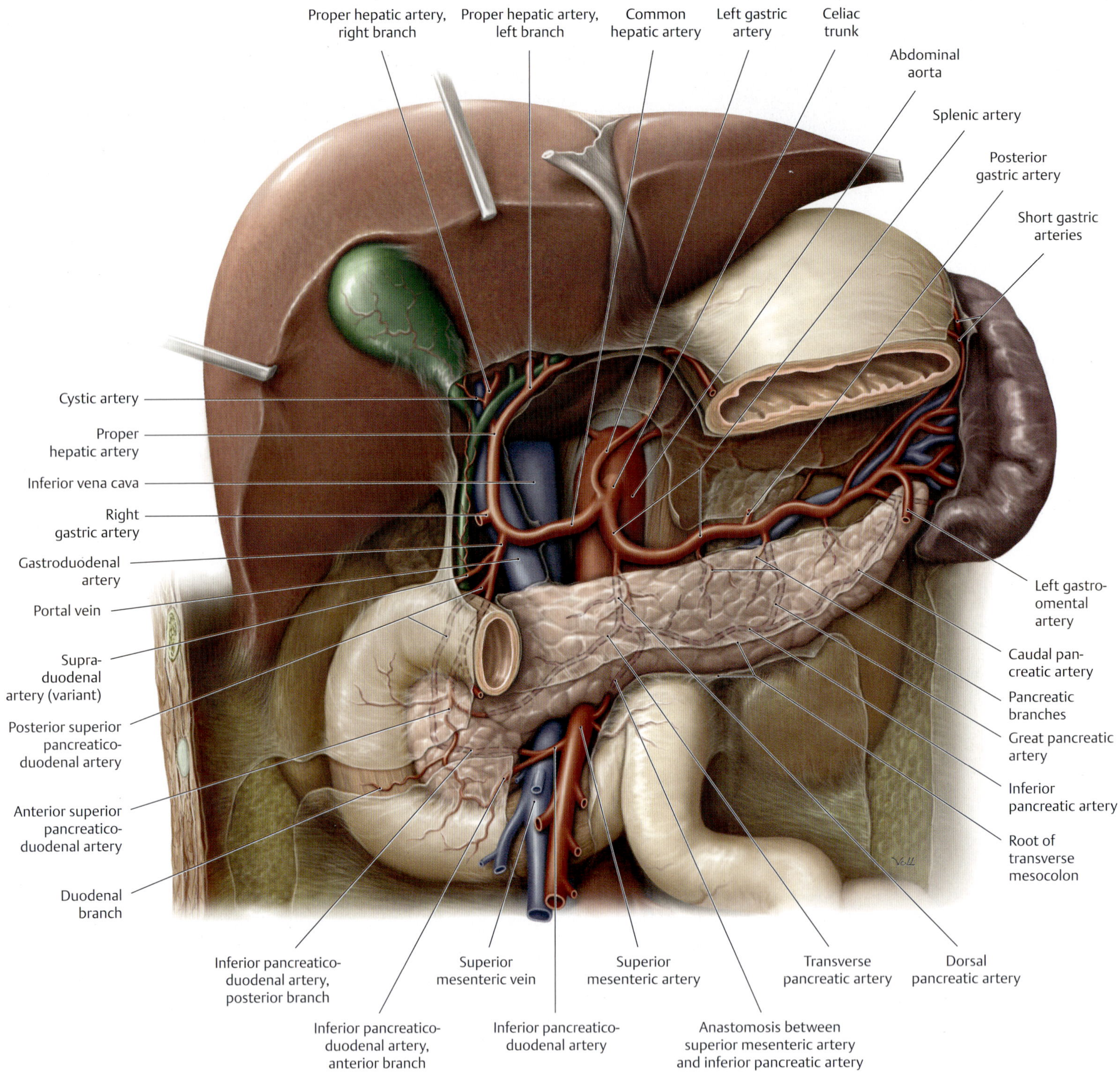

A Celiac trunk and arteries to the pancreas, duodenum, and spleen

Anterior view with the body of the stomach, pylorus, lesser omentum, and colon removed. For better exposure of the vascular structures, the parietal peritoneum has been partially removed.

The left gastric artery passes to the left and runs superiorly to the lesser curvature of the stomach. The proper hepatic artery in the hepatoduodenal ligament passes to the right and runs to the liver. Before reaching the spleen, the splenic artery gives off branches to supply blood to the pancreas (close to the spleen) and to the stomach via the left gastro-omental artery. The superior mesenteric artery (and vein) runs in an inferior direction and in close proximity to the head of the pancreas (while giving off branches to supply blood to the pancreas, see **C**). Pancreatic tumors may compress the artery and vein and restrict their blood flow. The celiac trunk is the uppermost of the three arteries that supply the organs of the digestive system (plus the spleen).

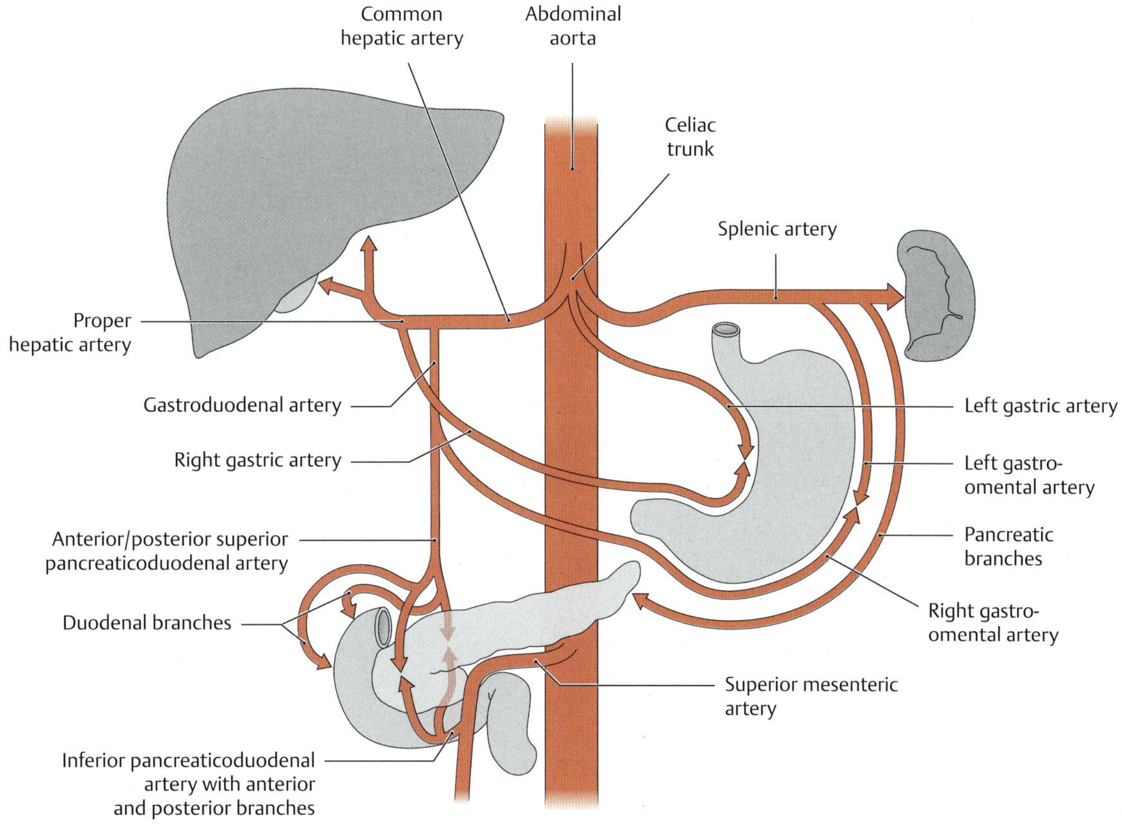

B Schematic overview of the distribution of the celiac trunk
Note: The pancreas is additionally supplied by branches from the superior mesenteric artery.

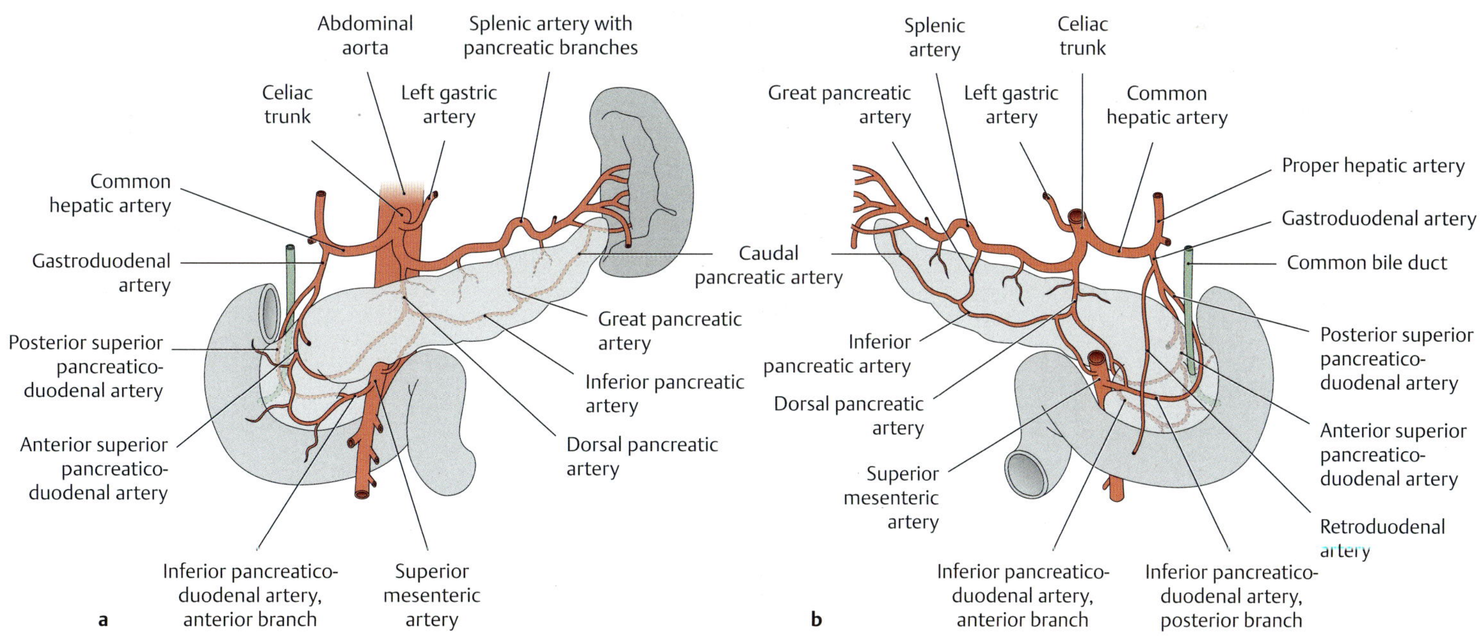

C Arterial supply to the pancreas
a Anterior view; **b** Posterior view. In **b**, the abdominal aorta has been removed to show the origins of the celiac trunk and superior mesenteric artery.
Note that the pancreas is supplied by branches from the celiac trunk as well as branches from the superior mesenteric artery. The superior and inferior arteries that supply the pancreas are arranged in an anastomosing system called the "pancreatic arcade." The largest of the anastomoses between the splenic artery and inferior pancreatic artery is called the great pancreatic artery.

3.22 Branches of the Superior Mesenteric Artery: Arteries Supplying the Pancreas, Small Intestine, and Large Intestine

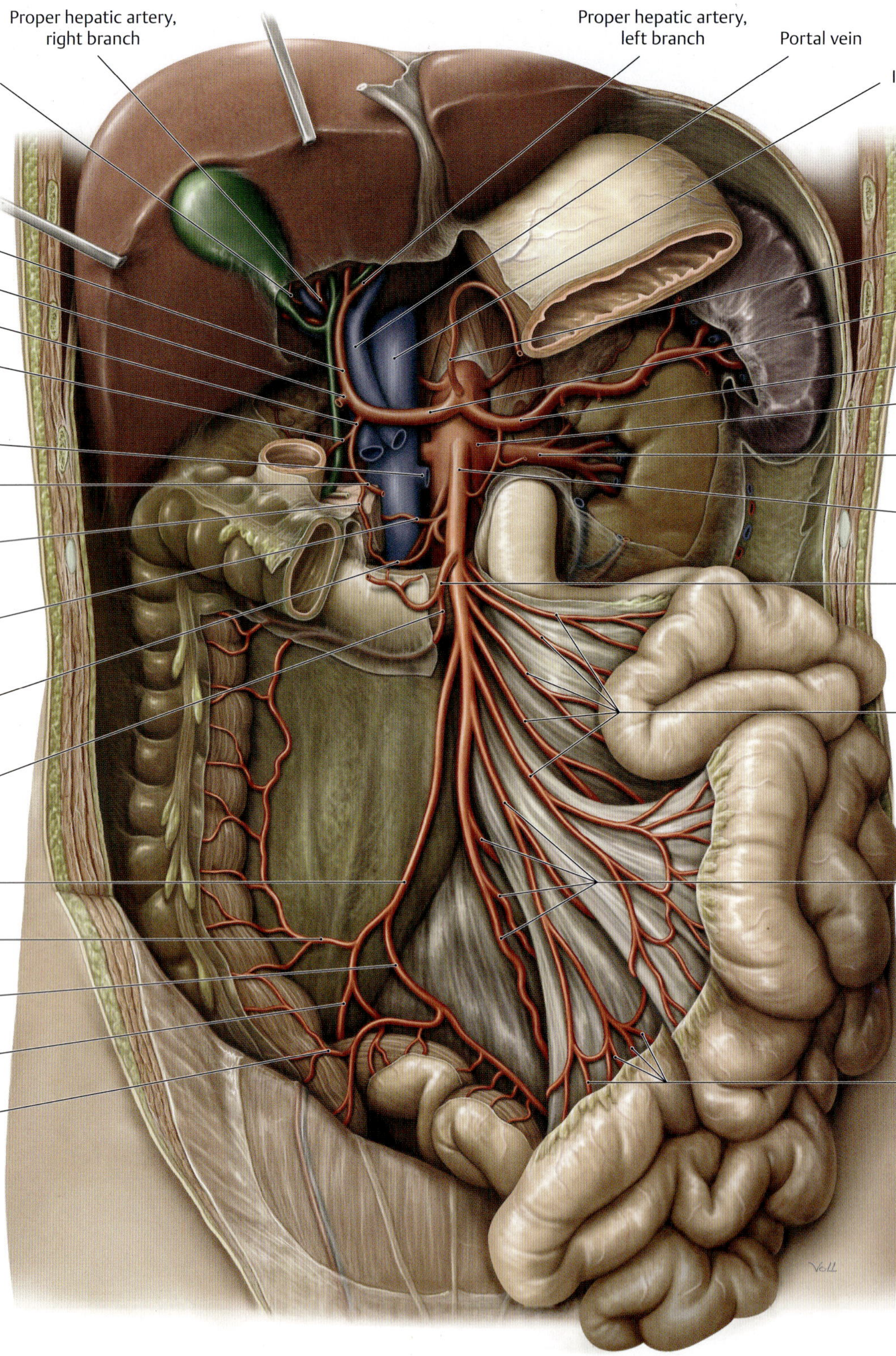

A Distribution of the superior mesenteric artery

Anterior view. For clarity, the stomach and peritoneum have been partially removed or windowed, leaving intact most of the retroperitoneal connective tissue below the transverse colon.

The superior mesenteric artery arises from the front of the abdominal aorta at the level of the first lumbar (L 1) vertebra. It passes anteriorly and inferiorly, distributing most of its numerous branches to the right side. Thus, it is clearly accessible to inspection and dissection only when the loops of small intestine are reflected to the left side, as illustrated here. This view also displays the series of arcades formed by the intestinal branches of the superior mesenteric artery (only one set of arches is present along the jejunum, but the arches increase distally and form multiple sets along the ileum). Straight arteries (vasa recta) extend from the arcades to the associated bowel segments. The superior mesenteric artery and its numerous branches supply the small intestine, portions of the pancreas (see p. 285), and a considerable part of the large intestine (see **C**), almost as far as the left colic flexure (not visible here). The trunk of the superior mesenteric artery passes over the duodenum and left renal vein (see **D**).

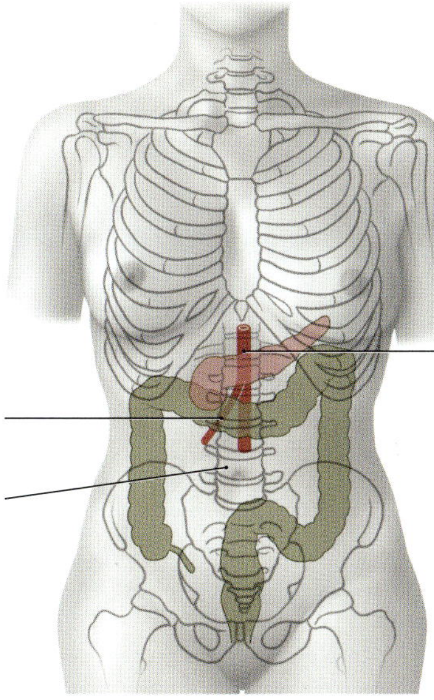

B Projection of the superior mesenteric artery onto the vertebral column and its relationship to the large intestine and pancreas

The superior mesenteric artery arises at the level of the first lumbar vertebra.

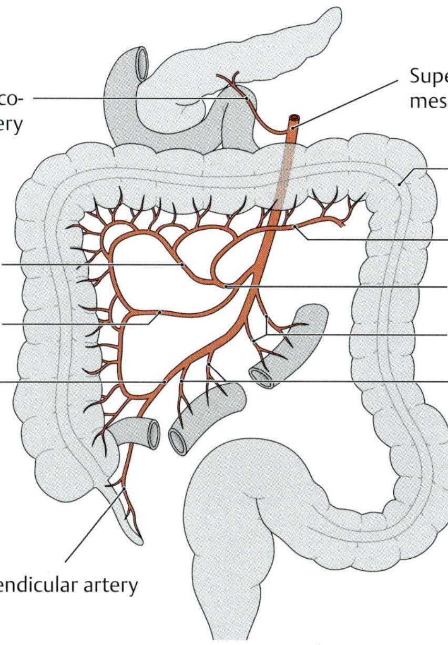

C Sequence of branches from the superior mesenteric artery (see also **E**)

Relationship of the superior mesenteric artery to specific organs. The territory of the *superior* mesenteric artery ends just proximal to the left colic flexure, at which point the supply by the *inferior* mesenteric artery begins (see p. 289). It is common for multiple anastomoses to exist between the two mesenteric systems (see p. 229).

Note: The diagram is highly schematic and does not incorporate the topographical relationships between the distinct structures.

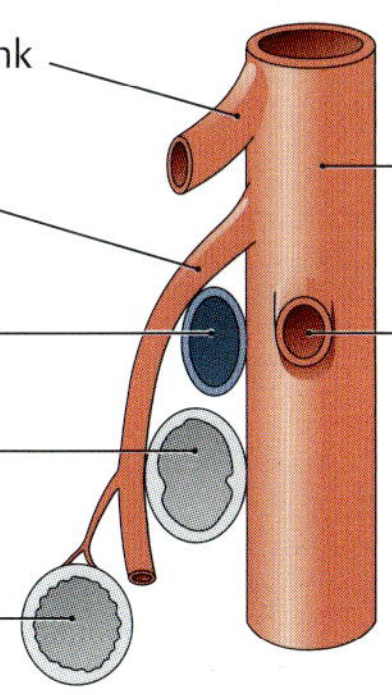

D Relationship of the superior mesenteric artery to the duodenum and left renal vein

Left lateral view.

Note: The superior mesenteric artery descends in front of the duodenum and left renal vein. The left renal vein lies within the aorticomesenteric angle, where it may become entrapped and compressed.

E Branches of the superior mesenteric artery, listed in the sequence of the organs they supply

- Inferior pancreaticoduodenal artery
- Jejunal and ileal arteries (approximately 14–20)
- Ileocolic artery with anterior and posterior cecal arteries and appendicular artery
- Right colic artery*
- Middle colic artery

The arteries to the small and large intestine form numerous arcades from which small straight arteries (vasa recta) pass through the mesentery to supply the various parts of the intestine.

* *Note:* The right colic artery varies in its origin. According to Lippert and Pabst (1985), as well as Kuzu et al. (2017), it arises directly from the superior mesenteric artery in only 40% of all cases. In 20% of all cases the right colic artery shares a common trunk with the middle colic artery, and in 15% of cases it arises directly from the ileocolic artery. In 25% of cases, the right colic artery is actually absent.

3.23 Branches of the Inferior Mesenteric Artery: Arteries Supplying the Large Intestine

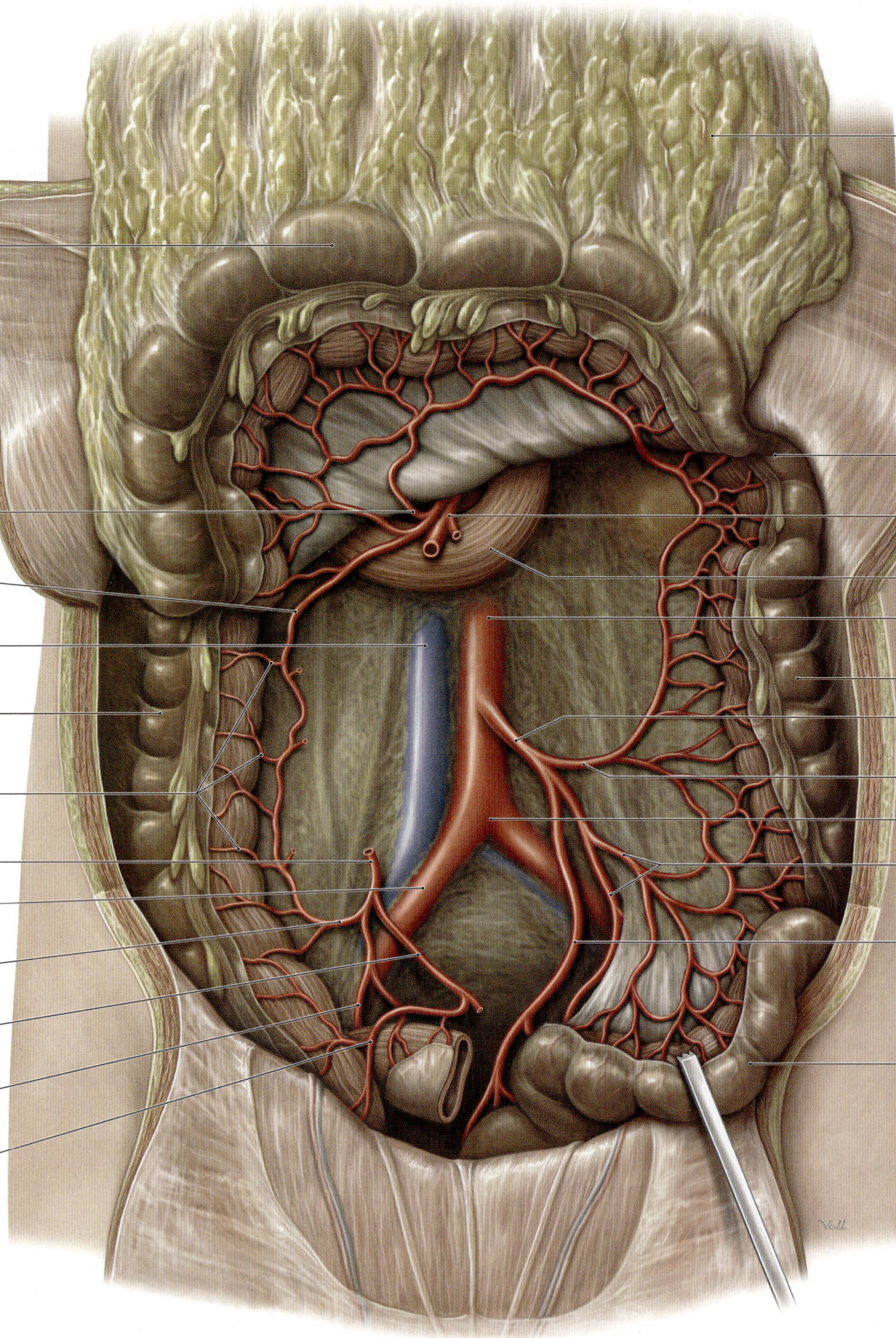

A Arterial supply to the large intestine from the superior and inferior mesenteric arteries

Anterior view. The jejunum and most of the ileum have been removed, and the transverse colon has been reflected superiorly. The peritoneum has been windowed or removed at several sites, leaving part of the retroperitoneal connective tissue in place. The inferior mesenteric artery arises from the abdominal aorta at the level of the L3 vertebra (see **B**) and descends toward the left side. Thus, it is clearly accessible to inspection and dissection only when the loops of small intestine are reflected to the right side (bowel loops have been removed here). This view also displays the numerous sets of arcades formed by the branches of the inferior mesenteric artery. This artery supplies the distal portions of the large intestine, starting approximately at the left colic flexure.

Note: The rectum is supplied by three arteries (see **D**), only one of which, the superior rectal artery, is visible in this dissection.

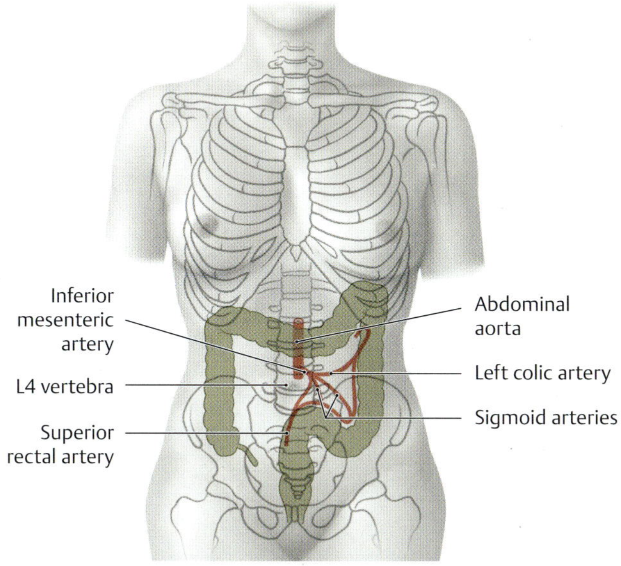

B Projection of the inferior mesenteric artery onto the vertebral column and its relationship to the large intestine

The inferior mesenteric artery branches from the abdominal aorta at the level of the L 3 vertebra.

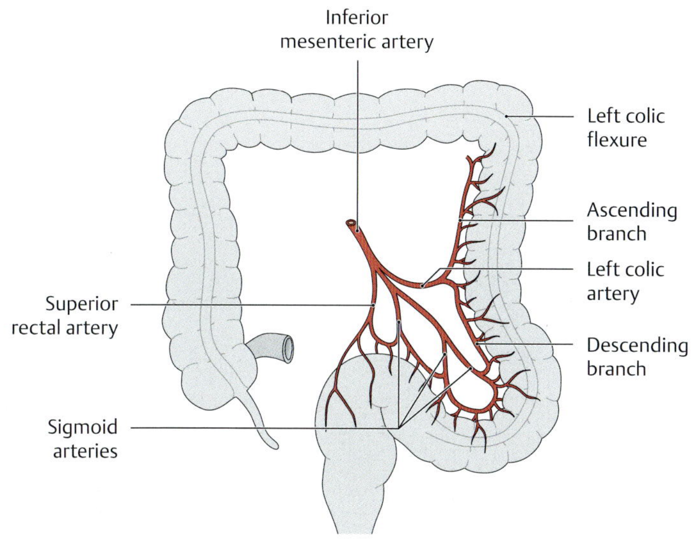

C Sequence of branches from the inferior mesenteric artery (see p. 229)

Left colic artery, sigmoid arteries (two or three), superior rectal artery. Note that the left colic flexure marks the approximate boundary between the blood supply by the superior and inferior mesenteric arteries.

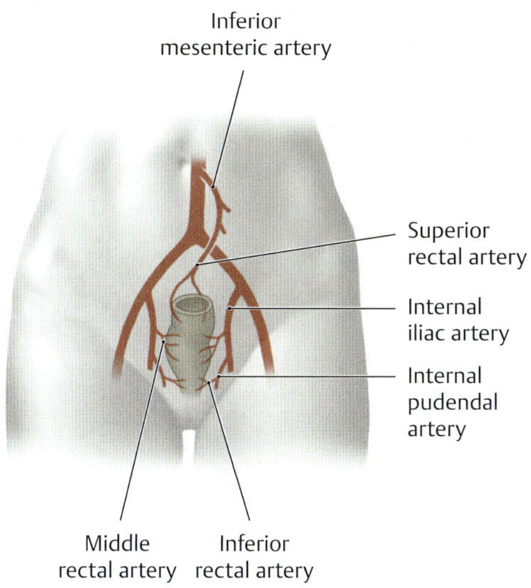

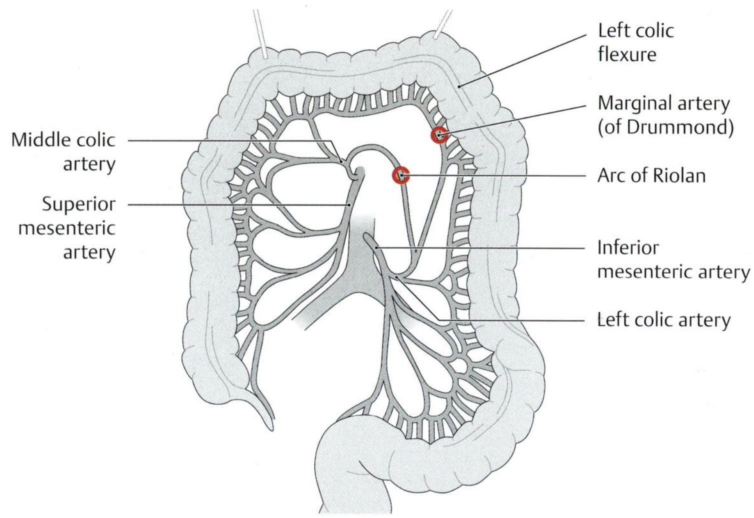

D Contribution of the inferior mesenteric artery to the rectal blood supply

The rectum is supplied by three different arteries or branches (see p. 291):

- The inferior mesenteric artery (or its branch, the superior rectal artery)
- The middle rectal artery (directly)
- The internal pudendal artery (or its branch, the inferior rectal artery)

The inferior mesenteric artery supplies most of the rectum from above, while the other two arteries supply the smaller, lower portions of the rectum.

E Shortcircuits between arteries of the large intestine

Shortcircuits between arteries of the large intestine have two consequences: Abnormally low blood flow in one artery can be compensated for via a shortcircuit with blood from an adjacent artery. The portion of the colon with the initially low flow can still be sufficiently supplied. When performing a resection of a portion of the colon, the supplying vessel is tied off and the shortcircuit disconnected to prevent blood loss via a neighboring vessel. Because of their size, two shortcircuits are described below:

- Riolan's arcade: a direct connection between the middle colic artery and the left colic artery (usually close to the trunk where the middle and left colic arteries arise from the superior and inferior mesenteric arteries, respectively);
- Marginal artery of Drummond: close to the margin of the intestinal tube, connects the arteries of the entire colon.

Such shortcircuits are referred to—often imprecisely—as anastomoses.

Due to the extensive anastomoses described above, occlusive arterial diseases are very rare in the region of the colon. Vascular obstruction leads to symptoms only if two of the three major vessels (celiac trunk, superior or inferior mesenteric arteries) are severely constricted. In that case, patients complain of upper abdominal pain approximately 15 minutes after eating. The pain is caused by ischemia resulting from vascular occlusion that follows an increase in oxygen demand by the colon after eating large meals. As a consequence, the patient eats only small portions (small meal syndrome) but more often. Because of the smaller portions, blood flow to the colon does not need to increase.

3.24 Branches of the Inferior Mesenteric Artery: Supply to the Rectum

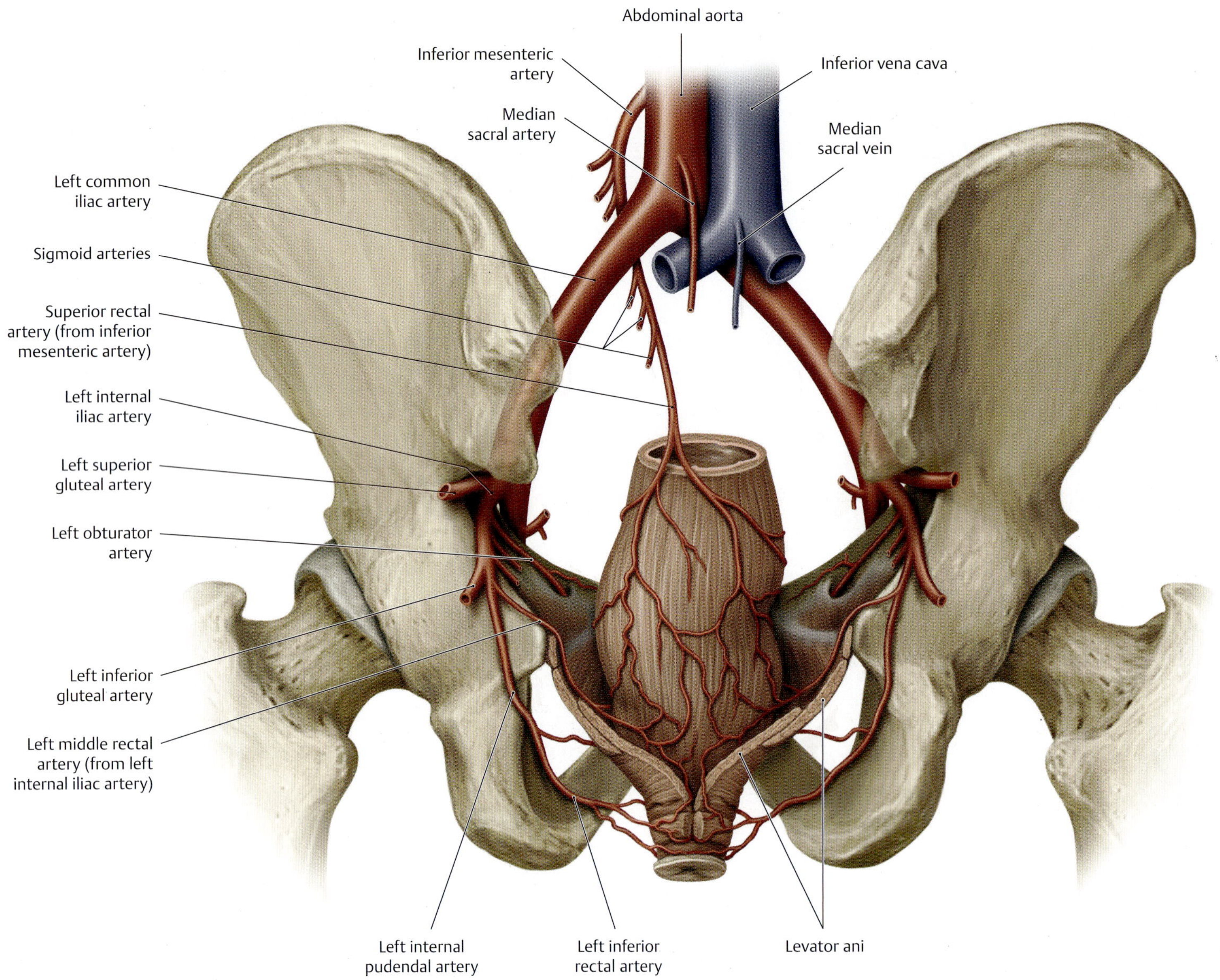

A Arterial supply of the rectum

Posterior view. For clarity, portions of the ilium are shown translucent. *Note:* The unpaired *superior* rectal artery (from the unpaired inferior mesenteric artery) divides into two branches on reaching the rectum. The right, sturdier branch further divides into two equally strong arterial branches. From these two or three major branches originate multiple collaterals that form anastomotic networks. The *middle* rectal arteries (from the internal iliac arteries) and the inferior rectal arteries (from the internal pudendal arteries) are paired owing to their origin from paired parent vessels. In females, it is not unusual for the middle rectal artery to arise from the uterine artery. The *inferior* rectal artery leaves the internal pudendal artery in the pudendal canal (*Alcock's canal*). The superior rectal artery approaches the rectum from above and posteriorly, also coming in contact with the peritoneal covering of the rectum (for clarity, not shown here). The course of this artery is also described as "peritoneal." It runs in the mesorectum where it further divides before it descends in the cavernous body of the rectum. The middle and inferior rectal arteries approach the rectum from the sides, the levator ani forming a well-defined partition between them: The middle rectal arteries pass to the rectum above that muscle, the inferior rectal arteries below it. Because the levator ani forms an essential part of the "pelvic diaphragm" (see p. 415), the course of the middle and inferior rectal arteries is also described as *supradiaphragmatic* and *infradiaphragmatic*, respectively. The rectal arteries frequently accompany the rectal veins for a considerable distance.

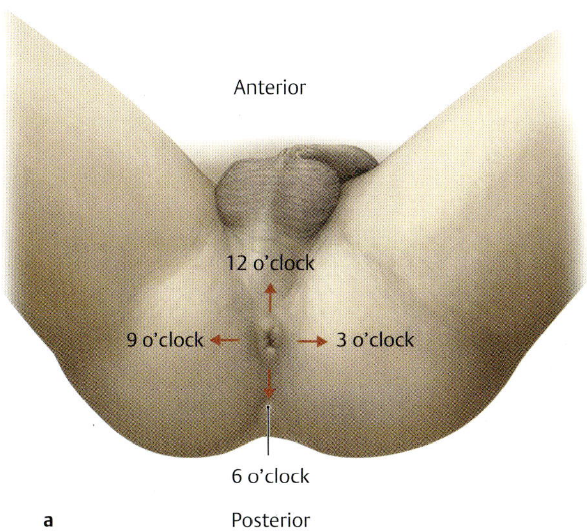

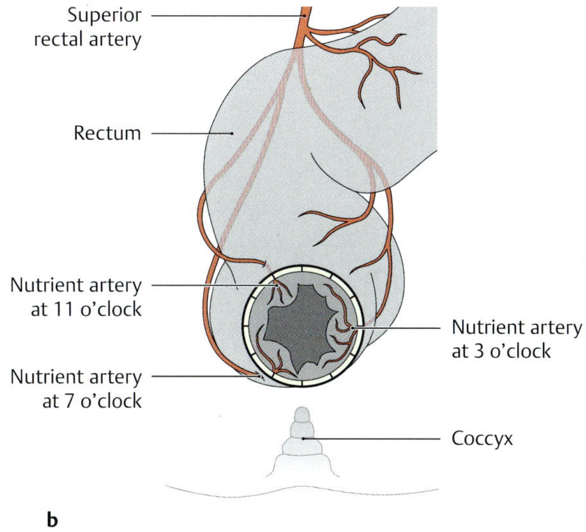

B Arterial supply of the cavernous body of the rectum (hemorrhoidal plexus)

a Caudal view with the patient supine in the lithotomy position and the examiner having a view of the perineum, clock face orientation is used. The hemorrhoidal plexus is a permanently distended cavernous body (see p. 259), which is supplied by three main branches (**b**) at the typical positions (3, 7, and 11 o'clock) where they form three major cushions (**c**) in the area of the anal columns. The three major vessels divide into four branches and form minor cushions (**d**) at the 1, 5, 6, and 9 o'clock positions. Together, these circular cavernous structures filled with blood serve as a very effective continence mechanism that ensures liquid- and gas-tight closure. The sustained contraction of the muscular sphincter apparatus inhibits venous drainage, and blood is allowed to drain from the cavernous body when the sphincters relax during defecation.

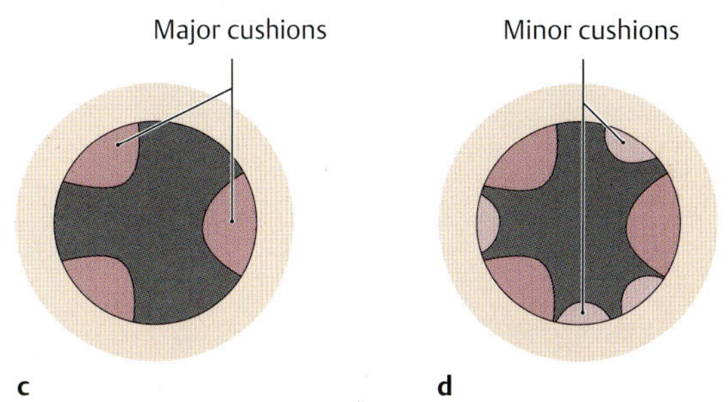

Note: Abnormal dilation (hyperplasia) of the hemorrhoidal plexus beyond the physiological range leads to hemorrhoidal disease, one of the most common proctological disorders (see p. 262f).

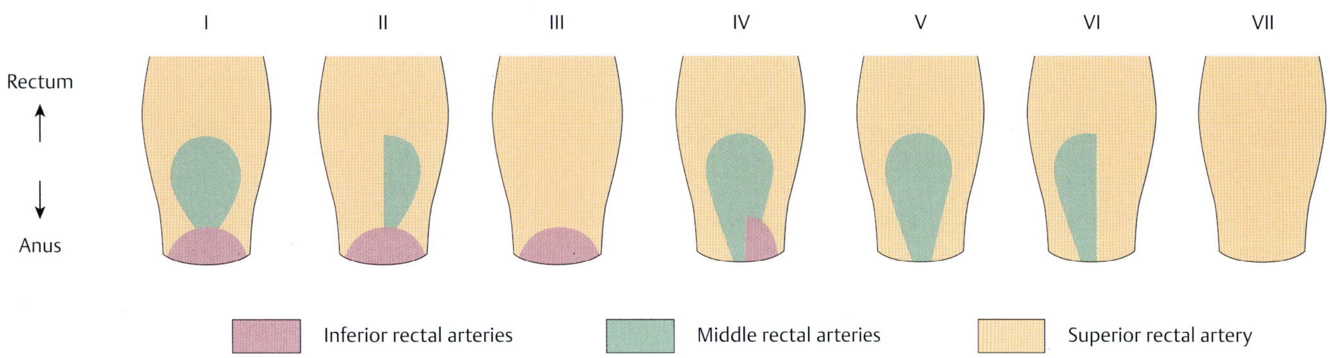

C Areas supplied by the rectal arteries

Schematic representation of the distinct types of arterial supply in the sagittally cut rectum. Rendered from radiographs obtained after the injection of radiographic contrast agent into the supplying arteries. View of the anterior wall of the splayed out colon.

There are 7 distinct patterns of arterial supply to the rectum (I–VII). The most common pattern is I (36% of cases). The upper three-quarters are supplied almost exclusively by the unpaired superior rectal artery, the lower one quarter is supplied by the smaller caliber middle rectal arteries (from the internal iliac arteries) and the inferior rectal arteries (from the internal pudendal arteries). All three arteries form extensive anastomoses.

Note: The common notion that the superior rectal artery supplies the upper-third of the rectum, the middle rectal arteries the middle-third, and the inferior rectal arteries the lower third, is thus incorrect.

3.25 Portal Vein: Venous Drainage of the Stomach, Duodenum, Pancreas, and Spleen

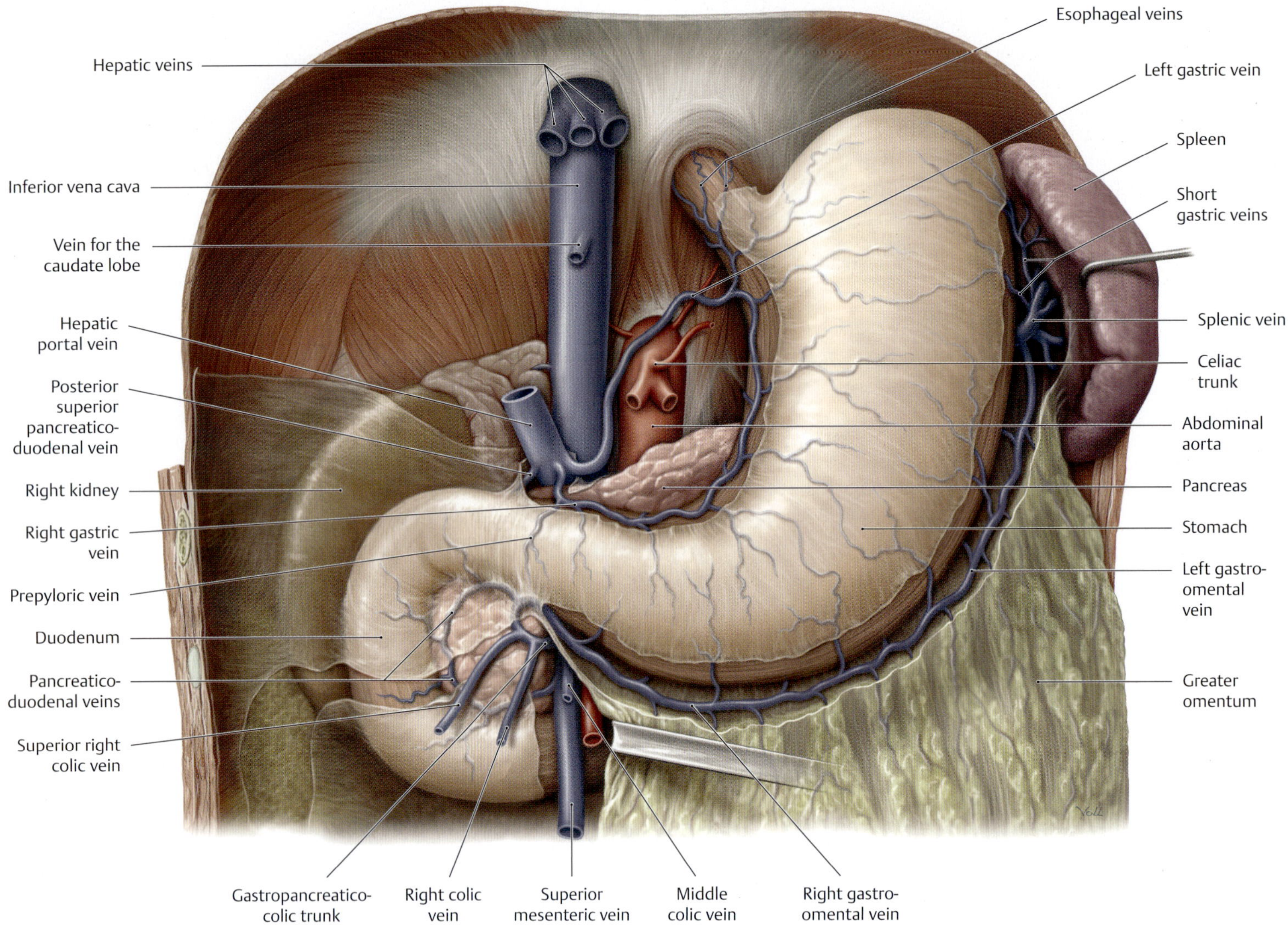

A Venous drainage of the stomach and duodenum

Anterior view. The liver and lesser omentum have been removed, and the greater omentum has been opened and retracted to the left. The stomach has been pulled slightly inferiorly, and the peritoneum has been removed or windowed at several sites to display the termination of the hepatic veins in the inferior vena cava and the communication of the gastric veins with the portal venous system.

Blood from the *lesser curvature of the stomach* generally flows directly into the portal vein, while blood from the *greater curvature* reaches the portal vein by way of the splenic vein and superior mesenteric vein. The lower portions of the duodenum drain chiefly to the superior mesenteric vein, while the upper portions usually drain directly to the portal vein. Variants are common, however.

Note how the esophageal veins drain into the portal vein by way of the left gastric veins. This is important in the portacaval collateral circulation (see **B** and p. 234).

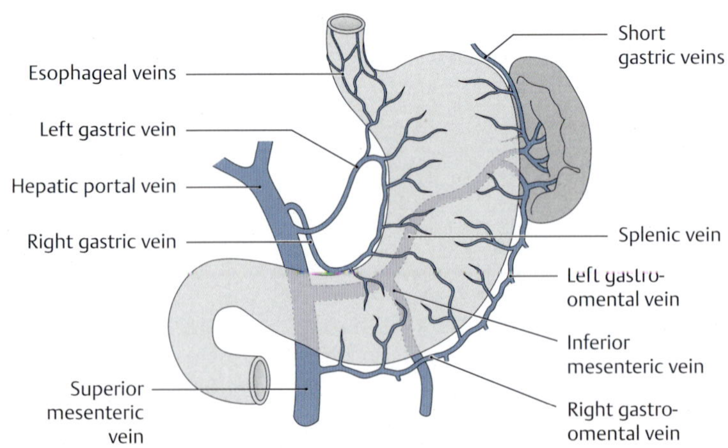

B Junction of the inferior mesenteric vein and splenic vein

Anterior view. This view, with the stomach translucent, demonstrates the site where the inferior mesenteric vein typically opens into the splenic vein behind the stomach.

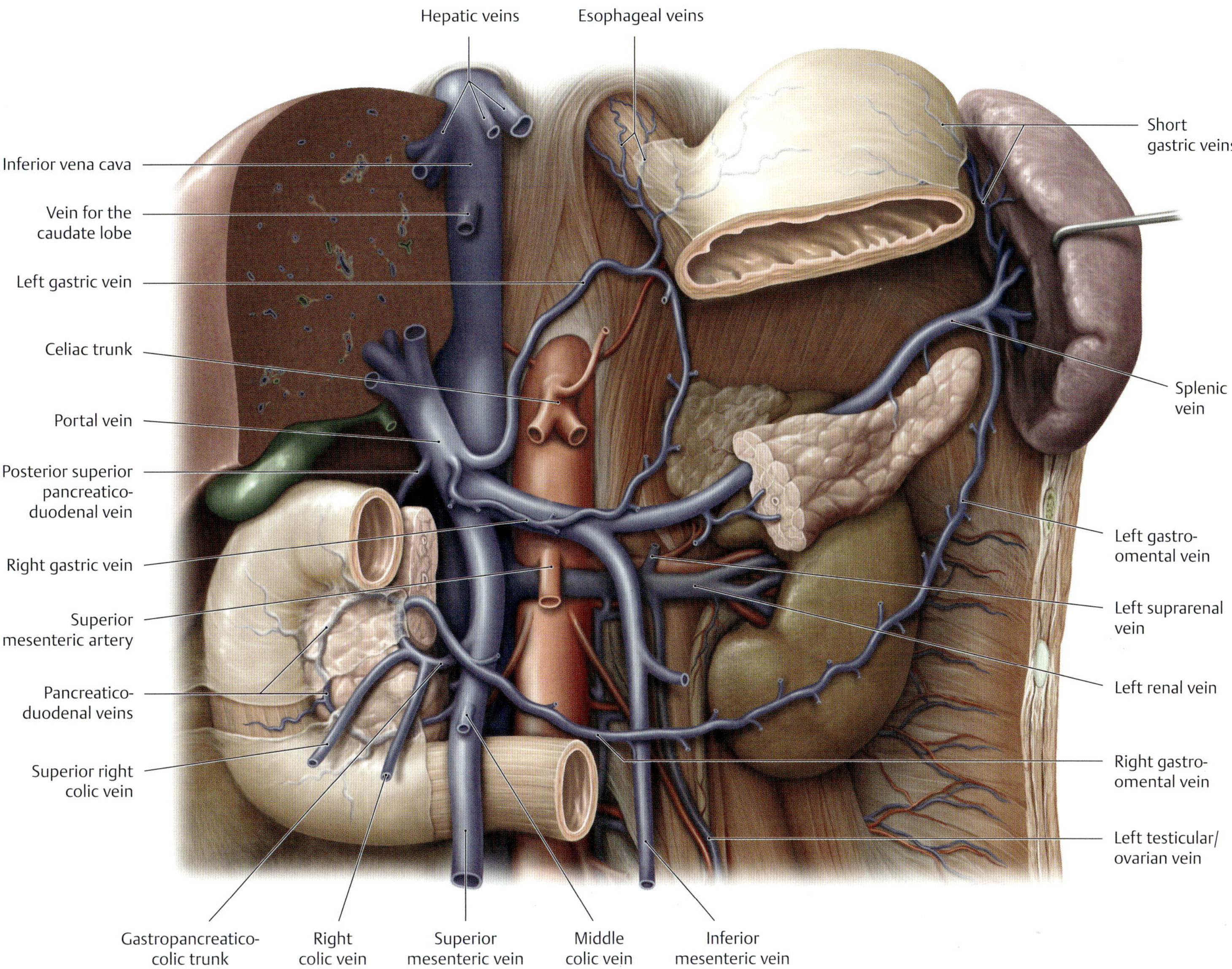

C Venous drainage of the pancreas and spleen
Anterior view. The stomach has been partially removed and pulled slightly inferiorly for better exposure, and most of the peritoneum has been removed. This dissection clearly shows how the portal vein is formed by the junction of the superior mesenteric vein and splenic vein near the liver. In 70% of cases the splenic vein receives the inferior mesenteric vein, as shown here, before uniting with the superior mesenteric vein (see also **B**).

Venous blood from the spleen is carried by the splenic vein *directly* to the portal vein, while blood from the *pancreas* takes various routes: Most of the pancreatic veins (mainly from the tail and body of the pancreas) open into the splenic vein. A few, along with the veins draining the stomach and ascending colon, open into the superior mesenteric vein via the gastropancreaticocolic trunk (see **D**).

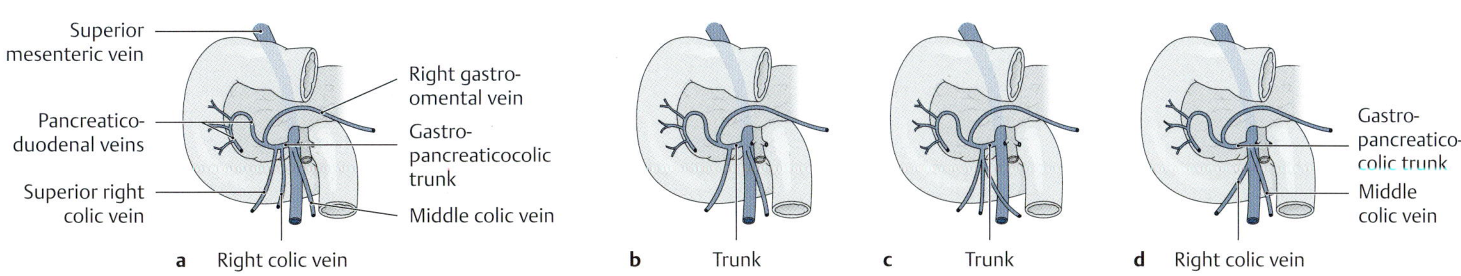

D Variants of the gastropancreaticocolic trunk (trunk of Henle)
a 45%; **b** 33%; **c** 11%; and **d** 11% of cases.
In 90% of cases, the venous gastropancreaticocolic trunk provides drainage of the ascending colon (right colic vein) and the right colic flexure (superior right colic vein) in addition to the stomach (right gastro-omental vein) and head of the pancreas/duodenum (pancreaticoduodenal veins). In 11% of cases, the gastropancreaticocolic trunk also receives the middle colic vein (**c**). The gastropancreaticocolic trunk drains into the superior mesenteric vein at the level of the uncinate process.
Note: The gastropancreaticocolic trunk is an important landmark for surgeons, particularly in operations on the head of the pancreas and the right colic flexure.

3.26 Superior and Inferior Mesenteric Veins: Venous Drainage of the Small and Large Intestine

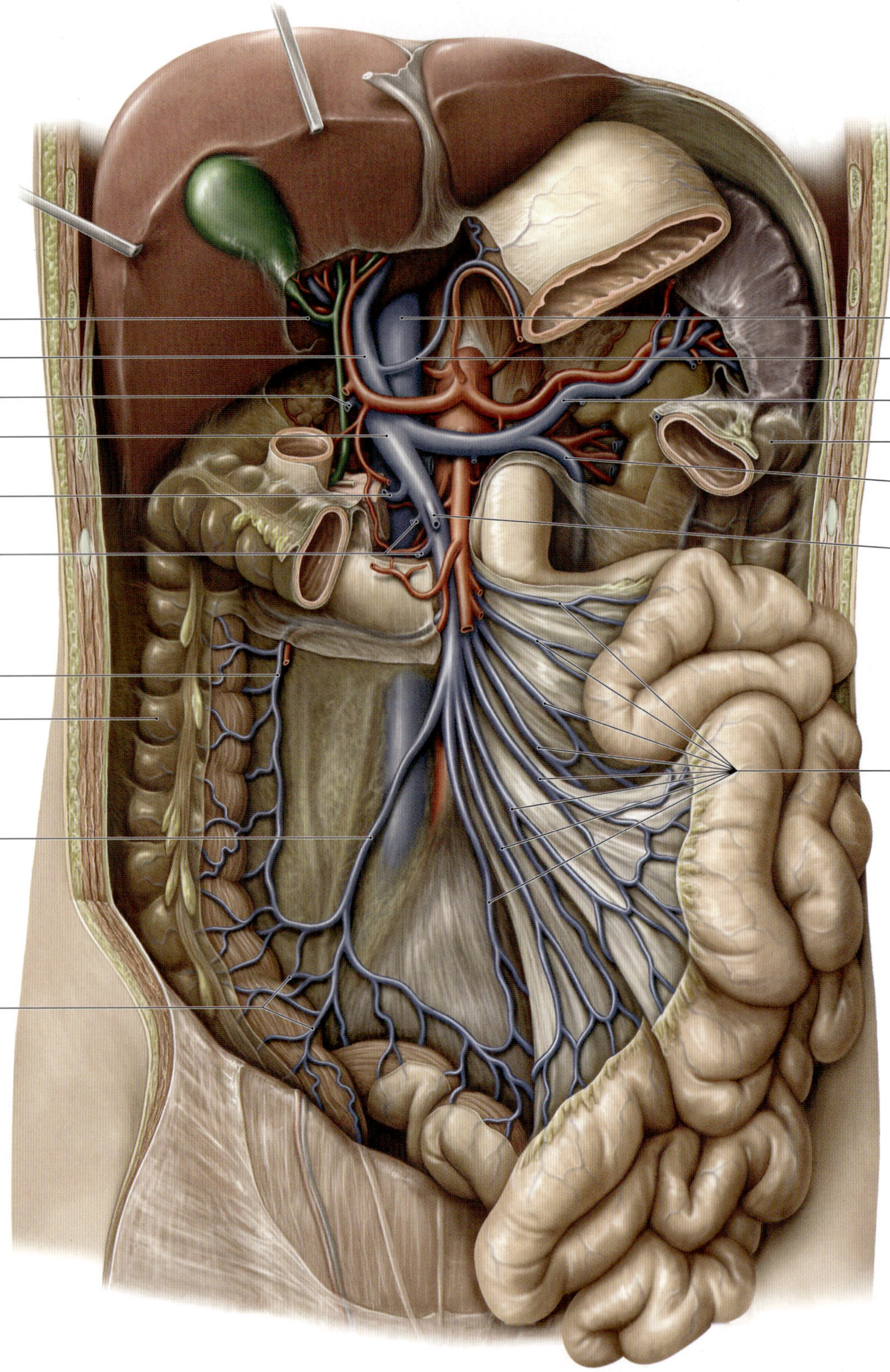

A Tributaries of the superior mesenteric vein

Anterior view. Most of the stomach has been removed, and the peritoneum has been removed or windowed at multiple sites, leaving some of the retroperitoneal connective tissue in place. The mesentery and transverse colon have been partially removed, and the loops of small intestine have been displaced to the left. The superior mesenteric vein unites with the splenic vein at the L 1 level to form the portal vein (see **B**, p. 292).

The small intestine drains exclusively into branches of the superior mesenteric vein. The superior mesenteric vein also collects blood from the cecum, appendix, ascending, and two-thirds of the transverse colon almost to the left colic flexure. From that point the colon is drained by the inferior mesenteric vein. As with the mesenteric arteries, multiple anastomoses are present between these two large veins. The superior mesenteric vein drains a much larger territory than the inferior mesenteric. Thus, the venous drainage of the small and large intestine follows the pattern of their arterial supply.

Note: The ascending colon, which is secondarily retroperitoneal, may also be drained by veins in the retroperitoneum (lumbar veins) that empty into the inferior vena cava. This is another example of a portacaval collateral pathway (see p. 234).

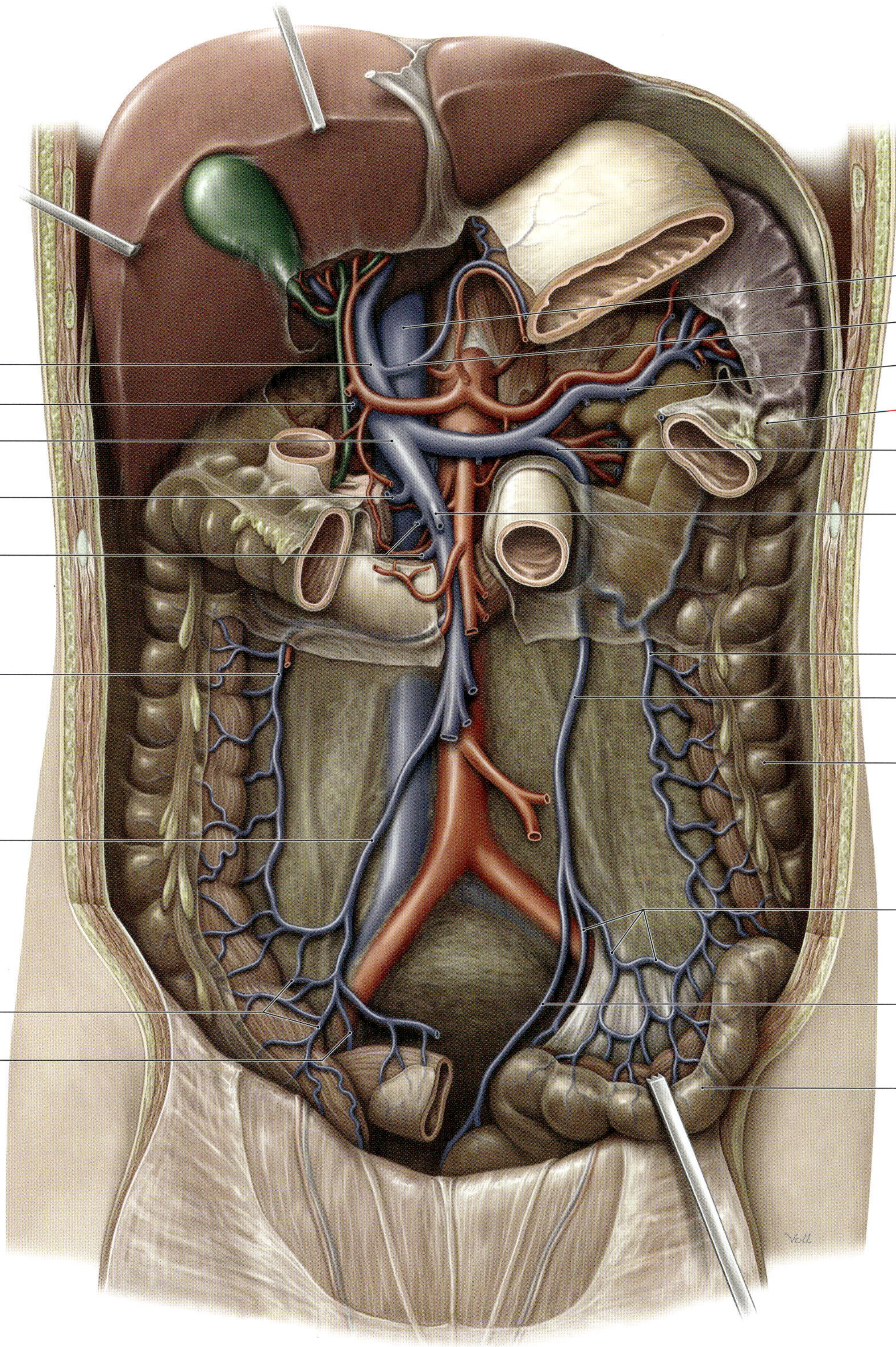

B Tributaries of the inferior mesenteric vein

Anterior view. Most of the stomach, pancreas, and small intestine have been removed. The peritoneum has been removed or windowed at several sites, leaving some of the retroperitoneal connective tissue in place.

The inferior mesenteric vein is formed by the union of the left colic vein, sigmoid veins, and superior rectal vein. Unlike the *superior* mesenteric vein, the *inferior* mesenteric vein runs separate from the artery and generally opens into the splenic vein behind the stomach and pancreas (see p. 293). Thus the inferior mesenteric vein returns blood *only from the large intestine*. The boundary between the territories of the superior and inferior mesenteric veins is usually located in the transverse colon near the left colic flexure, although multiple anastomoses exist between the two mesenteric veins.

The descending colon, which is secondarily retroperitoneal, may also be drained by veins in the retroperitoneum (lumbar veins), again establishing a portacaval collateral pathway.

Note: Blood from the *upper rectum* drains through the *superior* rectal vein to the inferior mesenteric vein before entering the *portal vein*. The *lower rectum* (not shown here) is drained by the middle and inferior rectal veins, which drain into the *inferior vena cava* by way of the iliac veins (see p. 296). A portacaval anastomosis may also be present in this region.

3.27 Branches of the Inferior Mesenteric Vein: Venous Drainage of the Rectum

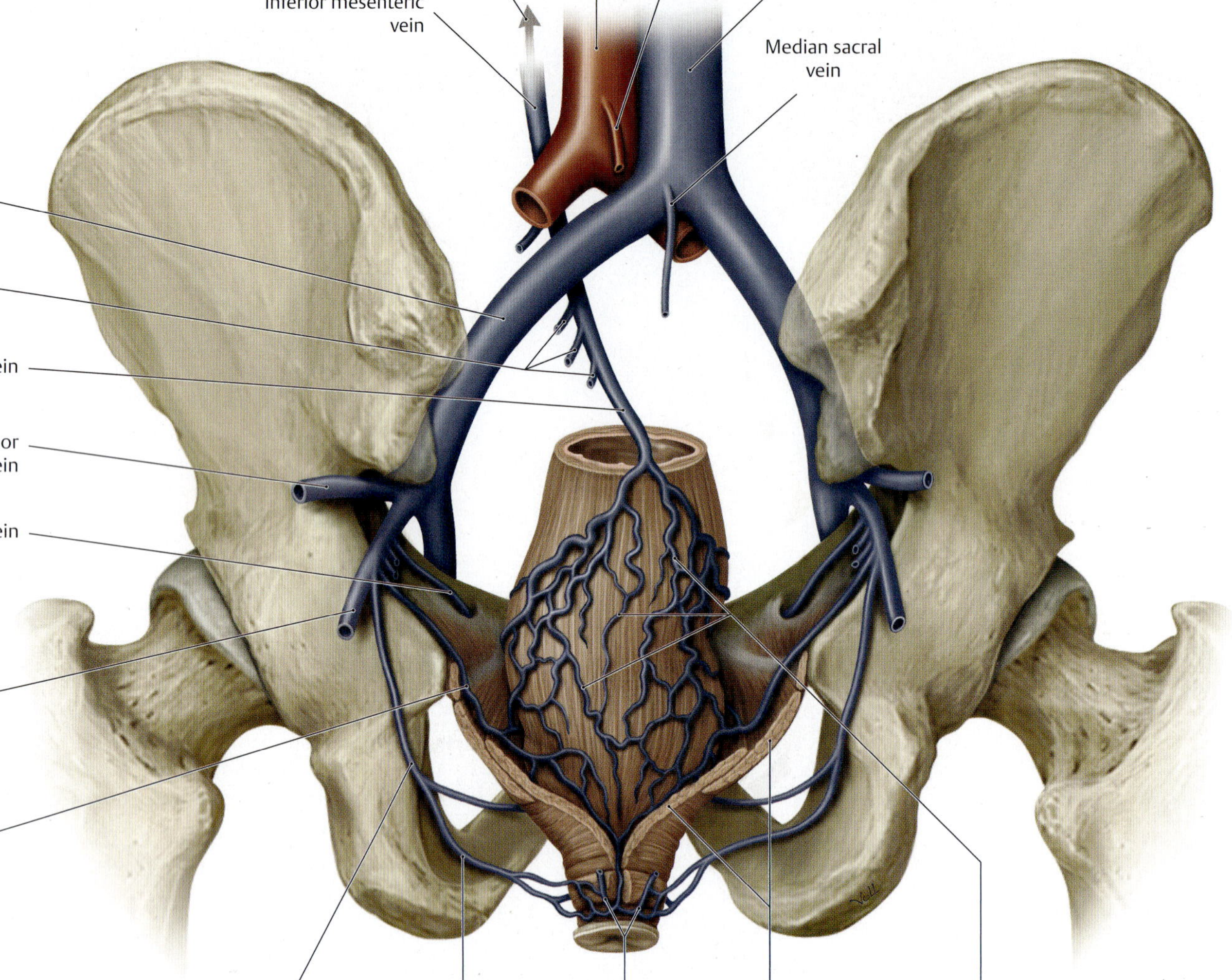

A Venous drainage of the rectum
Posterior view. Portions of the ilium are shown translucent for clarity.
Note: The unpaired *superior* rectal vein (to the unpaired inferior mesenteric vein) divides into two branches on reaching the rectum. By contrast, the *middle* rectal veins (to the internal iliac veins) and *inferior* rectal veins (to the internal pudendal veins) are paired owing to their termination in paired venous trunks.
Because the rectal veins accompany the corresponding arteries for some distance, their course is analogous to that previously described for the arteries: The superior rectal vein follows an abdominal route, while the middle and inferior rectal veins take supra- and infradiaphragmatic routes. The superior rectal vein drains to the hepatic portal system by way of the inferior mesenteric vein (see **B**).
Note: Tumors in the region drained by the *superior* rectal vein can metastasize through the portal venous system to the capillary bed of the liver (hepatic metastases), whereas tumors in the region drained by the *middle* and *inferior* rectal veins metastasize through the inferior vena cava to the capillary bed of the lung (pulmonary metastases). Note also the importance of these veins as portacaval collaterals (see **B**).

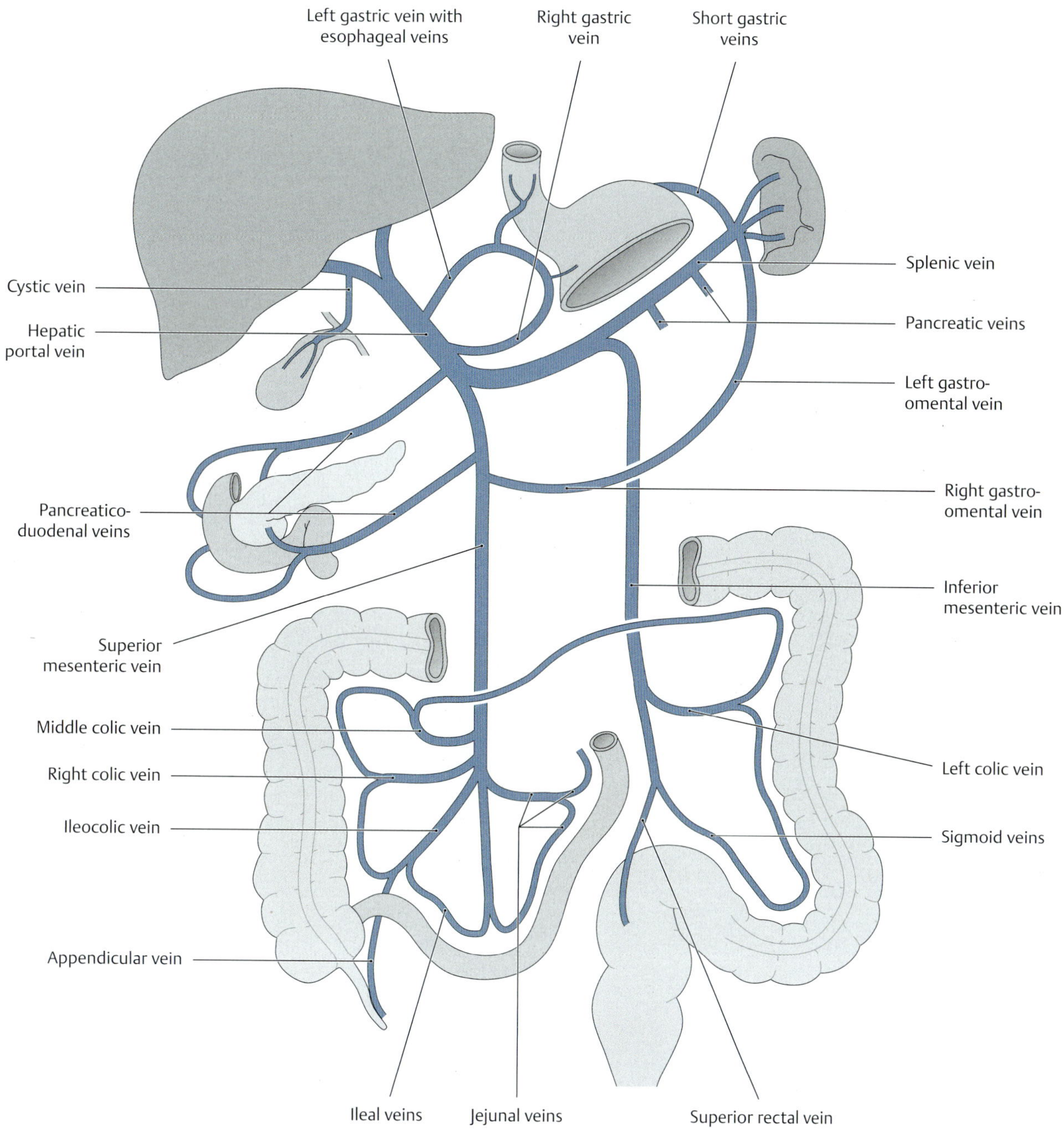

B Draining of the superior rectal vein into the portal vein (hepatic portal vein)

The rectum sends most of its venous drainage to the superior rectal vein, which drains into the portal hepatic vein. Particularly the upper two-thirds of the rectum are drained this way. However, venous blood of the lower third of the rectum is carried via the inferior and middle rectal veins to the internal iliac veins, which drain into the inferior vena cava. Along the perirectal veins (rectal venous plexus), numerous anastomoses exist between the two drainage areas (to the portal vein and to the inferior vena cava), which under certain circumstances (e.g., portal hypertension resulting from intrahepatic drainage disorders) may form a portacaval anastomosis.

Note: The rectal venous anatomy varies particularly in the lower third of the rectum, similar to the arterial anatomy. Blood from the rectal veins drains not only into the inferior vena cava but also into the portal vein and thus reaches the liver. This plays an important role in the rectal administration of drugs (e.g., in the form of suppositories). The idea is to bypass the liver and the first-pass-effect (intestinal drug absorption and presystemic elimination in the liver) to ensure systemic distribution of the drug throughout the entire body, which because of the variable venous anatomy of the rectum, is not guaranteed. Thus, there are varying degrees of absorption and systemic distribution of drugs that are administered rectally. Rectal delivery is particularly suited for children as an alternative to the often difficult to perform venipuncture.

3.28 Lymphatic Drainage of the Stomach, Spleen, Pancreas, Duodenum, and Liver

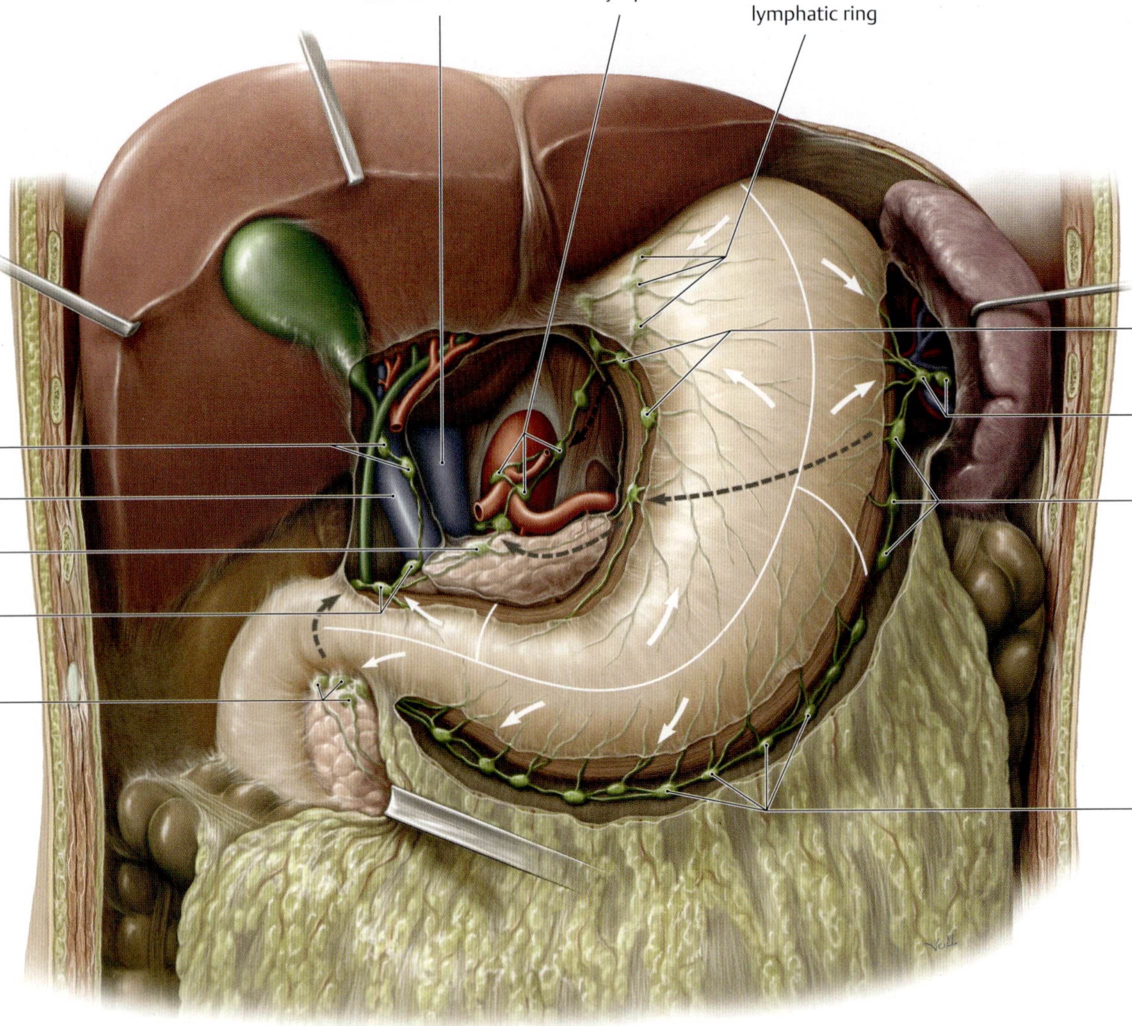

A Lymphatic drainage of the stomach
Anterior view. The lesser omentum has been removed, the greater omentum has been partially opened along the greater curvature of the stomach, and the liver has been retracted slightly superiorly. The following lymphatic pathways are important in this region:

- Drainage toward the **greater and lesser curvatures of the stomach**. Initial drainage is to the regional lymph nodes: the right and left gastric lymph nodes (toward the lesser curvature) or the right and left gastro-omental lymph nodes (toward the greater curvature, see white lines and arrows). These regional lymph nodes convey lymph either directly or indirectly to the celiac lymph nodes (indirectly by way of the pyloric and splenic nodes). From there the lymph drains to the intestinal trunk.
- Drainage from the **fundus and cardia**: initially to the inconstant (not always present) lymphatic ring of the gastric cardia, then to the intestinal trunk.

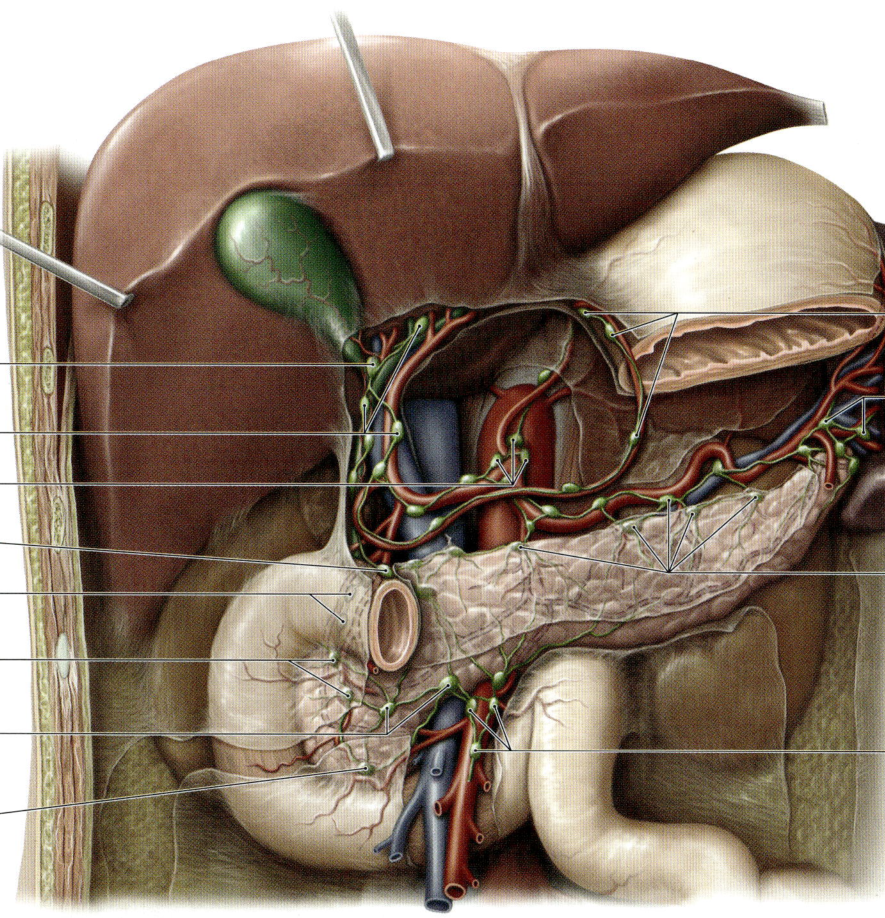

B Lymphatic drainage of the spleen, pancreas, and duodenum
Anterior view. Most of the stomach has been removed, the colon has been detached, and the liver has been retracted upward. The following lymph nodes and groups of nodes are important in this region:

- **Spleen:** drains initially to the *splenic lymph nodes*, then directly or indirectly to the *intestinal trunk* (the indirect route may be through the superior pancreatic lymph nodes alone or through the superior pancreatic nodes *and* the celiac nodes).
- **Pancreas:** drains initially to the *superior* and *inferior pancreatic lymph nodes*, then directly or indirectly (via the celiac nodes) to the intestinal trunk; *or* drains initially to the *superior and inferior pancreaticoduodenal lymph nodes* (mainly on the posterior side of the pancreas), then directly or indirectly via the superior mesenteric nodes to the intestinal trunk.
- **Duodenum:** The *upper portion* of the duodenum drains initially to the *pyloric lymph nodes* (see **C**), then to the superior pancreaticoduodenal lymph nodes and from there to the hepatic lymph nodes, or directly to the celiac nodes in some cases, before entering the intestinal trunk. The *lower portion* of the duodenum first drains to the *superior and inferior pancreaticoduodenal lymph nodes*, then directly to the intestinal trunk.

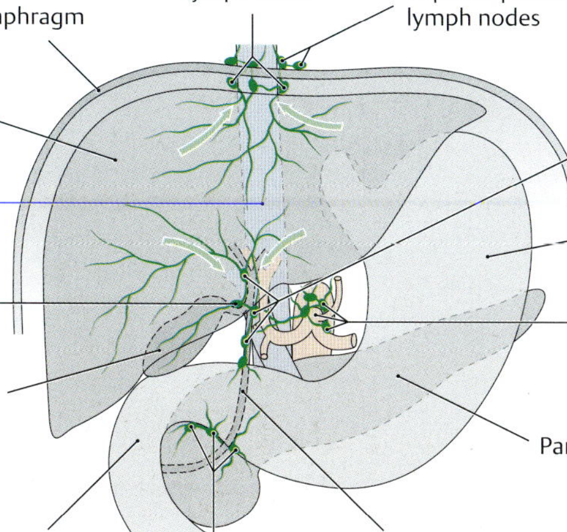

C Lymphatic pathways for the liver and biliary tract
Anterior view. The following lymphatic pathways are important in this region:
Liver and intrahepatic bile ducts (three drainage pathways):

- Most lymph drains inferiorly through the hepatic lymph nodes to the celiac lymph nodes and then to the intestinal trunk and cisterna chyli, or it may drain directly from the hepatic lymph nodes to the intestinal trunk and cisterna chyli.
- A small amount of lymph drains cranially through the inferior phrenic lymph nodes to the lumbar trunk.
- In some cases lymph drains through the diaphragm (partly through the caval opening and partly through muscular openings in the diaphragm) to the superior phrenic lymph nodes and then to the bronchomediastinal trunk.

Gallbladder: Lymph from the gallbladder drains initially to the cystic lymph node, then follows the pathway described above.
Common bile duct: Lymph from the bile duct drains through the pyloric lymph nodes (supra-, sub-, and retropyloric nodes) and the foraminal lymph node to the celiac nodes, then to the intestinal trunk.

3.29 Lymphatic Drainage of the Small and Large Intestine

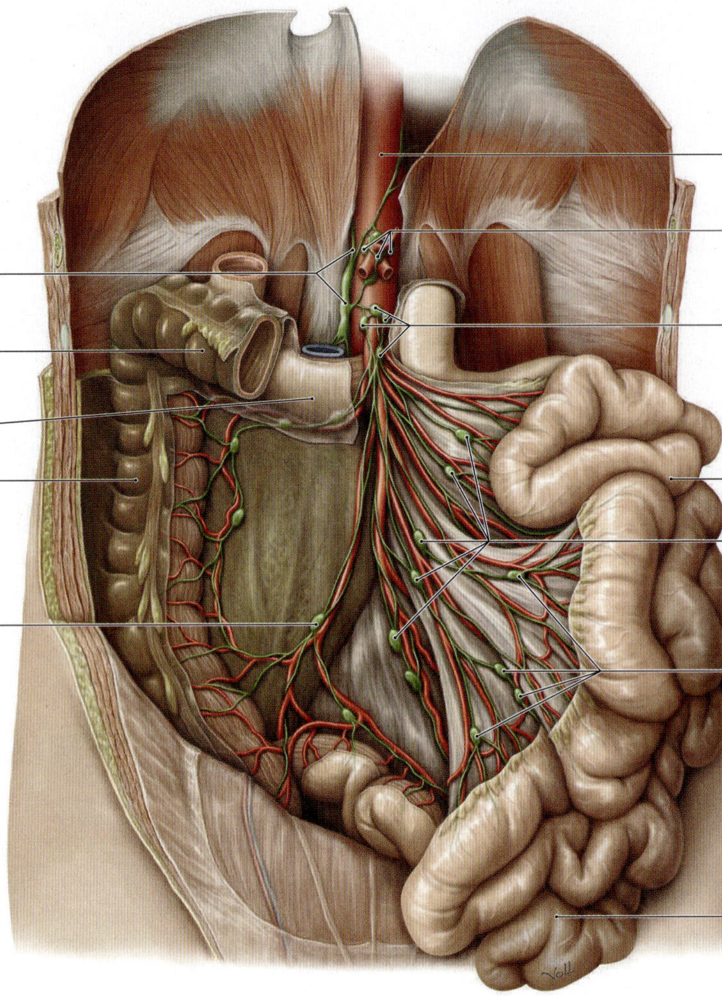

A Lymph nodes and lymphatic drainage of the jejunum and ileum
Anterior view. The stomach, liver, pancreas, and most of the colon have been removed. The lymph nodes of the small intestine are the largest group of lymph nodes in the human body, numbering approximately 100 to 150 nodes of greatly varying size. For clarity, the above drawing shows only a few lymph nodes that are representative of larger groups. Lymph from both the jejunum and ileum drains initially to regional lymph nodes (juxta-intestinal lymph nodes), then to the superior mesenteric lymph nodes, and finally to the intestinal trunk.
The lymph nodes and vessels in the *mesentery* basically follow the distribution of the arteries and veins. They are called "intermediate" because they are situated *between* visceral and collecting lymph nodes (the superior and inferior mesenteric lymph nodes). In patients with a malignant tumor, it is desirable to remove as many lymph nodes as possible along a drainage pathway to ensure the removal of any micrometastases that may be present in the nodes. In the case of the duodenum, this means that the resection should include not only the affected part of the duodenum but also the attached portion of the mesentery and the (intermediate) lymph nodes that it contains. Occasionally even the superior and inferior mesenteric lymph nodes are also removed.

B Lymphatic drainage of the intestine by segments
Lymph is collected in several plexuses (networks of lymphatic vessels and lymph collectors) in the intestinal wall and drained via lymphatic vessels in the mesentery (**a**). The lymphatic vessel in the mesentery drains the intestinal segment that is supplied by mesenteric arteries. Valves in the subserous collectors determine the direction of lymph flow and define the boundaries of the individual drainage segments in the intestinal wall toward the mesentery (**a**). The valves also prevent the lymph from spreading longitudinally along the intestine. This creates drainage segments along the intestinal wall and mesentery (**b**). Because of these segmental boundaries, it is rare for a tumor to spread extensively along the intestine by the lymphatic route.

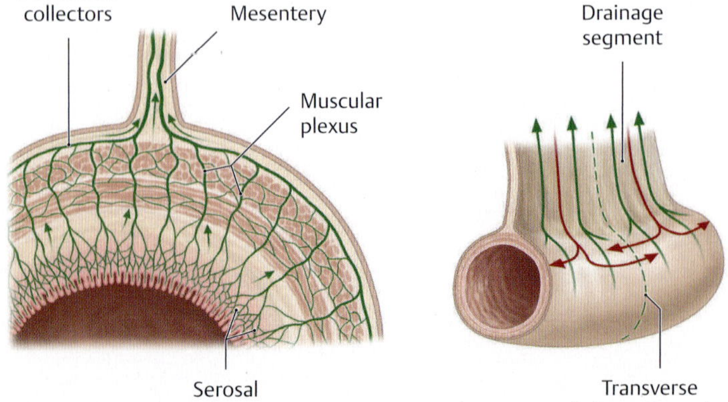

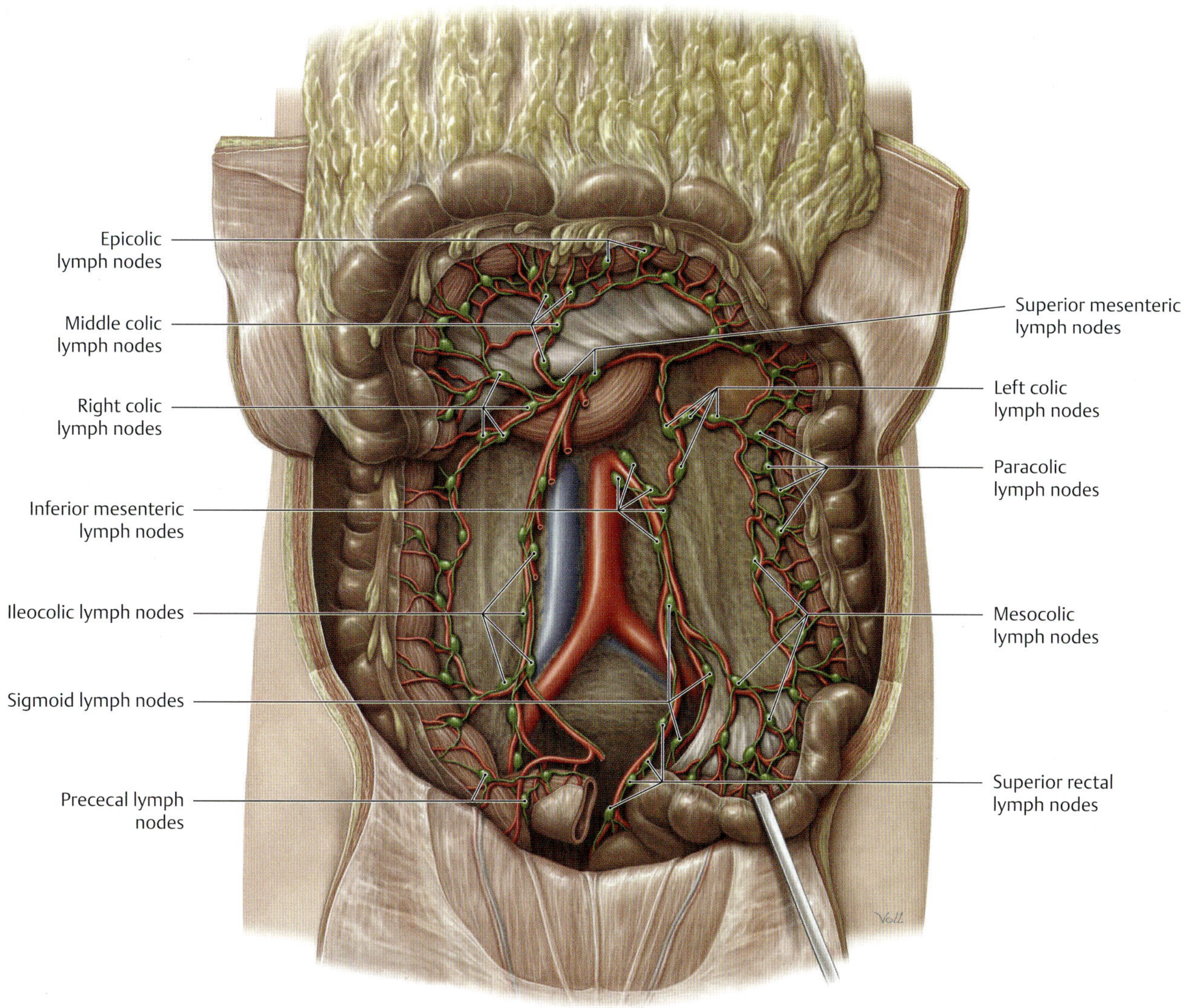

C Lymphatic drainage of the large intestine (modified from Földi and Kubik)

Anterior view. The transverse colon and greater omentum have been reflected superiorly. The following lymphatic pathways are important in this region:

- **Ascending colon, cecum, and transverse colon:** Lymph from these structures drains initially to the *right and middle colic lymph nodes*, then to the *superior mesenteric lymph nodes*, and finally to the *intestinal trunk*.
- **Descending colon:** Lymph from the descending colon drains initially to the regional lymph nodes, the *left colic lymph nodes*, then to the *inferior mesenteric lymph nodes*, and then drains into the intestinal trunk.
- **Sigmoid colon:** Lymph from the sigmoid colon drains initially to the sigmoid lymph nodes, then follows the pathway described for the descending colon (above).
- **Upper rectum** (see also **D**): Lymph from the upper rectum drains initially to the *superior rectal lymph nodes*, then follows the pathway described for the sigmoid colon (above).

Thus, a malignant tumor undergoing lymphogenous spread must negotiate several lymph node groups (all of which should be removed in tumor resections) before the malignant cells can reach the intestinal trunk and thoracic duct and finally enter the bloodstream. This long route of lymphogenous spread improves the prospects for a cure.

The lymph nodes of the large intestine can be classified *clinically* and *functionally* into more groups than by anatomical criteria alone: lymph nodes of the intestinal wall (epicolic group), lymph nodes near the intestine (paracolic group), lymph nodes at the origins of the three large intestinal arteries (central group), and lymph nodes at the origins of the mesenteric arteries (collecting lymph nodes). In standard anatomical nomenclature, the epicolic nodes are not distinguished as a seperate group, and the paracolic and central groups are considered collectively as mesocolic lymph nodes.

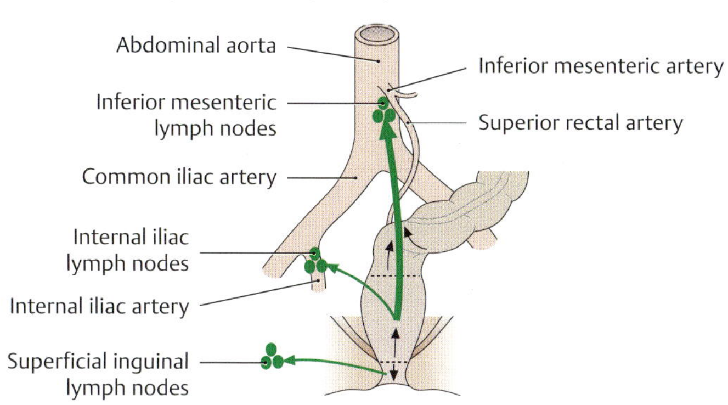

D Lymphatic drainage of the rectum

Anterior view. The rectum has three levels and three principal directions of lymphatic drainage (direct or indirect via the pararectal lymph nodes on the rectal wall):

- Upper level: through superior rectal lymph nodes (not shown here) to inferior mesenteric lymph nodes (→ intestinal trunk).
- Middle level: internal iliac lymph nodes (→ right and left lumbar trunks).
- Lower level:
  - Columnar zone: to internal iliac lymph nodes.
  - Cutaneous zone: through superficial inguinal lymph nodes to external iliac lymph nodes (→ lumbar trunks).

3.30 Autonomic Innervation of the Liver, Gallbladder, Stomach, Duodenum, Pancreas, and Spleen

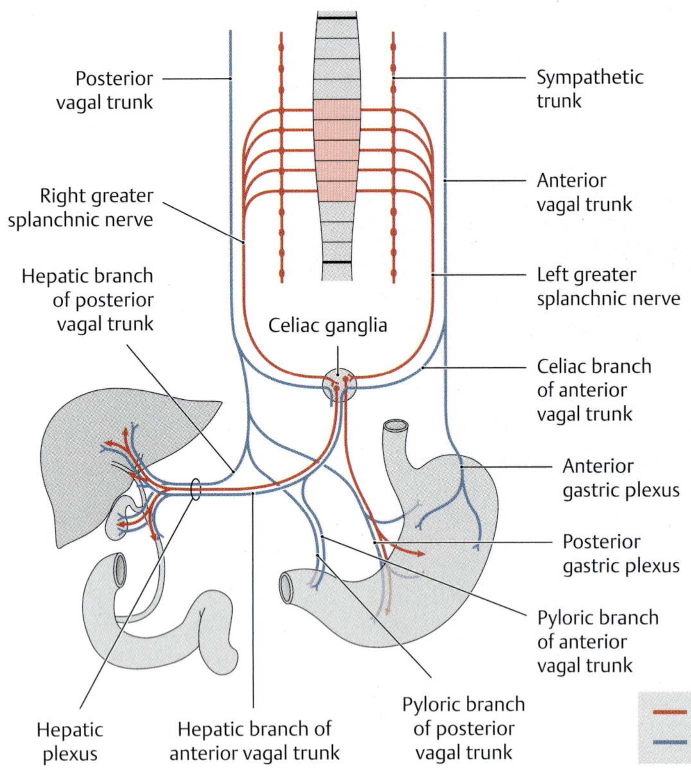

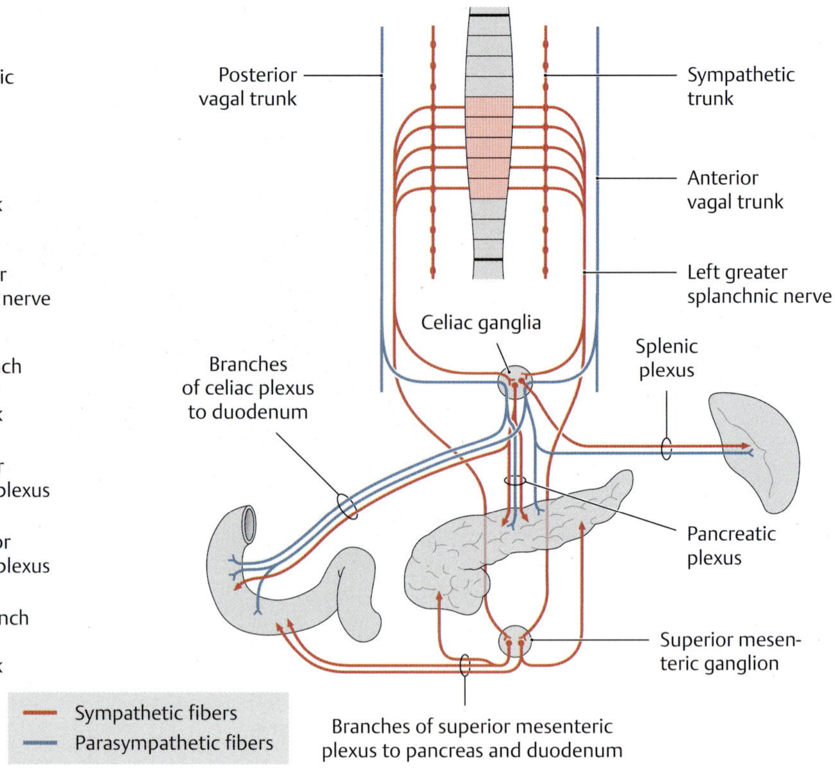

A Autonomic innervation of the liver, gallbladder, and stomach

These organs receive their **sympathetic supply** from the celiac ganglia. The *postsynaptic* fibers course with the branches of the celiac trunk, while the *presynaptic* fibers form the splanchnic nerves (mainly the greater splanchnic nerve) and synapse with the postsynaptic neuron in the ganglion. They receive their **parasympathetic supply** from the vagal trunks (presynaptic fibers). The *anterior* vagal trunk (preponderance of left vagus nerve fibers) terminates at the stomach, while the *posterior* vagal trunk goes on to supply large portions of the intestine. The anterior and posterior gastric plexuses are distributed to the anterior and posterior walls of the stomach. The synapse with the postsynaptic parasympathetic neuron occurs in small ganglia located directly on the stomach wall.

Sympathetic and parasympathetic fibers pass along the proper hepatic artery to the porta hepatis as the hepatic plexus. After dividing at the liver, this plexus also distributes fibers to the gallbladder and the intra- and extrahepatic bile ducts.

B Autonomic innervation of the pancreas, duodenum, and spleen

These organs receive their **sympathetic supply** from the celiac ganglia and superior mesenteric ganglion. The *postsynaptic* fibers pass along the branches of the celiac trunk and superior mesenteric artery. The *presynaptic* fibers form the greater and lesser splanchnic nerves. They receive their **parasympathetic supply** from the vagal trunks (mainly the posterior trunk).

Sympathetic and parasympathetic fibers course with the splenic artery to the spleen as the *splenic plexus*, and they course with branches of the splenic artery and superior mesenteric artery to the pancreas as the *pancreatic plexus*. The fibers to the duodenum reach that organ via the gastroduodenal artery, pancreaticoduodenal artery, and duodenal branches as part of the *superior mesenteric plexus*. The synapse with the second parasympathetic neuron occurs in small ganglia located near the organs.

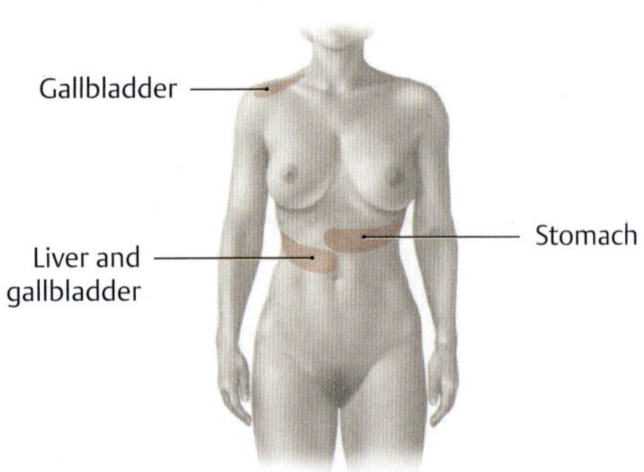

C Referred pain from the liver, gallbladder, and stomach

The Head zones (see p. 73) of the liver, gallbladder, and stomach extend from the right and left hypochondriac regions to the epigastric region. Gallbladder pain may also radiate to the right shoulder (C 4, phrenic nerve). (There are no Head zones associated with the duodenum and spleen.)

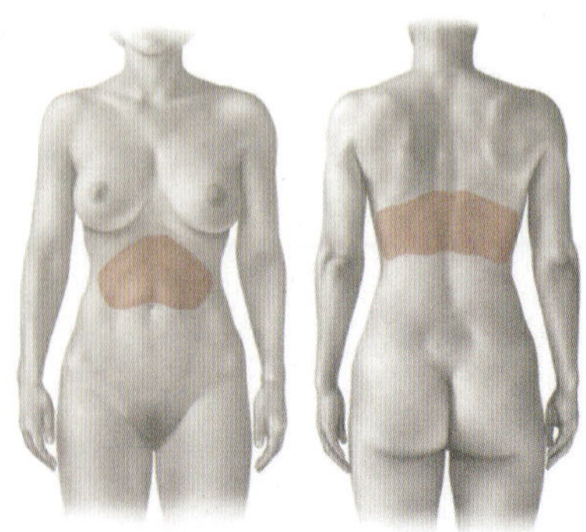

D Referred pain from of the pancreas

The Head zone of the pancreas girdles the abdomen. Pain due to pancreatic disease may be perceived not just in the upper abdomen but also in the back. The anterior Head zone overlaps with the zones of the liver and stomach.

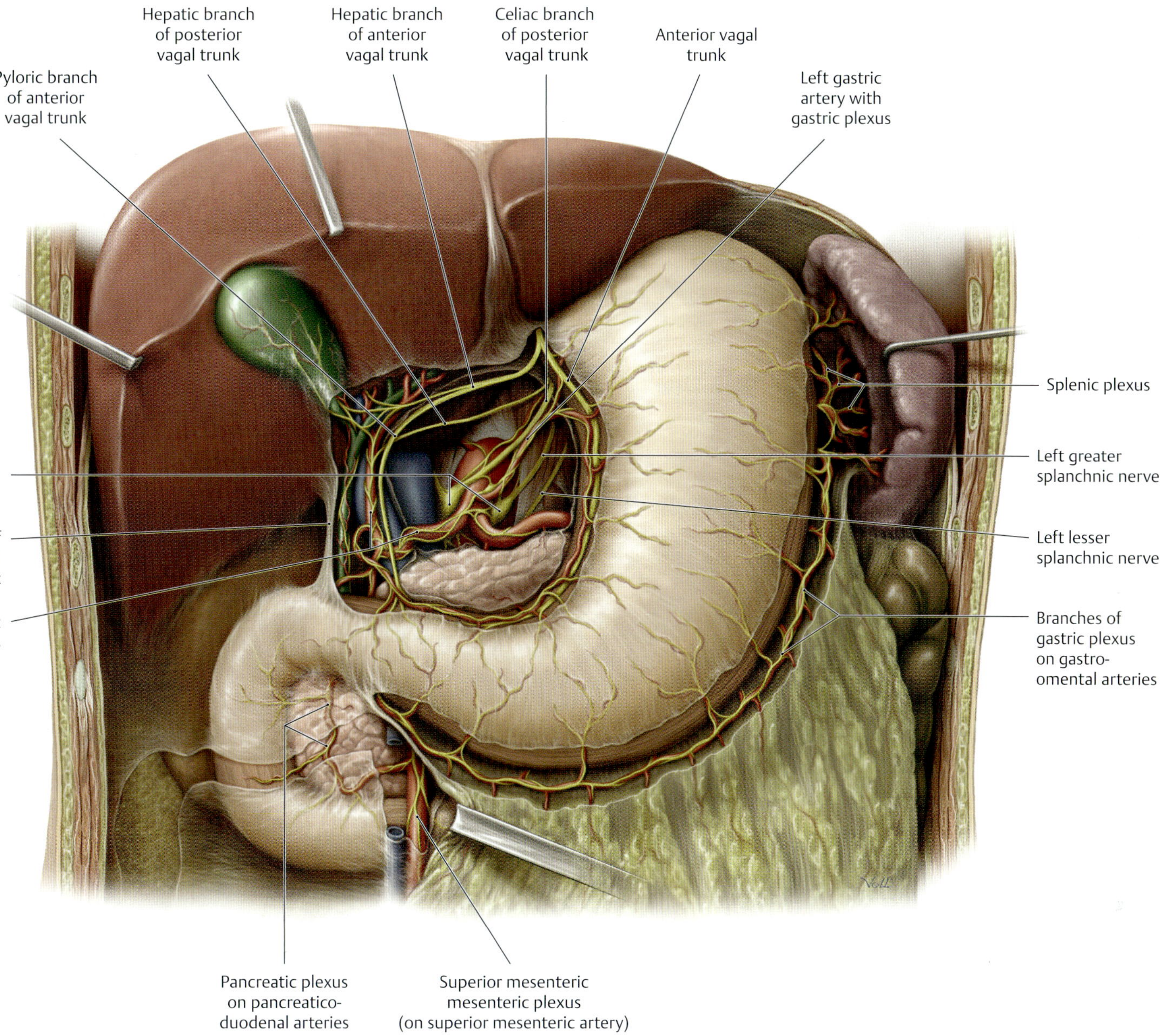

E Innervation of the liver, gallbladder, stomach, duodenum, pancreas, and spleen

Anterior view. The lesser omentum has been broadly removed, and the greater omentum has been opened. The ascending colon and part of the transverse colon have been removed. The retroperitoneal fat and connective tissue has been partially removed to improve the exposure. The visceral plexuses arising from the celiac ganglion mainly accompany the arteries as they pass to their target organs.

Note: The **pylorus** is generally supplied by separate pyloric branches that arise from the vagal trunks (parasympathetic supply) and often run initially with the hepatic branches.

The **liver and bile ducts** receive their autonomic supply from *parasympathetic* hepatic branches that join the *sympathetic* fibers in the hepatic plexus. The *hepatic plexus* accompanies the proper hepatic artery to the liver and gives off branches that supply the gallbladder and biliary tract. The **spleen** and **pancreas** receive autonomic fibers from the splenic and pancreatic plexuses. The **duodenum** derives part of its supply from the superior mesenteric ganglion and superior mesenteric plexus.

3.31 Autonomic Innervation of the Intestine: Distribution of the Superior Mesenteric Plexus

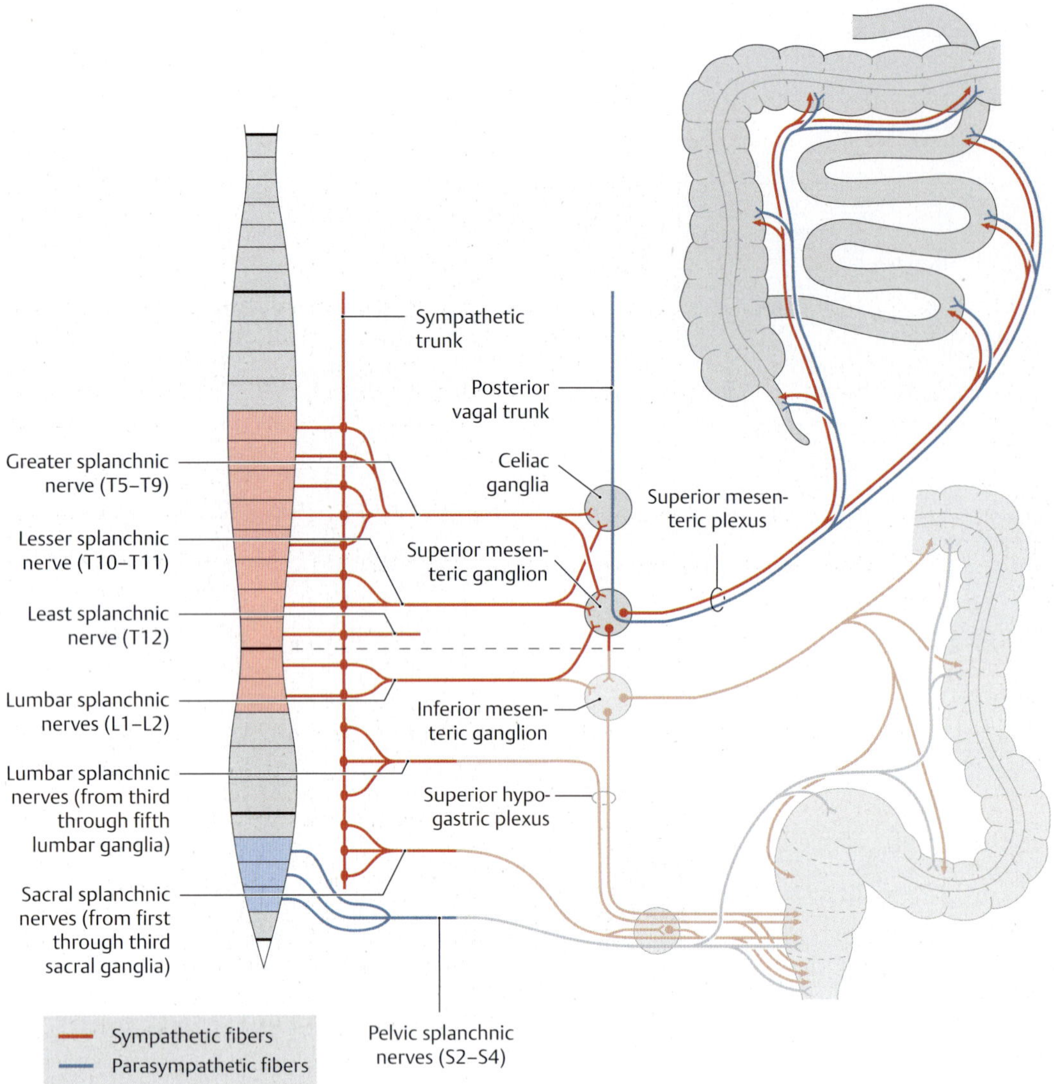

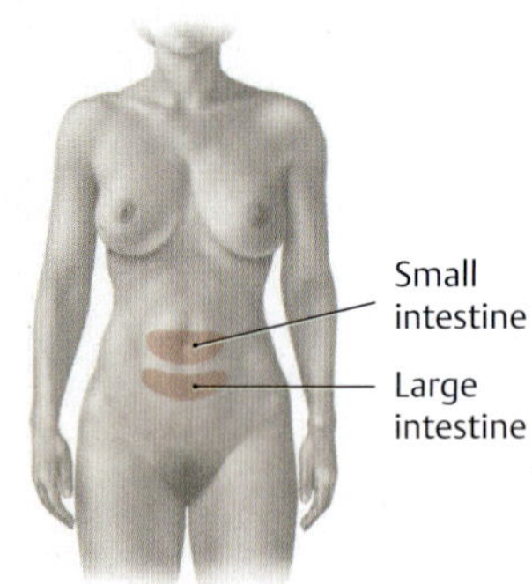

B Referred pain from the small and large intestine
In many cases the pain associated with intestinal diseases is not localized precisely to the bowel. Frequently the pain is projected to the color-shaded areas on the abdominal wall.

A Autonomic distribution of the superior mesenteric plexus
While a clear distinction is drawn between the small and large intestine topographically and histologically, autonomic innervation is based on the supply of a particular intestinal segment by a particular plexus, regardless of whether that segment is part of the small or large intestine. The main distinction to be made is whether the intestinal segment is supplied by the *superior* or *inferior* mesenteric plexus. This principle is illustrated in the above diagram:

Sympathetic innervation:

- The *jejunum, ileum, cecum, ascending colon*, and the *proximal two thirds of the transverse colon* are supplied by postsynaptic branches of the superior mesenteric ganglion via the superior mesenteric plexus, which is distributed to the various intestinal segments along the branches of the superior mesenteric artery.
- Similarly, the *distal third of the transverse colon*, the *descending colon, sigmoid colon*, and *upper rectum* are innervated by postsynaptic branches of the inferior mesenteric ganglion and the associated plexus, which is distributed along the branches of the inferior mesenteric artery.
- The *middle and lower rectum* are supplied by the lumbar and sacral splanchnic nerves via the inferior hypogastric plexus (the supply to the three levels of the rectum is shown on p. 306).

The superior mesenteric ganglion, then, provides **sympathetic** innervation to the entire small intestine and part of the large intestine, supplying by far the greater portion of the entire bowel.

The **parasympathetic innervation** of the small and large intestine is analogous to their sympathetic innervation.

- The *small intestine, cecum, ascending colon*, and *proximal two-thirds of the transverse colon* are supplied by the *vagal trunk* and its branches.
- The remaining *colon* and *rectum* are innervated by the *pelvic splanchnic nerves* from segments S2–S4 (see p. 306). Some of these nerves have their synapses in ganglion cells within the inferior hypogastric plexus and some in ganglion cells on the organ wall.

Thus, the vagal trunk (i.e., elements of the cranial part of the parasympathetic nervous system) provides **parasympathetic** innervation to the entire small intestine and part of the large intestine, supplying the greater portion of the entire bowel. A site on the transverse colon called the *Cannon-Böhm point* marks the boundary between the proximal and distal territories of the autonomic nervous system.

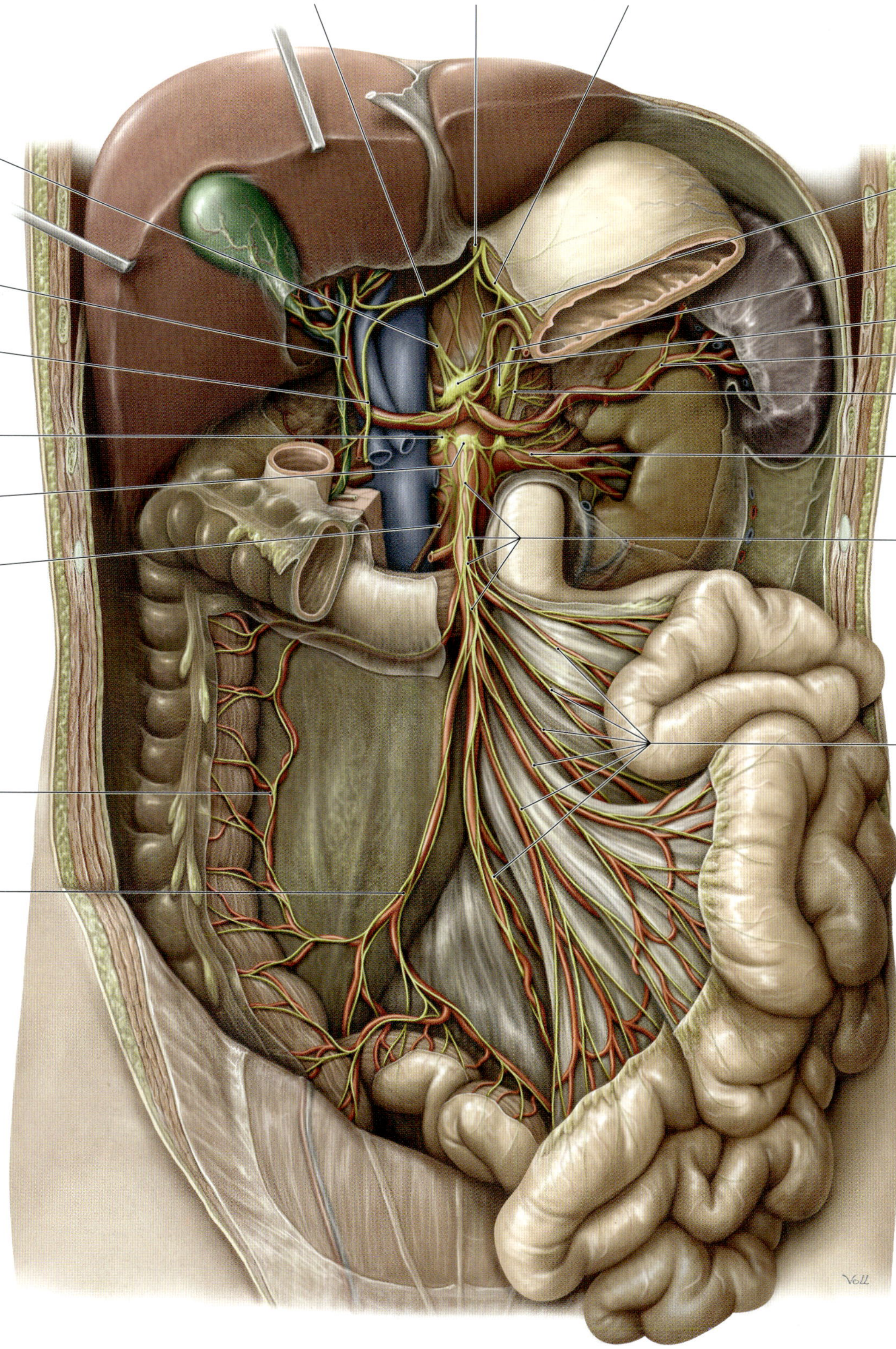

C Autonomic distribution of the superior mesenteric plexus to the intestine

Anterior view. The liver has been retracted superiorly, and the stomach and pancreas have been partially removed. Most of the distal part of the transverse colon has been removed, and all loops of small intestine have been reflected toward the left side.

The postsynaptic branches of the superior mesenteric ganglion (**sympathetic supply**) pass along the branches of the superior mesenteric artery in the mesentery as the superior mesenteric plexus, being distributed to the jejunum, ileum, cecum (and vermiform appendix), and the colon as far as the junction of the middle and distal thirds of the transverse colon. Past that point the bowel receives its sympathetic innervation from the inferior mesenteric ganglion (not visible here). **Parasympathetic innervation** from the jejunum to the distal third of the transverse colon is supplied by the vagal trunk and its branches. The innervation of the remaining colon and rectum is described on p. 306.

3.32 Autonomic Innervation of the Intestine: Distribution of the Inferior Mesenteric Plexus and Inferior Hypogastric Plexus

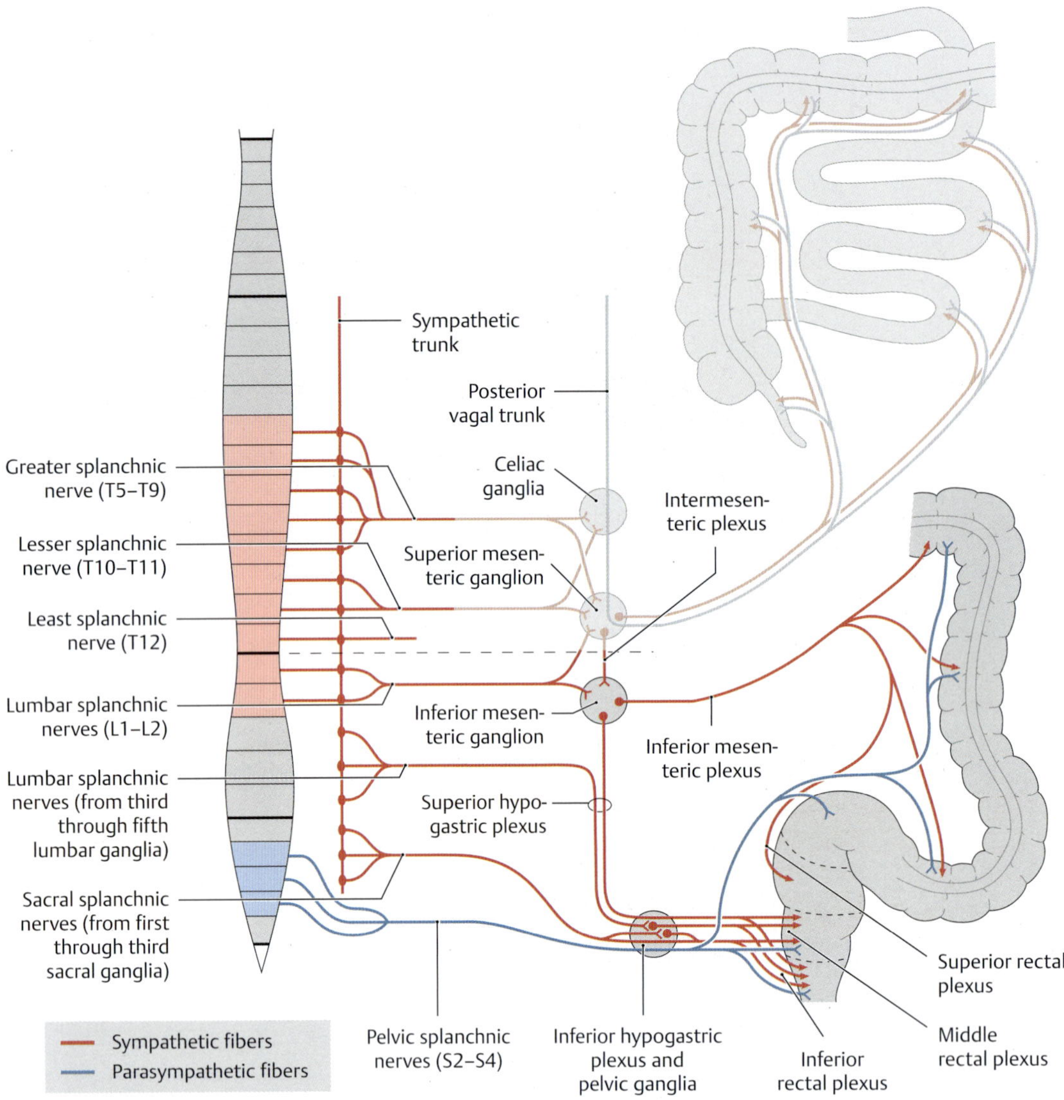

A Autonomic distribution of the inferior mesenteric plexus and inferior hypogastric plexus

Note: The autonomic innervation of the bowel is not divided anatomically between the small and large intestine. It is best understood in terms of the particular bowel segment that is supplied by a particular plexus (superior or inferior mesenteric plexus, inferior hypogastric plexus). Because this unit is concerned mainly with the distribution of the inferior mesenteric plexus and inferior hypogastric plexus (see also **C**), the regions supplied by these plexuses are highlighted in the above diagram. Further details on the innervation pattern are given on p. 241.

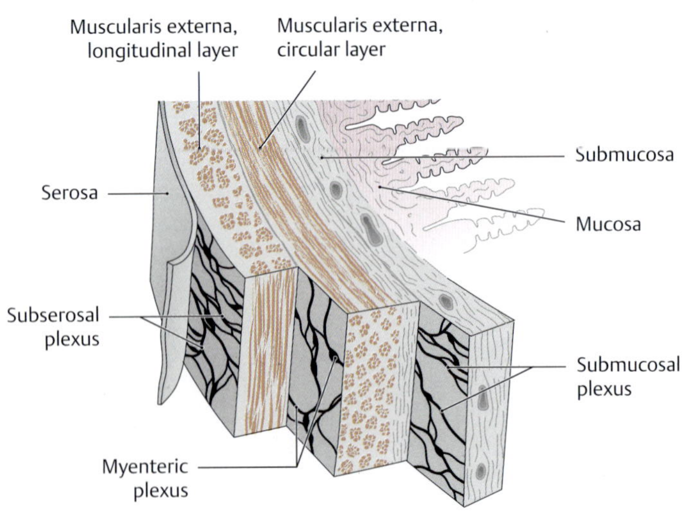

B Organization of the enteric plexus

The enteric plexus is the portion of the autonomic nervous system that specifically serves *all the organs of the gastrointestinal tract.* Located within the wall of the digestive tube (intramural nervous system), it is subject to both sympathetic and parasympathetic influences. Congenital absence of the enteric plexus leads to severe disturbances of gastrointestinal transit (e.g., Hirschsprung disease). The enteric plexus has basically the same organization throughout the gastrointestinal tract, although there is an area in the wall of the lower rectum that is devoid of ganglion cells (see p. 259). Three subsystems are distinguished in the enteric plexus:

- Submucosal plexus (Meissner's plexus)
- Myenteric plexus (Auerbach's plexus)
- Subserosal plexus

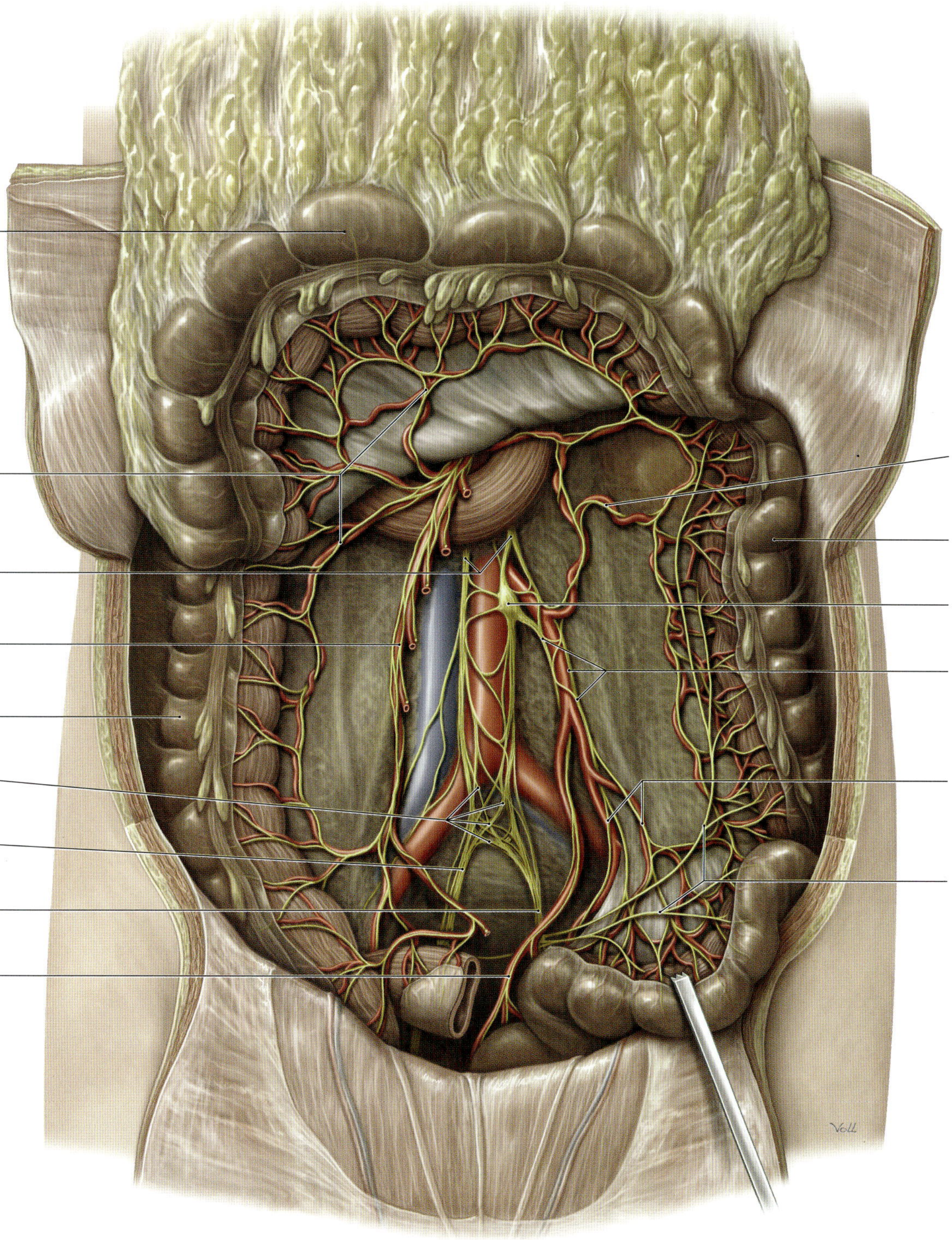

C Autonomic distribution of the inferior mesenteric plexus and inferior hypogastric plexus to the bowel

Anterior view. The jejunum and ileum have been removed, leaving a short ileal stump on the cecum. The transverse colon has been reflected superiorly, and the sigmoid colon has been retracted inferiorly.

Sympathetic innervation:

- The *cecum, vermiform appendix, ascending colon*, and *proximal two-thirds of the transverse colon* (plus all of the small intestine, not visible here) are supplied by postsynaptic branches of the superior mesenteric ganglion.
- The *distal third of the transverse colon, descending colon, sigmoid colon*, and *upper rectum* are supplied by postsynaptic branches of the inferior mesenteric ganglion, which follow the branches of the inferior mesenteric artery as the inferior mesenteric plexus.
- The *middle and lower rectum* (see p. 334) are supplied by the lumbar and sacral splanchnic nerves via the inferior hypogastric plexus (which follows the visceral branches of the internal iliac artery).

Parasympathetic innervation is also divided at the junction of the middle and distal thirds of the transverse colon:

- The *proximal* portion is innervated by the vagal trunk and its branches (i.e., the *cranial* part of the parasympathetic nervous system).
- The *distal* portion is innervated by the pelvic splanchnic nerves of segments S2–S4 and parts of the inferior hypogastric plexus (i.e., the *sacral* part of the parasympathetic nervous system; see also p. 243).

4.1 Overview of the Urinary Organs; the Kidneys in situ

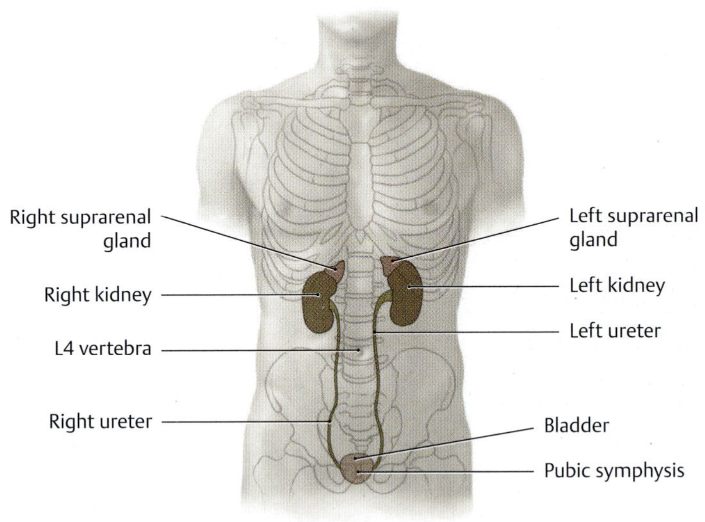

A Projection of the kidneys and other urinary organs onto the skeleton

Anterior view. The suprarenal glands are also shown to aid orientation. The kidneys are located next to the vertebral column and are high enough that they overlap the eleventh and twelfth ribs. The renal hilum is situated at the L 1/L 2 level. Usually the right kidney is somewhat lower than the left kidney due to the space occupied by the liver (see p. 402). The bladder is shown fully distended in the diagram. When empty, it is considerably smaller and is hidden behind the pubic symphysis. The ureters descend in the retroperitoneum and open into the bladder from the posterior side.

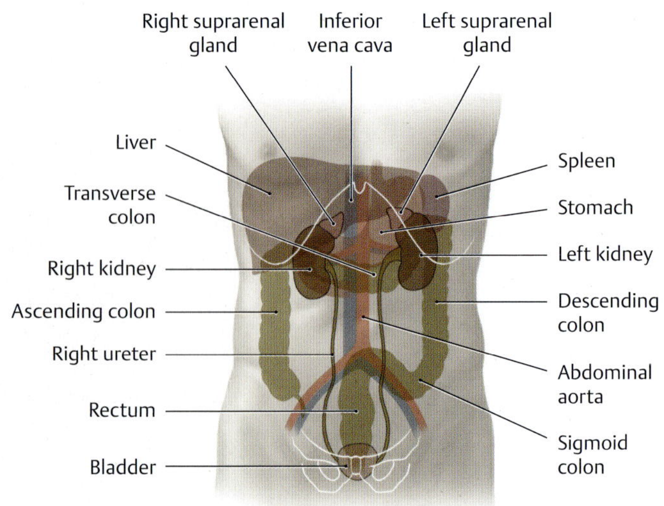

B Projection of the urinary organs onto the organs of the abdomen and pelvis

Anterior view. Owing to its large size, the liver displaces the right kidney slightly inferiorly. The bladder is shown in a fully distended state. It is anterior to the rectum in the male and anterior to the uterus (not shown here) in the female. Because of this relationship, marked distention of the rectal ampulla or enlargement of the uterus due to pregnancy exerts greater pressure on the bladder, creating an urge to urinate even when the bladder is not full. Urinary incontinence may develop due to pathological processes of longer duration, such as muscular tumors of the uterus (fibroids), or due to weakening of the bladder closure mechanism as a result of previous vaginal deliveries (descent of the muscular pelvic floor).

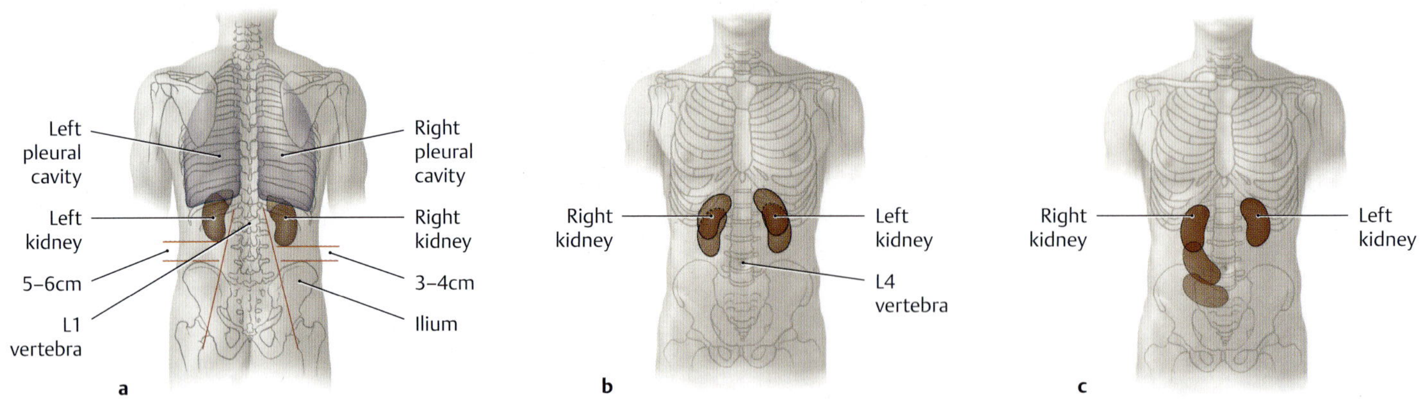

C Location of the kidneys, normal vs. pathological mobility

a Posterior view. The pleural cavities overlap the kidneys posteriorly owing to the convexity of the diaphragm.
Note that the right kidney is lower than the left kidney and is closer to the palpable iliac crest.

b, c Anterior view. The kidneys are located in the retroperitoneum just below the diaphragm. Hence they move passively with the diaphragm during respiratory excursions, moving inferiorly and slightly laterally during inspiration because of their oblique position (their inferior poles point away from the spine, see oblique red lines in **a**).

These passive movements may cause respiration-dependent pain in patients with renal disease. A *pathological* increase in renal mobility ("floating kidney," see **c**) results from atrophy of the fat capsule that normally surrounds the kidneys and keeps them in a stable position. A wasting illness (e.g., metastatic tumors of varying origin) may cause such severe fatty atrophy that the kidneys descend to a lower level in the abdomen. As they are still tethered by the ureter and vascular stalk, this descent may kink the renal vessels or ureter and interfere with renal blood flow or urinary outflow.

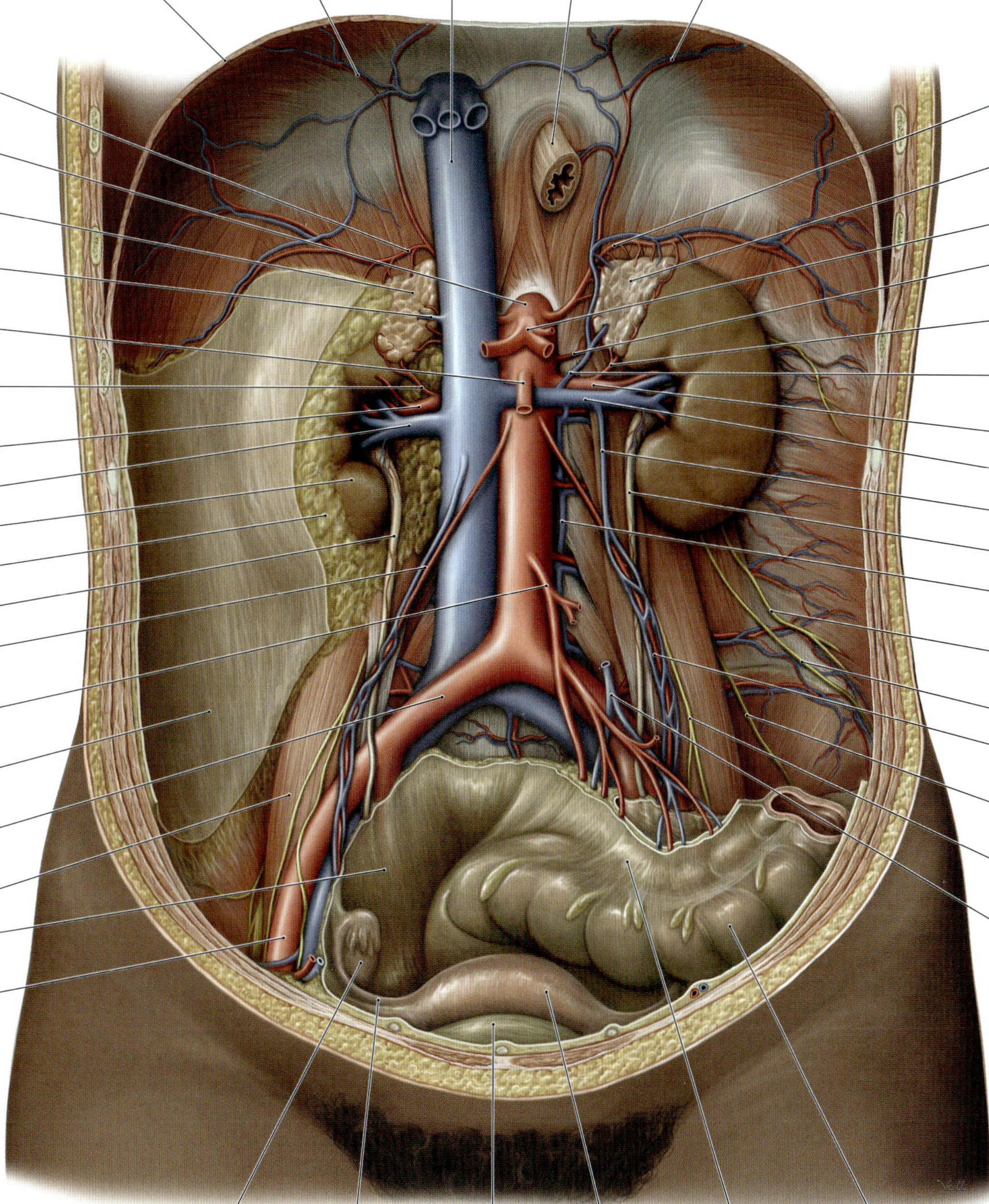

D The urinary organs in situ

Anterior view of an opened female abdomen. The spleen and gastrointestinal organs have been removed to the sigmoid colon, and the esophagus has been pulled slightly inferiorly. The fat capsule remains partially intact on the right side, removed on the left side. The kidneys and suprarenal glands are incorporated into the retroperitoneum by the structural fat of this capsule. The moderately distended bladder is just visible above the pubic symphysis in front of the uterus. The parietal peritoneum has been removed to provide a clear view into the retroperitoneum.

Note: The ureters pass behind the ovarian vessels and in front of the iliac vessels as they descend in the retroperitoneum. These sites represent clinically important constrictions of the ureter where a stone from the renal pelvis may become lodged (see **B**, p. 319).

In most cases the kidneys are not oriented parallel to the coronal plane. The renal hilum, where the blood vessels and ureter enter and leave the kidneys, is directed anteromedially (see **Ab**, p. 310). Also, the renal superior poles are closer together than the inferior poles, so that the kidneys appear slightly "tilted" toward the midline. Thus the renal hilum also points slightly downward.

4.2 Kidneys: Location, Shape, and Structure

A Position of the kidneys in the renal bed
Right renal bed. **a** Sagittal section at approximately the level of the renal hilum, viewed from the right side. **b** Transverse section through the abdomen at approximately the L 1/L 2 level, viewed from above.
The renal bed is located on each side of the spine in the retroperitoneum. It contains the kidneys, which are invested by a thin **organ capsule** (renal fibrous capsule), and the suprarenal glands, which are surrounded by the **perirenal fat capsule** that also encloses the kidneys. The fat capsule is thicker posteriorly than anteriorly.
Note: Swelling of the kidney (usually due to inflammation) may cause severe pain due to stretching of the fibrous capsule.
The fat capsule is surrounded by the **renal fascia**, which separates it from its surroundings by two layers:

- The anterior layer behind the parietal peritoneum (to which it is fused at some sites)
- The posterior layer, which is partially attached to the transversalis fascia and muscular fasciae on the posterior trunk wall

The renal fascia, and thus the renal bed, is open inferiorly and medially to allow passage of the ureter and renal vessels. It is closed laterally and superiorly by fusion of the fascial layers. Because of this arrangement, inflammatory processes that are adjacent to the kidney but within the renal fascia tend to spread to the contralateral side or inferiorly and may spread into the pelvis.
Note: The entire renal bed moves downward during inspiratory depression of the diaphragm, *indirectly* causing the kidney and suprarenal gland to move as well. This differs from the liver, which is attached to the diaphragm (bare area) and is *directly* moved by diaphragm excursions.

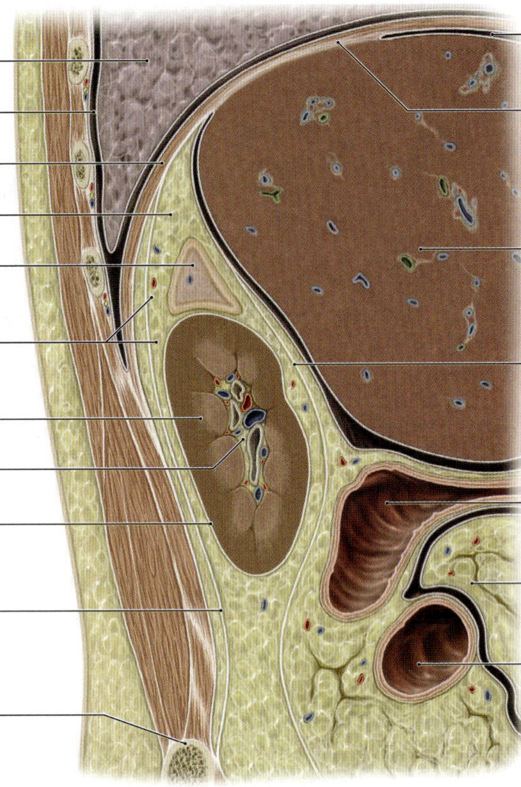

a

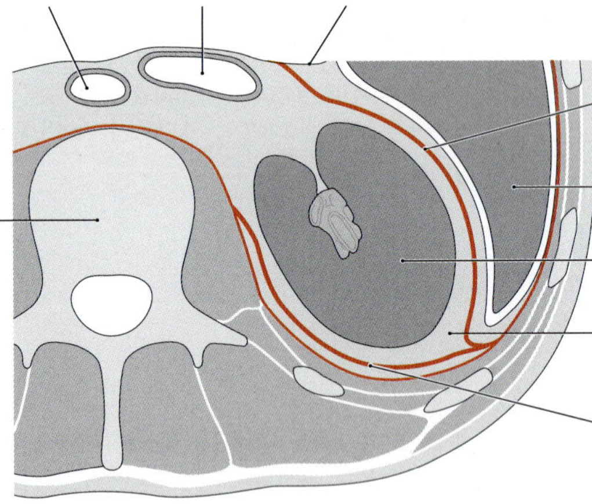

b

B Renal bed: fasciae and capsules of the kidneys

Renal fibrous capsule	Thin, firm connective-tissue capsule that closely invests each kidney
Perirenal fat capsule	Mass of fat that surrounds the kidneys and suprarenal glands and completely occupies the renal bed; it is thickest lateral and posterior to the kidneys
Renal fascia	Connective-tissue fascial sac that encloses the perirenal fat, portions of the abdominal aorta and inferior vena cava close to the kidney (see **Ab**), and the proximal ureter; subdivided into a thin anterior layer and a thick posterior layer (see **Aa**)

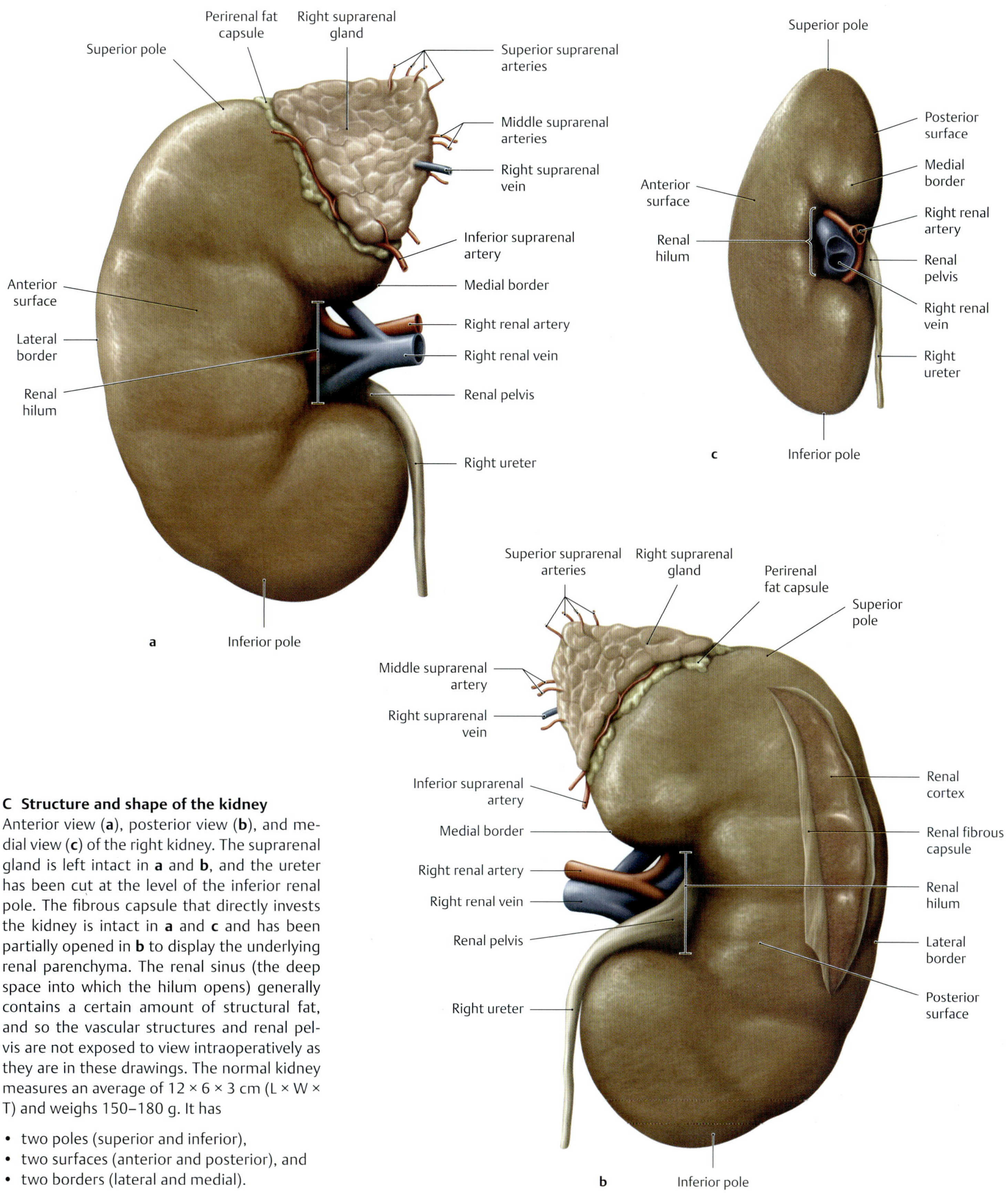

C Structure and shape of the kidney

Anterior view (**a**), posterior view (**b**), and medial view (**c**) of the right kidney. The suprarenal gland is left intact in **a** and **b**, and the ureter has been cut at the level of the inferior renal pole. The fibrous capsule that directly invests the kidney is intact in **a** and **c** and has been partially opened in **b** to display the underlying renal parenchyma. The renal sinus (the deep space into which the hilum opens) generally contains a certain amount of structural fat, and so the vascular structures and renal pelvis are not exposed to view intraoperatively as they are in these drawings. The normal kidney measures an average of 12 × 6 × 3 cm (L × W × T) and weighs 150–180 g. It has

- two poles (superior and inferior),
- two surfaces (anterior and posterior), and
- two borders (lateral and medial).

The medial border bears the renal hilum, where vascular structures and the ureter enter and leave the kidney. The shallow surface grooves result from the embryonic lobulation of the kidney. The hilar structures are usually arranged as follows from anterior to posterior (as shown in **c**): right renal vein, right renal artery, and right ureter.

Note: The renal artery is usually posterior to the renal vein because the right renal artery passes to the right kidney *behind* the inferior vena cava (where the renal veins terminate), while the left renal vein passes to the left kidney in *front of* the abdominal aorta (which gives origin to the renal arteries). The left renal artery may also loop around the left renal vein from above to occupy an anterior position. The ureter leaves the renal pelvis (see p. 312) below the vessels and is usually somewhat posterior in relation to the blood vessels.

4.3 Kidneys: Architecture and Microstructure

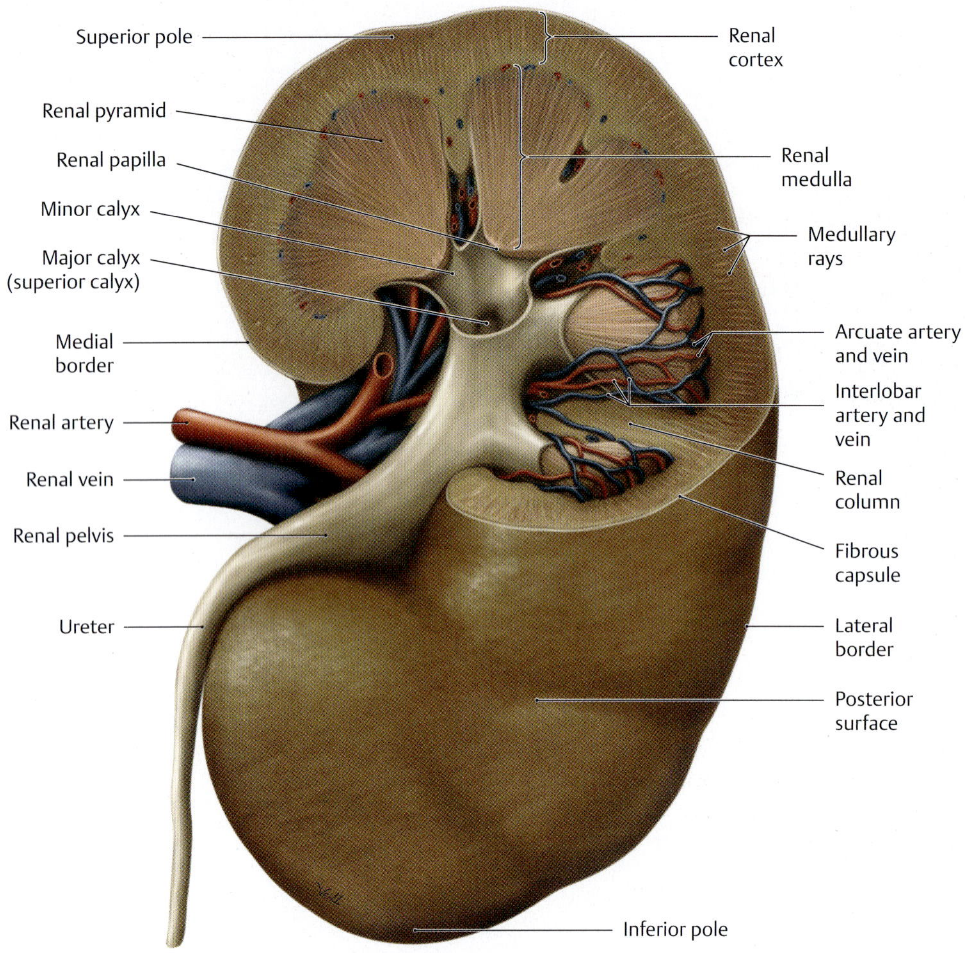

A Macroscopic structure of the kidney
Posterior view of a right kidney with the upper half of the kidney partially removed. The **renal parenchyma** consists of an outer cortex and inner medulla:

- The *renal cortex* is a relatively thin layer that lies beneath the fibrous capsule and forms columns (renal columns) that extend between the pyramids of the medulla. The cortex and columns contain approximately 2.4 million renal corpuscles (which contain the glomeruli, see **B**) as well as the proximal and distal renal tubules (see **C**).
- The *renal medulla* consists of approximately 10–12 renal pyramids. The bases of the pyramids are directed toward the cortex and capsule, while their apices converge toward the renal pelvis. The medulla mainly contains the ascending and descending limbs of the renal tubules.

The **renal pelvis** is described on p. 314.

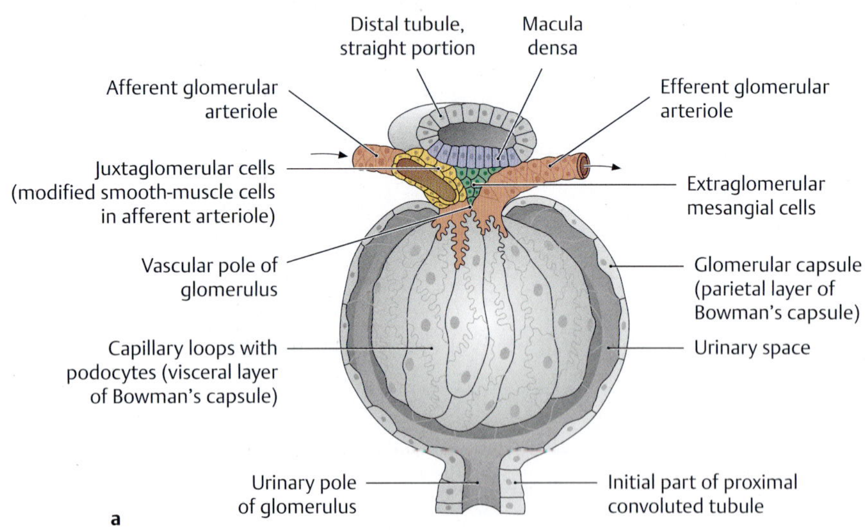

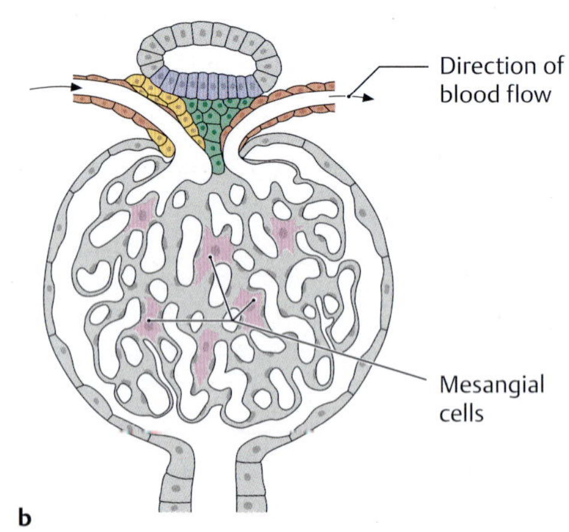

B Renal corpuscle
a With the capsule opened; **b** In section.
The renal corpuscle is the interface between the blood vessels and the excretory portion of the urinary tract (see **C**). It consists of a central convoluted vascular loop, the glomerulus, and a bulbous envelope lined by squamous epithelial cells, the *glomerular capsule* (Bowman's capsule). Blood enters the *glomerulus* at the vascular pole of the renal corpuscle by flowing through the *afferent* glomerular arteriole, and it leaves the glomerulus through the *efferent* glomerular arteriole. The primary urine is formed within the renal corpuscle and drains through a tubular system at the urinary pole of the glomerulus. The initial portion of this tubular system that is connected to the glomerular capsule is the proximal convoluted tubule (see **C**).
Note: Specialized cells at the vascular pole of the renal corpuscle regulate the blood pressure that is necessary for ultrafiltration.

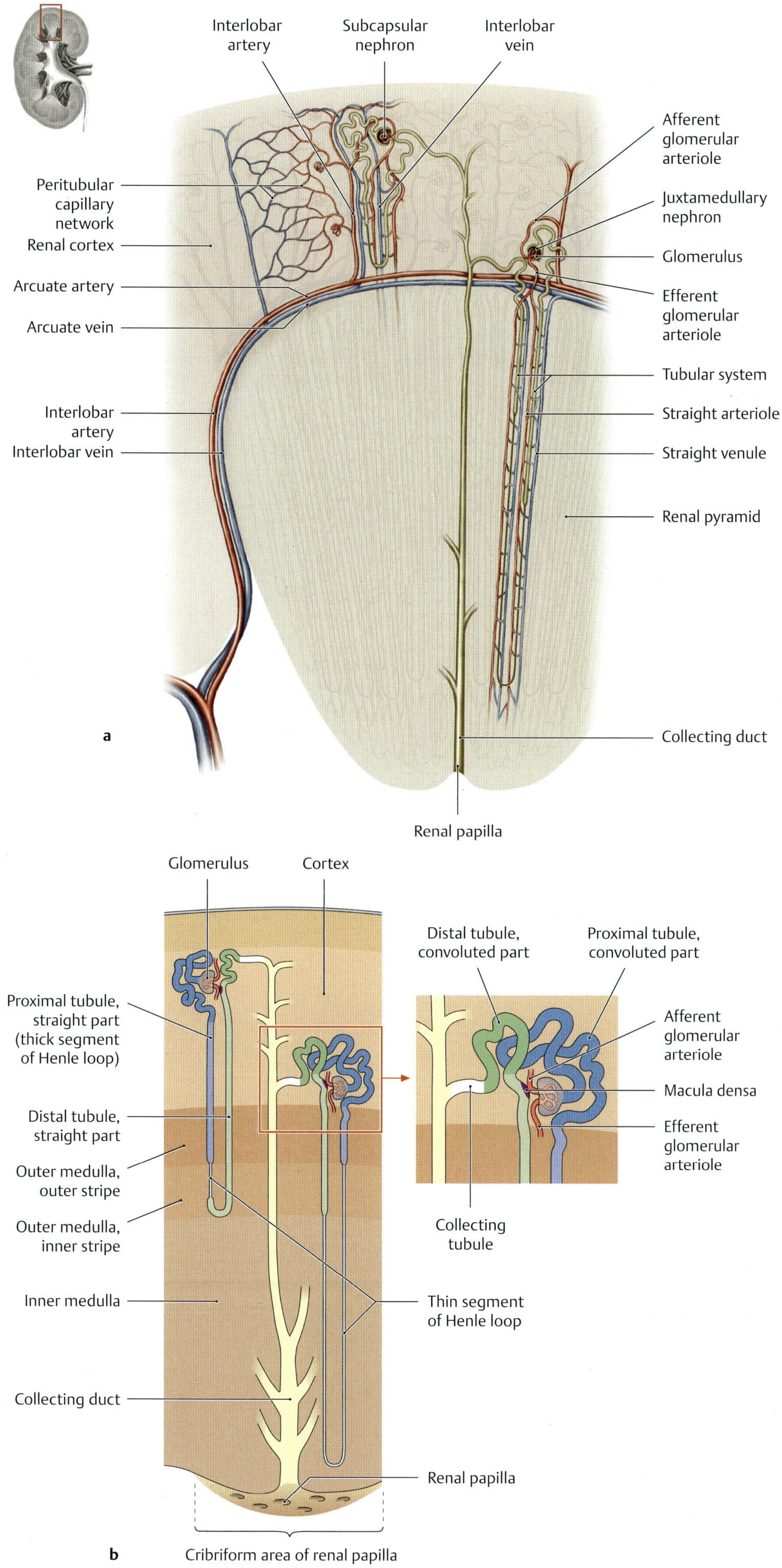

C Architecture of the renal vessels and intrarenal collecting system

a Renal vessels: Sectional view of a medullary pyramid with adjacent cortical areas. The intrarenal vascular and collecting systems are closely interrelated spatially and functionally. An ultrafiltrate from the blood (primary urine) drains into a microscopically small system of renal tubules. *Blood flow to the kidney* (**a**) is supplied by interlobar arteries that pass along the sides of the medullary pyramids from the renal hilum. Each interlobar artery supplies two adjacent medullary pyramids and the associated cortical zones (these branches are not shown). At the base of the pyramid, the interlobar artery gives rise to the arcuate artery, from which the interlobular arteries are distributed into the cortex as far as the fibrous renal capsule. The *afferent* glomerular arterioles that arise from an interlobular artery each supply one glomerulus. The *efferent* glomerular arterioles that emerge from the glomerulus are still carrying blood at a high oxygen tension; they supply the renal cortex or medulla.

b Intrarenal collecting system: The smallest functional unit of the kidney is the nephron, which consists of the renal corpuscle and renal tubules. Each nephron drains via a short connecting tubule into a collecting duct which collects the urine from about 10–12 nephrons. There are approximately 1 million nephrons, which process approximately 1700 liters of blood daily to form approximately 170 liters of *primary urine.* This primary filtrate enters the tubular system at the urinary pole of the renal corpuscle and reaches the renal papilla as the *final urine*, which drains into the calyceal system (approximately 1.7 liters/day). The *tubular system* consists of the proximal and distal tubules (each with a convoluted and straight portion) and an intermediate tubule (with descending and ascending limbs). The intermediate tubule and the adjacent straight portions of the proximal and distal tubules comprise the *loop of Henle*. While passing through the tubular system, substances contained in the filtrate (mainly water) are reabsorbed while other substances (e.g., ions) are secreted into the filtrate. This process yields the final urine, which passes through a collecting tubule into a collecting duct and drains through the renal papilla into the *caliceal system*. It is conveyed from the calyces and renal pelvis to the ureter by peristalsis.

4.4 Renal Pelvis and Urinary Transport

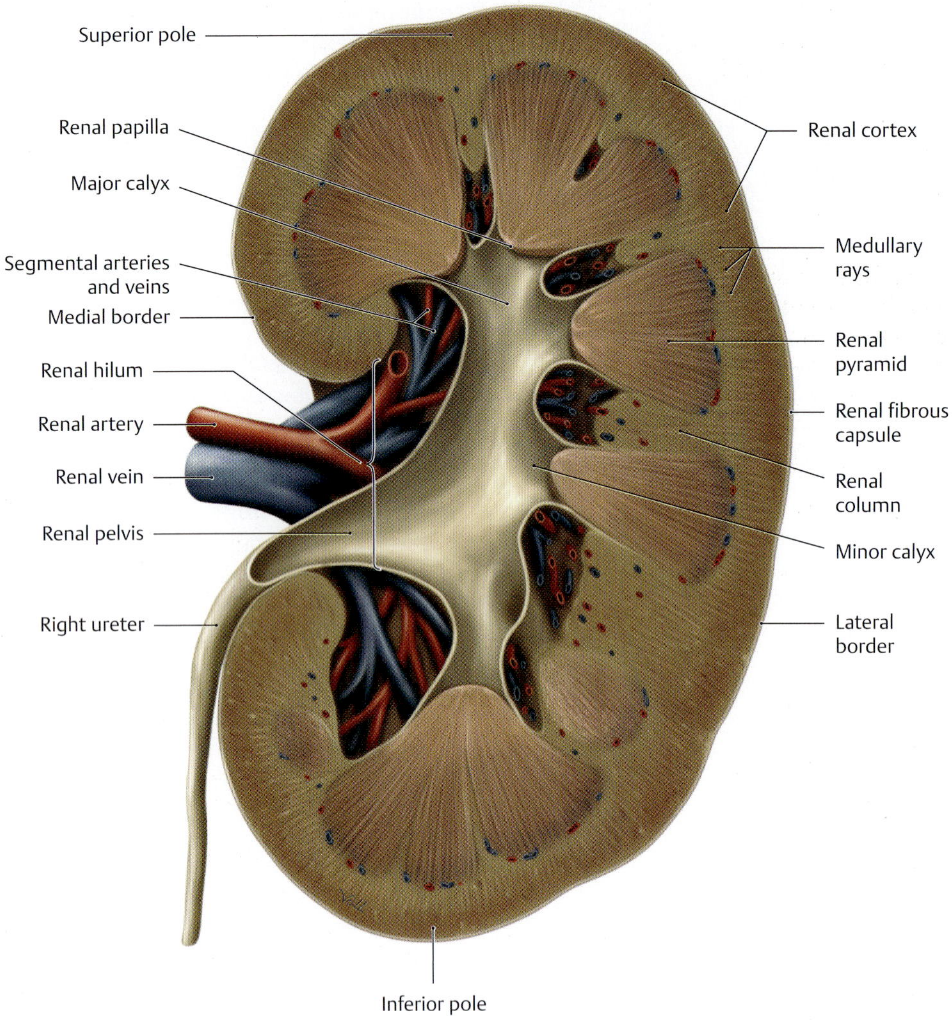

A Structure and shape of the renal pelvis
Mid-longitudinal section through a right kidney, posterior view. The renal pelvis lies posterior to the renal vessels and is continuous inferiorly with the ureter. It may vary in shape (see **B**). It is usually divided into two or three indistinctly separable larger (major) calyces, which further divide into smaller (minor) calyces. They encompass the tips of the renal papillae in such a way that urine drains from the papillae into the calyx without entering the renal parenchyma. Smooth-muscle fibers in the calyces, renal pelvis and ureter (for details about wall structure, see **D**), enable these structures to undergo peristaltic contractions (see **C**).
Note: Stones (see **C**, p. 319) that form in the calyces or renal pelvis may become so large that they more or less fill the cavity and assume its shape (caliceal stone, staghorn calculus).

B Variations in the shape of the renal pelvis
Anterior view of the left renal pelvis. The renal pelvis and ureter develop from an outgrowth of the mesonephric duct. This "ureteric bud" grows from the bony pelvis toward the renal primordium and unites with it. Branching extensions of the renal pelvis form the major and minor calyces. The major calyces in particular vary in number and shape: neighboring major calyces may fuse and "become incorporated" into the renal pelvis. The renal pelvis is found in basic forms along with transitional forms:

- Dendritic type (with extensive branching, also called linear) (**a**): very fine major calyces, narrow renal pelvis;
- Transitional form (**b**);
- Ampullary type (**c**): indistinct major calyces with wide renal pelvis; minor calyces arise "directly" from the renal pelvis.

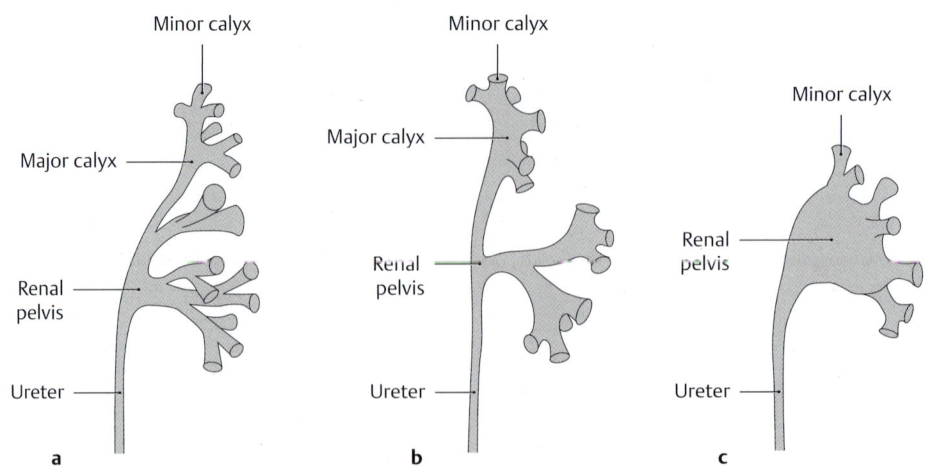

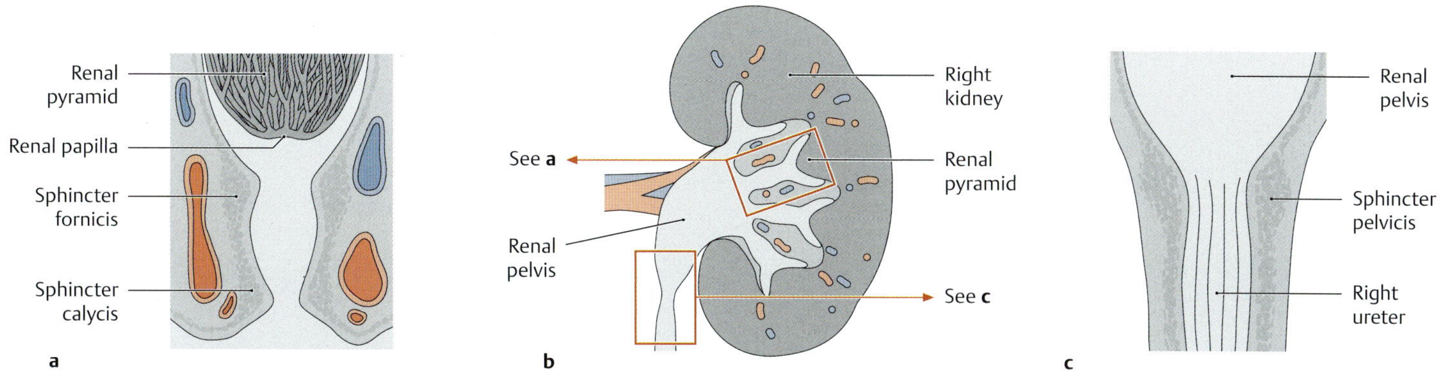

C Closure mechanisms of the renal calyces and renal pelvis; urinary transport

Schematic representation of a kidney (**b**) with magnified sections of a calyx (**a**) and renal pelvis (**c**) and a dynamic functional diagram of the calyx and pelvis during urinary transport (**d**). Urine is transported by an active mechanism. The smooth musculature of the sphincter fornicis and calycis (**a**) and the sphincter pelvicis (**c**) (the functional sphincter system) enables the wall of the renal calyces and pelvis to contract in segments. These contractions are continuous with the peristaltic waves of the ureter, with the result that the urinary tract is never patent over its entire length but is patent in some portions and closed in others (**d**). This maintains a distal flow of urine from the tip of the renal papilla into the calyx, through the renal pelvis, into the ureter, and on toward the bladder while preventing the reflux of urine into the kidneys.

Note: If this active transport process is impaired (e.g., by renal stones or drugs that inhibit the ureteral muscles), urine may reflux into the kidney and incite an inflammatory process in the renal pelvis. The papillae, calyces, and pelvis are often affected jointly by disease (e.g., inflammation) because of their close proximity to one another. One of the most common diseases is suppurative bacterial pyelonephritis (*pyelo-*, referring to the [renal] pelvis, from Gr. *pyelos*—trough, tub, or vat).

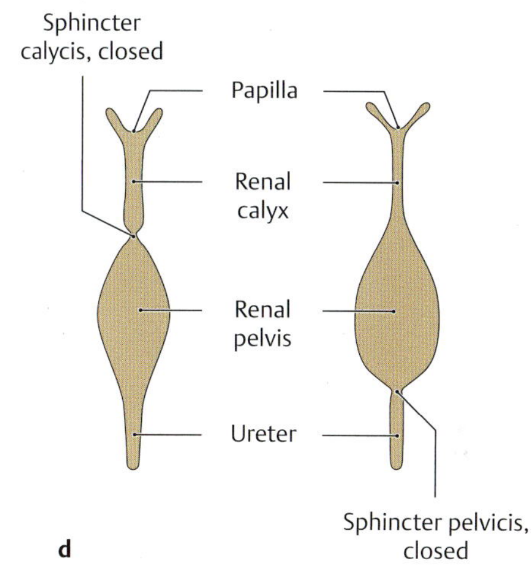

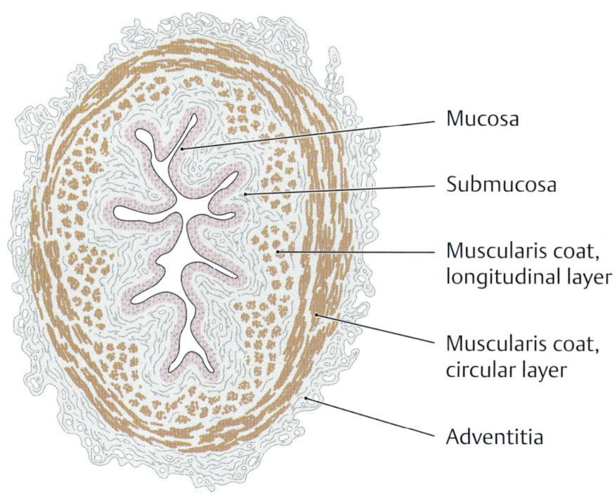

D Wall structure of the ureter

Transverse section through a ureter. A characteristic feature is the stellate lumen that appears in cross-section due to the longitudinal mucosal folds. As in the urethra and bladder, the ureteral mucosa consists of a transitional epithelium of varying height (see p. 323). The smooth muscle consists basically of a longitudinal and a circular layer. It is powerfully developed and shows a functionally spiral architecture (see **E**). When a renal stone enters the ureter, the smooth muscle in the ureteral wall undergoes powerful contractions in an effort to expel the stone, causing very severe pain (renal or ureteral colic). The colic may be relieved by drugs that suppress the activity of the parasympathetic nervous system, though this will also inhibit normal urinary transport to the bladder. The renal pelvis is structurally analogous to the ureter, including the stellate shape of its lumen.

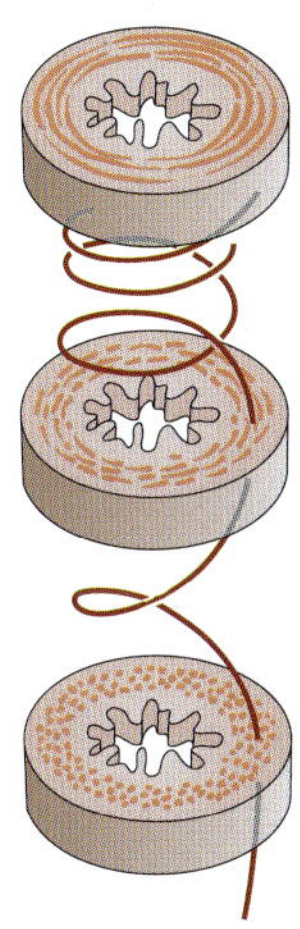

E Arrangement of the ureteral musculature

Schematic cross-sections at various levels of the ureter. The longitudinal and circular muscle layers of the ureter wall have a slightly oblique arrangement, forming a kind of spiral that propels urine toward the bladder by peristaltic contractions. Although the ureters are richly innervated, the peristaltic contractions are instigated by spontaneously depolarizing smooth-muscle cells in the walls of the renal pelvis. Peristaltic waves of contraction (with a speed of 2–3 cm/s) are propagated through direct electrical connections (gap junctions) between adjacent smooth-muscle cells. Autonomic motor innervation and local sensory reflexes serve to modulate this intrinsic activity. This mechanism may thus have some superficial similarities to the system that controls heartbeat.

4.5 Suprarenal Glands

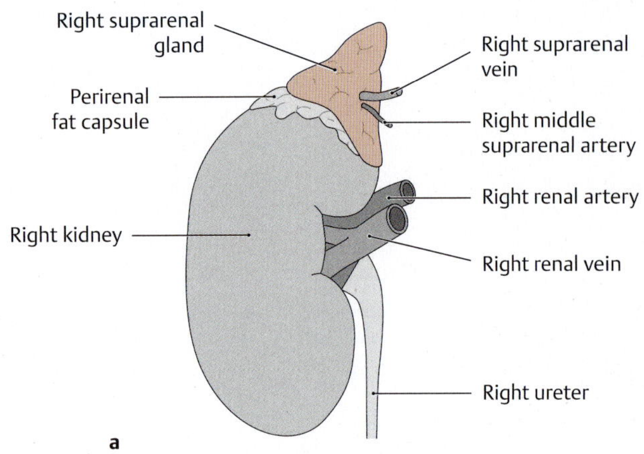

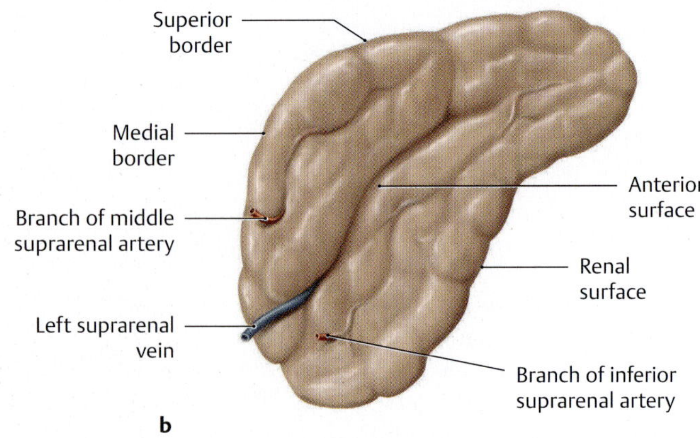

A Location and shape

a Location of the suprarenal gland on the right kidney. **b** Isolated left suprarenal gland, anterior view.

The renal surface of each suprarenal gland lies upon the superior pole of the associated kidney. A thin layer of fat separates the suprarenal gland from the *renal* fibrous capsule (making it easy to dissect the gland from the kidney). The *perirenal* fat capsule, however, encompasses both the kidney and the suprarenal gland.

Note: The entire suprarenal gland cannot be seen while in situ, and its true size is not appreciated until it has been detached from the kidney. Portions descend on the posterior surface of the kidney and are not visible in situ.

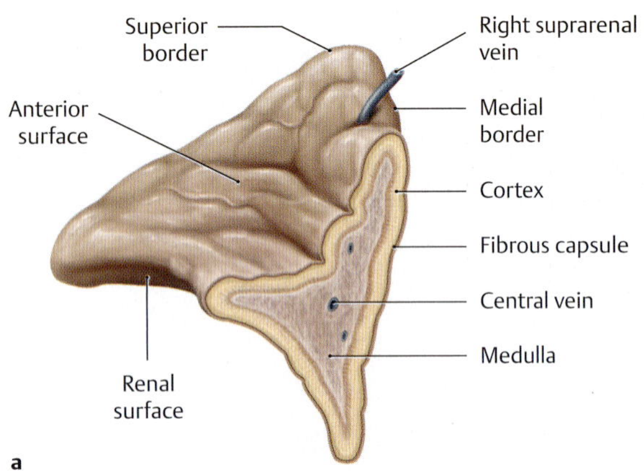

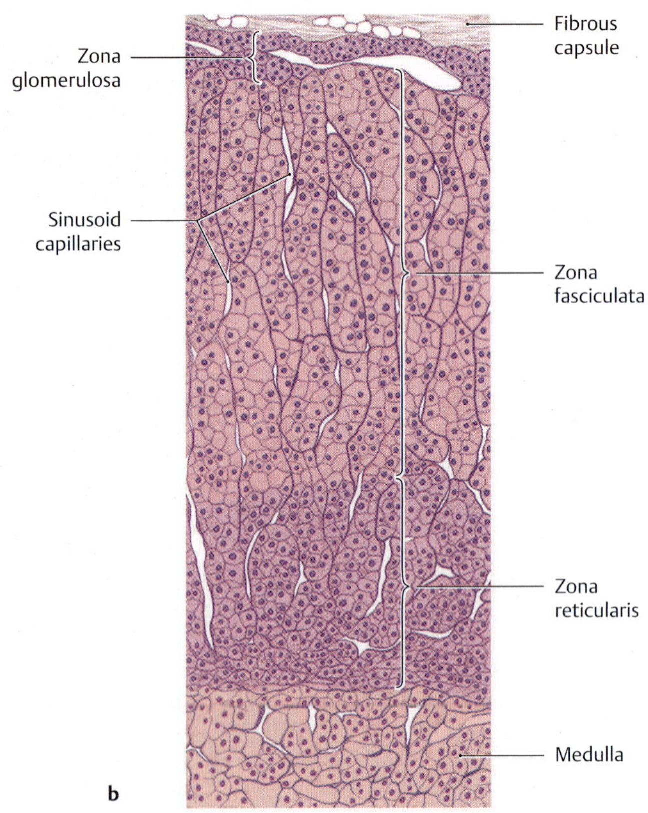

B Structure of the suprarenal gland

a Right suprarenal gland, cut open. **b** Histological section from a suprarenal gland.

The suprarenal gland consists of an outer cortex and an inner medulla (see **a**). The **cortex** is covered by a thin fibrous capsule and consists of three morphologically distinct zones (see **b**) in which adrenocortical hormones are produced and secreted into the bloodstream. These zones are, from outside to inside:

- Zona glomerulosa: mainly secretes mineralocorticoids (aldosterone)
- Zona fasciculata: mainly secretes glucocorticoids (hydrocortisone)
- Zona reticularis: sex hormones (estrogens and androgens)

Note: Loss or deficiency of both suprarenal cortices leads to Addison disease, while hyperfunction of the suprarenal cortex (or adrenocortical tumors) leads to Cushing syndrome.

The **suprarenal medulla** is essentially a completely different endocrine gland, of different origin, that happens to be anatomically (but also functionally) associated with the suprarenal cortex. The cortex is derived embryonically from mesoderm lining the posterior abdominal wall. The suprarenal medulla is, by contrast, a neural crest derivative, and thus has an ectodermal origin. The catecholamines epinephrine and norepinephrine are produced in the suprarenal medulla and are released into the bloodstream. From a (neuro)functional standpoint, the suprarenal medulla is less a gland than a *sympathetic ganglion:* presynaptic sympathetic neurons pass from the greater and lesser splanchnic nerves into the suprarenal medulla. Because the suprarenal glands are endocrine glands and sympathetic ganglia in one, they can secrete both epinephrine and glucocorticoids (cortisone) in response to stress.

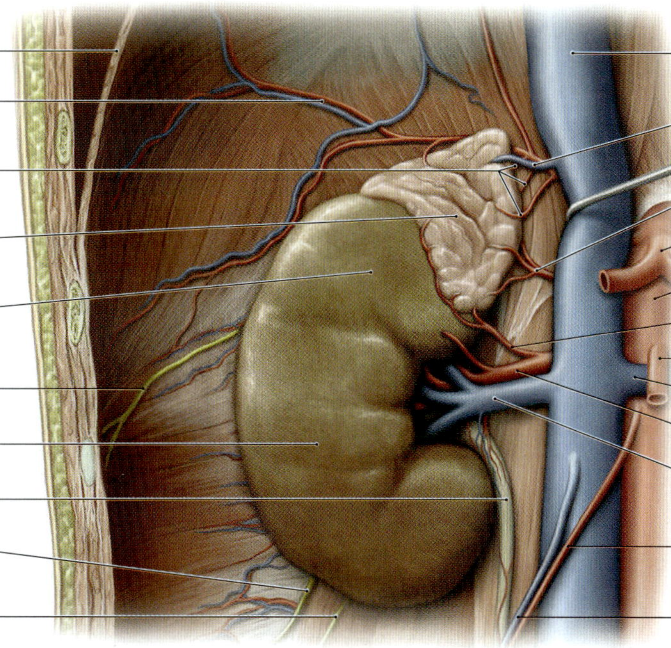

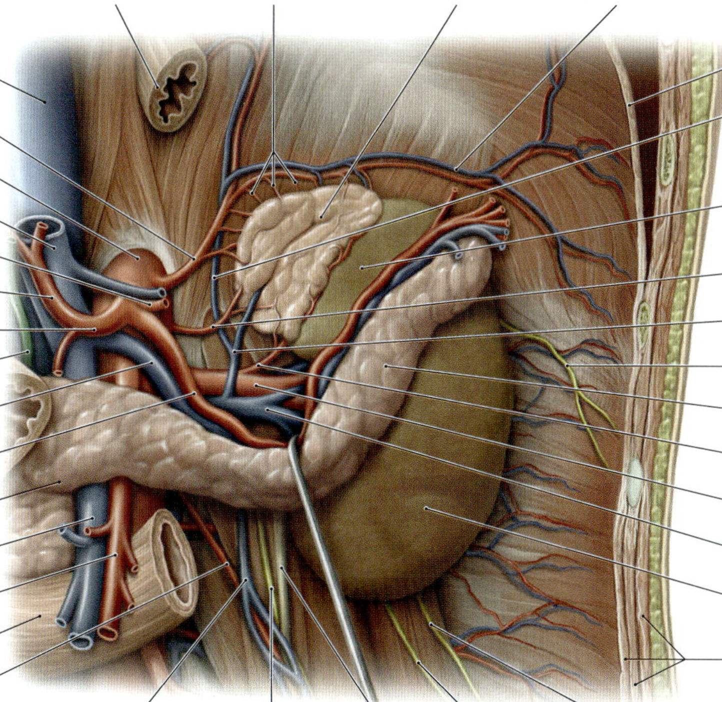

C Right and left suprarenal glands in situ

Anterior view of the right (**a**) and left (**b**) kidney and suprarenal gland with the perirenal fat capsule removed. To demonstrate the vessels behind the suprarenal gland, the vena cava has been retracted medially in **a** and the pancreas has been retracted inferiorly in **b**. The principal differences between the two suprarenal glands are as follows:

- The right suprarenal gland is often somewhat smaller than the left suprarenal gland, which frequently extends inferiorly to the renal hilum.
- The right suprarenal gland is pyramid-shaped while the large left suprarenal gland is more oblong. The right suprarenal gland is normally in contact with the inferior vena cava (retracted medially here), but the left suprarenal gland is *not* in contact with the abdominal aorta.
- The right suprarenal vein usually opens *directly* into the inferior vena cava, unlike the left suprarenal vein, which opens into the left renal vein.

Note: The suprarenal glands are richly vascularized because, as endocrine organs, they release their hormones directly into the bloodstream.

4.6 Ureters in situ

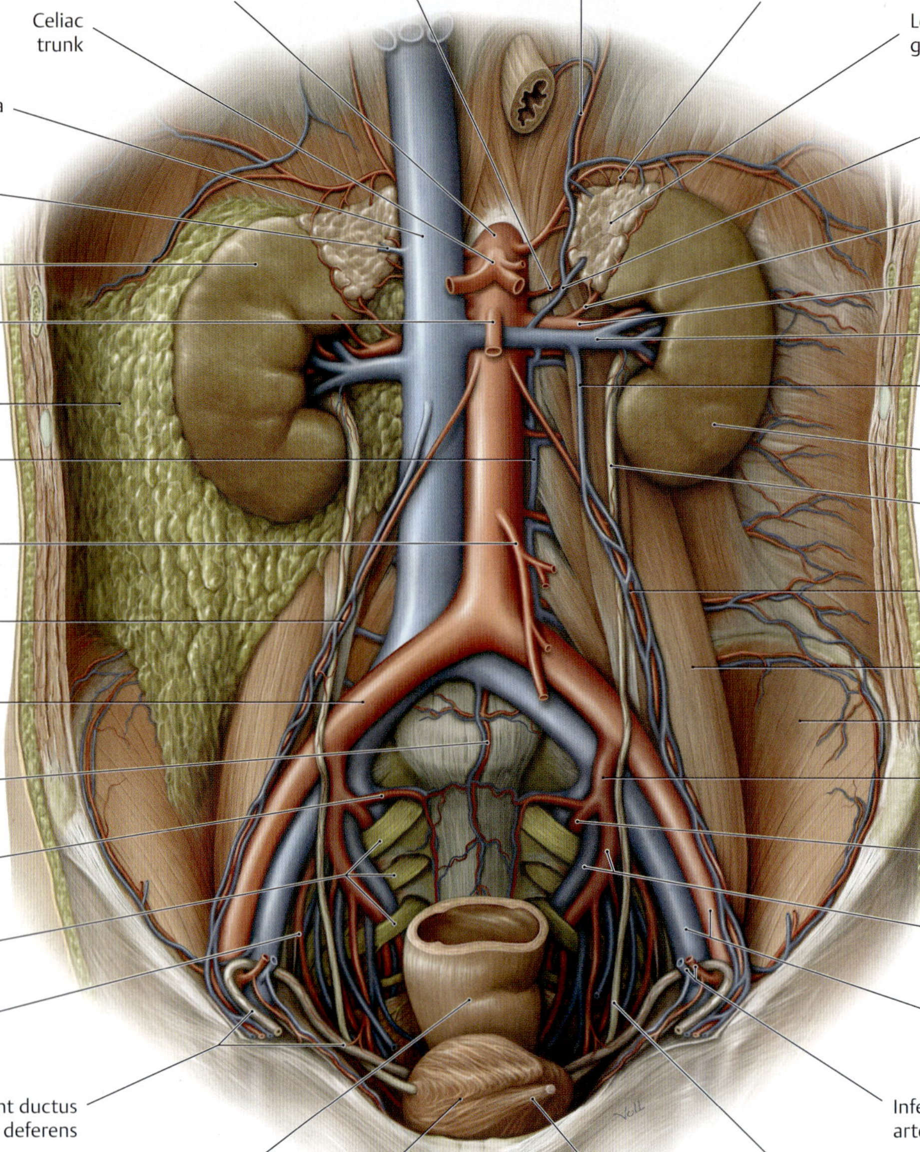

A Course of the ureter in the abdomen and pelvis

Anterior view, male abdomen. All organs have been removed except the urinary organs, suprarenal glands, and a rectal stump. The esophagus has been pulled slightly downward, and the fat capsule of the right kidney has been partially preserved. A prolongation of the renal pelvis, the ureter passes inferiorly and slightly anterior in the retroperitoneum for a length of approximately 26–29 cm. It opens into the posterior aspect of the bladder. *Anatomically*, the ureter consists of three parts:

- Abdominal part (from the renal pelvis to the linea terminalis of the bony pelvis)
- Pelvic part (from the linea terminalis to the bladder wall)
- Intramural part (passes through the bladder wall)

The ureter is also divided into three *clinical* segments, based more on the presence of a free segment and two organ-bound segments than on the anatomical boundary between the abdominal and pelvic parts:

- Renal segment (connected to the kidney)
- Lumbar segment (between the kidney and bladder)
- Vesical segment (in the bladder wall, corresponds anatomically to the intramural part)

The most common *congenital anomalies* of the ureter are duplication anomalies and clefts. They may allow urine to back up to the kidney (e.g., a cleft may allow reflux due to deficient vesicoureteral closure), producing an infection that ascends from the bladder to the renal pelvis (bacterial pyelonephritis).

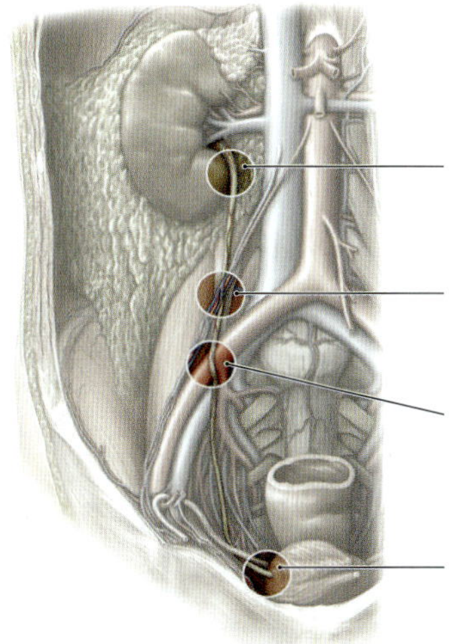

B Anatomical constrictions of the ureter

There are three normal *anatomical constrictions* where a stone from the renal pelvis is apt to become lodged:

- Origin of the ureter from the renal pelvis (ureteropelvic junction)
- Site where the ureter crosses over the external or common iliac vessels
- Passage of the ureter through the bladder wall (ureterovesical junction)

Occasionally a *fourth constriction* can be identified where the testicular or ovarian artery and vein pass in front of the ureter.

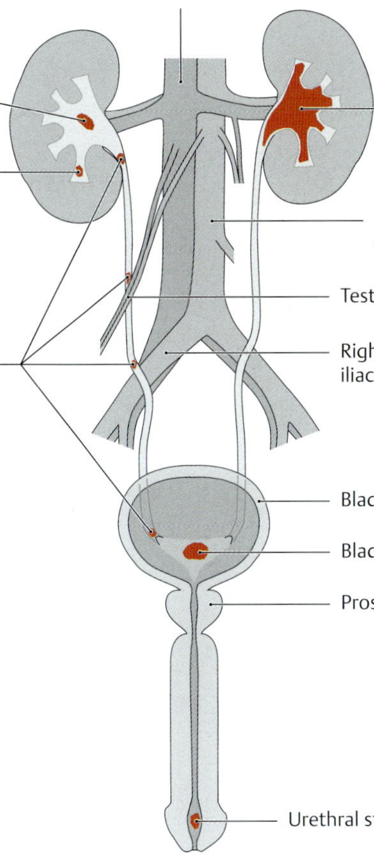

C Common sites of occurrence of urinary stones

When the solubility limit of certain compounds in the urine (e.g., uric acid) is exceeded, the compounds do not remain in solution but are precipitated to form crystallization nuclei. These calculi ("stones") may develop anywhere in the upper urinary tract and may migrate to various sites in any of the urinary organs (renal and renal pelvic stones, ureteral stones, bladder stones, urethral stones). Larger stones are particularly apt to become lodged in the ureter, often stimulating powerful waves of muscular contractions to expel the stone and causing excruciating pain (renal colic, ureteral colic).

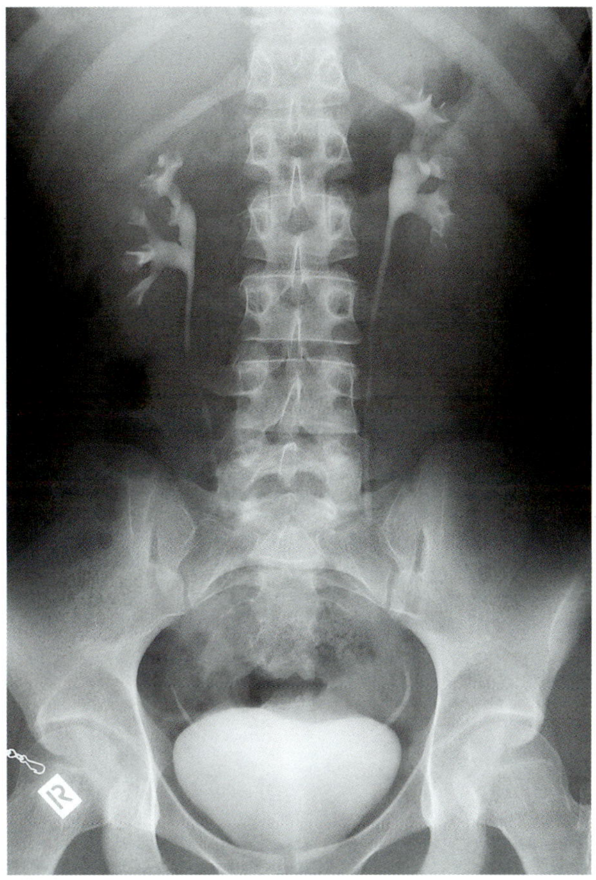

D Intravenous urography

With intravenous urography, which is a radiographic examination, iodinated contrast agent is injected and excreted by the kidneys. The test provides information about renal function, and pathological findings such as anomalies, cysts, urinary obstruction, urinary stones, tumors, etc. (from: Möller, T.B., E. Reif: Taschenatlas der Roentgenanatomie, 7th ed. Stuttgart; Thieme: 2021).

4.7 Urinary Bladder in situ

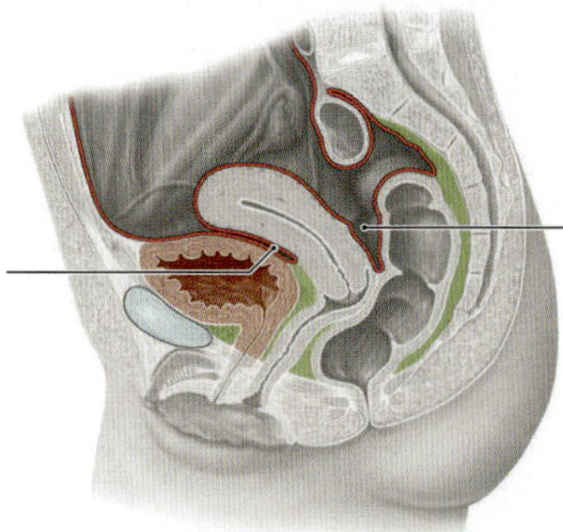

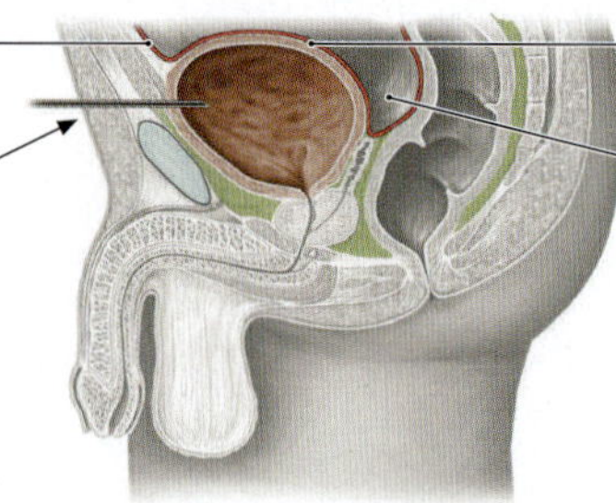

A Location and peritoneal covering of the female (a) and male (b) bladder
Midsagittal section, viewed from the left side. The bladder is shown slightly distended, raising the uterus to a slightly higher position. The peritoneum extends from the posterior surface of the anterior abdominal wall to the superior surface of the bladder and is reflected onto the organ posterior to the bladder, forming a peritoneal pouch. In the female, it forms the vesicouterine pouch; in the male, it forms the rectovesical pouch. Most of the bladder is loosely embedded in pelvic connective tissue.

Note: When the bladder is distended and thus enlarged, the upper part of the bladder, which is covered by urogenital peritoneum, is pushed so far cranially that the anterior wall of the bladder, which is embedded in the surrounding connective tissue and not covered with peritoneum, appears superior to the upper margin of the pubic symphysis (like a "sun rising on the horizon"). This provides an access route for percutaneous puncture of the distended bladder above the symphysis without having to enter the peritoneal cavity with the needle.

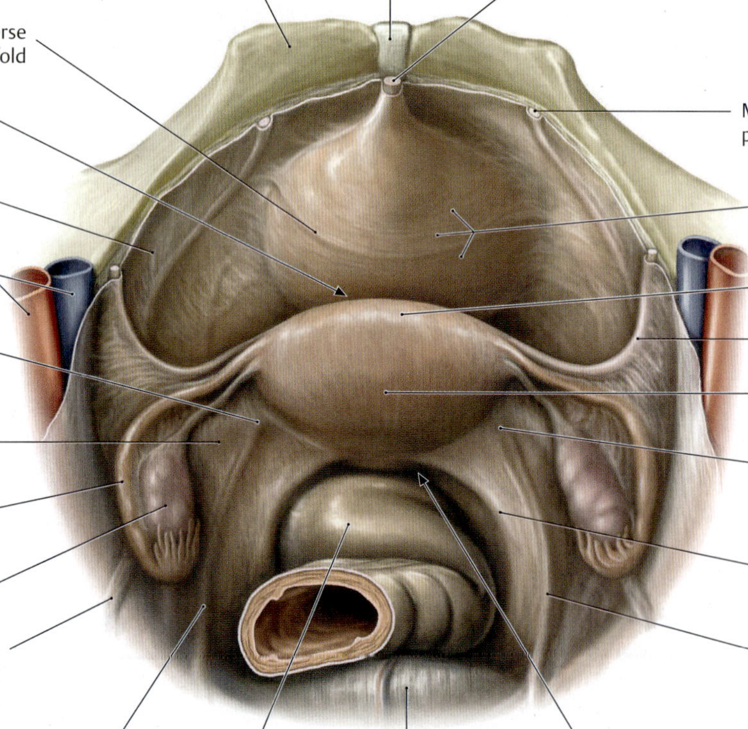

B Location of the bladder in the pelvis and on the pelvic floor
Superior view. The uterus is shown upright for clarity. Most of the large intestine has been removed, leaving the urogenital peritoneum intact. The transverse vesical fold, a peritoneal fold on the surface of the bladder, is effaced when the bladder is full (as shown here). In the female, the bladder lies inferior to the uterus and elevates it when distended. When the structures of the pelvic floor (levator ani and its fasciae) are weakened due to injuries sustained in a vaginal delivery, for example, they may allow the bladder to descend, resulting in incontinence.

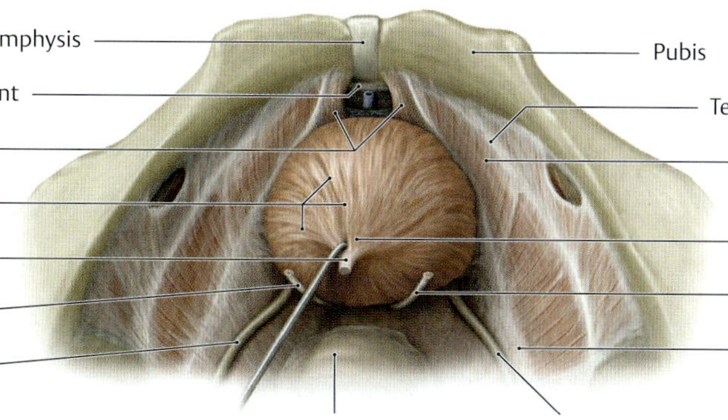

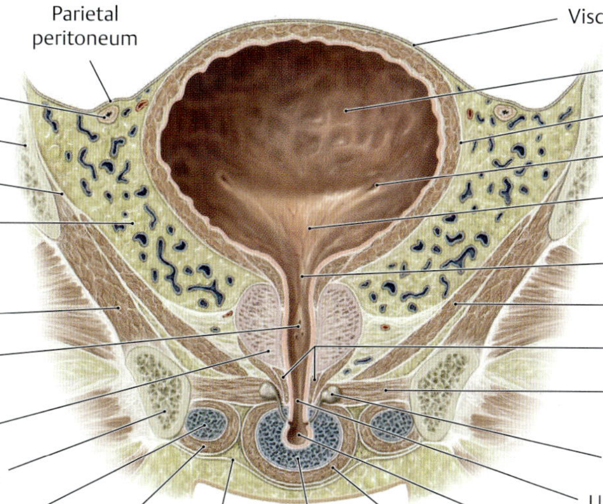

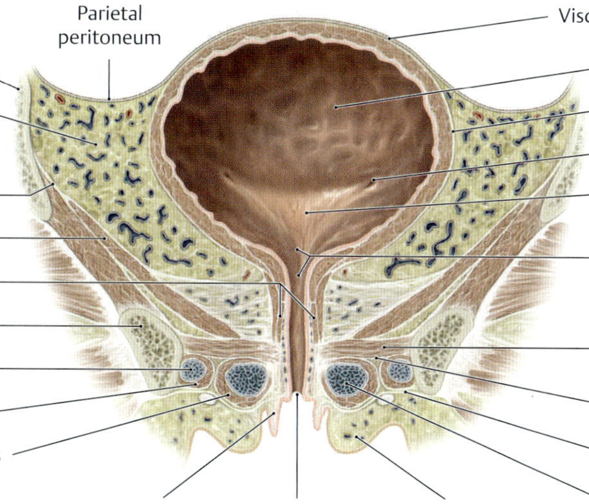

C Comparison of the location of the bladder in the male (a and b) and female (c)

a Superior view with the bladder pulled slightly posteriorly. Unlike in **B**, the urogenital peritoneum has been removed; the bladder has an almost spherical shape given that it is well distended.
The bladder is located on the muscular sheet of the pelvic diaphragm (lying principally upon the levator ani and its fascia = superior fascia of the pelvic diaphragm). This area of contact is smaller in the male than in the female because the lesser pelvis also contains the prostate.

b and **c slightly angled coronal section** with the bladder and urethra opened. The portions of the bladder not covered by peritoneum are integrated into the pelvis by a connective tissue space, which has a well-developed venous plexus. This plexus and the mobile visceral peritoneum allow for considerable changes in bladder size. Like the bladder itself, the initial portion of the urethra is surrounded by connective tissue, and in the male also by the prostate, which lies upon the deep transverse perineal muscle and the levator ani of the pelvic diaphragm.

4.8 Urinary Bladder, Bladder Neck, and Urethra: Wall Structure and Function

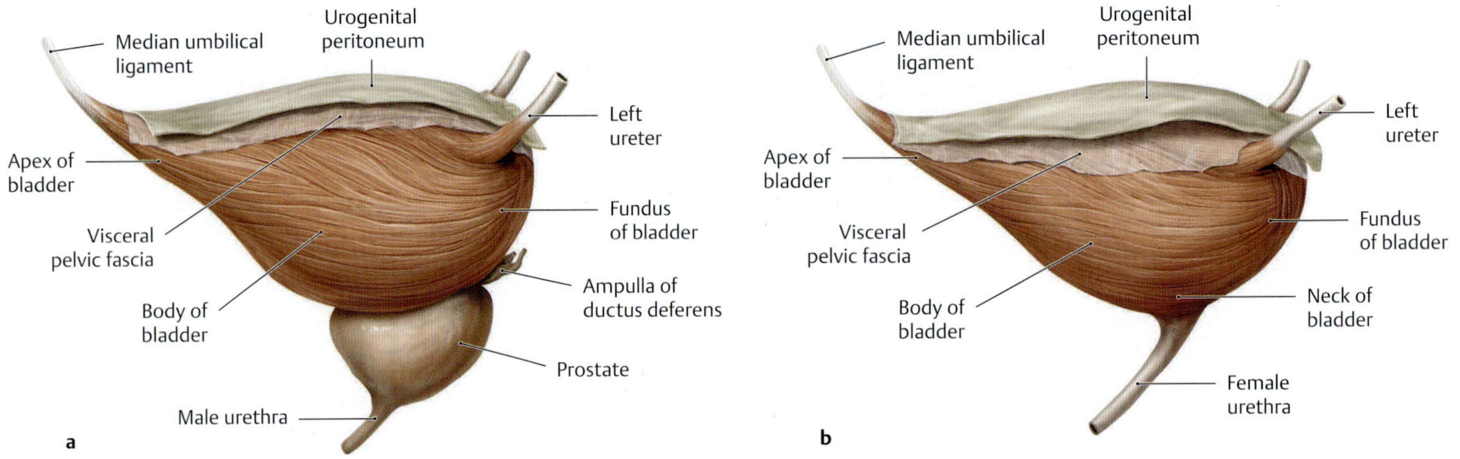

A External morphology of the bladder and urethra

Bladder in a male (**a**) and a female (**b**), viewed from the left side.

The bladder is a hollow muscular organ that collects urine produced by the kidneys and passes it to the urethra at the right time. The maximum bladder capacity is between 500 and 700 ml (females < males). The desire to urinate is already experienced when the bladder contains about 150–200 ml, and even less in pregnant women as the growing uterus increases pressure on the bladder. A normal bladder empties fully without retaining residual urine. The bladder is subdivided into the body of the bladder, the posterior base of the bladder, and the anterior apex of the bladder, which is continuous with the median umbilical ligament (obliterated urachus) at the inner surface of the anterior trunk wall. The two ureters, which enter the bladder dorsolaterally, open into the fundus of the bladder. The urethra begins at the ventrocaudal neck of the bladder.

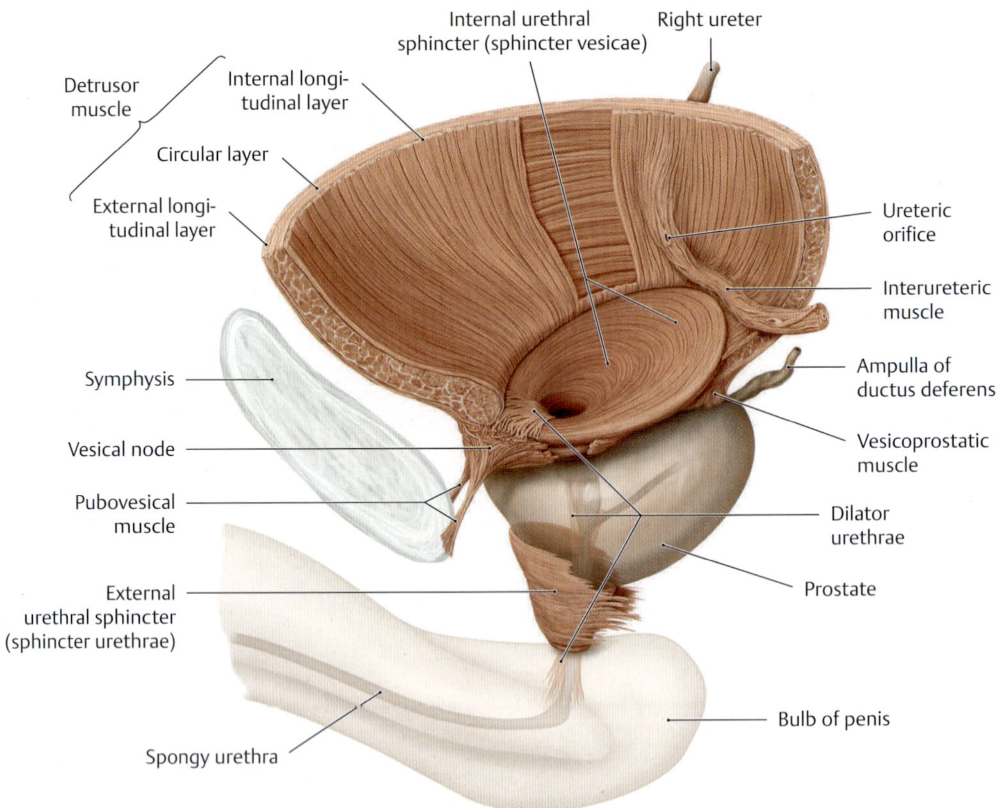

B Muscles of bladder and urethra

Bladder in the male, viewed from the left side.

The **main muscles of the bladder** are

- Detrusor muscle (bladder emptying) and
- Internal urethral sphincter (bladder closure).

The **main muscles of the urethra** are

- Dilator urethrae (urethral dilation) and
- External urethral sphincter (urethral closure).

According to Dorscher et al (2001), the detrusor and internal urethral sphincter are two morphologically separate muscles (see p. 324). The *detrusor* consists of three layers and is responsible for firmly affixing the bladder to the pelvis in the anterior-posterior direction. Fibers of its external longitudinal muscle layer extend *posteriorly* to the vesicoprostatic muscle (or vesicovaginalis muscle in the female) and in the area of the vesicle node *anteriorly* to the pubovesical muscle, which forms an important part of the ventral suspension apparatus (see p. 325). The middle and internal layers end posteriorly above the interureteric crest (see **C**). The internal sphincter is elliptical in shape in the male and circular in the female. Its only function is to close the bladder. Around its posterior circumference, the *internal sphincter* forms the morphological basis of the bladder trigone (see **C**).

The *dilator* (see p. 324) is a fan-shaped muscle that arises from the symphysis and the tendinous arch of the pelvic fascia (see p. 325). It extends posteriorly across the urethral opening and inferiorly at the anterior surface of the urethra, where it inserts on the bulb of penis or the vestibular bulbs. The *external sphincter* consists of an inner layer of smooth muscle fibers and an external layer of striated muscle fibers (for more details see **D**, p. 325).

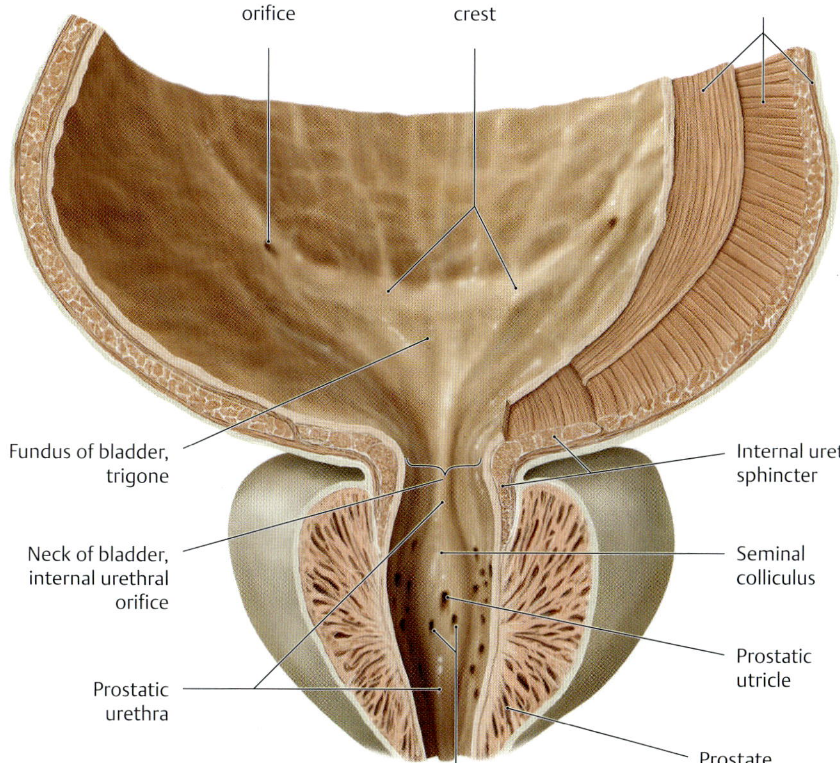

C Bladder neck, bladder trigone, and internal urethral orifice

Coronal section at the level of the urethral opening in the male, anterior view.

The interior of the bladder is lined with a relatively thick mucosal layer (urothelium and associated underlying connective tissue, see **D**). Except for at the bladder trigone, it is easily movable and is thrown into folds when the bladder is not distended. The bladder trigone is an area of smooth mucosa at the base of the bladder or at the bladder neck between the urethral opening and the two ureters, which enter the bladder on its dorsolateral aspect. In the upper border of the trigone is the interureteric crest, a ridge, produced by the interureteric muscle that extends between the orifices of the two ureters. Inferiorly, the internal urethral sphincter, shaped like an elliptical cylinder in the male and a circular cylinder in the female, surrounds the internal urethral orifice.

Note the slit-like ureteral orifice and the oblique transit of the ureter through the bladder wall. This obliquity creates a normal constriction in the intramural part of the ureter (see p. 319). The oblique course, the ureteral muscle, and the bladder-wall muscle provide for functional closure of the ureteral orifice and guard against reflux.

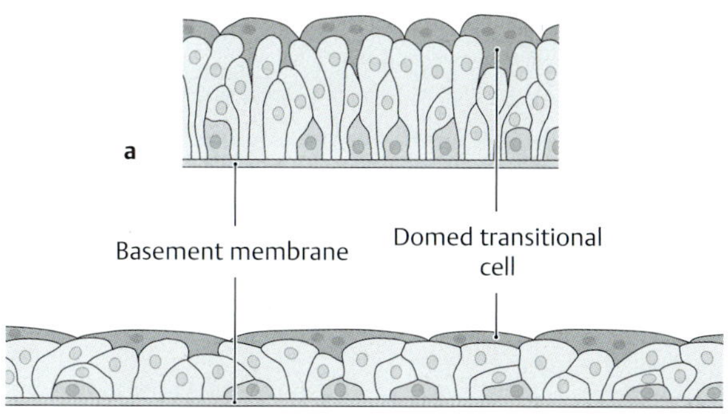

D Epithelium of the bladder mucosa

a Bladder empty: tall epithelium. **b** Bladder full: flattened epithelium.

Like almost all portions of the urinary tract (except the distal urethra), the bladder is lined by transitional epithelium (urothelium) whose height and stratification depend on the degree of distention of the urinary tract segment. The transitional epithelium basically consists of multiple cell layers. The conspicuous cells in the surface layer are called "transitional cells" because they change shape.

Note: The total thickness of the bladder wall (muscle plus mucosa) ranges from 2 to 5 mm in the full bladder and from 8 to 15 mm in the empty bladder.

E Emptying and closing the bladder: micturition and continence

Micturition is the process of emptying the bladder. The ability to hold urine with a full bladder is called *continence*. Coordinated interaction of muscular mechanisms for opening and closing the bladder is crucial for optimal bladder function. Involuntary (autonomic) and voluntary (pudendal nerve) control of the muscular apparatus of the bladder and the urethra play an important role in (cf. p. 334)

- Emptying the bladder completely during micturition,
- Protecting the ureteral orifice from reflux, and
- Maintaining urinary continence with a full bladder.

Emptying the bladder (micturition): activation of the sacral micturition center by a center in the brainstem (pontine micturition center); contraction of the detrusor muscle thereby raising the pressure within the bladder (supported by an increase in intraabdominal pressure, abdominal press); relaxation of the internal sphincter and contraction of the urethral dilator and pubovesical muscle, dilating the urethra (internal urethral orifice); simultaneous closure of the two ureteral orifices by the trigone muscles; relaxation of the external sphincter including both the smooth and striated muscle portions and detumescence of the submucosal venous plexus; voiding of the bladder occurs.

Closing the bladder (continence): structures responsible for maintaining continence primarily include the muscular mechanisms for closing the bladder and urethra (internal sphincter and external sphincter), the ventral suspension apparatus (see p. 325) and parts of the pelvic floor and perineal body. Optimal interaction of these distinct structures ensures continence.

Note: At rest, the urethra forms an angle between its posterior margin and the base of the bladder of 110–120 degrees (posterior vesicourethral angle) in both the male and female. An increased angle due to pelvic floor descent results in incontinence.

4.9 Functional Anatomy of Urinary Continence

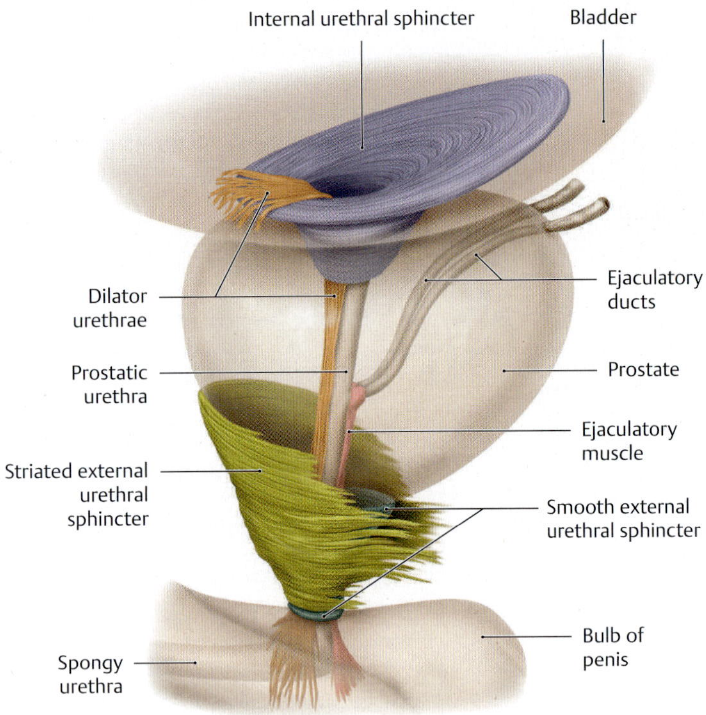

A Muscles of the bladder neck and proximal urethra in the male
According to Dorschner et al (2001) and Schwalenberg et al (2010), maintaining continence occurs by the interaction of distinct functional units including the anatomically correct positions of the sphincter muscles, tone of the urethral smooth and striated musculature, and a ventral suspensory mechanism at the level of the bladder neck. Dysfunction of one of these components may cause urethral hypermobility and result in incontinence. Two muscular systems are differentiated:

- **A system of sphincter muscles:**
  - internal urethral sphincter,
  - external urethral sphincter with smooth and striated muscle portions,
  - longitudinal urethral musculature with smooth ventral urethral musculature and dorsal longitudinal ejaculatory musculature.
- **A musculofibrous anchoring system in the pelvic floor:**
  - ventral vesicourethral suspension apparatus made up of pubovesical muscle, pubourethral and puboprostatic ligaments and the tendinous arch of the pelvic fascia from which the bladder neck is suspended;
  - perineal body (central tendon of the perineum) which counters and anchors the external urethral sphincter.

Note: Except for the dorsal longitudinal ejaculatory muscle, all structures are found in both males and females.

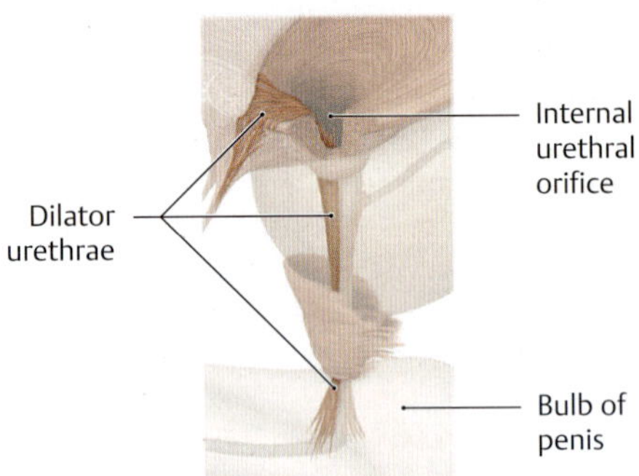

B Dilator urethrae
This is the ventral longitudinal urethral musculature. It is a fan-shaped muscle that arises from the symphysis and along the tendinous arch of the pelvic fascia (see **E**). It runs over the top of the ventral circumference of the internal urethral sphincter and through the internal urethral orifice. It extends inferiorly along the anterior surface of the urethra, where it inserts on the bulb of penis. The urethra is shortened and the internal urethral orifice is widened by the contraction of the longitudinal musculature. This allows initiation of micturition.

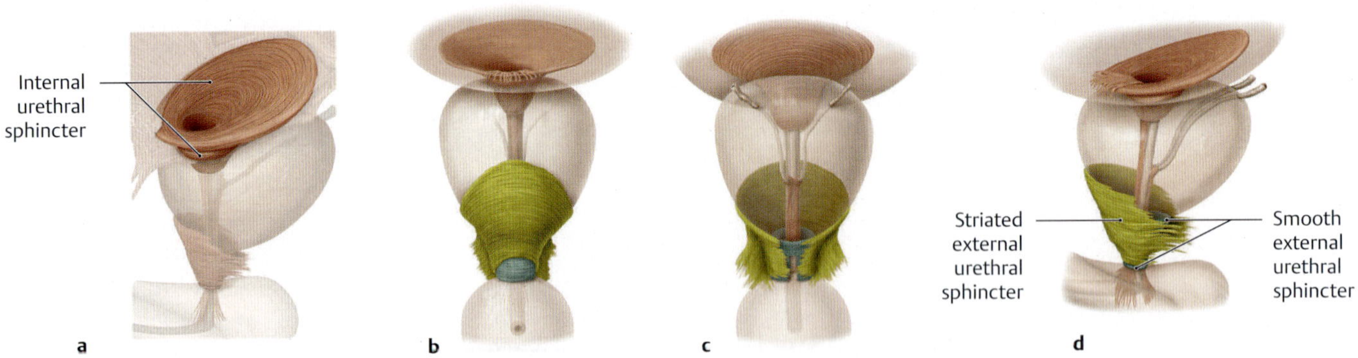

C Internal urethral sphincter and external urethral sphincter
a Internal urethral sphincter; **b–d** External urethral sphincter, anterior, posterior, and lateral views.
According to Dorschner et al. (2001), the internal sphincter is a distinct, independent functional sphincter. Its smooth musculature is not related to the detrusor or urethral musculature. Thus, it does not arise from the trigone or detrusor musculature. Generally, the internal sphincter is more distinct in the male than the female, in particular the urethral portion, which extends to the proximal urethra. One reason may be that in the male the internal sphincter ensures not only continence but also the effective closure of the bladder neck to prevent retrograde ejaculation (dual function). According to Dorschner et al. (see above), the external sphincter consists of

- an inner circular layer of smooth muscle, and
- an outer striated layer, which has an omega or horseshoe shape and a depression in its posterior surface.

Note: Numerous studies have shown that the striated external sphincter (like the internal sphincter) is an independent muscle and is not split off from the levator ani or the deep transverse perineal muscles.

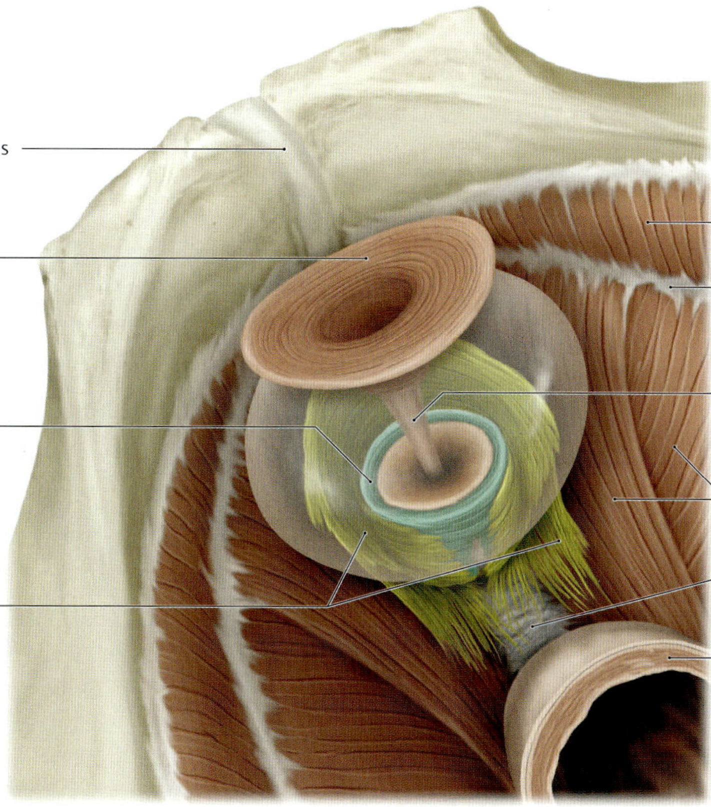

D Integration of the external urethral sphincter into its surroundings

Anteriorly and laterally, the outer portion of the external urethral sphincter borders the distinct venous plexus (see **E**) and is partially interspersed with veins. According to Wallner et al. (2009) and Schwalenberg et al. (2010) the lateral fibers of the external sphincter extends into the fascia of the levator ani. Additionally, it has been discussed whether its muscle fibers are anchored to the perineal body. As a result, when the external sphincter contracts, its fibers stretch to both sides of the levator ani, where it is dynamically anchored. Whereas the circular muscle fibers of the smooth external urethral sphincter exert light but permanent pressure on the membranous urethra, the striated external urethral sphincter, which receives somatic innervation, together with the perineal body and the levator ani are able to increase the urethral closure pressure (= improved continence) during pelvic floor contraction.

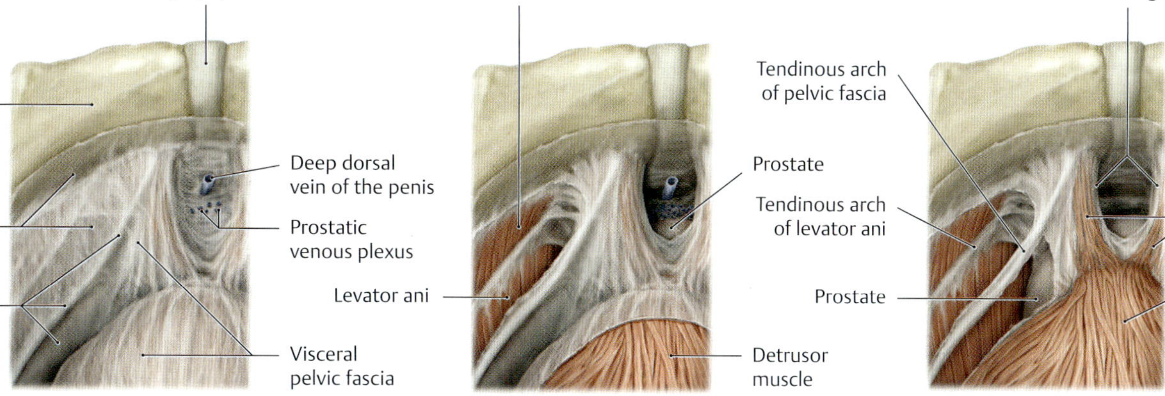

E Ventral vesicourethral suspension apparatus

Aside from the anterolateral stabilization of the vesicourethral junction, the most important function of the ventral suspension apparatus in the retropubic space is suspension of the bladder neck, which ensures continence (Schwalenberg et al. 2010). Essential components of the ventral suspension apparatus include the pubovesical muscles and the tendinous arch of the pelvic fascia, which is a thickened band of the pelvic fascia that extends from the pubic symphysis over the pelvic diaphragm to the ischial spine. There the visceral and the parietal layers (superior fascia of the pelvic diaphragm) merge. The tendinous arch of the pelvic fascia, partially due to its anterior extensions, serves as an additional aponeurotic insertion of the pubovesical muscles that extend as the continuation of the ventral outer longitudinal layer of the detrusor muscle on both sides of the symphysis to the pubic bone. The pubourethral and puboprostatic ligaments listed in the Nomina Anatomica are not ligaments in the proper sense. They are strong sheets of connective tissue of the visceral and parietal pelvic fascia and extend from the pubic symphysis to the bladder neck or prostate

Note: Protection and restoration of the structures of the ventral suspension apparatus as described above have led to a significant decrease in postoperative incontinence after surgery to remove the prostate.

4.10 Urethra

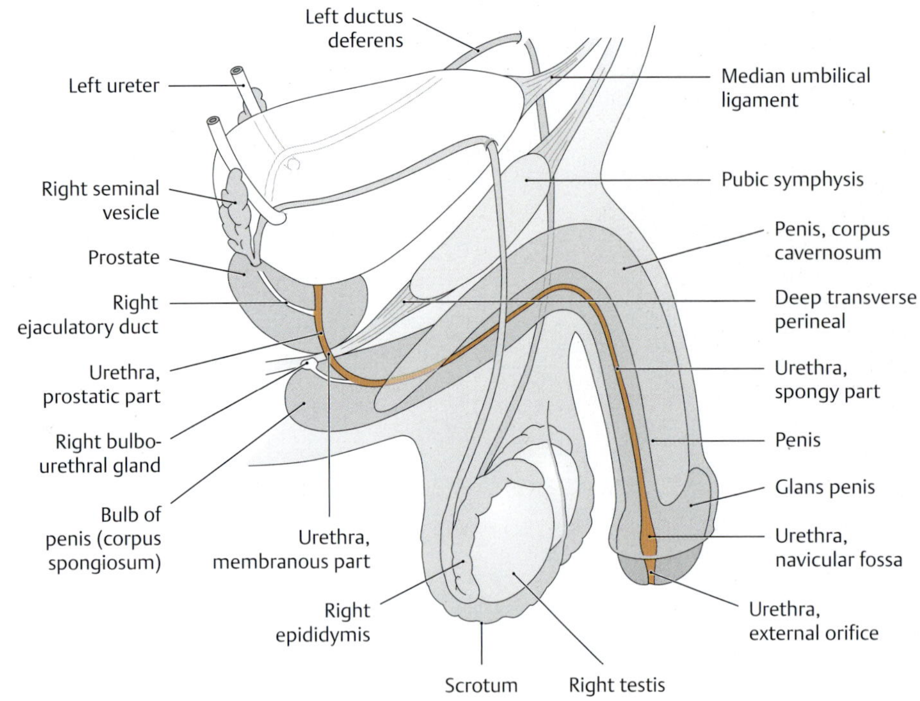

A Parts of the male urethra
Male urogenital system in the pelvis, viewed from the right side. Unlike the female urethra, the male urethra functions as a common urinary *and* genital passage. It has an average length of 20 cm and consists of four parts with three constrictions and three expansions (see **B**). The intramural part of the urethra in the bladder wall is not shown here. While the female urethra is essentially straight (see **E**), the male urethra presents two curves: *an infrapubic curve* and a *prepubic curve*. These curves are important in transurethral bladder catheterization (see **F**).

B Wall segments, constrictions, and expansions of the male urethra (see also **D**)

Wall segments	Constrictions and expansions
Internal urethral orifice	
Intramural part	First constriction: internal urethral sphincter
Prostatic part	First expansion
Membranous part	Second constriction: external urethral sphincter
Spongy part	Second expansion: ampulla Third expansion: navicular fossa
External urethral orifice	Third constriction

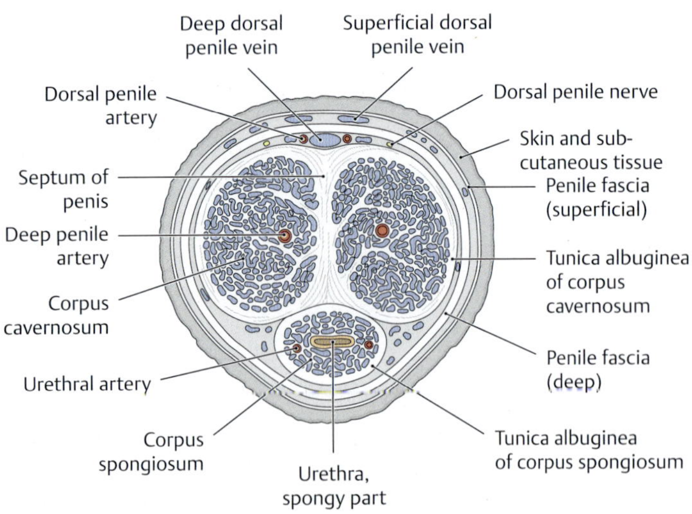

C Location of the male urethra in the penis
Transverse section through the penile shaft. The spongy part of the urethra is contained in the corpus spongiosum of the penis. The corpus spongiosum does not become completely hard even at maximum erection, ensuring that the urethra remains patent during ejaculation. The urethral lumen often presents a flattened rather than circular shape in cross-section, with the upper and lower walls touching.

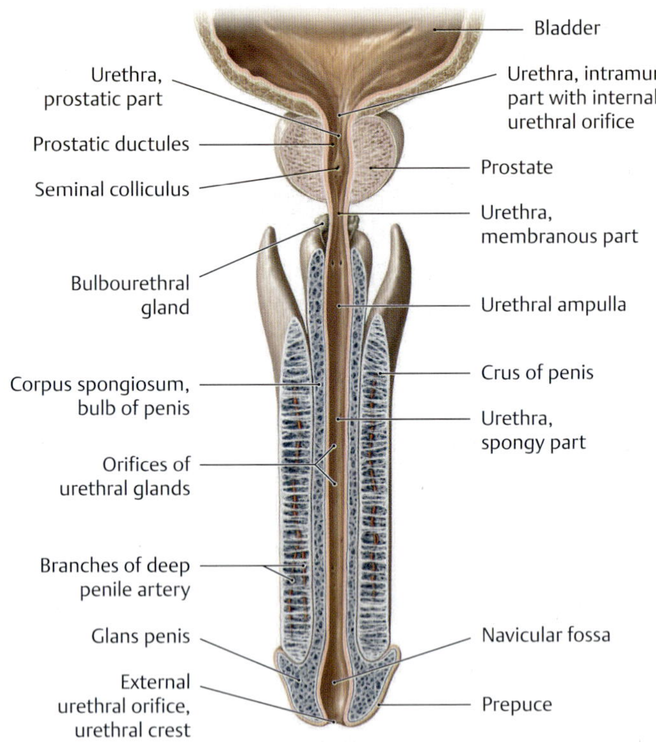

D Male urethra in longitudinal section
The whole length of the urethra has been cut open and displayed without curves, and all of the pelvic floor muscles have been removed. The four parts of the male urethra can be identified. The male urethra extends distally in the corpus spongiosum to its external orifice on the glans penis. The *prostatic* part of the urethra may be greatly narrowed in patients with benign prostatic enlargement (*prostatic hyperplasia*, see p. 356). This condition is often marked by incomplete voiding and the dribbling of urine after micturition. The residual urine left in the bladder may incite an (often bacterial in nature) inflammation of the bladder (cystitis).

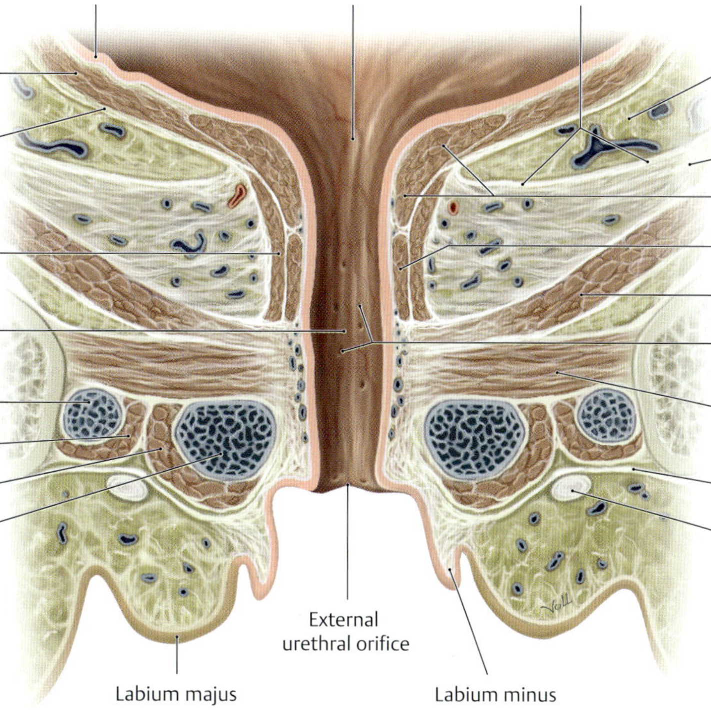

E Female urethra in longitudinal section

Coronal section tilted slightly posterior, anterior view. Unlike the male urethra, the female urethra is straight and only about 3–5 cm long. Thus it is much easier to catheterize than in the male. At the same time, the short length of the female urethra increases susceptibility to urinary tract infections.

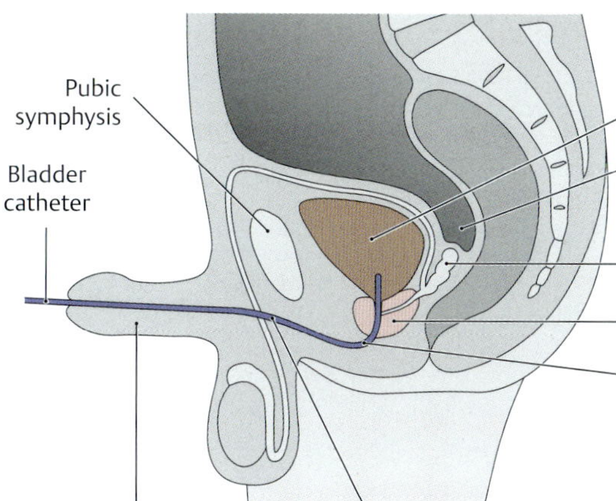

F Transurethral bladder catheterization in the male

The two curves of the male urethra (infrapubic and prepubic) and its three constrictions may pose an obstacle to transurethral catheterization. The prepubic curve can be straightened out somewhat by straightening the penile shaft.

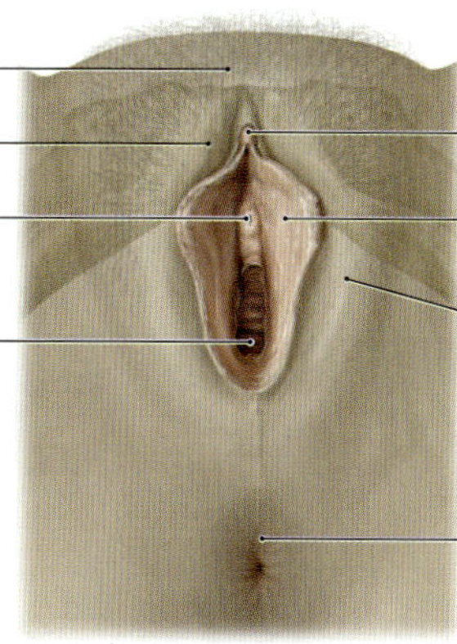

G External orifice of the female urethra

Viewed from below. The pubic bone (pubis) is shown in shadow to aid orientation. The external urethral orifice is located between the labia minora, anterior to the vagina. Despite its proximity to the female external genitalia, the female urethra functions exclusively as a urinary passage. The close topographical relationship of the urethra and external genitalia is important during embryonic development, however: both the urethra and the vagina initially have a common opening at the urogenital sinus and become separated only after further development. Failure of this separation results in an abnormal fistulous connection between the vagina and urethra, a *urethrovaginal fistula*. Even with normal embryonic development, the proximity of the urethra (which is physiologically germ-free) to the vagina (which is not a sterile zone) predisposes to bacterial inflammation of the urethra (urethritis). Given the short length of the female urethra, the infection can easily ascend to the bladder (cystitis).

4.11 Arteries and Veins of the Kidneys and Suprarenal Glands: Overview

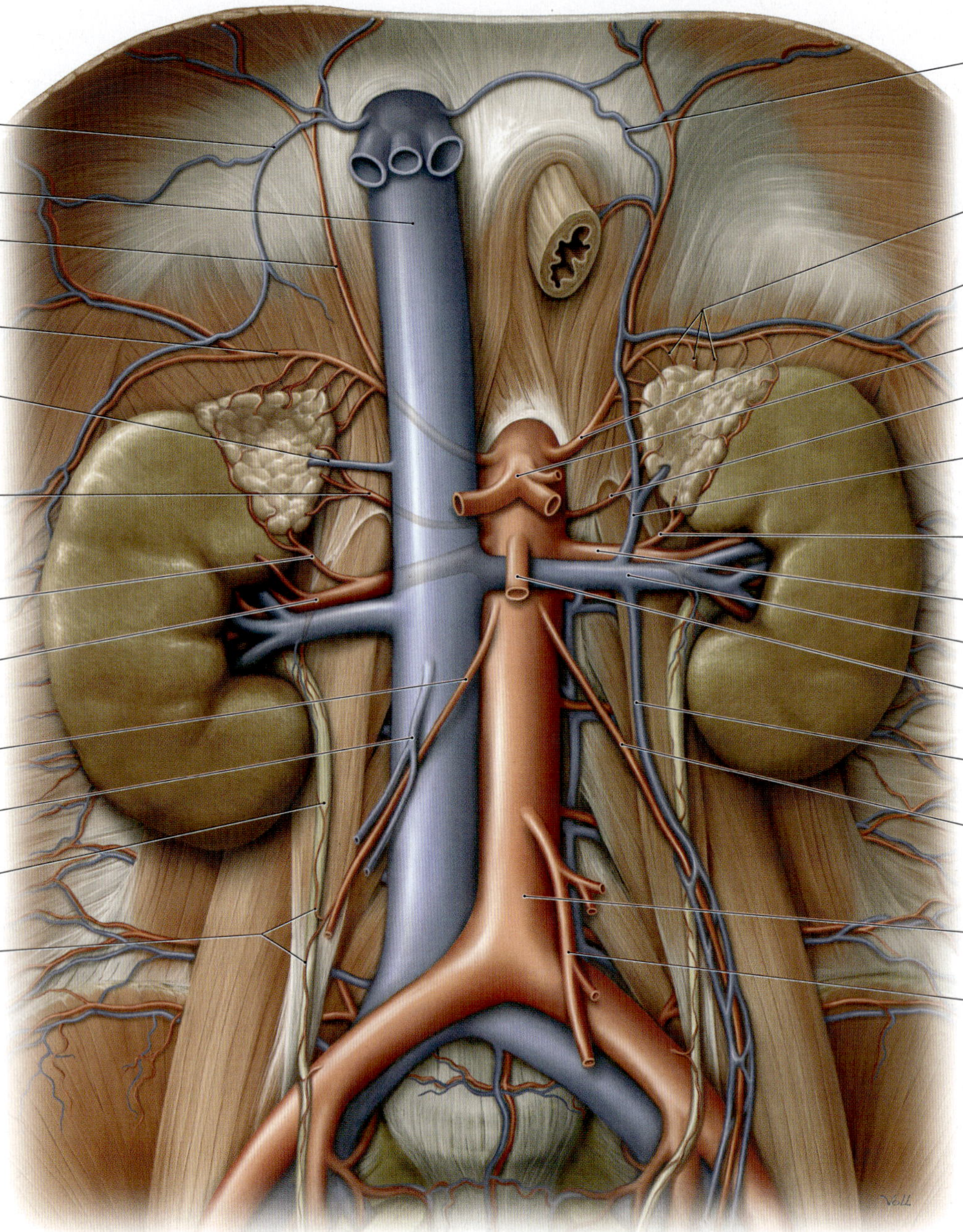

A Overview of the arteries and veins of the kidneys and suprarenal glands

Anterior view. The esophagus has been pulled slightly inferiorly, and the right kidney and suprarenal gland have been pulled away from the inferior vena cava to show the vascular anatomy of the suprarenal gland. The other abdominal organs have been removed.

Renal artery: The renal arteries branch from the sides of the abdominal aorta at the level of the L 1/ L 2 vertebrae (see **C**). The *right* renal artery runs *posterior* to the inferior vena cava (shown transparent in the drawing), and the *left* renal artery runs *posterior* to the left renal vein. Each renal artery divides into an anterior and posterior branch. The renal arteries give off inferior suprarenal arteries to the suprarenal gland, capsular (perirenal) branches to tissue surrounding the kidney and to the renal capsule (fibrous capsule and perirenal fat capsule, removed here for clarity), and ureteral branches to the upper portion of the ureter and the distal renal pelvis. Possible variants are illustrated in **E**, p. 331.

Suprarenal arteries: Superior, middle, and inferior suprarenal arteries (from the inferior phrenic artery, abdominal aorta, and renal artery, see above).

Renal vein: The renal vein on each side is generally formed by the union of two or three venous branches (variants are shown in **F**, p. 331). While the *left* renal vein receives the left suprarenal vein and left testicular or ovarian vein, the *right* renal vein opens directly into the inferior vena cava without receiving these tributaries (see also **D**). The renal vein also receives capsular branches from the renal fibrous capsule in addition to small branches from the renal pelvis and proximal ureter (not shown here).

Suprarenal veins:

Note: The three main arteries of the suprarenal glands (see above) are generally accompanied *by only one vein* (rarely two), the *suprarenal vein*. While the *left* suprarenal vein opens into the left renal vein, frequently anastomosing with the left inferior phrenic vein (as shown here), the *right* suprarenal vein empties directly into the inferior vena cava (see also **D**).

* The blood vessels supplying the bladder are discussed together with the neurovascular structures of the internal genital organs that are also located in the pelvis (see p. 364).

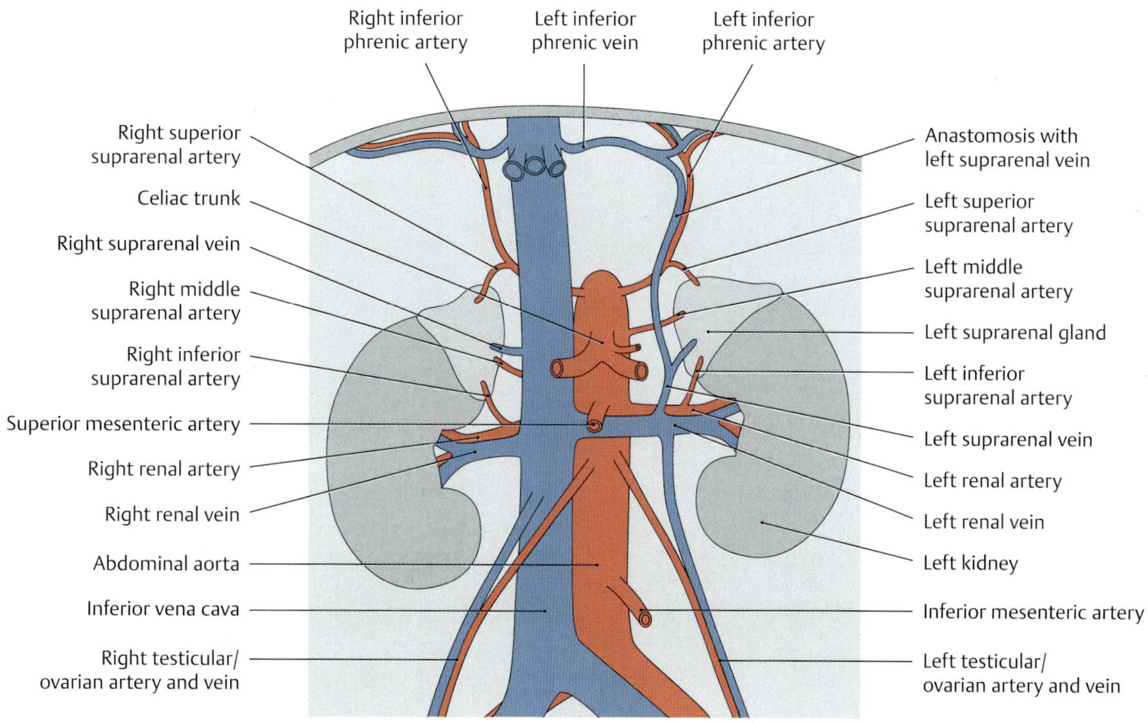

B Arteries and veins of the kidneys and suprarenal glands

Anterior view. The right kidney and suprarenal gland have been slightly retracted from the inferior vena cava to display their blood vessels more clearly.

It is evident in this diagram and in **A** that the suprarenal glands have a more complex vascular anatomy than the kidneys: More than 50 small branches may pass from the arterial trunks of the suprarenal glands (superior, middle, and inferior suprarenal arteries) into the glands.

Note that the three main arteries of the suprarenal glands are generally accompanied by only one vein, the suprarenal vein. This vessel opens *directly* into the inferior vena cava on the *right* side and into the renal vein on the *left* side (see **D**).

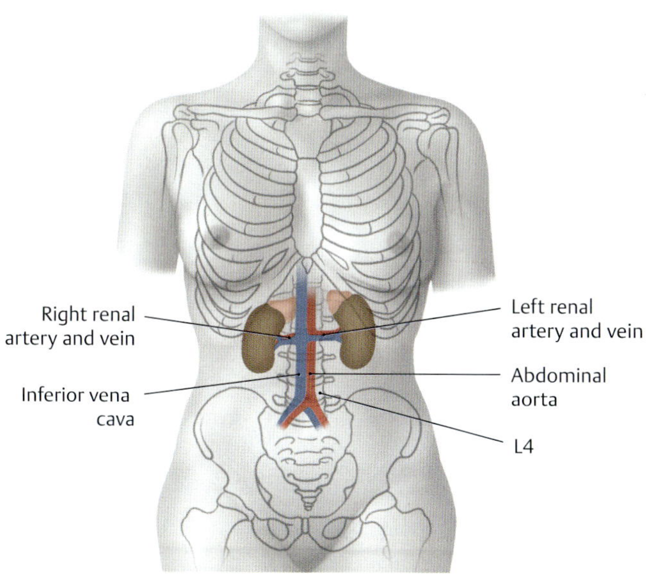

C Projection of the renal arteries and veins onto the vertebral column

The renal artery arises from the abdominal aorta at the L 1/L 2 level.

Note: The renal veins lie anterior to the arteries.

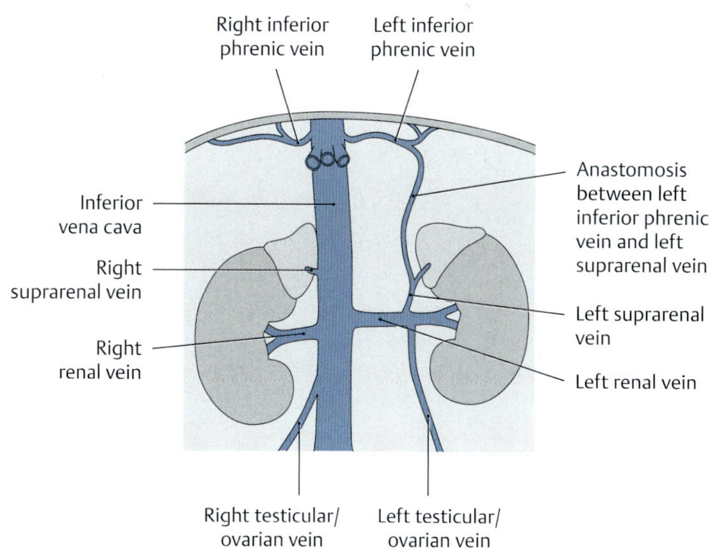

D Tributaries of the left renal vein

The renal vein has more tributaries on the left side than on the right. The *left* renal vein receives the left suprarenal vein (often anastomosing with the left inferior phrenic vein, see **A**) and the left testicular/ovarian vein, whereas the corresponding veins on the *right* side open *directly* into the inferior vena cava. Because of this arrangement, varicose dilations of the veins in the spermatic cord (varicoceles) are more common on the left side than on the right.

4.12 Arteries and Veins of the Kidneys and Suprarenal Glands: Variants

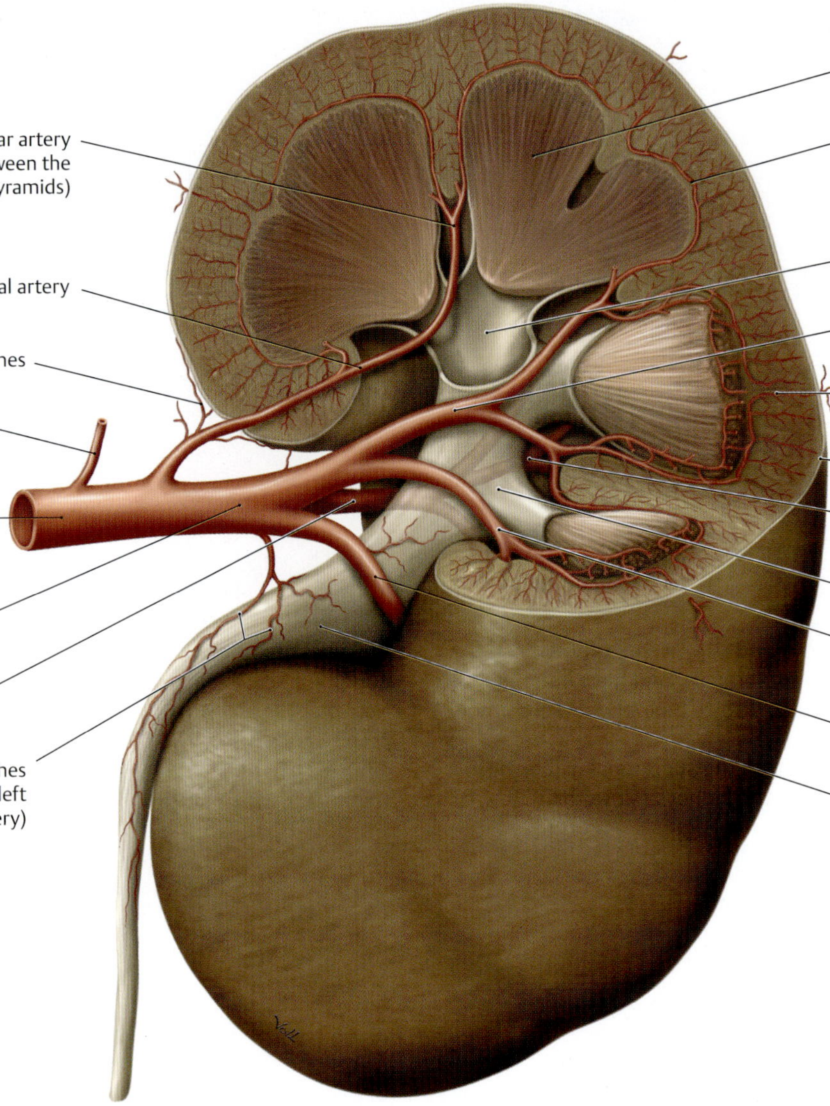

A Division of the renal artery into segmental arteries
Anterior view of the left kidney.
The main trunk of the renal artery divides into an anterior and posterior branch. The anterior branch divides further into four segmental arteries:

- Superior segmental artery
- Anterior superior segmental artery
- Anterior inferior segmental artery
- Inferior segmental artery

The posterior branch gives rise to only one segmental vessel, the posterior segmental artery.

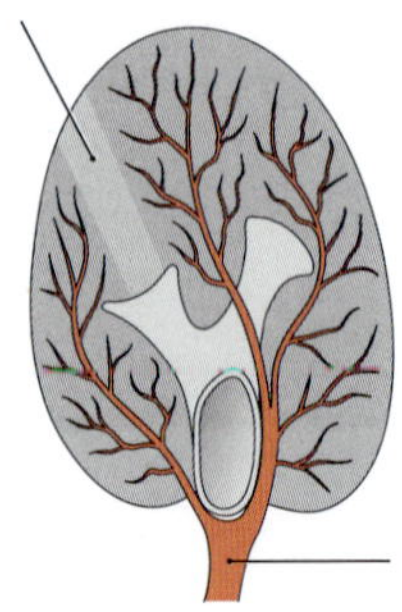

B "Avascular" zone in the kidney
Inferior view of the right kidney.
Between the posterior segment and anterior segments is a relatively avascular zone of the kidney, which otherwise is *very heavily vascularized*. This zone provides an important line of access for intrarenal surgery.

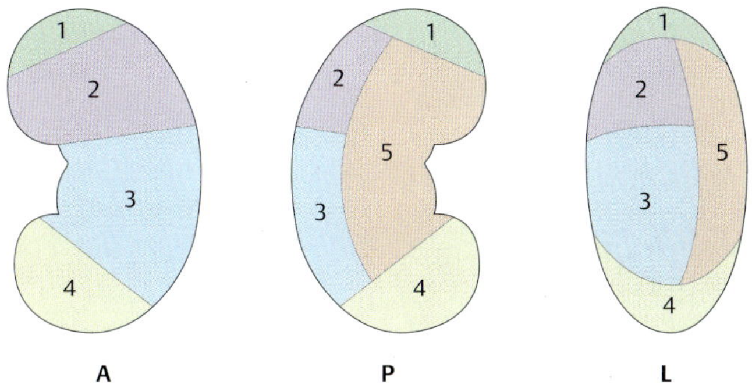

C Vascular segmentation of the kidney
Left kidney viewed from the anterior (A), posterior (P), and lateral (L) sides.
The renal artery and its branches divide the kidney into five segments:

1 Superior segment
2 Anterior superior segment
3 Anterior inferior segment
4 Inferior segment
5 Posterior segment

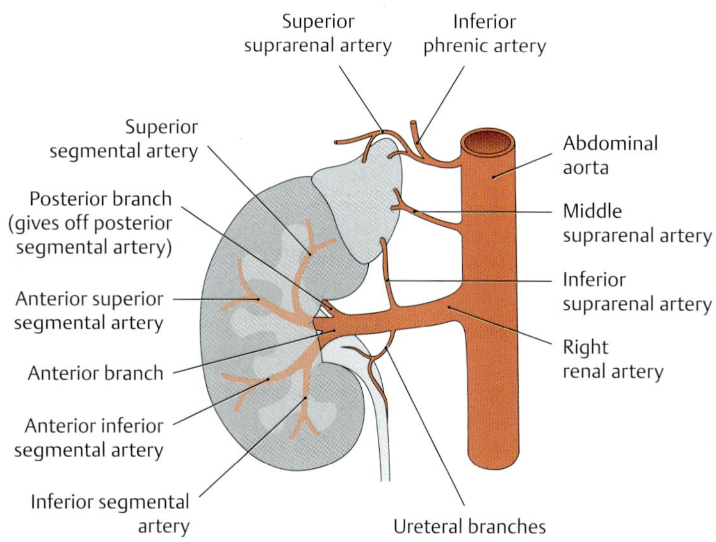

D Relationship of the renal arterial branches to the renal segments
Anterior view of the right kidney, demonstrating the origins of the renal artery, middle suprarenal artery, and inferior phrenic artery from the abdominal aorta.
Note the division of the renal artery into an anterior branch (anterior segments, superior and inferior segments) and a posterior branch (for the posterior segment, see also **A**). The upper part of the ureter is supplied by ureteral branches from the renal artery.

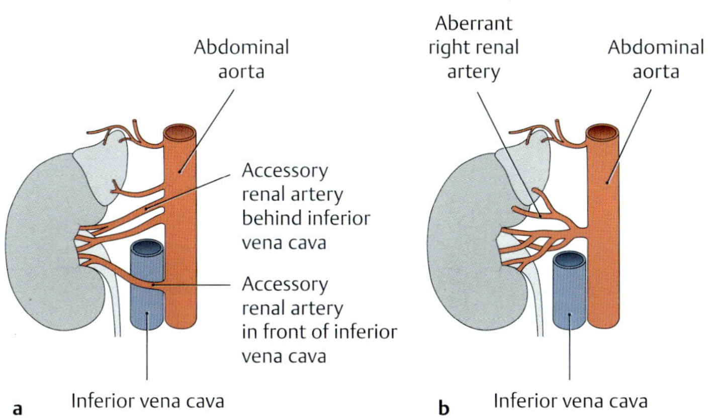

E Variants of the renal arteries
Anterior view of the right kidney.

a Two accessory renal arteries (one crossing in front of the inferior vena cava): Accessory renal arteries are extra arteries that pass from the abdominal aorta to the renal hilum. As a common variant with accessory renal arteries, the inferior suprarenal artery does not arise from the renal artery.
b An *aberrant* renal artery is one that does not enter the kidney at the renal hilum.

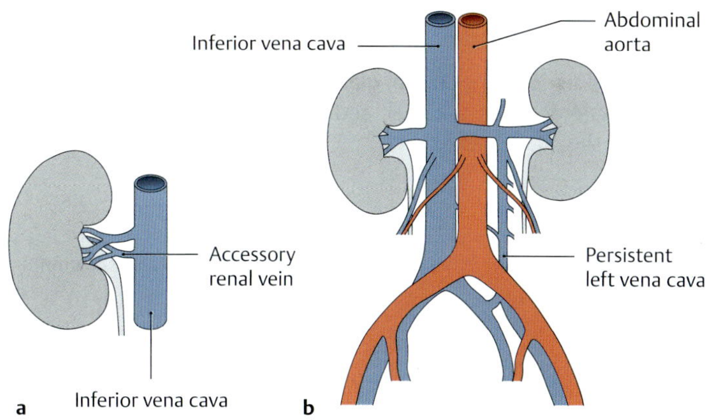

F Variants of the renal veins
Anterior view.

a Accessory (supernumerary) renal veins
b A left vena cava (persistent lower part of the supracardinal vein) ascends to the level of the left renal vein and opens into it.

4.13 Lymphatic Drainage of the Kidneys, Suprarenal Glands, Ureter, and Urinary Bladder

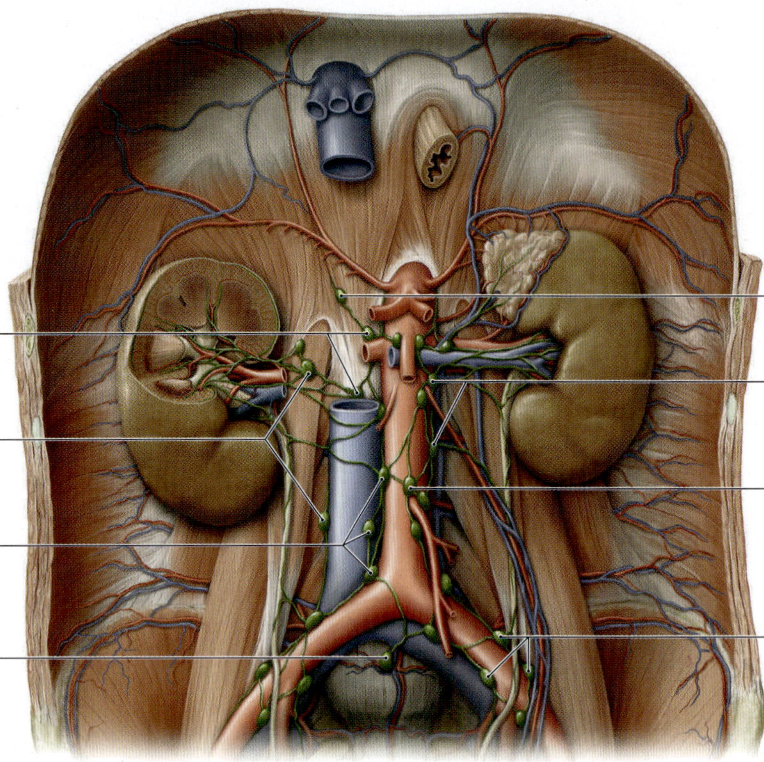

A Lymphatic drainage of the kidney, suprarenal gland, and ureter (abdominal part; the pelvic part is shown in **C**)
Anterior view. The following lymphatic pathways are important in this region (see also p. 237):

- **Right kidney and suprarenal gland:** drain to the *right lumbar lymph nodes* (lateral caval, precaval, and retrocaval lymph nodes, see **B**), then to the *right lumbar trunk*.
- **Left kidney and suprarenal gland:** drain to the *left lumbar lymph nodes* (lateral aortic, preaortic, and retroaortic lymph nodes, see **B**), then to the *left lumbar trunk*.
- **Ureter (abdominal part):** follows the pathway for the right and left kidneys and suprarenal glands (see also **C**).

The lumbar lymph nodes additionally function as collecting lymph nodes for the common iliac nodes.

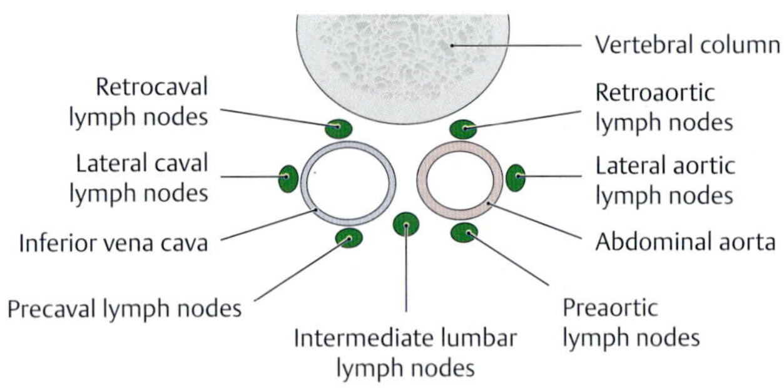

B Classification of the lumbar lymph nodes
Transverse section, viewed from above. The lumbar lymph nodes are distributed around the abdominal aorta and inferior vena cava. They are divided into three groups based on their relationship to these vessels:

- Left lumbar lymph nodes (around the aorta)
- Intermediate lumbar lymph nodes (between the aorta and inferior vena cava)
- Right lumbar lymph nodes (around the inferior vena cava)

These groups are further divided into subgroups (see legend of **A**).

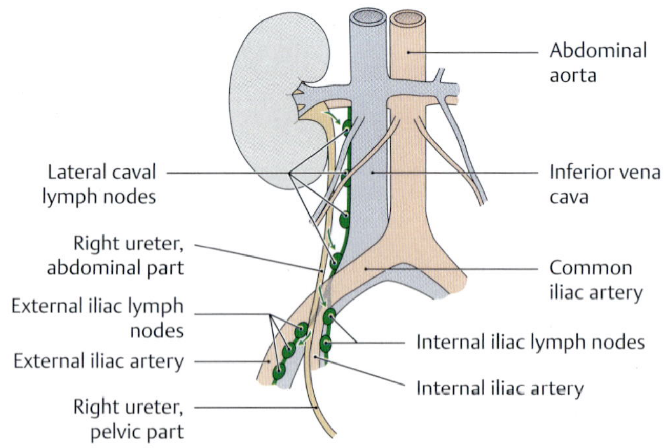

C Lymph nodes of the ureter
Anterior view of the right ureter.
The lymphatic drainage of the ureter is roughly divided into two levels:

- Abdominal part of the ureter: lumbar lymph nodes
  - Right: lateral caval lymph nodes (right lumbar lymph nodes)
  - Left: lateral aortic lymph nodes (left lumbar lymph nodes)
- Pelvic part of the ureter: external and internal iliac lymph nodes.

Both pathways empty into the lumbar trunks.

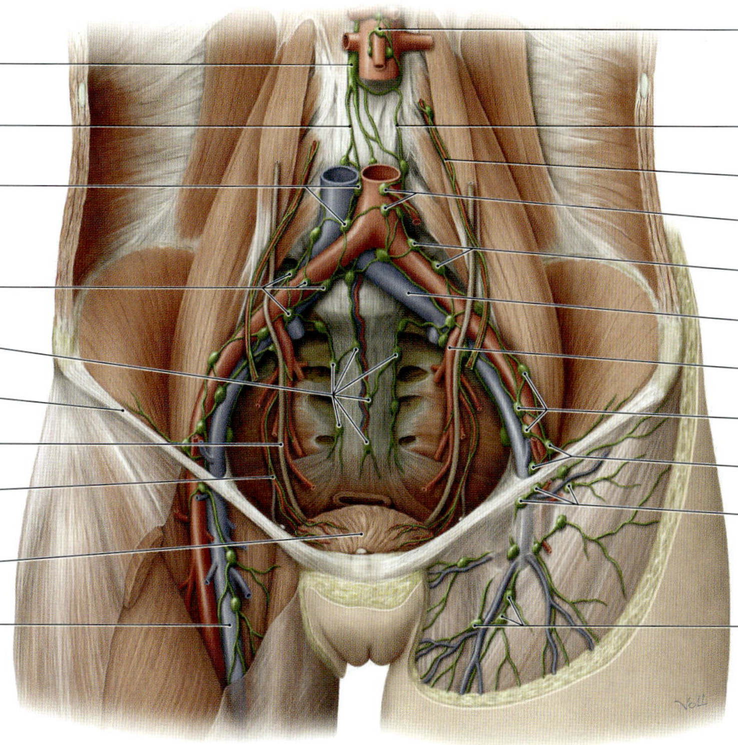

D Overview of the pelvic lymph nodes and the lymphatic drainage of the bladder

Anterior view of an opened female abdomen and pelvis. All organs have been removed except for the bladder and a small rectal stump, and the peritoneum has been removed. The bladder is distended, making it visible above the pubic symphysis. This drawing clearly shows the numerous parietal lymph nodes that are distributed around the iliac vessels in the pelvis (see **E**). Lymph from the bladder usually drains first to groups of visceral lymph nodes: the lateral vesical lymph nodes and the pre- and retrovesical lymph nodes (known collectively as the paravesical nodes). These nodes are embedded in the pelvic connective tissue surrounding the bladder and lie so deep within the pelvis that they are not visible here. Lymph from these visceral nodes drains directly or indirectly along two major pathways, reaching lymph nodes lateral to the abdominal aorta and inferior vena cava (lumbar lymph nodes) and finally entering the lumbar trunks. These pathways are illustrated in **F**.

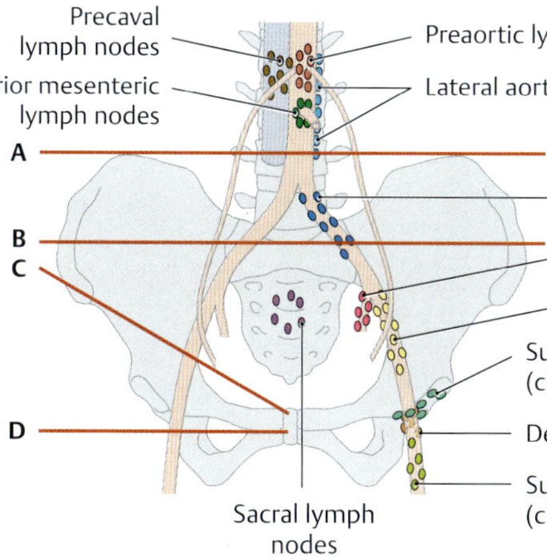

E Overview of the pelvic lymph nodes

The pelvic lymph nodes are distributed along major blood vessels and in front of the sacrum. The blood vessels are not visualized by lymphography (contrast radiography of the lymph nodes), however, and so the location of the pelvic lymph nodes must be determined by other means. One method is to use four reference lines based on skeletal landmarks:

- **A** Iliolumbar line: horizontal line tangent to the superior borders of the iliac crests
- **B** Iliosacral line: horizontal line through the center of the sacroiliac joint
- **C** Inguinal line: line along the inguinal ligament
- **D** Obturator line: horizontal line through the center of the obturator foramen

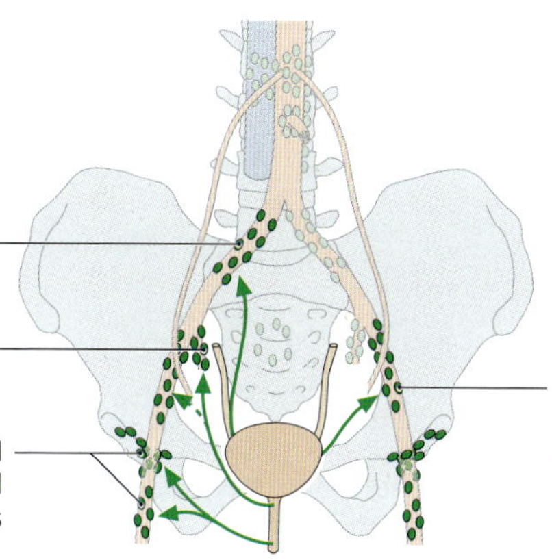

F Lymphatic drainage of the bladder and urethra

The **bladder** is drained by two principal pathways:

- Cranially along the visceral iliac vessels (see **D**)
- To the internal and external iliac lymph nodes (mainly at the base of the bladder)

Portions of the bladder near the internal urethral orifice are drained by the superficial and deep inguinal lymph nodes. The **urethra** drains chiefly to the deep and superficial inguinal lymph nodes (the latter mainly draining areas near the external urethral orifice). The proximal portions of the urethra are drained by the iliac lymph nodes, particularly the internal iliac nodes.

Note: The penis, like the urethra, is drained by the superficial and deep inguinal lymph nodes.

4.14 Autonomic Innervation of the Urinary Organs and Suprarenal Glands

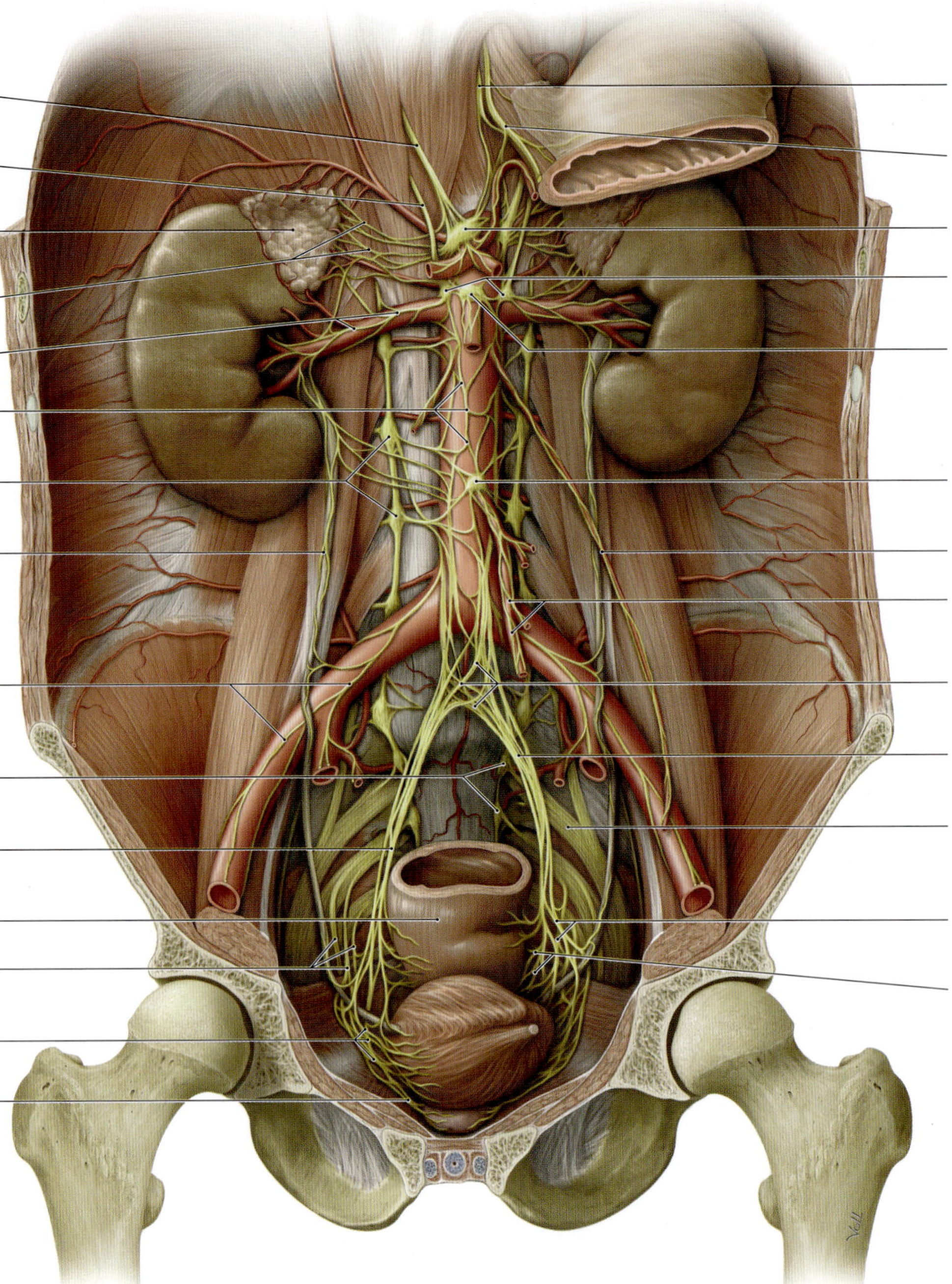

A Overview of the autonomic innervation of the urinary organs and suprarenal glands

Anterior view into an opened male abdomen and pelvis. The stomach has been largely removed and pulled slightly inferior with the esophagus for better exposure. The right kidney has been displaced slightly laterally, and the bladder has been straightened and retracted to the left. The pelvis has been sectioned in a coronal plane passing approximately through the center of the acetabula. The autonomic innervation of the urinary organs and suprarenal glands varies according to the location of the specific organ:

- The **kidneys in the retroperitoneum** and portions of the upper urinary tract (**proximal ureters**) receive *sympathetic* fibers initially from the lesser, least, and lumbar splanchnic nerves (see **B**), which synapse with the postsynaptic neuron in the aorticorenal or renal ganglia. The *parasympathetic* fibers originate from the posterior vagal trunk and partly from the pelvic splanchnic nerves (the plexuses are described in **B**).
- The **suprarenal cortex and medulla in the retroperitoneum** receive *sympathetic* fibers from the greater and lesser splanchnic nerves. They receive *parasympathetic* fibers from the posterior vagal trunk, which pass with the renal plexus to the suprarenal glands as the suprarenal plexus. The *sympathetic* autonomic innervation of the suprarenal medulla is exceptional in that the suprarenal medulla is supplied only by presynaptic sympathetic fibers from the suprarenal plexus. These axons directly innervate the suprarenal medullary cells. At present, there is no convincing evidence that the suprarenal medulla receives *parasympathetic* innervation.
- The **bladder, most of the abdominal part and pelvic part of the ureter** (and the **urethra**, not shown here) **in the pelvis** (see **D**) receive *sympathetic* fibers from the lumbar and sacral splanchnic nerves, and they receive *parasympathetic* fibers from the pelvic splanchnic nerves (S2–S4). The plexuses are shown in **D**.

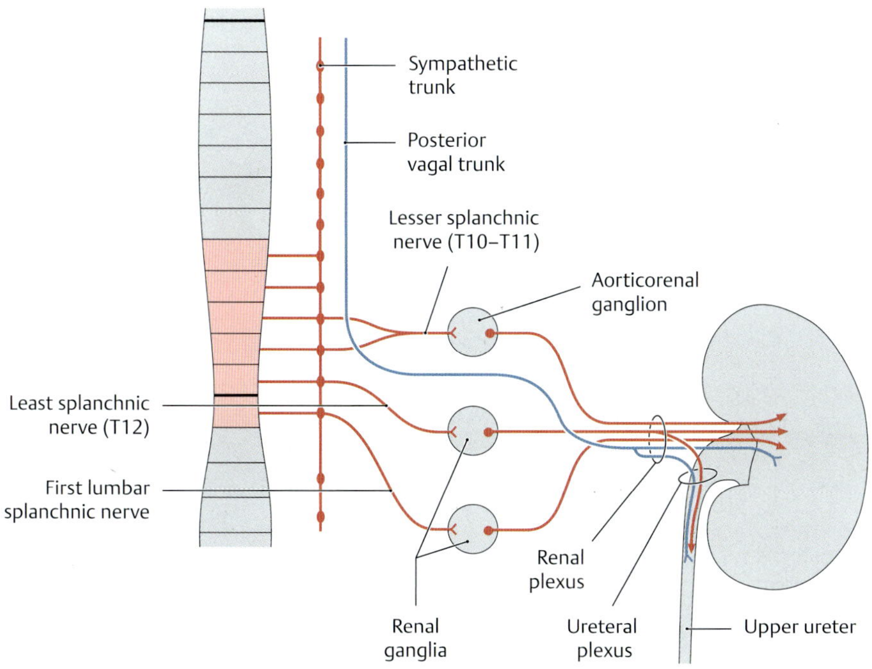

B Autonomic innervation of the kidney and upper ureter

The sympathetic fibers from the aorticorenal ganglia and renal ganglia combine with the parasympathetic fibers from the posterior vagal trunk to form the *renal plexus*, which passes to the kidney. Branches from that plexus form the *ureteral plexus*, which supplies the abdominal (upper) part of the ureter. The presynaptic sympathetic fibers come primarily from the thoracic splanchnic nerves.

Note: Due to their topographic proximity, the aorticorenal ganglia often merge with the celiac ganglia. Illustrations providing an overview, such as on page 70, often show the kidneys as receiving their innervation from the celiac ganglia. Functionally, however, the aorticorenal ganglia are separate and are thus separately mentioned in the schematic diagram.

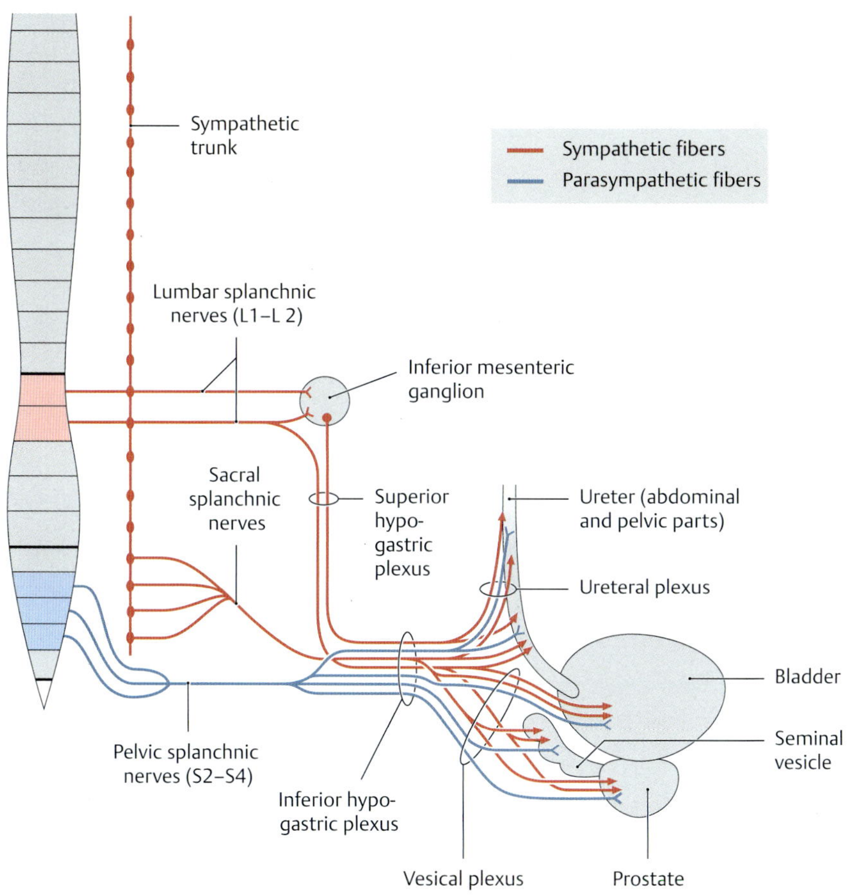

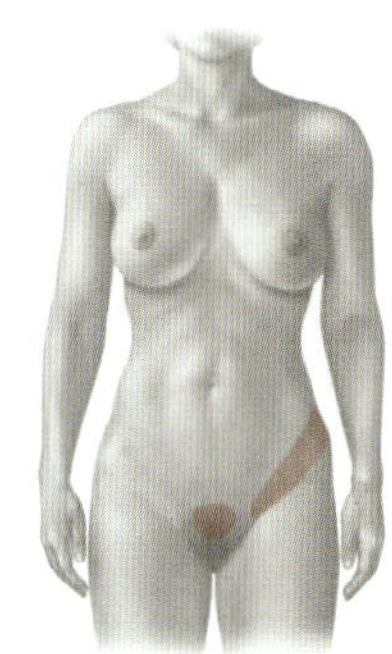

C Referred pain from the left kidney and bladder

Pain associated with diseases of the kidney and bladder (inflammation, calculi) may be perceived in these skin areas. Occasionally the pain radiates into the groin ("loin to groin pain").

D Autonomic innervation of the bladder and the abdominal and pelvic parts of the ureter

Sympathetic fibers from the lumbar and sacral splanchnic nerves pass with the parasympathetic fibers from the pelvic splanchnic nerves to the inferior hypogastric plexus. Branches from that plexus are distributed to form additional plexuses, including the vesical and ureteral plexuses that supply the bladder and ureter (its abdominal and pelvic parts). For the *parasympathetic* fibers, the synapse with the postsynaptic neuron is located entirely in the inferior hypogastric plexus (or organ wall). The *sympathetic* fibers synapse partly in the inferior mesenteric ganglion and partly in the inferior hypogastric plexus (see the fibers that continue from the superior hypogastric plexus to the inferior hypogastric plexus).

Note: With a complete transection of the spinal cord, the effect of higher CNS centers on the central parasympathetic neurons of S2–S4 (pelvic splanchnic nerves) is abolished. Because the pelvic splanchnic nerves initiate and control micturition, a complete cord lesion also causes problems of bladder control.

5.1 Overview of the Genital Tract

Classification of the genital organs

The genital organs of the male and female can be classified in various ways:

- Topographically (**A**) as
  - internal genital organs (internal genitalia) or
  - external genital organs (external genitalia)
- Functionally (**B**, **C**) as
  - organs for germ-cell and hormone production (gonads) or
  - organs of transport, incubation and copulation, plus accessory sex glands
- Ontogenically (see p. 62) as
  - the undifferentiated gonad primordium (develops into the gonads)
  - two undifferentiated duct systems (develop into the male and female transport organs, the female uterus, a portion of the female copulatory organ, and one of the accessory sex glands in the male)
  - the urogenital sinus and its derivatives (giving rise to the external genitalia of both sexes, the accessory sex glands, and portions of the copulatory organs)

A Male and female internal and external genitalia*

See also *Atlas of Anatomy, General Anatomy and Musculoskeletal System*, which includes a detailed discussion of the external genitalia as part of the trunk wall.

	Male	Female
Internal genitalia	Testis Epididymis Ductus deferens Prostate Seminal vesicle Bulbourethral gland	Ovary Uterus Uterine tube Vagina (upper portion)
External genitalia	Penis and urethra Scrotum and coverings of the testis	Vagina (vestibule only) Labia majora and minora Mons pubis Greater and lesser vestibular glands Clitoris

* The *female* external genitalia (pudenda) are known clinically as the *vulva*.

B Functions of the male genital organs

Organ	Function
Testis	Germ-cell production Hormone production
Epididymis	Reservoir for sperm (sperm maturation)
Ductus deferens	Transport organ for sperm
Urethra	Transport organ for sperm and urine
Accessory sex glands (prostate, seminal vesicles, and bulbourethral glands)	Production of secretions (semen)
Penis	Copulatory and urinary organ

C Functions of the female genital organs

Organ	Function
Ovary	Germ-cell production Hormone production
Uterine tube	Site of conception and transport organ for zygote
Uterus	Organ of incubation and parturition
Vagina	Organ of copulation and parturition
Labia majora and minora Clitoris	Copulatory organ
Greater and lesser vestibular glands	Production of secretions

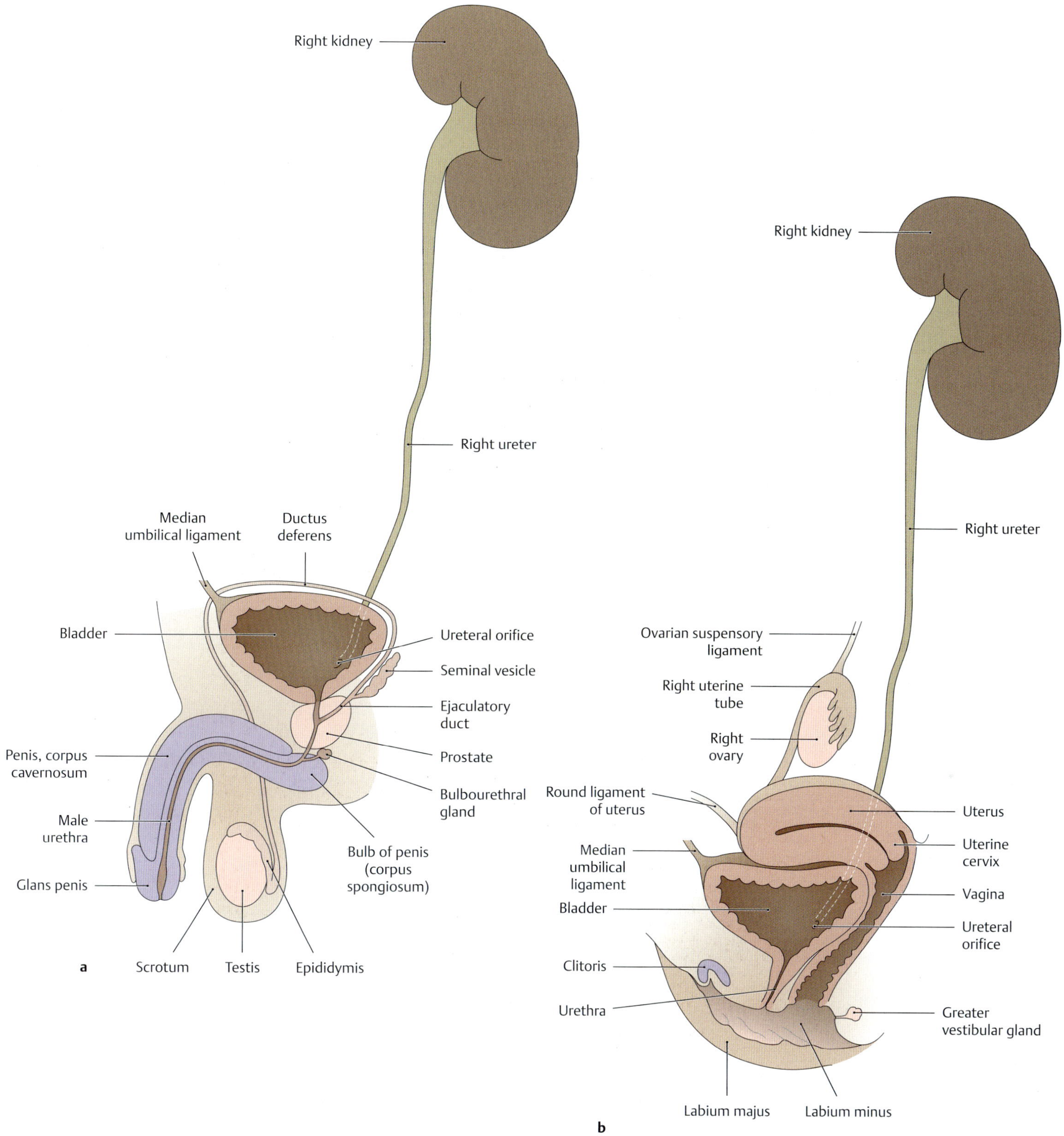

D Overview of the urogenital system

Schematic representation of the urogenital apparatus in the male and female, viewed from the left side. Unpaired pelvic organs and the external genitalia are shown in midsagittal section.

a In the **male**, the urinary and genital organs are closely interrelated functionally and topographically. The urethra passes through the prostata, which is derived embryologically from the urethral epithelium. All of the accessory sex glands (prostate, seminal vesicles, and bulbourethral glands) ultimately discharge their secretions into the urethra.

b In the **female**, the urinary and genital tracts are *functionally* separate from each other. *Topographically*, however, the anterior wall of the uterus is closely related to the vesicula urinaria. In the external genital region as well, the urethra is embedded in the paries anterior of the vagina.

For these reasons, the collective term *urogenital* system is generally used.

5.2 Female Internal Genitalia: Overview

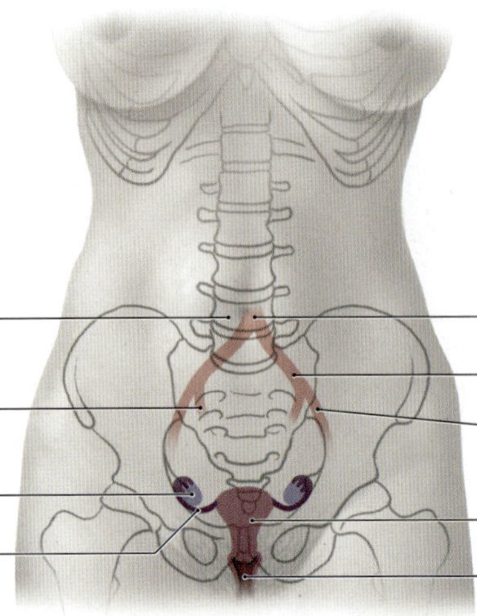

A Projection of the female internal genitalia onto the pelvis
Anterior view. The bifurcation of the abdominal aorta into the common iliac arteries is also shown to aid orientation. The uterus, like the vagina, is located in the pelvic midline while the ovaries are superior, lateral, and posterior to the uterus in the RLQ and LLQ. Each ovary occupies a fossa located just inferior to the division of the common iliac artery. The uterine tubes do not pass to the ovaries by the shortest route but circle around them from the lateral side, because both of the paramesonephric ducts (which develop into the uterine tubes) run lateral to the gonadal ridge in which the ovaries develop.

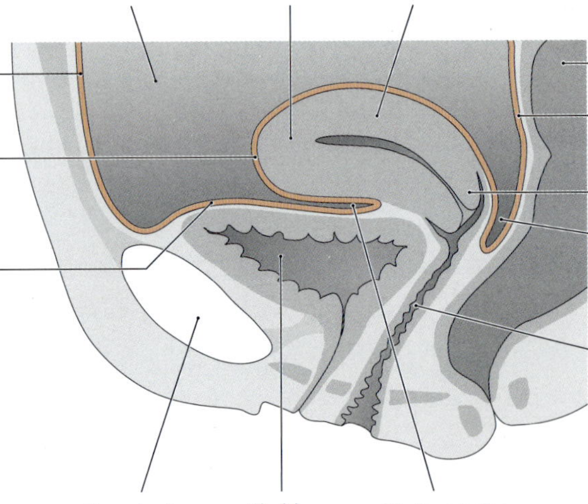

B Uterus and vagina: relationship to the pelvic organs
Midsagittal section through a female pelvis, viewed from the left side. The peritoneum has been outlined in color. The uterus directly overlies the bladder, and the rectum is posterior to the uterus. The fundus and corpus (body) of the uterus are covered by visceral peritoneum, which is reflected onto the bladder and rectum to form the vesicouterine pouch and rectouterine pouch. The peritoneum extends farther down the posterior wall of the uterus than its anterior wall, with the result that the *posterior* part of the uterine cervix and upper vagina is covered by peritoneum while the anterior part is not. The vagina is surrounded on all sides by pelvic connective tissue. This tissue is thickened anteriorly and posteriorly to form the vesicovaginal and rectovaginal septa.

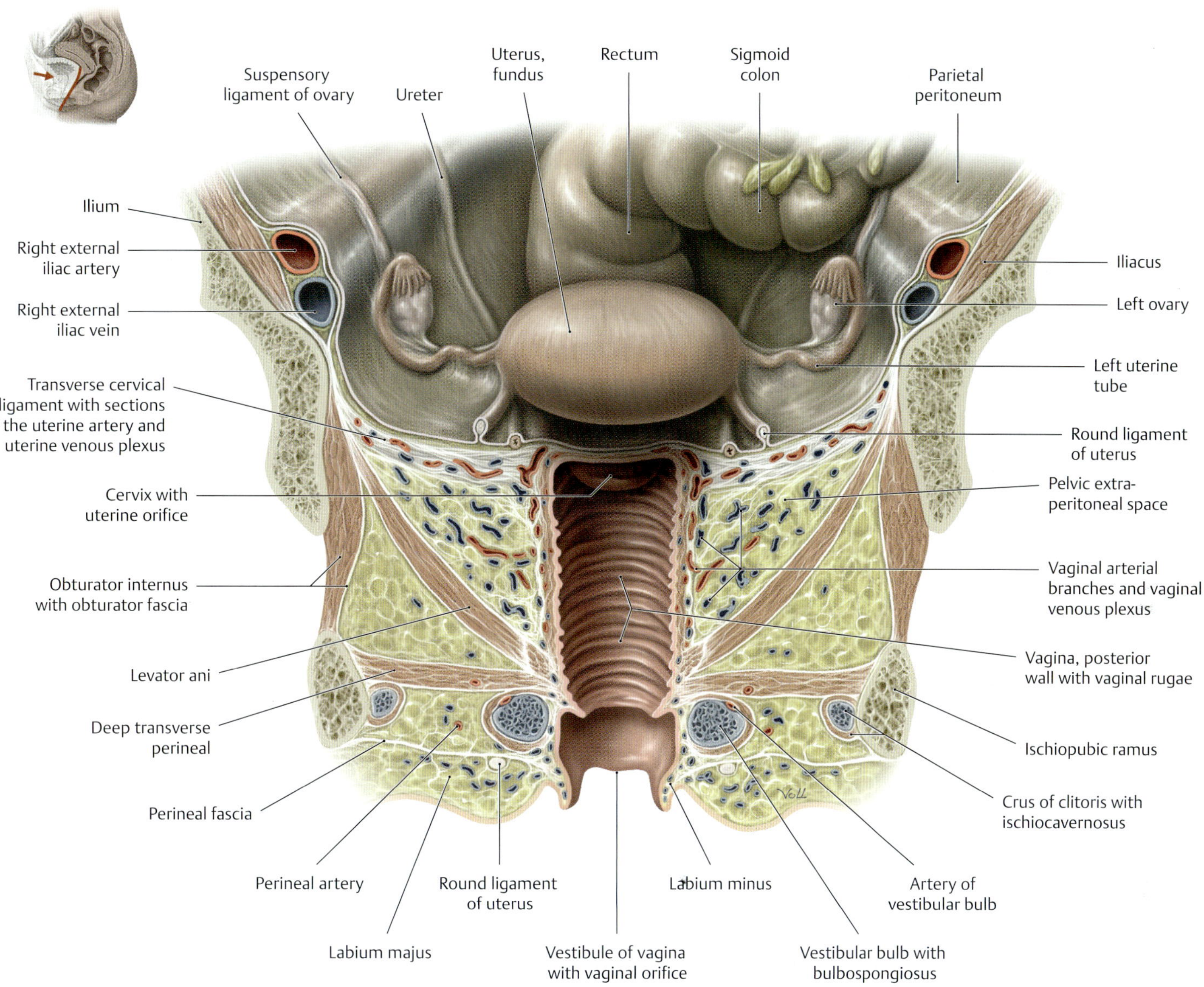

C The female genital organs in situ

Slightly angled coronal section, anterior view. The bladder, which lies anterior to the vagina and inferior to the uterine fundus (see **B**), is not shown. This illustration represents a compilation of multiple sections to provide a single integrated view. The uterine fundus, which is directed anteriorly owing to its anteverted and anteflexed position (see p. 344), projects out of the deeper plane of section toward the observer. Around the vagina is a connective-tissue space containing an elaborate venous plexus. This loose connective tissue allows for considerable expansion of the vagina during childbirth. The sections of arterial vessels are arterial branches to the vagina as well as sections of the inferior vesical arteries. See p. 414f for the subdivisions of the pelvic space and structure of the pelvic floor.

5.3 Female Internal Genitalia: Topographical Anatomy and Peritoneal Relationships; Shape and Structure

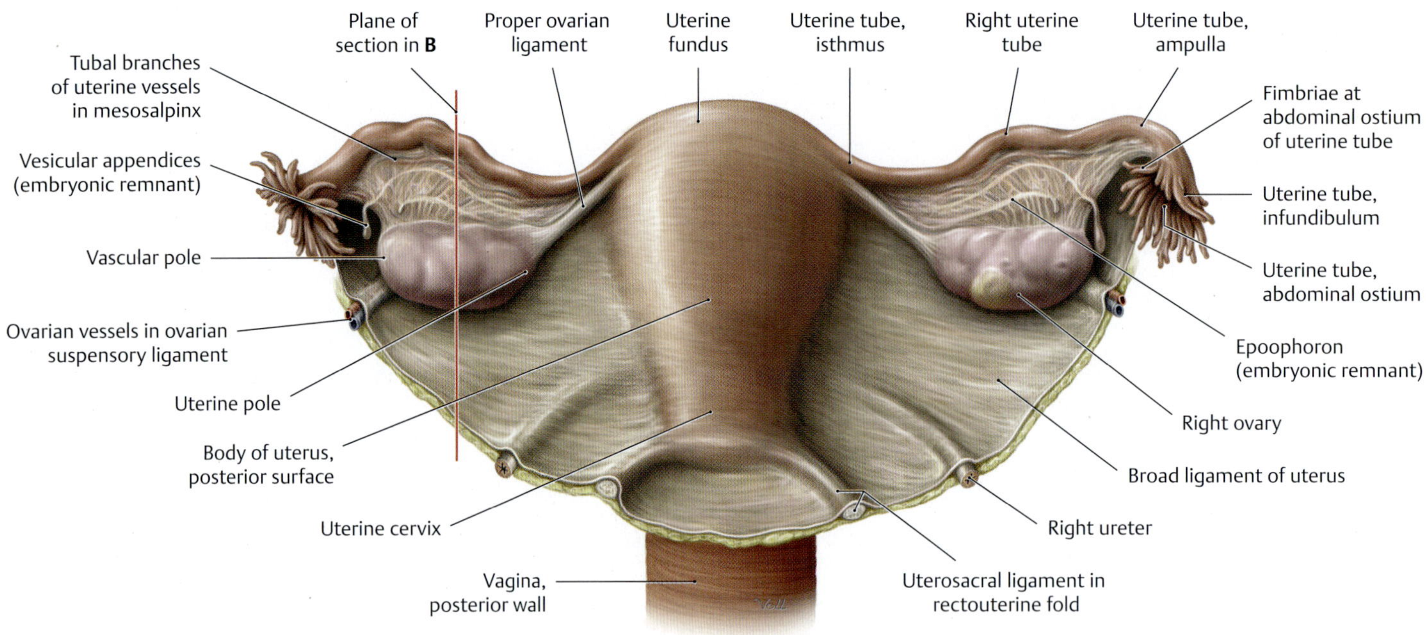

A Uterus and adnexa: topography and peritoneal relationships
Posterosuperior view of the uterus, adnexa, and the posterior surface of the uterine broad ligament. The uterine adnexa (ovary and uterine tube) are attached to the superior border and posterior surface of the broad ligament by folds of peritoneum (mesovarium and mesosalpinx, see **B**). The mesometrium, which follows the anteflexed position of the uterus, attaches the uterus to the pelvic sidewall and transmits the *uterine* vascular structures. The *ovary* receives its vascular supply through the ovarian suspensory ligament (these and other ligaments are reviewed in **C**).
Note: The ureters descend in the retroperitoneum to the base of the broad ligament and run forward between its layers to the bladder, passing inferior to the uterine artery (not visible here, see p. 369). This relationship must be duly noted in operations on the uterus and broad ligament (risk of ureteral injury).

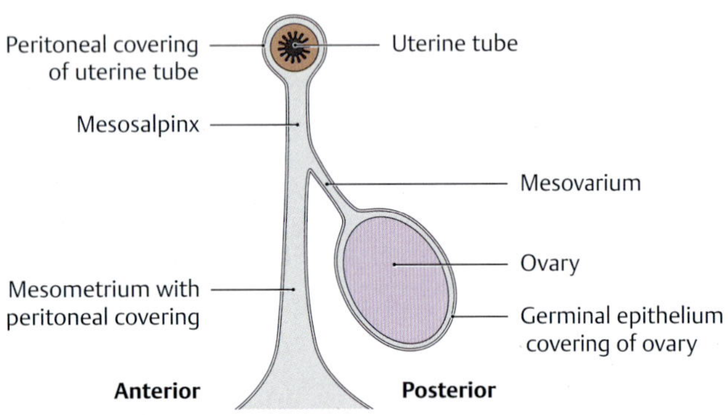

B Folds of peritoneum on the female genital organs
Sagittal section through the broad ligament of the uterus. The ovary, uterine tube, and much of the uterus (see **A**) are covered by peritoneum. The uterine tube is attached to the superior margin of the broad ligament by the mesosalpinx. The ovary is attached to the posterosuperior surface of the broad ligament by its own peritoneal structure, the mesovarium. These peritoneum-covered bands of connective tissue perform the same functions for the genital organs as the mesenteries do for the bowel and are named accordingly (see **C**): the mesovarium for the ovary, the mesosalpinx for the uterine tube (salpinx), and the mesometrium for the uterus. Collectively they form the broad ligament.

C Ligaments and peritoneal structures of the female genital organs

Broad ligament of uterus	Broad fold of peritoneum extending from the lateral pelvic wall to the uterus (transmits vascular structures to the internal genital organs). The ligament has three main parts that extend to specific organs: • Mesometrium = to the uterus • Mesosalpinx = to the uterine tube • Mesovarium = to the ovary The connective-tissue space between the two peritoneal layers of the broad ligament is known clinically as the parametrium
Transverse cervical ligament (cardinal ligament)	Transverse bands of connective tissue between the uterine uterina and pelvic wall (paracervix, see p. 416)
Round ligament of uterus	Distal remnant of the gubernaculum (embryonic cord in both sexes, guides the descent of the testis or ovary). Extends from the lateral angle of the uterus through the inguinal canal into the subcutaneous connective tissue of the labium majus and is not sectioned posteriorly in view **A**
Rectouterine fold	Peritoneum-covered fold of connective tissue between the uterus and rectum; often contains smooth muscle (rectouterine muscle)
Proper ovarian ligament	Proximal remnant of gubernaculum passing from the uterine pole of the ovary to the angle of the uterus with the uterine tube
Ovarian suspensory ligament	Fold of peritoneum stretching from the pelvic wall to the ovary; transmits the ovarian vessels

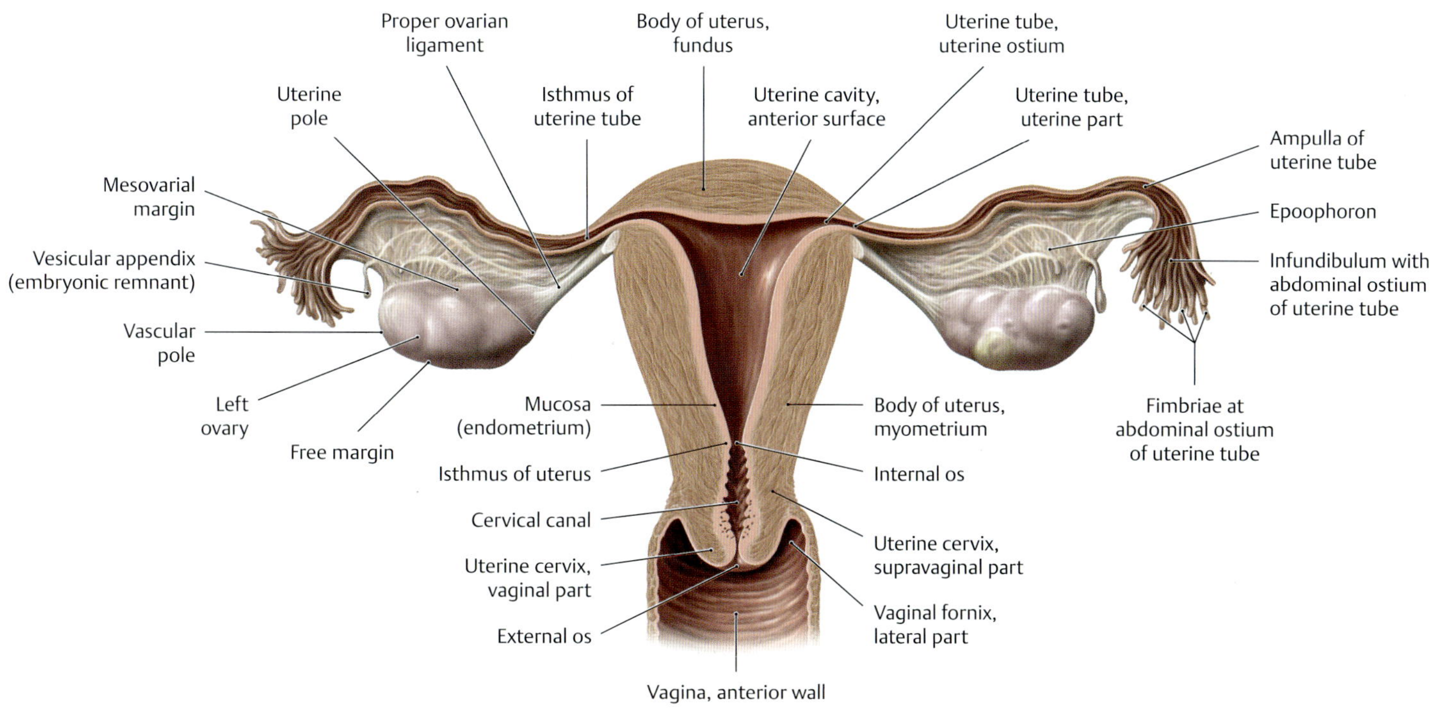

D Uterus and uterine tubes: shape and structure
Posterior view of a coronal section with the uterus straightened and the mesometrium removed. The uterus consists basically of the corpus (with the fundus) and cervix, the corpus being joined to the cervix by a narrow isthmus approximately 1 cm long. Macroscopically, the uterine isthmus is classified as part of the cervix but histologically it is lined by endometrium. The junction of the body of the uterus and cervix is located at the internal os of the uterus. The lumen of the uterus, called the uterine cavity, communicates with the vaginal lumen through the isthmus and cervical canal. It has a total length ("probe length") of 7–8 cm. The uterine cavity presents a triangular shape in coronal section. The uterine cervix is subdivided into a supravaginal part and vaginal part. The external os of the uterus is the opening in the vaginal part of the cervix that is directed toward the vagina. The vaginal part of the cervix projects into the vagina, forming recesses called the vaginal fornices. The uterine tube (total length approximately 10–18 cm) is subdivided from lateral to medial into the infundibulum, ampulla, isthmus, and uterine part. The abdominal ostium of the tube at the infundibulum is surrounded by fimbriae (the "fimbriated end") and opens into the peritoneal cavity. The ostium at the uterine end of the tube opens into the uterine cavity.

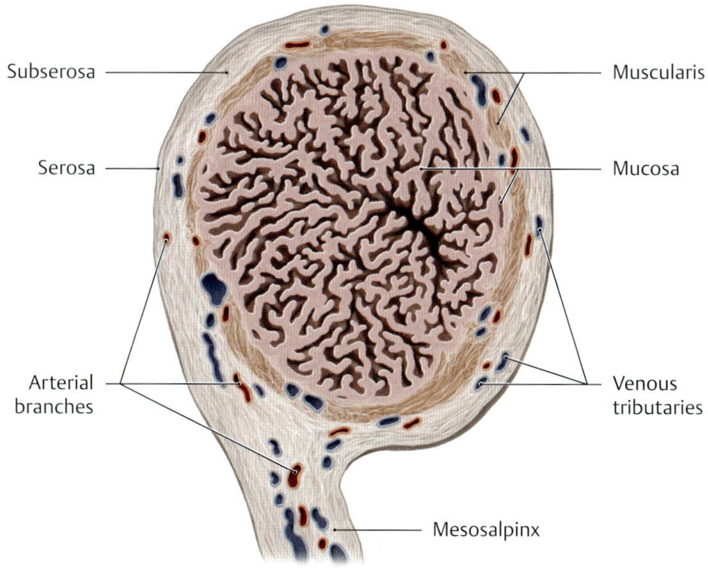

E Uterine tube in cross-section: wall structure
Cross-sectional view of the ampullary portion of a right uterine tube. The mesosalpinx extends inferiorly. The three wall layers are clearly distinguishable (wall thickness = 0.4–1.5 cm):

- The **mucosa** is raised into a great many folds that occupy most of the tubal lumen. These folds are of key importance in transporting the zygote to the uterus. Postinflammatory adhesions between the mucosal folds may hamper or even prevent transport of the fertilized ovum (see p. 352).
- The **muscularis** consists of several thin layers of smooth muscle that provide the uterine tube with its motility (see **B**, p. 350) and propel the zygote toward the uterus by a ciliated epithelium.
- The **serosa** (peritoneal covering) of the uterine tube is continuous with the mesosalpinx.

5.4 Female Internal Genitalia: Wall Structure and Function of the Uterus

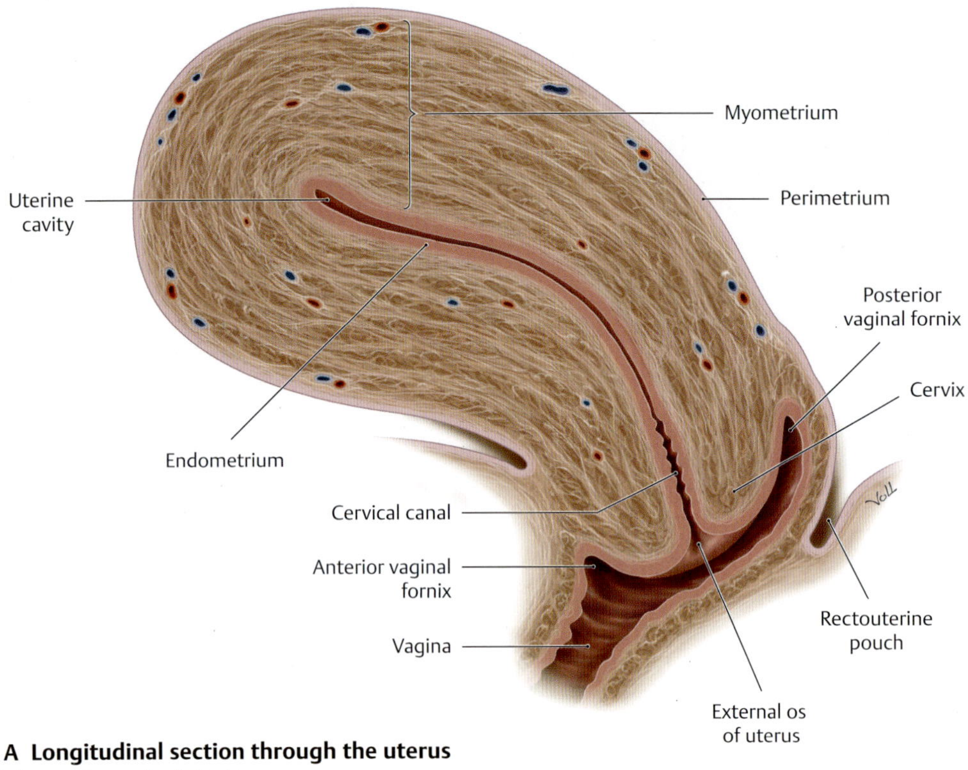

A Longitudinal section through the uterus
Viewed from the left side.

B Wall structure of the uterus

The uterine wall also consists of three layers from inside to outside:

- **Mucosa** or **endometrium** (see **D**): Single layer of columnar epithelium (epithelial layer) on a connective-tissue base (lamina propria)
- **Muscular coat** or **myometrium** (see **C**): Several smooth-muscle layers with a total thickness of approximately 1.5 cm
- **Serous coat** or **perimetrium**: Serosa covering the anterior and posterior sides of the uterine corpus and the posterior wall of the uterine cervix. The subserosa adjacent to the myometrium becomes adventitia in areas where the uterus lacks a peritoneal covering (e.g., at the attachment of the uterine broad ligament). of the uterine broad ligament).

C Layers of the myometrium (after Rauber and Kopsch)
The myometrium (tunica muscularis) of the uterus consists of three layers from outside to inside:

- **Supravascular layer:** thin outermost layer with criss-crossing lamellae; stabilizes the uterine wall
- **Vascular layer:** thick intermediate layer with a reticular pattern of muscle fibers; very vascular; the principal source for uterine contractions during labor
- **Subvascular layer:** thin innermost layer just below the endometrium; provides for functional closure of the uterine ostium of the uterine tube. Its contraction promotes separation of the uterine mucosa (shedding of the functional layer) during menses and separation of the placenta after childbirth.

The myometrium performs two seemingly contradictory functions: It must keep the uterus closed during pregnancy, but it must open the cervix during childbirth. To fulfill these functions, the individual muscle layers (see above) are equipped with longitudinal, oblique, and transverse or circular fibers. The circular muscle fibers are most abundant in the cervical region and serve to maintain closure of the cervix during pregnancy. The longitudinal and oblique muscle fibers are most abundant in the uterine body and fundus; they shorten the uterus and lower the fundus during childbirth. The myometrium blends with the circular fibers of the uterine tube muscles at the uterine fundus near the tubal ostium. Myometrial contractions are stimulated most effectively by the pituitary hormone oxytocin. These contractions occur not only during labor and delivery but also during menstruation, when they aid in expulsion of the uterine mucosa. Benign tumors of the myometrium (fibroids, myomas) may cause abnormalities of menstrual bleeding.

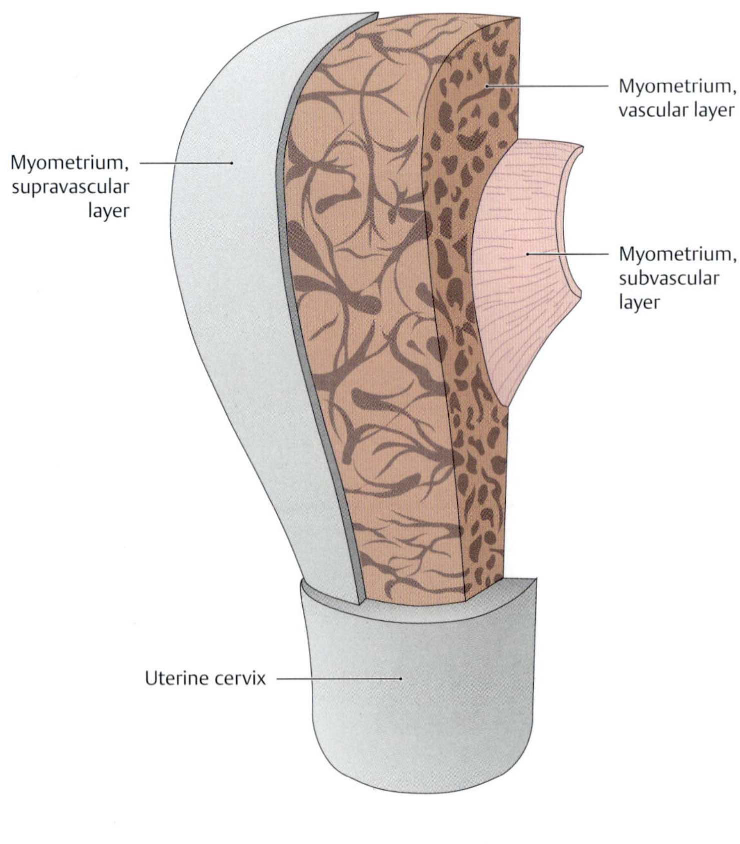

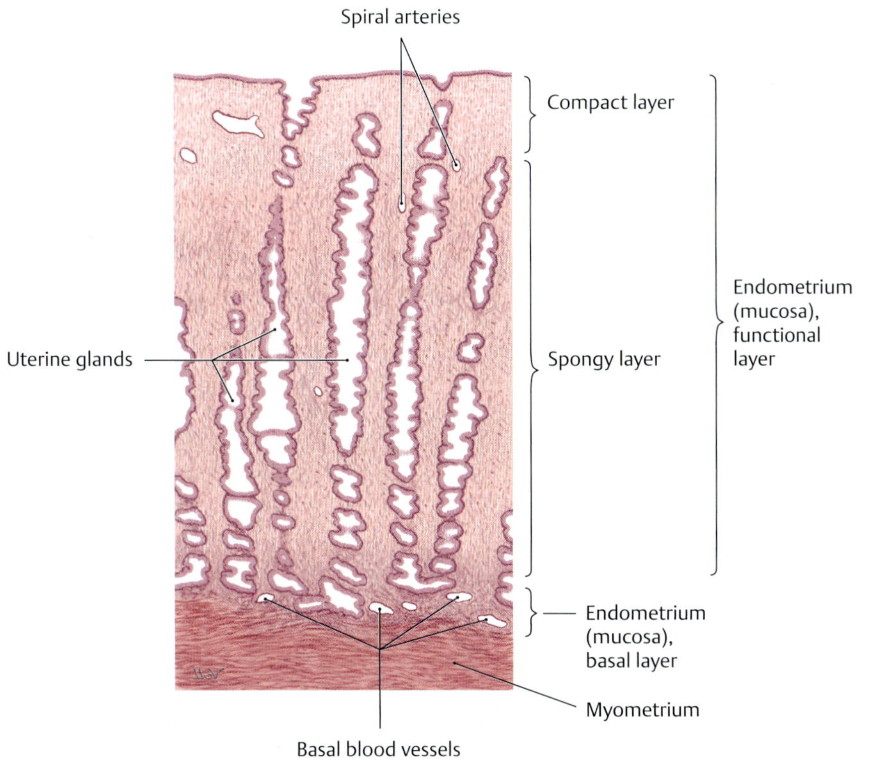

D Structure of the uterine mucosa (endometrium)

Structurally, the endometrium consists of a simple columnar epithelial cell layer and a lamina propria. The epithelial layer lines the uterine surface and encloses the tubular, coiled endometrial *uterine glands*. The lamina propria, which surrounds and supports the uterine glands, is made up of connective tissue (stroma) and the vessels embedded in it. The endometrium is *functionally* subdivided into a basal layer (stratum basale) and a functional layer (stratum functionale). The *basal layer* is approximately 1 mm thick, is largely exempt from the cyclical changes in the endometrium, and is not shed during menstruation. The *functional layer* varies in thickness at different phases of the ovarian cycle in women of reproductive age. It is shed at intervals of approximately 28 days during menstruation. It is thickest during the secretory phase of the ovarian cycle, at which time it consists of a superficial compact layer and a deeper spongy layer. It receives its blood supply from tortuous vessels called spiral arteries. While in this secretory state, the endometrium is most receptive to the implantation of a zygote. The mucosa of the uterine cervix does not participate in these cyclical changes.

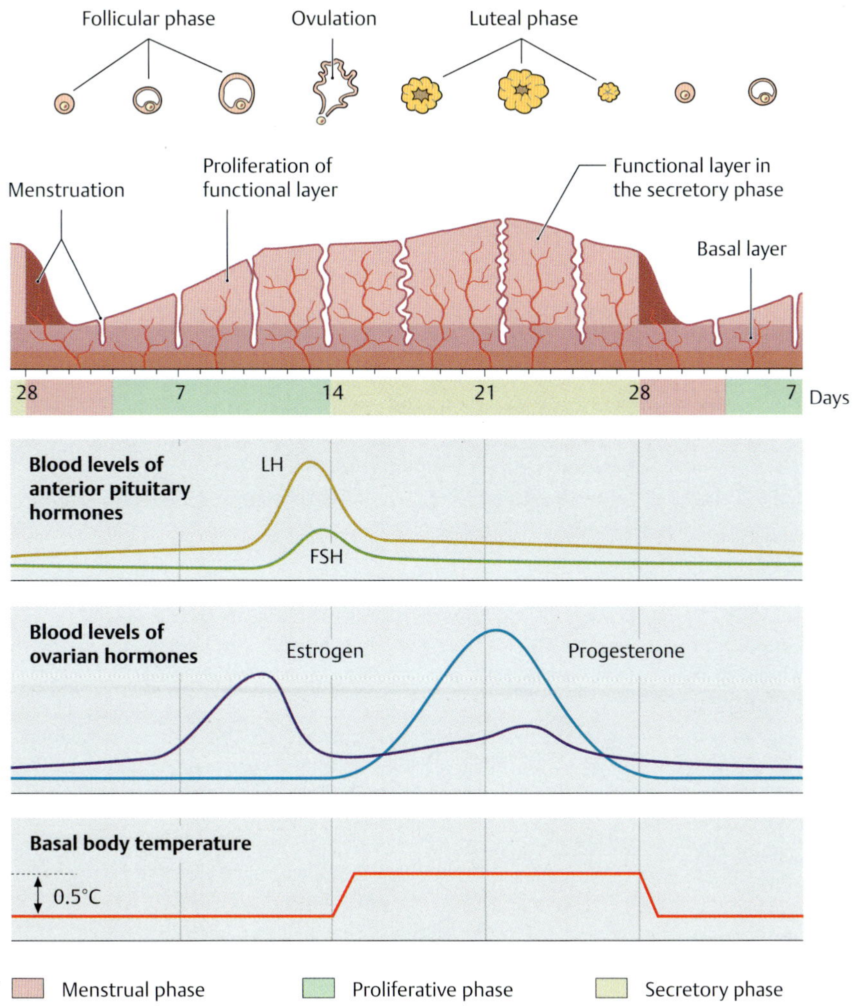

E Cyclical changes in the endometrium

The ovary secretes estrogens (e.g., estradiol) and progestins (e.g., progesterone) on a cyclical basis. Estrogens stimulate proliferation of the endometrium, while progestins induce its secretory transformation. The release of both hormones is controlled chiefly by the hormones FSH (follicle stimulating hormone) and LH (luteinizing hormone), which are secreted cyclically by the pituitary gland. While estrogens are produced by the ovarian follicle, progestins are produced in significant amounts only by the corpus luteum. If conception does not take place, the corpus luteum regresses and stops producing hormones. As a result of this, the functional layer of the endometrium breaks down and is expelled during menstruation. Estrogen production by a new, pituitary-stimulated ovarian follicle initiates a new cycle, which lasts an average of 28 days (1 lunar month). Ovulation usually occurs on day 14 of the cycle.

Note: For practical reasons, the first day of the menstrual period (which lasts about 4 days) is considered day 1 of the cycle, despite the fact that the cycle ends with menstruation. This is because the sudden onset of menstrual bleeding is easier to detect than its more gradual cessation. From the standpoint of the endometrium, however, the last day of the menstrual period (difficult to detect) marks the end of the cycle.

5.5 Female Internal Genitalia: Positions of the Uterus and Vagina

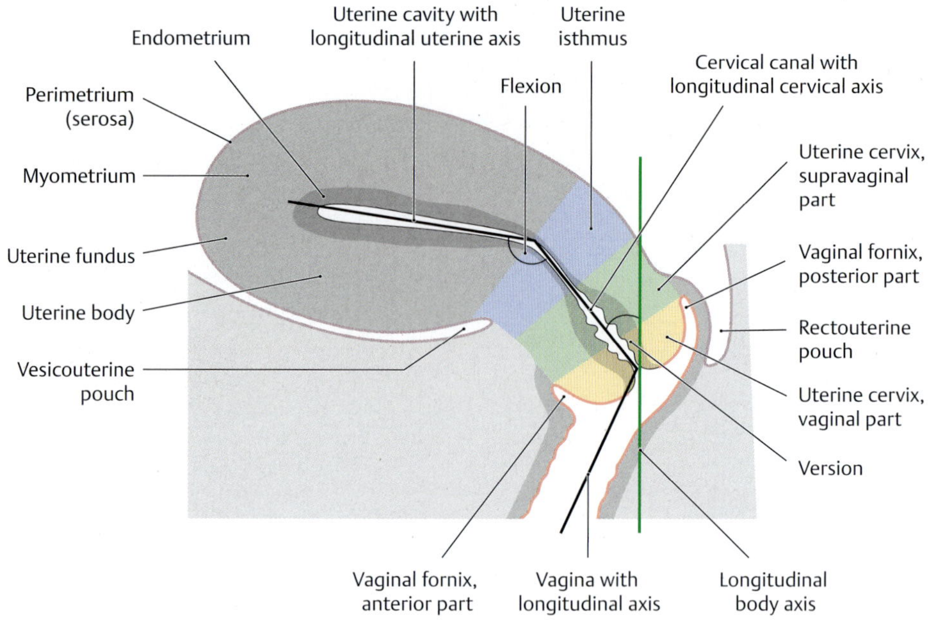

A Curvature and position of the uterus
Midsagittal section of the uterus and upper vagina, viewed from the left side.
Note the two angles that determine the normal anteversion and anteflexion of the uterus (see **D**). Posterior angulation and curvature of the uterus (retroflexion, retroversion) are considered abnormal. A retroverted uterus is more susceptible to descent because it is more closely aligned with the longitudinal axis of the vagina. Moreover, a retroverted uterus that enlarges during pregnancy may become immobile below the sacral promontory (L 5/S1 junction) and jeopardize the further course of the pregnancy by constraining uterine expansion.

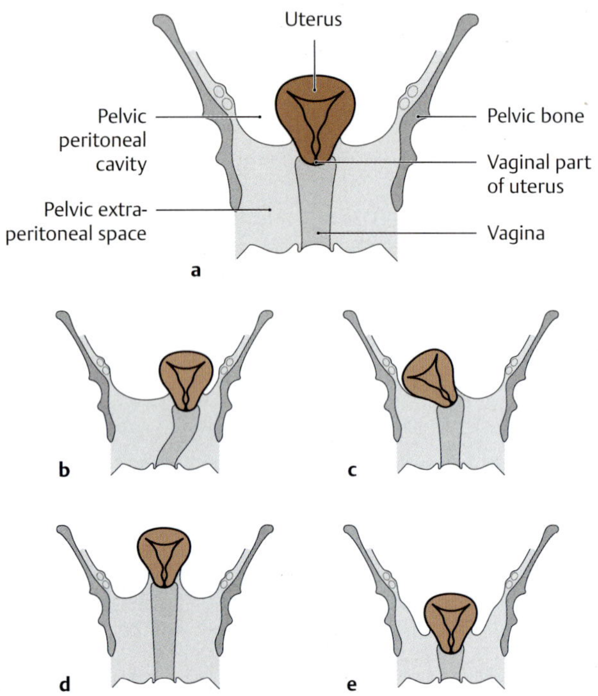

B Position and level of the uterus in the pelvis
Coronal section of the pelvis, anterior view. The uterus has been slightly straightened for clarity. Normally the uterus is located approximately in the median plane (**a**) with its vaginal part level with a line connecting the two ischial spines. The uterus may be displaced from this position to the left or right (sinistroposition or dextroposition, **b** and **c**) or may lie above or below the plane of the ischial spines (elevation or descent, see **d** and **e**). Anterior and posterior displacement (anteposition, retroposition) may also occur but are not illustrated here. Descent of the uterus usually results from a structural weakness of the pelvic floor (chiefly the levator ani, often after numerous vaginal deliveries). Displacement of the uterus may cause complaints and functional disturbances due to pressure on adjacent organs (bladder, rectum). Descent of the uterus may even cause the vaginal part of the uterus to protrude from the vagina (cervical prolapse).

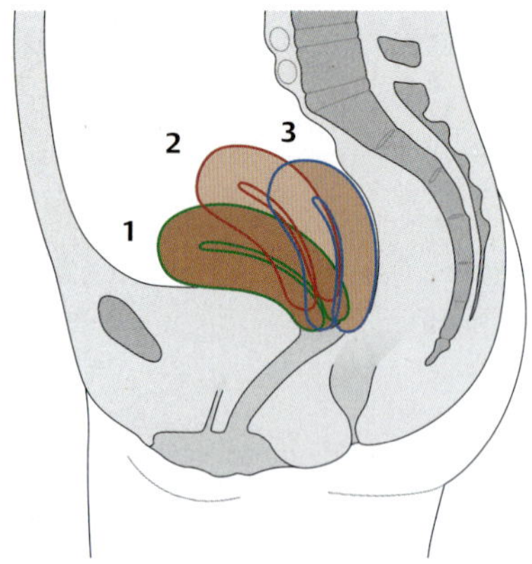

C Physiological changes in uterine position
Midsagittal section of the pelvis, viewed from the left side. Uterine position is directly affected by the varying degrees of bladder and rectal distention. **1** Bladder and rectum empty; **2** bladder and rectum full; **3** bladder full, rectum empty.

D Describing the position of the uterus in the pelvis
The position of the uterus in the pelvis can be described in terms of version, flexion, and position (angles are shown in **A**).

Version	Inclination of the cervix in the cavitas pelvis; defined by the angle between the cervical axis and the longitudinal axis of the body; the normal condition is *anteversion*
Flexion	Inclination of the corpus uteri relative to the cervix; defined by the angle between the longitudinal axes of the cervix and corpus uteri; the normal condition is *anteflexion*
Position	Position of the vaginal part of the uterus in the pelvic cavity; physiologically, the vaginal part of the uterus is at the level of the interspinous line at the center of the pelvis

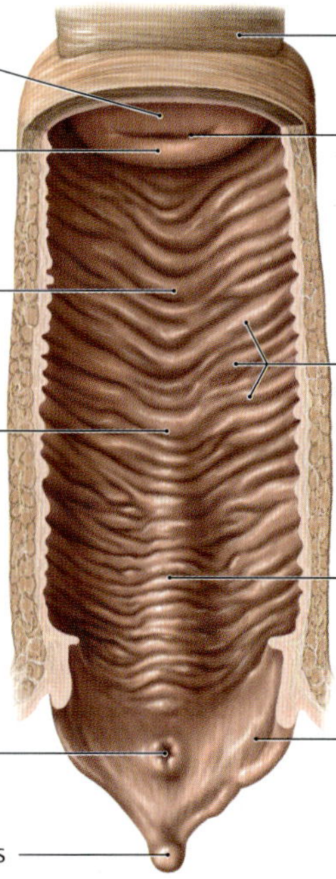

E Vagina
Posterior view. The vagina has been cut open along a coronal plane angled slightly posteriorly to display its anterior wall. The vaginal lumen presents an H-shaped cross section (see **F**), but the lumen in this dissection has been stretched open to a more circular shape (in situ the posterior and anterior walls are closely apposed). The vaginal mucosa has numerous transverse folds (rugae) as well as anterior and posterior ridges (vaginal columns) formed by the extensive venous plexus in the vaginal wall. The closely adjacent urethra raises the lower anterior wall of the vagina into a prominent longitudinal ridge (urethral carina).

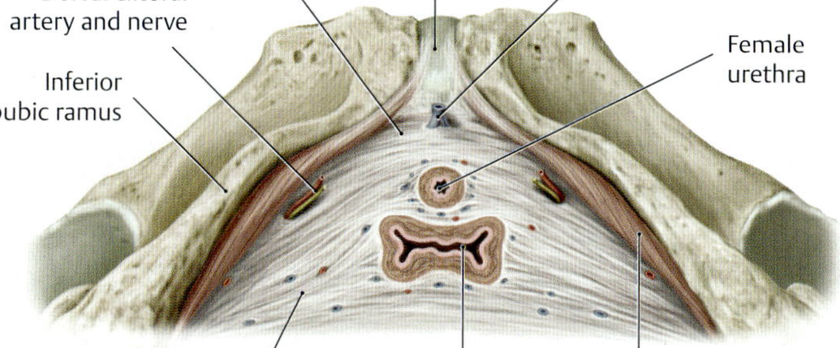

F Location of the vagina in the pelvic floor
This drawing illustrates the close proximity of the vagina and urethra. Muscular fibers from the deep transverse perineal encircle the vagina.

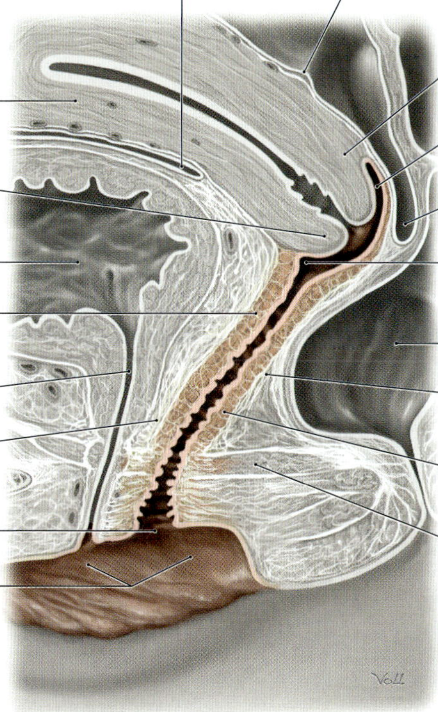

G Location of the vagina in the pelvis
Midsagittal section through a female pelvis, viewed from the left side. The longitudinal axis of the vagina is directed posterosuperiorly. The vagina is attached to the pelvic connective tissue anteriorly (vesicovaginal septum), posteriorly (rectovaginal septum), and laterally (not shown here). The vaginal fornix surrounds the vaginal part of the cervix, which itself is directed superiorly and anteriorly. The posterior fornix is significantly longer than the anterior fornix and projects further superiorly in the pelvis. The visceral peritoneum extends far down the posterior uterine wall, bringing the posterior part of the vaginal fornix into close proximity to the rectouterine pouch (cul-de-sac, the lowest part of the female peritoneal cavity).

5.6 Female Internal Genitalia: Epithelial Regions of the Uterus

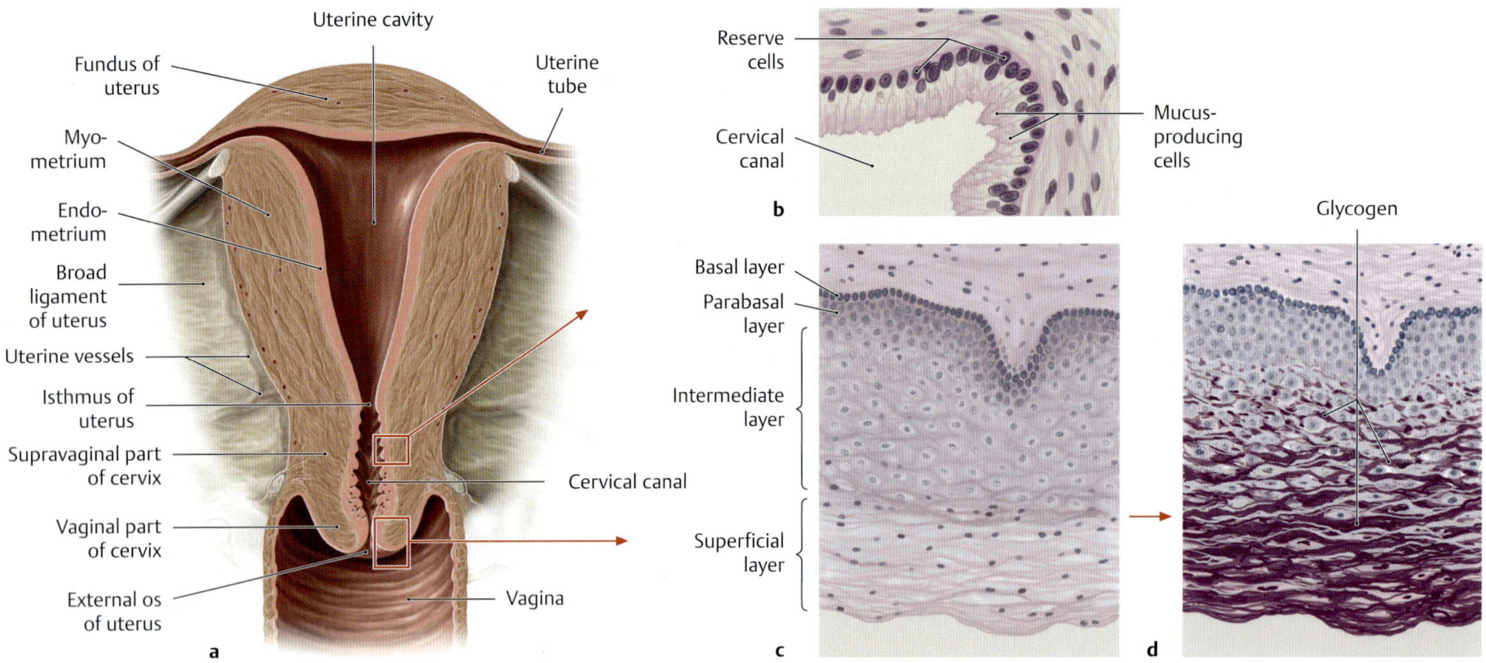

A Epithelial regions of the uterus

a Coronal section through uterus, anterior view; **b–d** Higher magnification of **a**: **b** Mucus-secreting columnar epithelium of the cervical canal; **c** Squamous epithelium of the vaginal part of cervix; **d** PAS method used to display glycogen (after Luellmann).

The cervix is the lower part of the uterus. It commences distal to the isthmus of the uterus as the *supravaginal* part of the cervix, which is the upper part of the cervix surrounded by connective tissue of the parametrium, and ends at its lower portion that extends into the vagina (*vaginal* part of cervix). At the level of the supravaginal part of the cervix the uterus is held in place by ligaments (mainly the cardinal ligament, cf. p. 416). The tubular lumen of the cervix is called the cervical canal. It is lined with mucosa and begins at the internal os and ends with the external os at the vaginal part of the cervix. The mucosal epithelium of the cervical canal is composed of a single layer of mucus-secreting columnar epithelium. A parallel arrangement of folds (palmate folds), which form crypts, gives the epithelium a rough appearance on the surface. The function of the reserve cells located at the base of the epithelium is to replenish the cervical epithelium. Unlike the one-layered cervical epithelium, the vagina is lined with stratified, nonkeratinized squamous epithelium, which depending on the hormonal situation in women may continue to the surface of the vaginal part of the cervix. The boundaries of the two epithelial layers can be either endo- or ectocervical (see **C**).

The stratified, nonkeratinized squamous epithelium lining the vagina (and vaginal part of cervix) is composed of up to 20 layers of cells and is made up of four tiers: basal, parabasal, intermediate, and superficial layers. Typically, cells of the two superficial-most layers contain abundant glycogen as a result of differentiation. The epithelium exhibits cyclical changes: whereas at the preovulatory stage, all layers are well developed, at the postovulatory stage cells of the superficial and intermediate layers desquamate and disintegrate. Glycogen that is released as a result nourishes lactic acid bacteria (lactobacillus acidophilus, Döderlein's bacillus), which inhabit the vagina. The transformation of glycogen into lactic acid leads to the acidic vaginal milieu (pH 4–5), which mainly in the second half of the menstrual cycle protects against pathogens (see **B**). The slightly alkaline cervical mucus has a similar effect as a physiologic barrier against infection. For much of the menstrual cycle, it has a stretchy texture and seals the cervical canal with a protective plug (barrier against ascending germs). The mucus is thin only at the time of ovulation and thus becomes penetrable by sperm.

B Defense mechanisms of the vagina and potential dysfunctions

The peritoneal cavity has an anatomical communication with the exterior of the body (via vagina–cervical canal–uterine cavity–uterine tube). This exposes the female to ascending infections, and this is why physiologic barriers against infection exist in the form of vaginal defense mechanisms. Dysfunction of these mechanisms may lead to gynecological inflammation and an increased risk of miscarriage.

Protection mechanism	Dysfunction due to
• Physiological acidic vaginal milieu with a pH 4–5 • Effect of estrogens: stimulates vaginal epithelium proliferation and differentiation (glycogen storage) • Effect of progestins: leads to desquamation of superficial and intermediate vaginal cells • Conversion of glycogen into lactic acid through lactobacillus acidophilus (Döderlein's bacillus)	• Elevated pH level: alkalizing effect of menstrual blood/cervical mucus • Lack of glycogen: lack of endogenous estrogen/progestins (childhood/old age/diseases) • Drugs: antibiotics disrupt vagina's normal flora • Exogenous effects: sex life, tampons, improper anal hygiene, using alkaline soaps • Infections: colpitis especially caused by chlamydia, trichomonads and fungi (candida albicans)

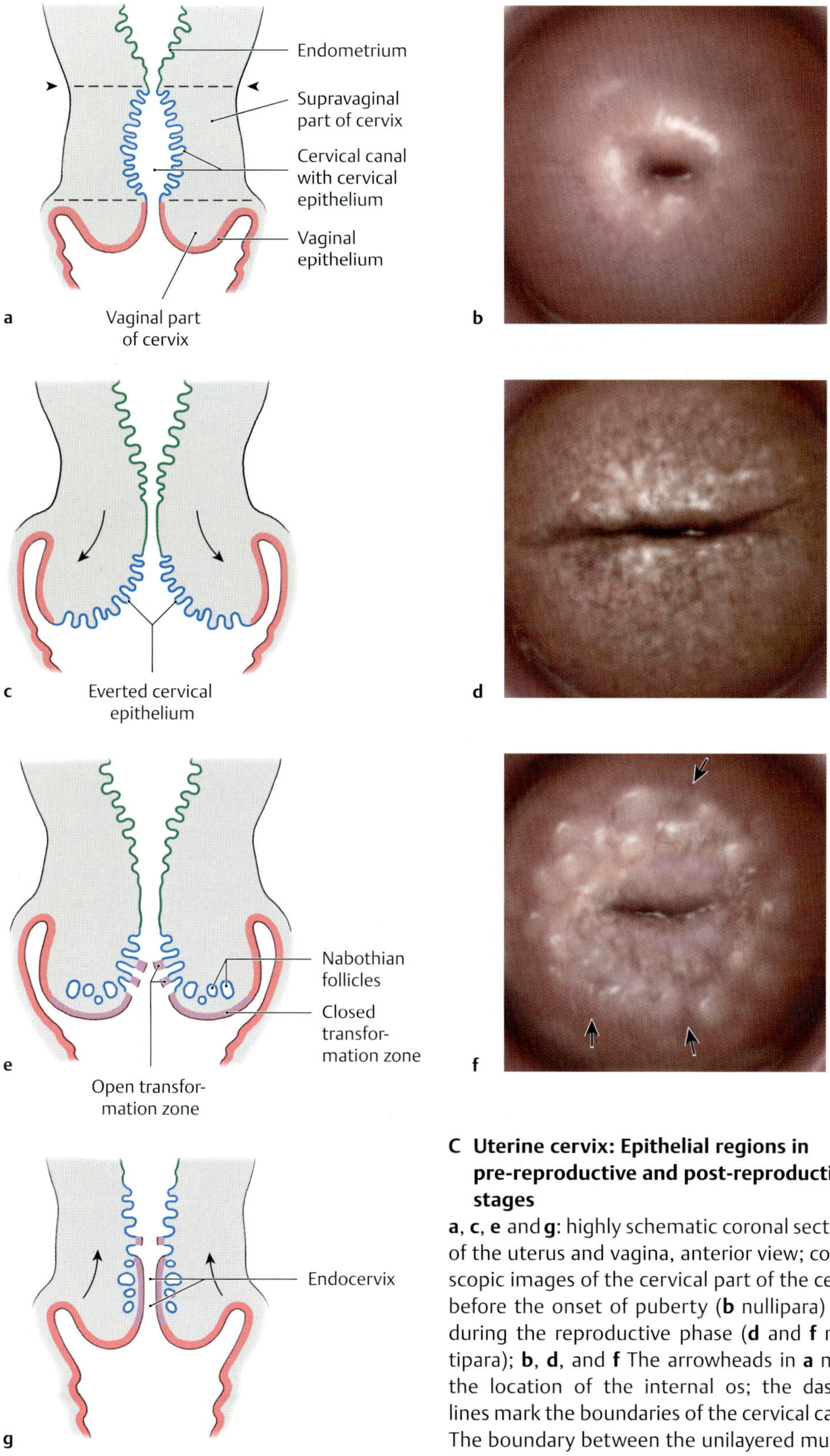

C Uterine cervix: Epithelial regions in pre-reproductive and post-reproductive stages

a, **c**, **e** and **g**: highly schematic coronal sections of the uterus and vagina, anterior view; colposcopic images of the cervical part of the cervix before the onset of puberty (**b** nullipara) and during the reproductive phase (**d** and **f** multipara); **b**, **d**, and **f** The arrowheads in **a** mark the location of the internal os; the dashed lines mark the boundaries of the cervical canal. The boundary between the unilayered mucus-secreting columnar epithelium (cervical epithelium) of the cervical canal and the stratified nonkeratinized squamous epithelium of the vaginal part of the cervix and the vagina varies according to the woman's hormonal status (see below). The visible portion of the uterus is called the ectocervix and the non-visible portion is called the endocervix.

Before the onset of puberty (a and b): Before the onset of the reproductive phase, the cervical part of the cervix is covered with squamous epithelium, the ecto-endocervical boundary is located within the cervical canal (above the external os), thus it is not visible from the vagina.

During the reproductive phase (c–f): in response to hormonal stimuli (estrogen) the cervical mucosa is everted and moves inside the vagina. It appears as a glandular field with a very rough surface on the ectocervix (**d**). The sharp boundary with the smooth pink-colored squamous epithelium of the vaginal part of the cervix is thus located outside of the external os and is clearly visible from the vagina. The eversion of the cervical glandular field is believed to be related to higher fertility (easier for spermatozoa to enter the cervix). The columnar endocervical epithelium, which has everted onto the ectocervix adjusts to the altered vaginal milieu (acidic milieu in contrast to alkaline milieu of the cervical canal) by converting to stratified nonkeratinized squamous epithelium (metaplasia). In this way, it is similar in structure and cyclic behavior to the regular squamous epithelium of the vaginal part of the cervix. As the mucus-secreting cervical epithelium transforms into squamous epithelium the columnar glands become sealed over (closed transformation zone in contrast to open transformation zone where the glands are not overgrown and occluded, arrows in **f** point to the "open" orifices) leading to the formation of macroscopically visible mucus-filled retention cysts (Nabothian cysts), which are not considered problematic. Squamous epithelium in the transformation zone may become malignant and contribute in pre-stages (precancerous) to squamous cell carcinoma formation (see p. 348 f).

During postmenopause (g): lower estrogen levels toward the end of the reproductive phase cause the relocation of cervical epithelium and the boundary of the endo-and ectocervix moves back into the cervical canal (similar clinical presentation to **b** although the cervix changes shape after vaginal delivery).

5.7 Female Internal Genitalia: Cytologic Smear, Conization; Cervical Carcinoma

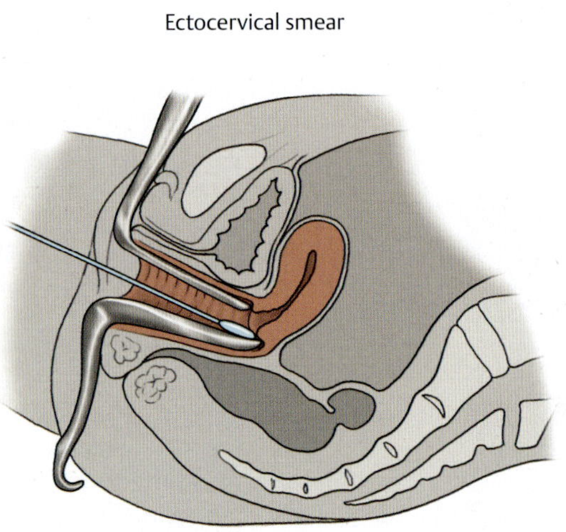

a

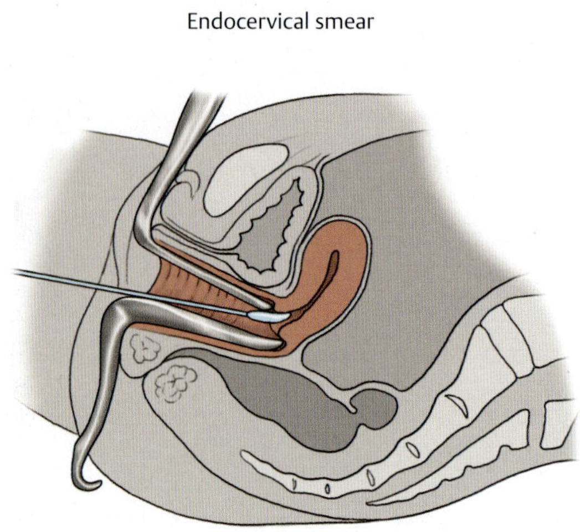

b

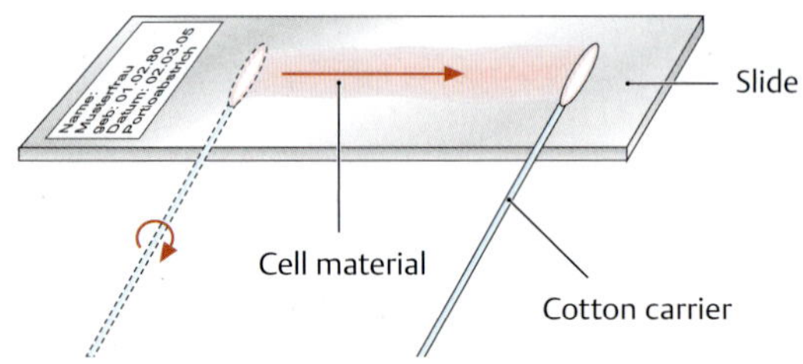

c

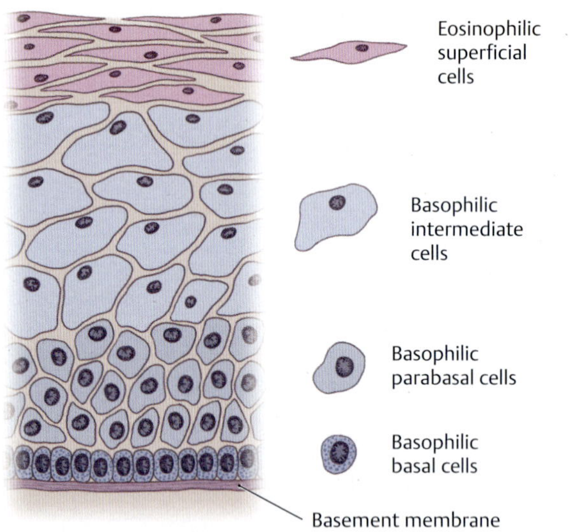

d

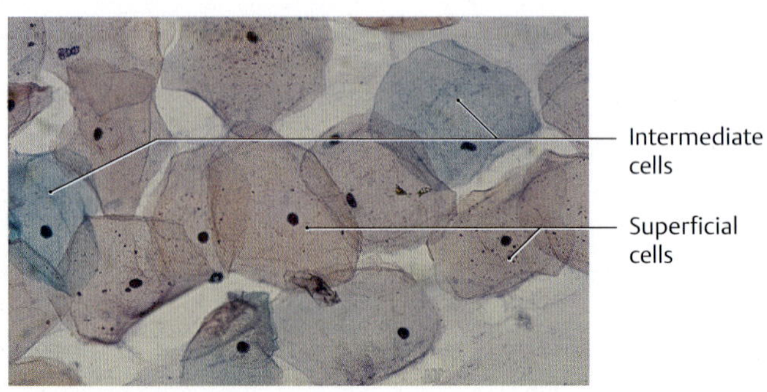

e

A Cytologic smear: cell morphology of vaginal and vaginal part of cervical epithelium; early detection of cervical cancer

a and **b** cytologic smears taken from the vaginal part of the cervix and the cervical canal, **c** transfer of smear material onto glass slide; **d** histological structure and cell morphology of the vaginal and cervical epithelium in the cytologic smear; **e** Pap staining of superficial and intermediate cells (**e** from Nauth H.F.: Gynäkologische Zytodiagnostik. 2nd ed. Stuttgart; Thieme: 2013).

Especially in the transformation zone of the uterine cervix, where with the onset of puberty the unilayered columnar epithelium of the cervix changes into stratified squamous epithelium (see p. 347), the squamous epithelium may undergo malignant transformation and turn into invasive squamous cell carcinoma. Because cervical cancer usually develops slowly over time, it is possible to detect it in its early stages with the help of cytologic smears. Thus, cytodiagnosis is one of the most important tools in early detection of cervical cancer (see **D**). Cytology testing is an obligatory part of the initial gynecologic examination and cancer screening (in Germany starting at the age of 20) and is also performed to evaluate suspicious changes in cervical tissue. The cytologic smear should always include cells from the uppermost epithelial layer, which if they are normal show signs of differentiation (see p. 346).

Two smears are taken routinely: the first one (**a**) must be taken at the surface of the vaginal part of the cervix (ectocervix), and the second one (**b**) from the cervical canal (endocervix). The smear material is taken with a cotton swab and transferred to a slide and fixed (**c**). After that, the *Papanicolaou method* (known as *Pap stain*) is used to stain the cervical smear and evaluate it for characteristics of cell differentiation (cell shape, nuclear shape, nucleus-plasma ratio, see **D**). Because structure, height and the degree of maturation vary with the hormonal status (menstrual cycle) of a woman, it is crucial to confirm at which point during the cycle the smear is taken. If it is taken during the follicular phase (effect of estrogen), it is dominated by eosinophilic superficial cells, which are stained red, and flat, basophilic intermediate cells with pyknotic nuclei, which are stained greenish-blue (**e**). This proliferative phase, during which the uppermost cell layer is constantly regenerated by cells from the basal layer, normally lasts about a week. The postovulatory phase is dominated by cell differentiation and desquamation. Hence, the epithelium is thinner in the second part of the menstrual cycle.

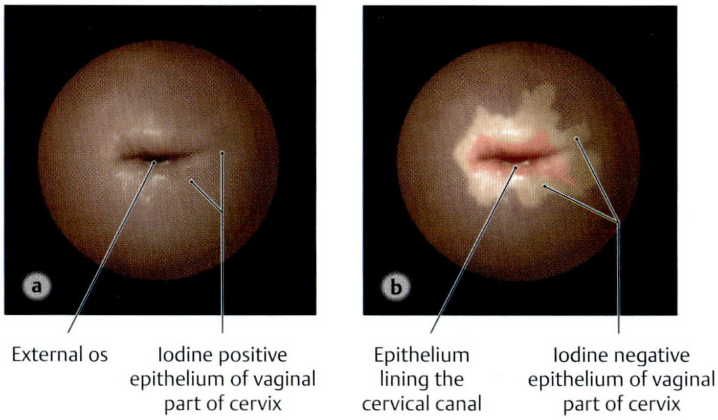

B Schiller's iodine test for localization of abnormal epithelial regions
a Normal vaginal cervical epithelium stained by iodine produces a dark brown color; **b** Iodine negative, insufficiently differentiated cervical epithelium.

After inserting a speculum into the vagina, the vaginal part of the cervix is initially examined macroscopically, if necessary with the help of a colposcope allowing a 6–40 fold magnification of the cervix. For the localization of abnormal areas, Schiller's iodine test utilizes the glycogen content of the surrounding normal squamous epithelium. To that end, iodine solution (Schiller's iodine test) is applied to the surface of the cervix. Normal squamous epithelium, regardless of whether it is autochthonous or metaplastic, takes on a dark brown color. However, insufficiently differentiated squamous epithelium with a high or low glycogen content turns only light brown or is iodine negative. Thus, the iodine-unstained areas correspond to the location of undifferentiated epithelium. Iodine-negative areas are not specific but combined with suspicious cytology results (see above cytologic smear) of the same area, point to epithelial abnormalities. Hence, Schiller's iodine test provides a method with which to assess the localization and expansion of cervical changes. Conization (see **C**) is used to remove affected areas.

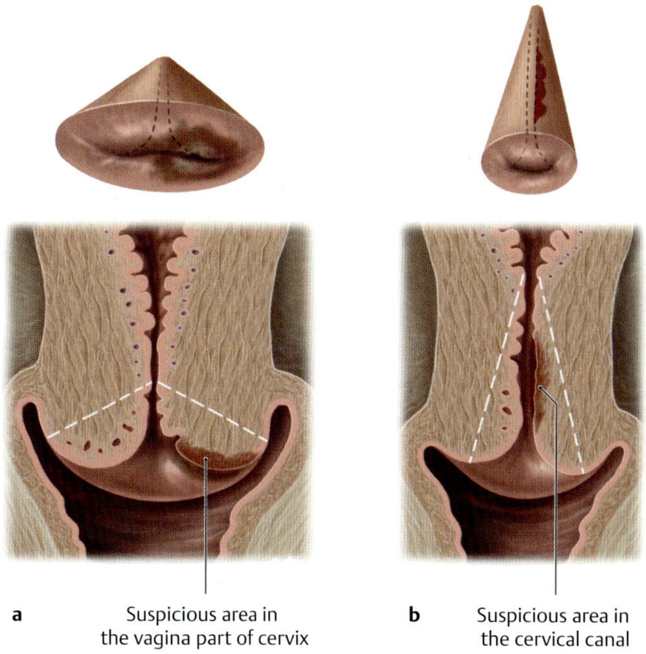

C Conization
For a histological examination of suspicious findings (iodine-negative areas, dysplastic cells in the smear), a *cone-shaped* wedge of uterine cervix tissue (*conization*) is removed while the patient is under anesthesia. In a sexually mature woman, abnormal epithelium is most likely found on the surface of the vaginal part of the cervix in the transformation zone. When removing a flat and broad wedge of tissue (**a**), this area is included. In postmenopausal women, atypical epithelial cells are usually found in the cervical canal. This area is included when removing a sharp cone of tissue (**b**).

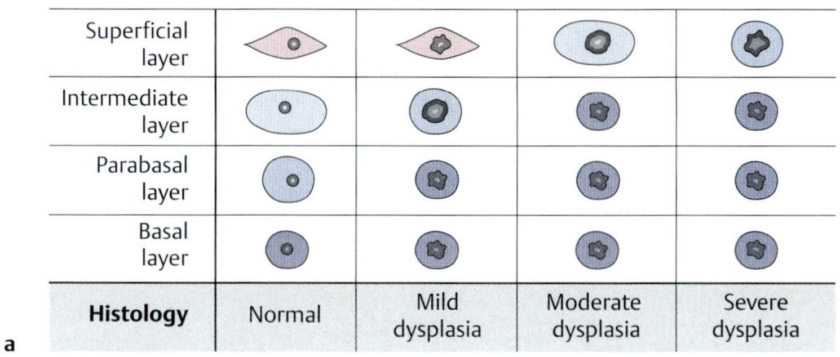

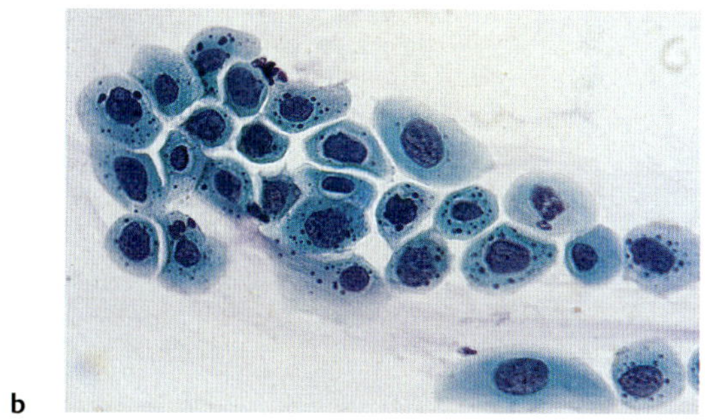

D Cervical carcinoma and its pre-stages
a Normal and dysplastic cells in the cytologic smear; **b** Parabasal squamous epithelial cells with atypical and polymorphous nuclei ("immature dyskaryotic cells") (from Nauth, H.F.: Gynäkologische Zytodiagnostik. 2nd ed. Stuttgart; Thieme: 2013).

Pre-stages of cervical carcinoma are initially confined to the epithelium, and the deeper layers have not yet been infiltrated (see below). Cellular changes that begin at the basal layer and progress to the superficial layer (cell shape, nuclear shape, nucleus-plasma ratio) are signs of increasing differentiation. They are not present when the cells only divide but don't mature (dysplasia = abnormal cells). Dysplastic cells often have enlarged hyperchromatic nuclei, so that the nucleus-plasma ratio shifts in favor of the nucleus. The cytologic smear helps to determine the different degrees of dysplasia, and thus the pre-stages of the cervical carcinoma (**a**). Based on the international classification, they are divided into stages of CIN (CIN = "cervical intraepithelial neoplasia"): mild dysplasia (CIN I); moderate dysplasia (CIN II) severe dysplasia/carcinoma in situ (CIN III). The more severe the dysplasia, the more likely the transformation into invasive carcinoma. In 50% of cases, mild dysplasia will spontaneously regress. In severe dysplasia (**b**), the atypical changes involve the full thickness of the epithelium and the regular stratification has been lost. However, the carcinoma has not yet perforated the basement membrane (carcinoma in situ). Invasion of the basement membrane is characteristic of an infiltrating growth pattern with subsequent metastasis. Approximately 20 % of intraepithelial changes have infiltrative growth patterns, with a latency period between formation of dysplasia and infiltration of more than 10 years.

Cervical carcinoma is the second leading cause of cancer-related deaths in women worldwide. Approximately 500,000 cases are diagnosed each year, and 350,000 die from it despite early detection and treatment. Infection (most commonly sexually transmitted) with certain types of the papilloma virus (HPV-16 and HPV-18) has been identified as one major pathogenetic factor. These viruses inactivate proteins that monitor cell growth (e.g., p53 and Rb). Recently, a vaccination against tumor-producing viruses has become available.

5.8 Female Internal Genitalia: Ovary and Follicular Maturation

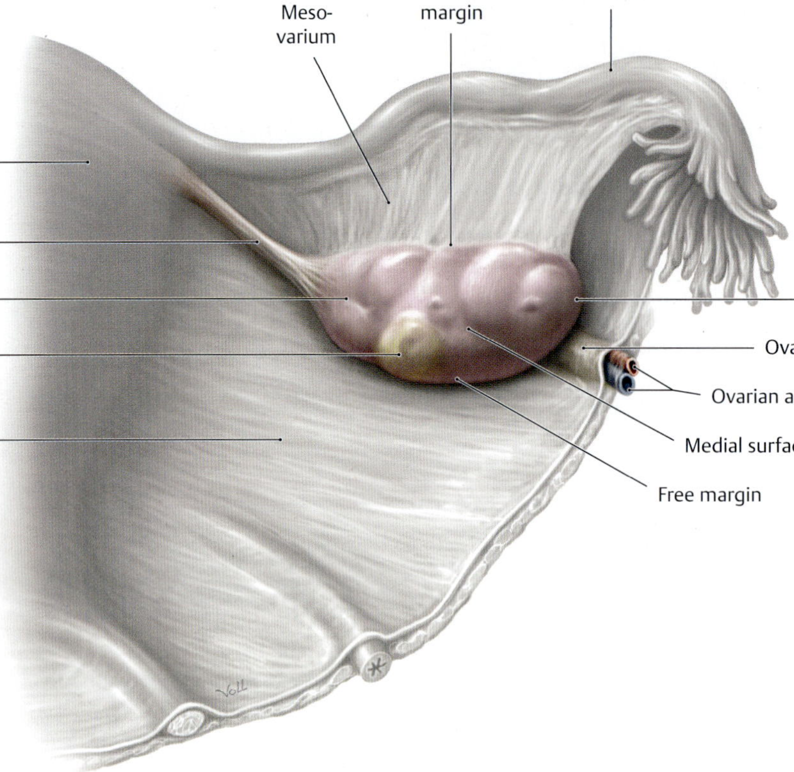

A Ovary

Posterior view of a right ovary, showing the peritoneal ligaments that transmit vessels to the ovary (ovarian suspensory ligament with the ovarian artery and vein, proper ovarian ligament with the ovarian branch of the uterine artery, and portions of the uterine venous plexus) along with part of the uterus, uterine tube, and broad ligament. The ovary is positioned such that it lies in the iliac fossa of the lesser pelvis.

Note: Given the dual vascular supply to the ovary from the upper abdomen (the vessels accompany the ovary during its developmental descent) and the blood supply to the uterus (close to the ovary), both vascular systems should be ligated during a hysterectomy.

In a woman of reproductive age, the ovary is 3–5 cm long and has the size and shape of a plum. It consists of a cortical and medullary zone (see **C**) and is surrounded by a tough collagenous capsule (tunica albuginea). The cortical zone contains follicles at varying stages of development. The follicles contain an oocyte surrounded by follicular epithelium and a connective-tissue mantle. Female hormones are not produced by the oocyte itself but by the cells that surround it. Although an intraperitoneal organ, the ovary is covered externally by germinal epithelium (on its tunica albuginea) and has a shiny surface.

Note: The visceral peritoneal covering of the ovary, a single-layered cuboidal epithelium that surrounds the tunica albuginea, has been referred to traditionally as "germinal epithelium," but it does not participate at all in the principal, reproductive function of the ovary—egg production—nor is it involved in replenishment of cells in the ovary itself. However, it is "germinal" in another, unfortunate way—90% of all malignant ovarian tumors are thought to originate in this cell layer.

B Ovum collection mechanism

Posterior view of a right ovary and uterine tube. Both the uterine tube and the ovary are motile. The tube derives its motility from its muscular wall and pulsations of adjacent vessels. Rotational and longitudinal movements of the tube make it easier for the fimbriated end of the tube to contact the entire ovary. The movements stop when the abdominal orifice of the tube has cupped the mound formed by a graafian follicle.

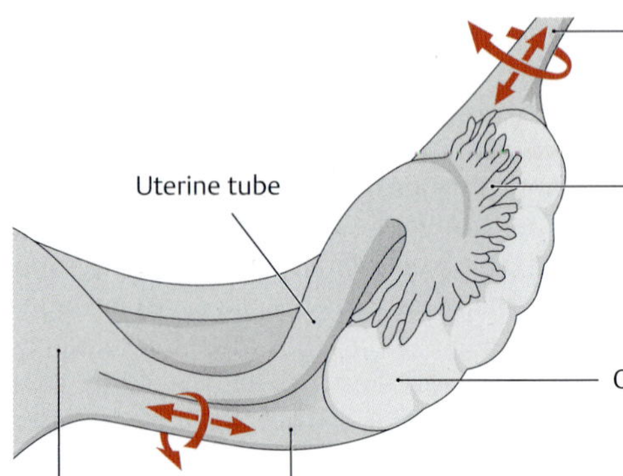

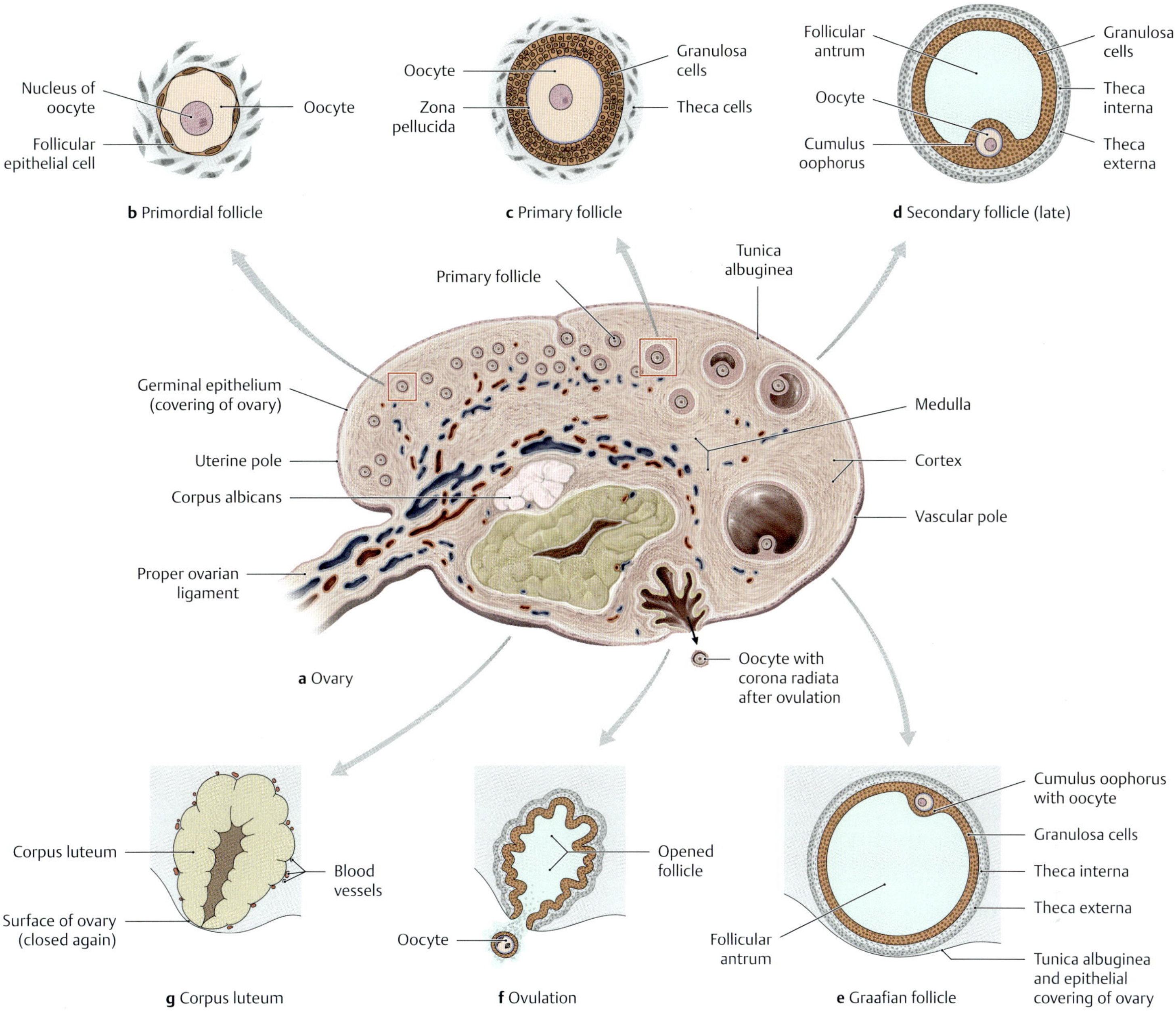

C Follicular maturation in the ovary
The sequence of follicular maturation is illustrated in a clockwise direction around the ovary. The follicular stages are not drawn to scale.

- **a Ovary:** Section through the ovary of an adult woman, demonstrating its structure and follicular stages. The central medulla is surrounded by a cortical region containing follicles at various stages of development. At the lower edge of the ovary, an oocyte is being released from a ruptured follicle (ovulation). After ovulation has taken place, the graafian follicle initially develops into a hormonally active corpus luteum and later regresses to form a white fibrous scar (corpus albicans).
- **b Primordial follicle:** Oocyte surrounded by a single layer of flat epithelial cells.
- **c Primary follicle:** When the single layer of epithelium around the oocyte becomes multilaminar but without an atrium, the follicle is called a primary follicle.
- **d Secondary follicle:** The epithelium (composed of granulosa cells) becomes stratified with an antrum present, and the epithelium and oocyte are separated from each other by a conspicuous zona pellucida. The fluid-filled spaces between the epithelial cells coalesce to form a single cavity (follicular cavity or antrum) containing follicular fluid. The connective tissue surrounding the follicular epithelium is organized into a theca externa and theca interna (hormone production), which are separated from the epithelium by a basement membrane.
- **e Graafian follicle:** Preovulatory follicle with a large follicular cavity. The oocyte is located on an eccentric hillock, the cumulus oophorus, together with a large aggregation of epithelial cells, the corona radiata.
  Note: The graafian follicle is approximately 2 cm in diameter—large enough to create a distinct bulge on the ovarian surface.
- **f Ovulation:** The follicle ruptures, and the oocyte is expelled with the cumulus oophorus cells into the peritoneal cavity. Generally the oocyte is caught by the fimbriated end of the uterine tube. Some spontaneous bleeding occurs into the follicular cavity.
- **g Corpus luteum:** This is a yellowish structure of very high hormonal activity formed by transformation of the graafian follicle. If the ovum is not fertilized, the corpus luteum involutes and degenerates during the menstrual cycle (becoming the corpus luteum of menstruation). If fertilization takes place, the corpus luteum persists (as the corpus luteum of pregnancy) during the first trimester in response to hormonal stimulation from the zygote, lasting until its hormonal function has been replaced by the placenta.

Note: A new follicle matures every 28 days. However, maturation of each individual follicle takes much longer.

5.9 Pregnancy and Childbirth

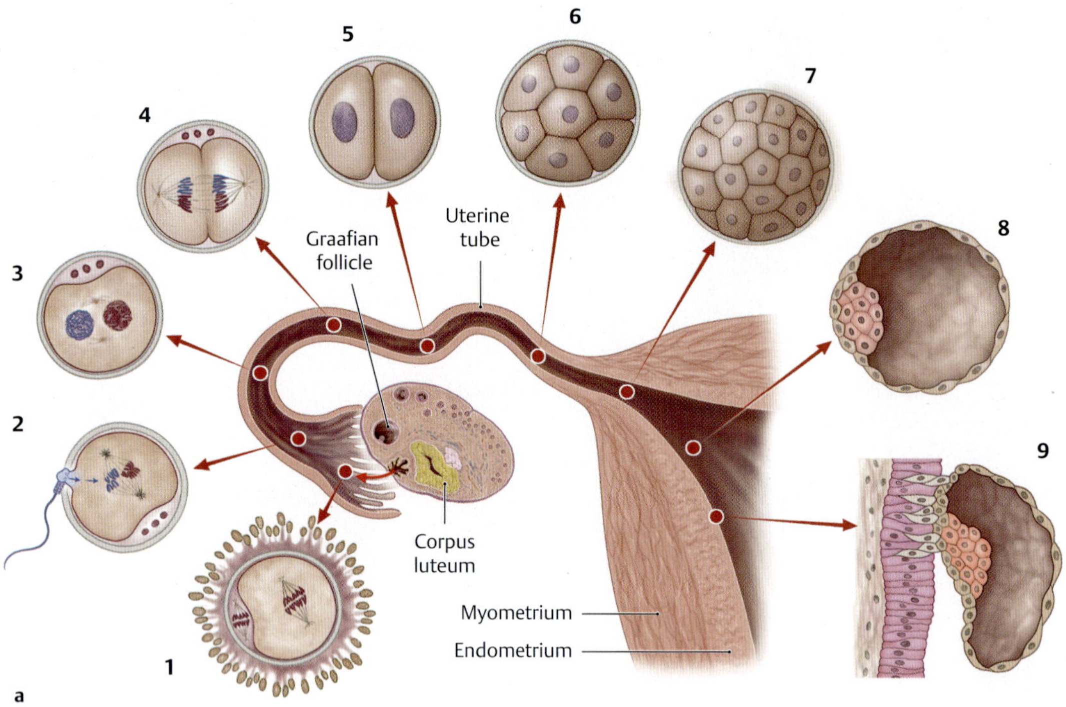

1 Ovum immediately after ovulation
2 Fertilization within approximately 12 hours
3 Male and female pronuclei, later forming a zygote
4 Initial division of zygote
5 Two-cell stage (30 hours)
6 Morula stage (third day)
7 Entry into uterine lumen (fourth day)
8 Blastocyst (fourth to fifth day)
9 Onset of implantation (fifth to sixth day)

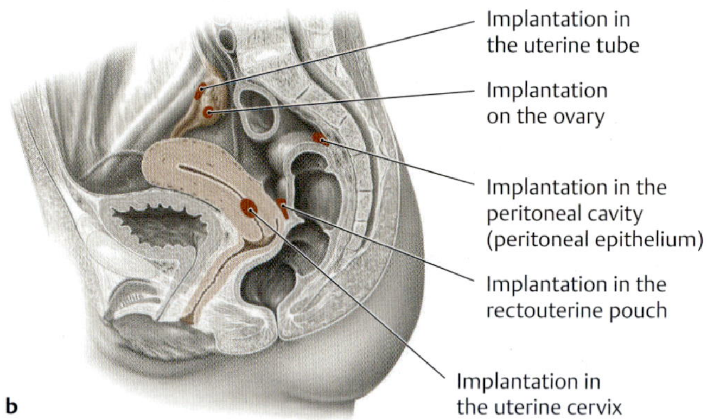

A Phases in the migration of the fertilized ovum and sites of ectopic pregnancy

a Phases in the migration of the fertilized ovum: Normally the zygote migrates to the uterus. The ovum is fertilized in the uterine tube, usually in its ampullary portion. Spermatozoa reach that site by a flagellating tail action that enables them to swim "upstream" against the flow of the ciliated epithelium (positive rheotaxis)—the same current that propels the zygote toward the uterine cavity. As it migrates through the uterine tube, the zygote undergoes various stages of development. On approximately the sixth day after ovulation, the blastocyst implants in the endometrium, which has been prepared by secretory transformation.

b Sites of ectopic pregnancy. Under abnormal conditions, a fertilized ovum may become implanted at various sites outside the uterine cavity:

- at sites close to the uterus (tubal pregnancy) or
- within the peritoneal cavity (abdominal pregnancy).

In a tubal pregnancy (e.g., caused by postinflammatory adhesions of the tubal mucosa that hamper zygote migration), there is a risk of tubal wall rupture due to the close confines of the tubal lumen, possibly causing a life-threatening hemorrhage into the peritoneal cavity.

B Levels of the uterus during pregnancy

a Anterior view; **b** Left lateral view.

The uterine fundus is palpable at different levels during the various lunar months of pregnancy (lunar month = a 28-day period).

Note: At the start of the 10th lunar month, the uterine fundus turns anteriorly and drops to a level that is slightly lower than in the 9th lunar month.

As term approaches, the greatly enlarged uterus presses against almost all the organs in the abdomen and pelvis. In the supine position the uterus may even compress the inferior vena cava, compromising venous return to the heart. In emergency situations, therefore, a pregnant patient should always be placed in the *left lateral decubitus* position to avoid vascular compression.

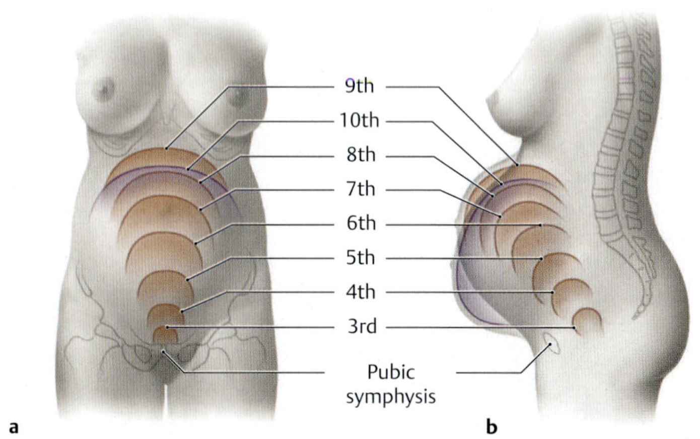

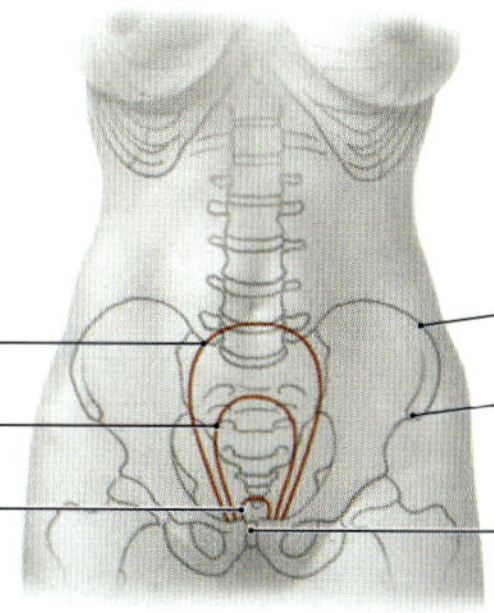

C Postpartum involution of the uterus

Anterior view. With normal postpartum involution of the uterus, the uterine fundus can be palpated and physically examined at various levels. Three palpable bony landmarks (the iliac crest, anterior superior iliac spine, and pubic symphysis) can be helpful in evaluating the level of the uterine fundus.

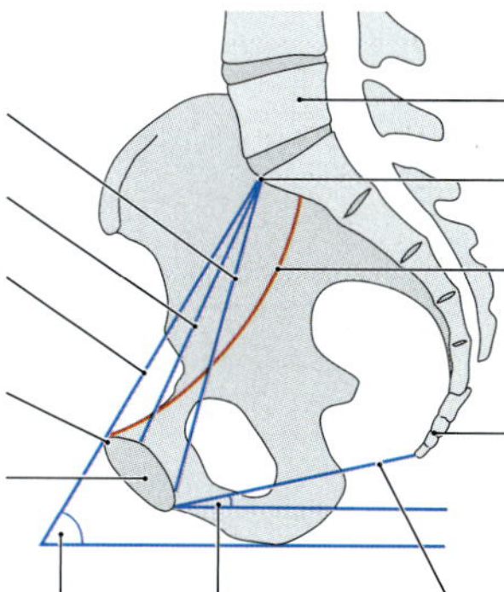

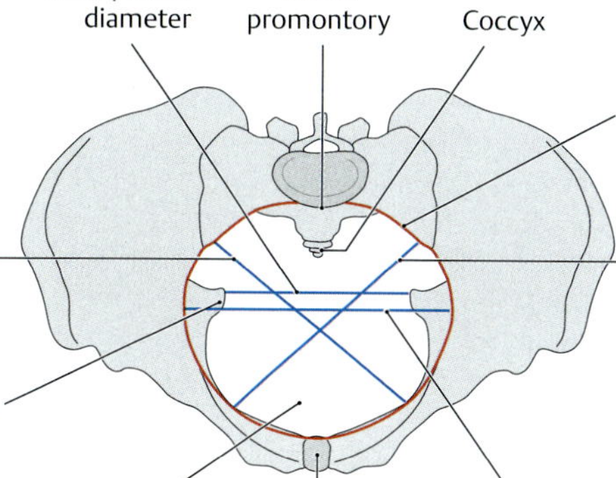

D Important obstetric pelvic dimensions: pelvic planes

a Midsagittal section of the female pelvis, viewed from the left side
b Superior view of a female pelvis.

During parturition, the fetus passes through various planes of the maternal pelvis. The pelvic dimensions of greatest clinical importance are sagittal (smallest anteroposterior diameter). The pelvis has its smallest sagittal diameter at the "true conjugate," which is the shortest distance from the posterior surface of the pubic symphysis to the sacral promontory. That distance should be at least 11 cm; if not, a normal vaginal delivery may be difficult or impossible. The most important fetal dimensions are cranial, particularly the greatest sagittal head diameter. The principal pelvic dimensions are reviewed in **E**.

E Internal dimensions of the female pelvis

Designation	Definition	Length
Conjugata vera obstetrica diameter (true conjugate)	Distance between the sacral promontory and the posterior border of the pubic symphysis	11 cm
Diagonal conjugate	Distance between the sacral promontory and the inferior border of the pubic symphysis	12.5–13 cm
AP diameter of pelvic outlet plane	Distance between the inferior border of the pubic symphysis and the tip of the coccyx	9 (+2) cm
Transverse diameter of pelvic inlet plane	Longest distance between the lineae terminales	13 cm
Interspinous diameter	Distance between the ischial spines	11 cm
Right (I) and left (II) oblique diameter	Distance between the sacroiliac joint at the level of the linea terminalis and the iliopectineal eminence on the opposite side	12 cm

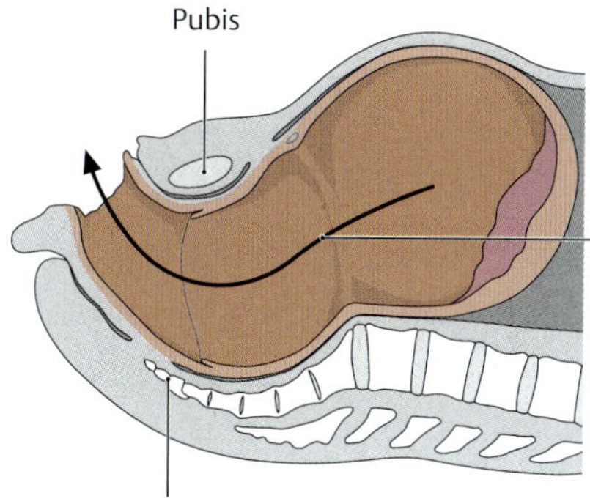

F Birth canal in the expulsion phase of labor (after Rauber and Kopsch)

The uterine cervix, vagina, and pelvic floor have been stretched open to form a "soft-tissue tube." The fetal head, which always rotates its greatest (sagittal) diameter to match the greatest diameter of the current pelvic plane, follows the line indicated. Most babies are delivered in the "occiput anterior" position, with the occiput pointing toward the pubic symphysis.

5.10 Male Genitalia: Accessory Sex Glands

A Accessory sex glands (prostate, seminal vesicles, and bulbourethral glands)

Posterior view of the bladder, prostate, seminal vesicles, and bulbourethral glands. The peritoneum and visceral pelvic fascia have been completely removed; stumps of both ureters and ductus deferentes have been left in place to aid orientation. Each of the **seminal vesicles** consists of a tube approximately 15 cm long that is coiled upon itself to a length of about 5 cm. The secretion from the seminal vesicles makes up approximately 70% of the volume of the ejaculate, is slightly alkaline (pH 7.4), and is very high in fructose (energy source for the spermatozoa). The term "seminal vesicle" is misleading in that the gland does not contain spermatocytes. The excretory duct of the seminal vesicle unites with the ductus deferens to form the ejaculatory duct, which passes through the prostate. The seminal vesicles develop from the epithelium of the mesonephric ducts and are situated lateral to the ductus deferentes, which also develop from the mesonephric ducts. The **bulbourethral glands** are embedded in the deep transverse perineal, and their approximately 2- to 4-cm-long ducts open into the posterior aspect of the urethra. They secrete a clear, watery fluid that prepares the urethra for the passage of the sperm. The prostate is described in **B**.

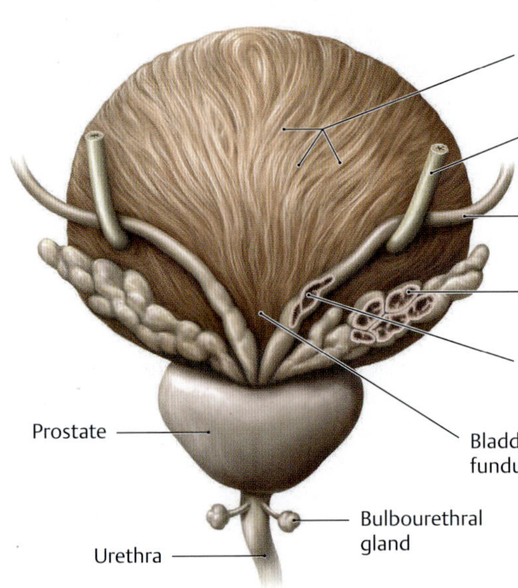

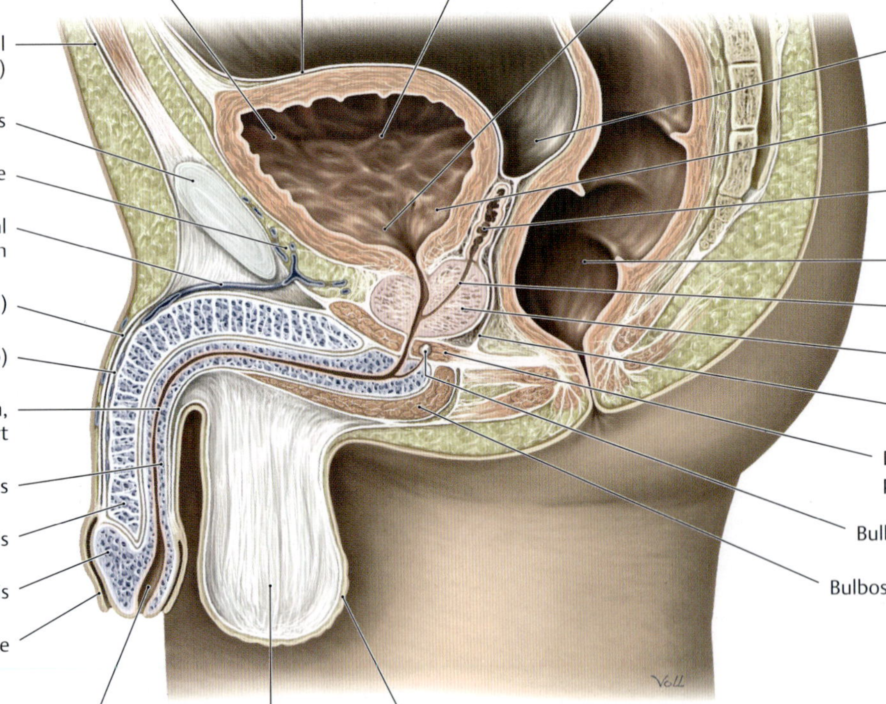

B The prostate in situ

Sagittal section through a male pelvis, viewed from the left side, with the bladder and rectum opened. This drawing is a composite from many planes to demonstrate the peritoneal relationships and the attachment of the seminal vesicle to the prostate and urethra. The paramedian ampulla of the ductus deferens has been straightened somewhat and projected into the sectional plane with the ejaculatory duct and left bulbourethral gland. The prostate is located at the bladder outlet and encircles the urethra (see **C**). It borders posteriorly on the anterior wall of the rectum, separated from it by connective-tissue fascia. The prostate has no contact with the peritoneum and lies entirely in the pelvic extraperitoneal space. By contrast, the tips of the seminal vesicles are frequently covered by visceral peritoneum.

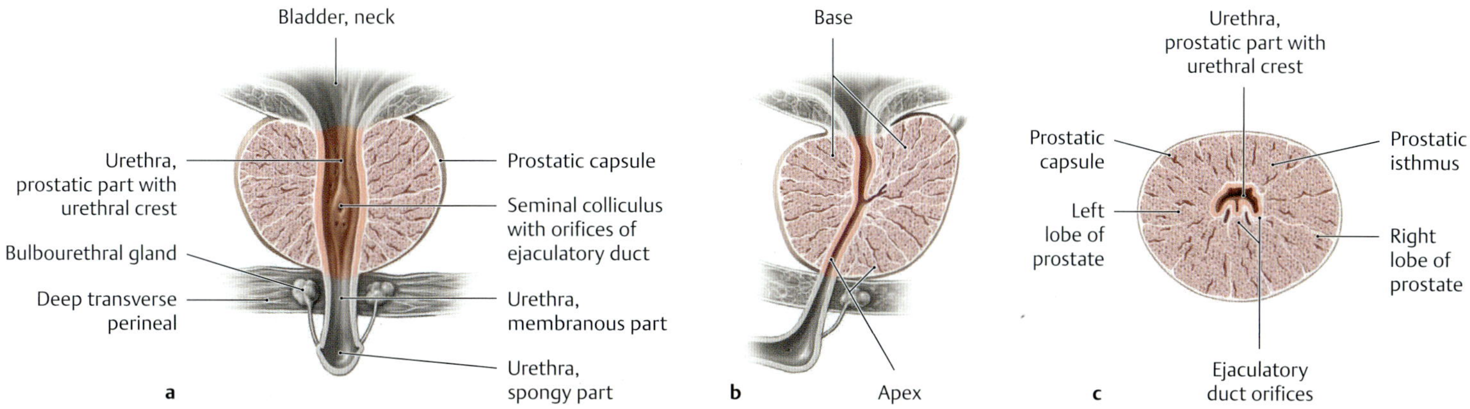

C Relationship of the prostate to the urethra

a Coronal section (anterior view), **b** sagittal section (left lateral view), and **c** transverse section (superior view) through the prostate and urethra.

The prostate is a chestnut-sized gland consisting of two lateral lobes (right and left) that are joined posteriorly by the median lobe and anteriorly by the prostatic isthmus. The entire gland is surrounded by a firm connective-tissue capsule (prostatic capsule). The prostate is a derivative of the urethral epithelium, appearing initially as a posterior epithelial bud that later grows to encircle the urethra (prostatic part). Histologically, the prostate is composed of 30–50 tubuloalveolar glands that open into the prostatic part of the urethra via approximately 20 excretory ducts. The prostatic secretion makes up approximately 30% of the volume of the ejaculate. It contains compounds that are important for active sperm motility. The secretion is colorless, watery, and slightly acidic (pH 6.4). It also contains a protein (prostate-specific antigen, PSA) whose serum levels are frequently elevated in patients with a prostatic malignancy.

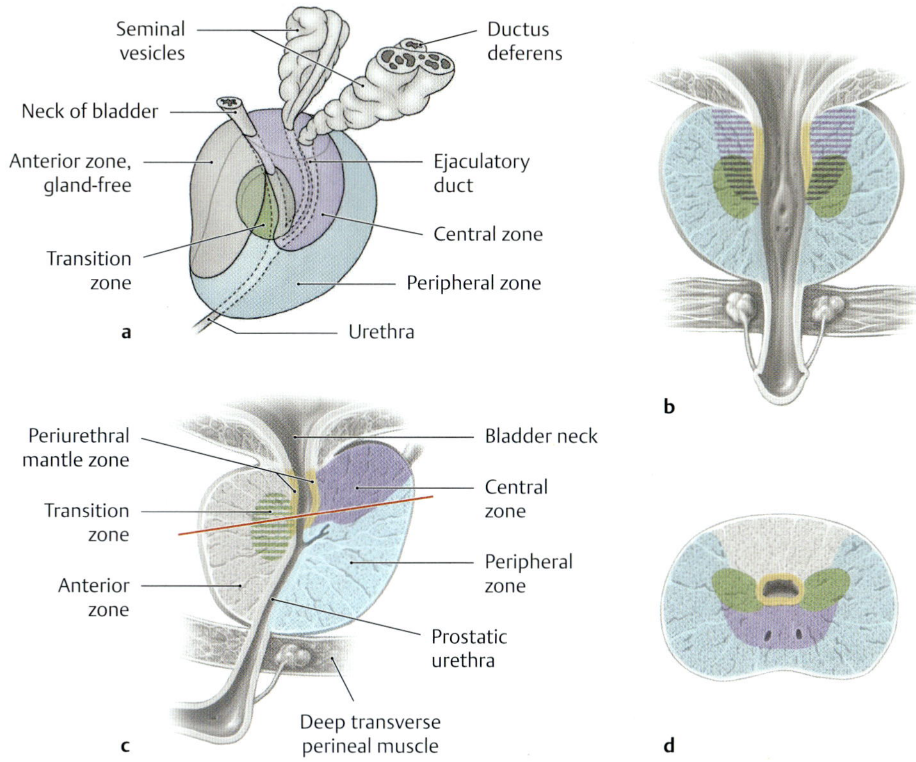

D Normal values for the male accessory sex glands

Prostate	
Sagittal diameter	ca. 2–3 cm
Width	ca. 4 cm
Thickness	ca. 1–2 cm
Glands	ca. 40 lobules
Duct system	ca. 20 ducts
Secretion	pH 6.4; enzyme-rich
Weight	ca. 20 g
Seminal vesicle	
Length – Coiled	ca. 3–5 cm
– Uncoiled	ca. 15 cm
Secretion	pH 7.4; fructose-rich
Bulbourethral gland	
Size	Pea-sized
Duct length	ca. 4 cm

E Clinical and histological division of the prostate into zones (after McNeal)

Schematic representation of the prostate (**a**) viewed in three sections: **b** frontal section, **c** sagittal section; **d** horizontal section.

The most commonly used system for anatomic division of the prostate is based on studies by McNeal. The prostatic urethra serves as a landmark and at the level of the seminal colliculus angles anteriorly (35 degrees) and divides into a proximal and a distal segment (**c** and **Cb**). At the level of the seminal colliculus lies the opening of the prostatic utricle (remnant of the paramesonephric ducts), on each side of which lie the openings of the ejaculatory ducts. The proximal urethral segment is surrounded like a cuff by the *periurethral zone*, which is flanked on each side by the *transition zone* that consists of two lobes that account for not more that 5% of the glandular tissue of the prostate. Behind it lies the wedge-shaped *central zone* that accounts for approximately 25% of the prostatic tissue. It is traversed by the ejaculatory ducts and the utricle. The *peripheral zone* extends posterolaterally and accounts for 70% of prostatic weight. Anterior prostate tissue consists of a fibromuscular stroma that lacks glands.

Note: Approximately 70% of prostatic carcinomas occur in the peripheral zone near the prostatic capsule. The most common site of benign prostatic hyperplasia is the transition zone, the volume of which increases significantly as a result (see p. 356).

5.11 Prostate Tumors: Prostatic Carcinoma, Prostatic Hyperplasia; Cancer Screening

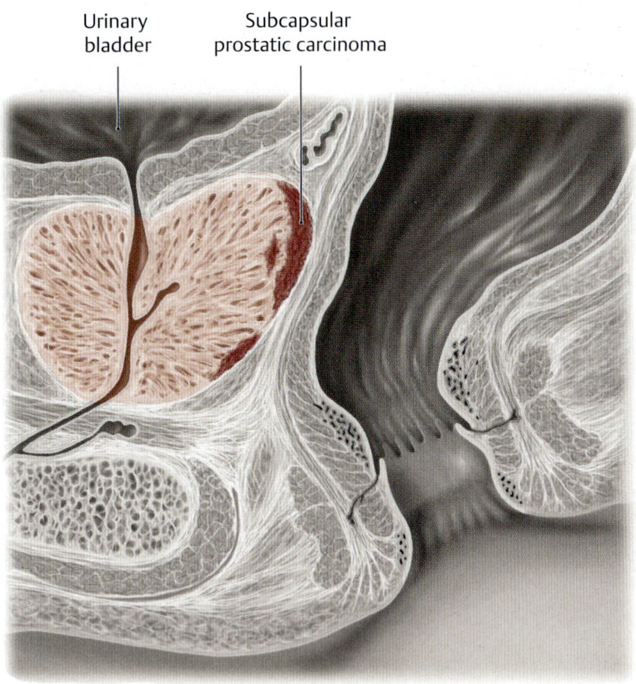

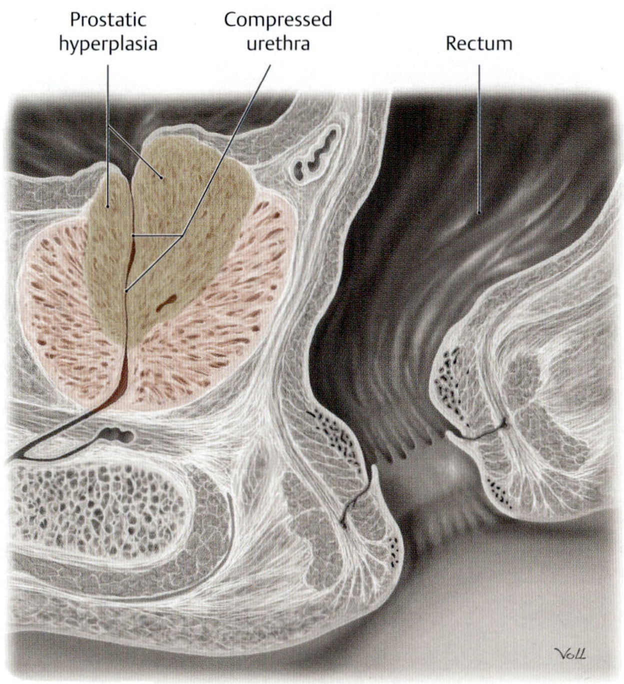

A Prostatic carcinoma

Prostatic carcinoma is the most common urological tumor in males, with 95 % of prostatic carcinomas occurring in males between the ages of 45 and 89. The average age at diagnosis is 70. In Germany, 50,000 males are diagnosed each year. It is the third most common cause of cancer related deaths (accounting for 10 % of deaths due to cancer). Prostatic carcinomas most often (85 %) grow in the peripheral zone of the prostate (see p. 355). Because of its predominantly peripheral location, typical symptoms appear only when the tumor has spread locally. Symptoms indicate bone metastases: back pain, sciatic nerve pain, and pulling pain in the pelvic region. In almost 50 % of patients who are diagnosed with a malignant prostate tumor, the cancer will metastasize which then signifies the incurable stage of the disease. Hence, screening for prostate cancer is crucial to improve the chances of survival. Currently, three tests are routinely performed as part of the screening (see **C**, **D**, and **E**):

- Measurement of prostate-specific antigen (PSA)
- Digital rectal examination (DRE)
- Transrectal ultrasound (TRUS)

Therapeutic concepts: Generally, treatment options are based on the stage of cancer at the time of diagnosis. Usually, a locally confined prostatic carcinoma is treated with surgery (radical prostatectomy) or radiation (e.g., brachytherapy). Because prostate cancers are testosterone-dependent, progressive tumors are often treated with antiandrogens. Testosterone secretion is reduced by suppressing GnRH secretion (GnRH = gonadotropin-releasing-hormone) with the help of synthetic GnRH analogs, which permanently occupy pituitary GnRH receptors (functional castration).

B Benign prostatic hyperplasia (BPH)

Benign prostatic hyperplasia is the most common type of prostatic tumor in older men. BPH is characterized by structural changes accompanied by the formation of nodules particularly in the transition zone (see p. 355), but also often in the peripheral zone, caused by cell proliferation (hyperplasia). Both glandular and stromal proliferation contribute to the hyperplasia (fibromuscular/glandular hyperplasia) and result in an enlarged transition zone and thus the entire prostate. The affected areas are mainly those immediately surrounding the urethra. Compression of the urethra leads to voiding dysfunction including reduction in micturition interval, weak urinary stream and resulting strained efforts to push urine out of the bladder, and pollakiuria (frequent passing of small volumes of urine). At advanced stages, increasing obstruction of the bladder outlet leads to bladder wall hypertrophy (trabeculated bladder), residual urine retention and backlog of urine accompanied by the bilateral dilation of the ureters and the calyceal system of the renal pelvis.

Diagnostic process: In addition to the patient's history (typical symptoms?) and rectal palpation (enlarged prostate, clearly defined prostate), transvesical and transrectal sonography is used to assess size and structural changes of the prostate and to measure the volume of residual urine. Uroflowmetry measures urine flow (normal values range from 15 to 40 ml/s). Prostate-specific antigen (PSA, see **D**) can be elevated just like with the presence of prostate cancer.

Treatment options: In addition to a "wait and watch" approach (hyperplasia sometimes comes to a standstill), more conservative methods are used to significantly alleviate symptoms (phytotherapy, antiadrenergic therapy, and anti-androgens hormonal treatment–testosterone-dependent hyperplasia). The most common surgical treatment is transurethral resection of the prostate. An electric loop is used to break off small pieces of tissue, which are flushed through the urethra.

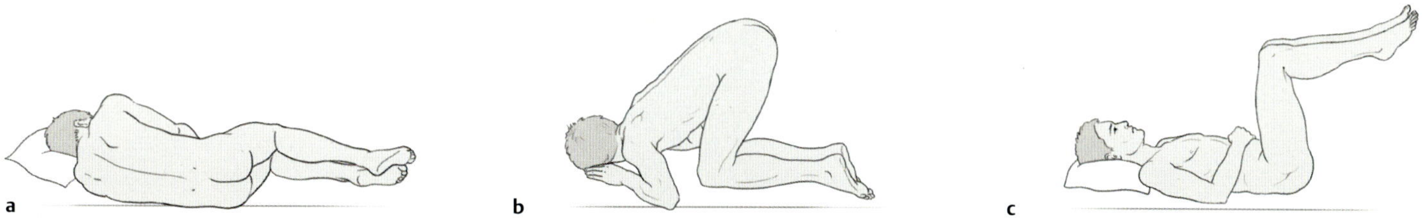

C Palpation of the prostate
a Left lateral position; **b** Knee-elbow position; **c** Lithotomy position; **d** Digital rectal palpation.
The digital rectal examination (DRE) of the prostate is an important screening test and should be performed yearly beginning at age 40. It can be done with the patient in the knee-elbow, lithotomy, or lateral position and starts with the inspection of the rectum. The prostate can be located at the anterior wall of the rectum 7–8 cm from the anus (**d**). Size, surface, and consistency of both lobes, the medial sulcus, the movability of the rectal mucosa, and the delineation from neighboring tissue are evaluated. The prostate is normally the size of a chestnut and its consistency is like the contracted thenar muscles of the thumb. With benign prostatic hyperplasia (see **B**) the prostate surface is smooth, despite being grossly enlarged, and the rectal mucosa is movable. Prostate cancer (see **A**), however, makes the gland hard and bumpy and reduces the mobility of the rectal mucosa. A soft, tender, ill-defined prostate is a sign of prostate infection.

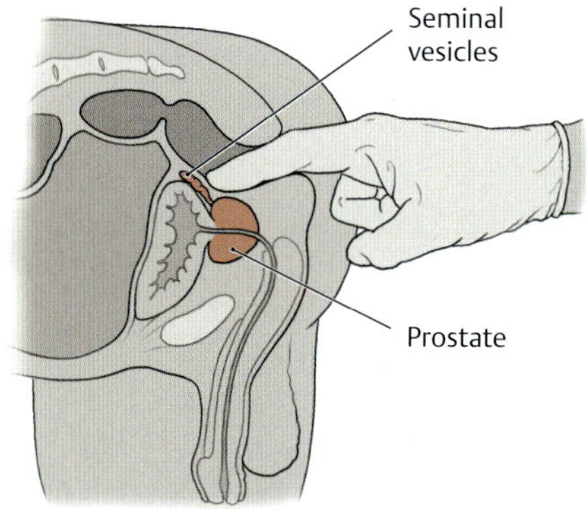

D Measurement of prostate-specific antigen (PSA)

Prostate-specific antigen (PSA) is a serine protease that is predominantly produced by the prostate epithelial cells, which are secretorially active. It contributes to the liquefaction of the viscous secretion of the seminal vesicles. Thus, PSA is a normal enzyme present in healthy men. Some of it enters the bloodstream and circulates freely (f-PSA) or in a complex formation (c-PSA). Normally, the serum level of total PSA is 4ng/ml, but it can vary for a specific individual. Because PSA formation rate in prostatic carcinoma cells can be up to 10 times higher than in normal cells, PSA values can be used as a tumor marker (although with some limitations). With slightly elevated levels (4–10 ng/ml), a prostatic carcinoma is detected in 25 % of cases, and in 50 % of cases with a greatly elevated level (greater than 10 ng/ml). Since other benign diseases (benign prostatic hyperplasia, chronic prostatitis), sporting activities (horse riding, bike riding) and simply straining on the toilet due to constipation can lead to elevated PSA levels, the value of PSA-based early detection of prostatic carcinoma is controversial.

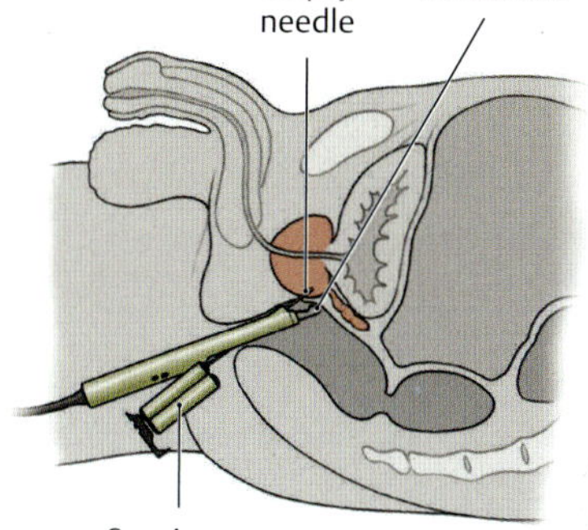

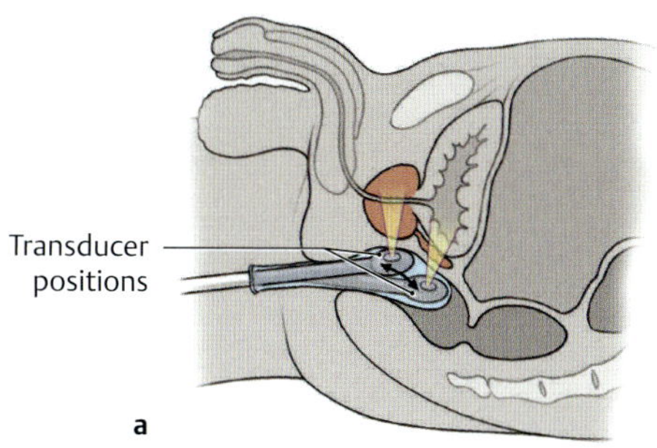

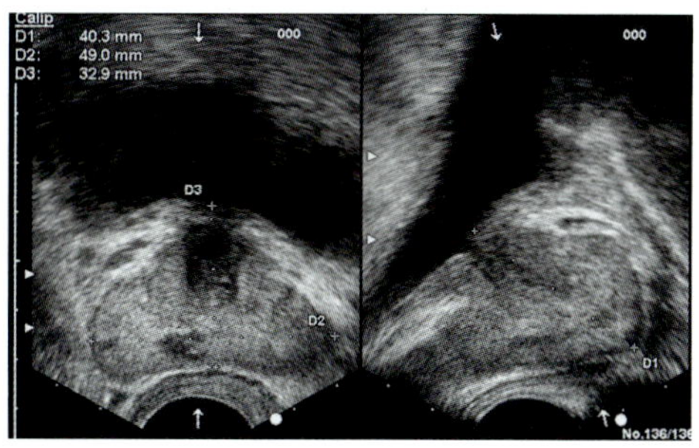

E Transrectal ultrasound (TRUS)
a Insertion of the ultrasound probe into the rectum; **b** Images of the prostate in transverse and sagittal section for the assessment of prostatic volume (from: Dietrich, CH.: Endosonographie, Lehrbuch und Atlas des endoskopischen Ultraschalls. Thieme, Stuttgart 2008).
Transrectal ultrasound or transrectal prostate sonography is a simple, quick and inexpensive procedure and thus the primary diagnostic imaging technique for evaluating the prostate. A gel-filled condom is placed over a probe, which is inserted into the rectum. This method allows for optimal coupling to the anterior wall of the rectum to minimize interference with air or feces. With a frequency of 7.5 MHz, high quality images can be taken at a depth of 1–5 cm from the surface of the prostate. To aid orientation, it is first displayed in transverse section. By turning the probe, the prostate can be evaluated in a sagittal section. Displaying the prostate in both sections helps to determine the exact size and thus volume of the prostate.

F Prostate biopsy guided by transrectal ultrasound (TRUS)
Ultrasound-guided transrectal trephine biopsy is performed to provide histological proof of prostatic carcinoma. The transrectal ultrasound is used to guide the biopsy needle either to systematically chosen areas of the prostate or to palpable lumps in suspicious areas. The needle, which is passed through the needle guide attached to the probe, is constantly visible on the ultrasound image. In this way, suspicious areas can be precisely located. In trephine biopsy usually 8–18 thin tissue cylinders are obtained, which will then be histologically assessed. The fact that a biopsy only evaluates parts of the prostate limits the conclusiveness of the results.

5.12 Male Genitalia: Scrotum, Testis, and Epididymis

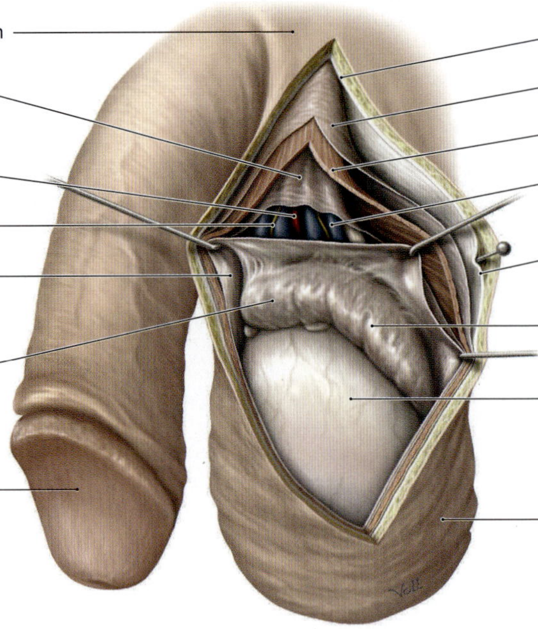

A The scrotum and coverings of the testis in situ

Left lateral view with the scrotum opened in layers. The testis is a paired organ having the approximate size and shape of a plum (see **D**). It is divided by fibrous septa into approximately 350 lobules. The layers of the scrotum and coverings of the testis are formed by the layers of the anterior abdominal wall during the developmental descent of the testis (see **E**). As the testis descends, it carries with it a finger-shaped process of peritoneum (vaginal process) through the inguinal canal; normally this process becomes obliterated and separated from the peritoneal cavity at the internal (deep) inguinal ring. Thus the peritoneum forms a closed sac within the scrotum (tunica vaginalis) composed of a visceral layer and a parietal layer. An abnormal collection of serous fluid in the space between the two peritoneal layers (hydrocele) may exert pressure on the testis, causing clinical complaints. Occasionally, however, the peritoneal process remains patent and gives rise to a congenital indirect inguinal hernia.

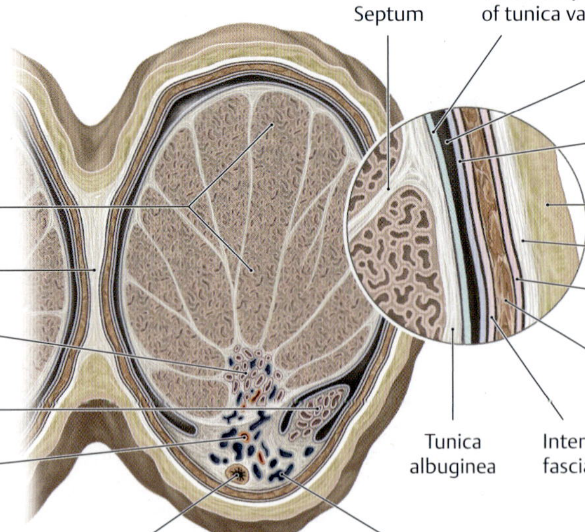

B Scrotum and coverings of the testis in cross-section

Transverse section through the right testis, viewed from above. The magnified view shows the various layers that make up the coverings of the testis. The testis is surrounded by a firm fibrous capsule, the tunica albuginea. Fine connective-tissue septa radiate inward from the tunica albuginea to the testicular mediastinum, subdividing the testis into approximately 350–370 lobules that contain the seminiferous tubules (see **C**). The seminiferous tubules are the sites where the spermatocytes develop (spermatogenesis). Groups of cells embedded in the interstitial connective tissue produce testosterone.

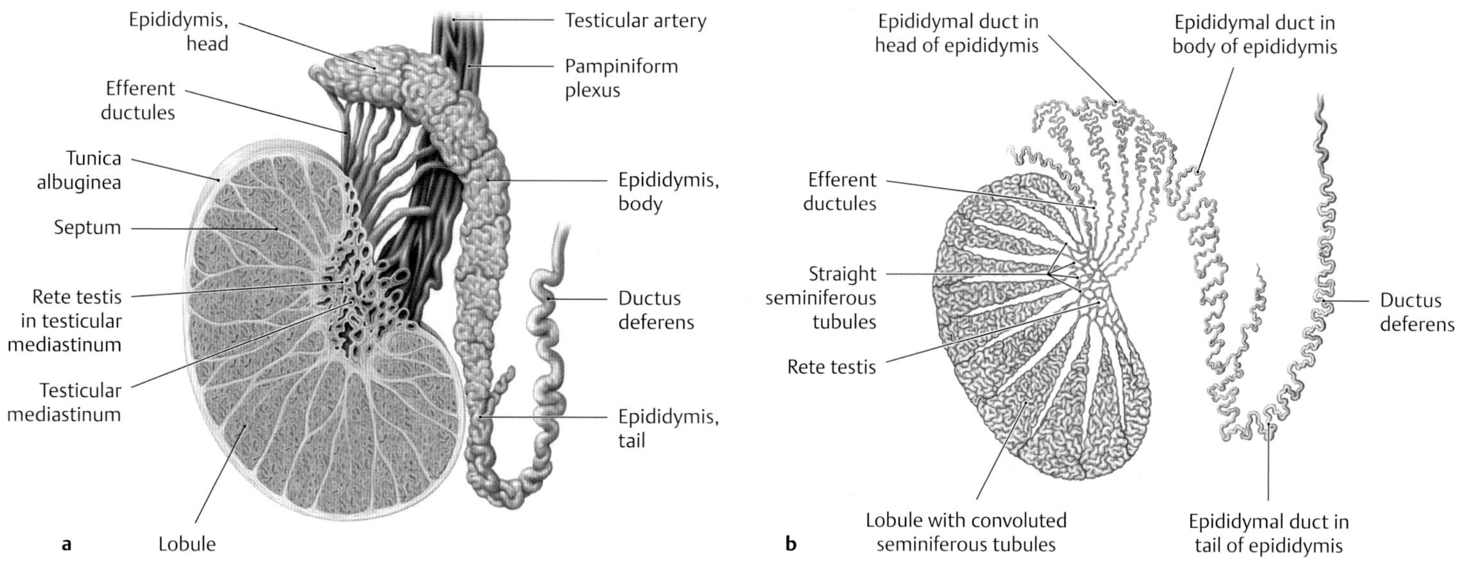

C Structure of the testis and epididymis
Left lateral view of the left testis and epididymis. The testis has been sectioned in the sagittal plane, and the epididymis has been elevated from the testis. The wedge-shaped lobules of the testis contain the **seminiferous tubules** (convoluted seminiferous tubules, approximately 3 cm long coiled, 20 cm long uncoiled), where the sperm develop. The tissue between the convoluted seminiferous tubules contains the interstitial (Leydig) cells, which produce androgens, principally testosterone. The convoluted tubules continue into the straight seminiferous tubules, which continue into the rete testis, a network of anastomosing epithelium-lined channels. The rete testis is connected to approximately 12 efferent ductules, which open into the epididymis. Attached to the posterior aspect of the testis, the epididymis is the organ of storage and maturation for the spermatozoa. The head of the **epididymis** consists mostly of the efferent ductules, while its body and tail consist of the highly convoluted epididymal duct (approximately 6 m long when unraveled). In the head of the epididymis, the efferent ductules open into the epididymal duct, which is continuous at its caudal end with the ductus deferens.
Note: The testis and epididymis lie inside the scrotum and outside the abdominal cavity because the temperature within the body cavity is too high for normal spermatogenesis. Thus, failure of the testis to descend normally into the scrotum (i.e., an inguinal testis) is frequently associated with infertility.
The formation and maturation of spermatocytes in the testis, the migration of spermatozoa in the epididymis, and their final storage in the caudal part of the epididymal duct takes approximately 80 days.

D Normal values for the testis and epididymis

Testis	Epididymis
Weight ca. 20 g Length ca. 4 cm Width ca. 2 cm 350–370 testicular lobules Approximately 12 efferent ductules	Length of epididymal duct – Uncoiled ca. 6 m – Coiled ca. 6 cm

E Coverings of the testis and layers of the abdominal wall
The inguinal canal is an evagination of the abdominal wall. As a result, the anatomical layers of the abdominal wall have their counterparts in the layers of the scrotum and testicular coverings.

Layers of the abdominal wall	Coverings of the spermatic cord and testis
• Abdominal skin and membranous (deep) layer of superficial fascia	→ Scrotal skin with tunica dartos
• External oblique fascia	→ External spermatic fascia
• Internal oblique muscle and fascia	→ Cremaster muscle and its fascia
• Transversalis fascia	→ Internal spermatic fascia
• Peritoneum	→ Tunica vaginalis: parietal layer and visceral layer

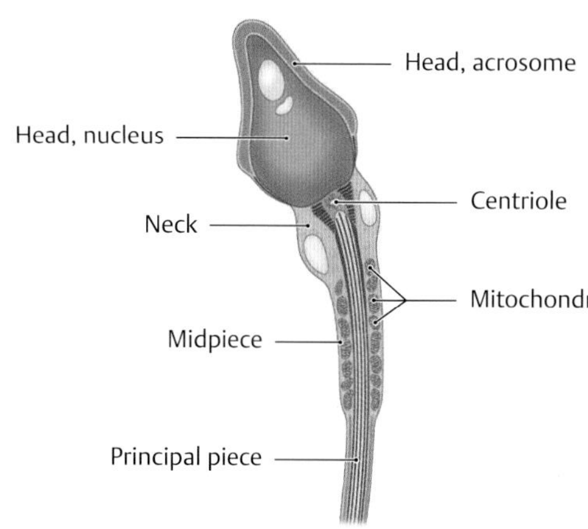

F Ultrastructure of a mature spermatozoon
It takes approximately 80 days for a spermatic stem cell (spermatogonium) to develop into a mature spermatozoon. The spermatogonia are formed in the convoluted seminiferous tubules, while final maturation takes place in the epididymis. The ultrastructural features of the spermatozoon, which is approximately 60 µm long (with tail), include the following:

- The *head* with the acrosome and nucleus
- The *tail* (flagellum), which contains the axonema (axial filament) and consists of several parts:
  - Neck
  - Midpiece
  - Principal piece
  - End piece (not shown here)

5.13 Male Genitalia: Seminiferous Structures and Ejaculate

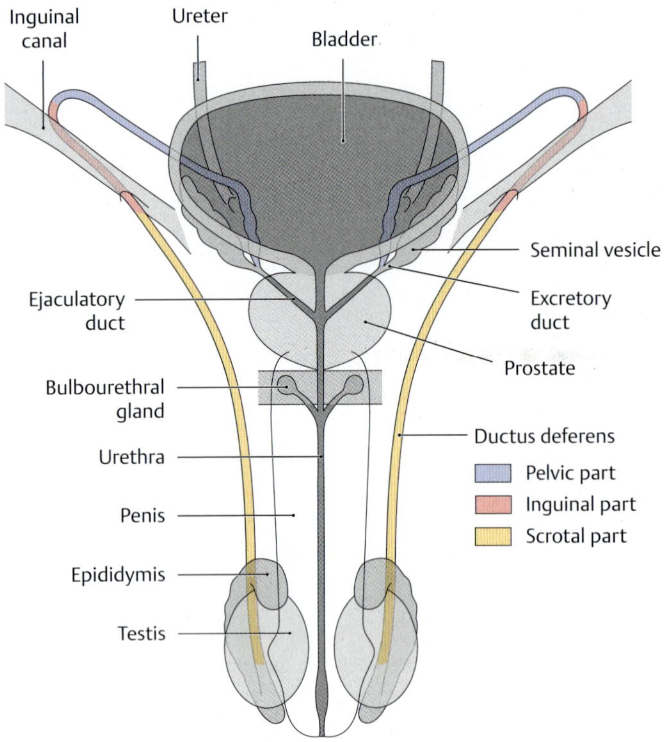

A Overview of the seminiferous structures

Anterior view of the male reproductive tract. The bladder is also shown to aid orientation.

Note: The male urethra serves as a common urinary and genital passage. The ductus deferens and the duct of the seminal vesicle join to form the ejaculatory duct, which opens into the urethra (see **C**).

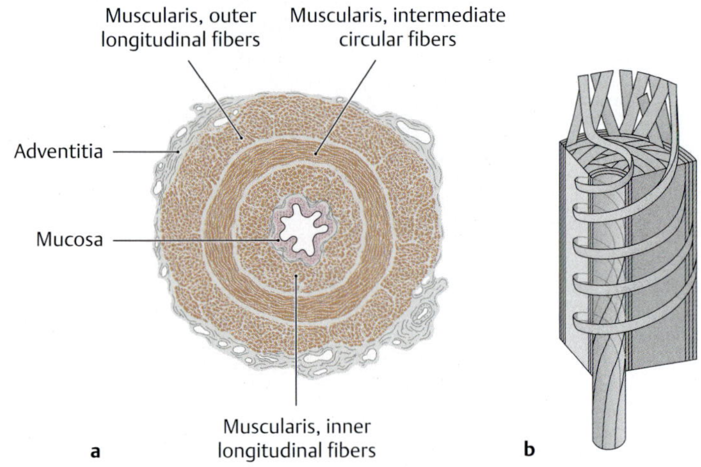

B Wall structure and musculature of the ductus deferens

a Wall structure of the ductus deferens, cross-section through the lumen. The ductus deferens (vas deferens) is approximately 40 cm long and 3 mm in diameter. It arises in continuity with the epididymal duct at the caudal end of the epididymis. Its function is to transport the sperm suspension rapidly toward the urethra during ejaculation. It is equipped for this task with powerful smooth muscle fibers that appear to be arranged in three layers (longitudinal, circular, and longitudinal; see **b**). Facing the lumen of the ductus deferens is a simple columnar epithelium. Close to the epididymis the epithelium becomes pseudostratified, and many cells bear stereocilia (nonmotile cellular projections).

b Musculature of the ductus deferens, three-dimensional representation of the muscle fiber pattern. The smooth muscle of the ductus deferens appears to have a three-layered arrangement when viewed in cross-section. Actually, however, the muscle fibers are arranged in a continuous pattern that spirals around the duct lumen in turns of varying obliquity. The smooth-muscle fibers of the ductus deferens have an extremely rich sympathetic innervation, as ejaculation is triggered by the sympathetic nervous system.

C Site of spermatogenesis and pathway of sperm transport

The seminiferous structures in the strict sense consist of the efferent ductules, epididymal duct, and ductus deferens.

Testis	• Convoluted seminiferous tubules (spermatogenesis) • Straight seminiferous tubules • Rete testis • Efferent ductules
Epididymis	
• Head	• Efferent ductules (open into epididymal duct)
• Body	• Epididymal duct
• Tail	• Epididymal duct (opens into ductus deferens)
Inguinal canal and pelvic cavity	• Ductus deferens
Prostate	• Ejaculatory duct (union of ductus deferens and duct of seminal vesicle)
Pelvic floor and penis (corpus spongiosum)	• Urethra

D The ejaculate (normal values and terminology)

The ejaculate consists of spermatozoa and seminal fluid, which comes mainly the seminal vesicles (approximately 70 %) and prostata (approximately 30 %).

Quantity	2–6 ml
pH	7.0–7.8
Sperm count	ca. 40 million spermatozoa/mL (40–50 % of which show vigorous motility; at least 60 % are structurally normal)
Length of spermatozoa	ca. 60 µm
Normospermia	Normal ejaculate
Aspermia	No ejaculate
Hypospermia	< 2 mL of ejaculate
Normozoospermia	Normal sperm count (see above)
Azoospermia	No spermatozoa
Oligozoospermia	< 20 million spermatozoa/mL
Necrozoospermia	All spermatozoa are motionless
Teratozoospermia	> 60 % of spermatozoa are structurally abnormal

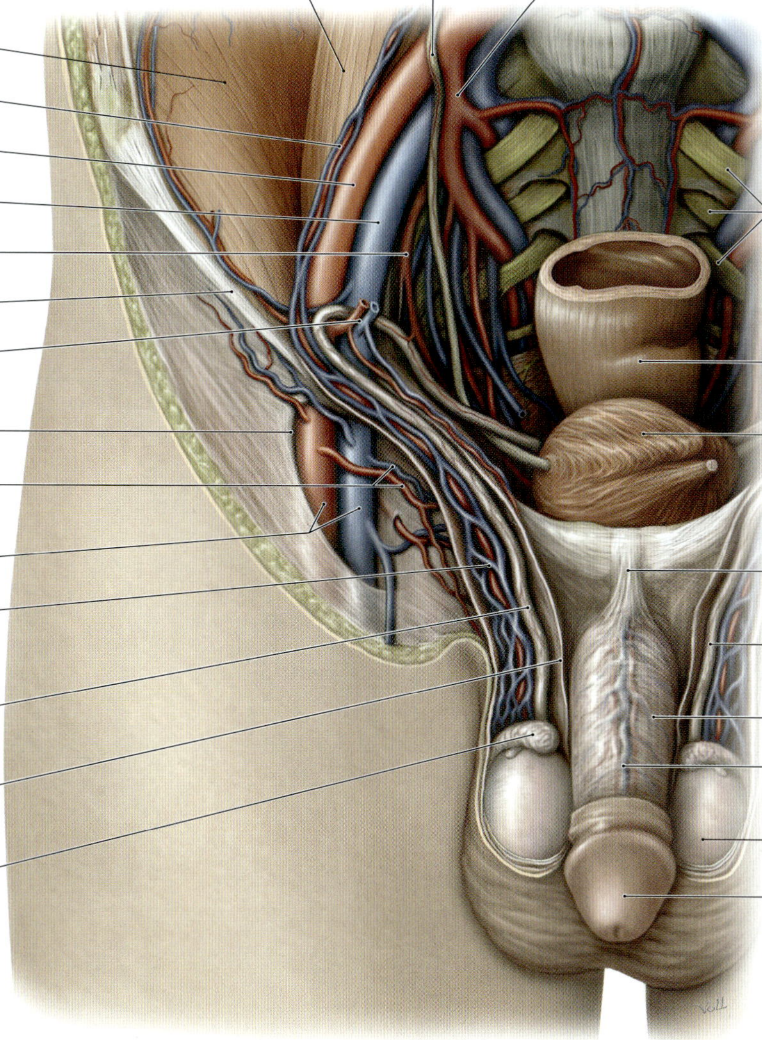

E The spermatic cord in situ
Anterior view. The inguinal canal has been opened on both sides, and the coverings of the spermatic cord have been opened anteriorly to show the course of the ductus deferens. The inguinal canal is markedly larger in the male than in the female due to the presence of the spermatic cord. This larger canal and the larger inguinal ring predispose the male to the herniation of abdominal viscera through the inguinal canal (inguinal hernia).
Note: The ductus deferens passes lateral to the inferior epigastric artery and vein. This relationship should be noted in operations on the inguinal ring to avoid vascular injury.

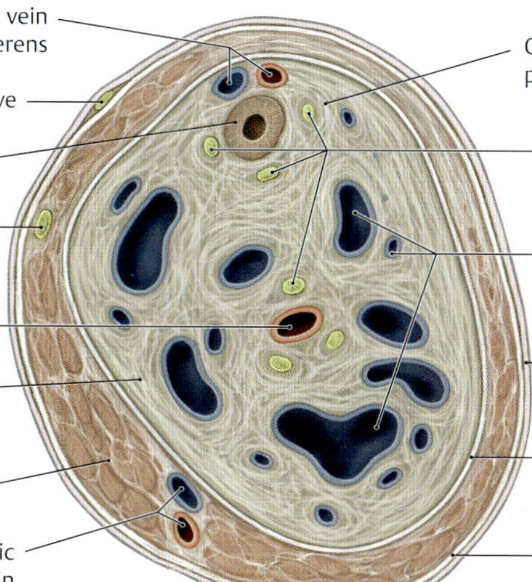

F Contents of the spermatic cord
Transverse section through the spermatic cord to display the wall layers of the cord and the arrangement of its contents. Even a normally developed venous network (pampiniform plexus) may be affected by abnormal varicose dilation about the testis (varicocele, due for example to a venous outflow obstruction) and may raise the temperature of the testis, leading to decreased fertility.
Note: The pampiniform plexus drains into the testicular vein. The right testicular vein opens into the inferior vena cava, while the left testicular vein runs close to the inferior pole of the kidney and enters the renal vein at almost a 90° angle. Thus, it is more common for varicoceles to develop on the left side than on the right side in response to a condition that obstructs testicular venous flow (mass on the lower renal pole, vein entering at a hemodynamically unfavorable angle).

5.14 Branches of the Internal Iliac Artery: Overview of Arteries Supplying the Pelvic Organs and Pelvic Wall

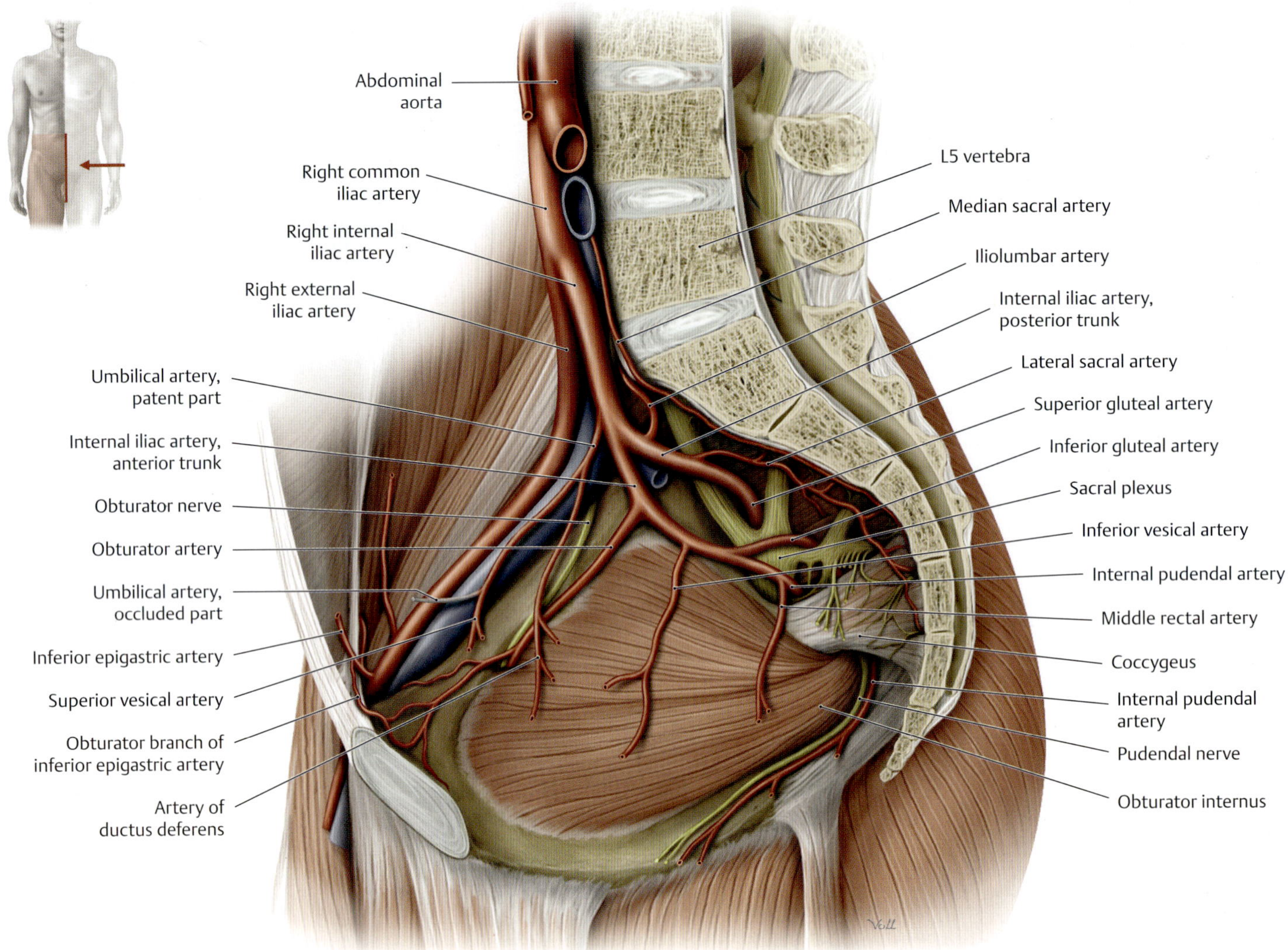

A Branches of the right internal iliac artery in the male pelvis
Sagittal section viewed from the left side, idealized, the pelvic organs have been removed.
The internal iliac artery arises from the common iliac artery. In 60 % of cases it divides anterior to the piriformis (see **D**) into an anterior and posterior trunk. The anterior trunk gives off visceral branches and also parietal branches to the pelvic wall, while the posterior trunk gives off branches only to the pelvic wall. The sequence of the branches is shown in **C**.
Note the relationship of the internal iliac artery and its branches to the sacral plexus. Several branches of the internal iliac artery "disappear" behind this nerve plexus.

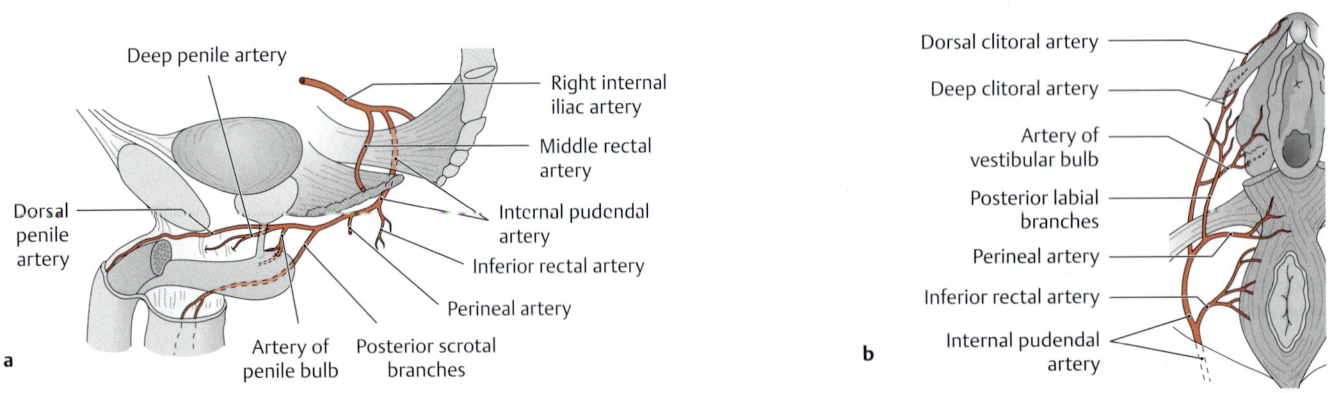

B Course and branches of the right internal pudendal artery on the pelvic floor
The internal pudendal artery is only partially visible in **A**. This diagram illustrates its further course.

a Course of the artery in the male (same perspective as in **A**);

b Course of the artery in the female. The course of the internal pudendal artery is analogous to its course in the male pelvis. An inferior view is shown to supplement the lateral view in **a**, and because this view is important in surgical procedures on the female pelvic floor.

C Sequence of branches of the internal iliac artery

Each internal iliac artery supplies the walls and organs of the pelvis with five parietal branches and five or six visceral branches (→ = "gives off").

Parietal branches (pelvic walls)	
Iliolumbar artery to the lateral pelvic wall	→ *Lumbar branch* → *Spinal branch* → *Iliac branch*
Lateral sacral artery to the posterior pelvic wall	→ *Spinal branches*
Obturator artery to the medial thigh and lateral pelvic wall	→ *Pubic branch* → *Acetabular branch* → *Anterior branch* → *Posterior branch*
Superior gluteal artery to the gluteal region	→ *Superficial branch* → *Deep branch*
Inferior gluteal artery to the gluteal region	→ *Accompanying artery of sciatic nerve*

Visceral branches (pelvic organs)	
Umbilical artery patent part gives off	→ *Artery of ductus deferens* → *Superior vesical artery (to the bladder)*
Inferior vesical artery to the bladder fundus	→ *Prostatic branches*
Uterine artery to the uterus, uterine tubes, vagina, and ovaries	→ *Helicine branches* → *Vaginal branches* → *Ovarian branch* → *Tubal branch*
Vaginal artery May arise as a separate branch from the internal iliac artery (as noted here) or, more commonly, from the inferior vesical artery or uterine artery ("vaginal azygos artery")	
Middle rectal artery to the rectal ampulla and levator ani	→ *Vaginal branches (f)* → *Prostatic branches (m)*
Internal pudendal artery (included with the visceral branches because it gives off the inferior rectal artery)	→ *Inferior rectal artery (to the terminal rectum, etc.)* → *Perineal artery* → *Posterior scrotal branches (m), posterior labial branches (f)* → *Urethral artery* → *Artery of vestibular bulb (f), artery of penile bulb (m)* → *Dorsal clitoral artery (f), dorsal penile artery (m)* → *Deep clitoral artery (f), deep penile artery (m)* → *Perforator arteries of penis*

D Arterial pathways in the pelvic wall

Medial view of right hemipelvis showing the pelvic apertures that transmit the arteries and corresponding veins. There are a total of six pathways, whose landmarks are the piriformis, sacrospinous ligament, sacrotuberous ligament, inguinal ligament, and obturator membrane (see also **E**).

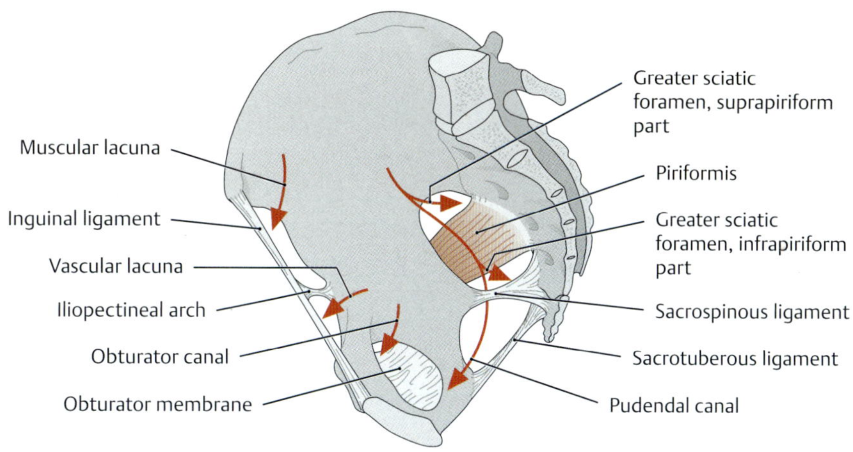

E Neurovascular tracts on the pelvic wall

There are six major neurovascular tracts on the pelvic walls, four of which (*) contain branches from the internal iliac artery.

Tract	Neurovascular structures transmitted
Posterior	
① Greater sciatic foramen, suprapiriform part* (above the piriformis)	Superior gluteal artery and vein, superior gluteal nerve
② Greater sciatic foramen, infrapiriform part* (below the piriformis)	Inferior gluteal artery and vein, inferior gluteal nerve, sciatic nerve, internal pudendal artery and vein, pudendal nerve, posterior femoral cutaneous nerve
On pelvic floor	
③ Pudendal canal*	Internal pudendal artery and vein, pudendal nerve
Lateral	
④ Obturator canal*	Obturator artery and vein, obturator nerve
Anterior	
⑤ Muscular lacuna (posterior to inguinal ligament, lateral to iliopectineal arch)	Femoral nerve, lateral femoral cutaneous nerve
⑥ Vascular lacuna (posterior to inguinal ligament, medial to iliopectineal arch)	Femoral artery and vein, lymphatic vessels (the femoral artery is a branch of the external iliac artery), femoral branch of genitofemoral nerve

5.15 Vascularization of the Male Pelvic Organs

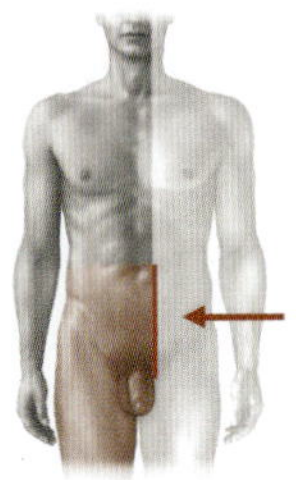

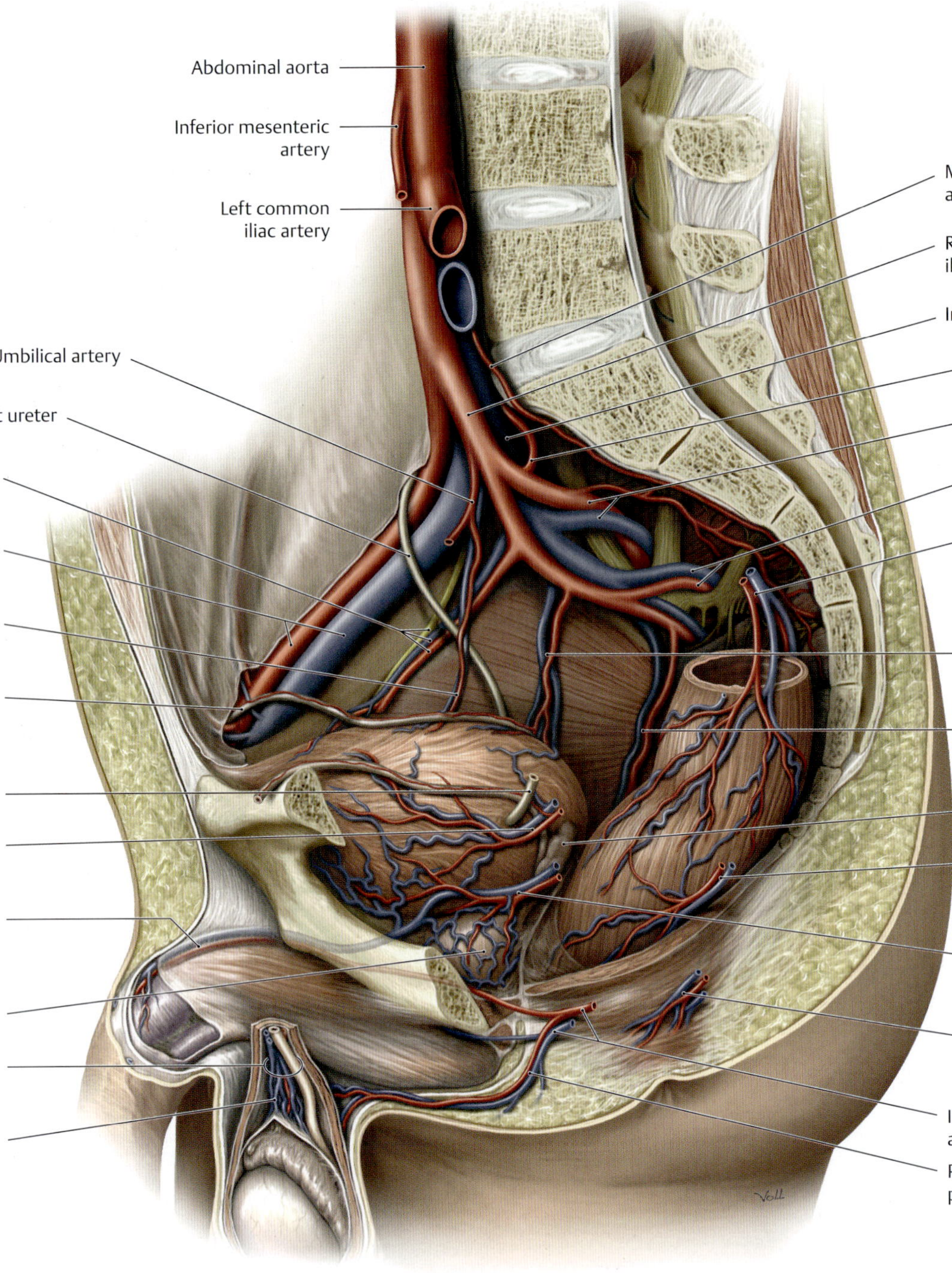

A Arterial supply and venous drainage of the pelvic organs in the male (overview)

Right hemipelvis (compiled from multiple sagittal sections) viewed from the left side, idealized. The pelvic organs derive their **arterial supply** from the visceral branches of the internal iliac artery. Their **venous drainage** is by corresponding veins (often running parallel to the arteries), which drain to the internal iliac vein. The veins, unlike the arteries, are frequently multiple on each side of the pelvis and are often expanded near the organs to form large plexuses. The main differences in the arterial supply and venous drainage of the pelvic organs in the male and female are based on the copious blood supply to the uterus and vagina in the female: The uterus and vagina are supplied by their own major vessels. In the male, however, the accessory sex glands are supplied by smaller branches arising from the vessels of nearby organs (bladder, rectum).

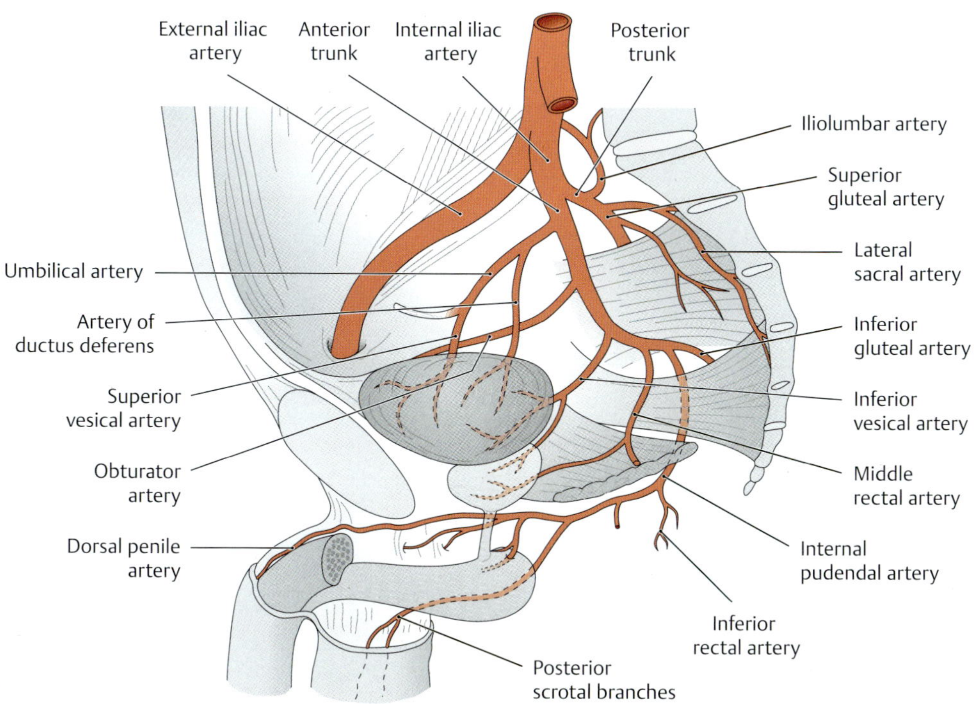

B Sequence of branches of the right internal iliac artery and their projection onto the male pelvis

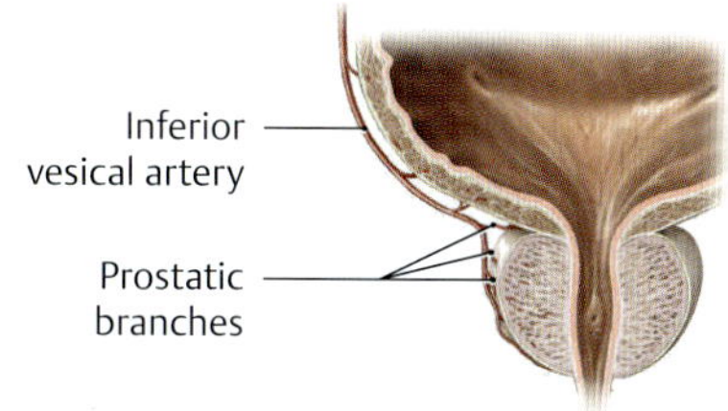

D Arterial supply of the prostate

Coronal section, anterior view. Most prostatic branches arise from the inferior vesical artery, and a smaller number arise from the middle rectal artery (not shown here). The prostatic branches ramify into a great many branchlets outside the organ capsule of the prostate.

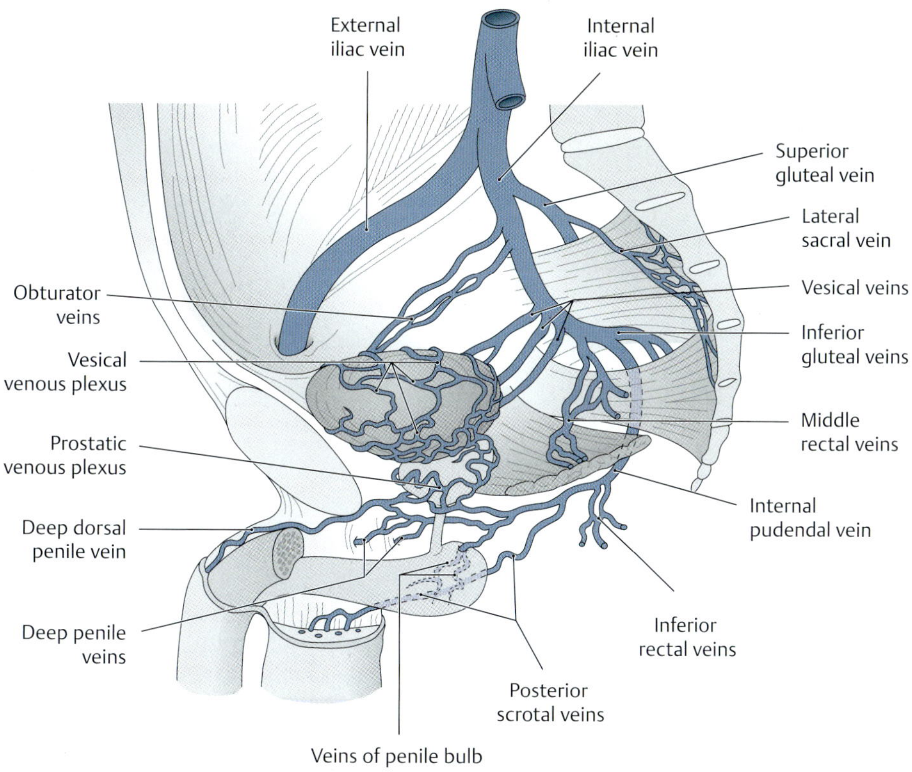

C Venous drainage of the bladder and male genitalia

Large venous plexuses around the bladder (vesical venous plexus) and prostate (prostatic venous plexus) drain through the vesical veins to the internal iliac vein. An anastomotic connection between the prostatic venous plexus and vertebral venous plexus (not shown here, aids venous drainage of the vertebral column and spinal canal) creates a route by which tumor cells from a prostatic carcinoma may metastasize to the spine (which may first come to clinical attention as back pain).

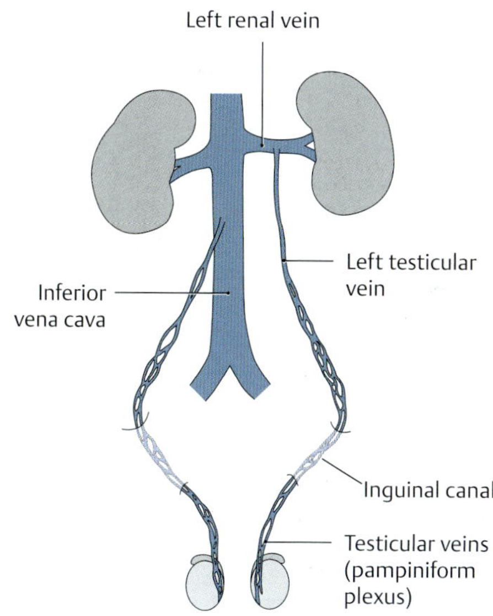

E Asymmetric venous drainage of the right and left testes

Venous blood from the testis and epididymis flows into the testicular veins in the area of the mediastinum testis. Especially distally, these veins form an elongated venous network called the pampiniform plexus. The plexus surrounds branches of the testicular artery and runs with it through the inguinal canal into the retroperitoneum where the *right* testicular vein opens into the inferior vena cava and the *left* testicular vein empties into the left renal vein. The asymmetric venous drainage is of clinical significance: The left testicular vein opens into the left renal vein at a right angle. This creates a physiological constriction that can obstruct outflow from the left testicular vein, which can result in enlargements called varicoceles (see p. 361) of the left testicular vein and thus of the pampiniform plexus. As a result, the pampiniform plexus can no longer perform its "thermostat" function (cooling of blood to the testis in the testicular artery) leading to hyperthermia, which affects the fertility of the left testis.

5.16 Vascularization of the Female Pelvic Organs

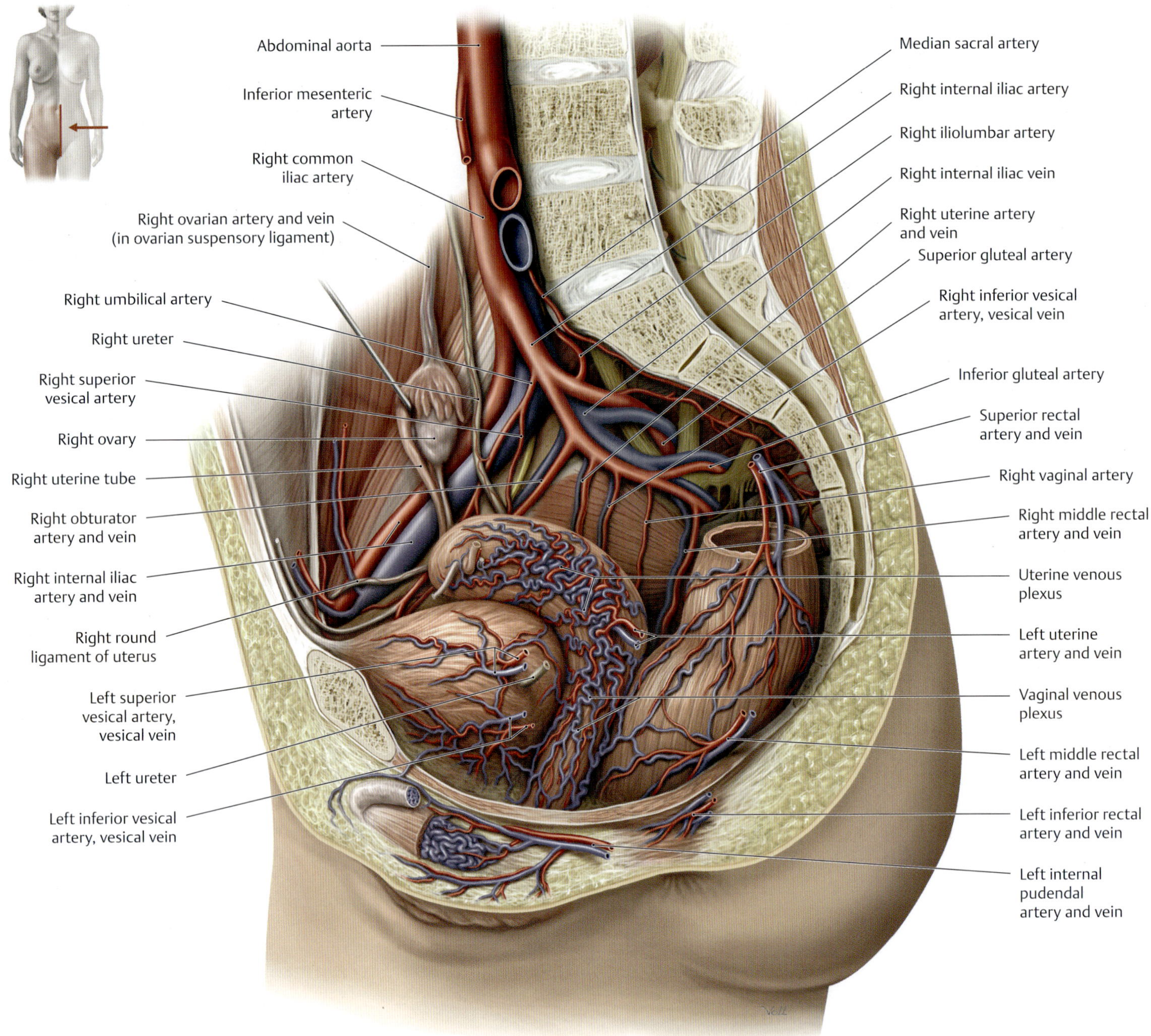

A Arterial supply and venous drainage of the pelvic organs in the female (overview)
Female pelvic organs viewed from the left side.

Arterial supply: The uterus is supplied by the uterine artery, which gives off a tubal branch and an ovarian branch. The bladder receives its blood supply from the superior and inferior vesical arteries. The rectum receives supply from the middle rectal artery, a branch of the internal iliac artery, and from the inferior rectal artery, which arises from the internal pudendal artery. The internal pudendal artery also supplies the pelvic floor and the external female genital organs. A characteristic of the ovary is that it has two sources of blood supply: because the ovaries descend during embryonic development, they drag their vascular structures (ovarian artery and vein) with them from the upper abdomen into the pelvic region (there the ovarian artery gives off a tubal branch to the uterine tube) where the ovarian artery anastomoses with the uterine artery. The uterine artery runs in the broad ligament to the uterus where it crosses the ureter (see p. 369). The uterine artery reaches the uterus at the junction of the corpus and cervix. There it often gives off a vaginal branch and from this point ascends in a torturous manner to the fundus of the uterus. This torturous course enables the uterine artery to elongate during pregnancy when the uterus enlarges.

Venous drainage: The uterus is drained by the uterine plexus into the uterine vein, which runs a course analogous to the artery. The uterine vein empties into the internal iliac vein. The right ovarian vein carries blood from its corresponding ovary directly to the inferior vena cava while the left ovarian vein drains into the left renal vein before reaching the inferior vena cava. The bladder drains through the vesical veins. Parts of the rectum that are supplied by branches of the internal iliac artery drain through same-named veins into the internal iliac veins.

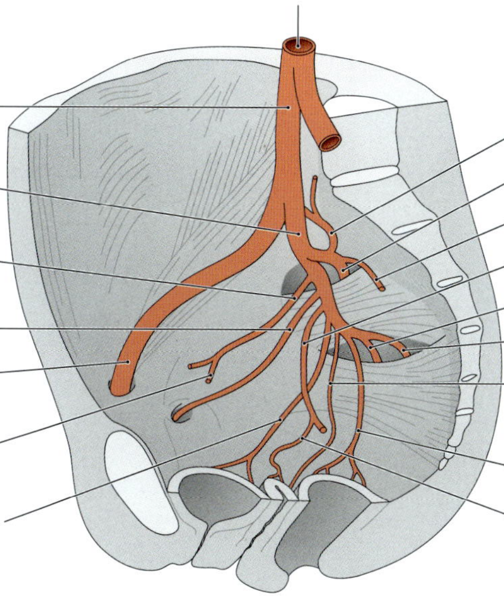

B Sequence of branches of the internal iliac artery in the female pelvis

Left lateral view. The vessels to the uterus and vagina mark the principal difference from the vasculature of the male pelvis (see also **B**, p. 365). The **uterus** receives a large vessel, the uterine artery, which usually arises separately from the internal iliac artery (the analogous vessel in the male, the artery of the ductus deferens, usually branches from the umbilical artery). The uterine artery *may* also arise from the middle rectal artery, which is larger in those cases. The arterial supply to the **vagina** is also subject to variation. The vagina may be supplied by a separate vaginal artery branching from the internal iliac artery or by a vaginal branch arising from either the uterine artery or the inferior vesical artery.

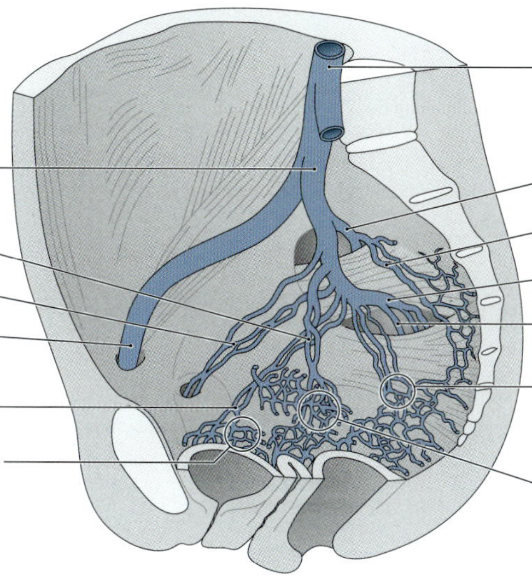

C Venous drainage of the organs of the female pelvis

Left lateral view showing the right internal iliac vein. The female pelvic organs are generally drained by four plexuses (see also **Ac**, p. 368):

- Vesical venous plexus (vesical veins)
- Vaginal venous plexus (vaginal veins)
- Uterine venous plexus (uterine veins)
- Rectal venous plexus (rectal veins)

The middle and inferior rectal veins drain to the internal iliac vein. The superior rectal vein drains into the inferior mesenteric vein. (The superior and inferior rectal veins are not shown here.)

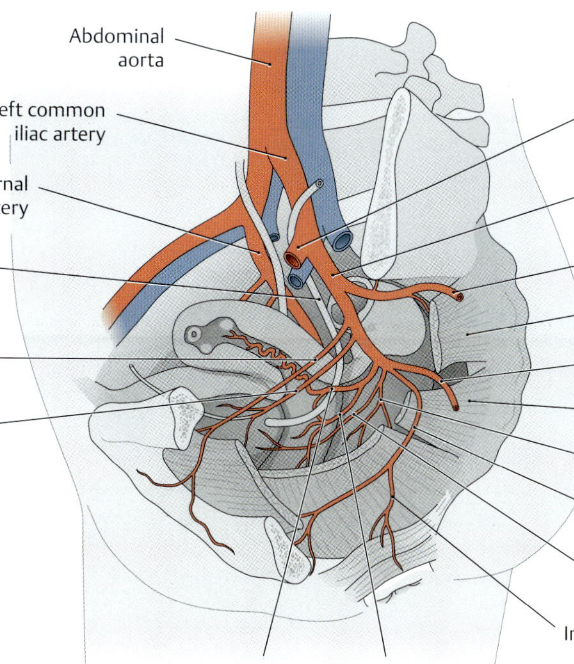

D Arterial supply of the uterus, vagina, and bladder

View into the pelvis from the left side. The uterine broad ligament has been cut open to display the branches of the left internal iliac artery.

Note: The serpentine course of the uterine artery along the uterine body is particularly well demonstrated in this lateral view. The origins of the uterine artery and vaginal artery are subject to considerable variation.

5.17 Vascularization of the Female Internal Genitalia and Urinary Bladder

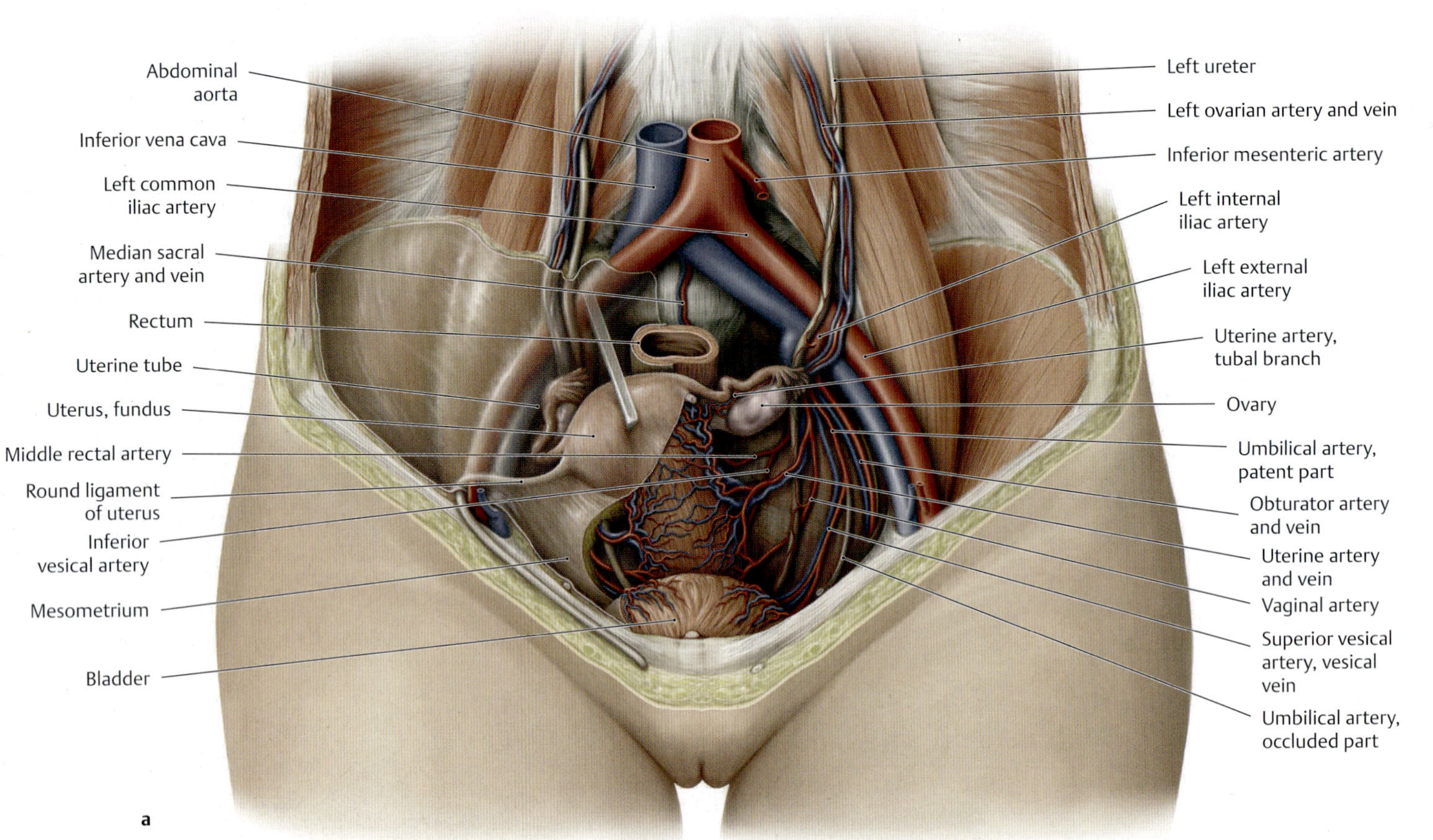

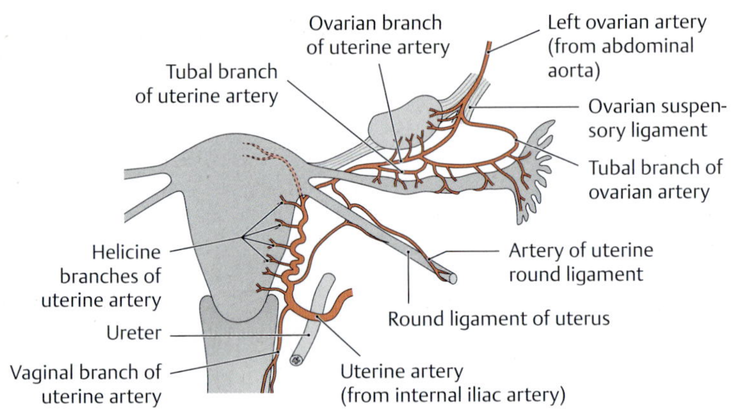

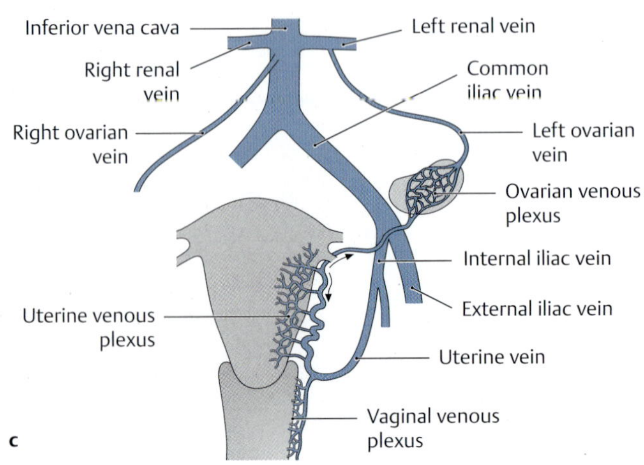

A Vascularization of the female internal genital organs
a Overview; all of the peritoneum has been removed on the left side and most has been removed on the right side; the uterus has been straightened and tilted to the right; **b** Arterial supply; **c** Venous drainage.
The female internal genital organs are supplied by two large arteries or their branches:

- Ovary: receives its arterial supply from two sources: predominantly from the ovarian artery as well as from the ovarian branch of the uterine artery (see ovarian arcade below)
- Uterus: from the uterine artery
- Uterine tube: from one branch each of the ovarian and uterine arteries

The two large arteries arise from different trunks: the ovarian artery usually originates from the abdominal aorta (for variants see **C**), the uterine artery from the internal iliac artery (visceral branch).
Note the ovarian arcade (see **b**), which needs to be noted during surgery: It is formed by the ovarian artery and the ovarian branch of the uterine artery.

The female genital organs are drained by two large veins or venous plexuses:

- Uterus: by the uterine venous plexus and partially by the vaginal venous plexus that empty into the internal iliac vein
- Ovary: on the right side by the ovarian vein directly into the inferior vena cava, and on the left side into the left renal vein before reaching the inferior vena cava; by the ovarian venous plexus: venous anastomosis between ovarian vein and uterine vein (plexus drains into both veins)

Arteries and veins run within the peritoneum: the ovarian artery and vein in the ovarian suspensory ligament, and the uterine artery and vein in the broad ligament.

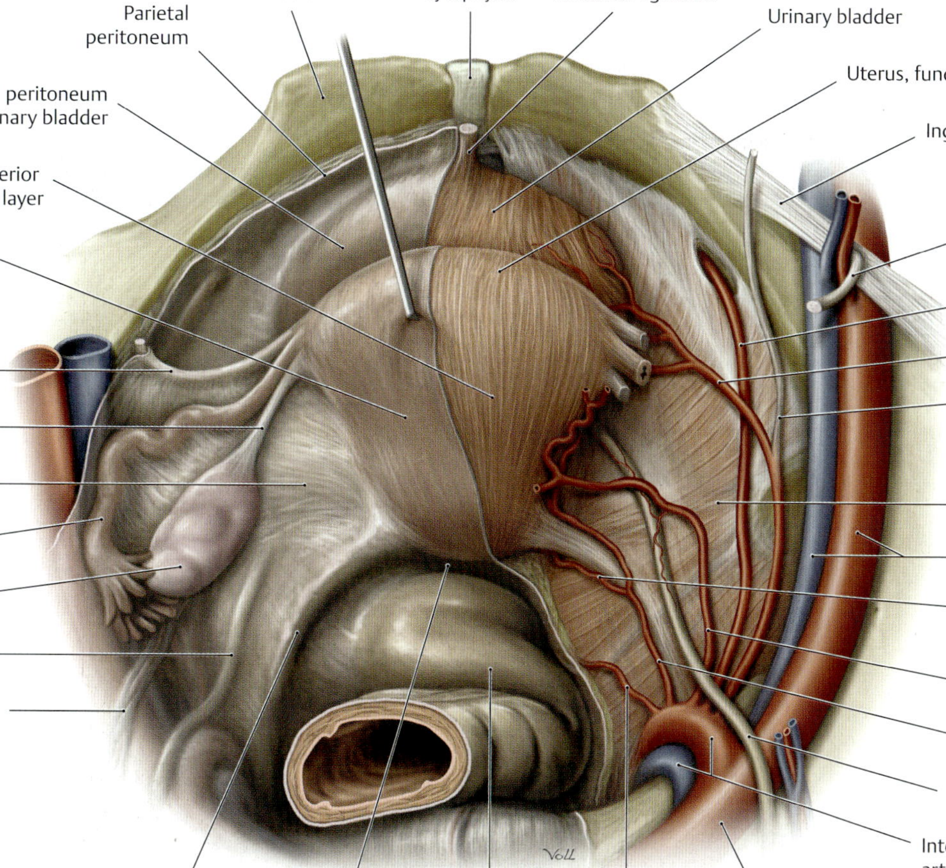

B Relationship of the uterine artery and ureter

a superior view looking into the pelvis, most of the peritoneum has been removed on the right side, the large intestine has been detached so that only a rectal stump is visible; **b** left lateral view of left uterine artery and left ureter.

The uterine artery runs in the broad ligament (in **a** removed on the right side and left in situ on the left side for clarity) to the uterus. There the ureter crosses inferior to the uterine artery (the ureter is thus susceptible to injury during operations on the uterus).

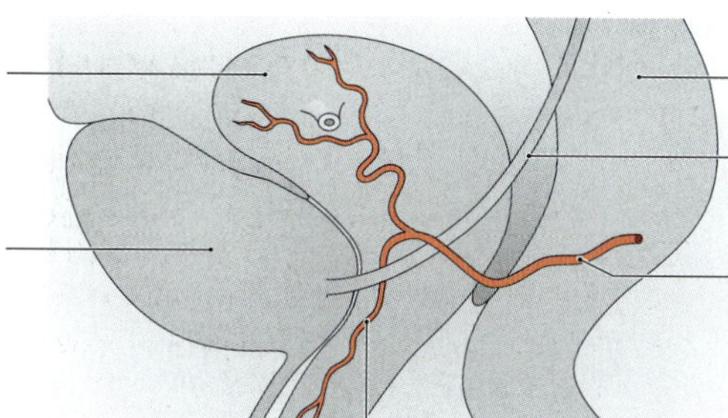

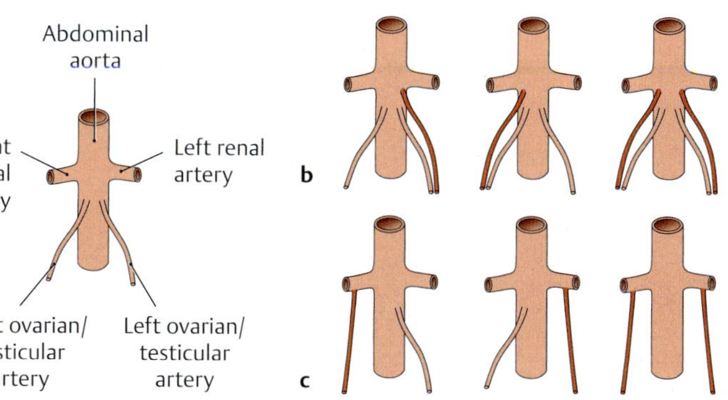

C Variants in the origin of the ovarian and testicular arteries (after Lippert and Pabst)

a Typical case: The ovarian or testicular arteries arise from the abdominal aorta (approximately 70 % of cases).
b Accessory vessels are present (approximately 15 %).
c The arteries arise from the renal artery (approximately 15 %).

5.18 Lymphatic Drainage of the Male and Female Genitalia

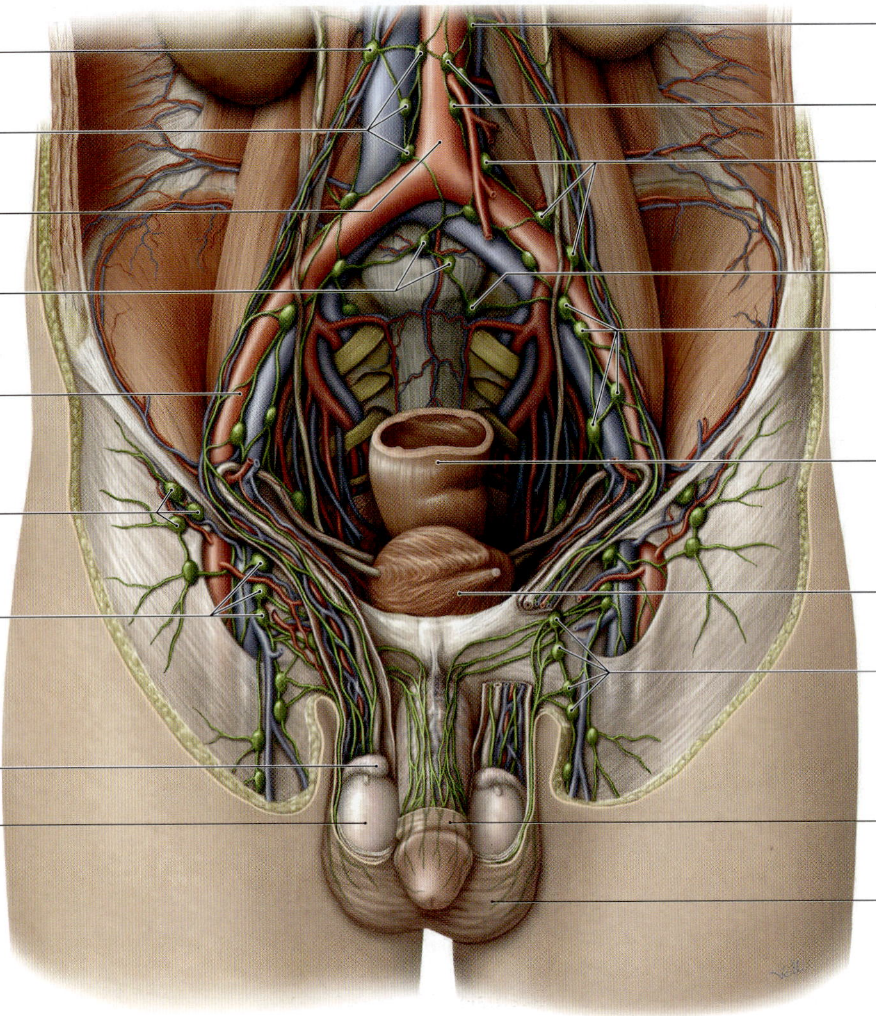

A Lymph nodes and lymphatic pathways of the male internal and external genitalia

Anterior view. All portions of the gastrointestinal tract have been removed except for a rectal stump. The peritoneum has been removed, and the bladder has been pulled slightly to the left. The *external genitalia* consist of the penis and scrotum, while the testis and epididymis (despite their location) are included with the *internal genitalia* because of their embryonic origin, along with the prostate and seminal vesicles. (The lymphatic drainage of the prostate, testis, and epididymis is described in **B**.)

Note: The lumbar lymph nodes that drain the *testis and epididymis* are located farther from these organs than most "visceral lymph nodes." As with the ovary, this results in a long drainage pathway from the testis and epididymis to the lumbar nodes. Metastases from a testicular malignancy are most frequently encountered in the lumbar lymph nodes. The *external genitalia* are drained by the superficial and deep inguinal lymph nodes. The lymphatic vessels on the dorsum of the penis are connected by anastomoses that allow for bilateral lymphatic drainage. Because of this bilateral arrangement, a malignant tumor on the right side of the penis may metastasize to the right *and* left inguinal lymph nodes.

B Lymphatic drainage of the testis, epididymis, and accessory sex glands

All lymph from the male genitalia is ultimately channeled by various groups of parietal lymph nodes to lumbar nodes distributed around the abdominal aorta and inferior vena cava (see pp. 237 and 239). The following specific drainage pathways are available:

Testis and epididymis: long, direct drainage pathway along the testicular vessels to the right and left lumbar lymph nodes

Ductus deferens: to the iliac lymph nodes (the external more than the internal)

Seminal vesicle: internal and external iliac lymph nodes (same pathway as the ductus deferens)

Prostate (multiple pathways): external iliac lymph nodes; along the vesicular vessels to the internal iliac lymph nodes; sacral lymph nodes (and on to the lumbar nodes).

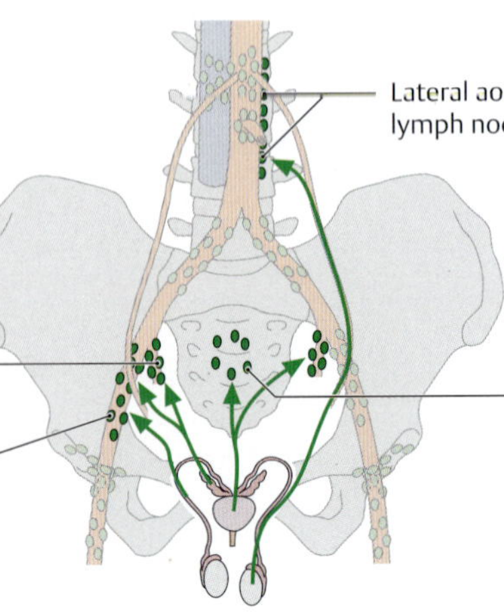

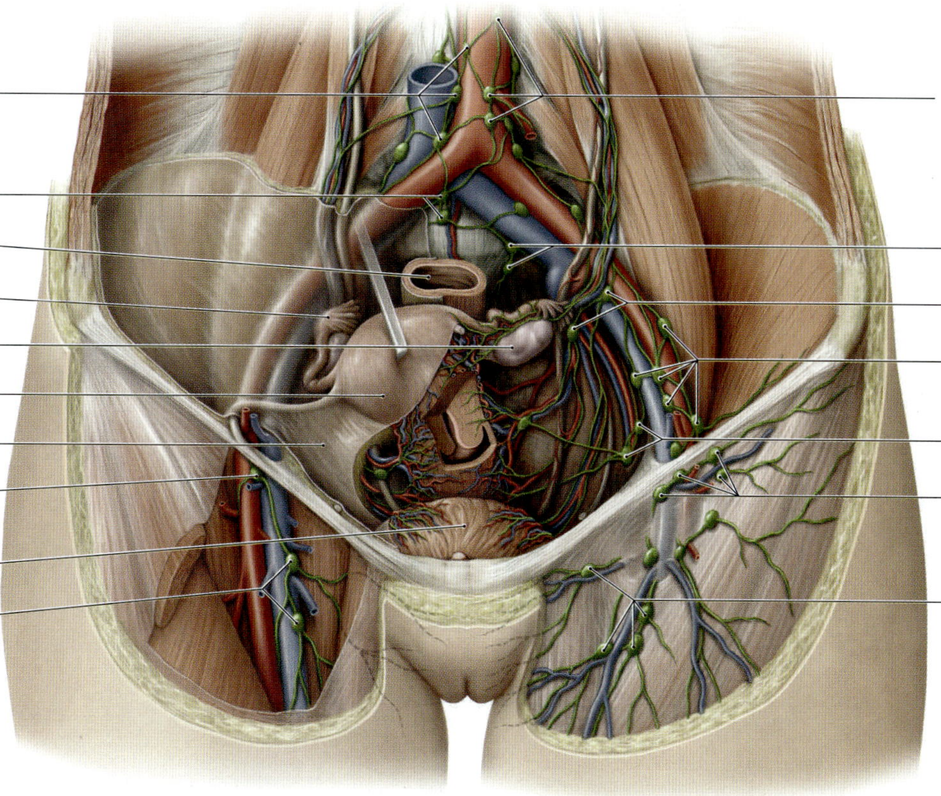

C Lymph nodes and lymphatic pathways of the female internal and external genitalia

Anterior view. The uterus is retracted to the right. The broad ligament has been removed on the left side and partially opened on the right side to display the numerous lymphatic vessels that traverse the ligament. For clarity, the drawing shows only isolated lymph nodes within certain groups of nodes. *Lymph from the internal genitalia* in the female pelvis drains principally to the iliac and lumbar lymph nodes, while *lymph from the external genitalia* drains mainly to the inguinal lymph nodes. The inguinal lymph nodes are divided by clinical criteria into a horizontal tract and vertical tract. It is believed that the *external* genitalia are drained mainly by the vertical tract.

Note: The ovary, though located in the pelvis, drains to the lumbar lymph nodes. A large portion of the lymphatic vessels of the uterus course within the broad ligament. Consequently the lymphogenous spread of malignant uterine tumors takes place along that ligament, proceeding laterally toward the pelvic wall.

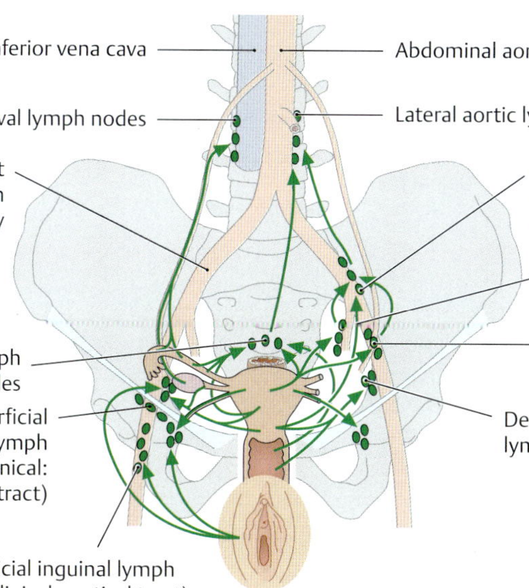

D Lymphatic drainage of the female genitalia

All of the genitalia are drained by various groups of parietal lymph nodes, which ultimately drain to lumbar nodes distributed around the abdominal aorta and inferior vena cava (see pp. 237 and 239).

External genitalia (and lowest portions of the vagina): superficial and deep inguinal lymph nodes, plus an accessory route (not shown) directly to the iliac lymph nodes

Internal genitalia:

- Ovary, uterine fundus, and (mainly distal) portions of the uterine tube: long drainage pathway to the lumbar lymph nodes around the abdominal aorta and inferior vena cava
- Uterine fundus and body and (mainly proximal) portions of the uterine tube: sacral lymph nodes, internal and external iliac lymph nodes
- Uterus (cervix) and middle and upper portions of vagina: inguinal lymph nodes

Note: Small visceral lymph nodes for the uterus and vagina (parauterine and paravaginal lymph nodes, not shown here) are embedded in regional pelvic connective tissue close to the organs they serve.

5.19 Autonomic Innervation of the Male Genitalia

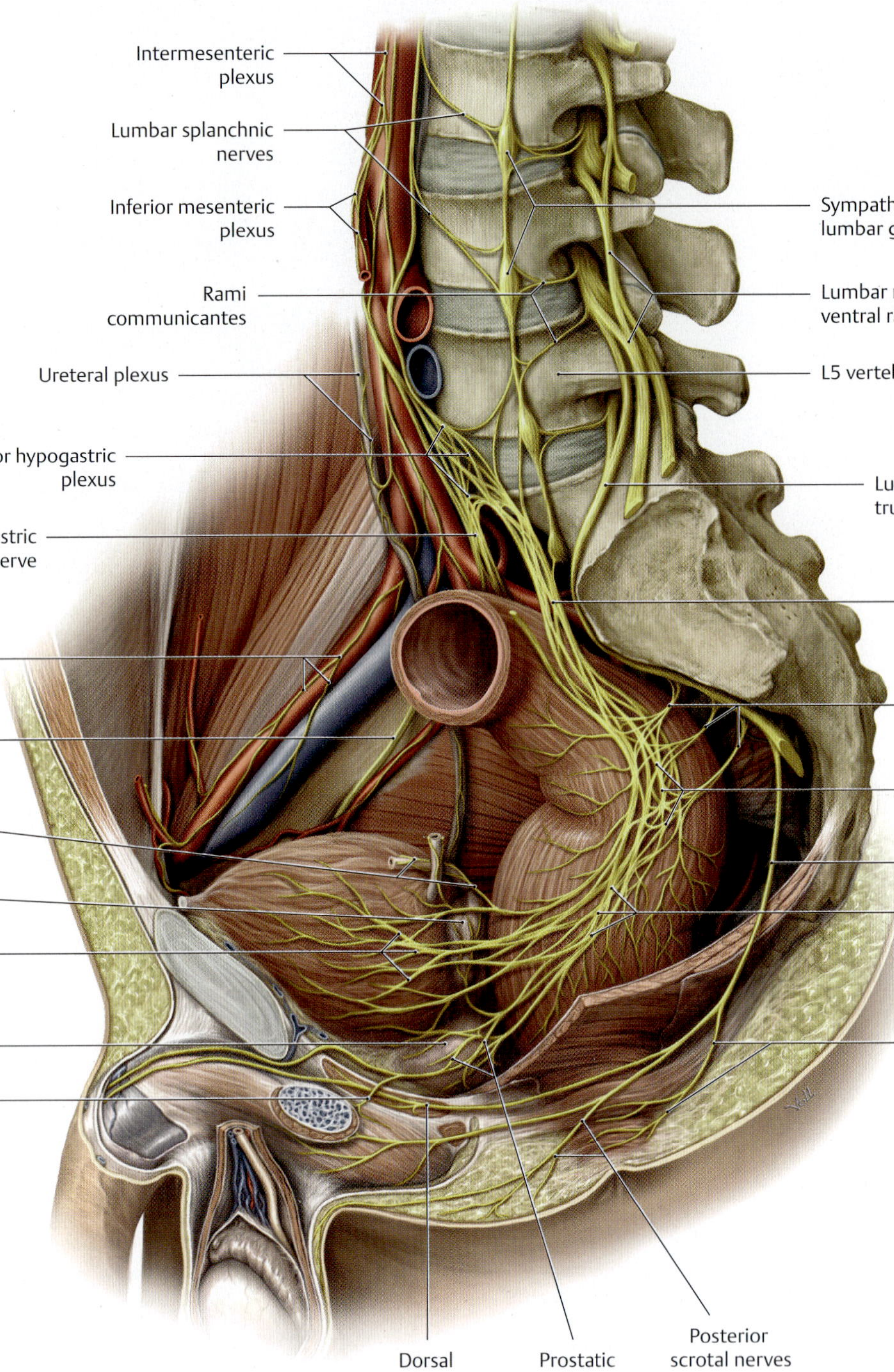

A Overview of the autonomic innervation of the male genitalia
Opened male pelvis viewed from the left side. This drawing is a composite from many planes of section to show the three-dimensional relationships more clearly. The *sympathetic* fibers that supply the testis and epididymis form the lesser, least, and lumbar splanchnic nerves. Those that supply the accessory sex glands (prostate, seminal vesicle, and bulbourethral glands), penis, and ductus deferens arise from the lumbar and sacral splanchnic nerves. The *parasympathetic* supply to the male genitalia is much more modest than the sympathetic supply; it arises predominantly from the pelvic splanchnic nerves (see **B**). Sympathetic and parasympathetic fibers join to form the *inferior hypogastric plexus*, which also receives the hypogastric nerves (arise from the division of the superior hypogastric plexus). The paired inferior hypogastric plexuses, which give origin to the plexuses that supply the urinary organs (see p. 241), then divide into multiple plexuses that innervate the genital organs (see **C**).

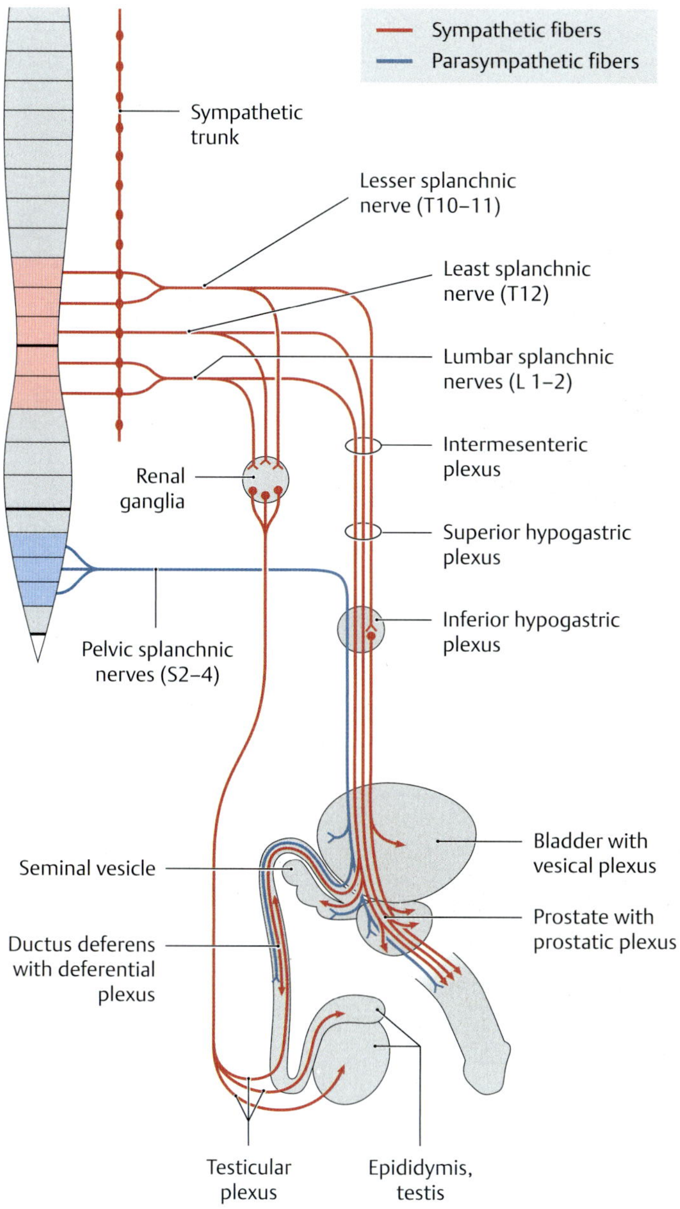

B Details of the autonomic innervation of the male genitalia

- The **accessory sex glands (prostate, seminal vesicle, and bulbourethral glands)** receive their autonomic innervation from the prostatic plexus, which branches from the inferior hypogastric plexus (also believed to carry pain fibers).
- The **penis** also receives its autonomic innervation from branches of the prostatic plexus and from the cavernous nerves of the penis (see **A**). In both cases the synapse with the postsynaptic neuron occurs in the ganglion cells of the inferior hypogastric plexus.
- The **ductus deferens** is supplied mainly by the deferential plexus, which also branches from the inferior hypogastric plexus and to a lesser degree from the testicular plexus that runs along the testicular artery.
- The **testis**, because of its developmental descent, receives most of its autonomic innervation from the testicular plexus (sympathetic fibers along the testicular artery, which synapse in the renal ganglia). The testicular plexus also gives off fibers to the epididymis. Both organs receive a smaller amount of autonomic innervation from the inferior hypogastric plexus (not included in **C**).

C Autonomic innervation of the male genitalia

First neuron	Peripheral course (sympathetic and parasympathetic)	Target organ	Effect
Sympathetic:			
T10–T12 (lesser and least splanchnic nerves)	Via renal ganglia to testicular plexus	• Testis • Epididymis	• Vasoconstriction
L1–L2 (lumbar and sacral splanchnic nerves)	Via superior hypogastric plexus and inferior hypogastric plexus to prostatic plexus and to	• Prostate • Bulbourethral glands and seminal vesicle	• Stimulate secretions
	Deferential plexus	• Penis (partly) • Ductus deferens	• Ejaculation • Deferential plexus
Parasympathetic:			
S2–S4 (pelvic splanchnic nerves)	Via inferior hypogastric plexus to prostatic plexus, continuing to the cavernous nerves of the penis	• Penis, erectile tissues	• Erection

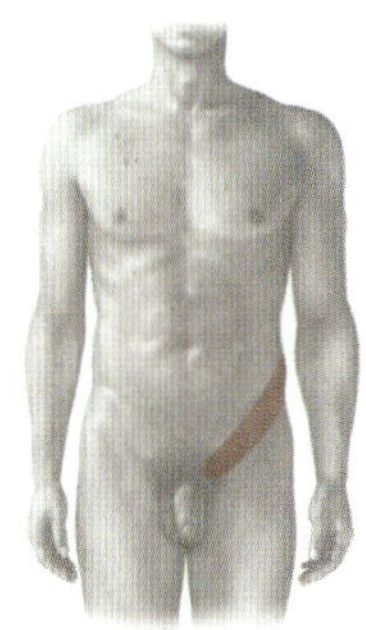

D Referred pain from the male gonads

The pain associated with diseases of the testis (e.g., inflammation) may be referred to this skin area. Gonadal pain, like intestinal pain, is not perceived at the anatomical location of the organ.

5.20 Autonomic Innervation of the Female Genitalia

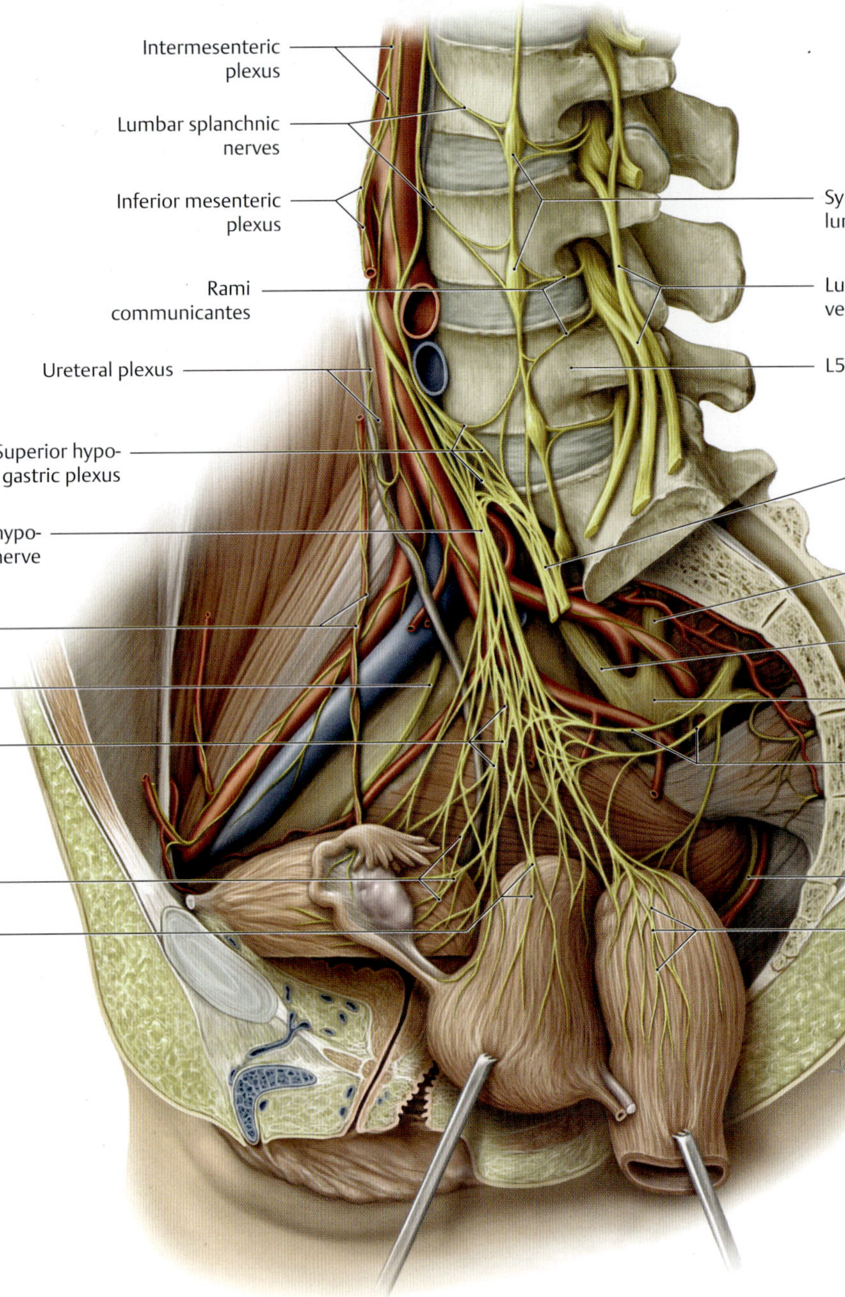

A Overview of the autonomic innervation of the female genitalia
An opened female pelvis viewed from the left side, with the rectum and uterus reflected. This drawing is a composite from multiple planes of section to show the three-dimensional relationships more clearly.
The *sympathetic* fibers for the uterus, uterine tubes, and ovaries arise predominantly from the lesser, least, and lumbar splanchnic nerves. The *parasympathetic* fibers arise from the pelvic splanchnic nerves.
Note: The fibers that are distributed to the ovary synapse mainly in the renal ganglia because as the ovary undergoes its developmental descent, it carries its autonomic supply from the abdomen with it. The fibers then continue on to the ovarian plexus, which also receives fibers from the superior mesenteric plexus. This is analogous to the innervation of the testis via the renal ganglia and the superior and inferior mesenteric plexus and testicular plexus in the male.

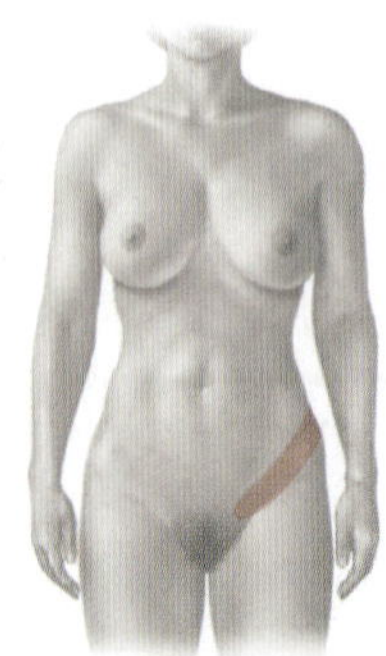

B Referred pain from the female gonads
The pain associated with ovarian diseases (e.g., inflammation) may project to these skin areas and may not be perceived within the organ itself.

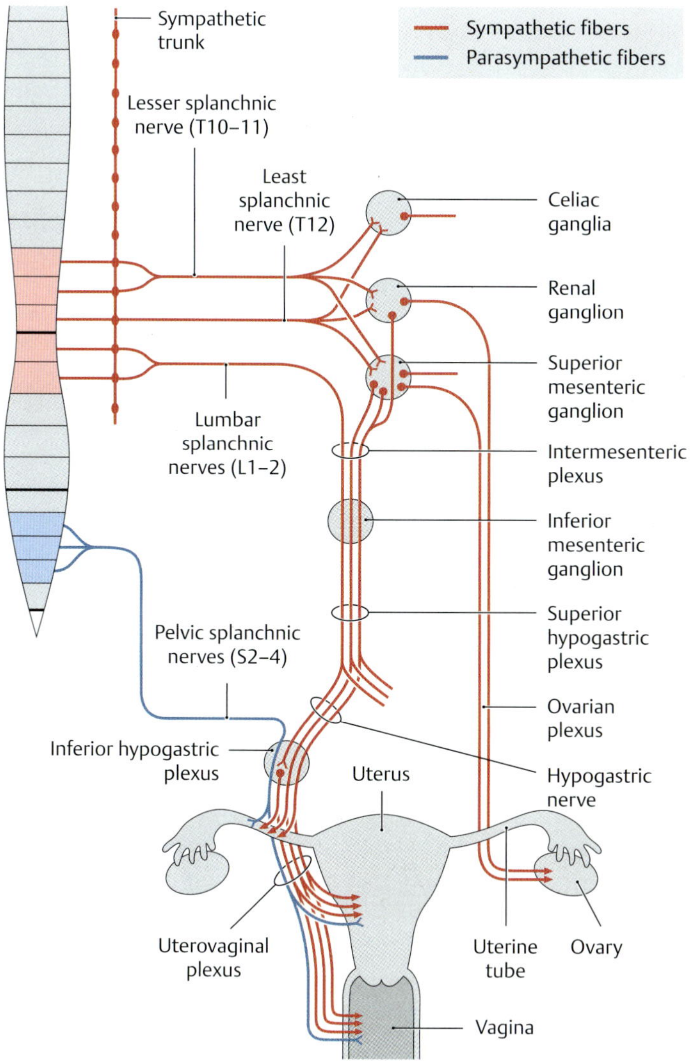

C Autonomic innervation of the female genitalia

Because of the developmental descent of the **ovary**, its nerve supply extends a considerable distance along the ovarian artery in the ovarian suspensory ligament (the ovarian plexus, which arises from the abdominal aortic plexus via the renal ganglia—analogous to the innervation of the testis via the testicular plexus).

The **uterus, uterine tube,** and **vagina** receive their autonomic innervation from the inferior hypogastric plexus. The *sympathetic* portion is derived from the lesser, least, and lumbar splanchnic nerves, which synapse partly in the mesenteric ganglia and partly in the ganglion cells of the inferior hypogastric plexus. The *parasympathetic* fibers are derived from the pelvic splanchnic nerves (S2–S4), which synapse in the inferior hypogastric plexus or in/on the organ wall. Branches from the inferior hypogastric plexus form the prominent uterovaginal plexus (of Frankenhauser) located on both sides of the uterus. The ovary may receive additional autonomic innervation along the uterine tube from the inferior hypogastric plexus.

D Autonomic innervation of the female genitalia

First neuron	Peripheral course (sympathetic and parasympathetic)	Target organ	Effect
Sympathetic:			
T10–T12 (lesser and least splanchnic nerves)	Via renal ganglia and superior mesenteric ganglion to ovarian plexus	• Ovary	• Vasoconstriction
L1–L2 (lumbar splanchnic nerves)	Via superior hypogastric plexus, hypogastric nerves, and inferior hypogastric plexus to uterovaginal plexus	• Uterus • Uterine tube • Vagina • Vagina	• Contraction (in uterus, depends on hormone status) • Vasoconstriction
Parasympathetic:			
S2–S4 (pelvic splanchnic nerves)	Inferior hypogastric plexus to uterovaginal plexus, continuing to cavernous nerves of clitoris	• Uterus, Uterine tube • Vagina • Clitoris	• Vasodilation • Transudation • Erection

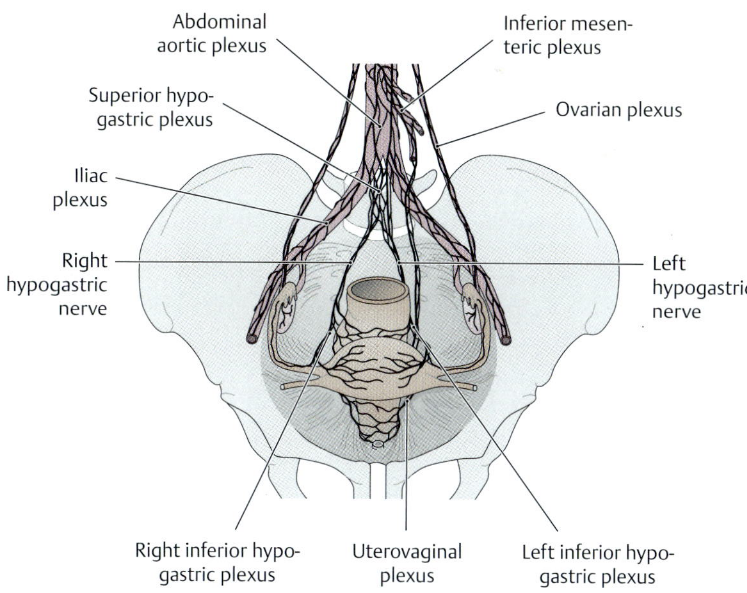

E Overview of the autonomic plexuses in the female pelvis

Anterior view.

Note the division of the of the superior hypogastric plexus into two *hypogastric nerves*, which are continuous with both *inferior hypogastric plexuses*. The latter then give off individual visceral plexuses to the rectum, uterus, vagina, and bladder (see **A**).

The ovary is supplied chiefly by the ovarian plexus, which runs along the ovarian artery in the ovarian suspensory ligament. Thus, the autonomic supply of the female pelvis corresponds to that in the male, although the plexuses in the female pelvis are more strongly developed due to the very rich nerve supply of the uterus.

6.1 Surface Anatomy, Topographic Regions, and Palpable Bony Landmarks

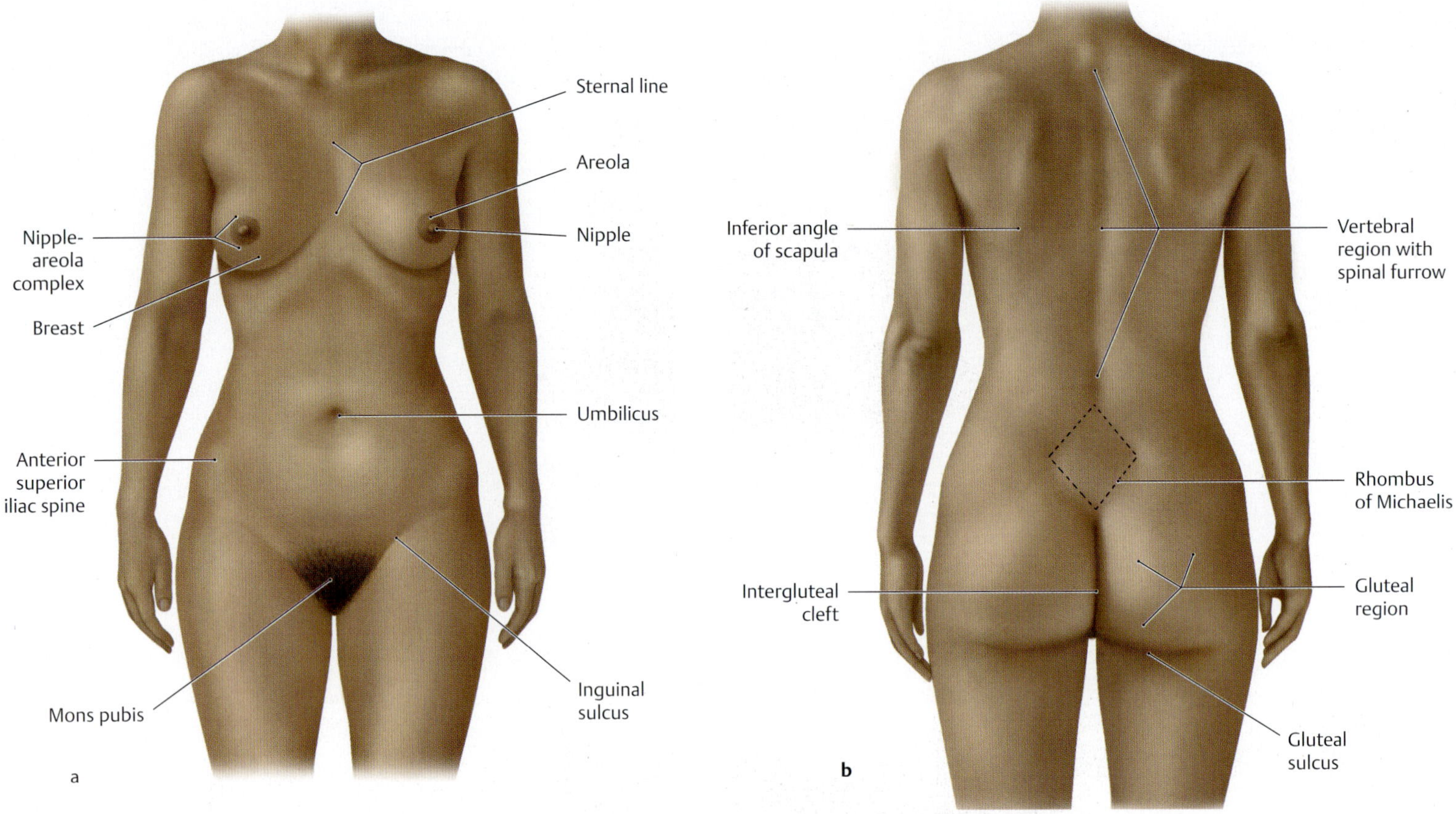

A Surface anatomy of the female
a Anterior view; **b** Posterior view.

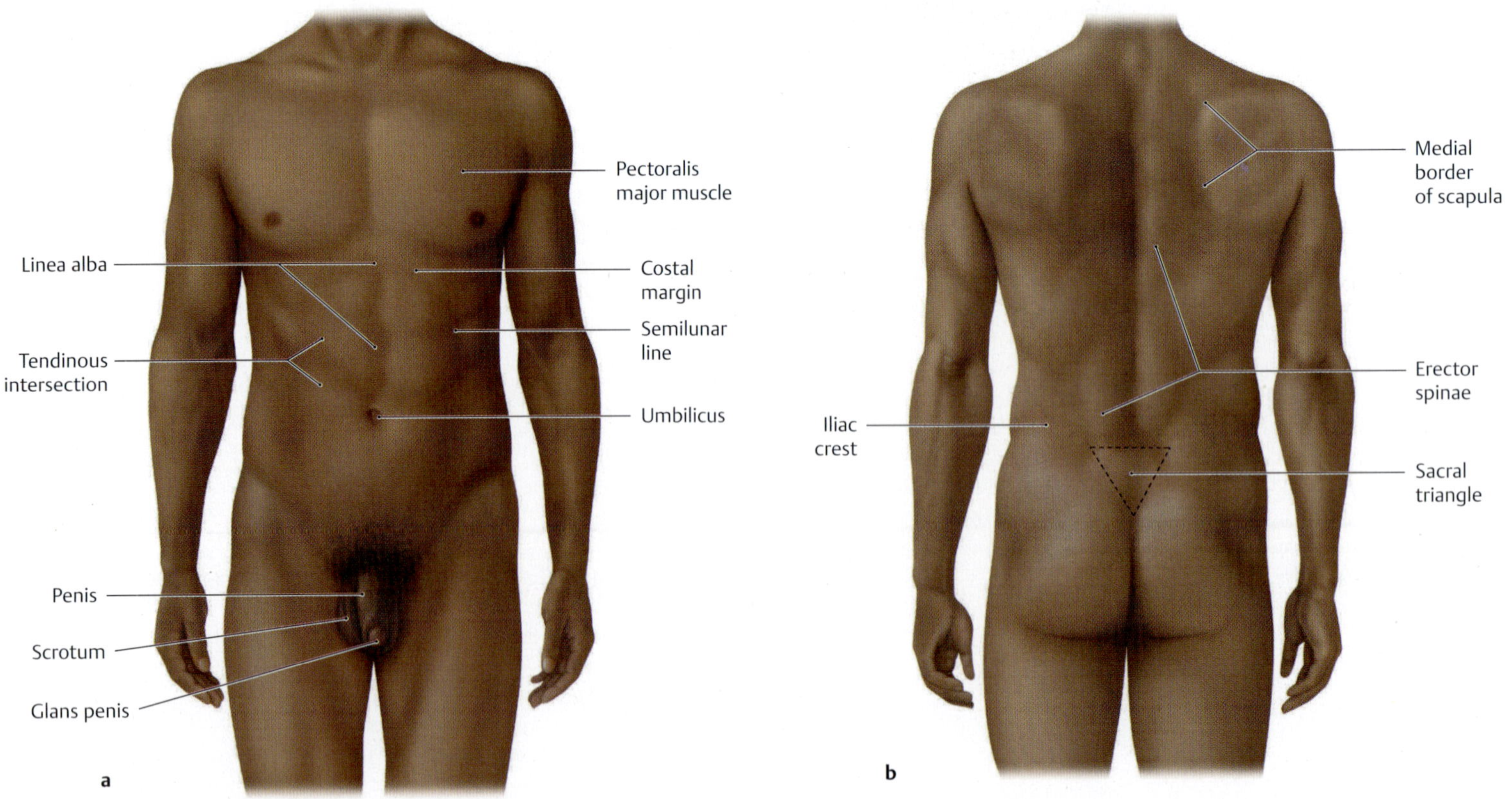

B Surface anatomy of the male
a Anterior view; **b** Posterior view.

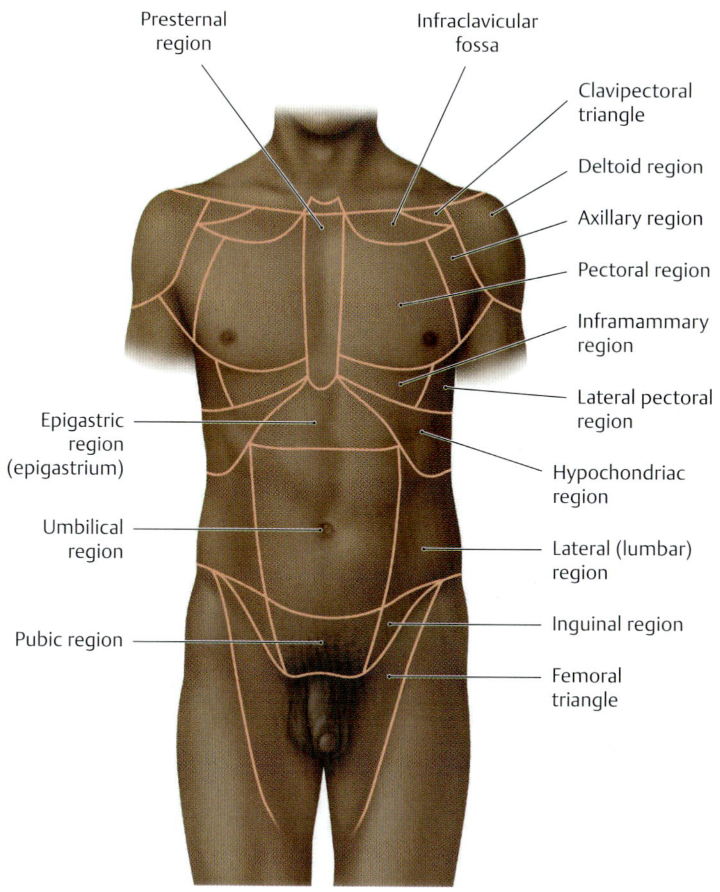

C Thoracic and abdominal regions
Anterior view.

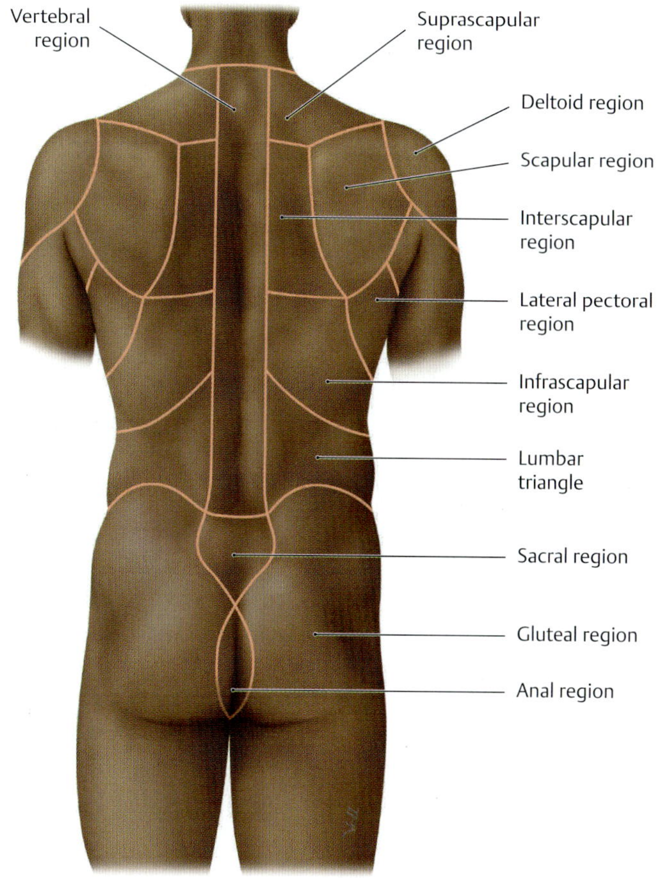

D Back and gluteal regions
Posterior view.

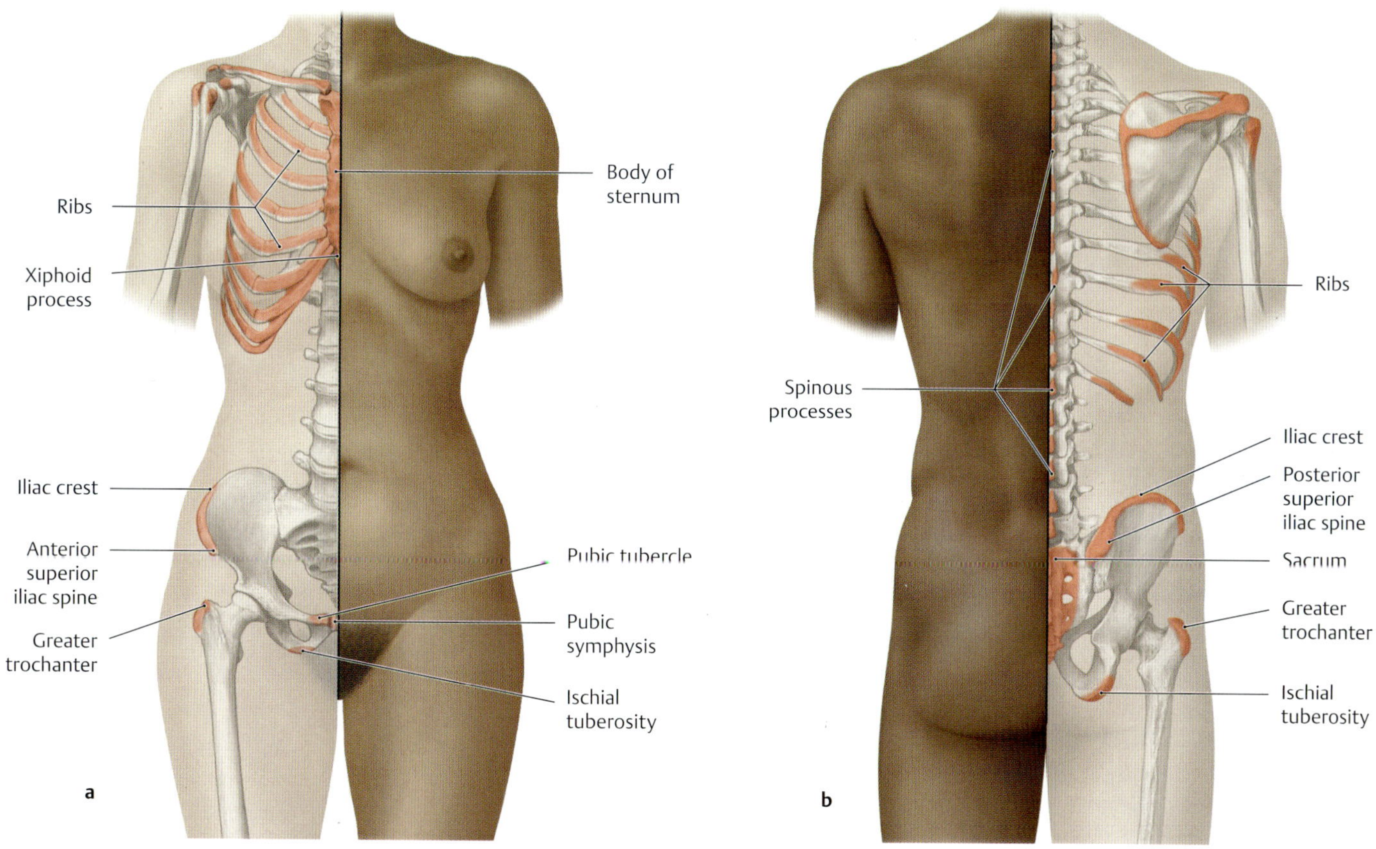

E Body surface contours and palpable bony landmarks of the trunk
a Anterior view; **b** Posterior view.

6.2 Location of the Abdominal and Pelvic Organs and their Projection onto the Trunk Wall

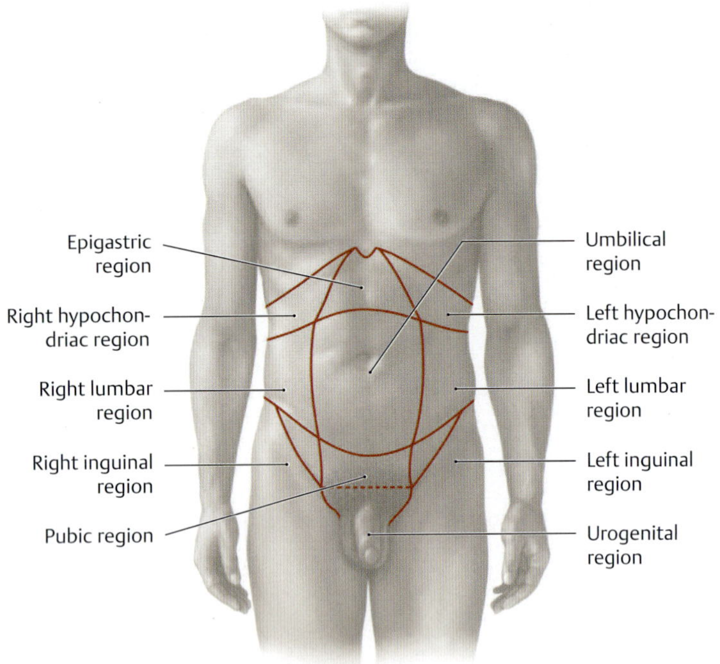

A Regions of the anterior trunk wall

Three levels can be identified on the abdominal wall from above downward: the epigastrium, mesogastrium, and hypogastrium. Each level consists of three regions:

- The median region of the epigastrium is the *epigastric region*. It is flanked laterally by the right and left hypochondriac regions.
- The median region of the mesogastrium is the *umbilical region*, which is bounded laterally by the right and left lumbar regions.
- The median region of the hypogastrium is the *pubic region*, which is flanked by the right and left inguinal regions. The pubic region is bounded inferiorly by the *urogenital region*.

The levels of the abdomen are defined by horizontal planes that are determined by palpable bony landmarks (see **C**).

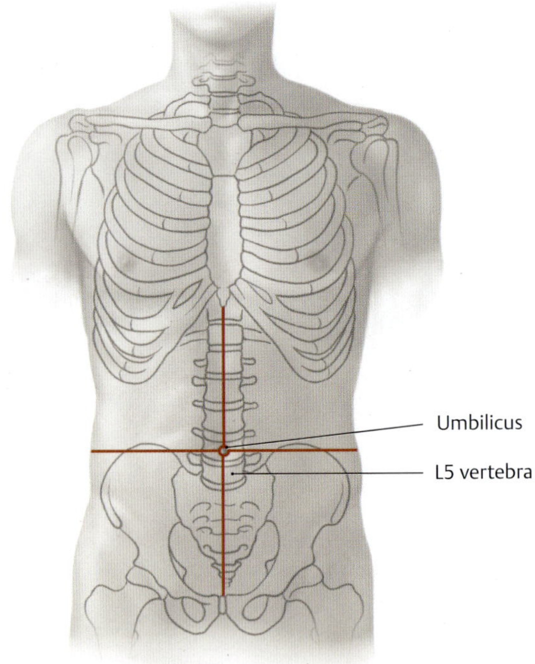

B Quadrants of the anterior trunk wall

The quadrants of the anterior trunk wall are centered on the umbilicus, which lies at the level of the L 3–4 vertebral body and are named right and left upper and lower quadrant (RUQ, LUQ, RLQ, LLQ).

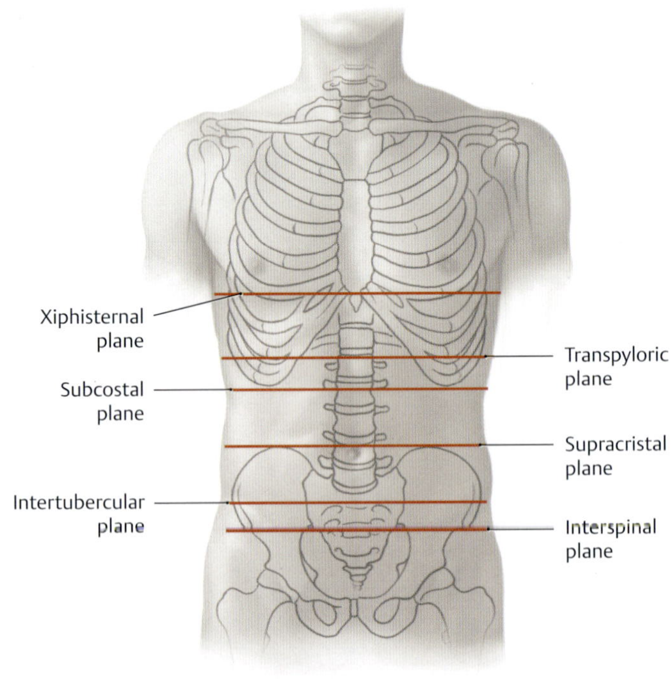

C Horizontal (transverse) planes in the anterior trunk wall

The anterior trunk wall is divided transversely by the following imaginary planes of section:

- **Xiphisternal plane:** passes through the synchondrosis between the xiphoid process and body of the *sternum*.
- **Transpyloric plane:** plane midway between the jugular notch of the sternum and the superior border of the pubic symphysis. Located at the level of the L 1 vertebra, it divides the anterior trunk wall into upper and lower halves. The pylorus of the stomach is generally located slightly *below* this plane.
- **Subcostal plane:** passes through the *lowest points of the costal arch* of the tenth rib at the level of the L 2 vertebral body. It marks the boundary between the epigastrium and mesogastrium (see **A**).
- **Supracristal plane:** usually passes through the body of the L 4 vertebra, connecting the *highest points on the iliac crests*.
- **Intertubercular plane:** connects the *iliac* tubercles and passes through the L 5 vertebral body. The intertubercular plane marks the boundary between the mesogastrium and hypogastrium.
- **Interspinal plane:** connects the two *anterior superior iliac spines*.

Note: The three upper planes are variable in their location, which depends on the position and shape of the thoracic cage. The key variables are respiratory position, age, sex, and constitutional type.

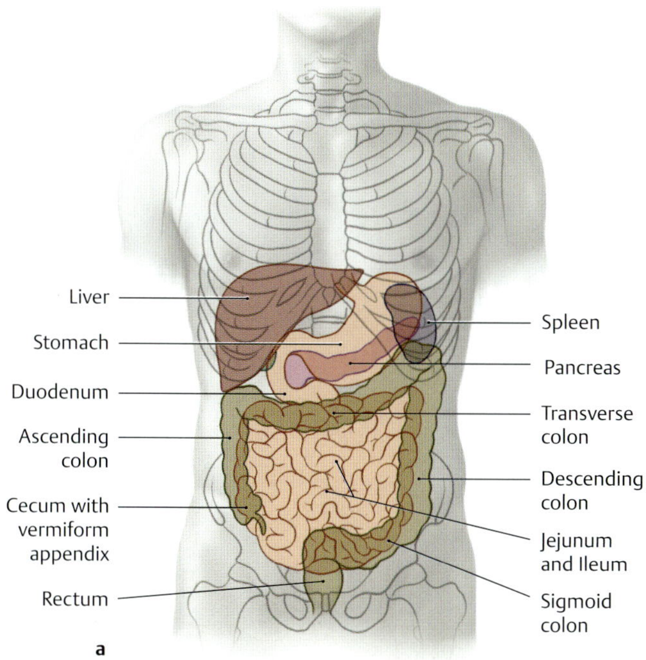

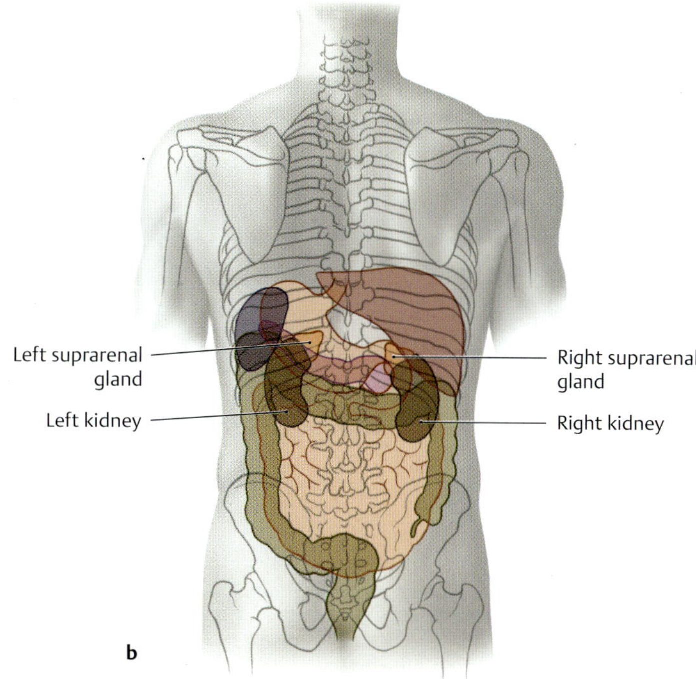

D Projection of the abdominal and pelvic organs onto the trunk wall

a Anterior trunk wall; **b** Posterior trunk wall.

The surface projection of organs on the trunk wall depends on body posture, age, constitutional type, sex, nutritional state, and respiratory position.

Note the overlap of the abdominal and thoracic cavities: Perforating injuries of the abdominal cavity that involve the liver, for example, may also involve the pleural cavity ("multicavity injury"). The projections of individual organs are shown in **E**.

E Projection of anatomical structures in the abdomen and pelvis onto the vertebral column

The spinal notation refers to vertebral bodies.

T 7	Superior border of the liver
T 12	Aortic hiatus
L 1	• Transpyloric plane (generally the pylorus is at or below this plane) • Gallbladder fundus • Renal hilum • Superior part of the duodenum • Pancreas (neck) • Origin of the celiac trunk • Origin of the superior mesenteric artery • Attachment of the transverse mesocolon • Spleen (hilum)
L 1/2	• Origin of the renal arteries
L 2	Duodenojejunal flexure
L 3	Origin of the inferior mesenteric artery
L 3/4	Umbilicus
L 4	Aortic bifurcation
L 5	Origin of the inferior vena cava from the common iliac veins
S 3	Upper (cranial) border of the rectum

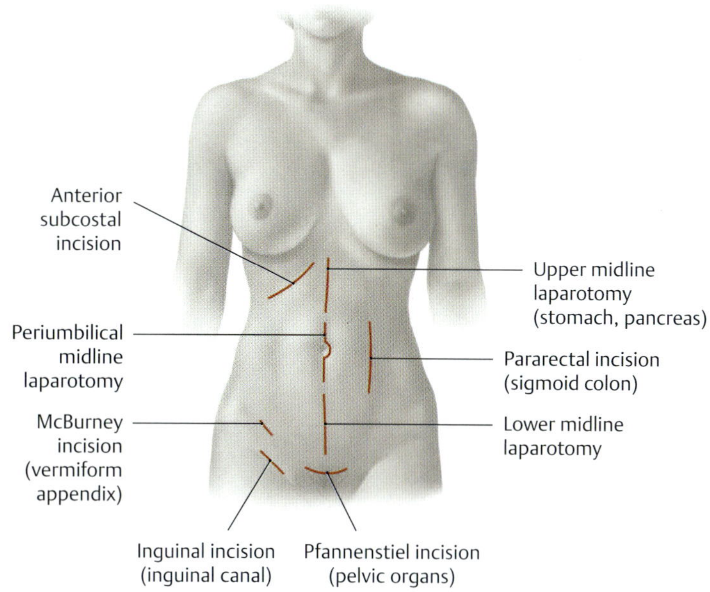

F Placement of surgical skin incisions in the anterior abdominal wall

Note: The periumbilical midline incision passes around the left side of the umbilicus to avoid cutting the remnant of the umbilical vein on the *right* side (the ligamentum teres of the liver, see p. 271). This umbilical vein remnant is generally but not always obliterated, and injury to the vessel, if it is still patent, may cause significant bleeding.

The McBurney incision is also called the *gridiron incision* because it changes direction in different planes of the trunk wall. The muscles of the trunk wall can be divided less traumatically by tailoring the direction of the cut to the prevailing fiber direction of the various muscle layers.

6.3 Topography of the Opened Peritoneal Cavity (Supracolic Part and Infracolic Part)

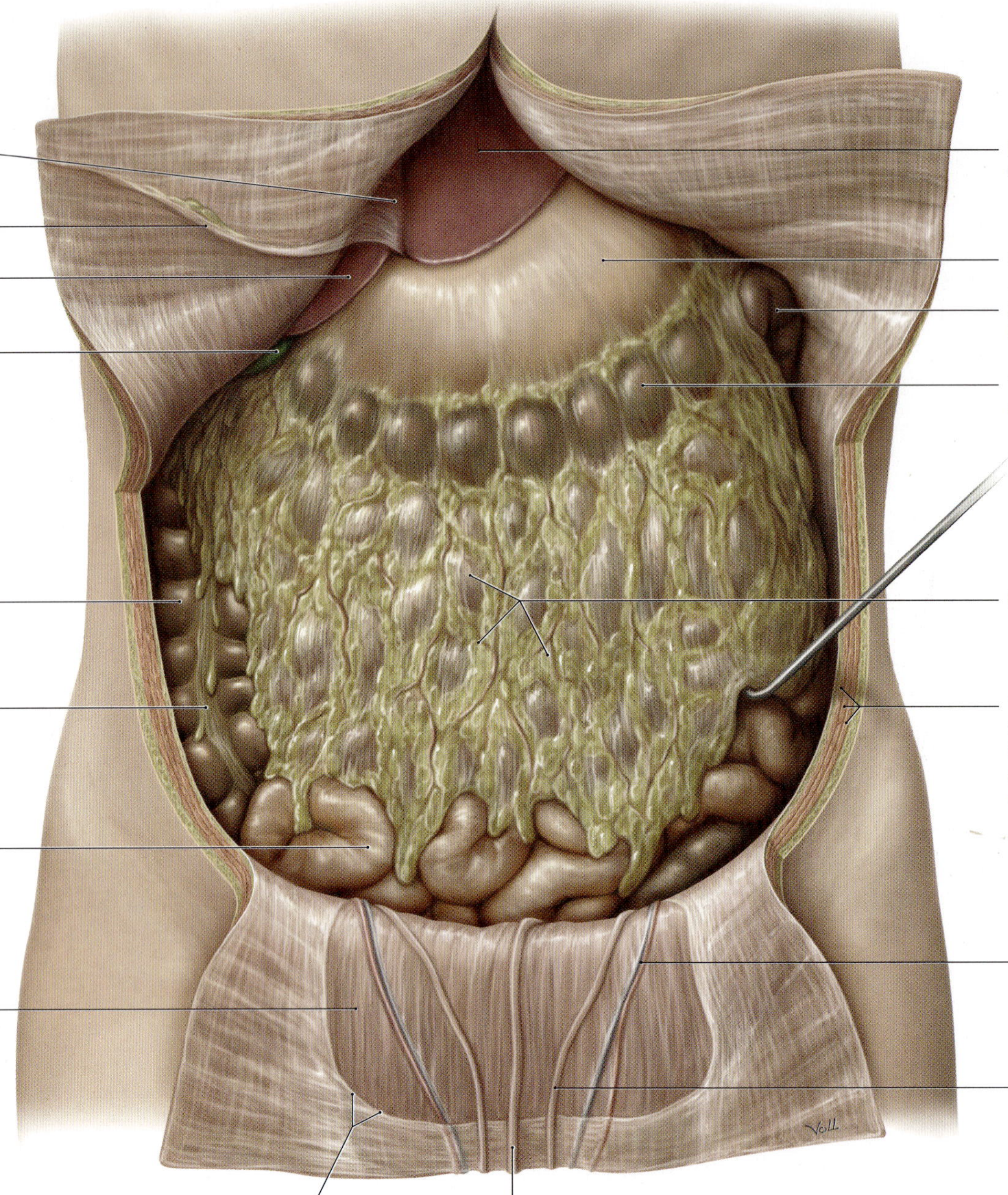

A The greater omentum in situ

Anterior view. The layers of the abdominal wall have been opened and retracted to display the greater omentum in its normal anatomical position. The greater omentum is draped over the loops of small intestine, which are visible only at the inferior border of the omentum. The greater omentum is an apron-like fold of peritoneum suspended from the greater curvature of the stomach and covering the anterior surface of the transverse colon. It develops from the embryonic dorsal mesogastrium, which becomes greatly enlarged to form a peritoneal sac suspended from the greater curvature. The greater omentum is relatively mobile, and is subject to considerable variation. Not infrequently, adhesions form between the greater omentum and the peritoneal covering of organs, especially as a result of local inflammation. While these adhesions help contain the spread of inflammation, they also limit the mobility of the organ to which the omentum is adherent. Peritoneal adhesions may undergo fibrotic changes over time, forming tough bands of scar tissue that may cause extrinsic narrowing and obstruction of organs such as the small intestine. In many cases the greater omentum also assumes importance as a lymphoid organ through the secondary acquisition of lymph nodes. The lesser omentum is described on p. 382.

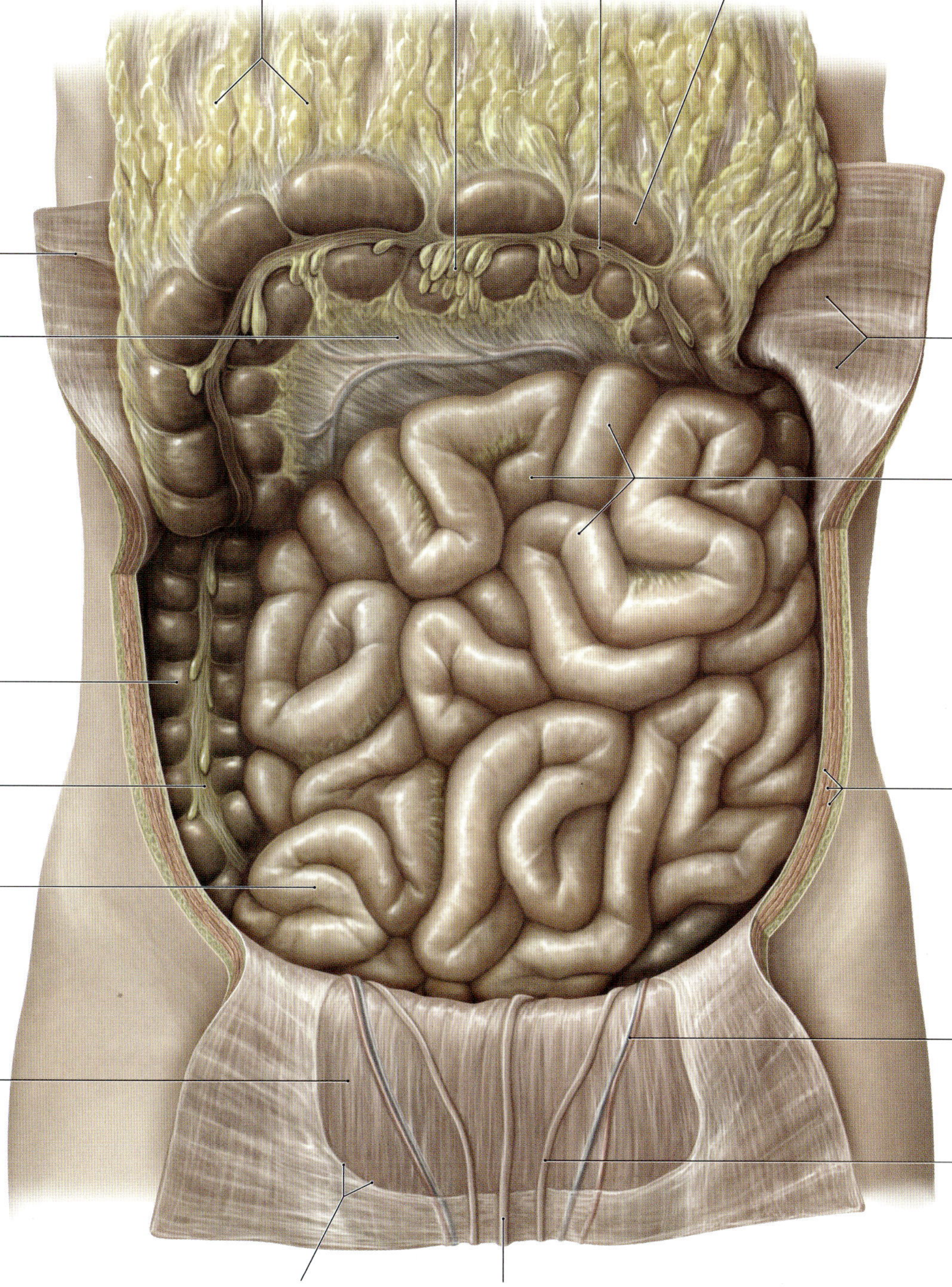

B Dissection with the greater omentum reflected superiorly and the small intestine in situ

Anterior view. The greater omentum has been reflected superiorly, carrying with it the transverse colon, to demonstrate how the intraperitoneal part of the small intestine is framed by the colon segments. The transverse mesocolon divides the peritoneal cavity into a *supracolic* part and an *infracolic* part (see **B**, p. 224).

The large epithelial surface area of the peritoneum is important clinically:

- With bacterial infection (caused by external trauma or the seepage of septic material from an inflamed appendix), pathogenic microorganisms can easily spread within the peritoneal cavity, where bacterial toxins are readily absorbed and carried into the bloodstream. As a result, bacterial peritonitis (inflammation of the peritoneum) generally constitutes a very serious and life-threatening condition.
- Localized inflammations may result in peritoneal adhesions and scar tissue bands (see **A**).
- The large surface area can be utilized for *peritoneal dialysis* in patients with renal failure: A dialysis solution instilled into the peritoneal cavity can absorb waste products from the blood through the peritoneum, allowing them to be removed from the body.

6.4 Drainage Spaces and Recesses within the Peritoneal Cavity

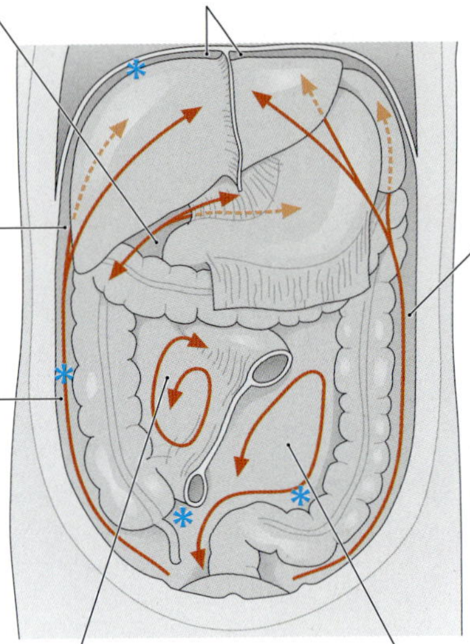

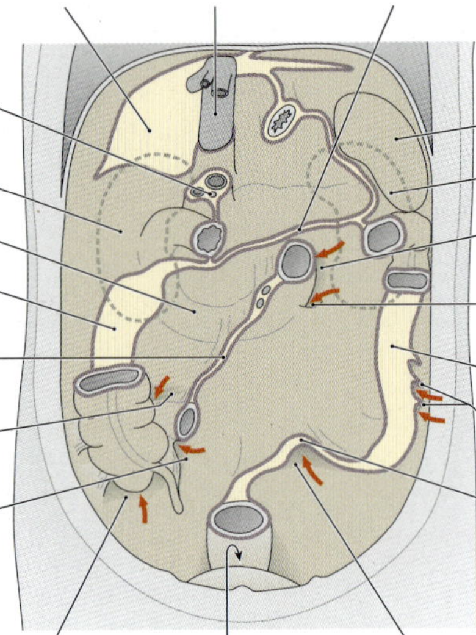

A Drainage spaces and recesses within the peritoneal cavity

a Anterior view with the greater omentum and small intestine removed; preferred metastatic sites (see blue stars);

b Posterior wall of the peritoneal cavity, anterior view. The mesenteric roots and sites of organ attachment create partially bounded spaces (recesses or sulci). Peritoneal fluid released by the peritoneal epithelium (transudate) can flow freely within these spaces.

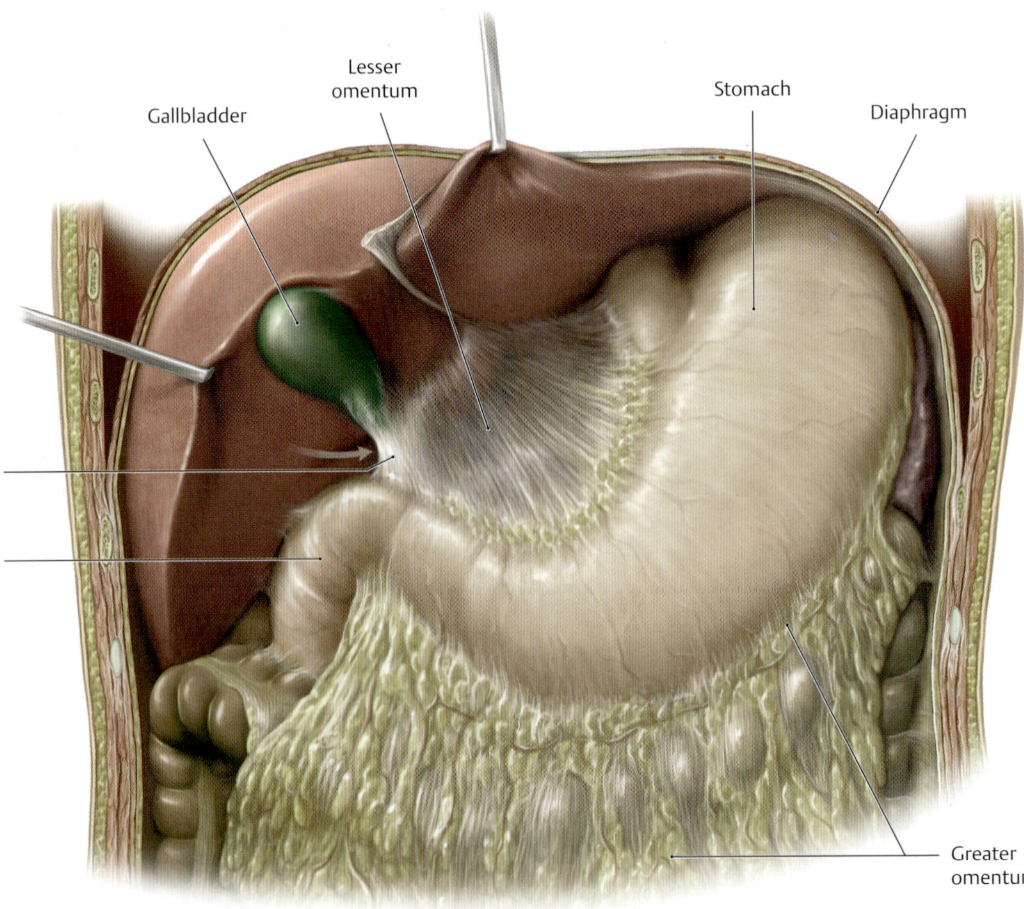

B Upper abdomen

Anterior view of the upper abdomen; the liver has been lifted to better display the subhepatic recess. The arrow points to the omental foramen, the opening into and out of the omental bursa behind the lesser omentum.

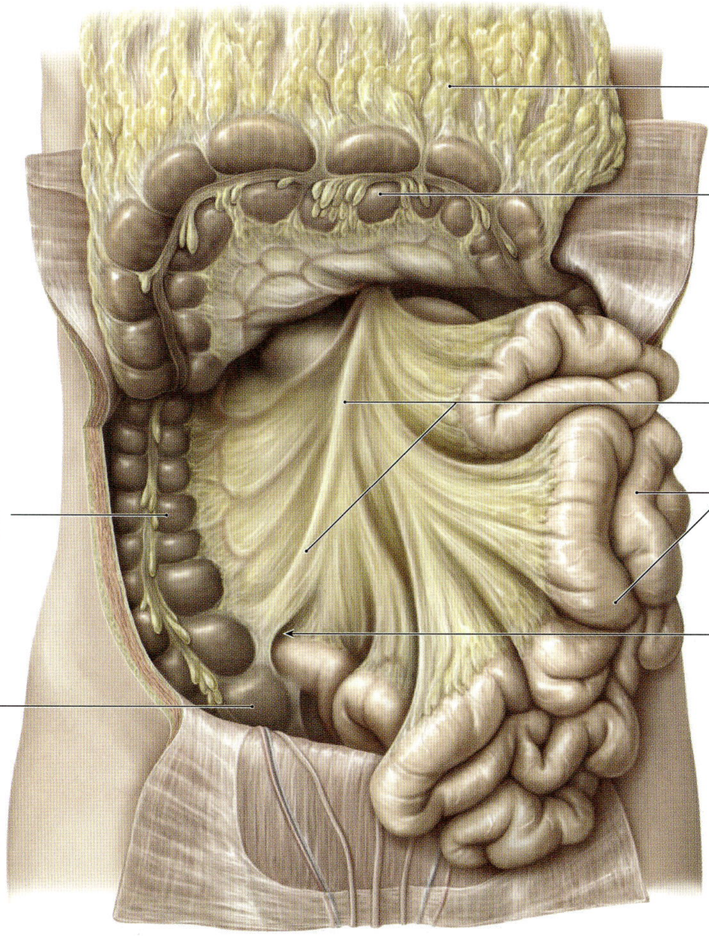

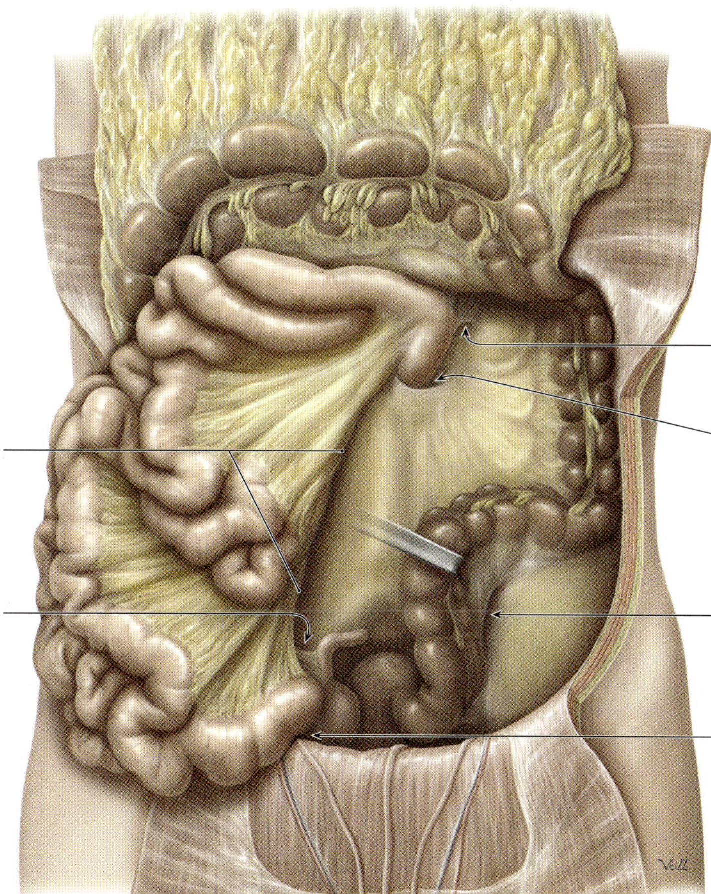

C Recesses in the posterior wall of the peritoneal cavity

Anterior view of a male abdomen and pelvis. Because the peritoneum extends between organs, it forms recesses and sulci (see also **A**). In a sense, the omental bursa may be considered the largest recess in the peritoneal cavity (see p. 386).

Note: The individual recesses are located between an organ and the wall of the peritoneal cavity or between organs. Freely mobile loops of the small intestine may become entrapped in these recesses ("internal hernia") hindering the passage of the intestinal contents and potentially causing a life-threatening bowel obstruction ("mechanical ileus").

6.5 Overview of the Mesenteries

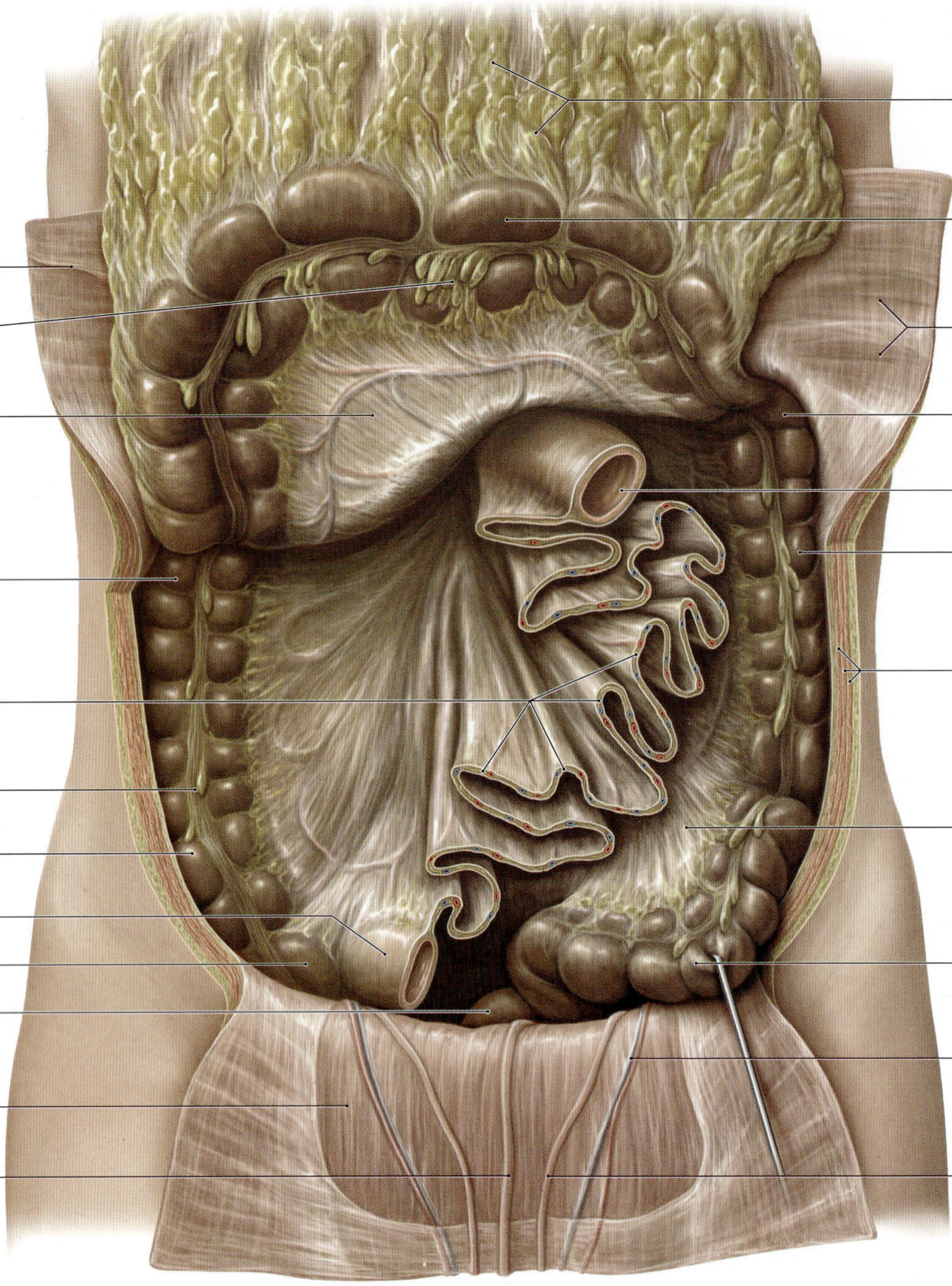

A Overview of the mesenteries with the greater omentum reflected superiorly and the small intestine removed

Anterior view. The transverse colon and greater omentum have been reflected superiorly and the intraperitoneal small intestine has been removed, leaving short stumps of jejunum and ileum. Three principal mesenteries are distinguishable in relation to the small and large intestine (the formation of the mesenteries is described on p. 42):

- The mesentery of the small intestine (the mesentery proper)
- The transverse mesocolon
- The sigmoid mesocolon (called also the mesosigmoid)

The origins of the mesenteries are shown in **B**. *Smaller mesenteries* are found on the vermiform appendix (*mesoappendix*) and rarely the upper part of the rectum (*mesorectum*, see **C**).

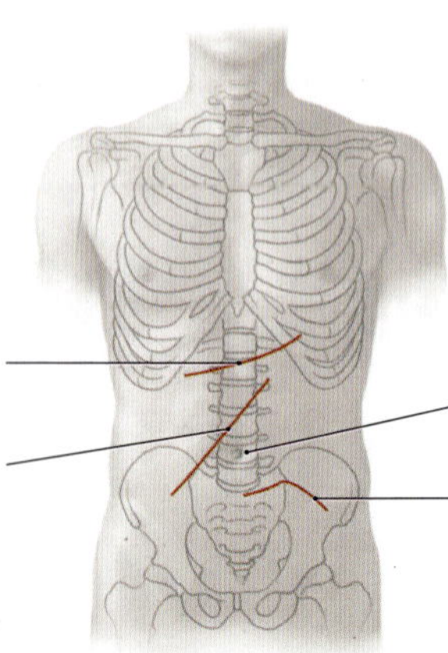

B Projection of the mesenteric roots onto the skeleton

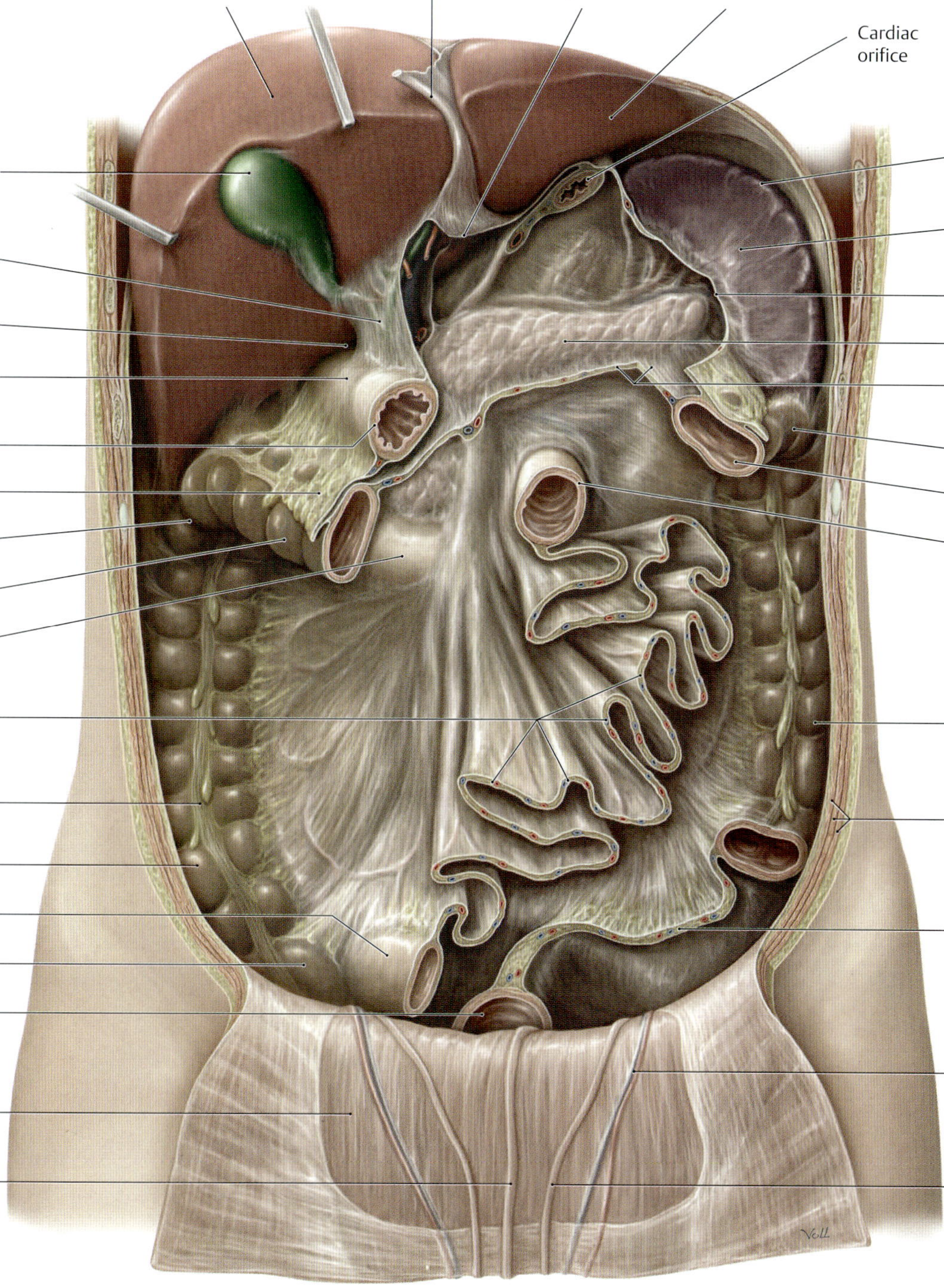

C Overview of the mesenteries* with the greater omentum removed

Anterior view. The mesenteries have been exposed by removing the stomach, jejunum, and ileum, leaving short stumps of small intestine. The liver has been reflected superiorly to display one part of the lesser omentum: the hepatoduodenal ligament, which connects the liver to the pylorus and duodenum. The other part of the lesser omentum, the hepatogastric ligament (peritoneal fold between the liver and lesser curvature of the stomach), has been removed with the stomach, opening the anterior wall of the omental bursa. Most of the transverse colon and sigmoid colon have been removed to display the roots of the transverse mesocolon and sigmoid mesocolon.

Note: The ascending and descending colon become attached to the posterior wall of the peritoneal cavity during the fourth month of embryonic development. The mesenteries of the ascending and descending *colon* become fused to the posterior wall of the peritoneal cavity. The *transverse* mesocolon crosses over the duodenum, whose mesentery also fuses to the posterior wall of the peritoneal cavity during embryonic development (see p. 46). The transverse mesocolon necessarily passes over this "retroperitoneal portion" of the duodenum because of its attachment to the posterior wall of the peritoneal cavity. Developmentally, almost all of the mesenteries are *dorsal* mesenteries. Only upper abdominal organs like the stomach and liver have ventral mesenteries.

* "Mesentery" in the broad sense refers to any of the peritoneal folds attached to the small and large intestine. "Mesentery" in the strict sense refers specifically to the mesentery of the jejunum and ileum, and consequently the terms "mesojejunum" and "mesoileum" are not used.

6.6 Topography of the Omental Bursa

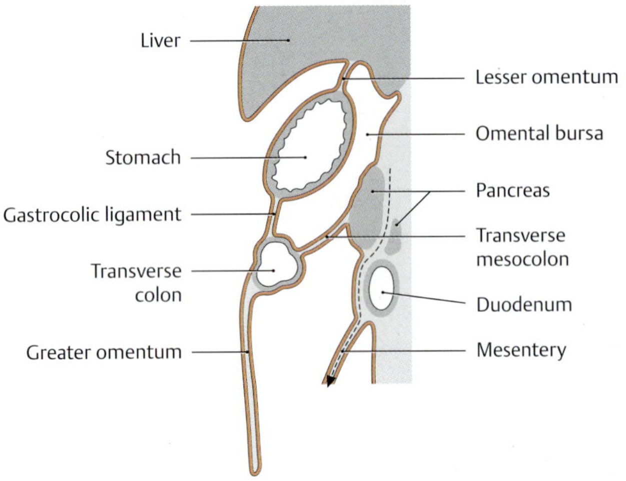

A Shape and location of the omental bursa in sagittal section
Left lateral view. The omental bursa is the largest potential space in the peritoneal cavity. It is located behind the lesser omentum and stomach. *Note:* As the stomach rotates during embryonic development, the omental bursa comes to lie posterior to the stomach. The pancreas, which migrates into the retroperitoneum secondarily, thus forms part of the posterior wall of the bursa, which provides a route for gaining surgical access to that organ. As the stomach rotates in the clockwise direction (viewed from the front), its lesser curvature points to the right and also superiorly, simultaneously displacing the liver superiorly and to the right. As a result of this, the omental bursa comes to lie partially posterior to the liver.

B Boundaries of the omental bursa

Anterior	Lesser omentum, gastrocolic ligament
Posterior	Pancreas, aorta (abdominal part), celiac trunk, splenic artery and vein, gastropancreatic fold, left suprarenal gland, superior pole of left kidney
Superior	Liver (with caudate lobe), superior recess of omental bursa
Inferior	Transverse mesocolon, inferior recess of omental bursa
Left	Spleen, gastrosplenic ligament, splenic recess of omental bursa
Right	Liver, duodenal bulb

C Surgical approaches to the omental bursa (see **A**)

- Through the omental foramen (natural opening, see **E**)
- Between the greater curvature of the stomach and the transverse colon through the gastrocolic ligament
- Through the transverse mesocolon after elevating the transverse colon (inferior approach)
- Between the lesser curvature of the stomach and the liver (through the lesser omentum)

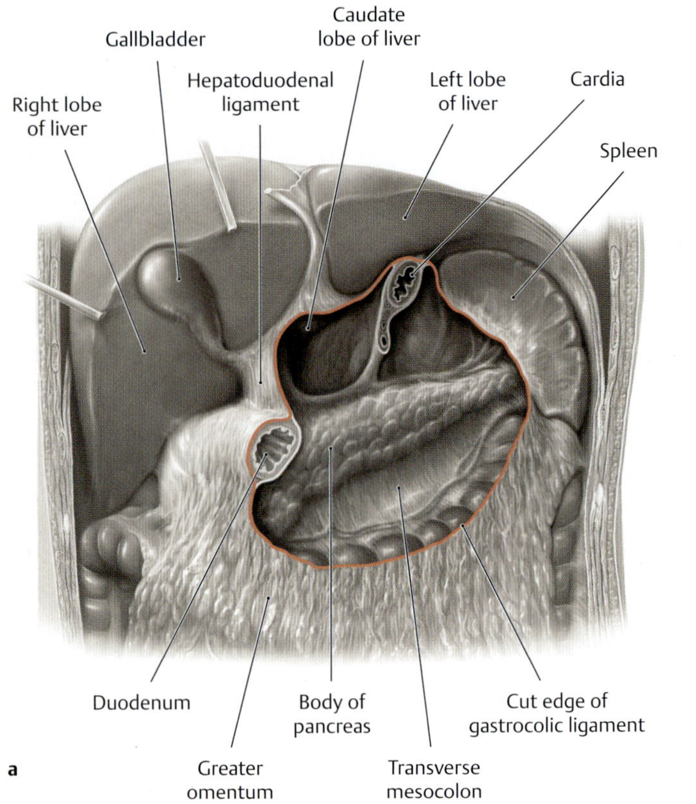

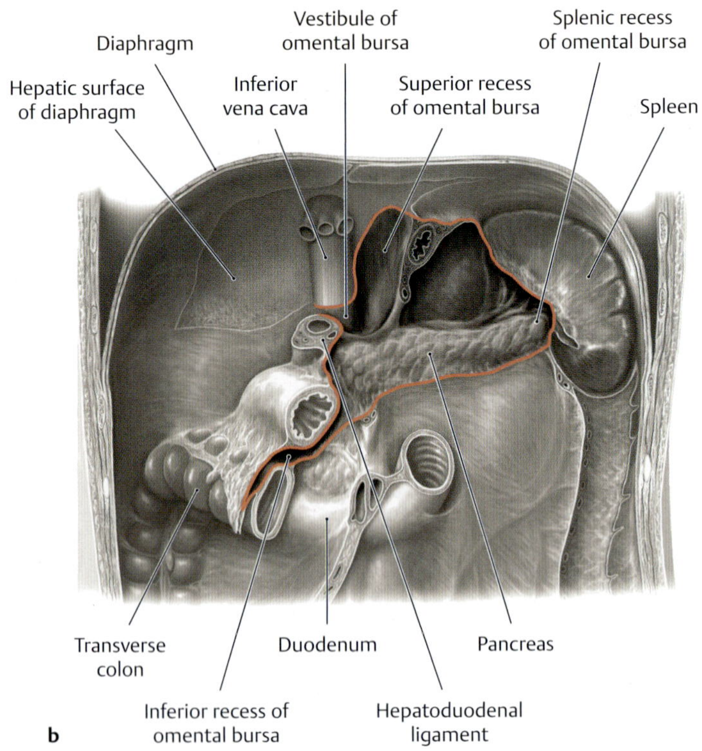

D Omental bursa, anterior view
a Boundaries of the omental bursa, also the shape and location of the gastric bed
b Structure of the posterior wall of the omental bursa

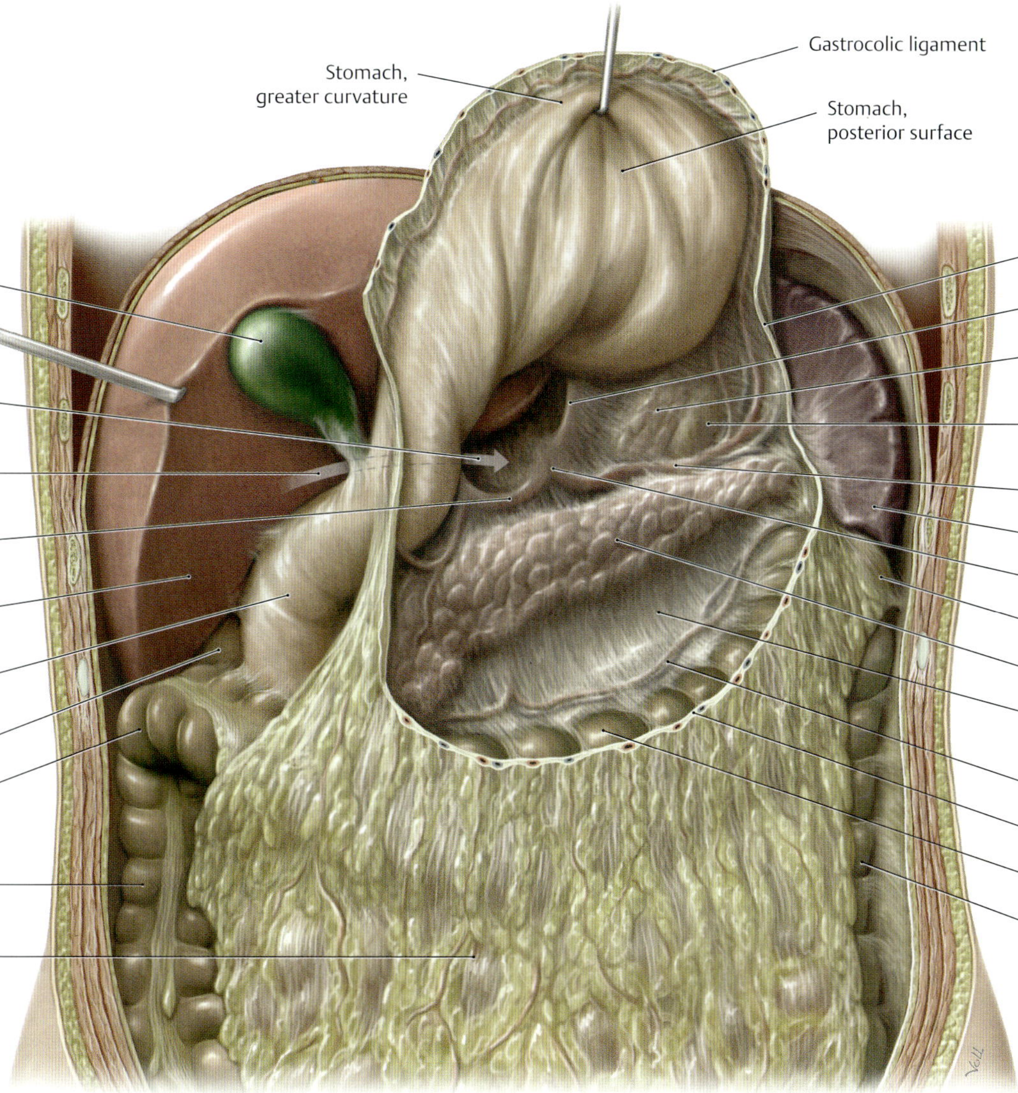

E Omental bursa in the upper abdomen

Anterior view. The gastrocolic ligament has been divided, the stomach has been reflected superiorly (surgical approach), and the liver has been retracted superolaterally. The *omental foramen* (arrow) is the only natural orifice of the omental bursa (opens posterior to the hepatoduodenal ligament). The *vestibule of the omental bursa* lies just past the foramen and forms the initial portion of the bursa cavity.

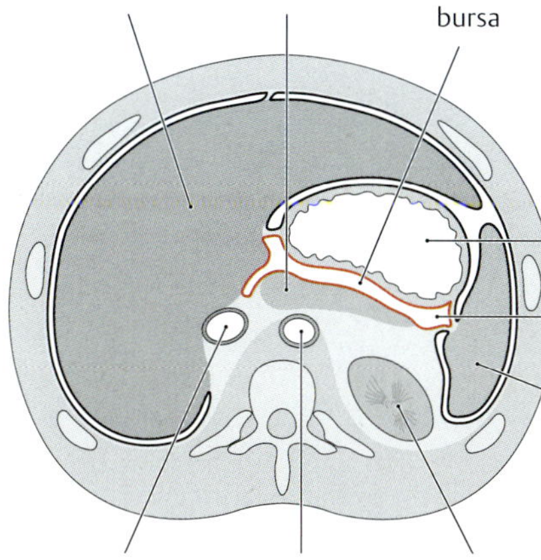

F Transverse section through the omental bursa

Schematic section through the abdomen at the T 12/L 1 level, viewed from below.

Note the walls and recesses that result from the formation of the bursa during the embryonic rotation of the stomach. Because the initial upper right portion of the embryonic body cavity moves posteriorly as part of the 90° rotation of the stomach, structures that were formerly posterior (spleen) move to the left side while structures that were formerly anterior (liver) move to the right side. Recesses in the omental bursa extend close to these organs (see **B**).

6.7 Topography of the Upper Abdominal Organs: Liver, Gallbladder, Duodenum, and Pancreas

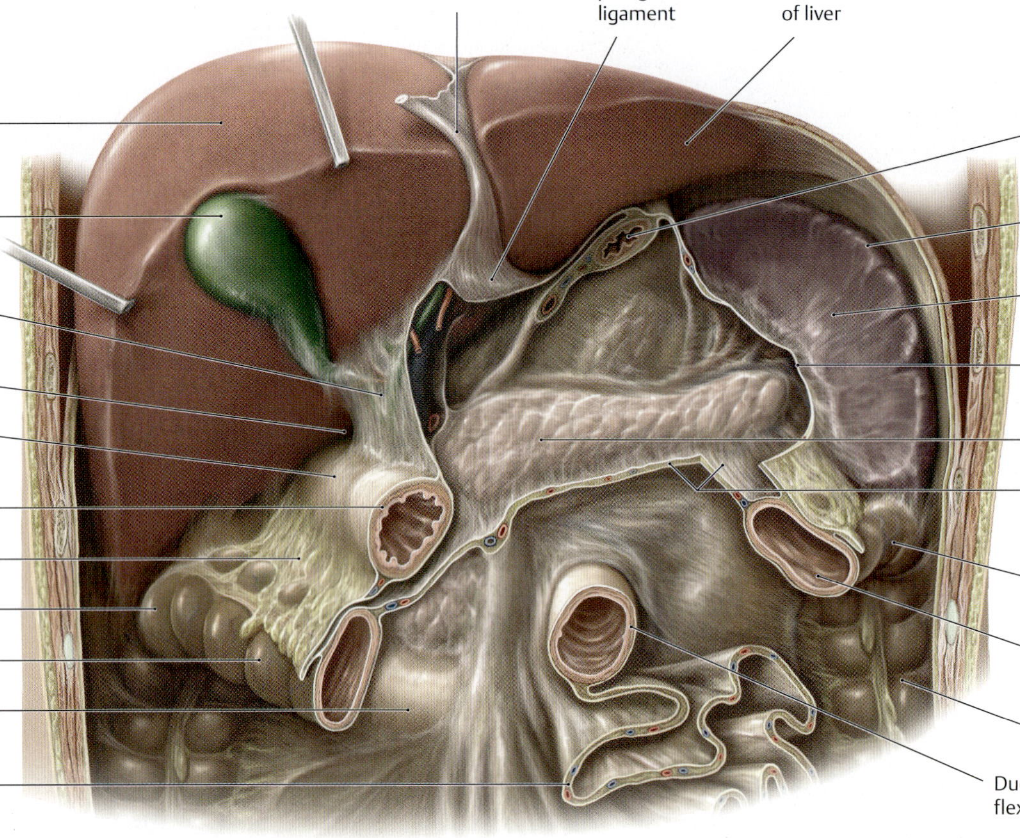

A Location of the liver and gallbladder
Anterior view, the stomach and small intestine have been removed, leaving a short stump of the jejunum. Most of the transverse colon has been removed. The liver has been lifted for better exposure of parts of the lesser omentum, hepatoduodenal ligament and pancreas (for the contents of the hepatoduodenal ligament see **Eb**).

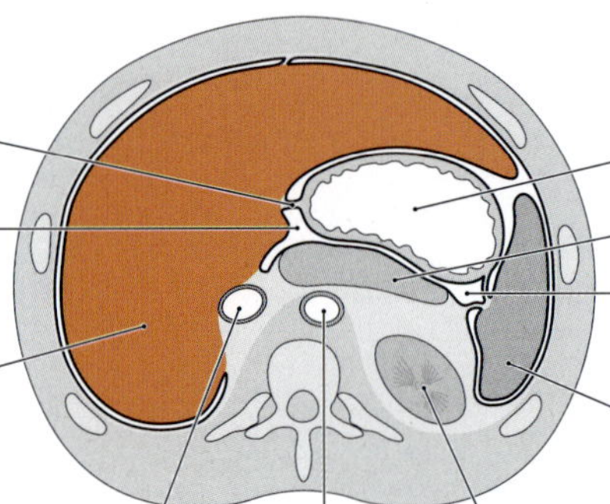

B Position of the liver
Transverse section through the abdomen at approximately the T 12/L 1 level, viewed from below. The liver is intraperitoneal except for the "bare area," which is not visible here. The left lobe of the liver extends into the LUQ, where it is anterior to the stomach. The peritoneal fold between the liver and the lesser curvature of the stomach (lesser omentum) can be seen. Portions of the liver form the right boundary of the omental bursa.

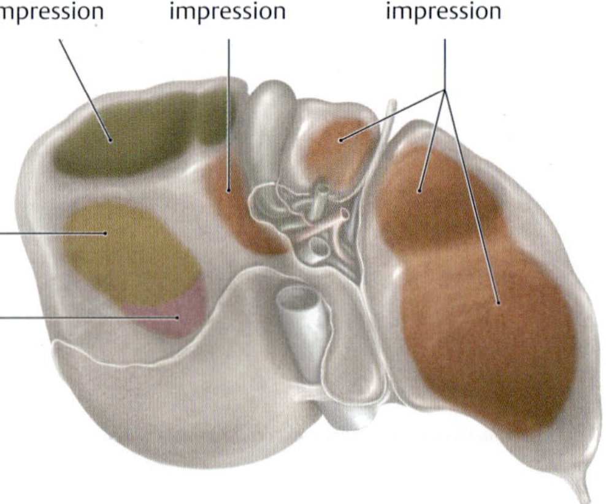

C Areas of contact with other organs
View of the visceral surface of the liver.
Note: Impressions from organs that are in direct contact with the liver are visible only on a liver that has been hardened in place by a chemical preservative ("fixation"). An unfixed liver from a cadaver that has not been chemically preserved is so soft that generally it will not show organ impressions. Diseases of the liver may easily spread to other organs, and vice versa, at areas of contact with adjacent organs (extensive owing to the size and topography of the liver).

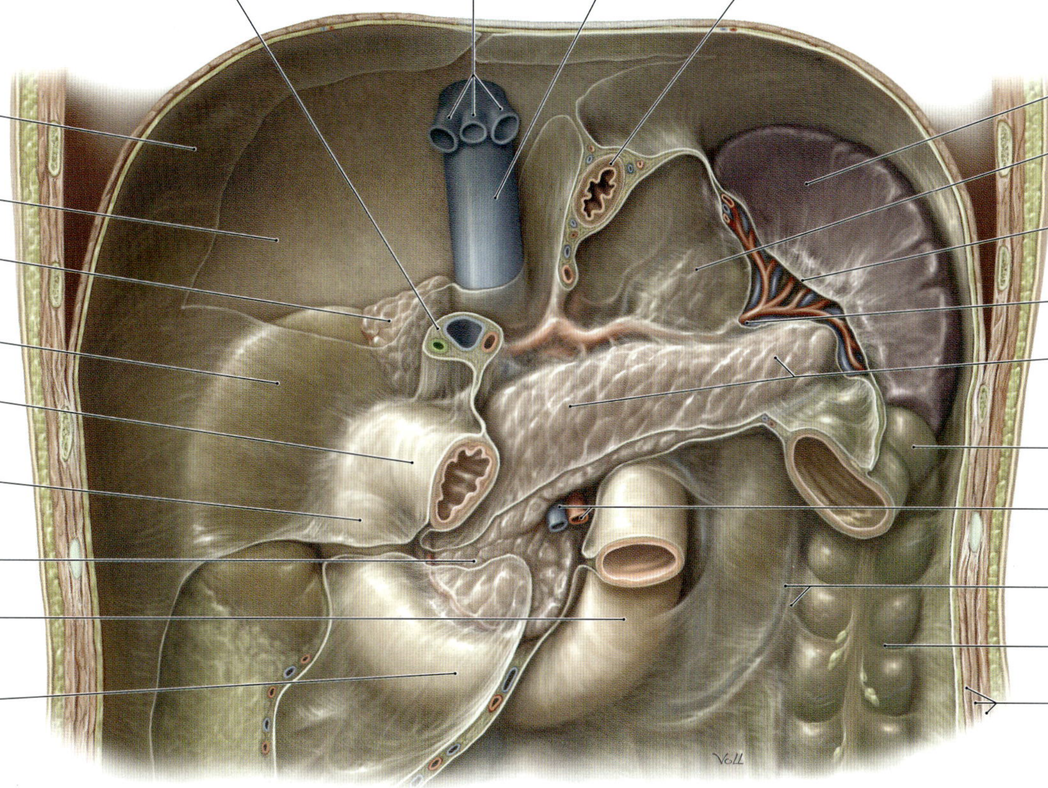

D Location of duodenum and pancreas
Anterior view; the liver, stomach and small intestine have been removed, leaving the duodenum and a very small stump of the jejunum. The ascending and transverse colon have been removed to expose the right kidney, pancreas, and duodenal loop. The *secondarily* retroperitoneal descending colon is left in situ. The pancreas and duodenum are also secondarily retroperitoneal (for peritoneal relationships see p. 225). Both kidneys and suprarenal glands, located in the retroperitoneal space, are visible through the parietal peritoneum. The kidneys and suprarenal glands are *primarily* retroperitoneal. The intraperitoneal spleen is located in the left upper quadrant in a compartment called the splenic niche.
Note: The root of the (intraperitoneal) transverse mesocolon crosses anterior to the duodenum and pancreas.

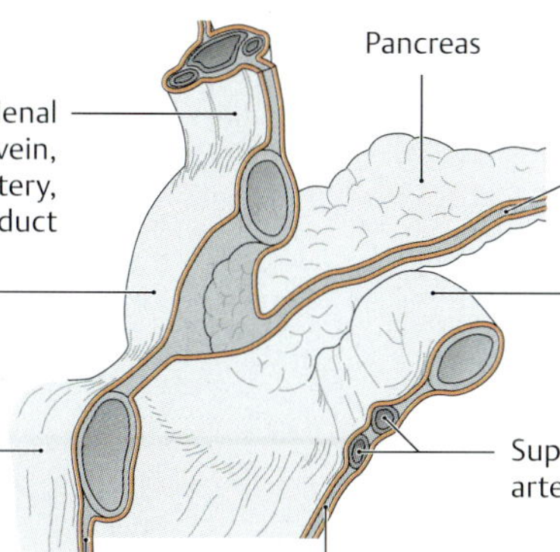

a

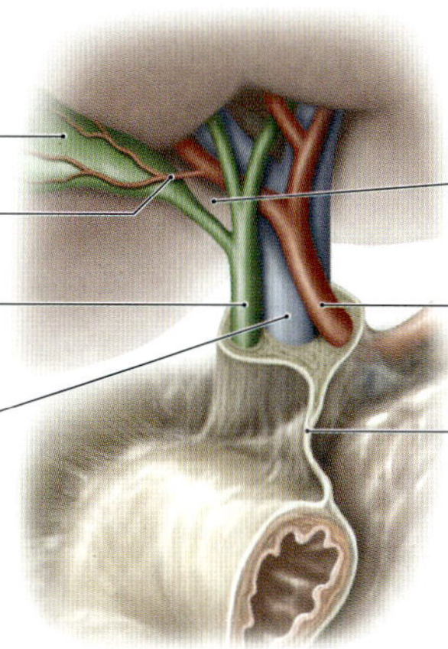

b

E Peritoneal relationships of the duodenum and pancreas; Contents of the hepatoduodenal ligament

a Peritoneal relationships of the duodenum and pancreas, anterior view. The root of the transverse mesocolon crosses over the descending part of the duodenum and the pancreas.

b Contents of the hepatoduodenal ligament. The hepatoduodenal ligament is part of the lesser omentum and connects the liver with the pylorus and superior part of the duodenum. It contains the hepatic portal vein, the proper hepatic artery, and the common bile duct.

6.8 Topography of the Upper Abdominal Organs: Stomach and Spleen

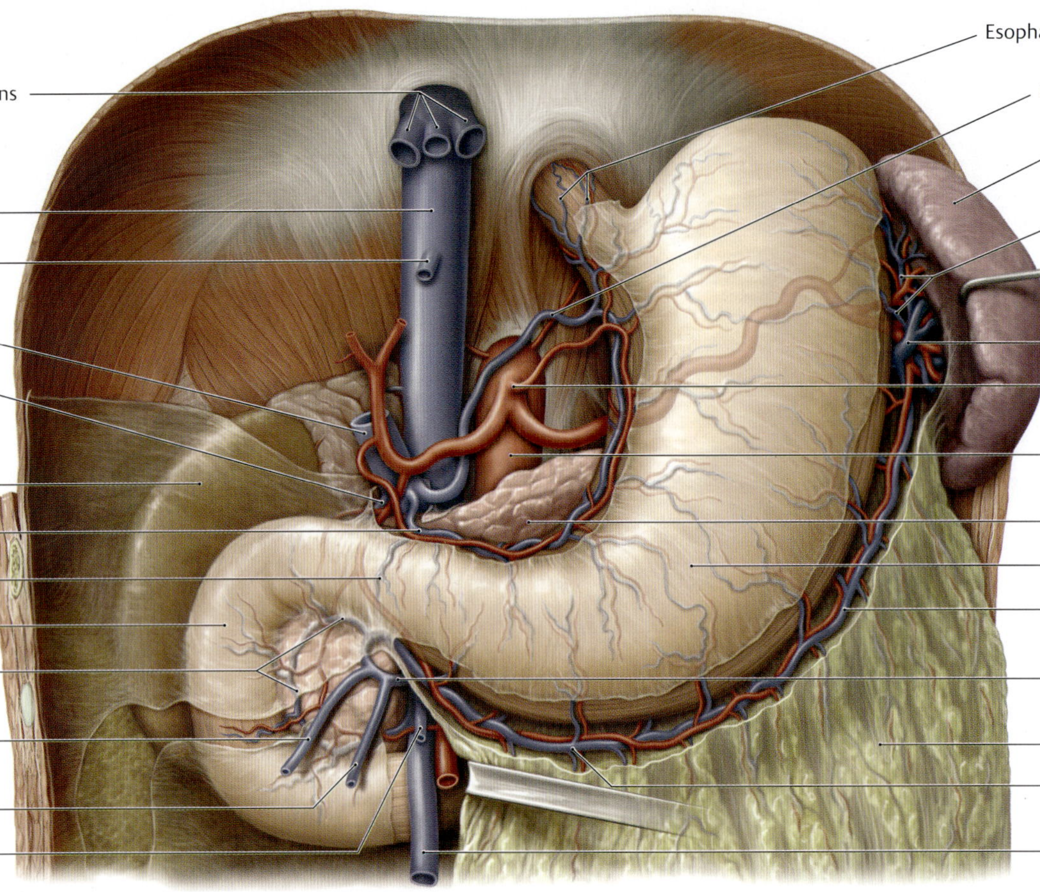

A Location of the stomach and spleen
Anterior view. The liver and lesser omentum have been removed, the greater omentum has been opened and retracted to the left, and the stomach pulled slightly downward for better exposure. At several sites, the peritoneum has been removed or windowed for better exposure of the opening of the hepatic veins into the inferior vena cava and the opening of the veins of the stomach into the hepatic portal vein at the margin of the hepatoduodenal ligament (here completely opened). The spleen is retracted from its "niche" and lies close to the fundus and greater curvature of the stomach. The intraperitoneal stomach covers most of the retroperitoneal pancreas. The greater omentum, a remnant of the dorsal mesogastrium, is suspended from the greater curvature of the stomach. The stomach is partially shown transparent to display the splenic artery that extends behind the stomach from the celiac trunk to the spleen.

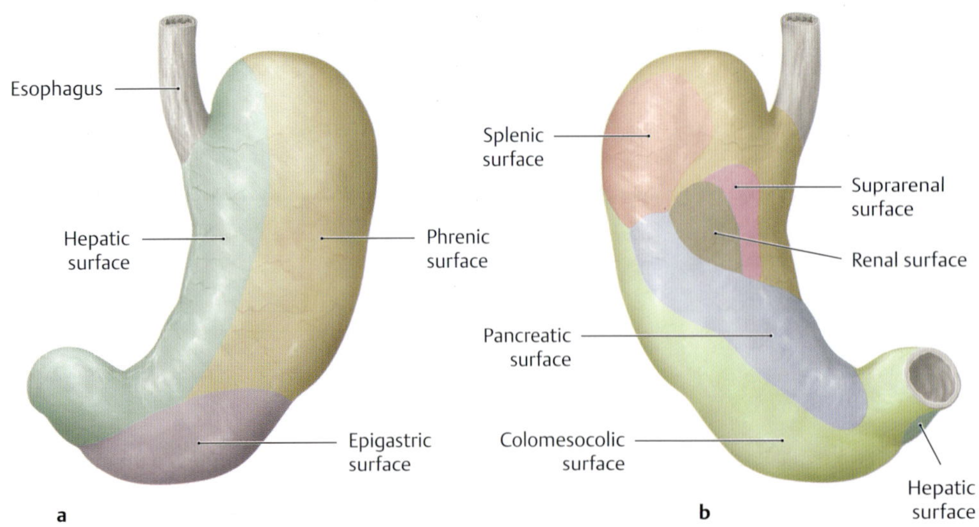

B Areas of contact with adjacent organs
a, b Anterior and posterior views of the stomach walls. Because the stomach is intraperitoneal, it is very mobile relative to adjacent organs. But since the stomach is in close contact with other organs, lesions that penetrate the stomach wall (ulcers, malignant tumors) may spread to nearby organs or may cause adhesions to develop between the stomach and adjacent organs.

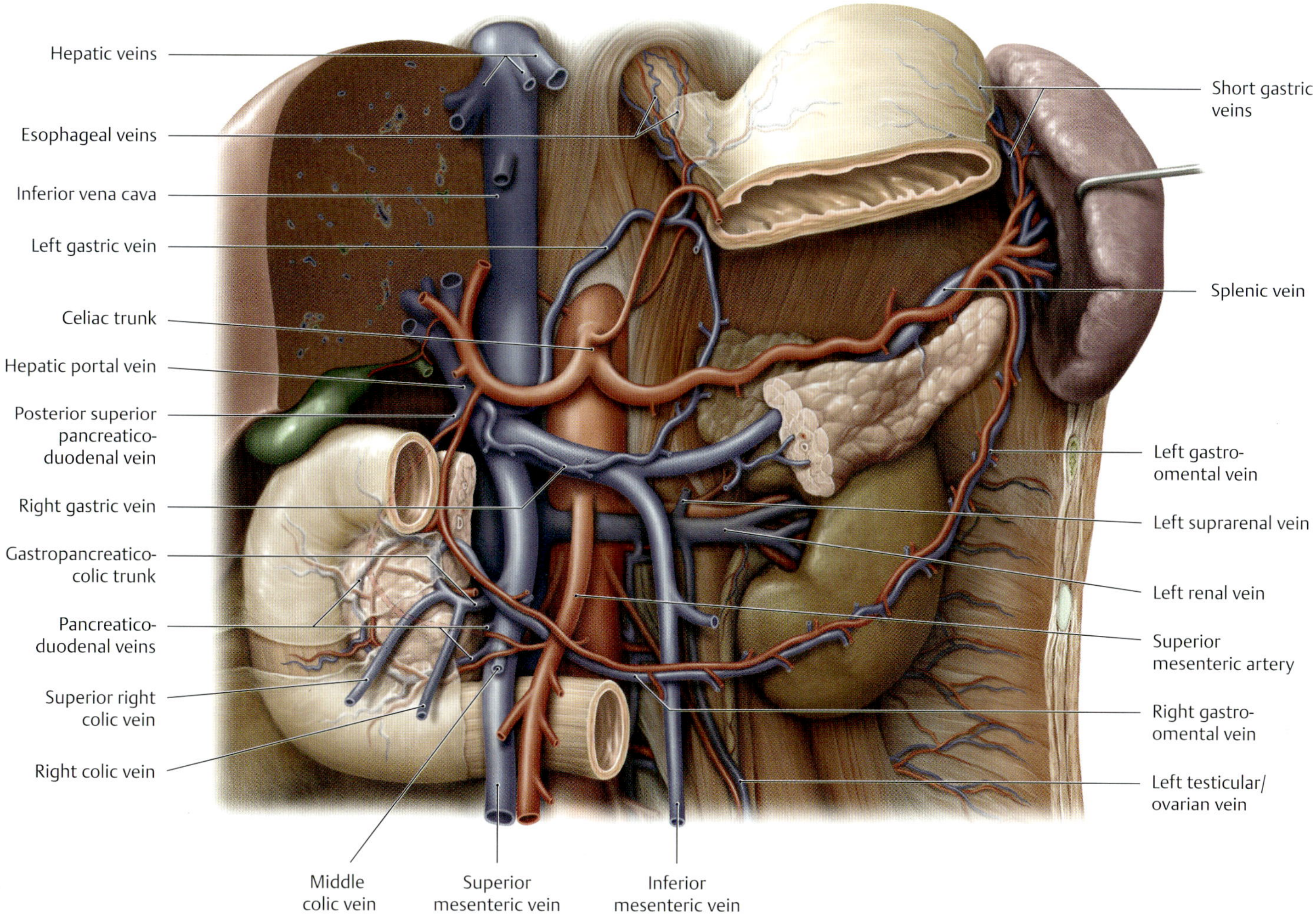

C Location of the pancreas, spleen, and major vessels
Anterior view. The stomach has been partially removed and pulled slightly downward, and most of the intestines have been removed leaving only the duodenum. The spleen has been lifted from its bed and retracted anterolaterally toward the fundus of the stomach. Part of the pancreatic body has been resected. Most of the peritoneum has been removed, and retroperitoneal fat and connective tissue have been cleared away.

The secondarily retroperitoneal pancreas crosses over the upper pole of the left kidney that also lies in the retroperitoneal space. The diagram shows that the displayed retroperitoneal organs are not arranged in a coronal plane but oriented anterior to posterior. The most anterior organ in the right upper quadrant is the duodenum. Posterior to the duodenum lies the pancreas that is oriented transversely in the right and left upper quadrants. The most posterior organs are the two kidneys (here only the left kidney is clearly visible, the right kidney is covered by the duodenum and the head of the pancreas).

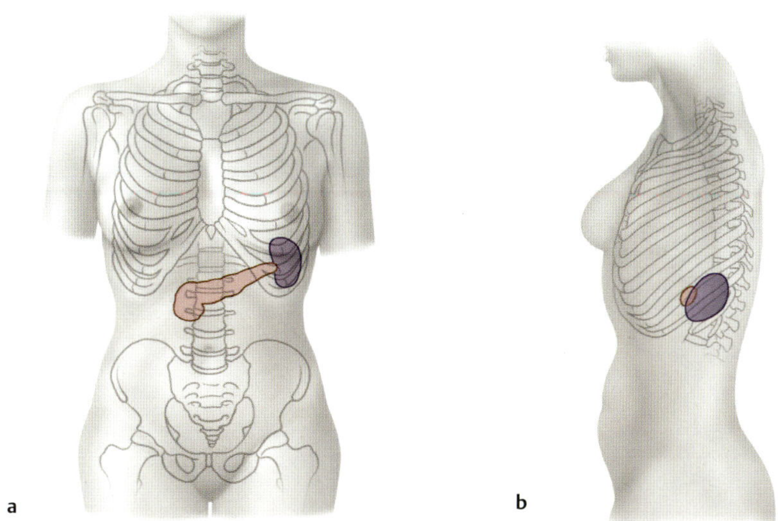

D Projection of the pancreas and spleen onto the skeleton
Anterior (**a**) and left lateral (**b**) views.
The body of the pancreas is located at the L 1/L 2 level, its head extends a little lower. The body along with the tail of the pancreas is directed upward and to the left (almost to T 12). The spleen is located in the left upper quadrant. Its longitudinal axis follows the line of the tenth rib. The tail of the pancreas seems to touch the spleen. It only "seems" to touch it because the pancreas lies retroperitoneal and the spleen lies intraperitoneal. Thus, they are separated by the peritoneal cavity.
Note in particular how far posterior the spleen is located as shown in (**b**). Just like the liver, the spleen touches the posterior wall of the peritoneal cavity.

6.9 Cross-Sectional Anatomy of the Upper Abdominal Organs

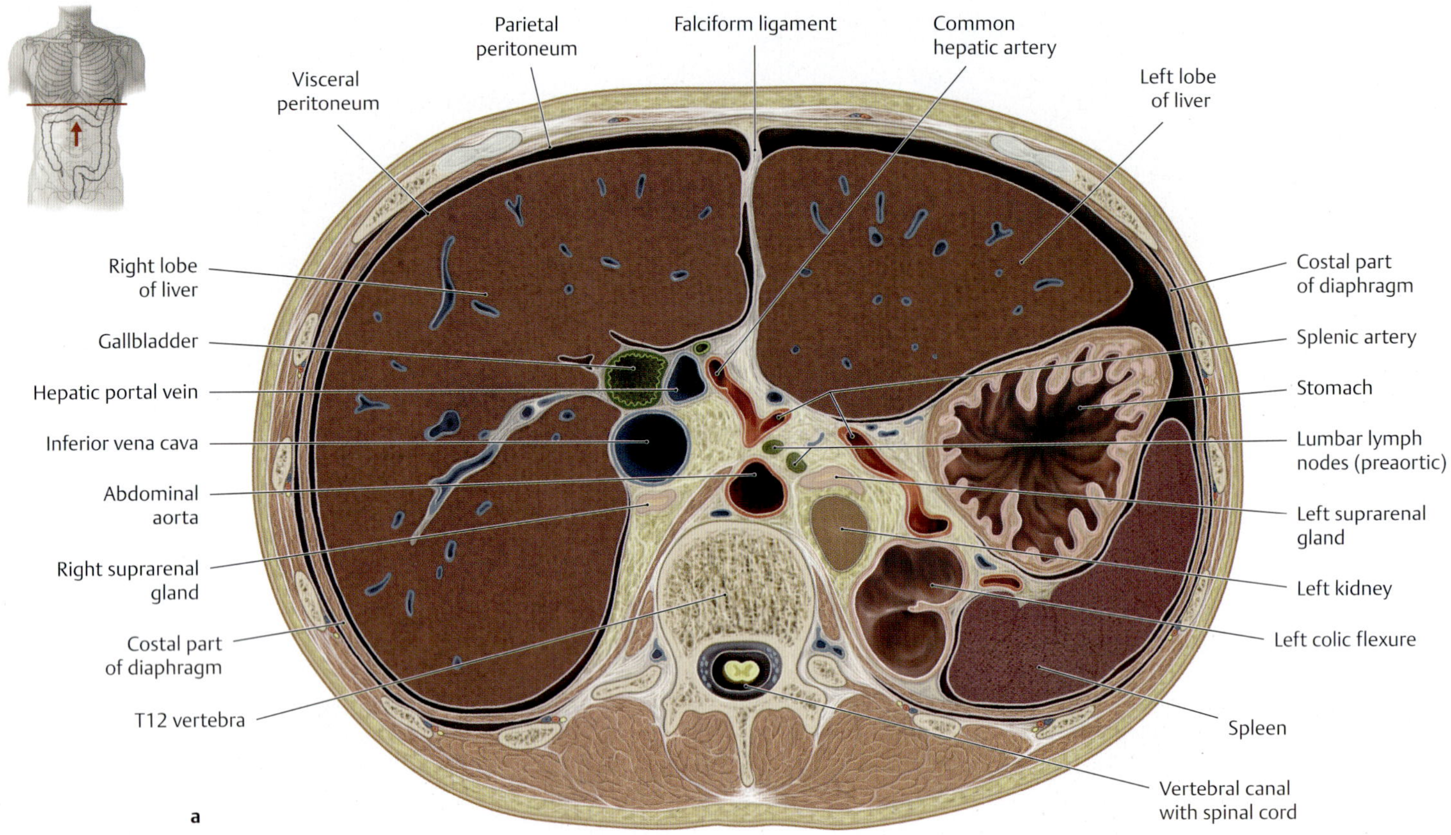

a

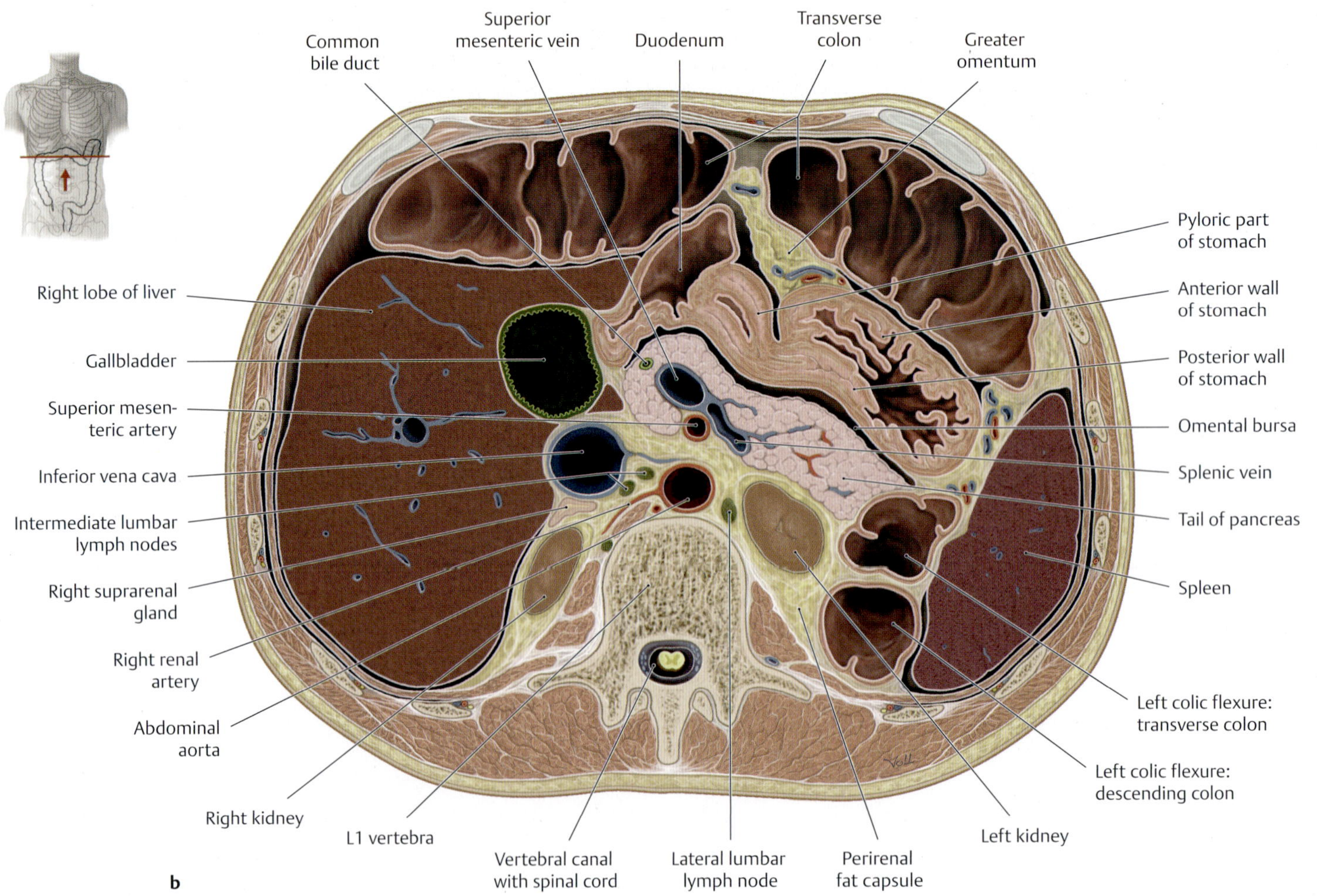

b

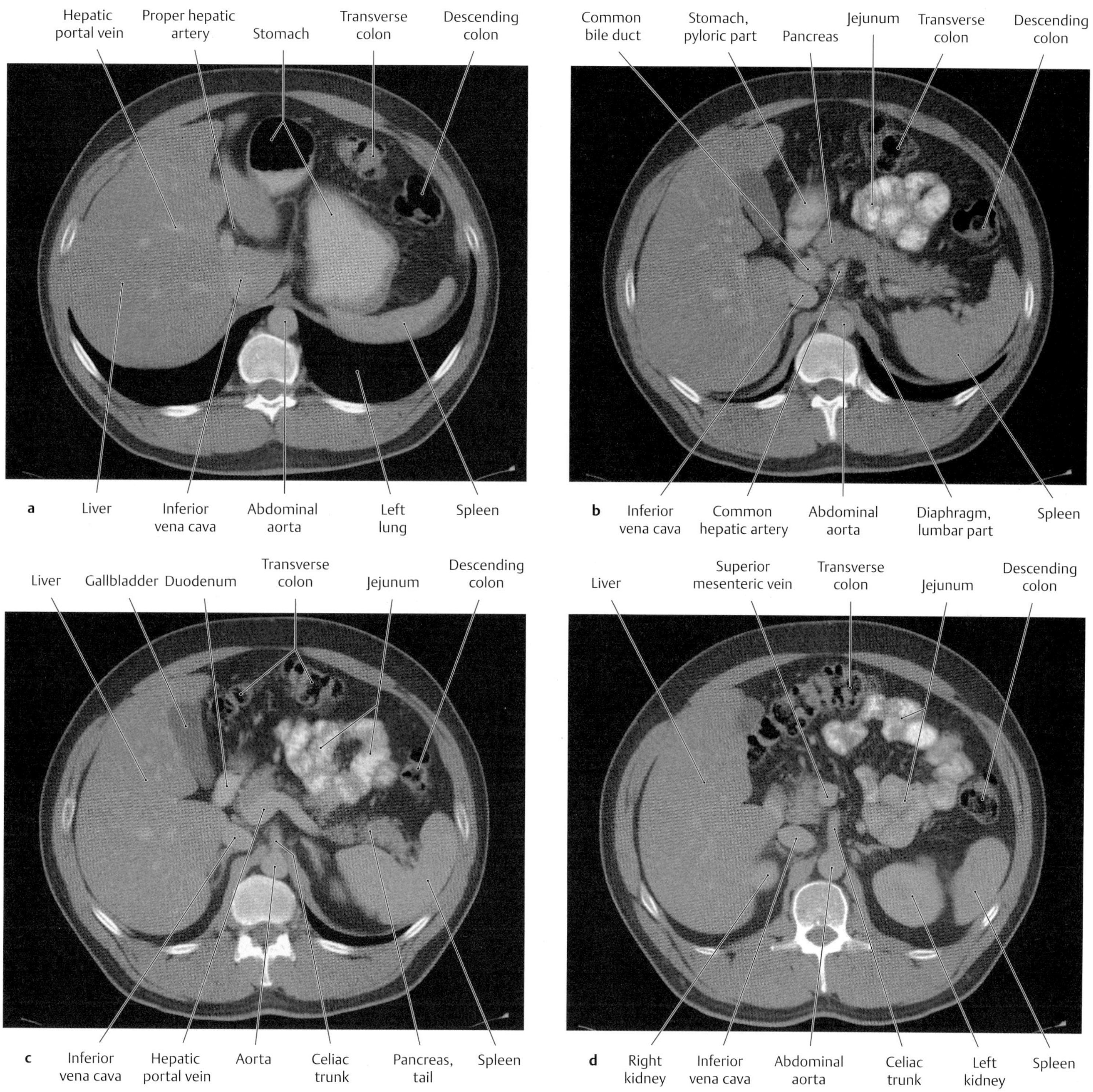

B Abdominal computed tomography
Axial scans of the upper abdominal organs at the T11 level (**a**), T12 level (**b**), and L1 level top (**c**) and bottom (**d**); all are caudal views (from: Möller T, Reif E. *Taschenatlas der Schnittbildanatomie, Band II: Thorax, Abdomen, Becken*. 2nd ed. Stuttgart: Thieme; 2019).

Note: The pancreas is normally located at the L 1/2 level between the exit of the celiac trunk (see **b**) and the superior mesenteric artery (see **c**) from the abdominal aorta.

A Transverse sections through the abdomen
a At the T 12 level; **b** At the L 1 level, inferior views.
The level that most organs occupy in the body is dependent on age, posture, constitutional type, nutritional state, and respiration. Thus, a section at a certain level may show considerable variation, especially in the organs that just border the plane of section. A section at the T 12 level (**a**) passes only through the left kidney, which is more superior than the right kidney (the right kidney is more inferior because of the liver and is below the plane of section). However, both suprarenal glands are visible, and the position of the right kidney can be inferred at the T 12 level from the location of the right suprarenal gland. At the L 1 level, the section almost always passes through both kidneys (see **b**).

6.10 Topography of the Small and Large Intestine

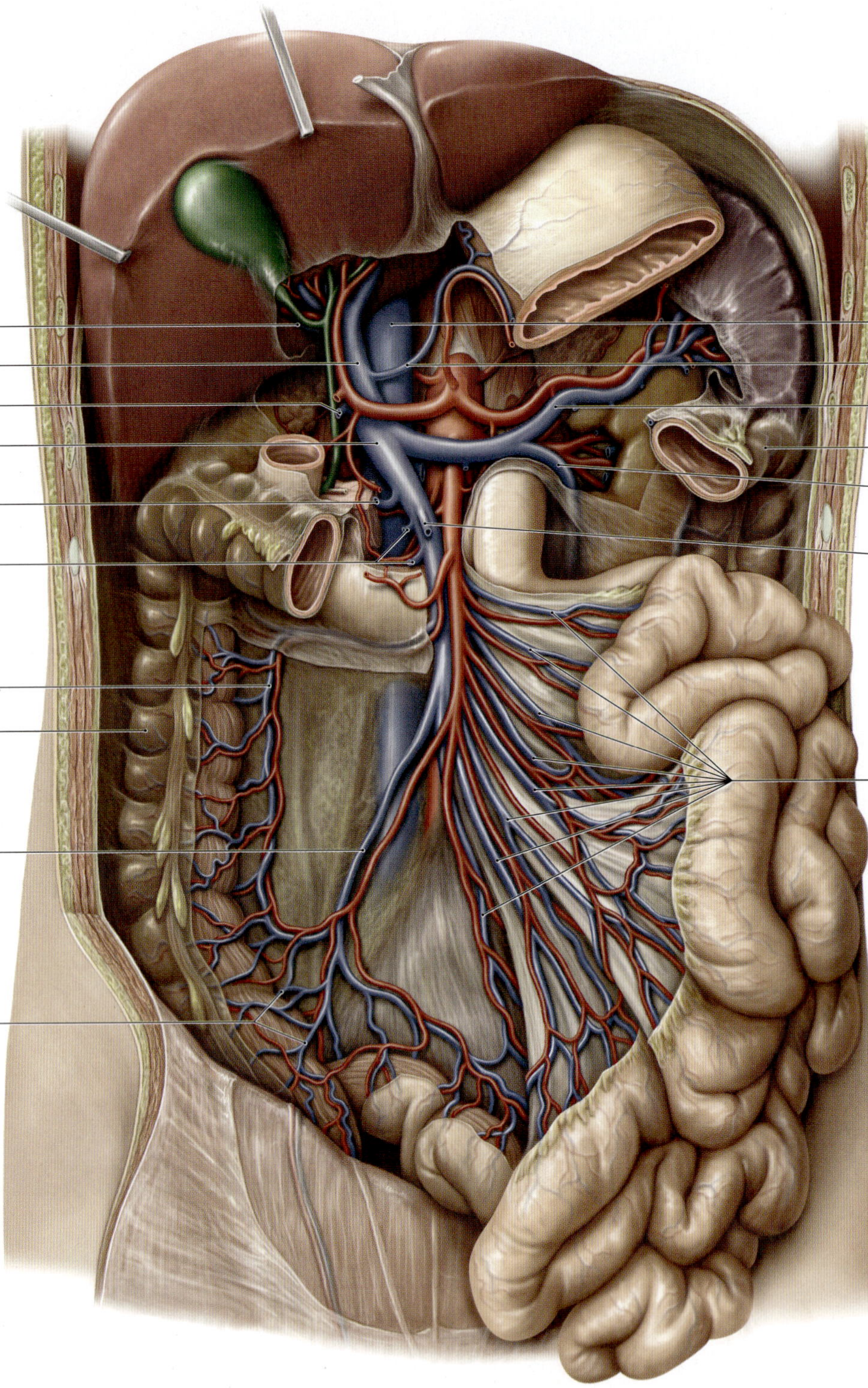

A Location of the small intestine

Anterior view of the opened abdomen. The liver has been lifted, most of the stomach and the transverse colon have been removed, and the pancreas has been largely resected.

The small intestine is the longest individual organ. Its location varies to such a degree that pointing out its relation to palpable bony landmarks is not useful. Reference points are useful only for the initial and terminal segments of the small intestine. The initial segment is the duodenum, a C-shaped loop that lies secondarily retroperitoneal in the right upper quadrant inferior (and slightly posterior) to the liver, approximately at the L 1–3 level. The duodenum is crossed by the transverse mesocolon. The terminal part of the small intestine is the ileum at the junction of the cecum with the ascending colon. The ileum is located in the right lower quadrant slightly inferior to the iliac crest. Most of the jejunum and ileum (both completely intraperitoneal) lie in the form of coils in the lower abdomen between the transverse mesocolon and the pelvic inlet within a "frame" formed by the colon. The jejunum and ileum are covered by the greater omentum (here removed) and are located more anterior than the duodenum (anterior layer of the abdomen). In this view, the mesentery has been largely removed to expose the numerous jejunal and ileal arteries and veins.

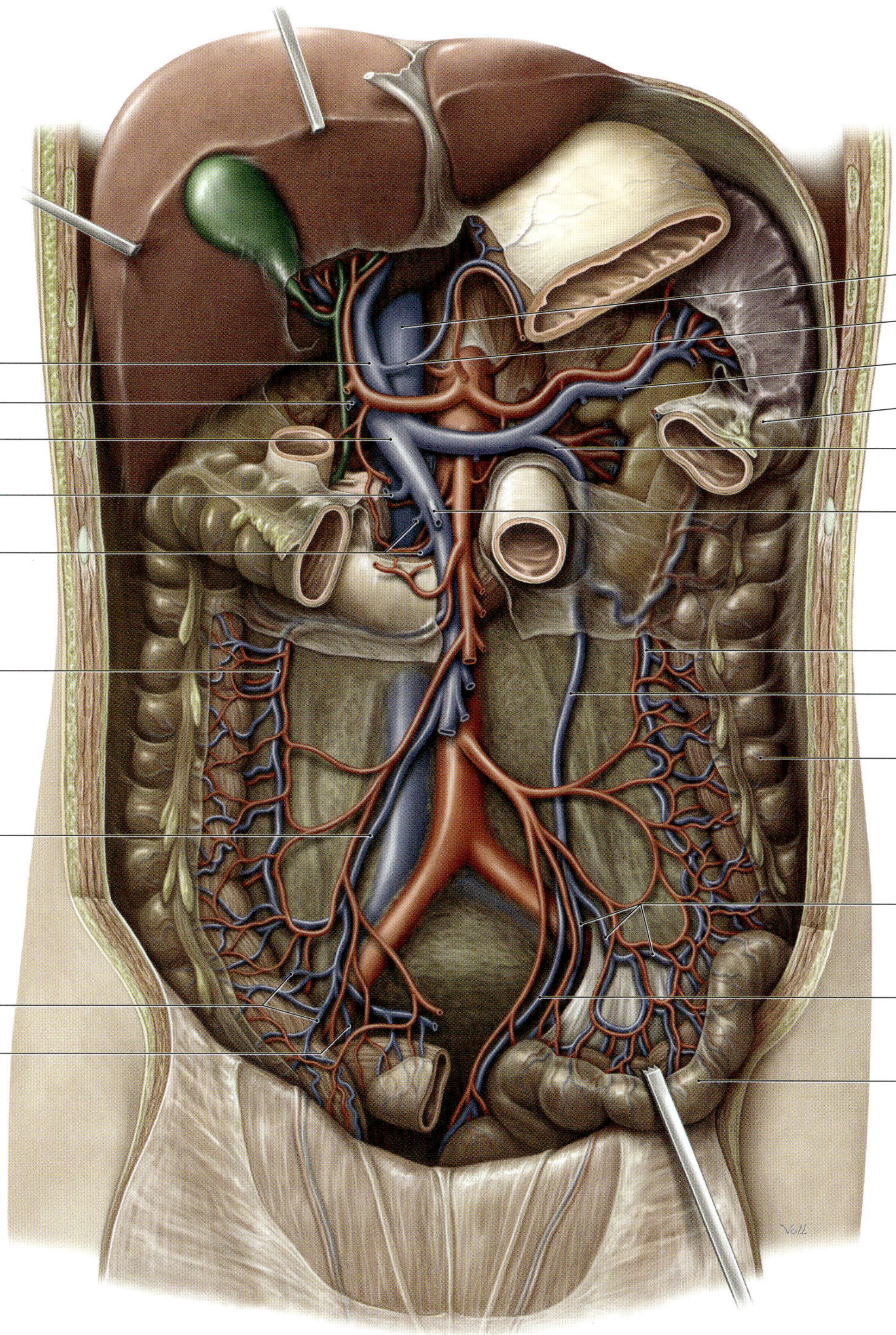

B Location of the large intestine

Anterior view of the opened abdomen. The liver has been lifted, most of the stomach and the transverse colon have been removed, the pancreas has been largely resected, and the small intestine has been removed leaving only the duodenum and a small stump of the jejunum and ileum. By removing a large area of the peritoneum, the neurovascular structures running to the ascending and descending colons are made visible.

The large intestine forms a frame around the small intestine. Its location also varies, but to a lesser degree than the small intestine:

- The ascending and descending colons (both secondarily retroperitoneal) are along the right and left sides,
- The transverse colon (intraperitoneal) runs horizontally across the border between the upper and lower abdomen,
- The sigmoid colon is at the pelvic brim in the left lower quadrant, and
- The rectum and anal canal (retro- or subperitoneal) are in the pelvis anterior to the sacrum.

Using bony landmarks make sense only as reference points to define the location of the rectum that extends in front of the sacrum from the junction between S 2 and S 3 to the pelvic floor. Because of the colon's proximity to the liver (right colic flexure, or hepatic flexure) and spleen (left colic flexure, or splenic flexure) they also serve as topographic reference points. If the abdomen is divided into layers from anterior to posterior, the intraperitoneal transverse colon is located in the anterior layer, and the retroperitoneal portions of the ascending and descending colons are located in the middle layer. However, the descending colon lies significantly more posterior than the ascending colon.

6.11 Diagnostic Imaging of the Small and Large Intestine: Plain-Film Abdominal Radiographs and Double-Contrast Studies

A Standing abdominal radiograph
Depending on the medical problem, images of the gastrointestinal tract may be obtained using conventional X-rays (with or without the administration of a contrast medium), computerized tomography (CT and MRI) or sonography. Left lateral decubitus or standing abdominal radiographs are employed to detect the presence of free gas within the peritoneal cavity, which may indicate perforation of a hollow organ, or to look for fluid levels in the intestinal lumen if ileus is suspected. (Photos from: Reiser M, Kuhn F, Debus J, eds. *Duale Reihe Radiologie*. 4th ed. Stuttgart: Theme; 2017.)

- **a** Standing abdominal image - normal findings: the diaphragm is clearly defined (arrows) with no evidence of free gas under the domes of the diaphragm. Under normal physiologic conditions, small quantities of gas are present (intestinal gases or gastric bubble);
- b Mechanical ileus after right hemicolectomy: proximal to the site of stenosis, greatly distended coils of the ileum are visible as well as air-fluid levels at different heights in the remaining colon. The pattern of distribution of the air-fluid levels may indicate the site of obstruction (see **c**);
- c Schematic representation of radiologic findings in cases of mechanical ileus showing the different levels at which the obstruction has occurred: I duodenal ileus demonstrating the 'double-bubble' characteristic, **II** high and **III** deep small intestine ileus (no presence of gas in colonic frame), **IV** large intestine ileus with air-fluid levels located along the course of the colon.

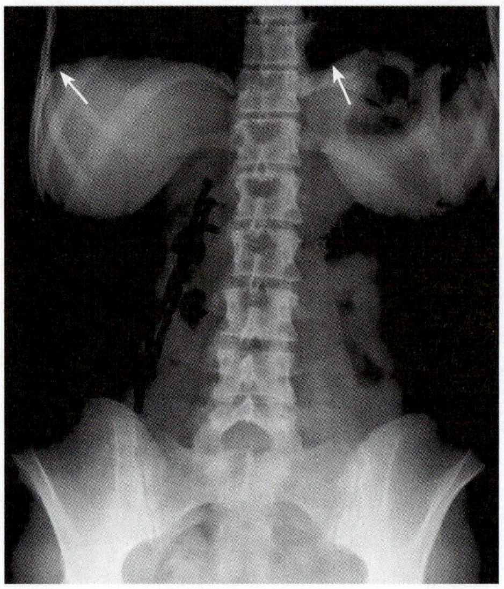
a

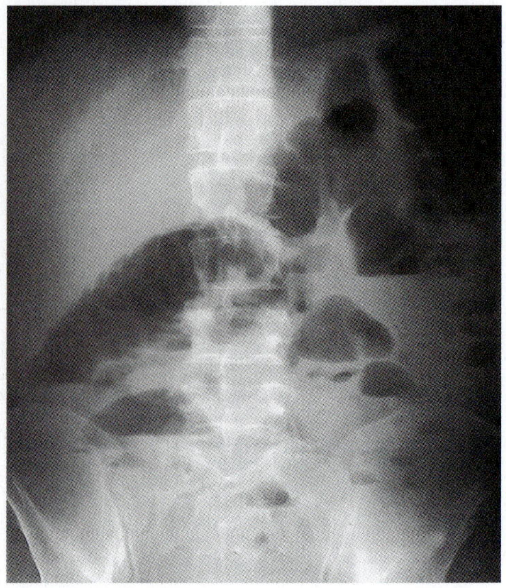
b

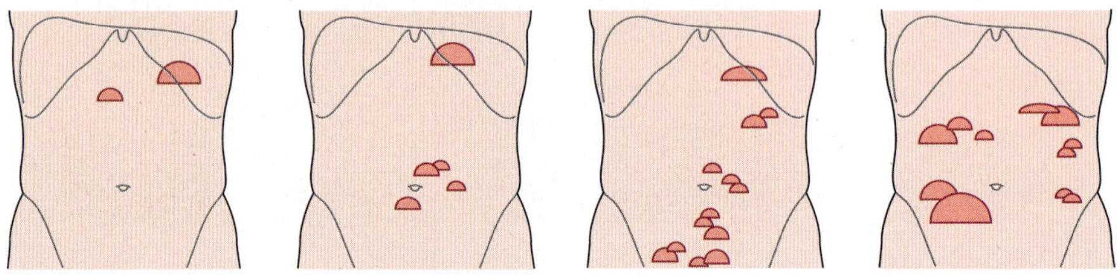
c I II III IV

B Double-contrast radiograph of the small intestine
Double-contrast radiograph of the small intestine in the anteroposterior projection (X-ray source in front of the patient, film-screen combination behind the patient). Anterior view (source: Universitätsmedizin Mainz; Klinik und Poliklinik für Diagnostische und Interventionelle Radiologie). In a double-contrast study, air is instilled into the bowel through a tube and a radiopaque liquid contrast medium (barium sulfate) is administered to provide an exceptionally high-contrast image. This technique guarantees high morphological resolution and is sensitive in detecting mucosal changes. The image to the right illustrates a normal double-contrast study. The transversely oriented circular folds of the small intestine are defined with great clarity.

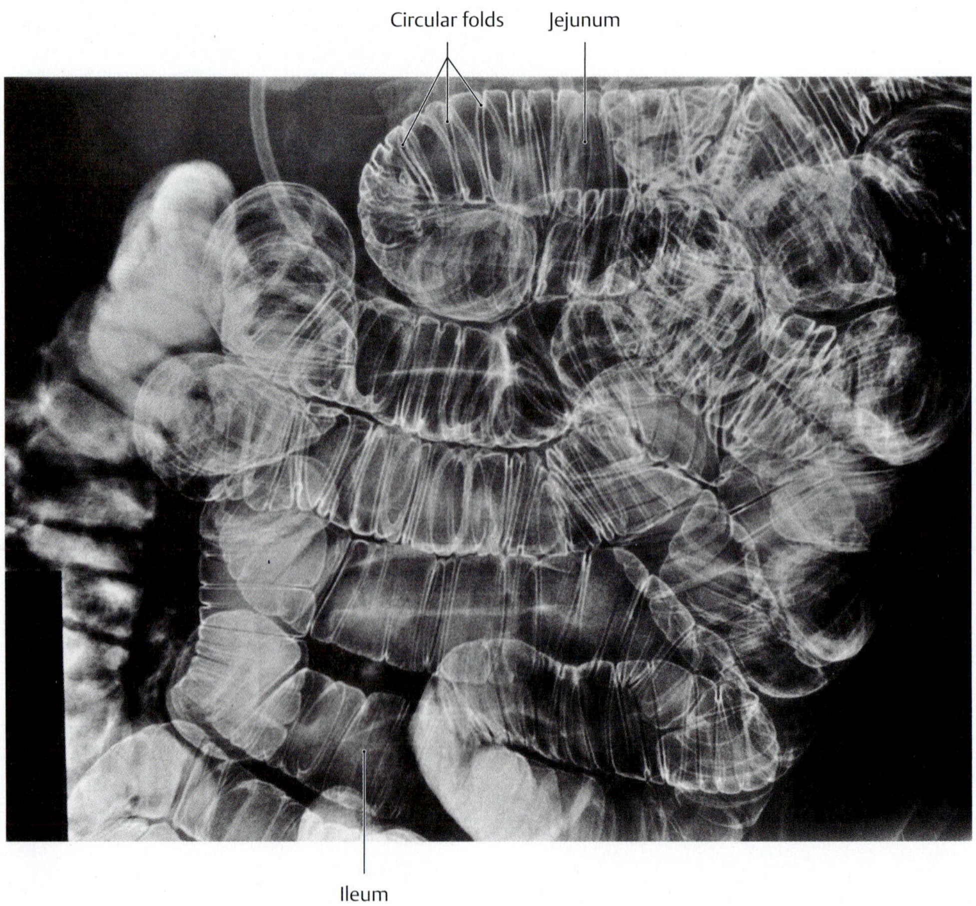

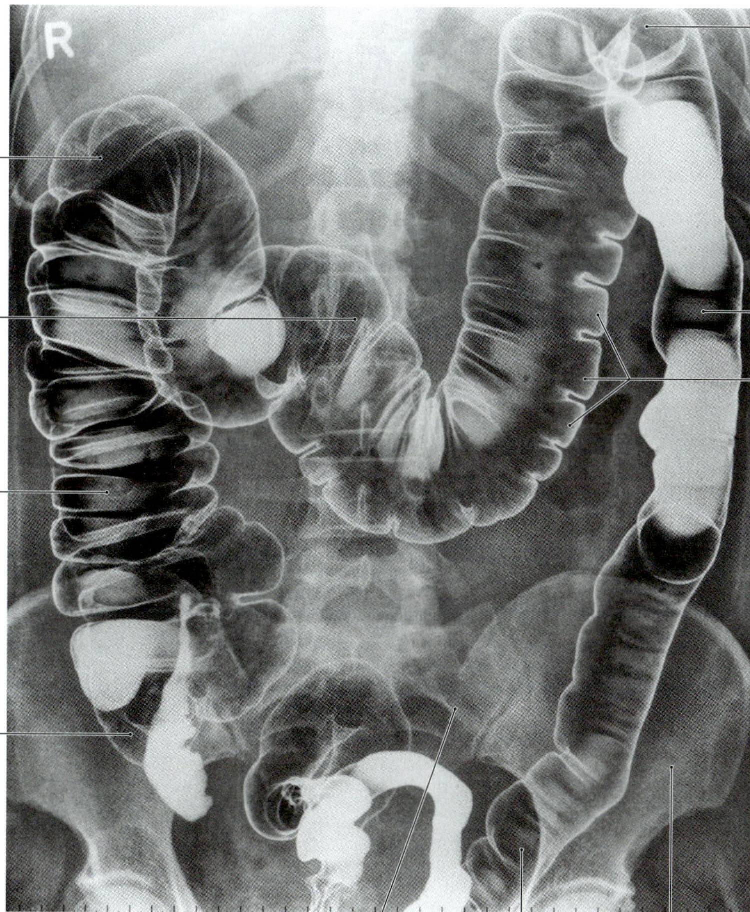

a

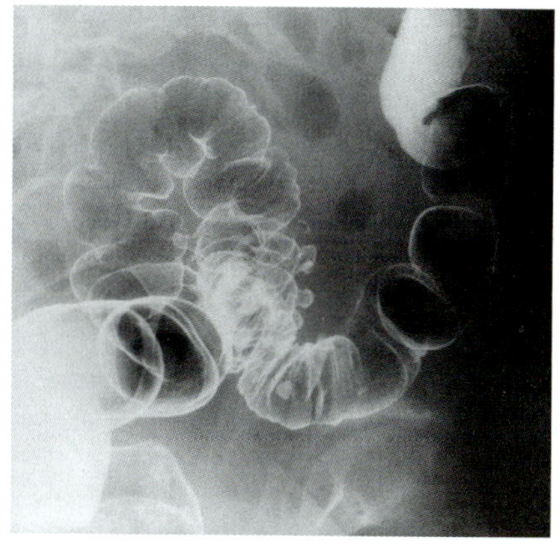

b

C Radiographic appearance of the large intestine

AP double-contrast radiograph of the large intestine (anterior view); **a** Normal findings (source: Universitätsmedizin Mainz; Klinik und Poliklinik für Diagnostische und Interventionelle Radiologie); **b** Multiple sites of outpouching in sigmoid diverticulosis (source: Reiser M, Kuhn F, Debus J, eds. 3rd ed. Stuttgart: Thieme; 2011). In **a** the individual segments of the colon with the haustra are clearly visible. The radiopaque contrast agent has not spread entirely uniformly; whitish areas of low transparency and of various sizes indicate accumulations of contrast agent.

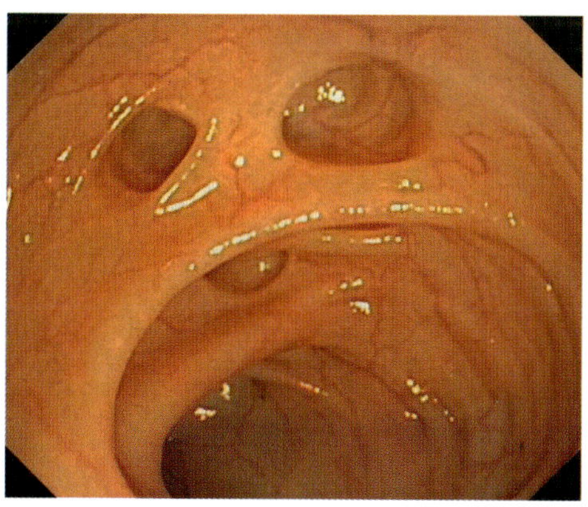

a

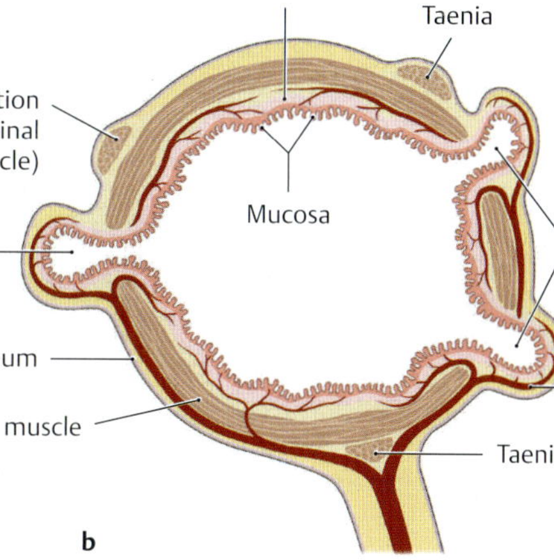

b

D Colonic diverticula

a Colonoscopic view of several diverticula at the right colic flexure (source: Messmann H, editor. *Lehratlas der Koloskopie.* 2nd ed. Stuttgart: Thieme; 2014); **b** Schematic cross section of the colon showing the location of the diverticula at the sites where the vasa recti pass through the ring musculature.

Viewed on colonoscopy, colonic diverticula are sacciform, serosa-covered sites of outpouching in the wall of the colon (**a**). These are usually pseudodiverticula, i. e., not all layers of the wall of the colon are involved in the outpouching rather only the mucosa and submucosa (**b**). Diverticula usually occur at preexisting weak points in the intestinal wall, that is where the intramural vessels, the vasa recta, are located (see **b**). The most common location is the sigmoid colon, accounting for nearly 90% of all cases. In Germany nearly one-third of all people over age 65 have diverticula and 80% of them are asymptomatic (= **diverticulosis**). Twenty percent of people with diverticula develop symptoms such as pain or diarrhea (= **diverticular disease**). Inflammation of the diverticula (= **diverticulitis**) can lead to severe complications such as abscess or fistula formation, diverticular bleeding, perforation of the diverticulum, and constriction of the intestinal wall. Pathogenetic factors include such things as advanced age, genetic predisposition (hereditary connective tissue disease), and a low-fiber diet with high meat consumption. Neuromuscular changes in the intestinal wall that may possibly lead to disturbances in intestinal motility have also been discussed. The precise diagnosis of diverticulitis is made by clinical examination with imaging modalities, ideally colon ultrasound and computed tomography (see p. 398).

6.12 Diagnostic Imaging of the Small and Large Intestine: Intestinal Ultrasound, Computed Tomography, and MR Enterography

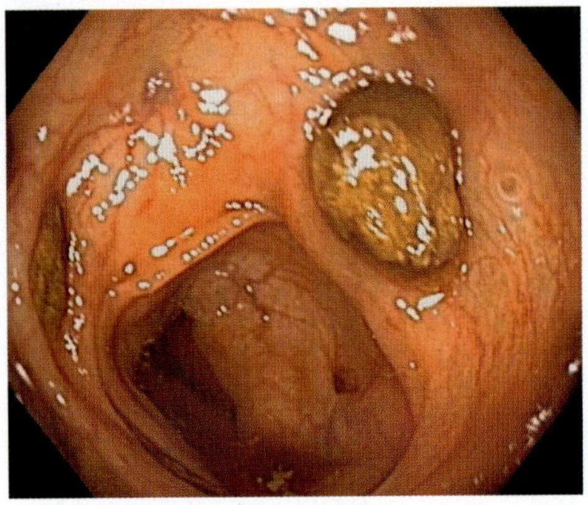

a

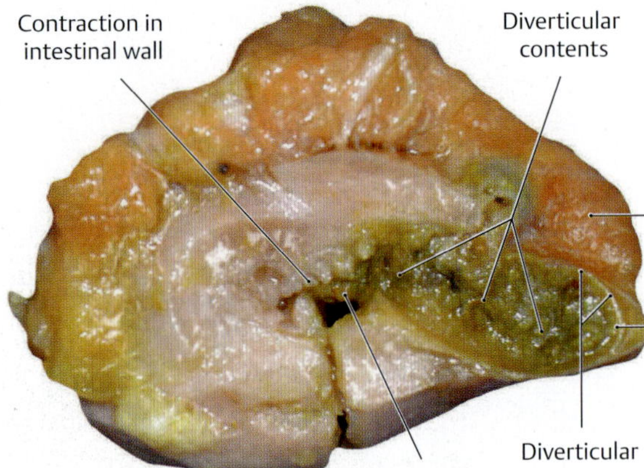

b

A Colonoscopic macropathologic findings of stool-filled diverticula of the intestinal wall

a Residual stool in a diverticulum of the intestinal wall can be identified by how it impairs visualization of the lumen of the diverticulum. Residual stool poses several different problems. It remains in the diverticulum because it often cannot empty through the narrow neck of the diverticulum. There it hardens and remains a constant source of pathogens. Together with the compression of vascular structures and especially the vasa recta (see p. 397) which can lead to ischemia, this increases the risk of bacterial inflammation of the diverticular mucosa. As the wall of the diverticulum is thin (only a mucosal layer, no muscular layer) and is covered at its apex only by serosa and epiploic fat (**b**), it is easily perforated, thus compromising the intestinal wall. Pathogens can then escape into the pericolic tissue and the abdominal cavity, leading to peritonitis and later sepsis as well (original images: **a** Messmann H, editor. *Lehratlas der Koloskopie*. 2nd ed. Stuttgart: Thieme; 2014; **b** Imke Weyers, M.D., Institut für Anatomie, Univerität Lübeck).

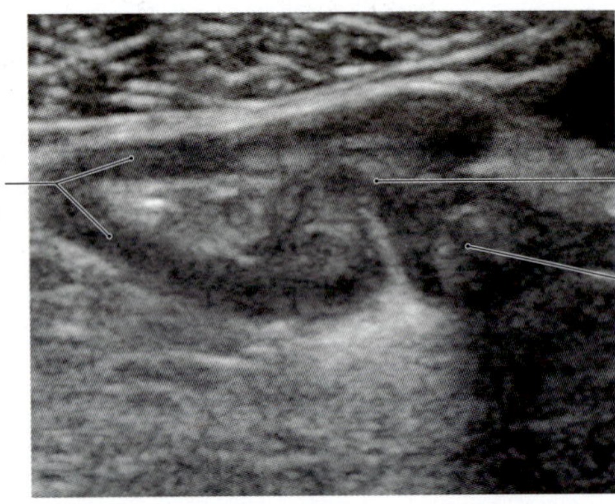

B Diverticulitis: sonographic findings of an inflamed diverticulum

Ultrasound is the imaging study of choice for evaluating acute diverticulitis. Colonoscopy would increase the risk of diverticular perforation, and ultrasound as a noninvasive modality is on the whole less of a burden on the patient. Additionally, intestinal ultrasound is particularly helpful in evaluating chronic inflammatory disorders as the inflammation leads to thickening of the intestinal wall which is well visualized on ultrasound images. The close proximity of the sigmoid colon and descending colon to the abdominal wall also facilitates the sonographic diagnosis (from: Seitz K, Braun B, editors. *Sonografie kompetent*. Stuttgart: Thieme; 2016).

Note the hypoechoic thickening of the wall indicative of hypertrophy of the circular muscle layer, the mucosa and submucosa protruding at the neck of the diverticulum, and the hardened fecal mass (fecalith) within the diverticular lumen.

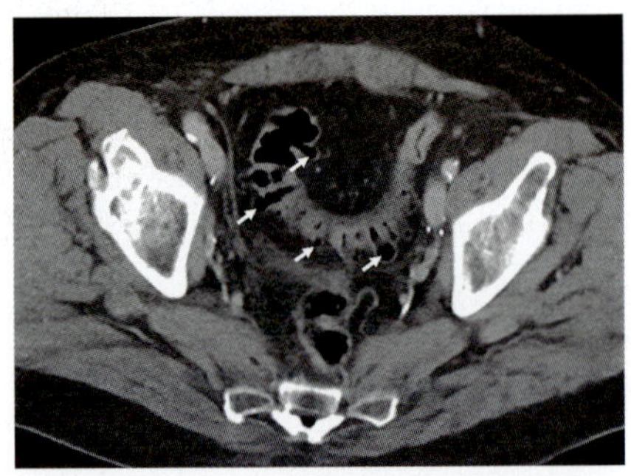

a

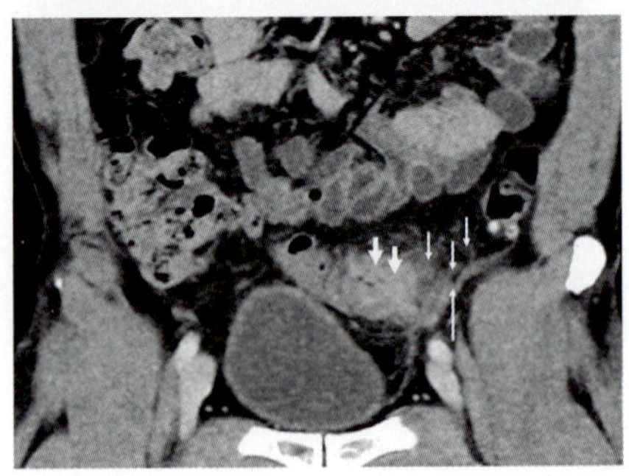

b

C Computed tomography in diverticulosis and diverticulitis in the sigmoid colon

a Diverticulosis (axial reconstruction); **b** Diverticulitis (coronal reconstruction). The CT examination is generally performed with the patient's rectum filled with contrast agent and where possible with additional intravenous contrast agent. In diverticulosis, the diverticula appear as small air-filled evaginations of the intestinal wall (arrows). Thickening of the intestinal wall with increased uptake of contrast agent (short thick arrows) and hyperemia with increased density of the pericolic fatty tissue (short thin arrows) are signs of diverticulitis. CT is superior to ultrasound in detecting complications such as a covered perforation or abscess (from: Reiser M, Kuhn F, Debus J, eds. *Duale Reihe Radiologie*. 4th ed. Stuttgart: Thieme; 2017).

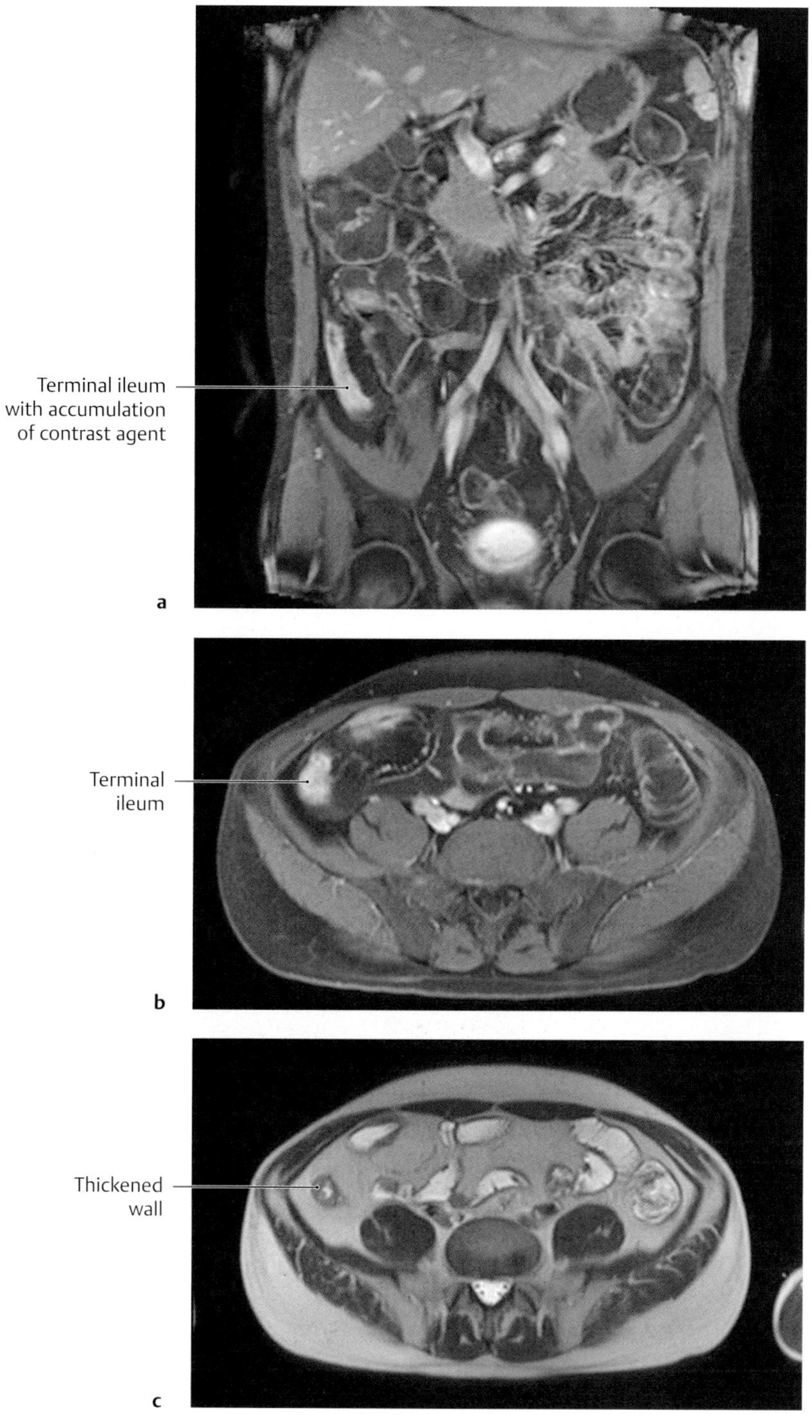

D MR Enterography in a patient with Crohn's disease

a T1-weighted, fat-saturated coronal MR image; **b** T1-weighted, fat-saturated axial image; **c** T2-weighted axial image. On T1-weighted MR images fatty tissue is hyperintense, that is bright. The fat saturation technique masks it. This makes it easier to see the structures of interest, here in Crohn's disease the small intestine. On both T1-weighted images a large volume of contrast agent is seen to have accumulated in the terminal ileum. This suggests inflammation of this segment of the intestine. On the T2-weighted image, fluid appears hyperintense, that is bright. This means that the edematous thickening of the intestinal wall due to inflammation in the affected segment is particularly well visualized.

MR enterography is primarily suitable for diagnosing chronic inflammatory intestinal disorders (such as Crohn's disease located primarily in the small intestine and ulcerative colitis located primarily in the large intestine, see **E**). The modality produces no ionizing radiation and the contrast agent and a preparation to dilate the intestine are administered orally. This means that patients better tolerate the frequent follow-up examinations required in chronic disorders. Diagnosable disorders include primarily early mucosal changes and signs of inflammation (shown here) and, in the chronic stage, fibrotic stenosis as well as rare neoplasms of the small intestine. (aus: Referenz Gastroenterologie. Riemann J, Fischbach W, Galle P et al., Hrsg. Stuttgart: Thieme; 2019).

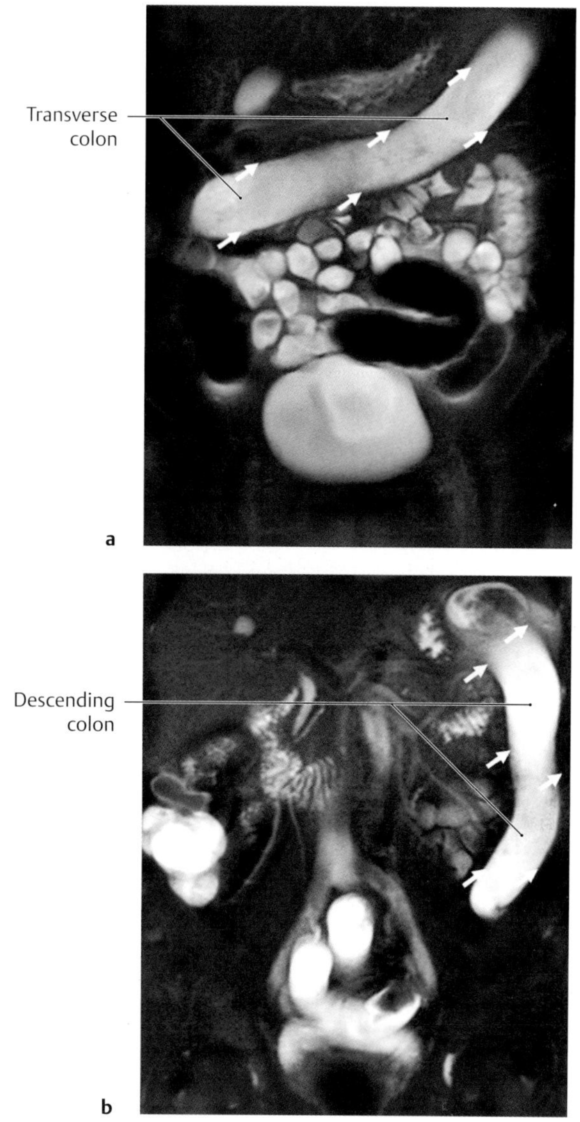

E MR Enterography in a patient with chronic ulcerative colitis

Coronal T1-weighted MR images in various planes: **a** At the level of the transverse colon; **b** At the level of the descending colon (from: Reiser M, Kuhn F, *Debus J, eds. Duale Reihe Radiologie.* 4th ed. Stuttgart: Thieme; 2017). Both segments of the colon show increased uptake of contrast agent and a smoothly demarcated wall structure (white arrows). In the chronic stage as in this example, this structure is particularly prominent and resembles the inner tube of a bicycle tire. The smooth wall is the result of loss of haustration that occurs in ulcerative colitis (fibrosis of the intestinal wall due to inflammation with resulting retraction). The mucosa and submucosa exhibit inflammatory changes. Ulcerative colitis begins in early adulthood, usually in the rectum, and continuously expands proximally. The course of the disease is chronic and generally episodic; its etiology is unclear. Initial symptoms include abdominal pain and bloody mucoid diarrhea. The risk of developing colonic carcinoma is increased (from: Riemann J, Fischbach W, Galle P et al., eds. *Referenz Gastroenterologie.* Stuttgart: Thieme; 2019).

6.13 Topography of the Rectum

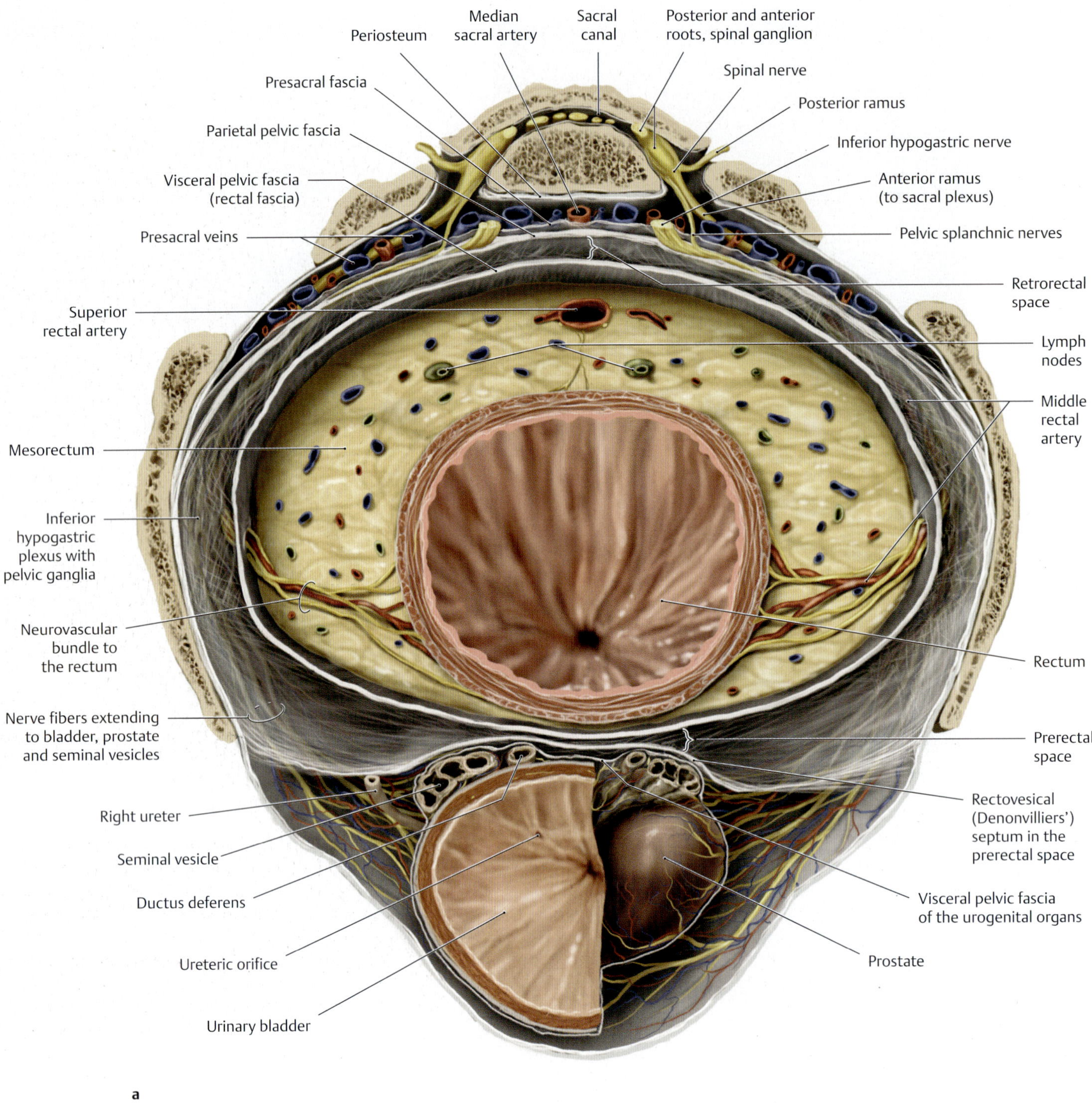

A Perirectal area with mesorectal fascial envelope
(with the collaboration of Wedel and Stelzner)
Male pelvis; **a** Transverse section at the level of the lower third of the bladder, viewed from above; **b** Midsagittal section, viewed from the left side; **c** Schematic representation of the perirectal region (transverse section, viewed from above).

Continence-maintaining operations, for example, total mesorectal excision (TME), play an increasingly important role in rectal cancer surgery (see p. 267). Of particular significance for the surgical treatment of rectal carcinoma are the mesorectal fascial envelopes, which divide the perirectal area and protect the neurovascular structures supplying the rectum and other pelvic organs. These fascial envelopes are derived from the transversalis fascia that continues into the pelvis as the pelvic fascia. Its visceral layer covers the pelvic organs and its parietal layer covers the bony and muscular pelvic wall. At the sites where the organs are attached to the pelvic floor, the fascial layers merge. One important compartment is the mesorectum, consisting of perirectal connective tissue and fat (also known as the rectal adventitia). It contains the superior rectal vessels and the rectal lymphatic vessels and their lymph nodes. Thus, the mesorectum is an area where rectal cancer can typically spread. The visceral pelvic fascia, which surrounds the mesorectum (and is commonly known as rectal fascia) abuts anteriorly and posteriorly against avascular and nerve-free slit-like spaces (retrorectal and prerectal spaces). Opening of these spaces allows for a posterior and anterior mobilization of the rectum during the TME procedure (see p. 267). Further posteriorly lies the parietal pelvic fascia (also known

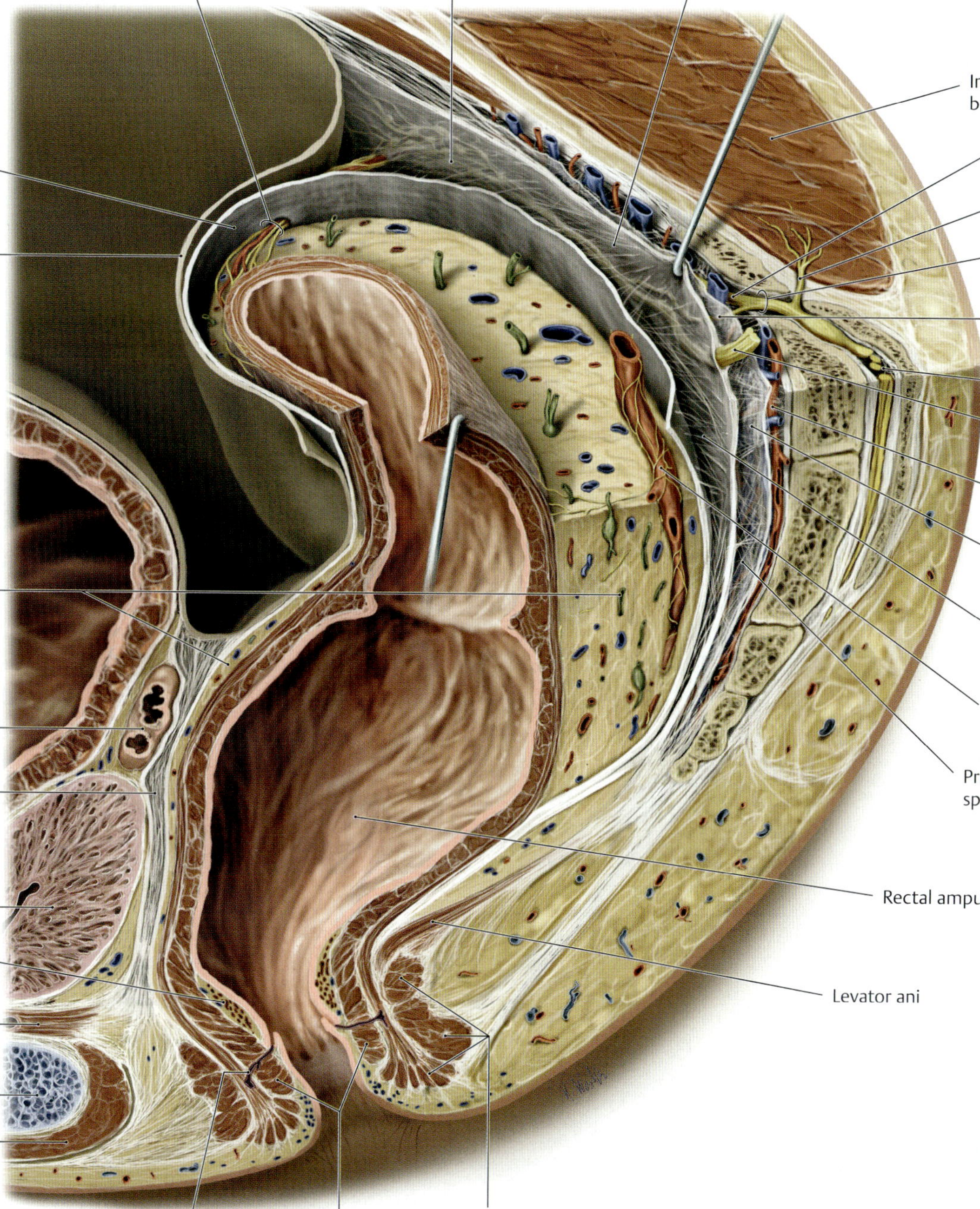

b

as Waldeyer's fascia). It encloses two bundles of sympathetic nerves (the left and right hypogastric nerves), which run laterally (see **c**). After receiving parasympathetic contributions from the pelvic splanchnic nerves, which arise from sacral spinal nerves in the area of the pararectal fascia, the hypogastric nerves together with the middle rectal artery approach the lateral wall of the rectum. Prominent venous plexuses (presacral veins) run between the parietal pelvic fascia and sacral periosteum in the presacral space. Anteriorly, the mesorectum is bounded by the rectovesical (Denonvilliers') septum of the urogenital organs, which particularly in males consists of a distinct plate of connective tissue at the level of the prostate and the seminal vesicles.

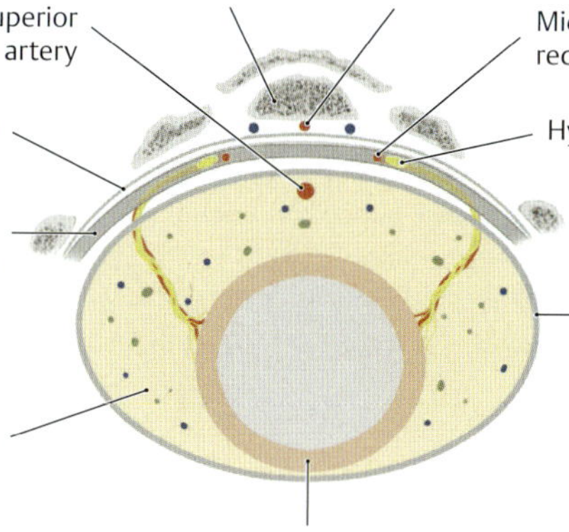

c

6.14 Retroperitoneum: Overview and Divisions

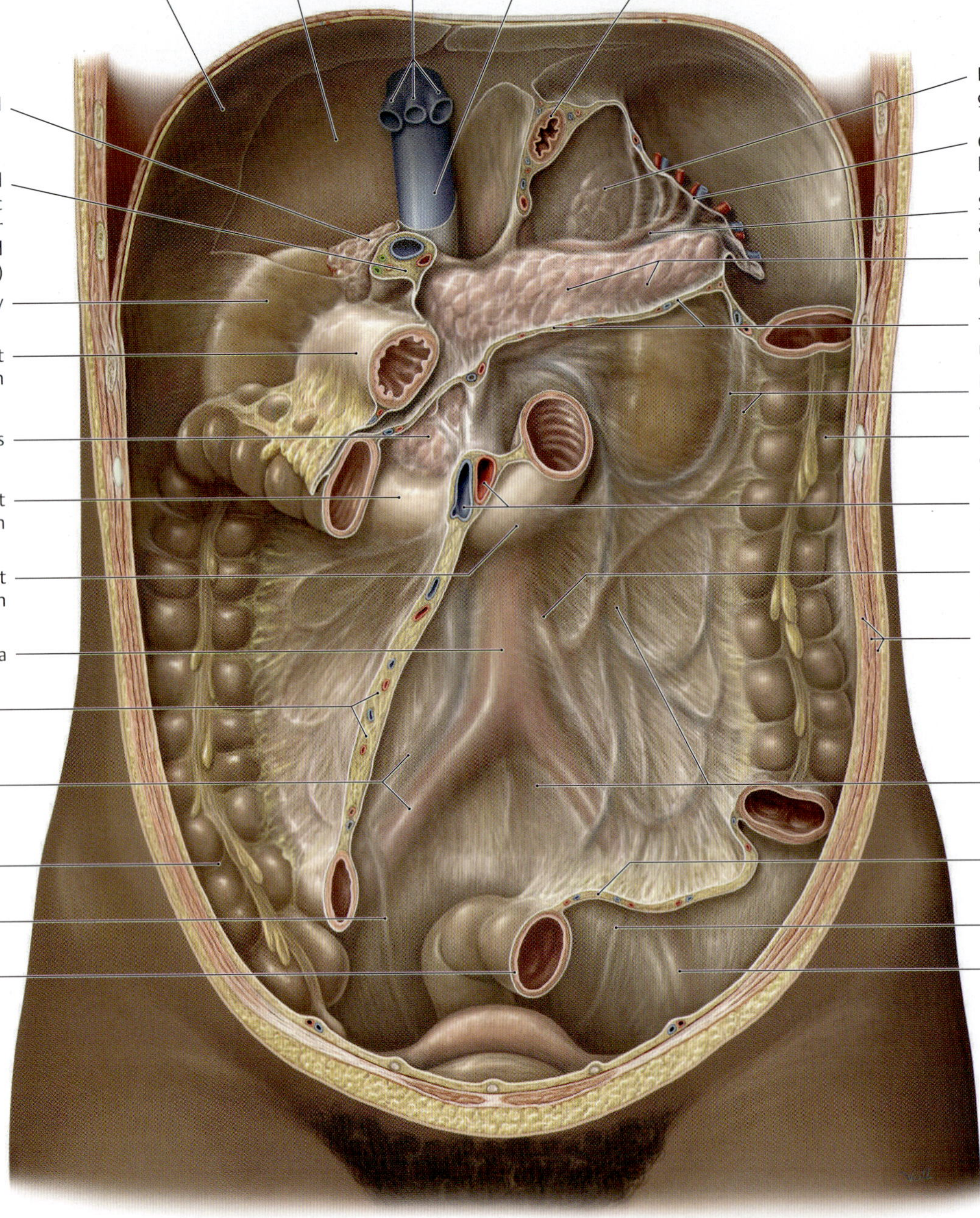

A Overview of the retroperitoneum

Anterior view of a female abdomen and pelvis. Most of the stomach, spleen, small intestine, transverse colon, and sigmoid colon (intraperitoneal organs) have been removed. The stump of the esophagus at the cardiac orifice is visible to provide an anatomical landmark.

Note: Some of the retroperitoneal organs are fully integrated in that space, having formed in the retroperitoneum: the kidneys, suprarenal glands, great vessels, and nerves. Other structures form in the peritoneal cavity and migrate to the retroperitoneum secondarily (the pancreas and duodenum, see **B**). Their visceral peritoneum becomes fused to the parietal peritoneum of the posterior wall, and they retain a peritoneal covering on their anterior surface. The primary retroperitoneal organs do not have a peritoneal covering because they are fully integrated into the retroperitoneal connective tissue.

B Organs and neurovascular structures in the retroperitoneum

Organs	Vessels	Nerves
Primarily retroperitoneal (or extraperitoneal): • Right and left kidneys • Right and left suprarenal glands • Right and left ureters *Secondarily retroperitoneal:* • Pancreas • Duodenum: descending and horizontal parts, some of the ascending part • Ascending and descending colon • Variable: portions of the cecum • Rectum to the sacral flexure	(all primarily retroperitoneal) • Aorta (abdominal part) and its branches • Inferior vena cava and its tributaries • Ascending lumbar veins • Portal vein (before coursing in the hepatoduodenal ligament) and its tributaries • Lumbar, sacral, and iliac lymph nodes, lumbar trunks, cisterna chyli	(all primarily retroperitoneal) • Branches of the lumbar plexus (iliohypogastric, ilioinguinal, genitofemoral, lateral femoral cutaneous, femoral, and obturator nerves) • Sympathetic trunk • Autonomic ganglia and plexuses

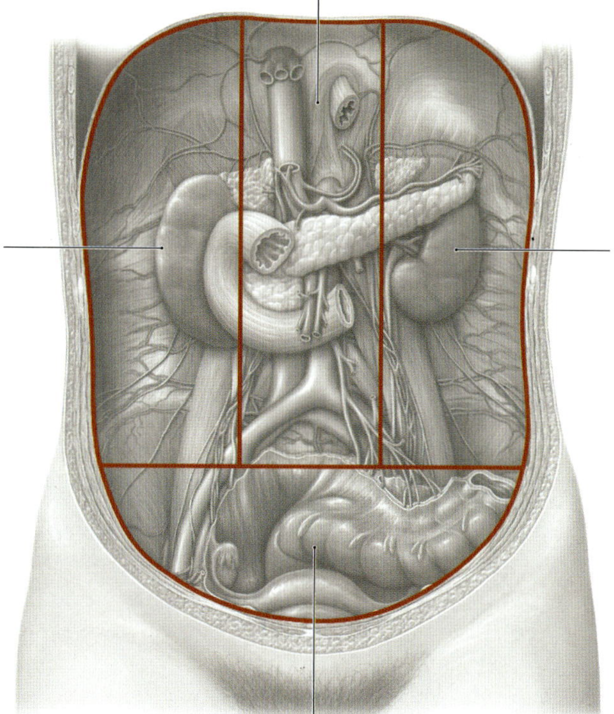

C Zones of the retroperitoneum
The retroperitoneum, like other body cavities, can be divided into zones based on clinical criteria. This type of classification is useful for evaluating what organs may be jointly affected by disease or injury due to their proximity to each other, even if they belong to entirely different functional systems. The retroperitoneum is divided into three zones:

Zone 1: central retroperitoneum with the duodenum and great vessels
Zone 2: left and right flank regions with the kidneys, ureters, ascending colon, and descending colon (omitted here to give a clearer view of the other organs)
Zone 3: pelvic region (corresponding to the hypogastrium) with the bladder, distal ureters, rectum, and internal genitalia

6.15 Retroperitoneum: Peritoneal Relationships

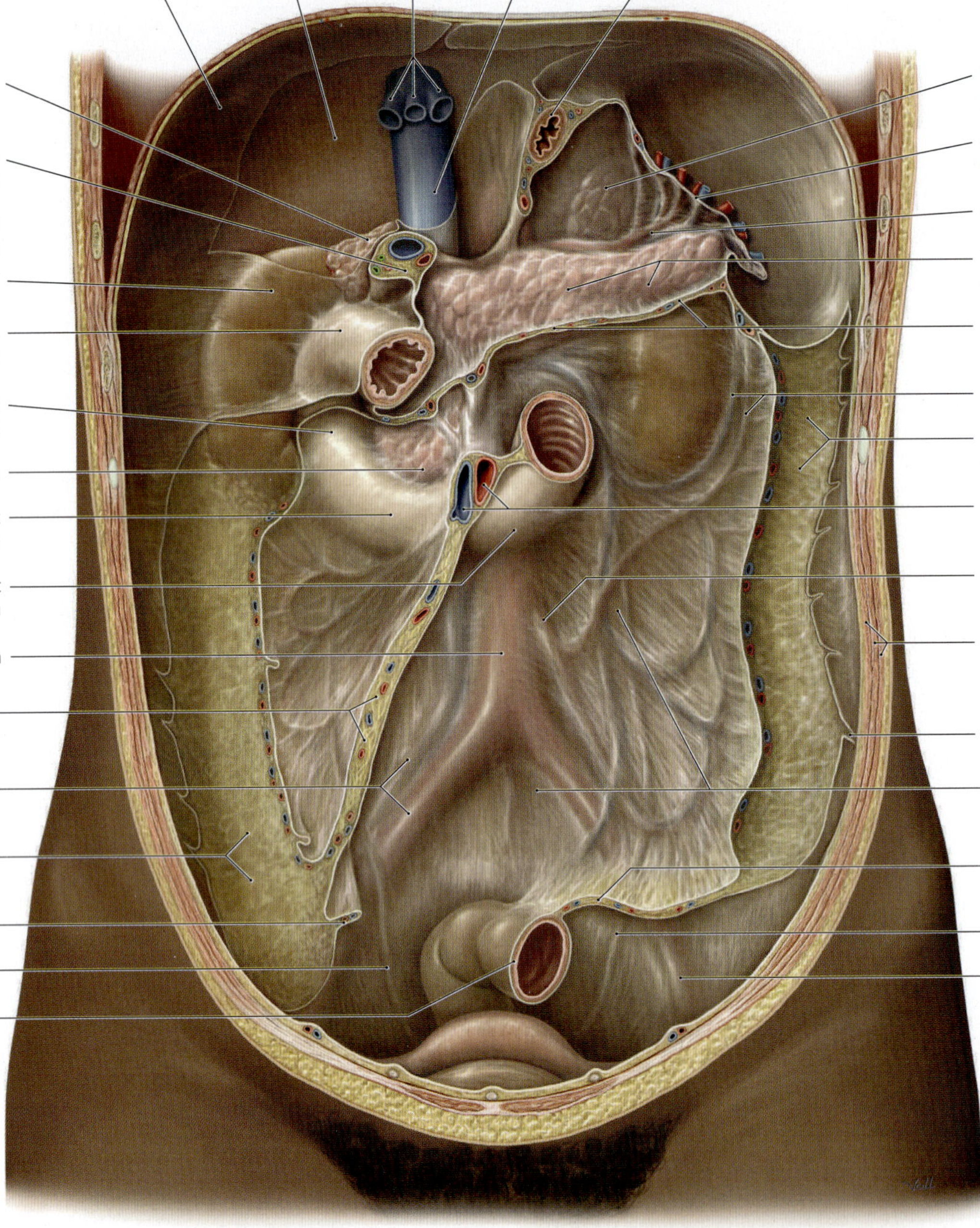

A Peritoneal relationships on the posterior wall of the peritoneal cavity

Anterior view of the opened thorax and abdomen. All of the intraperitoneal organs have been removed to display the retroperitoneum (retroperitoneal space). The posterior wall of the peritoneal cavity also forms the anterior wall of the retroperitoneum. Unlike the anterior wall of the peritoneal cavity, which consists largely of muscles and fasciae, much of the posterior wall is formed by the organs in the retroperitoneum, which are visible through the parietal peritoneum in this dissection. For clarity, the retroperitoneal connective tissue and fat have been thinned out to display the course of the retroperitoneal vessels and the ureter (where it crosses in front of the iliac vessels) (see **C**). The hepatic surface of the diaphragm is devoid of peritoneum and corresponds to the bare area of the liver. The ascending and descending colon (removed here for clarity) are attached by connective tissue to the posterior wall of the peritoneal cavity, so they are also located in the retroperitoneum (see p. 402). In this specimen, the area of attachment of the ascending colon extends further inferiorly to the pelvis than usual. The transverse mesocolon, like the transverse colon, is located anterior to the duodenum (i.e., is intraperitoneal). The migration of these organs during embryonic development is described on p. 42f. The sigmoid mesocolon crosses anterior to the left iliac vessels and left ureter.

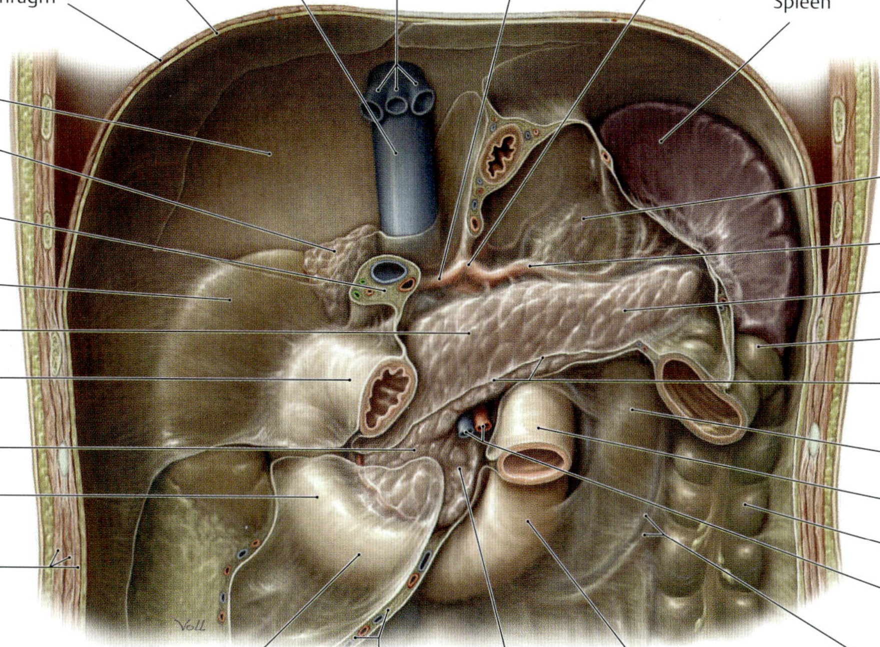

B Retroperitoneum
Anterior view. All intraperitoneal organs have been removed except for the spleen and a short stump of the jejunum (both of which have been left in place to aid orientation). The retroperitoneal ascending colon has also been removed; and to better display the kidneys, the retroperitoneal connective tissue is only hinted at.
The retroperitoneal organs "shine" through the peritoneum. The root of the transverse mesocolon crosses over the right kidney, duodenum and pancreas. From a superior to inferior direction, the root of the mesentery crosses the head of the pancreas. During retroperitonealization, the descending colon migrates so far to the posterior body wall, that it comes to lie almost in a coronal plane with the left kidney. The intraperitoneal spleen lies in its own small compartment located in the upper quadrant in close vicinity to the tail of the pancreas, descending colon, and left kidney. However, the spleen is separated from these organs by the peritoneal cavity.

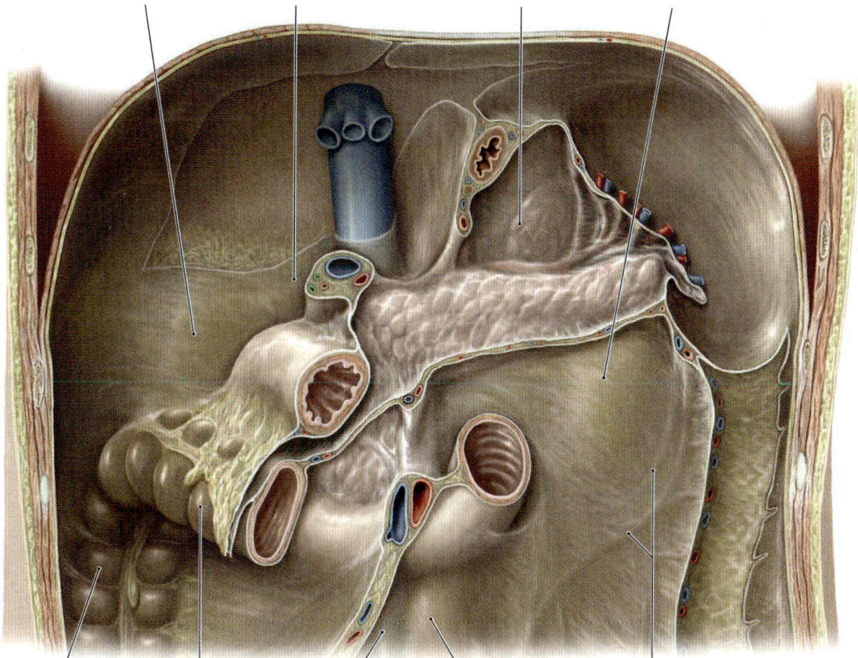

C Transperitoneal view of the retroperitoneum
Anterior view. The intraperitoneal organs have been removed except a small part of the transverse colon. The retroperitoneal descending colon has also been removed. The connective tissue and fat in the retroperitoneum are of normal volume in this dissection. The kidneys form in the retroperitoneum during embryonic development and are embedded in the retroperitoneal fat and connective tissue. Thus the kidneys, like the great vessels, are obscured by the anterior wall of the retroperitoneum and are visible only as bulges behind the parietal peritoneum. Additionally, the anterior layer of the renal fascia is interposed between the kidneys and the parietal peritoneum (see p. 310). Because the pancreas is secondarily retroperitoneal, it is not fully integrated into the retroperitoneal fat and connective tissue. Being attached to the posterior wall of the peritoneal cavity "only" by fusion of the peritoneal layers, the pancreas can be seen with much greater clarity. Although its anterior surface is covered by peritoneum, that layer is more translucent than the retroperitoneal connective tissue and fat.

6.16 Retroperitoneum: Organs of the Retroperitoneum

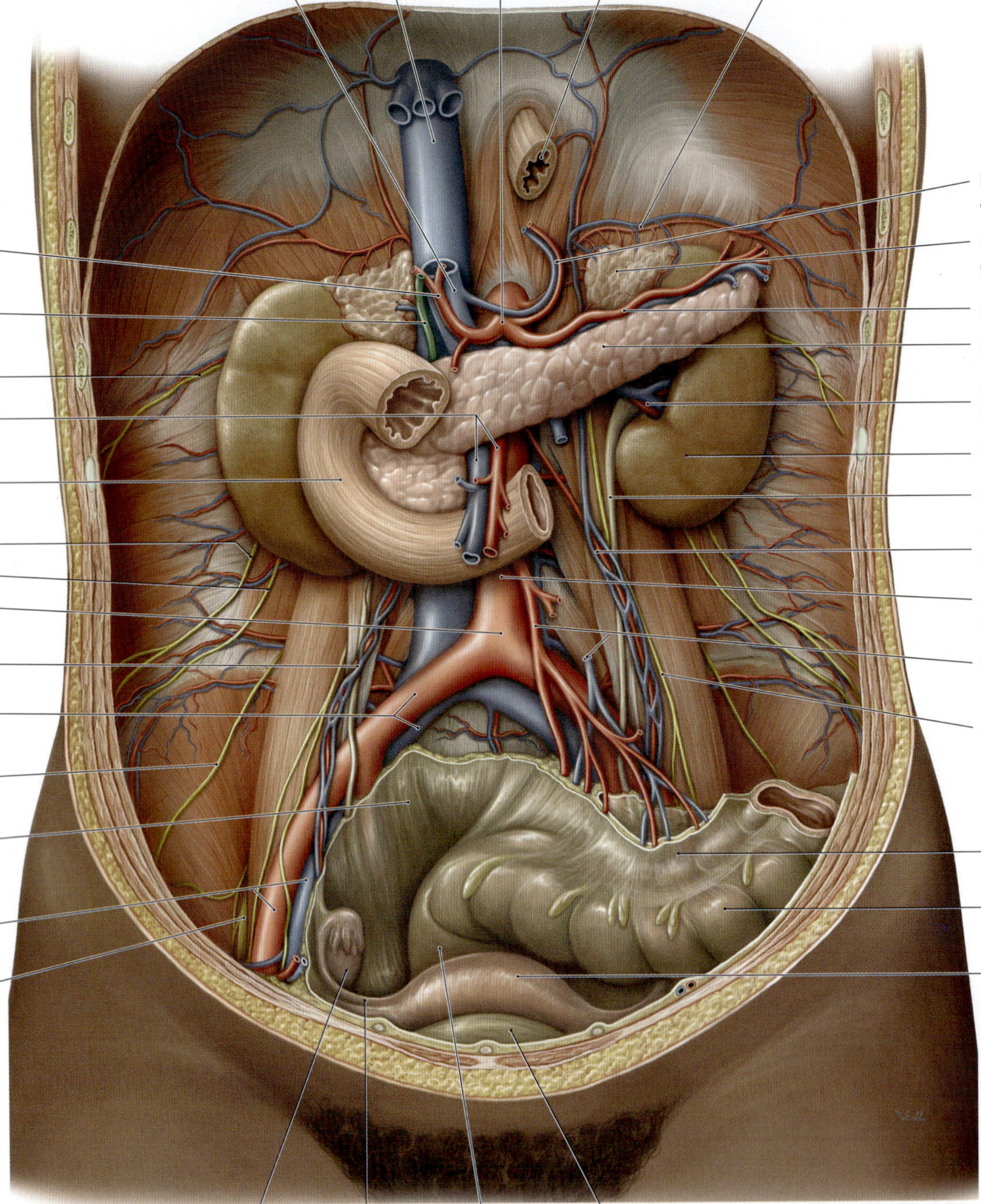

A Retroperitoneal organs, anterior view

Organs of the upper retroperitoneum, anterior view. Intraperitoneal organs except for the sigmoid colon have been removed; the uterus and adnexa as well as the subperitoneal bladder have been left in place to aid orientation. Retroperitoneal segments of the colon, parietal peritoneum, and retroperitoneal connective tissue have been completely removed; thus leaving peritoneum only in the area of the mentioned pelvic organs. The posterior wall of the abdominal cavity with its neurovascular structures is visible. The most dominant structures are the major retroperitoneal vascular trunks, the abdominal aorta and inferior vena cava, anterior or lateral to which the organs in the retroperitoneal space are located.

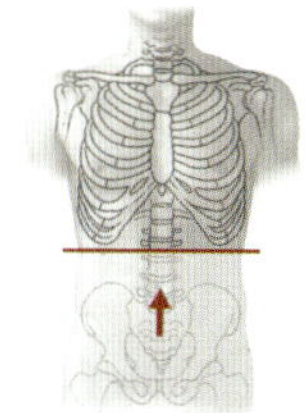

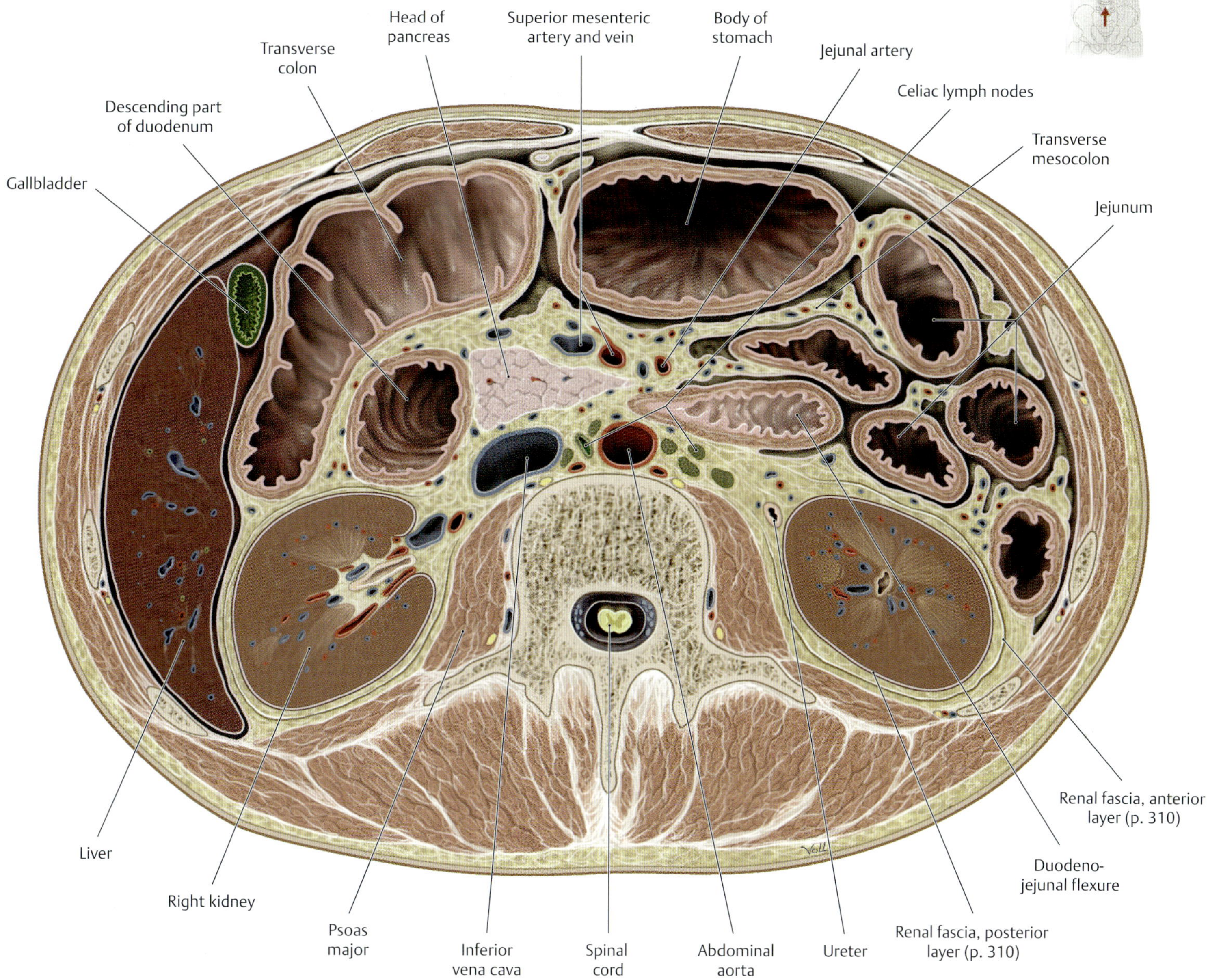

B Retroperitoneal organs in transverse section
Transverse section through the abdomen approximately at the L 1 level, inferior view.

This transverse section shows the relative positions of the organs in the retroperitoneal space from anterior to posterior:

- the duodenum with the head of the pancreas are located most anteriorly,
- the tail of the pancreas (not visible here because it is above the sectional plane) lies posterior to the head of the pancreas as the pancreas runs obliquely backward,
- the two kidneys are located most posteriorly.

Between the "duodenum–pancreas plane" and the plane of the kidneys lie the major retroperitoneal vascular trunks; the aorta is located anterior to the vertebral column and the inferior vena cava is situated anterior and slightly right of the vertebral column. It is clearly visible how the liver with the peritoneal cavity extends slightly behind the right kidney, and that the descending colon and left kidney lie almost in the same horizontal plane. It is clear how the kidneys are embedded in the retroperitoneal fat and connective tissue of the perirenal fat capsule.

6.17 Retroperitoneum: Location of the Kidneys

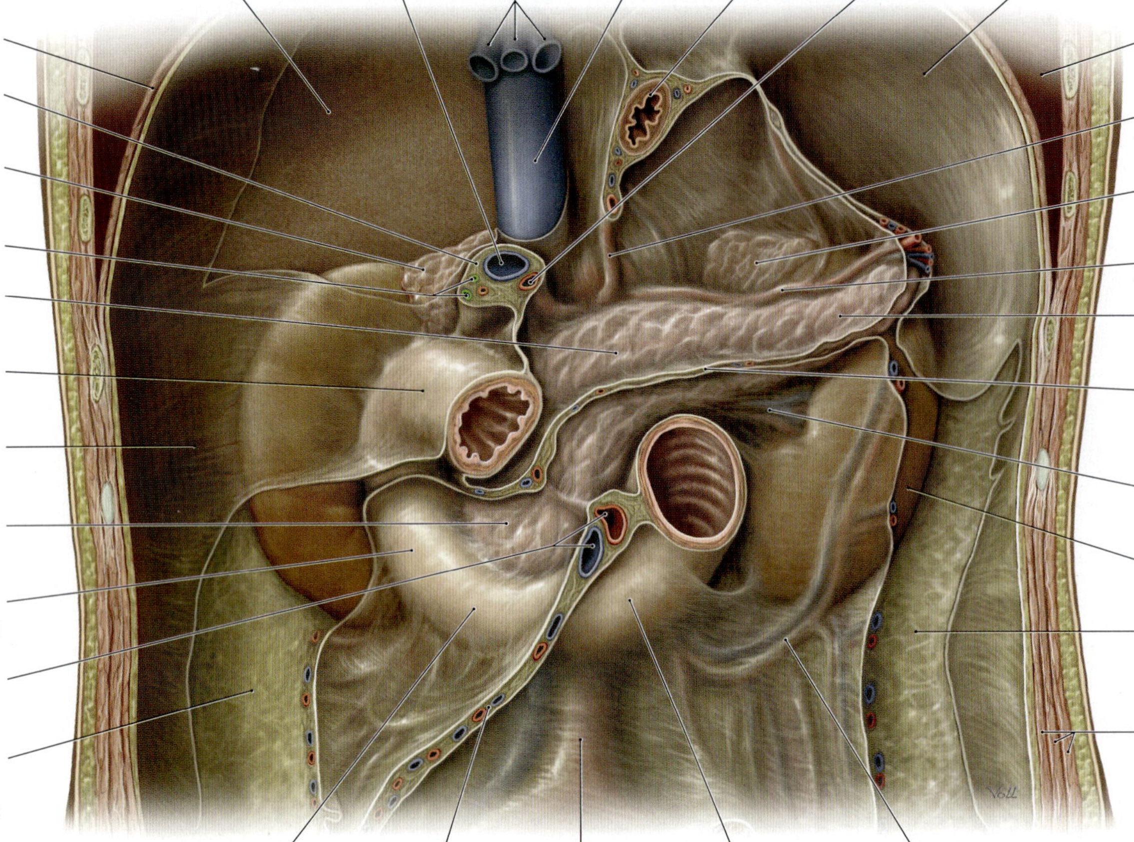

A Topographical relations of the kidneys in the retroperitoneum
Anterior view. All of the intraperitoneal organs and secondarily retroperitoneal portions of the colon (ascending and descending colon) have been removed, leaving the duodenum and pancreas in place. Most of the fat capsule anterior to the kidneys has also been removed. Both kidneys are overlapped by the attachments of the ascending and descending colon on the posterior wall of the peritoneal cavity and by the root of the transverse mesocolon. Because the pancreas, parts of the duodenum, and the left and right colic flexures are *secondarily* retroperitoneal, they are in close *proximity* to the primarily retroperitoneal kidneys but are still separated from them by the fat and connective tissue of the fat capsule (see **B**).

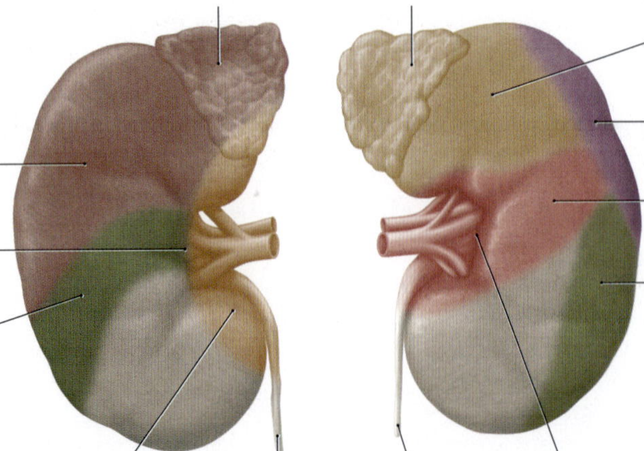

B Areas of renal contact with abdominal and pelvic organs
Anterior view. The suprarenal glands (also shown for clarity) are very close to the kidneys but do not touch them, being separated from the renal surface by the perirenal fat capsule. The *anterior surfaces* of the kidneys are related to numerous abdominal organs. The *retroperitoneal* organs are separated from the kidneys (also retroperitoneal) by the fasciae of the renal bed. The kidneys are additionally separated from the *intraperitoneal* organs by the peritoneum. As a result, surrounding organs do not form impressions on the kidneys, which are relatively firm and stable in their dimensions, and the areas of renal contact with other organs are important in terms of topographical anatomy but have little clinical importance.

C Proximity of the kidneys to the iliohypogastric and ilioinguinal nerves

a Neurovascular structures on the anterior side of the posterior trunk wall. Lumbar fossa on the right side after removal of the anterior and lateral trunk wall, all the fasciae, the peritoneum and the intra- and retroperitoneal organs except for the right kidney. The inferior vena cava has been partially removed. Anterior view.
b Posterior view of the right kidney. The renal fat capsule and parts of the posterior trunk wall have been removed.
c Skin areas supplied by the iliohypogastric and ilioinguinal nerves to which pain is referred.

After removal of trunk wall layers, the proximity of the kidneys to the iliohypogastric and ilioinguinal nerves can be seen. Both are branches of the lumbar plexus from T 12 and L 1, positioned lateral to the lumbar spine (see **a**). These nerves supply motor innervation to the muscles of the trunk wall and sensory innervation to skin areas on the lateral and anterior abdominal wall. If an abnormally enlarged kidney exerts pressure on the iliohypogastric and ilioinguinal nerves, pain is referred to the skin areas shown in **c**. The distance between the kidney and subcostal nerve is usually large enough so that it is not compressed by renal enlargement.

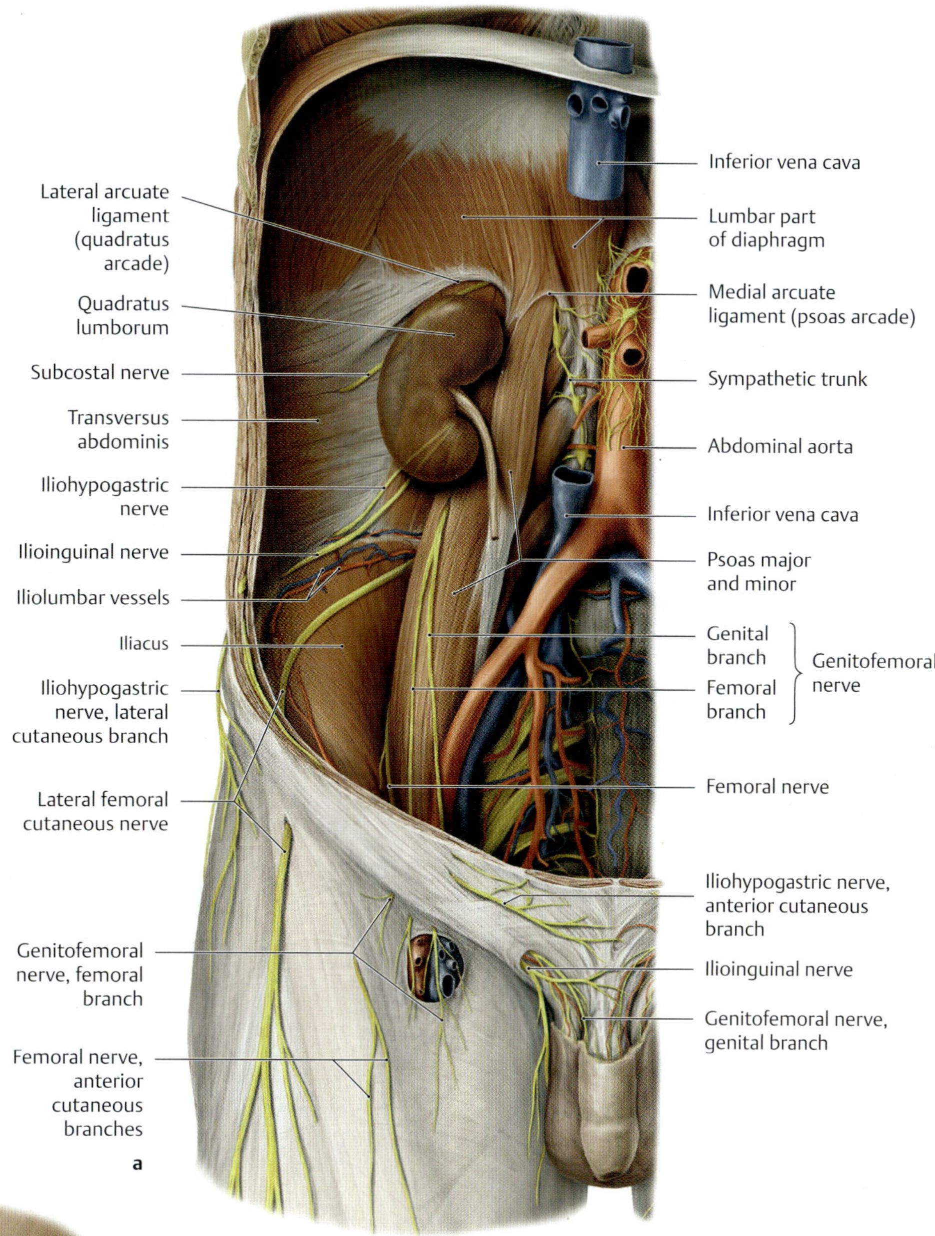

a

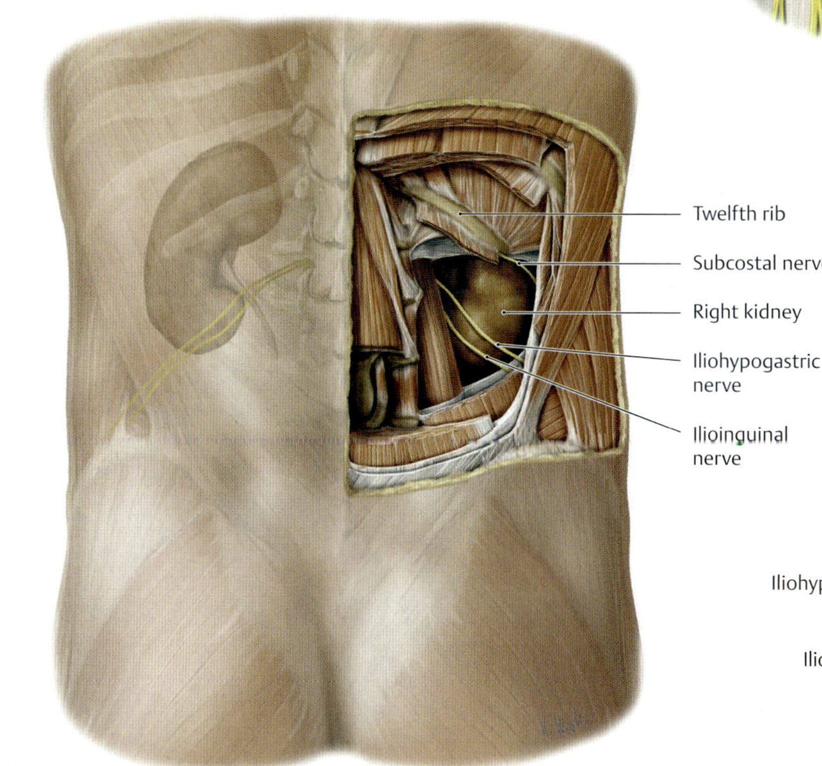

b

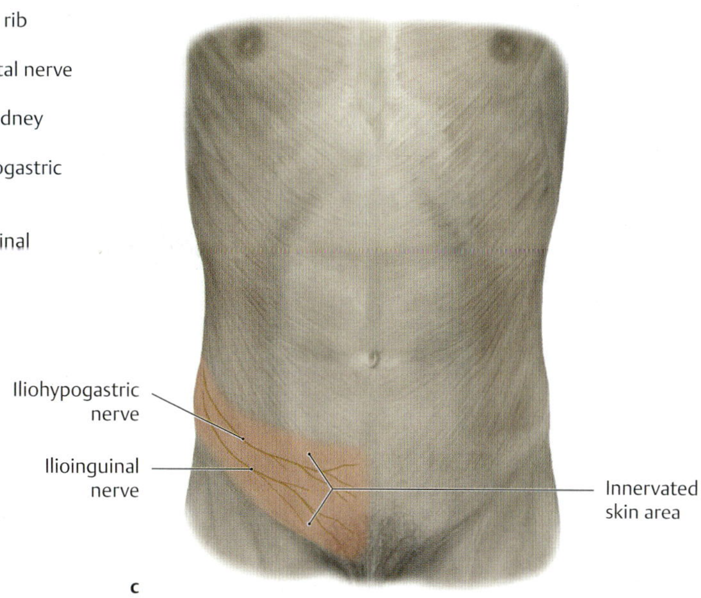

c

6.18 Peritoneal Relationships in the Anterior Abdominal Wall

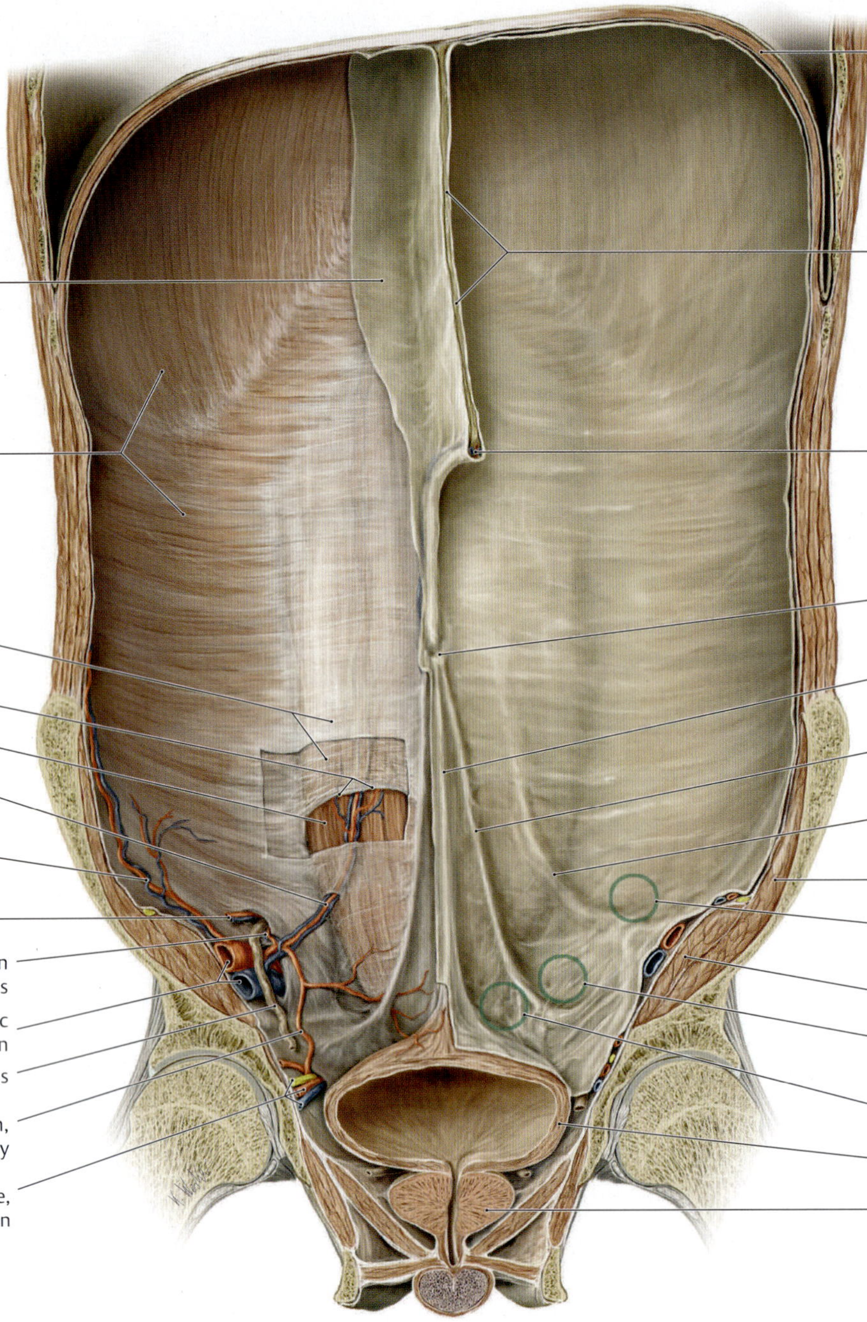

A Peritoneal relationships on the posterior surface of the abdominal wall

Posterior surface of the anterior abdominal wall, viewed from the posterior aspect. The peritoneum on the left side has been removed to display the contents of the peritoneal folds (umbilical folds). They are formed by the peritoneum that covers structures on the posterior surface of the anterior trunk wall. The parietal peritoneum lying between the folds raised by these structures forms shallow depressions called fossae.

Peritoneal folds (umbilical folds):

- One median umbilical fold: This is where the parietal peritoneum covers the median umbilical ligament, which is the obliterated urachus (remnant of the allantois that is obliterated during embryonic development).
  Note: Incomplete obliteration of the urachus may lead to umbilical fistulae in postnatal life.
- Two medial umbilical folds: sites where the parietal peritoneum covers the umbilical artery (the portion of the artery that becomes occluded at birth)
- Two lateral umbilical folds: sites where the parietal peritoneum covers the inferior epigastric artery and vein

Each of the *paired umbilical* arteries consists of a proximal patent part (which gives rise to the superior vesical artery and, in males, the branch to the ductus deferens) and a distal occluded part. The *unpaired umbilical vein* is usually obliterated to form the round ligament of the liver.

Peritoneal fossae:

- Two supravesical fossae
- Two medial inguinal fossae (posterior to the superficial inguinal ring)
- Two lateral inguinal fossae (in which the deep inguinal ring is located)

Note: The *deep inguinal ring* (internal inguinal ring) is a structural weak point in the abdominal wall which forms the entrance to the inguinal canal. This canal provides a path for the descent of the testis during normal development, but also creates a potential route for the herniation of abdominal viscera (indirect inguinal hernia) (see **B** and **C**).

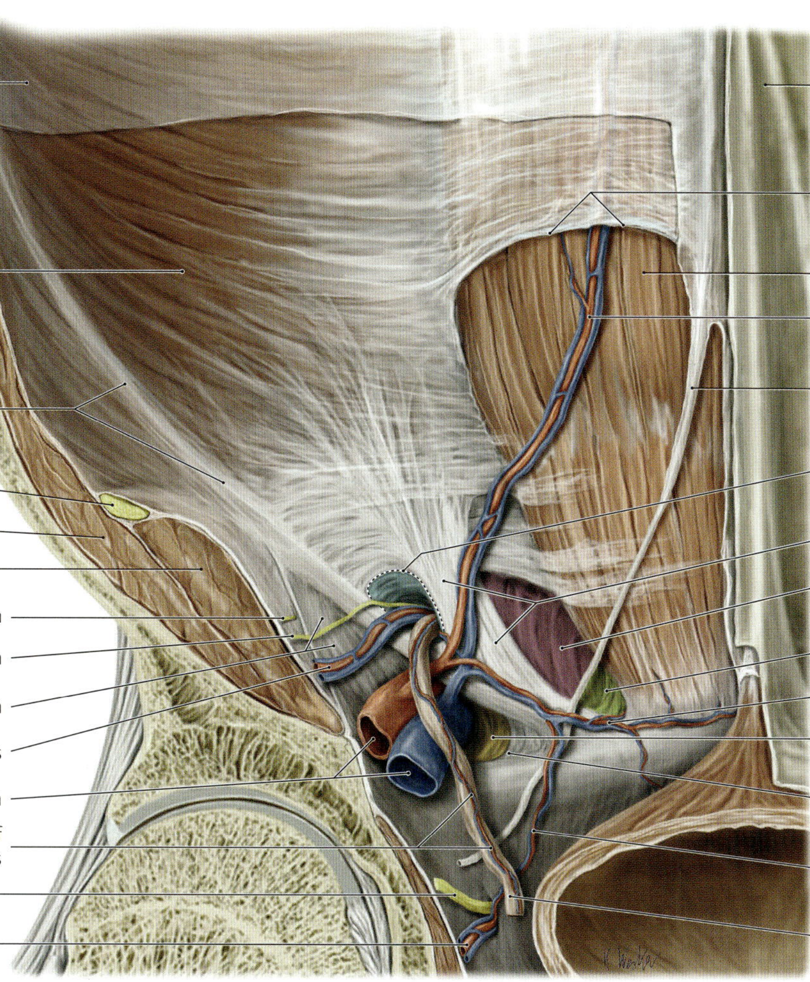

B Internal hernial openings in the male inguinal and femoral region

Detail from **A,** posterior view. For better exposure of the hernial openings, the peritoneum and transversalis fascia have been partially removed. The internal hernia openings (see **C**) for indirect and direct inguinal hernias, femoral hernias and suprapubic (supravesical) hernias are color-coded.

C Overview of internal and external openings of abdominal hernias

Above the inguinal ligament, the median, medial, and lateral umbilical folds (see **A**) form three weak spots on each side of the abdominal wall where indirect and direct inguinal hernias and suprapubic hernias typically occur. Another weak spot is located *below the inguinal ligament* and medial to the femoral vein in the vascular lacuna. There the femoral ring is covered only by compliant connective tissue, the femoral septum, which is permeated by numerous lymphatic vessels.

Internal opening	Hernia	External opening
Above the inguinal ligament:		
Supravesical fossa	Supravesical hernia	Superficial inguinal ring
Medial inguinal fossa (Hesselbach's triangle)	Direct inguinal hernia	Superficial inguinal ring
Lateral inguinal fossa (deep inguinal ring)	Indirect inguinal hernia	Superficial inguinal ring
Below the inguinal ligament:		
Femoral ring	Femoral hernia	Saphenous opening (fossa ovalis)

6.19 Peritoneal Relationships in the Lesser Pelvis

A Paramedian section through the lesser pelvis (= sectional plane slightly lateral from the midline)

a Female pelvis; **b** Male pelvis, both viewed from the right side.

Most of the connective tissue in the pelvic extraperitoneal space has been removed accounting for the apparently empty spaces between the organs. The bladder is well distended here so that the part of the bladder not covered by peritoneum is partially above the pubic symphysis (site of suprapubic bladder puncture).

Whereas the peritoneal cavity in the male is completely closed, in the female the abdominal end of the patent uterine tube creates a potential opening to the outside. The cervical mucus plug creates a germ-proof seal that protects the lesser pelvis from ascending infections.

The peritoneum forms pouches in the lesser pelvis of both males and females, the recto*uterine* pouch (between the uterus and rectum) in the female and the recto*vesical* pouch (deepest part in the pelvis between the bladder and rectum) in the male. Their specific shape depends on the degree of distention of the uterus and rectum or bladder and rectum. Generally, the rectouterine pouch is deep and the rectovesical pouch is shallow. The rectouterine pouch (pouch of Douglas) is the deepest point in the female peritoneal cavity (see **B**). This space is clinically significant because it can be accessed for puncture or ultrasound procedures by going through the vagina.

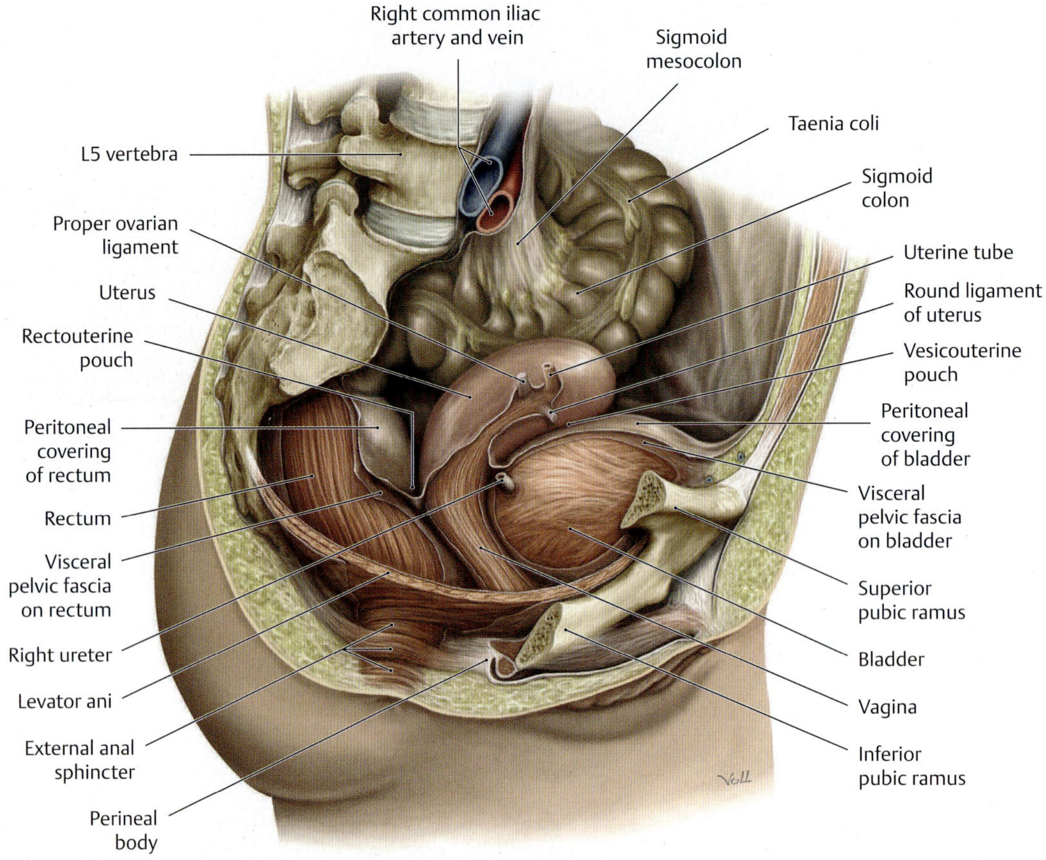

a

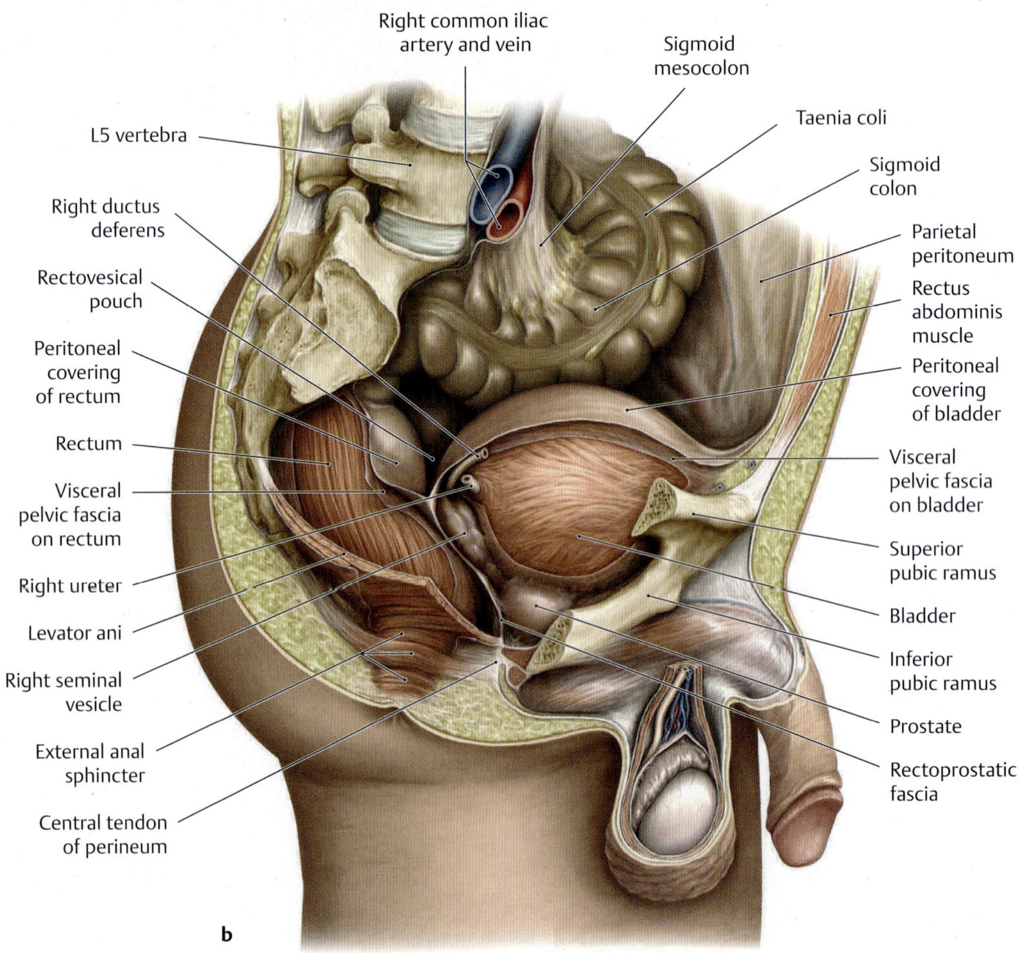

b

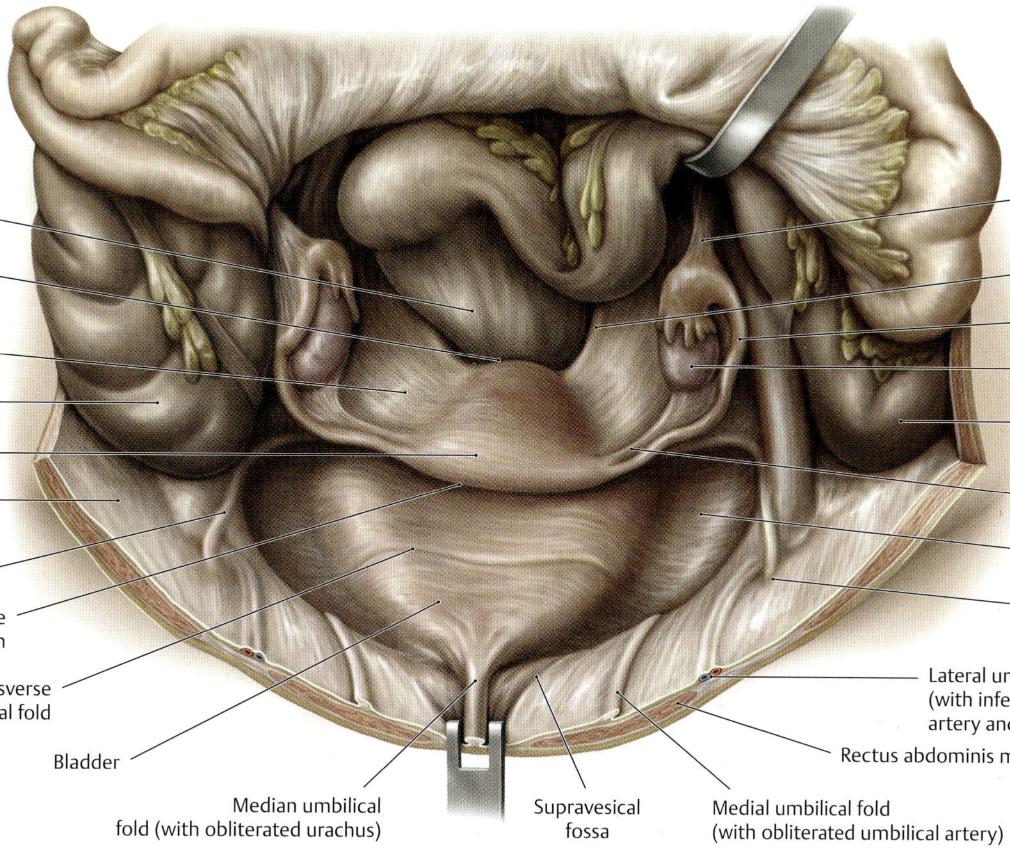

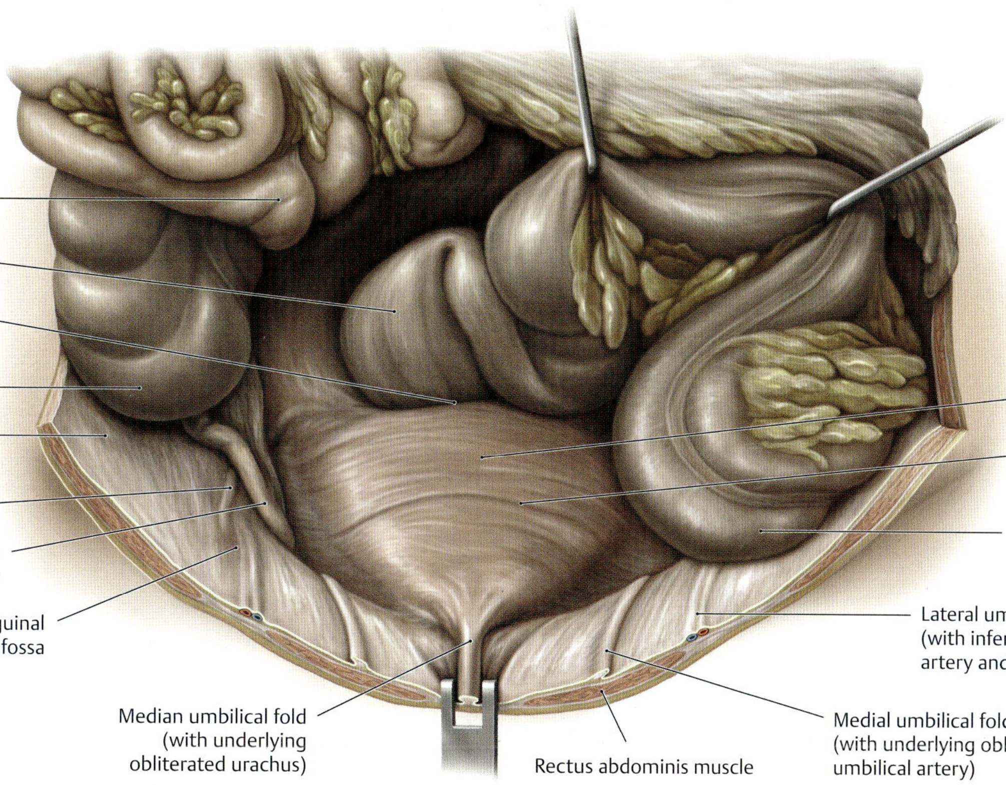

B Lesser pelvis, anterosuperior view

a Female pelvis, **b** Male pelvis. Loops of the small intestine and parts of the large intestine have been retracted laterally to show the bladder and rectum.

The parietal peritoneum is reflected onto the surface of the bladder and then continues onto the anterior wall of the rectum, or in the female to the uterus and the anterior wall of the rectum (the upper part of which is covered by peritoneum). The posterior wall of the bladder and lower parts of the rectum are not covered by peritoneum.

Note: On the surface of the relatively empty bladder, as shown here, the peritoneum forms a transverse crease called the transverse vesical fold. It disappears when the bladder is full. For the umbilical folds see p. 410. In the female, the peritoneum covers most of the uterus and parametrial connective tissue (parametrium) except for the uterine cervix, not visible here. As intraperitoneal organs, the ovaries and uterine tubes are covered by peritoneum. In the male, the peritoneum also covers the ductus deferens, which passes through the anterior wall via the inguinal canal.

6.20 Topography of Pelvic Connective Tissue, Levels of the Pelvic Cavity, and the Pelvic Floor

A Subdivision of the lesser pelvis by spaces and fasciae
Transverse (**a** and **b**) and midsagittal (**c** and **d**) sections through the (connective tissue of the) pelvis, anterosuperior and lateral views.
Spaces: The lesser pelvis consists of the *pelvic peritoneal cavity and pelvic extraperitoneal space* (see p. 9). The latter is further divided by the levator ani muscle into an upper and lower part, creating the three levels of the lesser pelvis (see **B**). The spaces are filled by connective tissue of variable density*. Topographically, based on the relationship to the peritoneum and pelvic wall, the extraperitoneal space can be subdivided into

- the retropubic space: between the bladder and pubic symphysis;
- the retroinguinal space: behind the inguinal region and below the peritoneum;
- the retroperitoneal space: between the peritoneum and sacrum (the continuation of the retroperitoneum of the abdomen).

Fasciae: The *pelvic fascia* consists of parietal fascia (covering the structures of the pelvic wall) and visceral fascia (covering the pelvic organs). The *connective tissue of the visceral fascia* is thickened at sites between and around the organs and is continuous with the adventitia or capsule of the pelvic organs:

- Rectoprostatic fascia or rectovesical septum (Denonvilliers' fascia) (male pelvis, located between the rectum and bladder)
- Rectovaginal fascia: rectovaginal septum (female pelvis, located between the rectum and vagina)

The *connective tissue* around the organs is also thickened and generally transmits the neurovascular bundles that supply the organs.

- Lateral rectal ligament (in pararectal fascia)
- Lateral ligament of the bladder (in paravesical fascia)
- Pubovesical ligament
- Transverse cervical ligament (in inferior parametrium)

* The extraperitoneal space is mostly filled by loose fatty connective tissue (sliding layer of connective tissue, mainly for the pelvic organs). At specific sites, the connective tissue is thickened and resembles dense, fibrous connective tissue (the entire parietal pelvic fascia and parts of the viscera pelvic fascia, as well as ligaments such as the cardinal ligament, which differ in character from the ligaments of the musculoskeletal system).

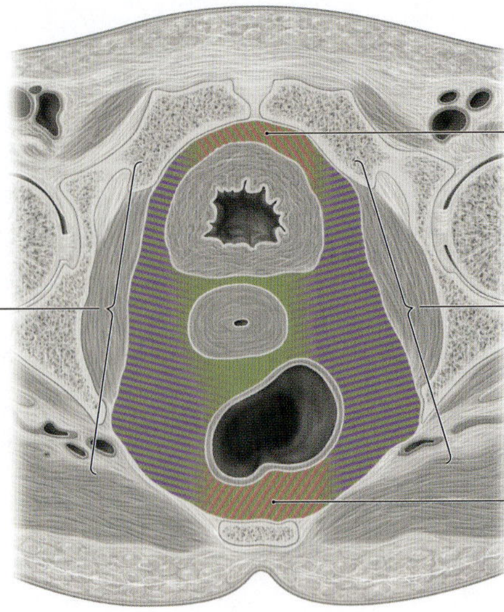

a

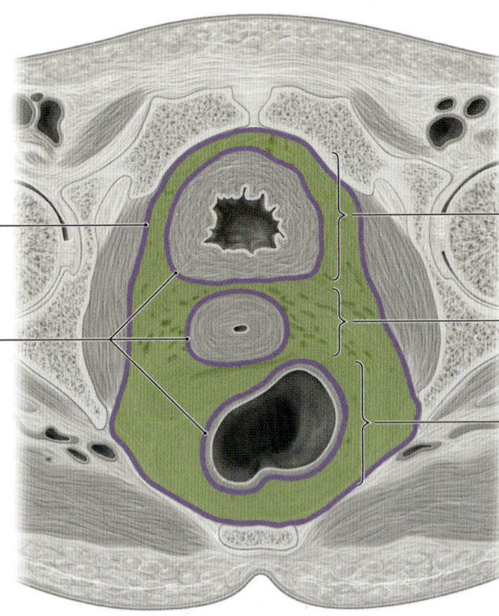

b

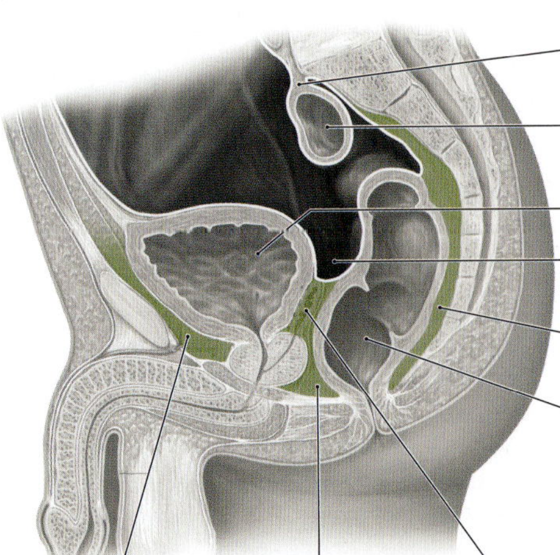

c

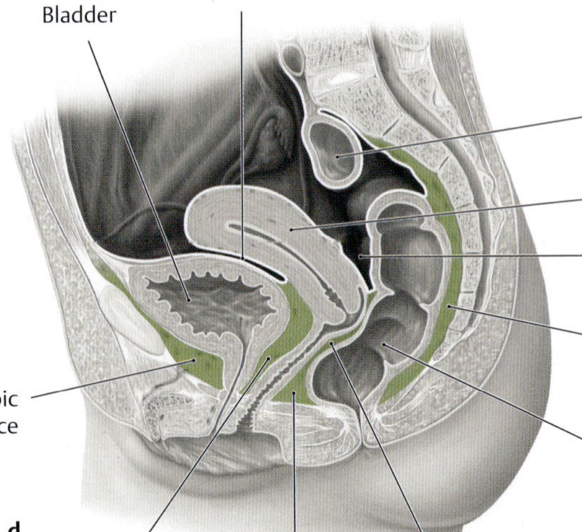

d

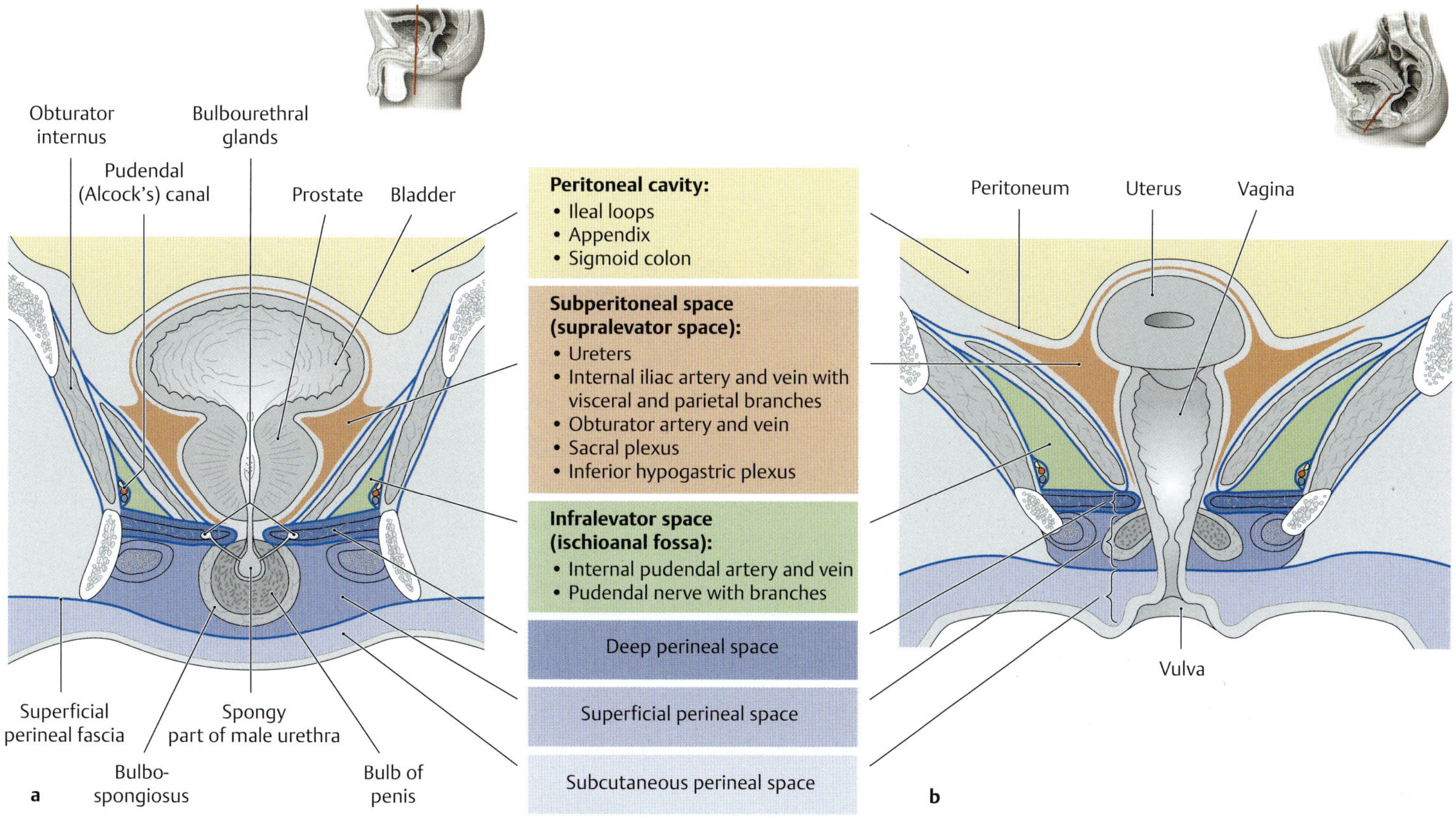

B Levels of the pelvic region and structures located in each level
Coronal section (for exact location of sectional planes see insets above) through a male (**a**) and female (**b**) pelvis. In addition to the levels of the pelvic region, the perineal spaces (deep, superficial, and subcutaneous) located below the pelvic region, are also outlined in color.

C Structure of the pelvic floor
The pelvic floor is composed of three muscle and connective tissue plates that are also divided into three levels:

- **Upper layer:** pelvic diaphragm
- **Middle layer:** urogenital diaphragm
- **Lower layer:** sphincters and erectile muscles of the urogenital and intestinal tracts

The funnel-shaped pelvic diaphragm is mainly formed by the levator ani and its superior and inferior muscular fasciae (superior and inferior fasciae of the pelvic diaphragm). The urogenital diaphragm is a fibromuscular connective tissue sheet that stretches horizontally between the ischiopubic rami and is mainly formed by the deep transverse perineal muscle and its superior and inferior muscular fasciae (superior and inferior fasciae of the urogenital diaphragm). The sphincters and erectile muscles include the bulbospongiosus, ischiocavernosus, external urethral sphincter, external anal sphincter, and their individual muscular fasciae.
The term "*urogenital diaphragm*" has become obsolete in current anatomic nomenclature. It included: deep and *superficial transverse perineal muscles* and the *superior* and *inferior urogenital diaphragmatic fasciae*. The superior fascia is no longer defined; the inferior fascia is referred to as the *perineal membrane*. Its expansion along the anterior margin of the deep transverse perineal muscle is referred to as the *transverse perineal ligament*.

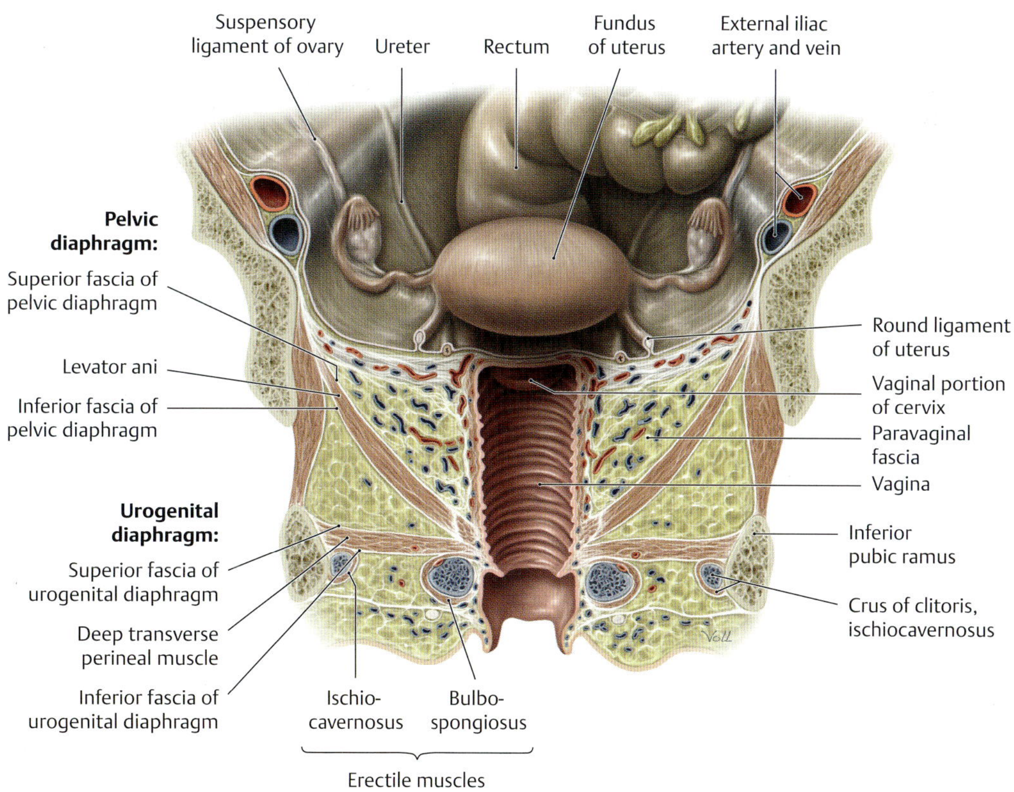

6.21 Suspensory Apparatus of the Uterus

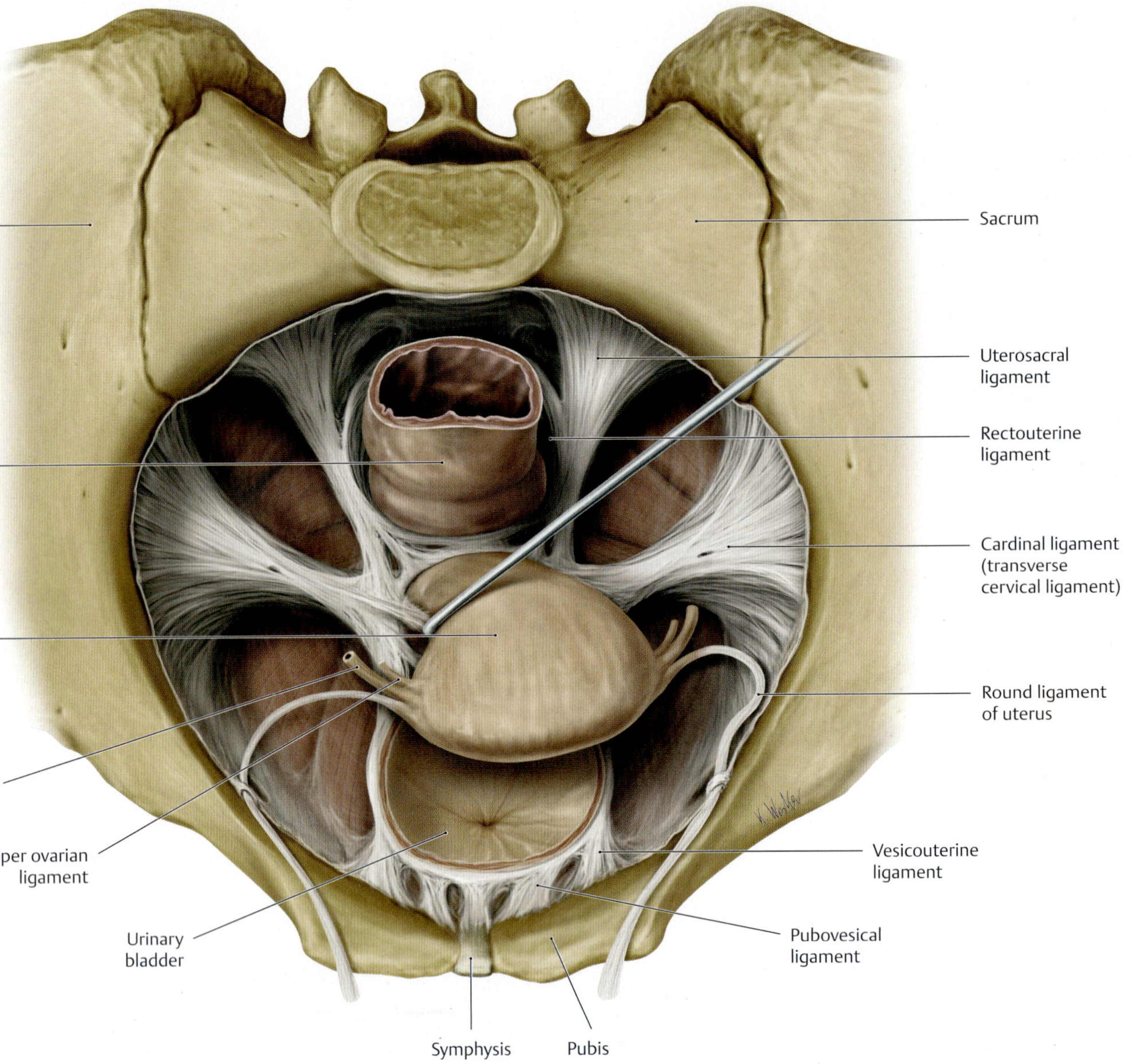

A Suspensory apparatus of the uterus

Location and function: The suspensory apparatus of the uterus is located in the subperitoneal connective tissue in the lesser pelvis and consists of band-like structures of dense fibrous parts of the pelvic connective tissue (see p. 414). The uterus is mainly anchored at the uterine cervix by tissue strands that extend in both the sagittal and transverse directions. Like the neck of a bottle turned upside down, the isthmus or supravaginal part of the cervix is clasped and attached to the lesser pelvis. In this way, the vaginal part of the cervix lies on the interspinal line. This is referred to as the *normal position of the uterus*. Generally, the suspensory apparatus permits physiological mobility of the uterus so it can adjust to the distention of surrounding organs. When the bladder is full the uterus becomes more erect. When the rectum is full the uterus is pushed forward. If the bladder and rectum are both full the uterus is elevated.

Components: The strongest supporting structure is the *cardinal ligament* (Mackenrodt's ligament) also known as the transverse cervical ligament, a fibrous layer in the parametrium. It fans out from the fascia of the lateral pelvic wall to the supravaginal part of the cervix. This fibrous apparatus keeps the uterus suspended in a position that is secured by the muscles of the pelvic floor. In the sagittal direction, the uterus is anchored by band-like structures extending between the pubic symphysis and sacrum. By running between bladder and uterine cervix as well as rectum and uterine cervix, these connective tissue fibers (*pubovesical ligament, vesicouterine ligament, uterosacral ligament, and rectouterine ligament*) anchor the organs. The round ligament arises at the uterine horns and runs along the inguinal canal to the labia majora where it is anchored. It has smooth muscle cells and holds the uterus forward in its typical position (anteversion–anteflexion, see p. 344).

Note: Intraperitoneal changes in uterine position are mostly congenital. However, tumors, inflammatory processes, and shortening of the suspensory ligaments can also influence uterine position. After childbirth, the uterus may assume a retroverted–retroflexed position (due to temporary overstretching of the uterine support system). As the body returns to its nonpregnant condition, the uterus returns to its normal position.

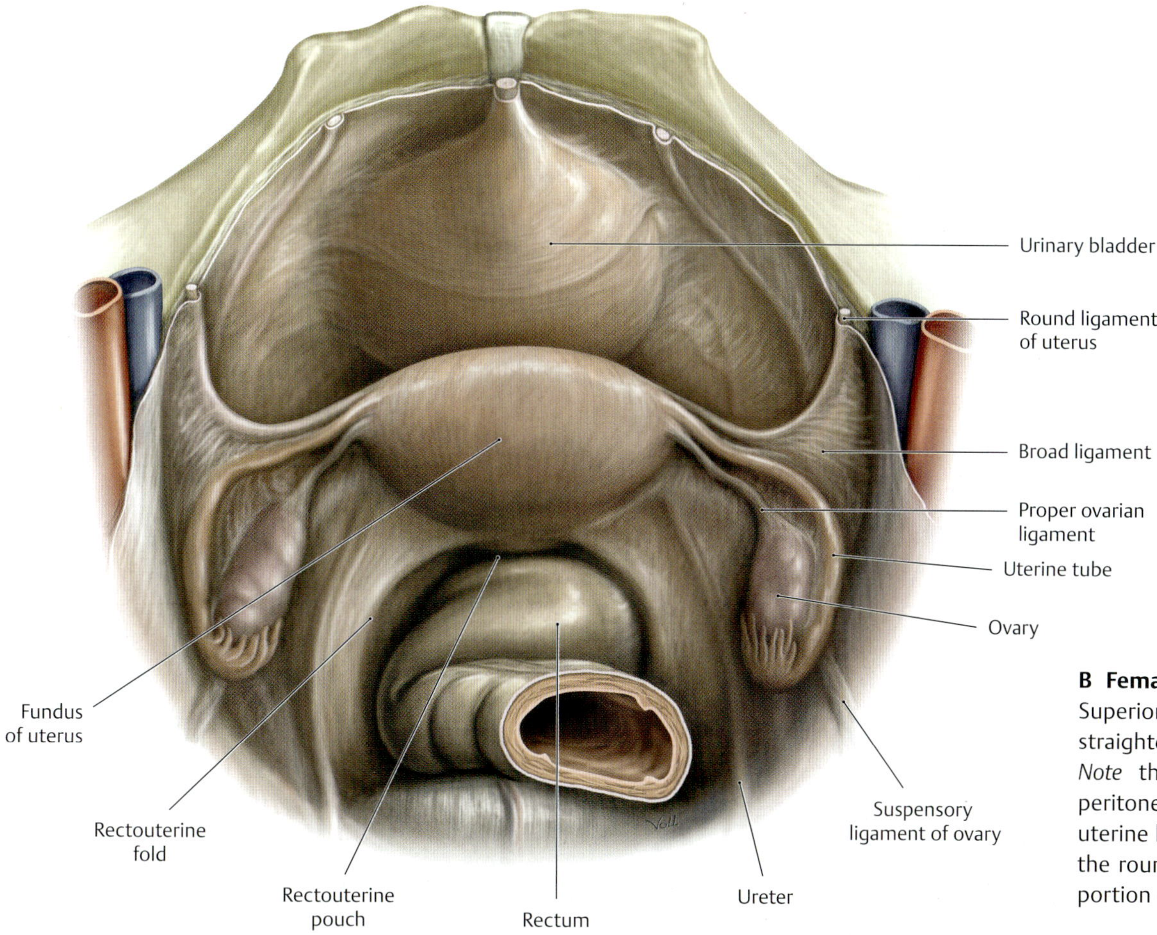

B Female pelvis in situ
Superior view, the uterus has been straightened for clarity.
Note the rectouterine fold as a peritoneal ridge over the rectouterine ligament, and the course of the round ligament in the superior portion of the broad ligament.

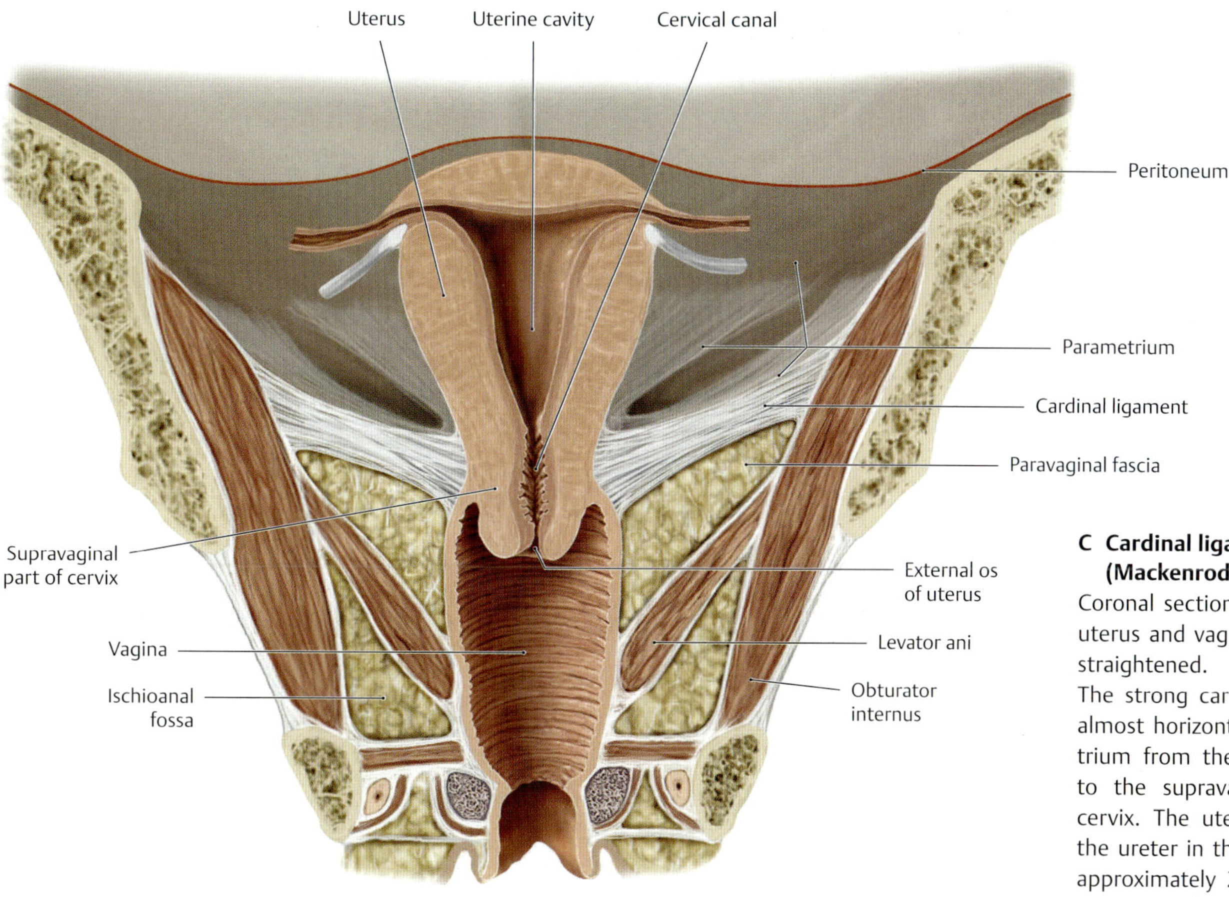

C Cardinal ligament (Mackenrodt's)
Coronal section at the level of the uterus and vagina, with the uterus straightened.
The strong cardinal ligament runs almost horizontally in the parametrium from the lateral pelvic wall to the supravaginal part of the cervix. The uterine artery crosses the ureter in the cardinal ligament approximately 2 cm lateral to the supravaginal part of the cervix (see p. 369).

6.22 Female Pelvis in situ

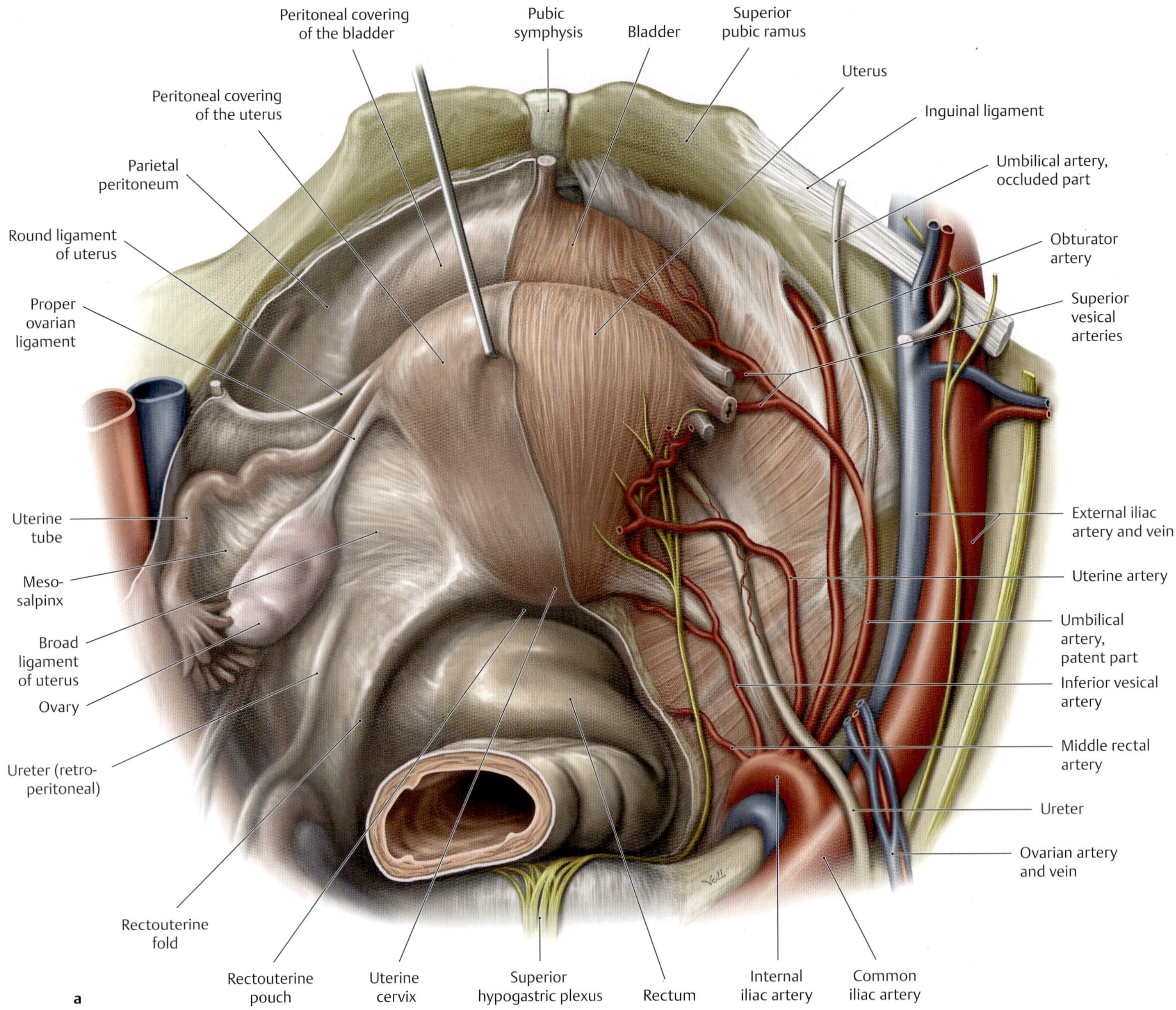

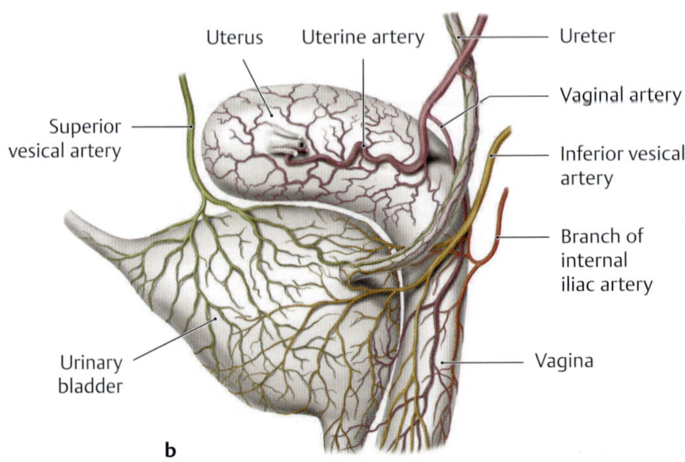

A Female pelvis in situ

a Posterosuperior view; the peritoneum covering the uterus, bladder and lateral and posterior walls of the pelvis has been partially removed, and the uterus pulled slightly anteriorly. The broad ligament (part of the parametrium, see p. 414), right ovary and uterine tube have been removed. *Note:* The ureter crosses inferior to the uterine artery approximately 2 cm lateral to the uterine cervix.

b Schematic representation of the blood supply to the female urogenital tract, left lateral view.

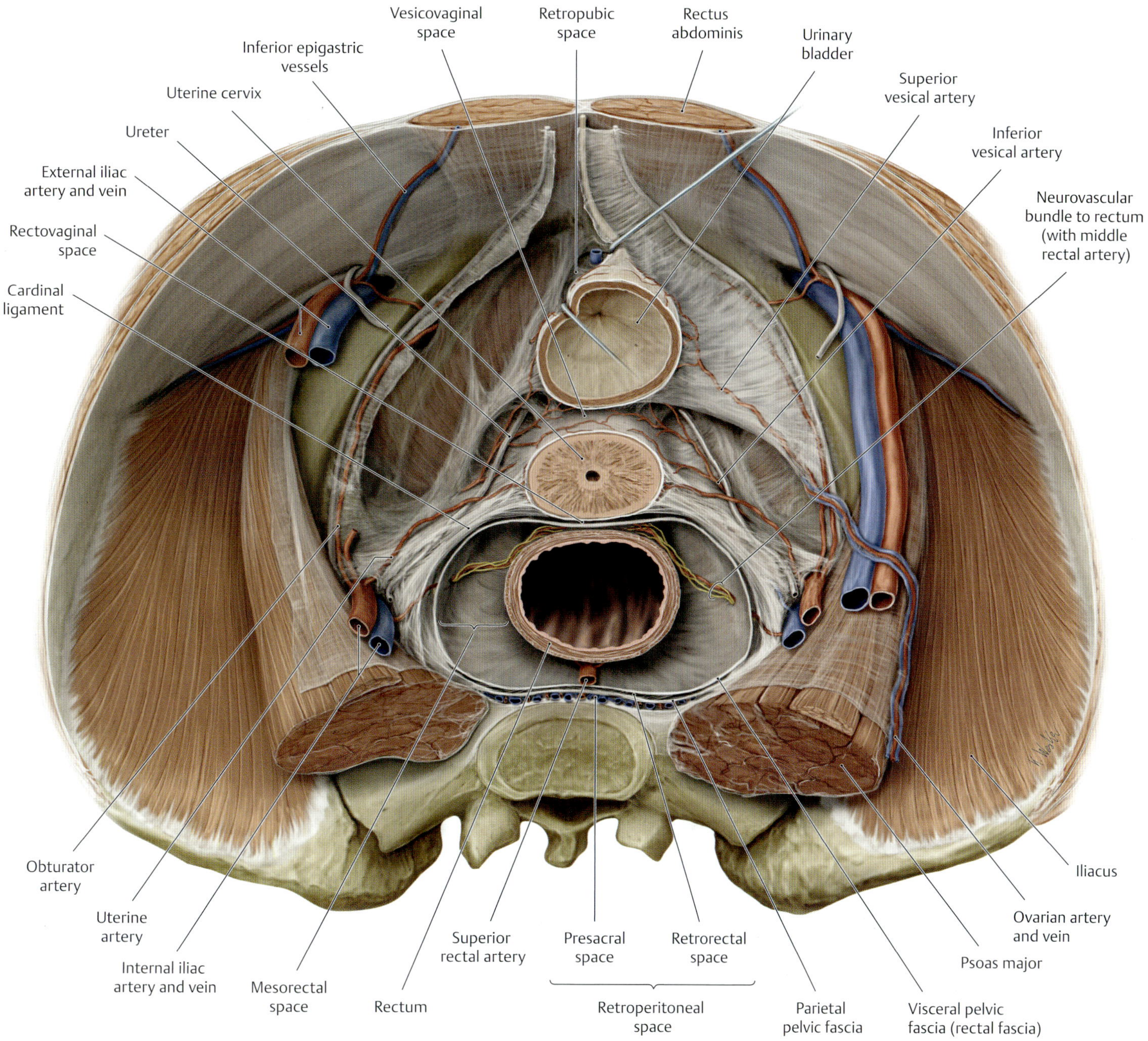

B Female pelvis in situ, superior view

Transverse cut of pelvic cavity; numerous structures have been removed for clarity. The uterus and adnexa have been removed, and the bladder and rectum have been opened superiorly. Vessels have been transected cranially so that the pelvic spaces are clearly visible:

- Retropubic space in front of the bladder
- Vesicovaginal space between bladder and uterus
- Rectovaginal space between uterus and rectum
- Retroperitoneal space (with retrorectal and presacral spaces) behind the rectum

For better exposure of the neurovascular bundle (middle rectal artery and nerve fibers of the inferior hypogastric plexus) running to the rectum, the mesorectal adipose tissue (cf. p. 400) between the rectum and rectal fascia has been completely removed. It can be clearly seen that the uterine artery runs lateral to the uterine cervix in the cardinal ligament (see p. 416), at the base of the broad ligament, and crosses the ureter 2 cm lateral to the cervix.

6.23 Male Pelvis in situ

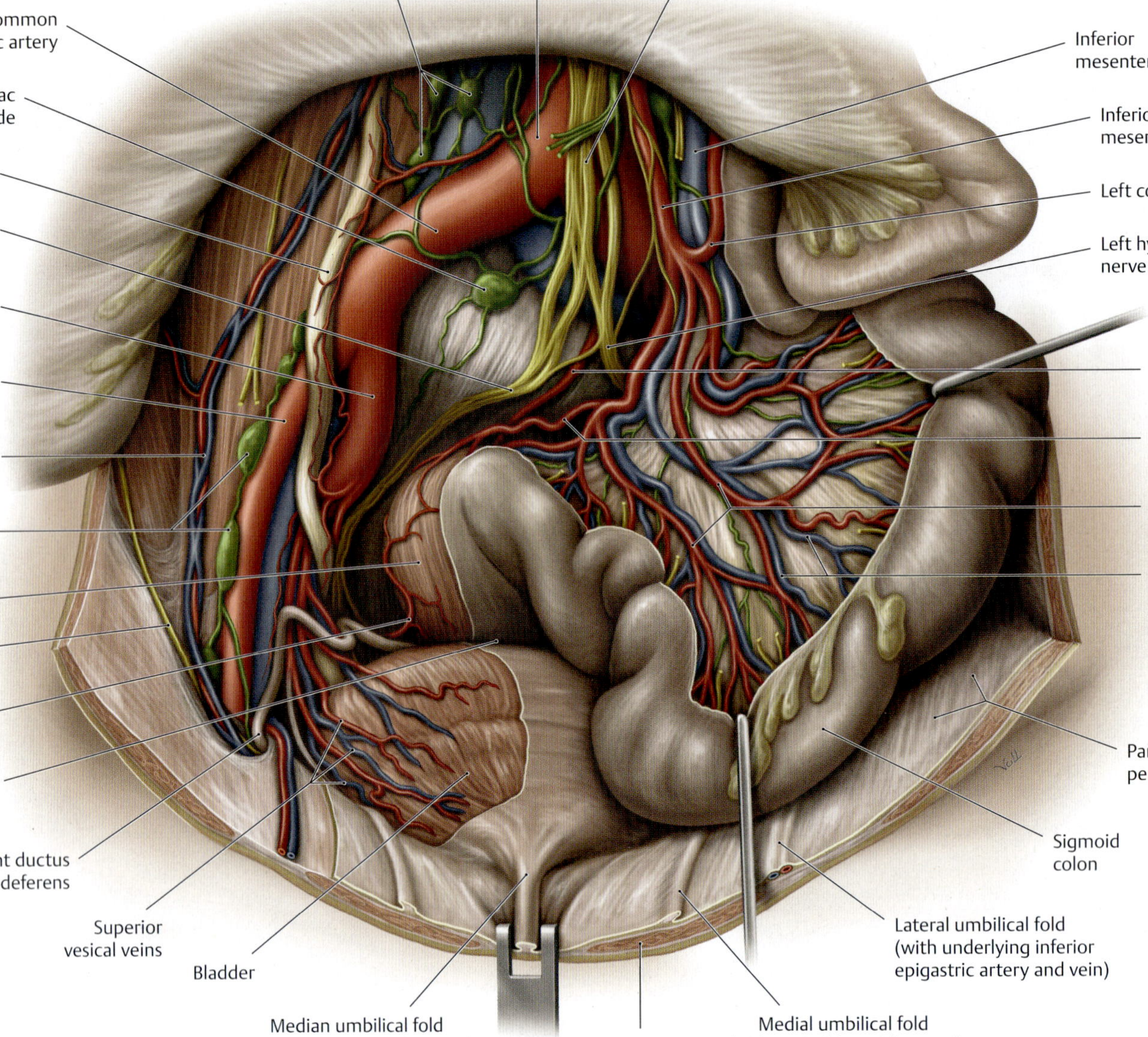

A Male pelvis in situ, anterosuperior view
The sigmoid colon has been retracted anterolaterally and upward; and wide areas of peritoneum covering the sigmoid mesocolon, rectum, bladder, and lateral and posterior pelvic walls have been removed to expose the underlying structures. Lymph nodes and autonomic nerve plexuses are shown schematically for clarity. In the male pelvis, the peritoneum is reflected from the bladder to the rectum to form the rectovesical fossa (pouch).

B Pelvic fasciae, mesorectum and course of the neurovascular bundle (see right page)

a Anterosuperior view of the male pelvis, the upper two-thirds of the rectum and bladder have been removed.
Clearly visible are the mesorectal adipose tissue together with the superior rectal artery, which runs in it, and the fascial envelope (rectal fascia or visceral layer of the pelvic fascia, cf. p. 400), which surrounds the mesorectum. Bilateral neurovascular bundles extend anteriorly between the visceral and parietal layers of the pelvic fascia. Both form an inferior hypogastric plexus, a network of sympathetic (inferior hypogastric nerves) and parasympathetic (pelvic splanchnic nerves) nerves and ganglia (pelvic ganglia). The nerve fibers together with the middle rectal artery extend from the plexus to the rectum, and together with the vesical arteries to the prostate, seminal vesicles, and bladder.

b Sagittal section through male pelvis, pelvic connective tissue and most of the pelvic fascia have been removed; viewed from the left side.
The rectum and its mesorectal fascial envelope (rectal fascia/visceral layer of the pelvic fascia) has been unfolded to show the location of the inferior hypogastric plexus and the course of the neurovascular bundle on its lateral side between the fascial layers. Part of the rectovesical septum has been left in place between the bladder, seminal vesicles, prostate, and rectum (cf. p. 400).

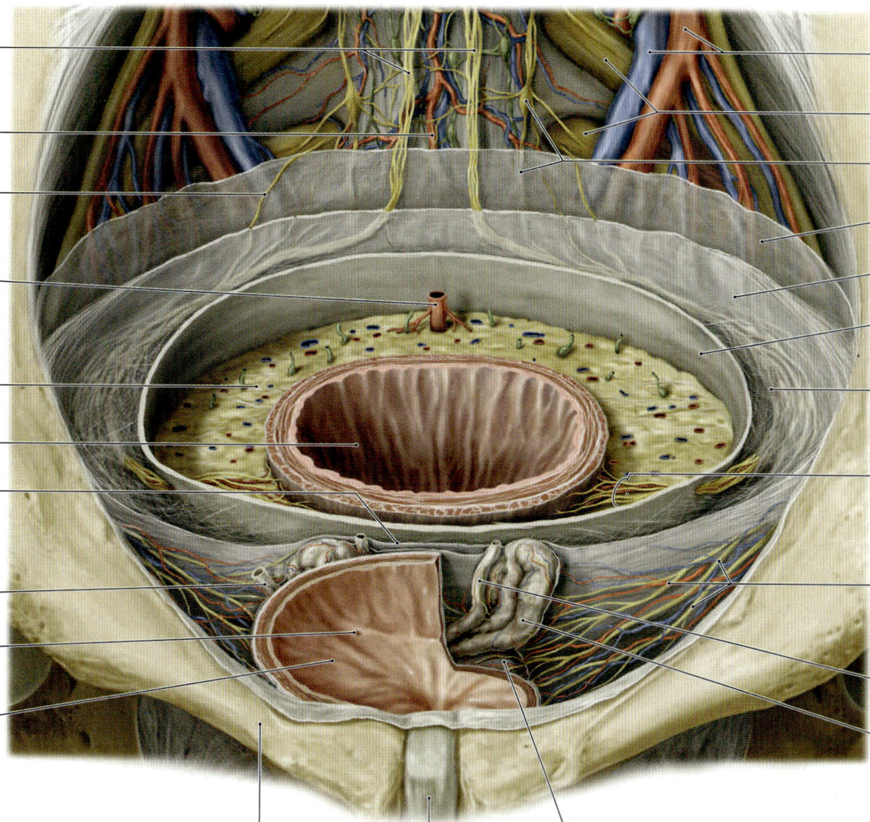
Inferior hypogastric nerves
Median sacral artery
Pelvic splanchnic nerves
Superior rectal artery (branching off the inferior mesenteric artery)
Mesorectum
Rectum
Rectoprostatic fascia of Denonvilliers
Right ureter
Ureteric orifice
Urinary bladder
Superior pubic ramus
Symphysis
Prostate
Internal iliac artery and vein
Sacral plexus
Sacral ganglia
Presacral fascia
Parietal pelvic fascia
Visceral pelvic fascia (rectal fascia)
Inferior hypogastric plexus (intrafascial)
Neurovascular bundle to rectum (with middle rectal artery)
Neurovascular bundle to the urogenital organs
Ductus deferens
Seminal vesicle

a

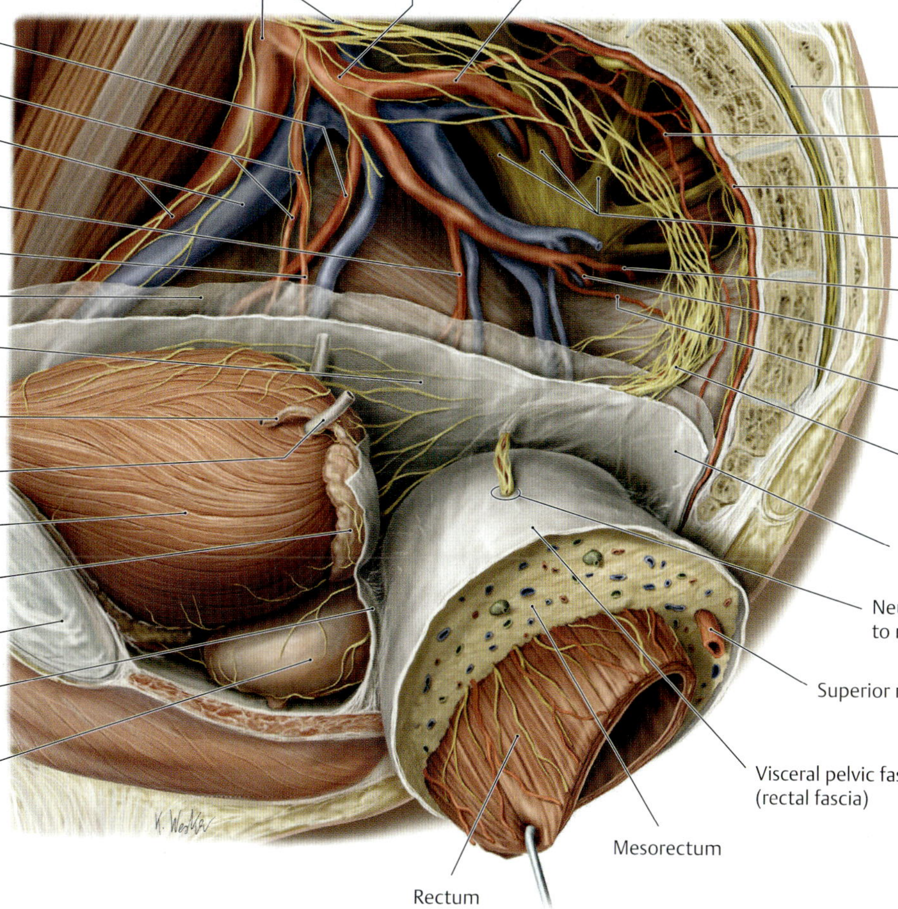
Common iliac artery and vein
Internal iliac artery
Superior gluteal artery
Obturator artery
Umbilical artery
External iliac artery and vein
Inferior vesical artery
Superior vesical artery
Presacral fascia
Artery of ductus deferens
Ductus deferens
Ureter
Urinary bladder
Seminal vesicle
Pubic symphysis
Rectoprostatic fascia of Denonvilliers
Prostate
Sacral canal
Lateral sacral artery
Median sacral artery
Sacral plexus
Inferior gluteal artery
Internal pudendal artery
Middle rectal artery
Inferior hypogastric plexus
Parietal pelvic fascia
Neurovascular bundle to rectum
Superior rectal artery
Visceral pelvic fascia (rectal fascia)
Mesorectum
Rectum

b

6.24 Cross-Sectional Anatomy of the Female Pelvis

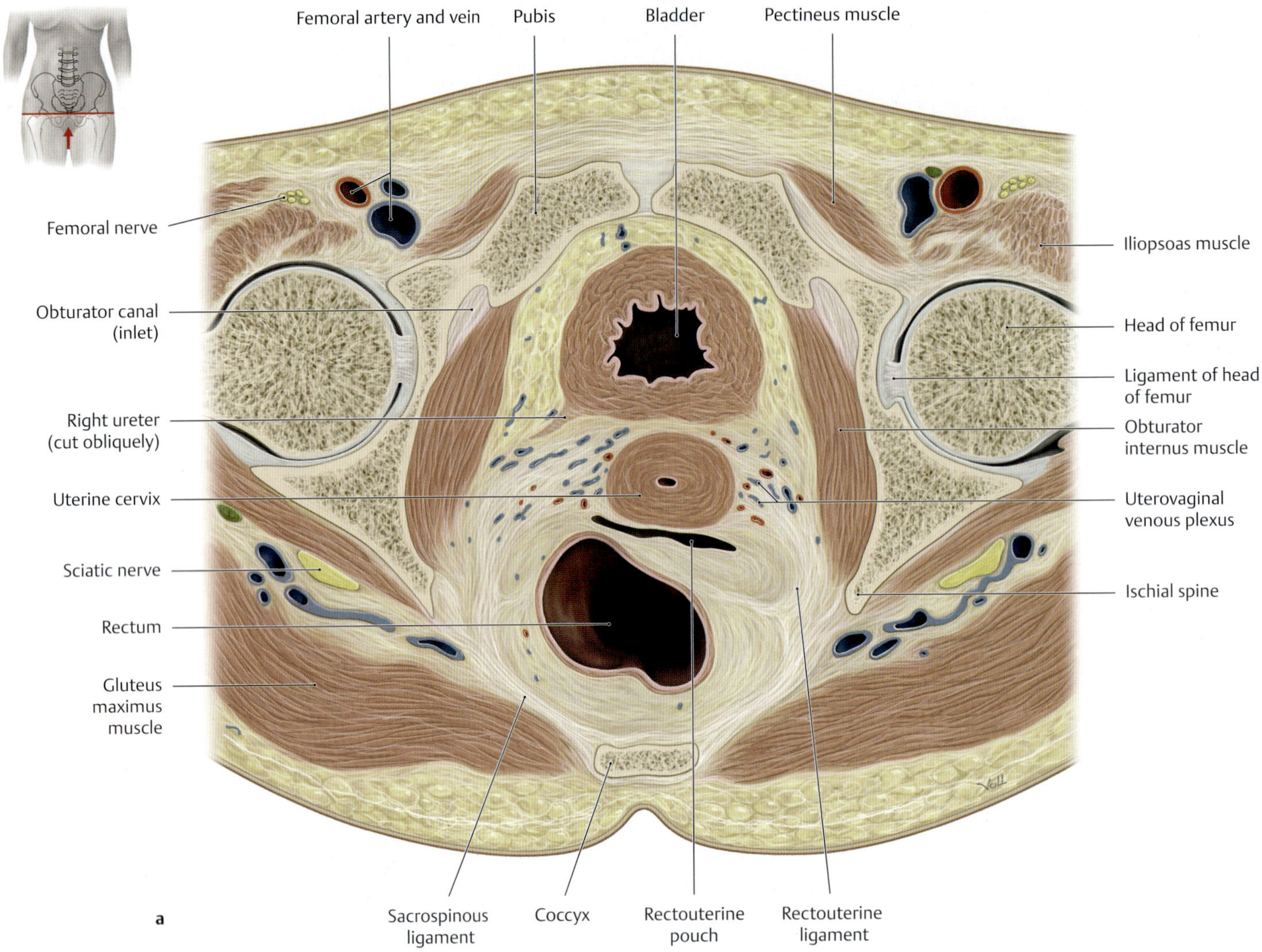

a

A Location of the female pelvic organs in transverse section

a Section through the female pelvis at the superior border of the pubic symphysis. The section cuts the bladder just below the ureteral orifices. Posterior to the bladder is a section of the uterine cervix, and behind that is the rectum (separated from the cervix by the base of the rectouterine pouch). As in the male pelvis, connective tissue is distributed around the bladder and rectum. Additional connective tissue is found around the cervix, representing a downward prolongation of the transverse cervical ligament. A venous network, the uterovaginal venous plexus, is embedded in the connective tissue and is cut at numerous sites in the section above. This plexus provides venous drainage for the uterus and vagina.

Note: Peritoneal pouches exist in front of and behind the uterus: the vesicouterine pouch anteriorly and the rectouterine pouch posteriorly. The section shown here cuts the pelvis at the level of the rectouterine pouch (cul-de-sac). The vesicouterine pouch does not extend as inferiorly and terminates above the plane of section. As a result, the area between the cervix and bladder in this section is occupied by connective tissue (formerly called the "vesicovaginal septum").

b **MRI of the pelvis, transverse scan** (from Hamm, B. et al.: MRT von Abdomen und Becken, 2nd ed. Thieme, Stuttgart 2006). The image shows the low-signal intensity cervical stroma (arrows), which surrounds the narrow high-signal intensity cervical canal.

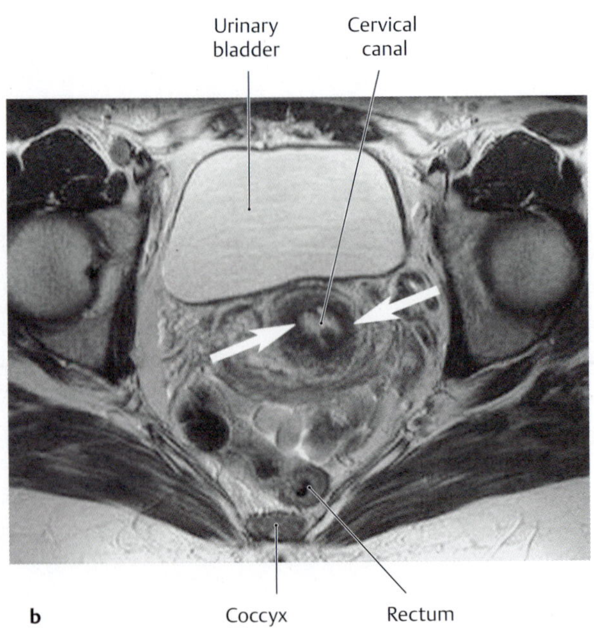

b

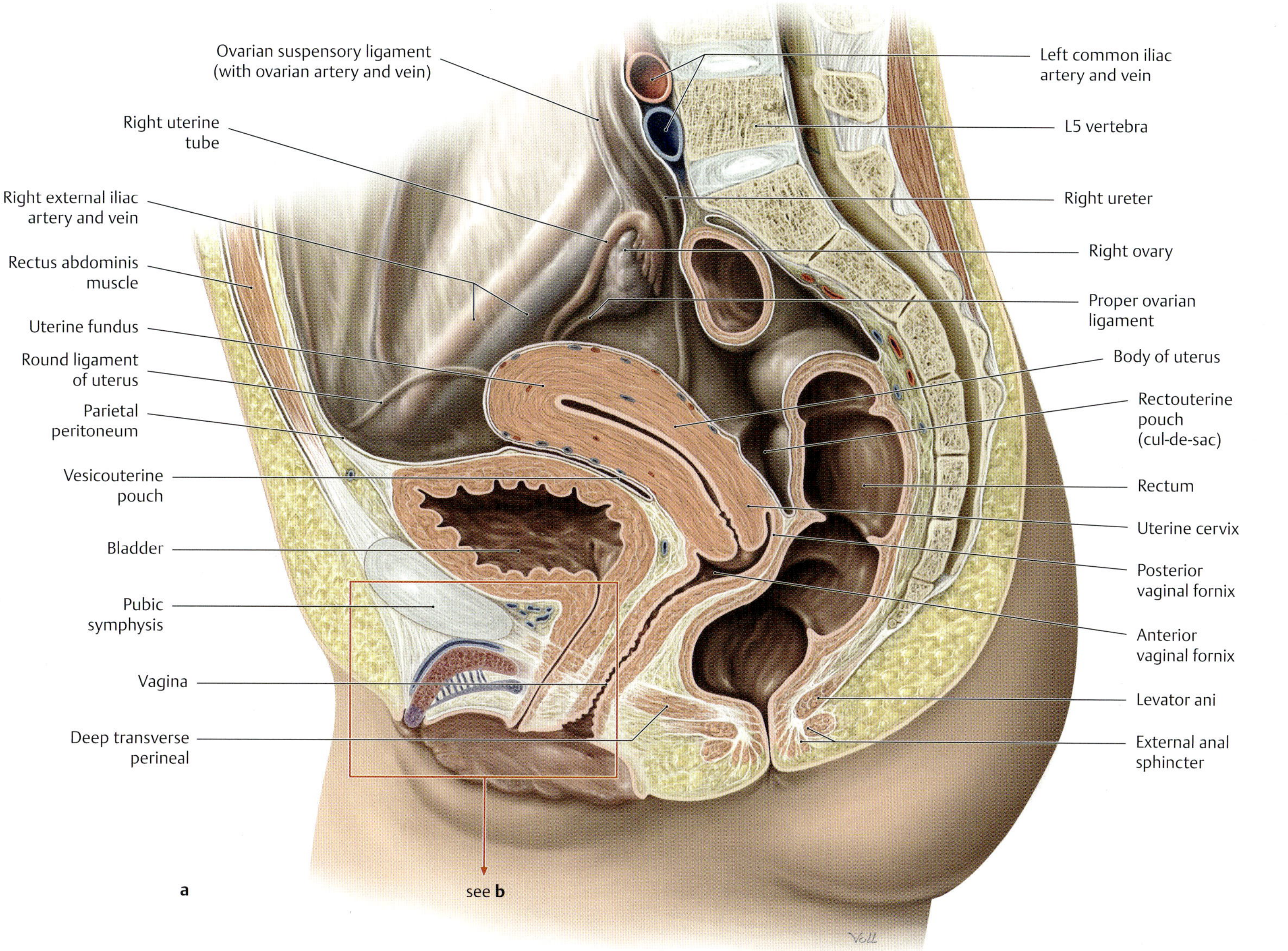

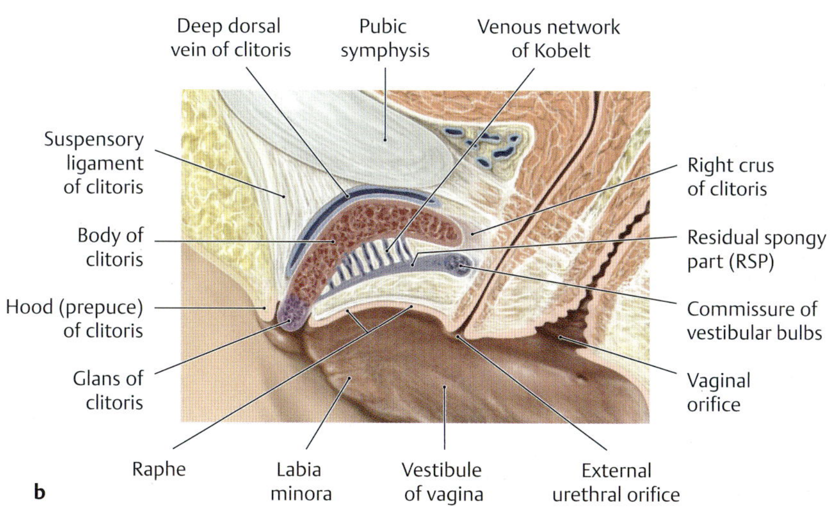

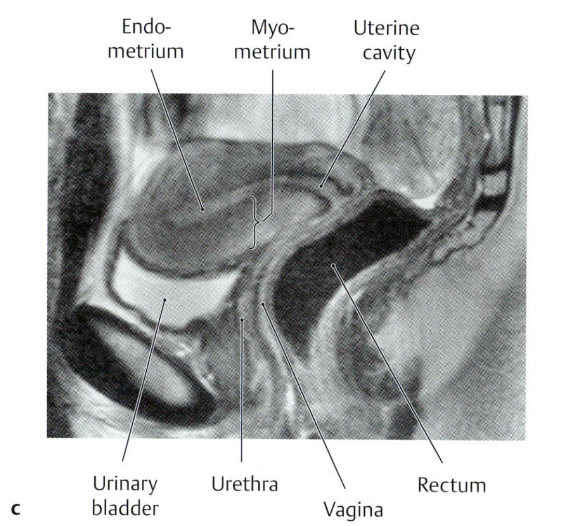

B Position of the female pelvic organs on a median sagittal section

a Left view; small and large intestine except for the sigmoid colon and rectum have been removed.

b Detail of **a**.

Note: In the female, the uterus and its network of ligaments, occasionally referred to as the genital plate, lie between the urinary bladder and rectum. This characteristically changes the peritoneal anatomic relationships in the pelvis compared with the male: As in the male, the female peritoneum extends from the anterior wall of the peritoneal cavity to the surface of the urinary bladder, but from there it continues on to the anterior wall of the uterus. Because the uterus typically occupies an anteflexed and anteverted position on the bladder, the peritoneum between the bladder and uterus forms a deep but narrow recess, the vesicouterine pouch (see p. 320).

c MRI of the pelvis, sagittal section (from: Hamm B. et al. MRT von Abdomen und Becken. 2nd ed. Stuttgart: Thieme; 2006). Uterus during the first half of the menstrual cycle (proliferation phase) with a narrow endometrium and relatively hypointense myometrium.

6.25 Cross-Sectional Anatomy of the Male Pelvis

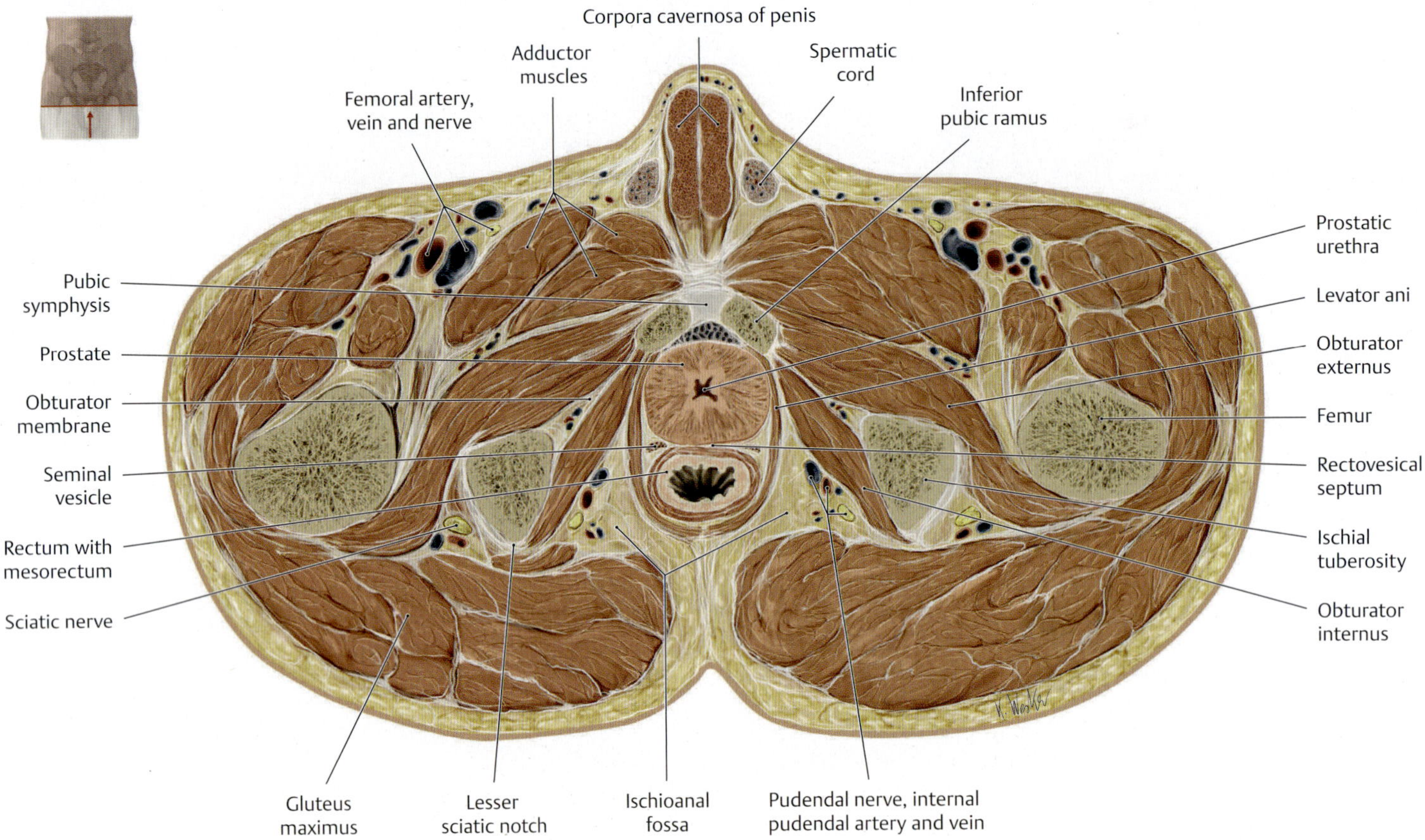

A Location of the male pelvic organs in transverse section
Section through the male pelvis at the level of the prostate, inferior view. The diagram shows the location of the prostate posterior to the inferior pubic rami and the pubic symphysis. Behind the prostate lie the sectioned seminal vesicles. The rectovesical septum, an anteriorly oriented layer of connective tissue, extends between the prostate and rectum. It acts as a border between the mesorectum and the urogenital organs. Laterally and posteriorly, the levator ani borders the ischioanal fossa.

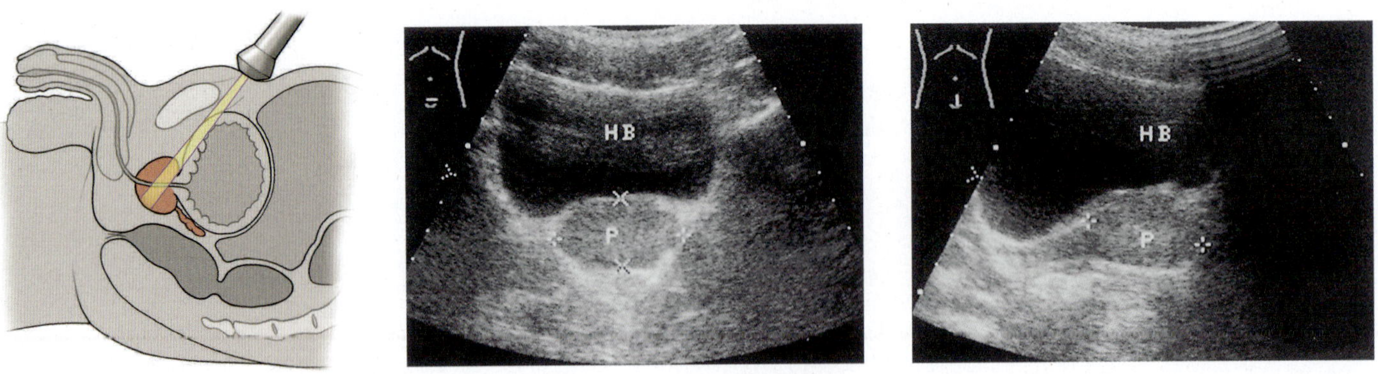

a b c

B Transvesical sonography of the prostate
a Schematic midsagittal section through the male pelvis to show suprapubic probe positioning, viewed from the left side; **b** Normal findings of the prostate imaged in the transverse plane; **c** Sagittal section through the prostate (from: Reiser M, Kuhn F, Debus J, eds. *Duale Reihe Radiologie*. 4th ed. Stuttgart: Theme; 2017).
Transvesical imaging of the prostate (P) is possible only when the bladder (HB) is sufficiently distended. Unlike transrectal sonography of the prostate, which allows for a differentiated assessment of the organ structure and facilitates proof that cancer has started to spread (see p. 356), suprapubic transvesical sonography provides a three-dimensional image of the organ (transverse, sagittal and frontal planes) and measurement of the volume by using the formula V = 0.523 × a × b × c.

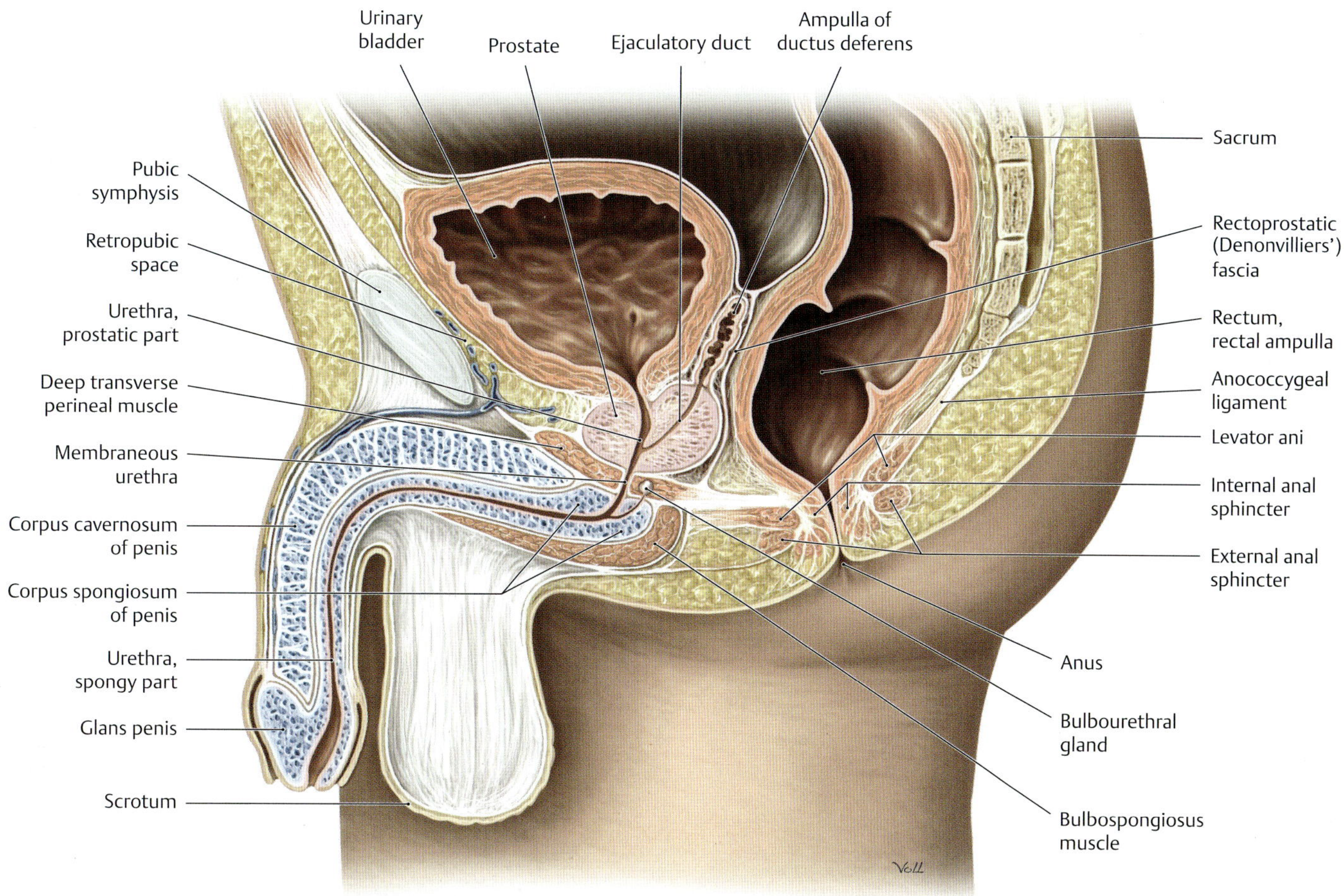

C Location of the male pelvic organs in sagittal section
Midsagittal section, viewed from the left.
The diagram shows the size and location of the bladder when it is significantly distended. When the bladder is empty, it is considerably smaller and lies behind the pubic symphysis and the peritoneum forms a transverse ridge on the surface of the bladder called the transverse vesical fold. The peritoneum extends from the bladder to the anterior wall of the rectum and forms a small recess, the rectovesical pouch (lowest part of the male peritoneal cavity). The peritoneum does not reach the prostate.
Note the two curvatures of the rectum in the sagittal plane (sacral flexure and perineal flexure) and the rectovesical septum (rectoprostatic fascia) along the posterior border of the prostate and seminal vesicles.

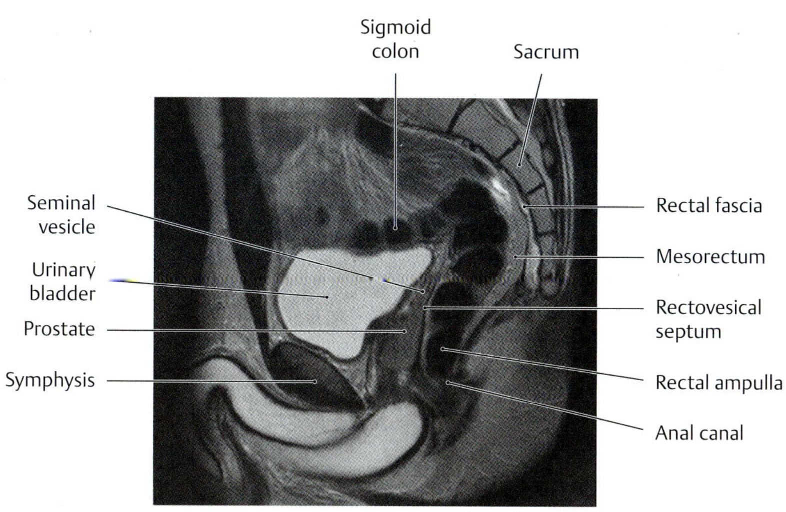

D Sagittal MRI scan of the male pelvis (T2-weighted TSE sequence)
Note: On T2-weighted MRI scans, the perirectal fat tissue of the rectum (mesorectum) is hyperintense. The mesorectal fascia (rectal fascia = visceral layer of pelvic fascia), which surrounds the mesorectum can be demonstrated as a fine low-signal intensity line (from Hamm, B. et al.: MRT von Abdomen und Becken, 2nd ed. Thieme, Stuttgart 2006).

D Neurovascular Supply to the Organs

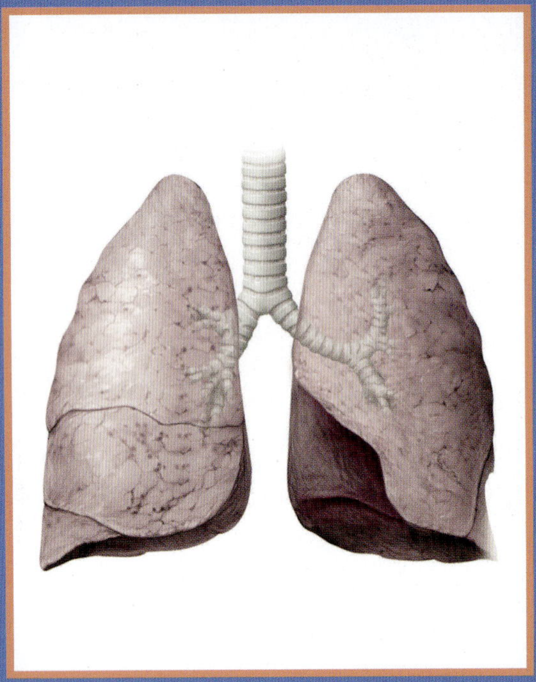

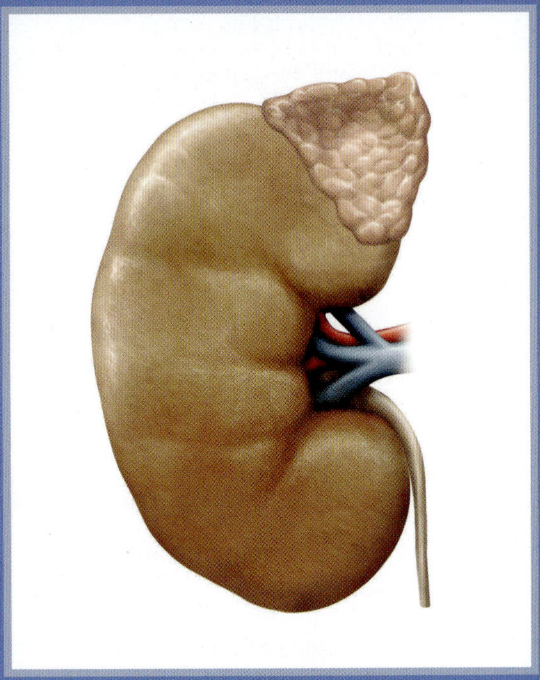

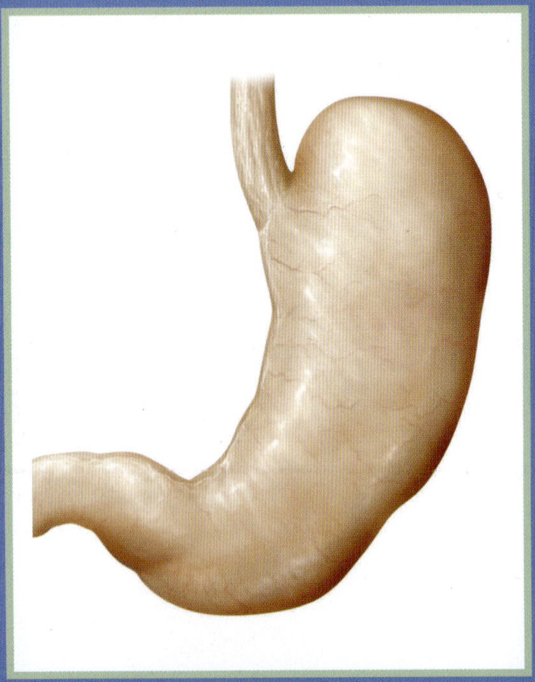

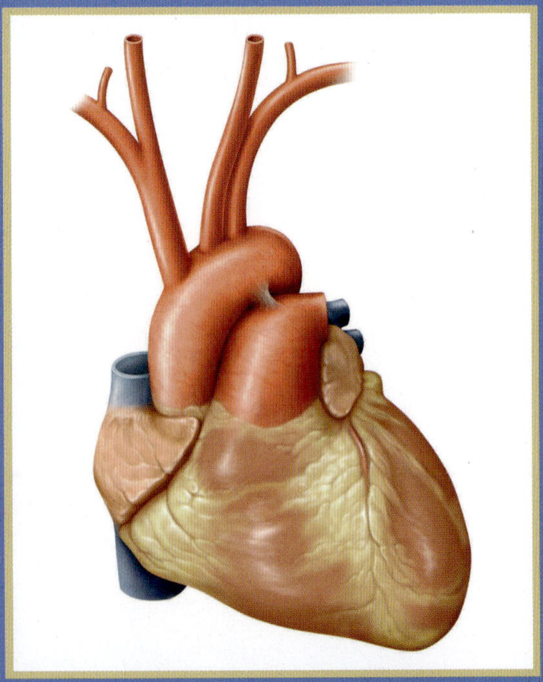

HOW TO USE THIS CHAPTER

Each of the sections in this chapter reviews the neurovascular supply to an organ or group of organs in a schematized form. The following subgroups are distinguished in the diagrams:

- Arterial supply (red)
- Venous drainage (blue)
- Lymphatic drainage (green)
- Innervation (yellow)

THE SCHEMATICS CAN BE USED IN VARIOUS WAYS:

- Reviewing for a test: The student can quickly obtain a basic grasp of neurovascular structures and pathways.
- Looking up a specific structure: The diagrams make it easy to locate and identify a particular neurovascular supply.
- Understanding complex anatomy by appreciating the basic neurovascular supply to an organ in the diagrams and then referring back to the more complex anatomical relationships shown in earlier chapters.

Points to keep in mind when using the schematics:

- They reflect a simplified, idealized view.
- Topographical anatomy is ignored, and the structures are not drawn to scale.
- Organs that are in close proximity to each other but are supplied by different groups of neurovascular structures are shown in separate diagrams.
- By and large, variants are disregarded.
- In cases where the neurovascular supply is bilaterally symmetrical, only one side is shown.

1.1 Thymus

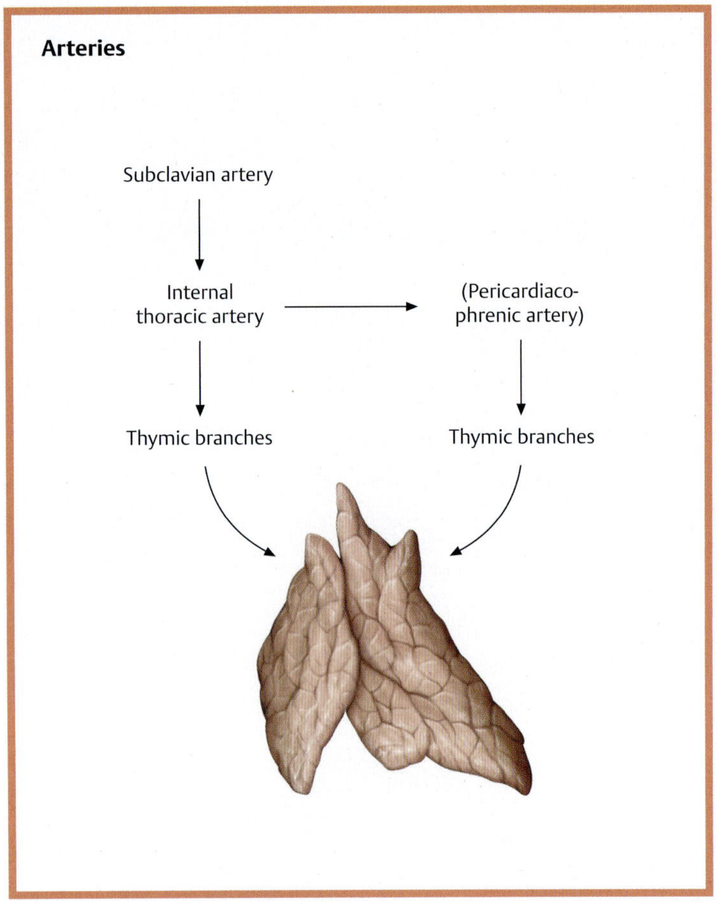
Arteries
Subclavian artery
Internal thoracic artery
(Pericardiaco-phrenic artery)
Thymic branches
Thymic branches

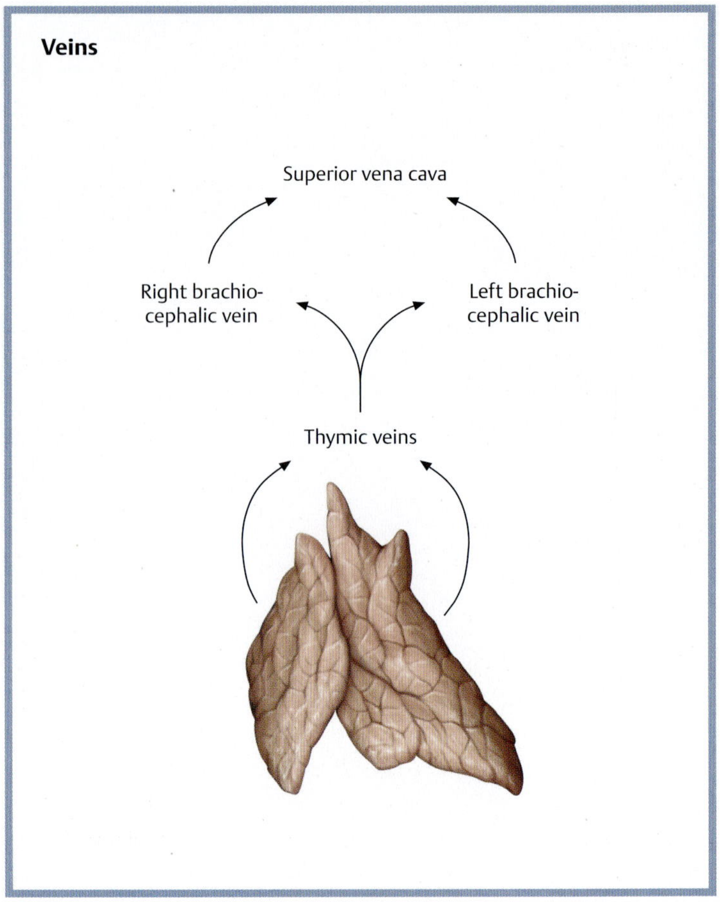
Veins
Superior vena cava
Right brachio-cephalic vein
Left brachio-cephalic vein
Thymic veins

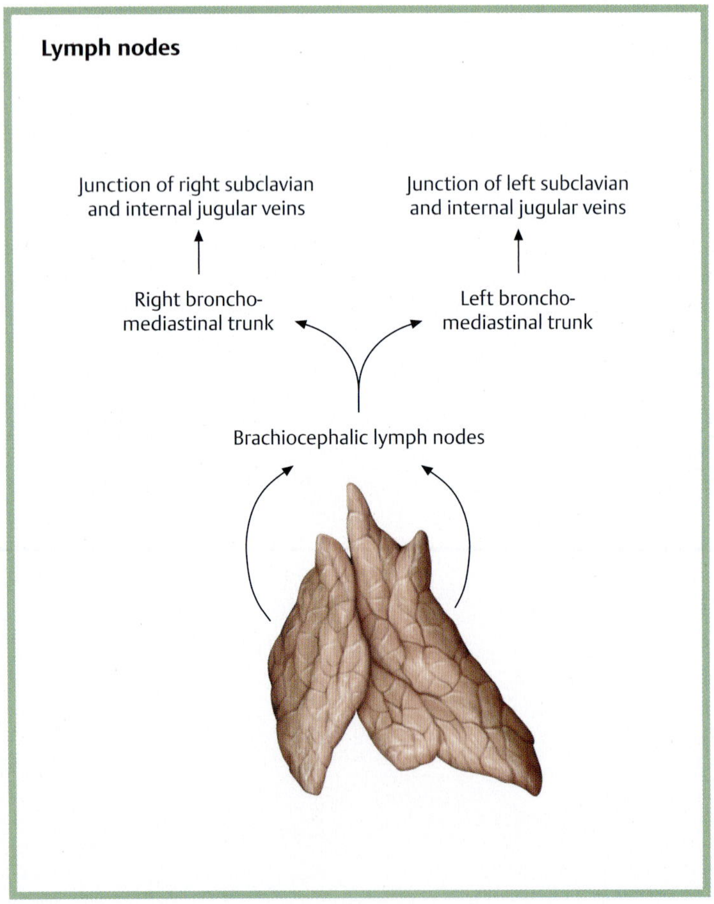
Lymph nodes
Junction of right subclavian and internal jugular veins
Junction of left subclavian and internal jugular veins
Right broncho-mediastinal trunk
Left broncho-mediastinal trunk
Brachiocephalic lymph nodes

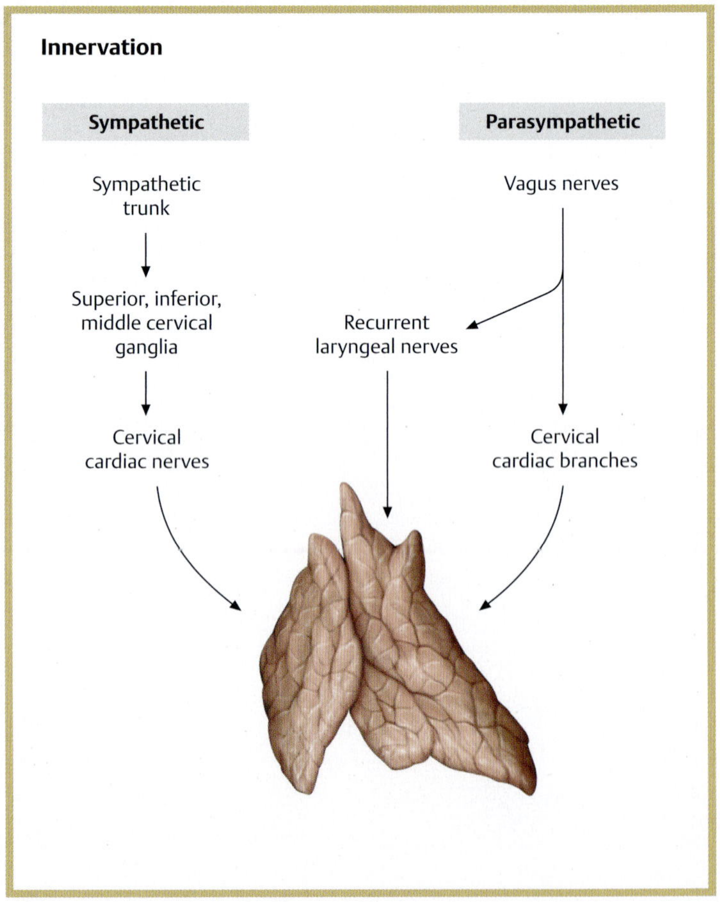
Innervation
Sympathetic
Parasympathetic
Sympathetic trunk
Vagus nerves
Superior, inferior, middle cervical ganglia
Recurrent laryngeal nerves
Cervical cardiac nerves
Cervical cardiac branches

1.2 Esophagus

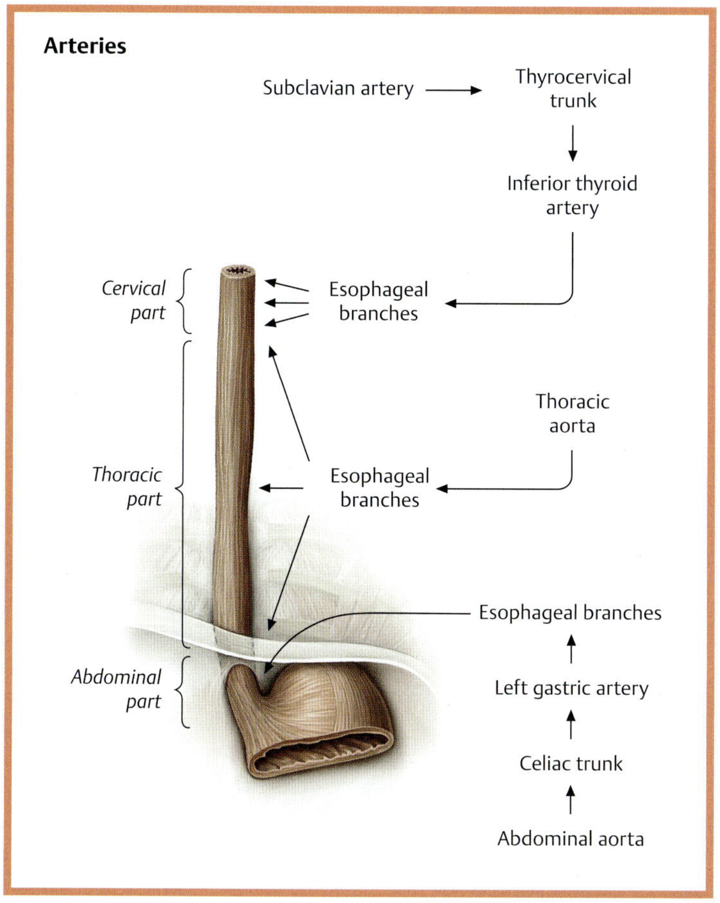

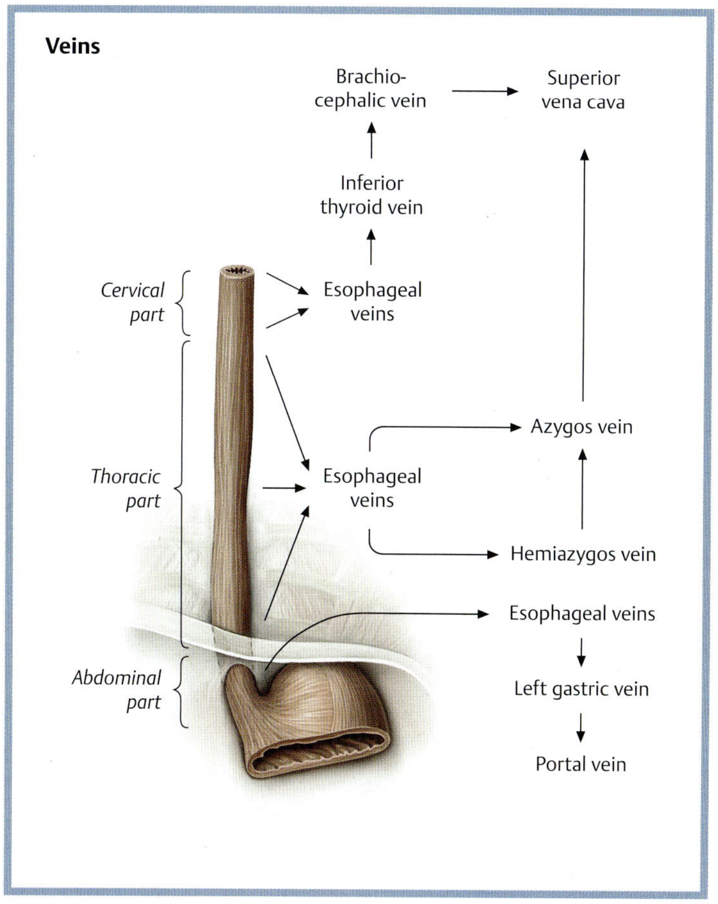

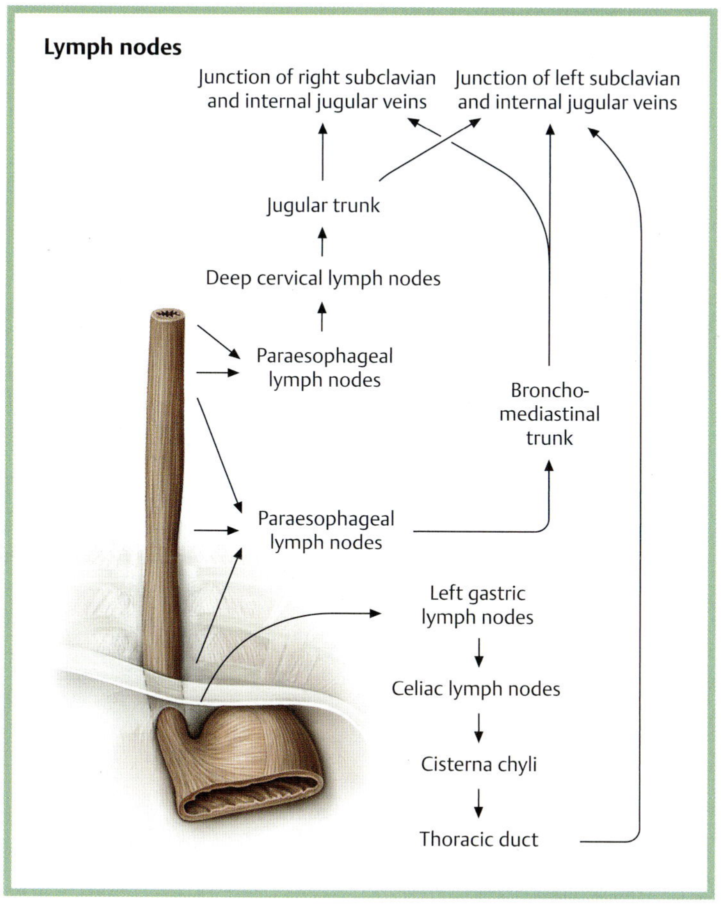

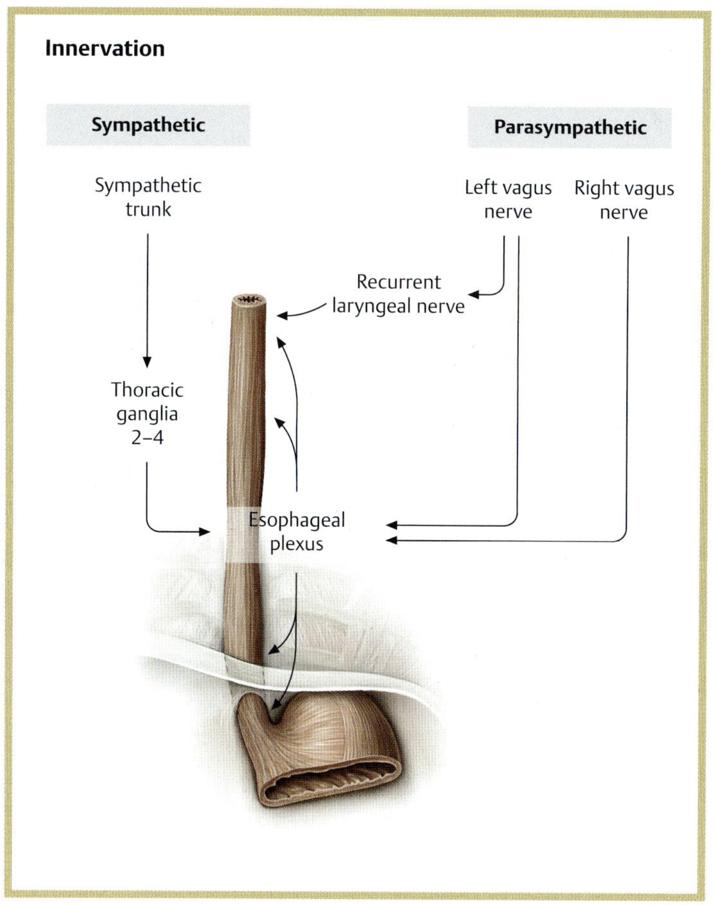

1.3 Heart

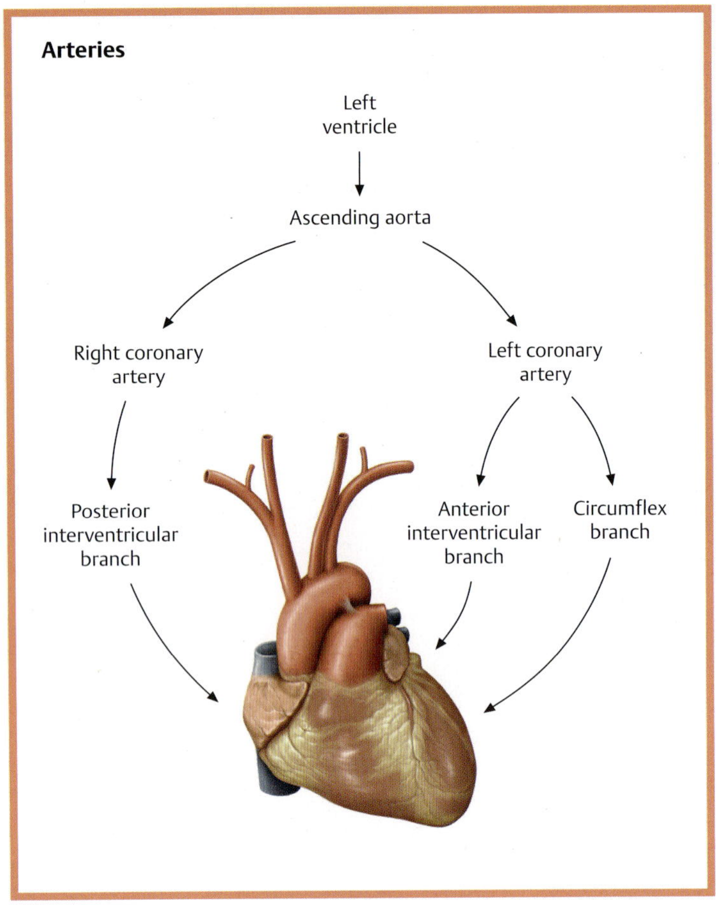
Arteries
Left ventricle
Ascending aorta
Right coronary artery
Left coronary artery
Posterior interventricular branch
Anterior interventricular branch
Circumflex branch

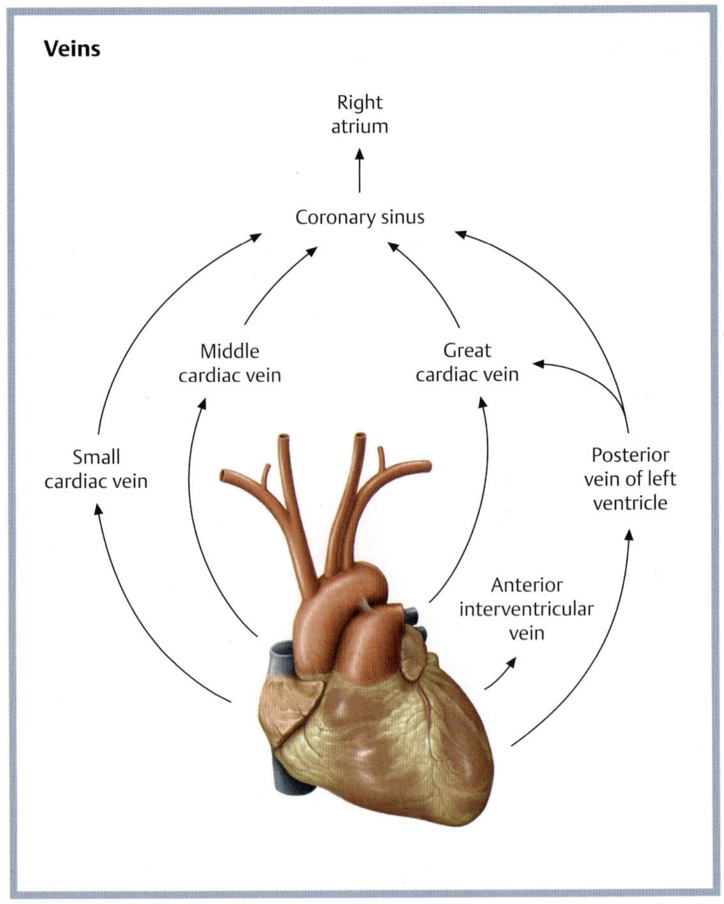
Veins
Right atrium
Coronary sinus
Middle cardiac vein
Great cardiac vein
Small cardiac vein
Posterior vein of left ventricle
Anterior interventricular vein

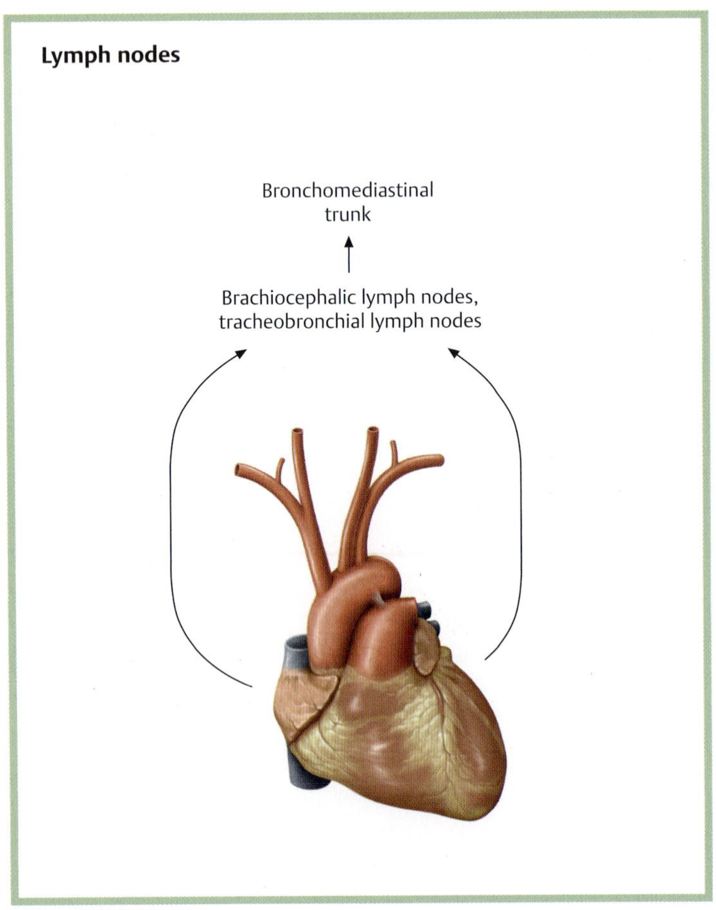
Lymph nodes
Bronchomediastinal trunk
Brachiocephalic lymph nodes, tracheobronchial lymph nodes

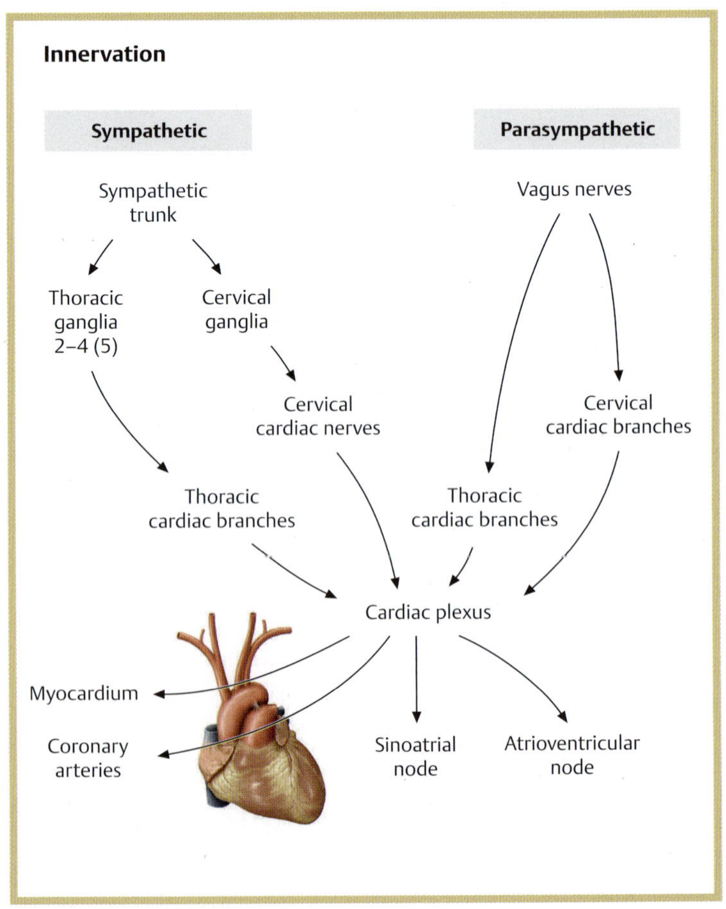
Innervation
Sympathetic
Parasympathetic
Sympathetic trunk
Vagus nerves
Thoracic ganglia 2–4 (5)
Cervical ganglia
Cervical cardiac nerves
Cervical cardiac branches
Thoracic cardiac branches
Thoracic cardiac branches
Cardiac plexus
Myocardium
Coronary arteries
Sinoatrial node
Atrioventricular node

1.4 Pericardium

Arteries

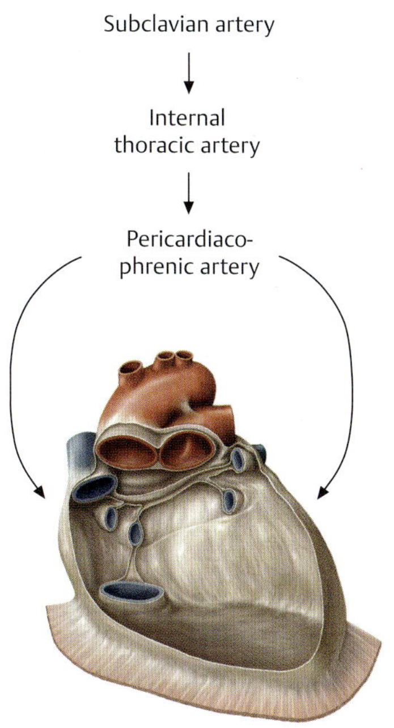

Veins

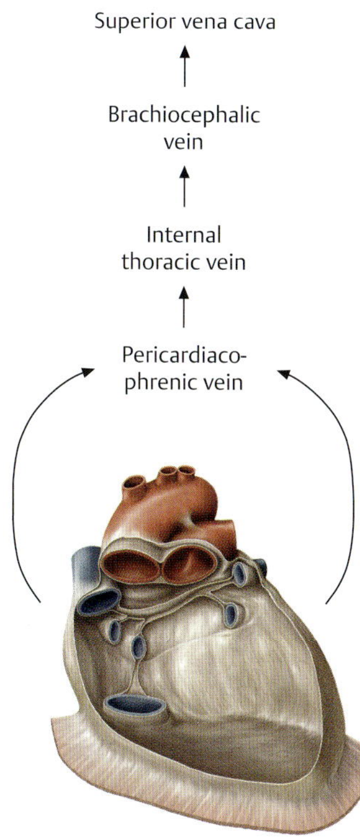

Lymph nodes

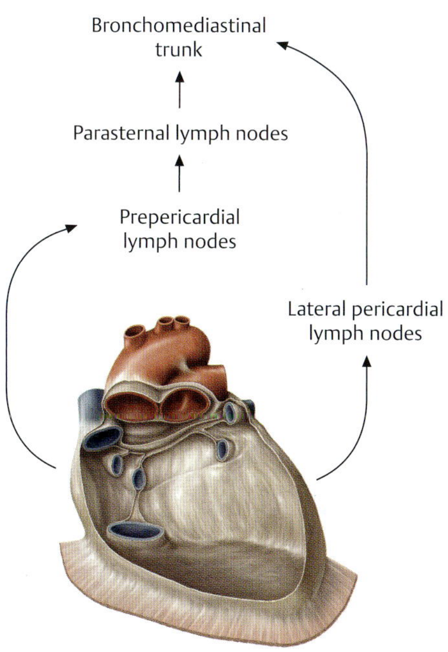

Innervation

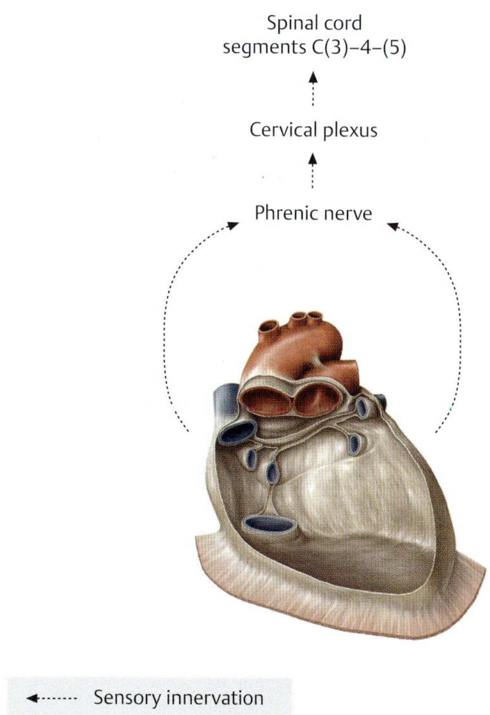

1.5 Lung, Bronchi, and Trachea

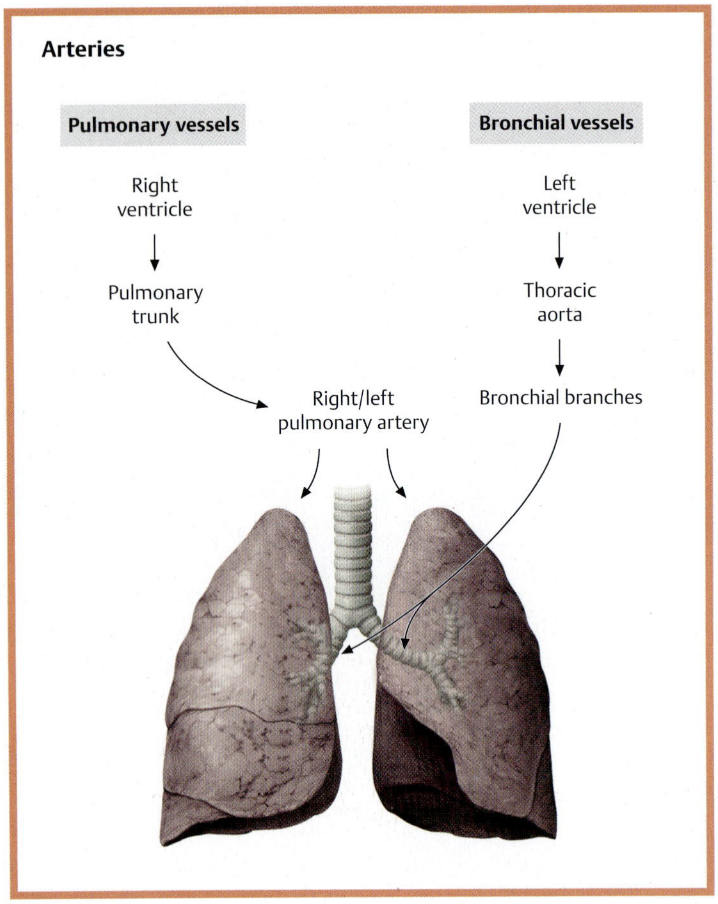

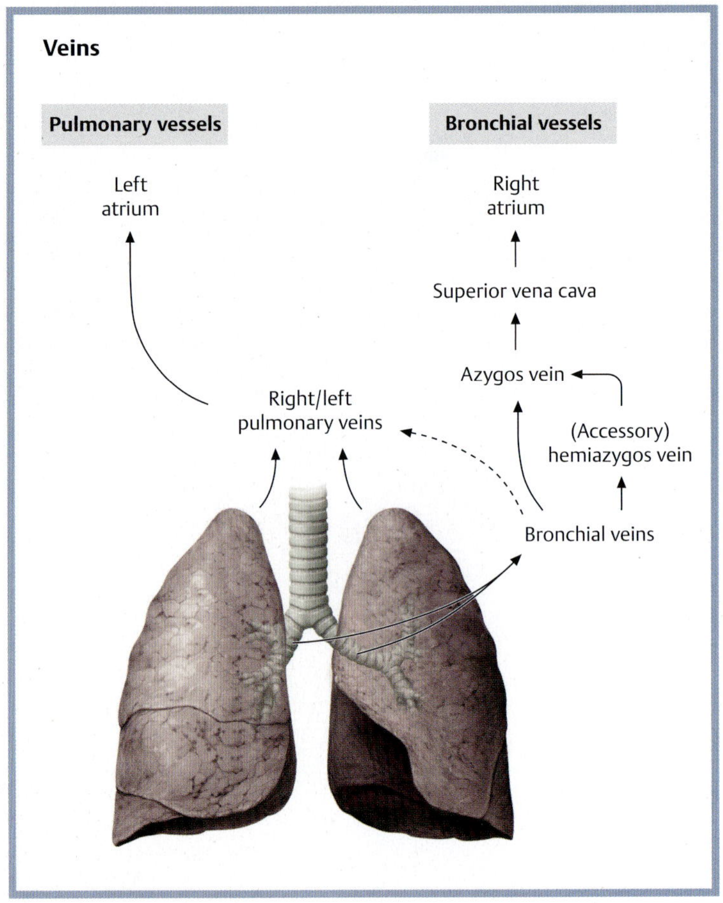

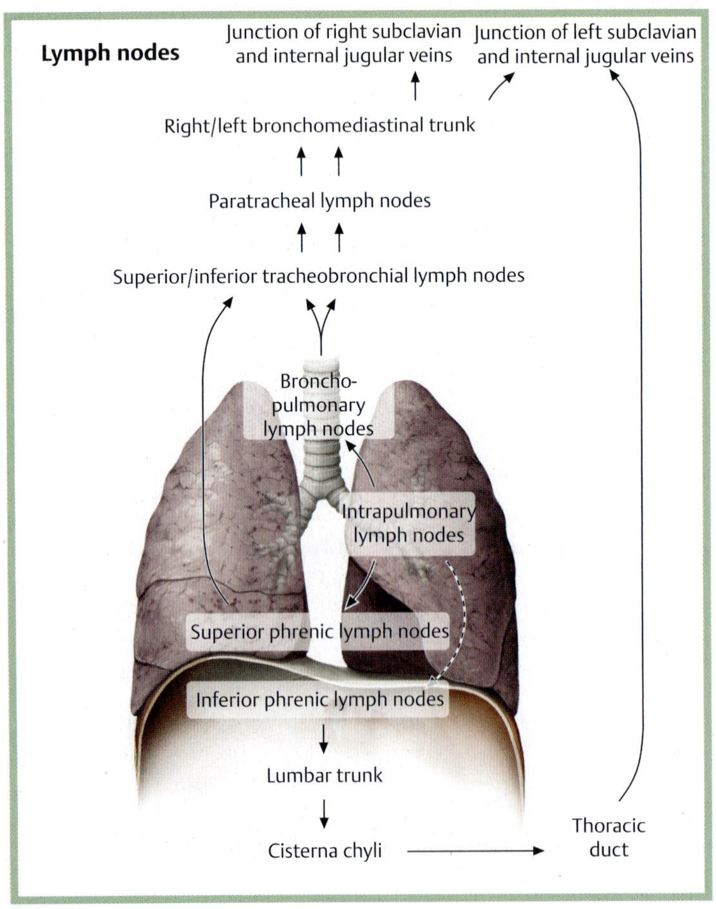

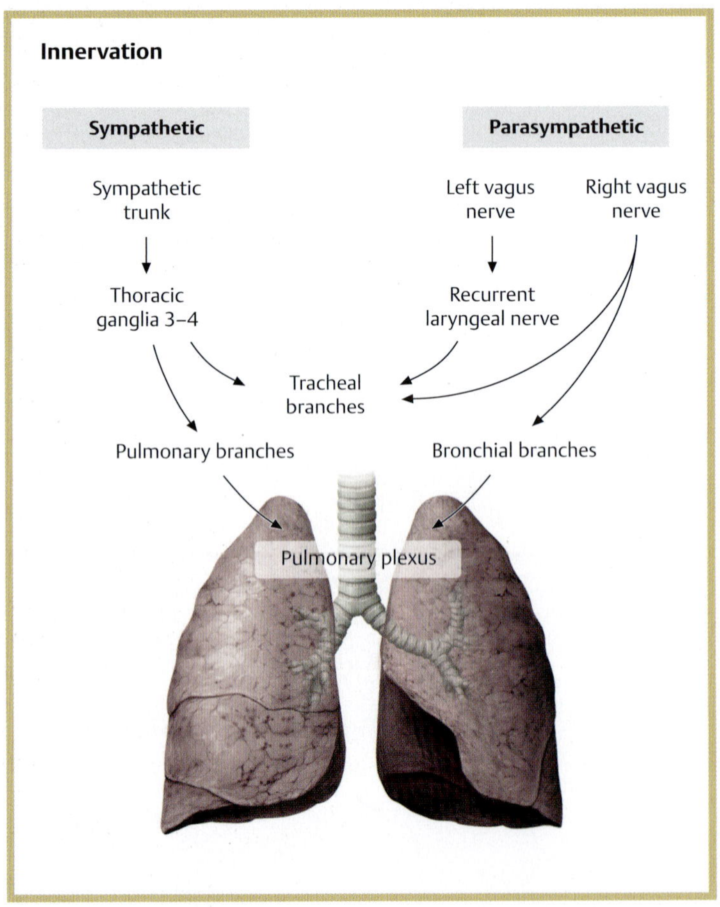

1.6 Diaphragm

Arteries

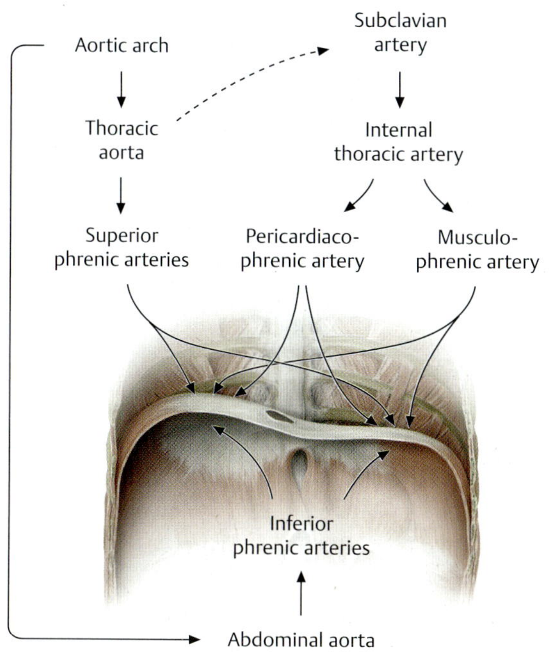

Veins

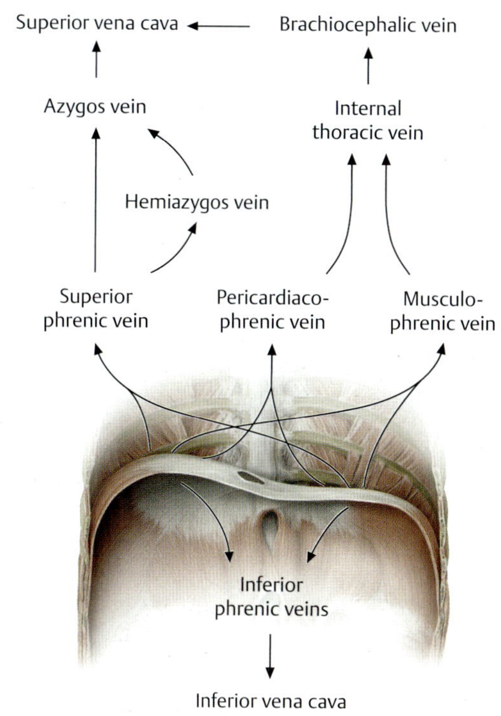

Lymph nodes

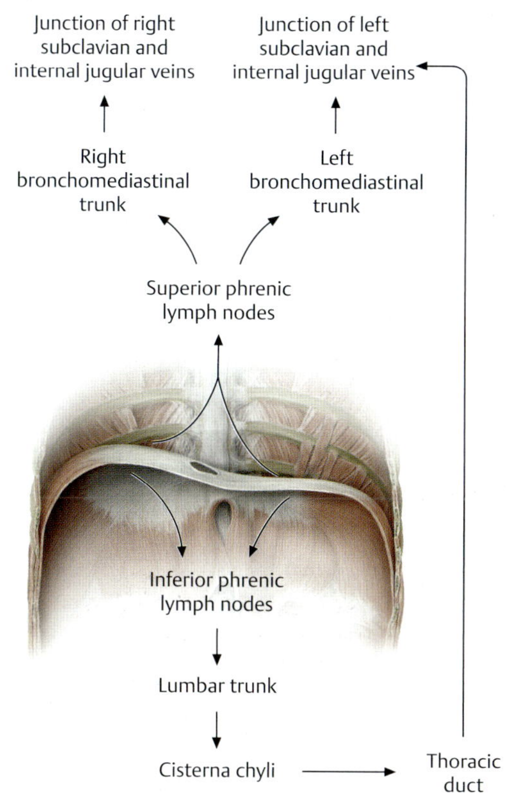

Innervation

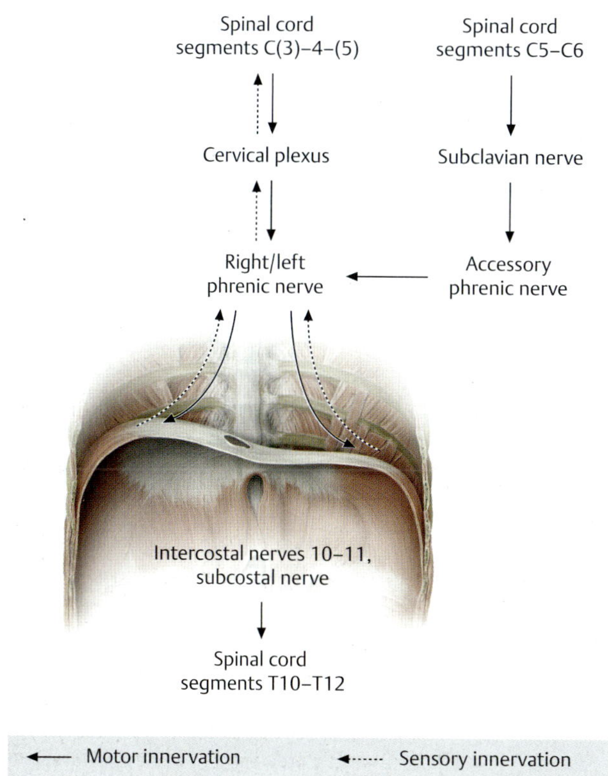

1.7 Liver, Gallbladder, and Spleen

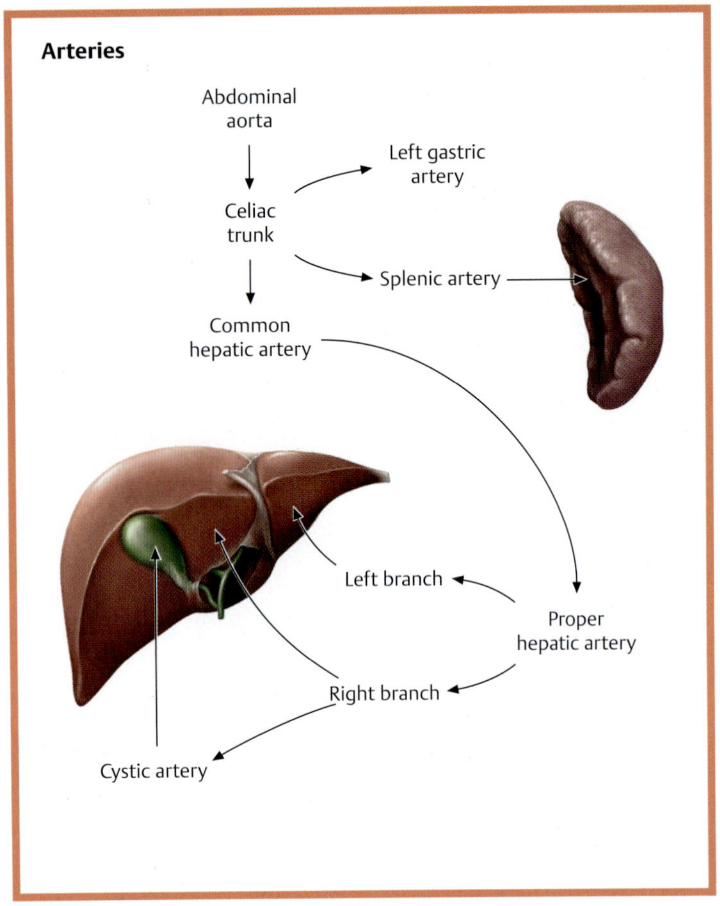

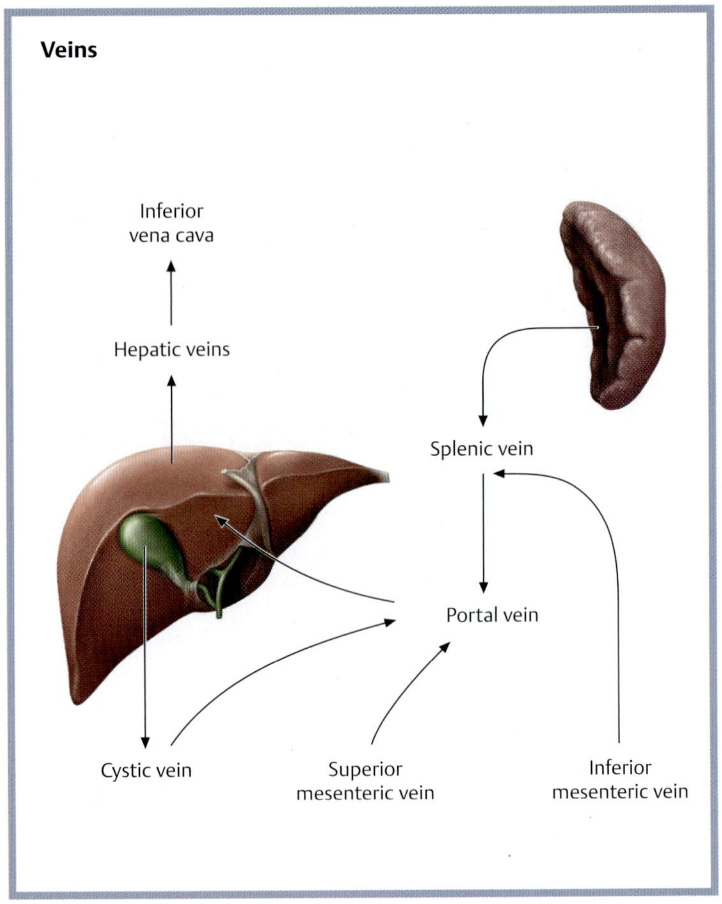

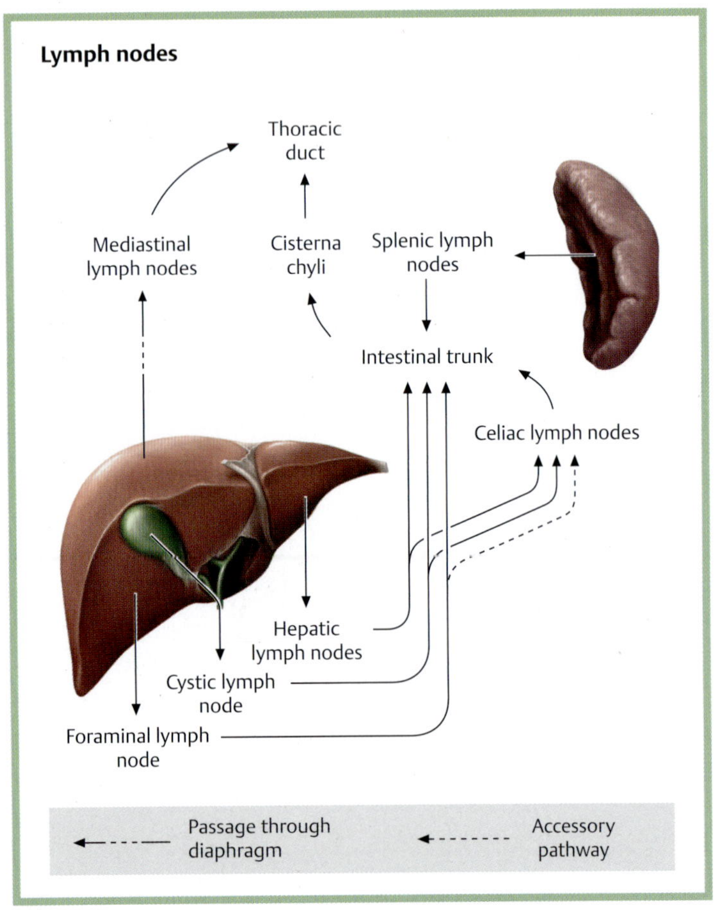

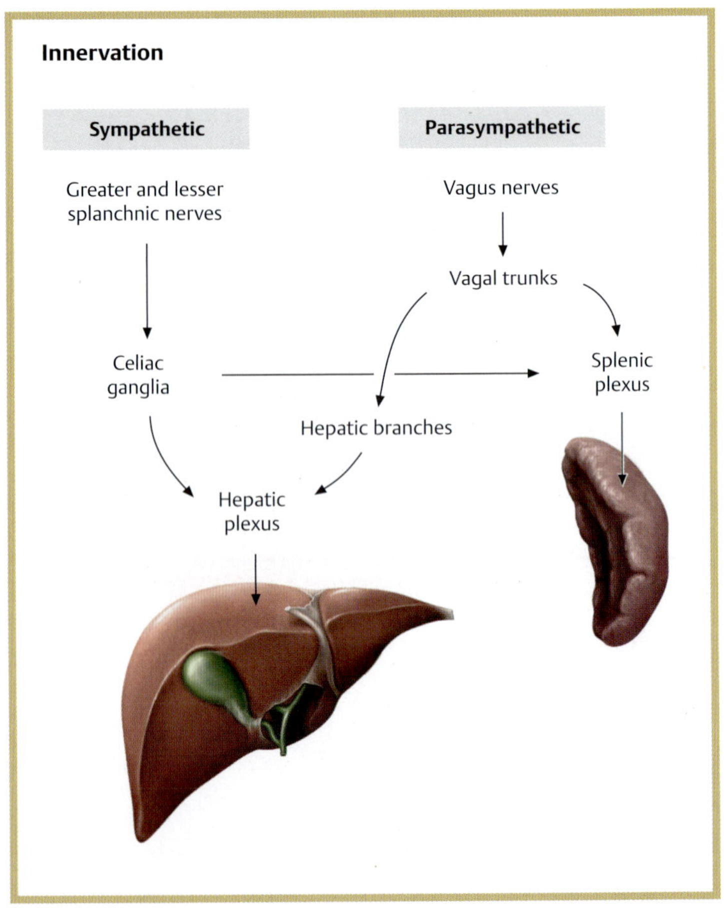

1.8 Stomach

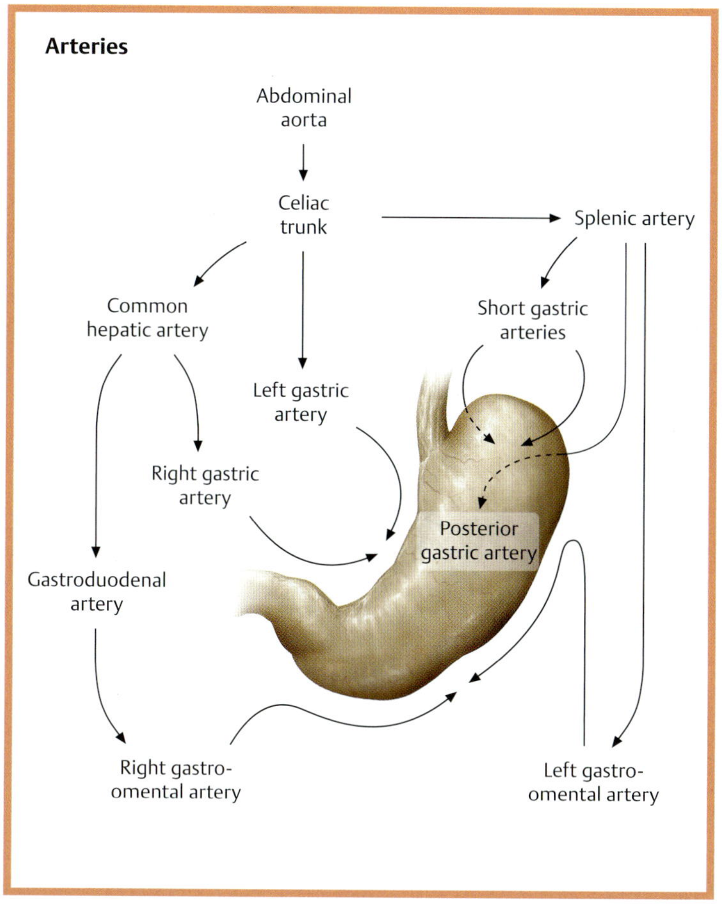
Arteries
Abdominal aorta
Celiac trunk
Splenic artery
Common hepatic artery
Short gastric arteries
Left gastric artery
Right gastric artery
Posterior gastric artery
Gastroduodenal artery
Right gastro-omental artery
Left gastro-omental artery

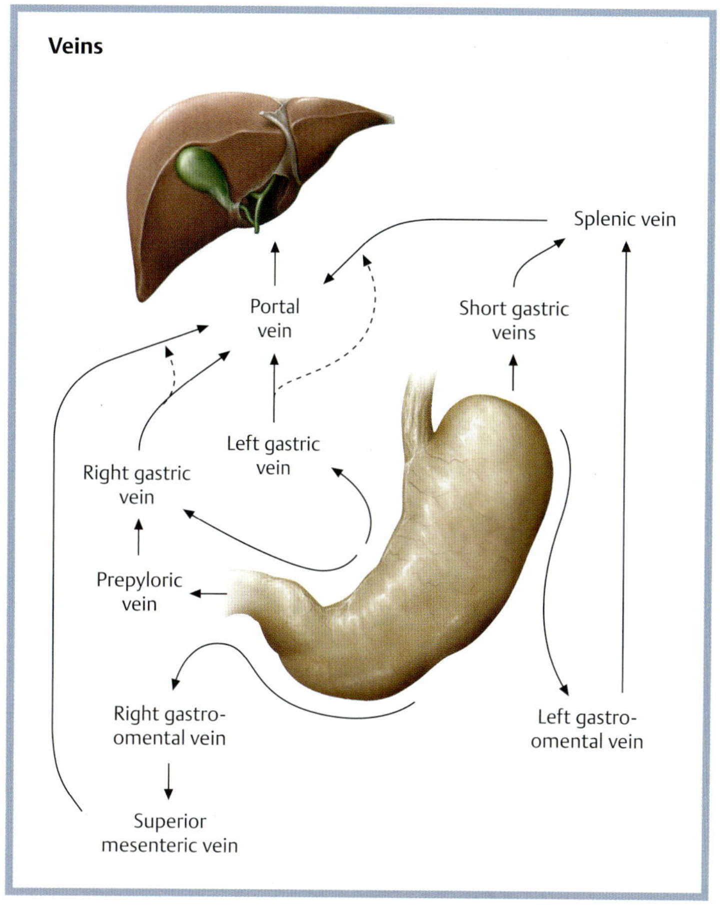
Veins
Splenic vein
Portal vein
Short gastric veins
Left gastric vein
Right gastric vein
Prepyloric vein
Right gastro-omental vein
Left gastro-omental vein
Superior mesenteric vein

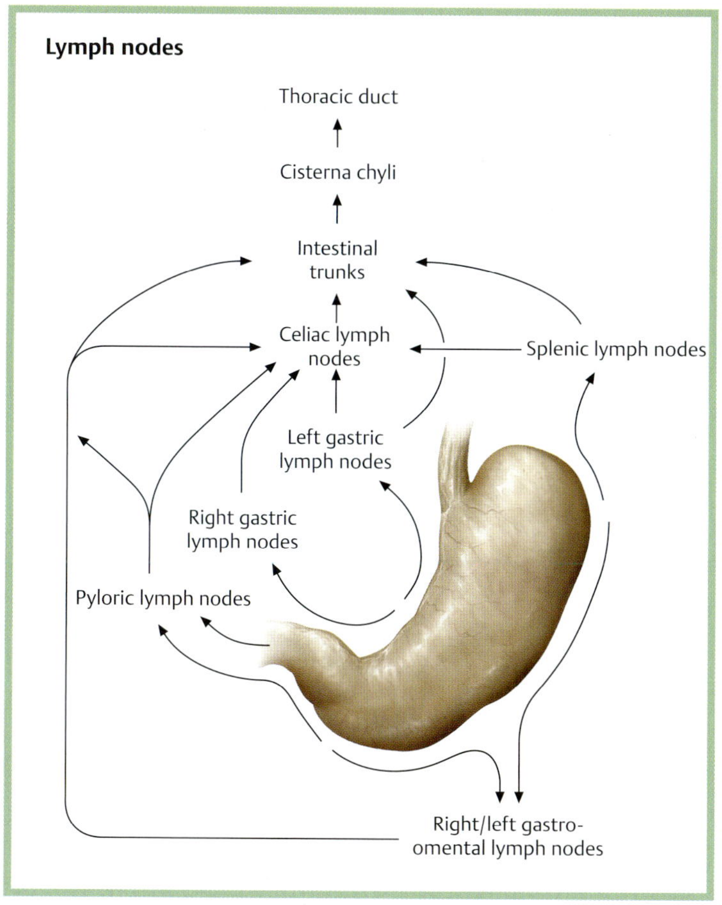
Lymph nodes
Thoracic duct
Cisterna chyli
Intestinal trunks
Celiac lymph nodes
Splenic lymph nodes
Left gastric lymph nodes
Right gastric lymph nodes
Pyloric lymph nodes
Right/left gastro-omental lymph nodes

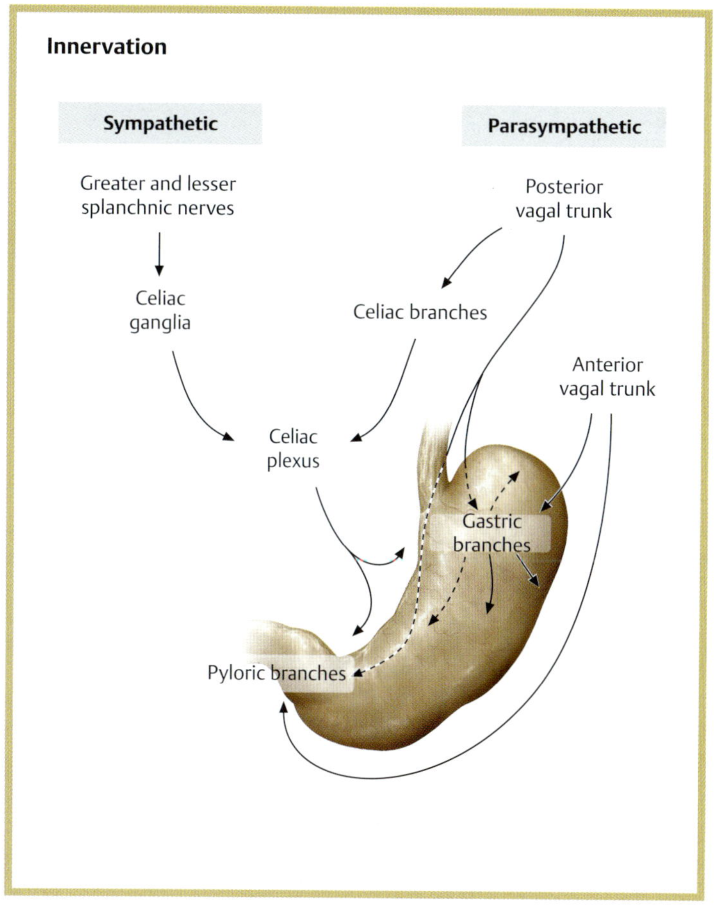
Innervation
Sympathetic
Parasympathetic
Greater and lesser splanchnic nerves
Posterior vagal trunk
Celiac ganglia
Celiac branches
Anterior vagal trunk
Celiac plexus
Gastric branches
Pyloric branches

1.9 Duodenum and Pancreas

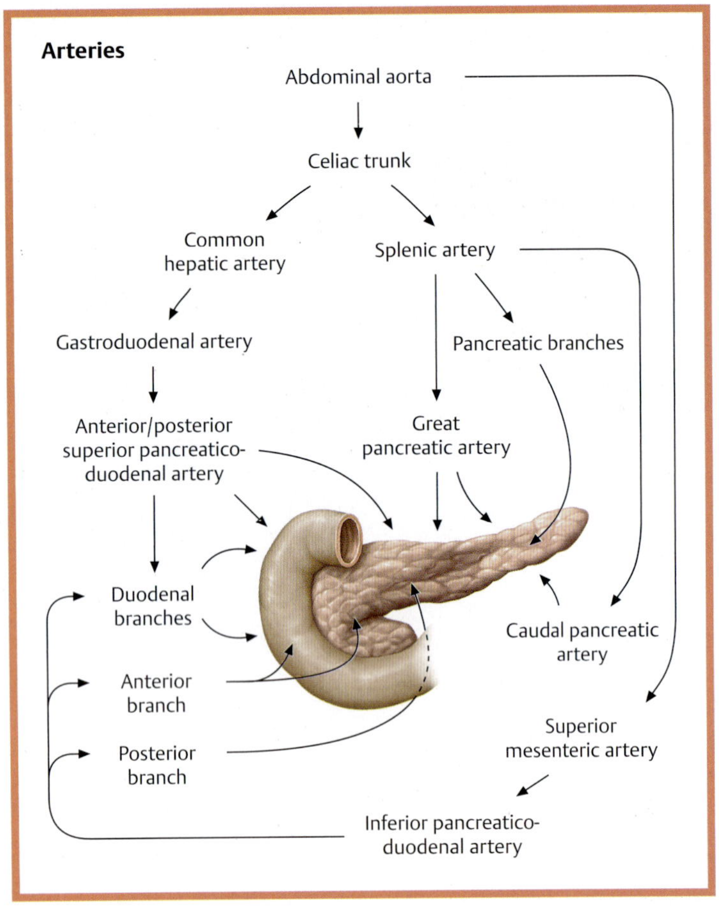

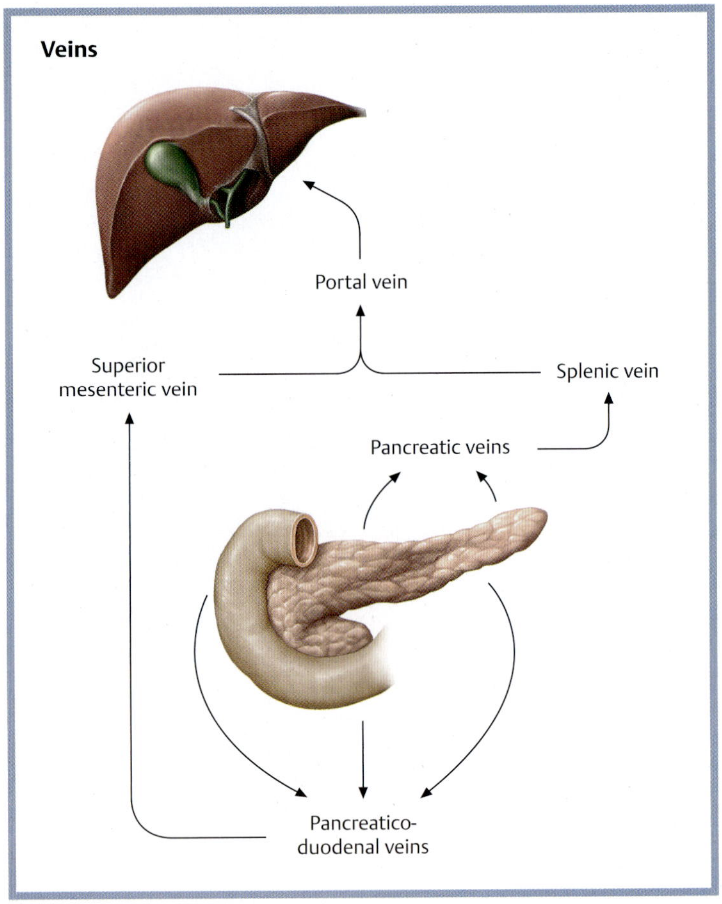

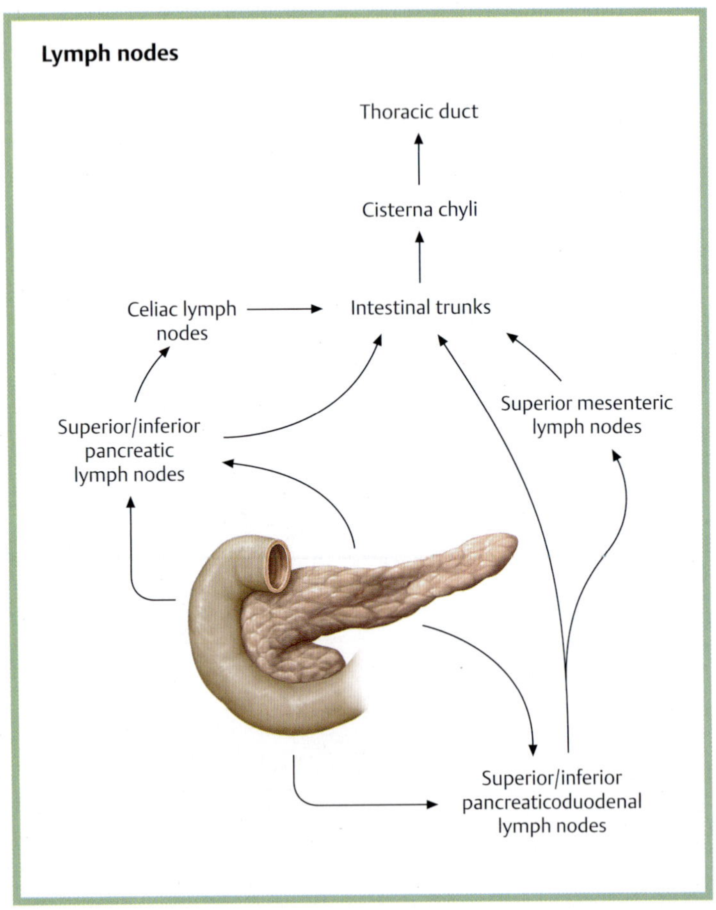

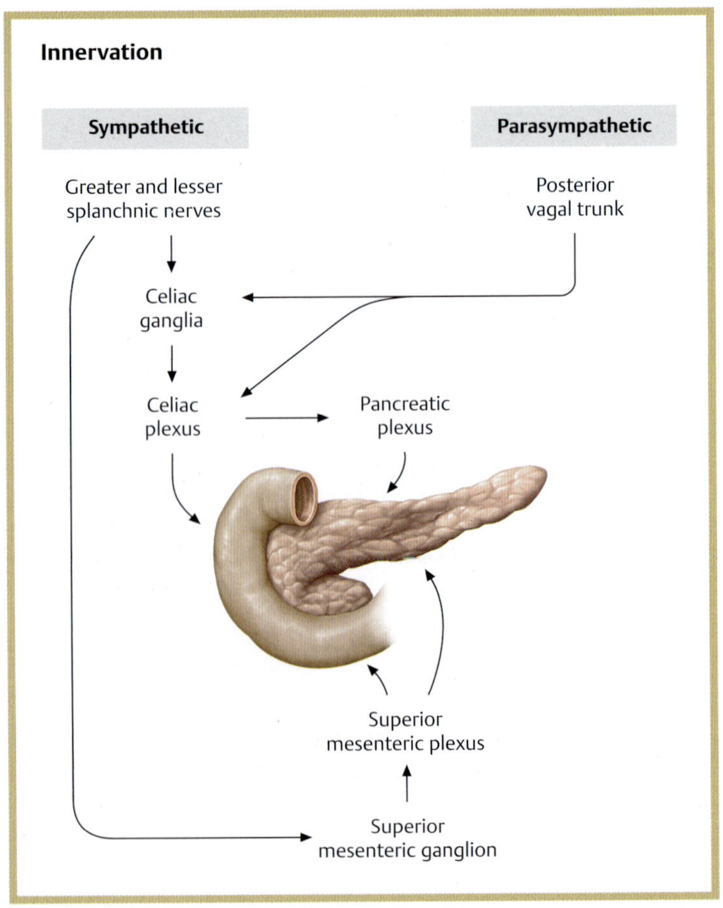

1.10 Jejunum and Ileum

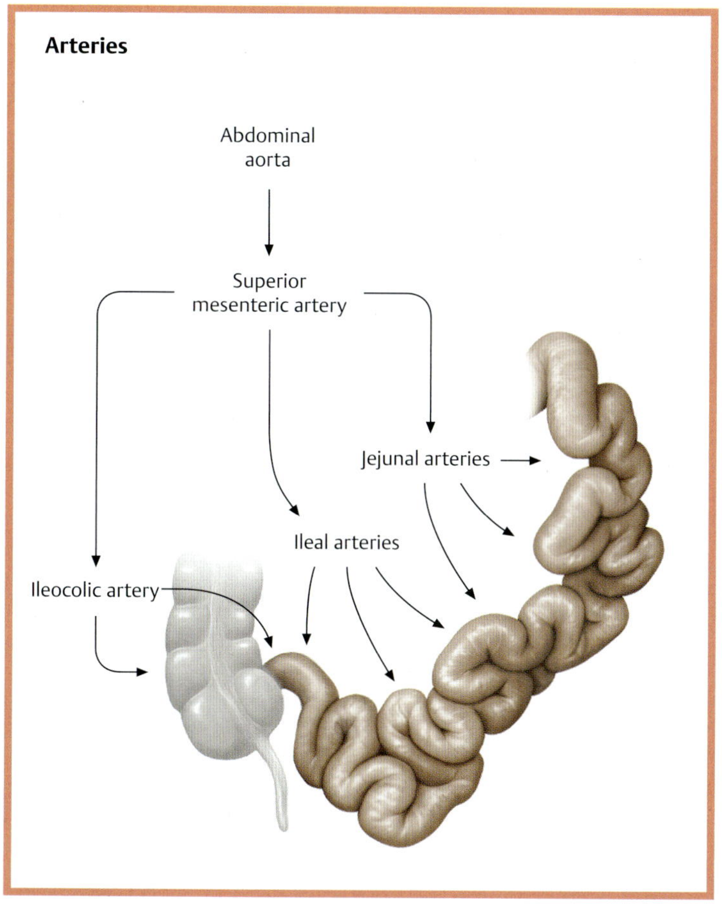

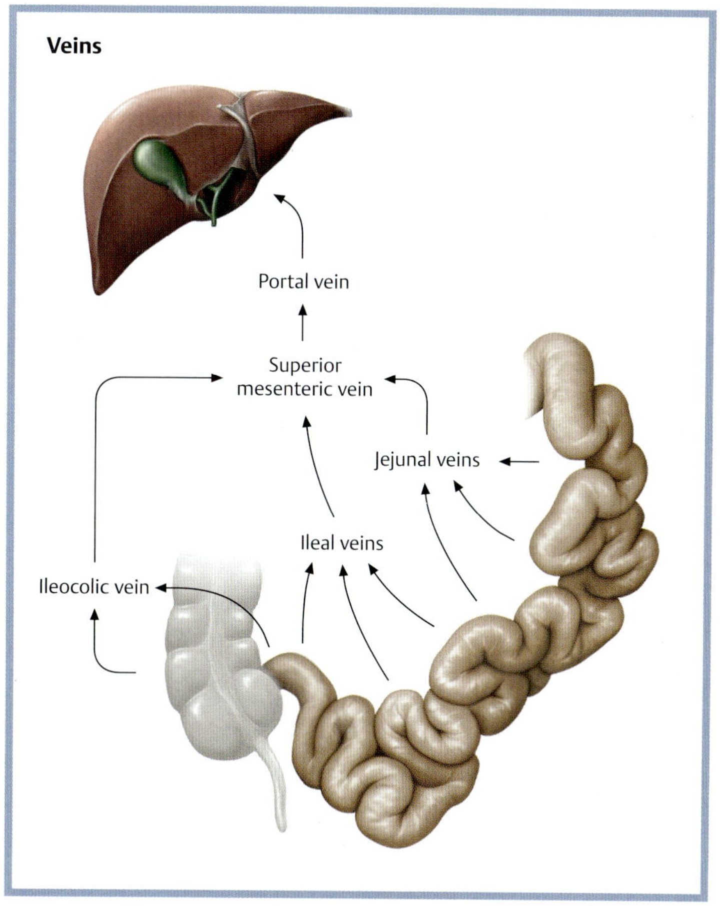

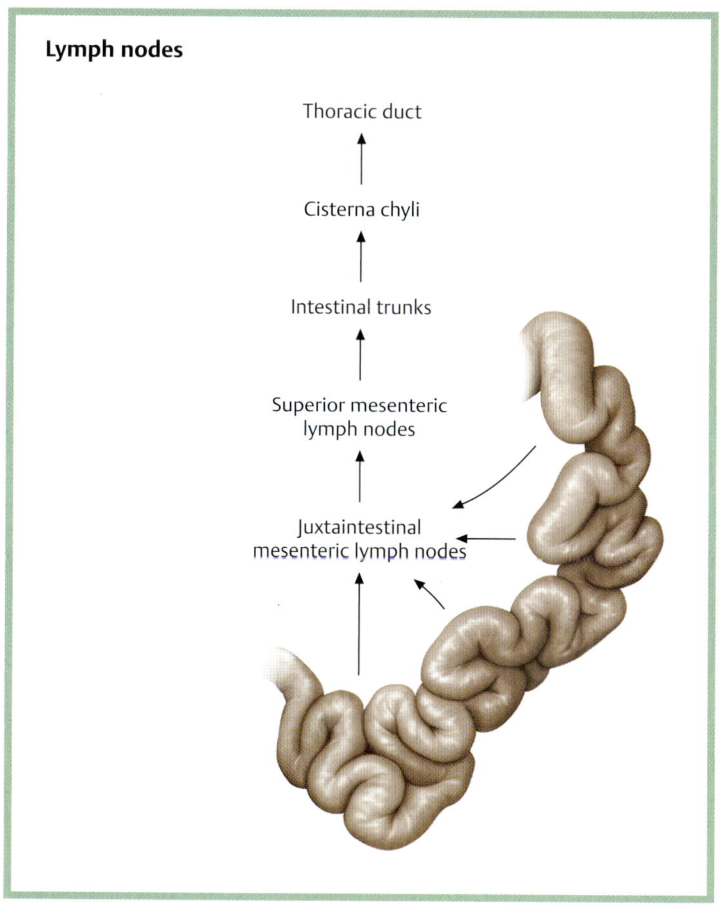

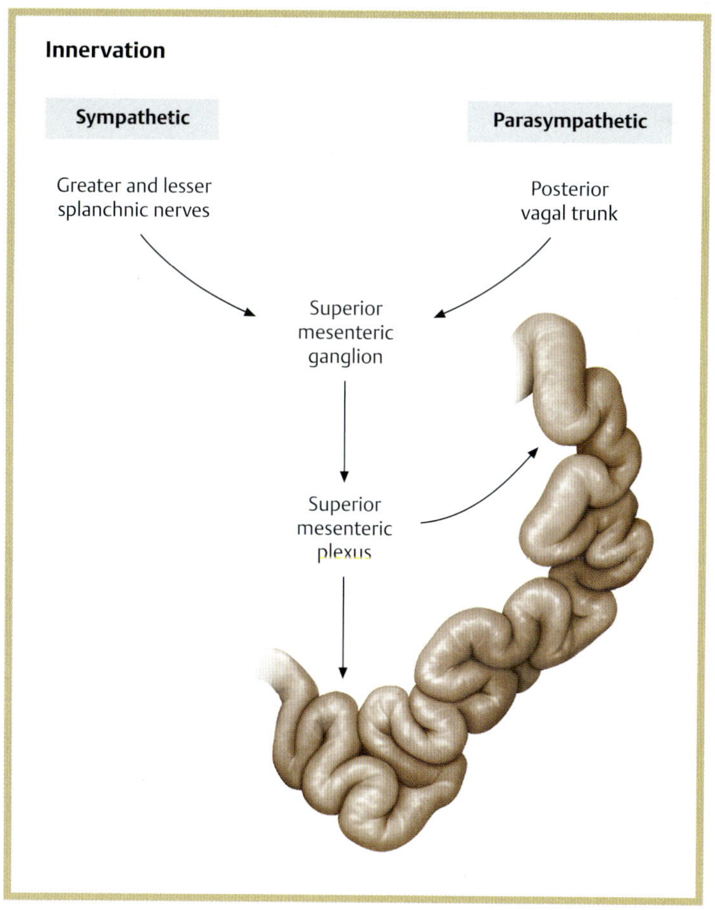

1.11 Cecum, Vermiform Appendix, Ascending and Transverse Colon

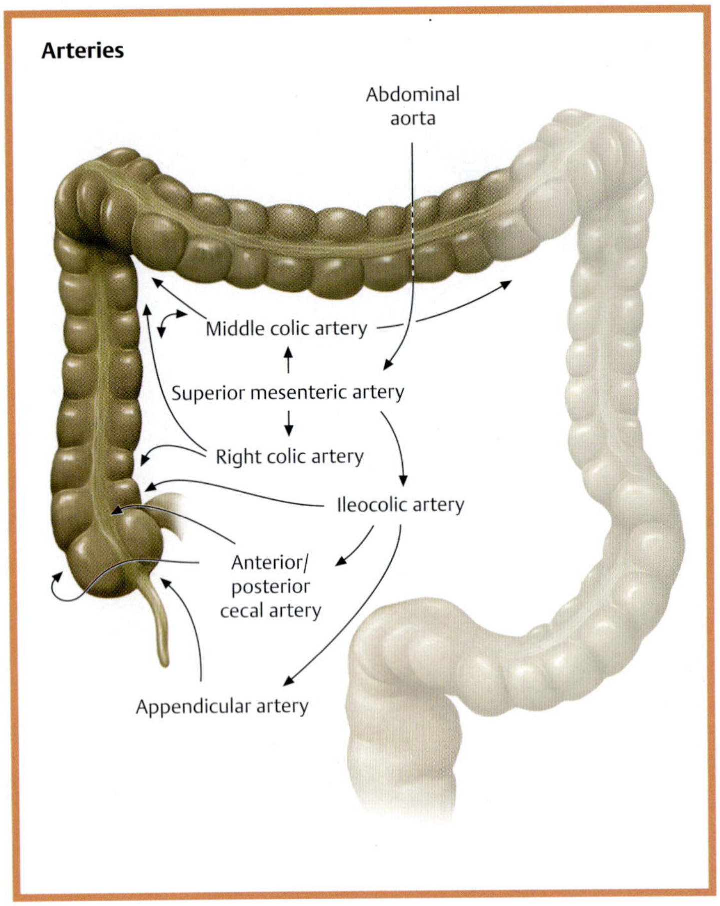

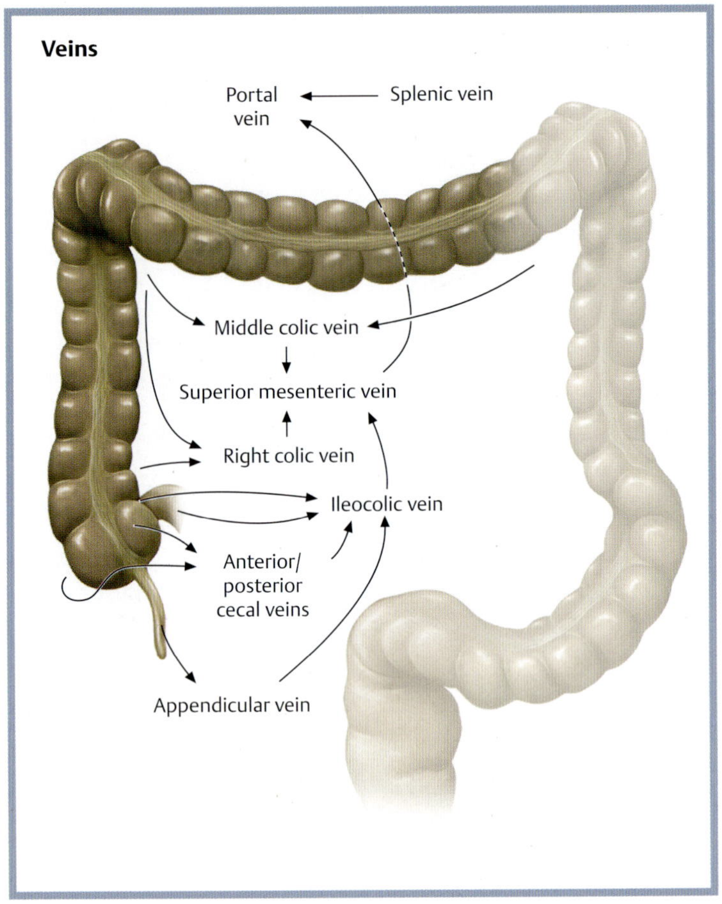

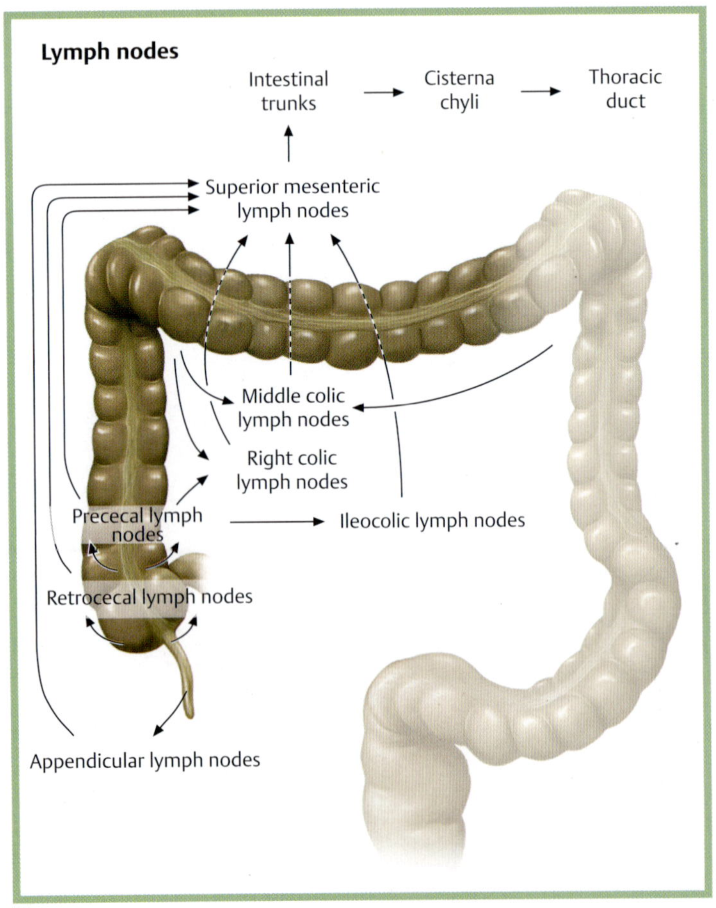

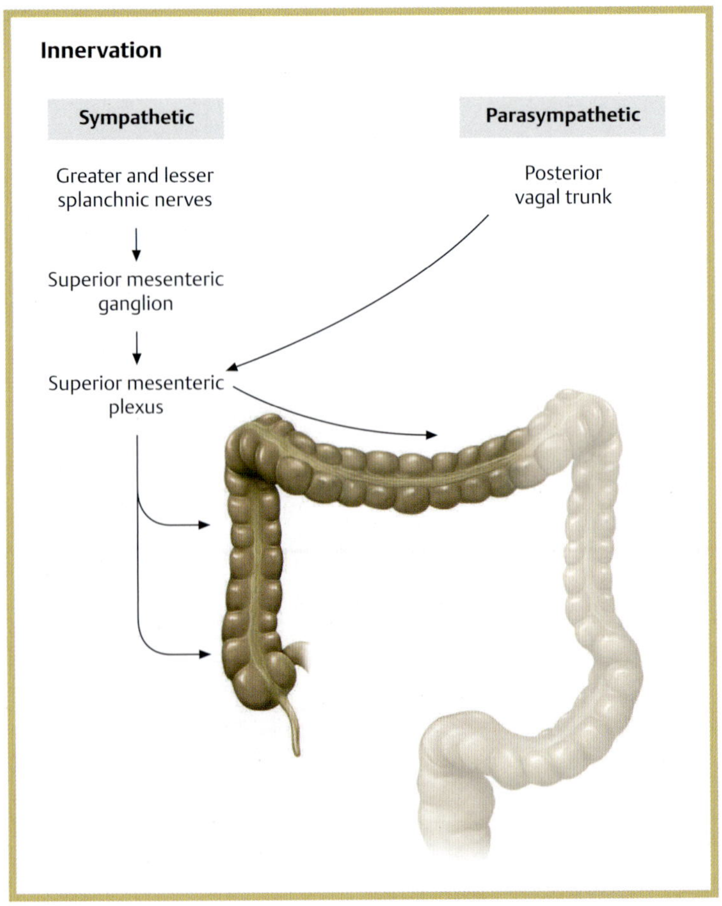

1.12 Descending Colon and Sigmoid Colon

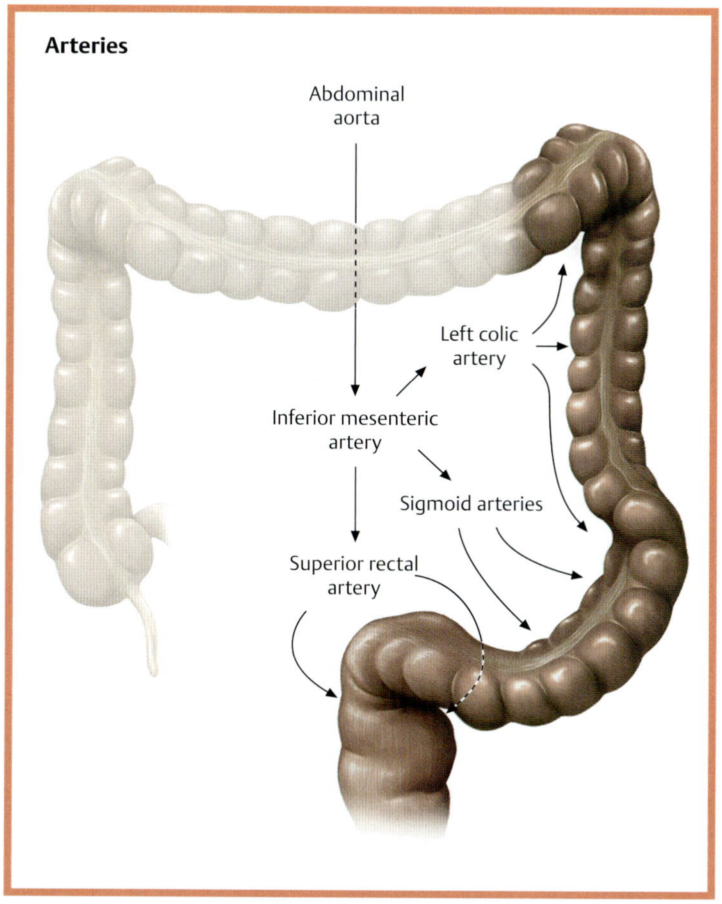

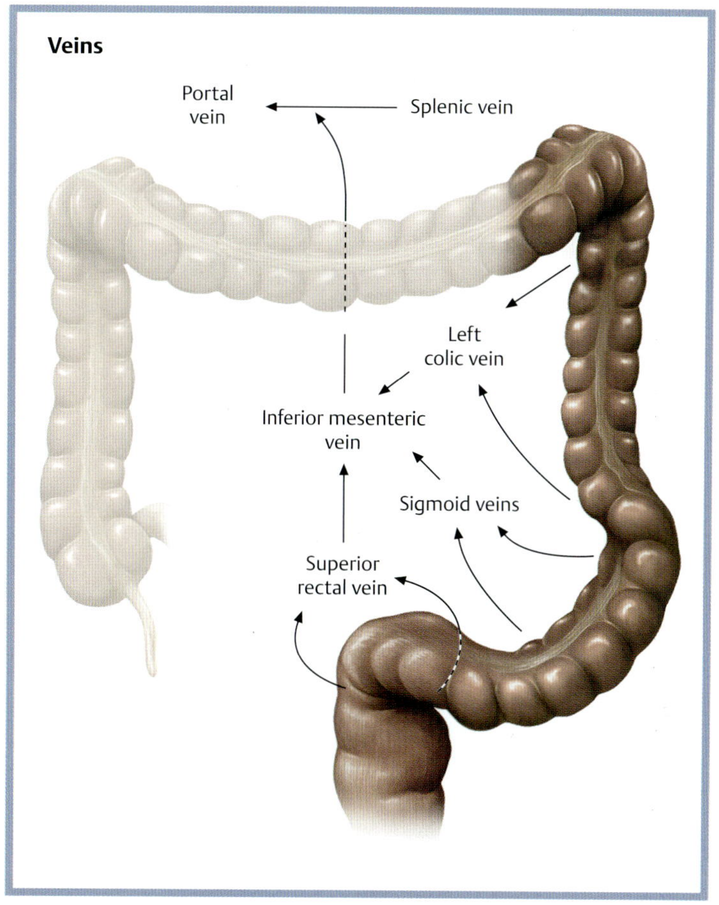

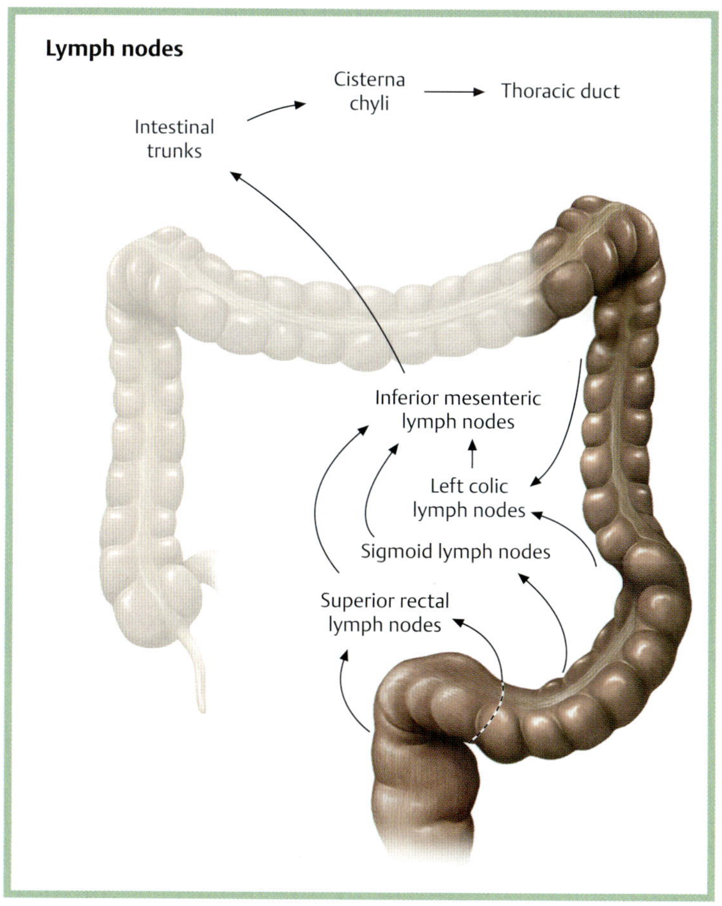

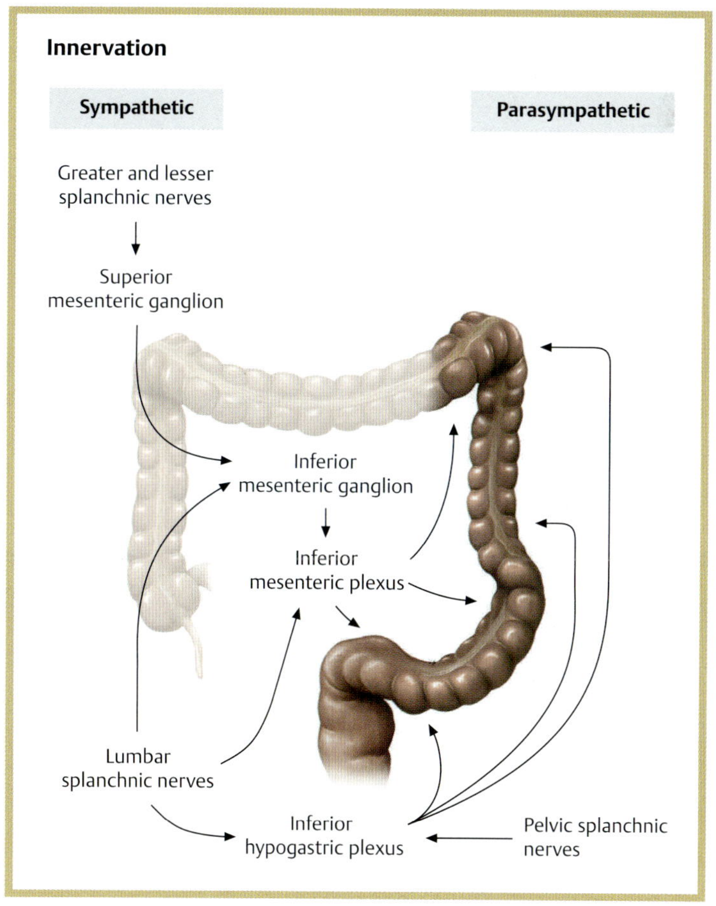

1.13 Rectum

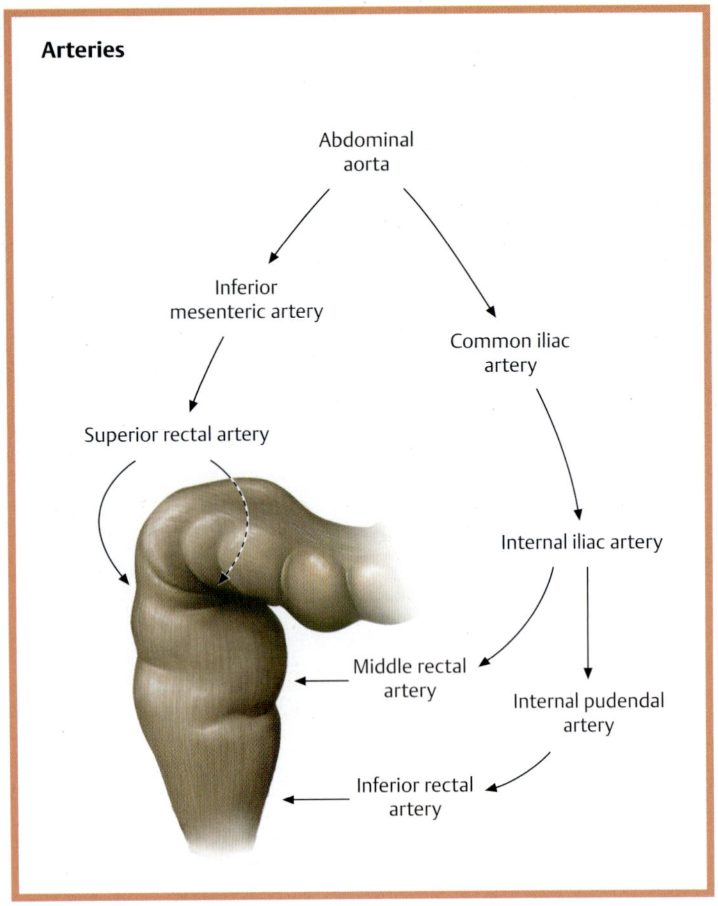
Arteries
Abdominal aorta
Inferior mesenteric artery
Common iliac artery
Superior rectal artery
Internal iliac artery
Middle rectal artery
Internal pudendal artery
Inferior rectal artery

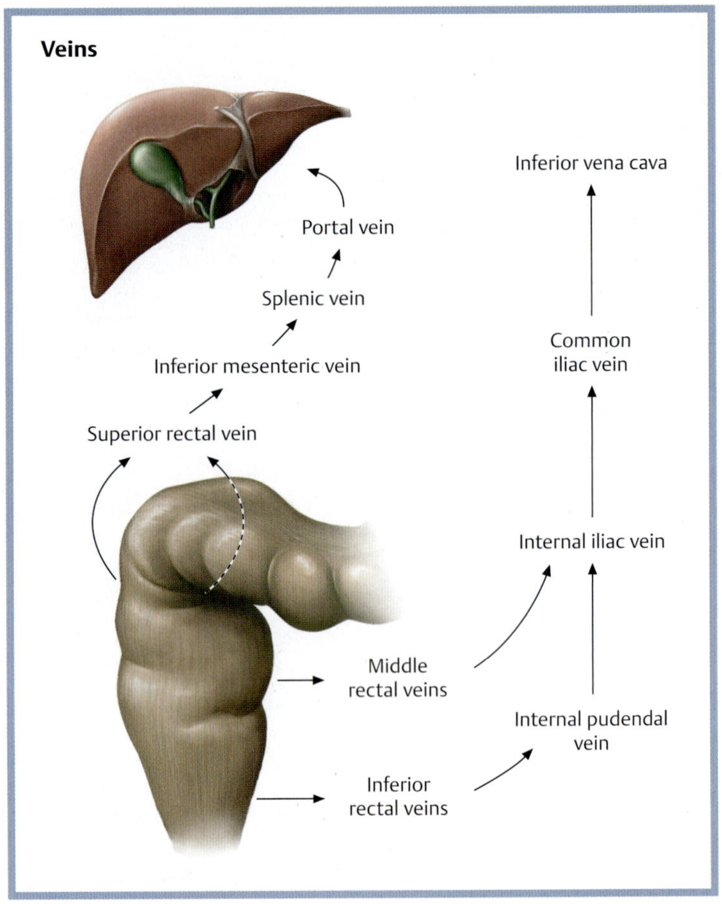
Veins
Inferior vena cava
Portal vein
Splenic vein
Inferior mesenteric vein
Common iliac vein
Superior rectal vein
Internal iliac vein
Middle rectal veins
Internal pudendal vein
Inferior rectal veins

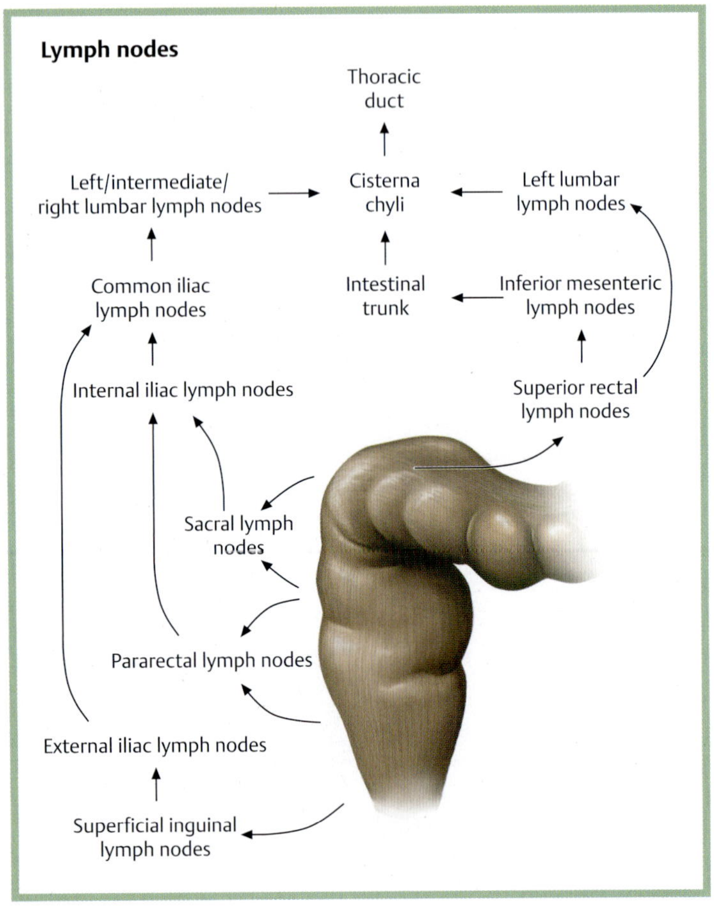
Lymph nodes
Thoracic duct
Left/intermediate/ right lumbar lymph nodes
Cisterna chyli
Left lumbar lymph nodes
Common iliac lymph nodes
Intestinal trunk
Inferior mesenteric lymph nodes
Internal iliac lymph nodes
Superior rectal lymph nodes
Sacral lymph nodes
Pararectal lymph nodes
External iliac lymph nodes
Superficial inguinal lymph nodes

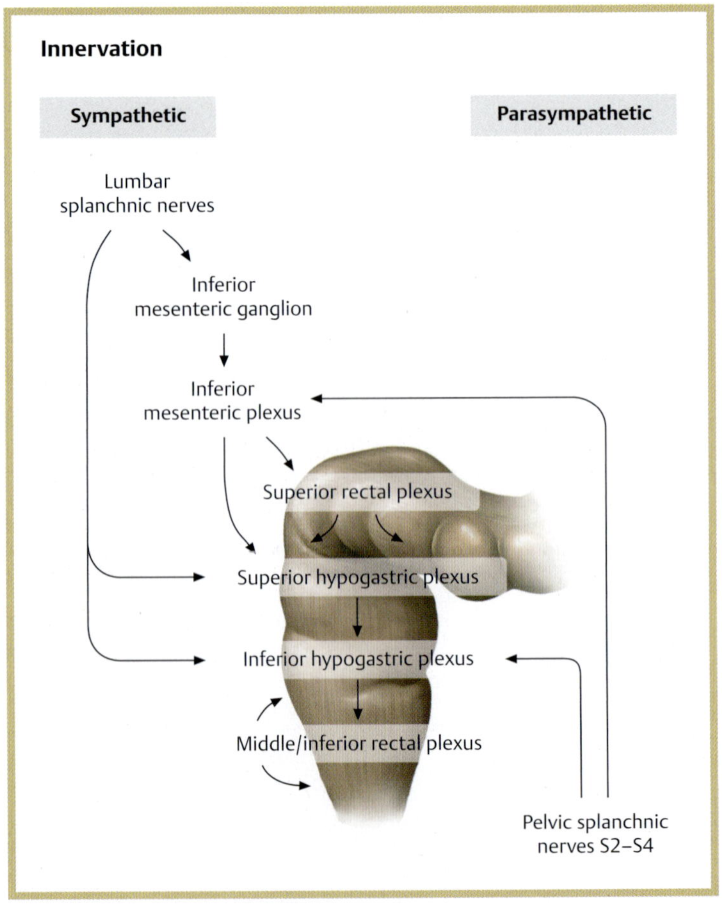
Innervation
Sympathetic
Parasympathetic
Lumbar splanchnic nerves
Inferior mesenteric ganglion
Inferior mesenteric plexus
Superior rectal plexus
Superior hypogastric plexus
Inferior hypogastric plexus
Middle/inferior rectal plexus
Pelvic splanchnic nerves S2–S4

1.14 Kidney, Ureter, and Suprarenal Gland

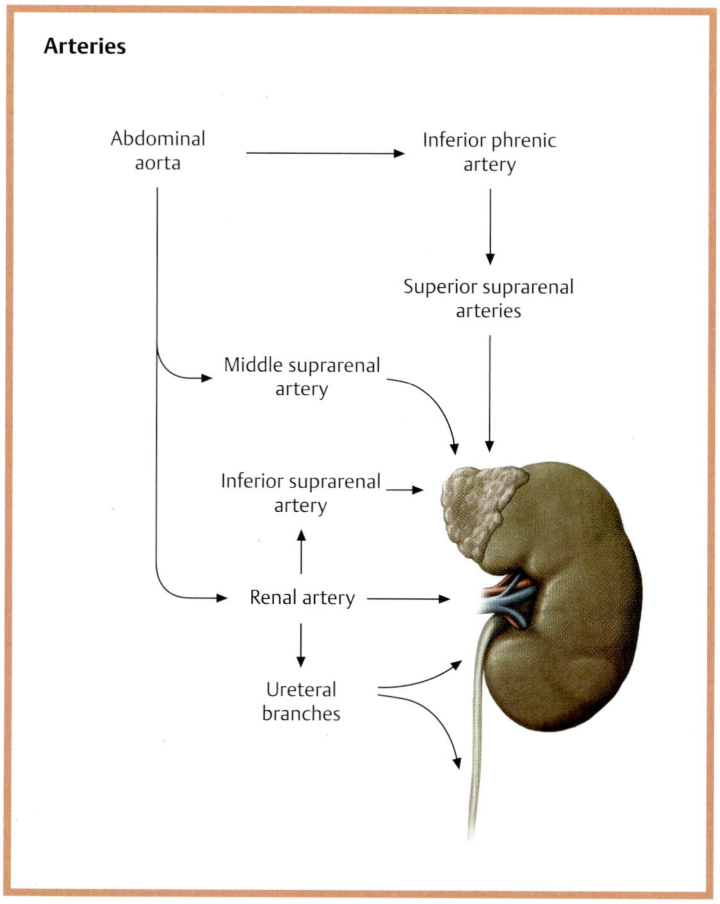

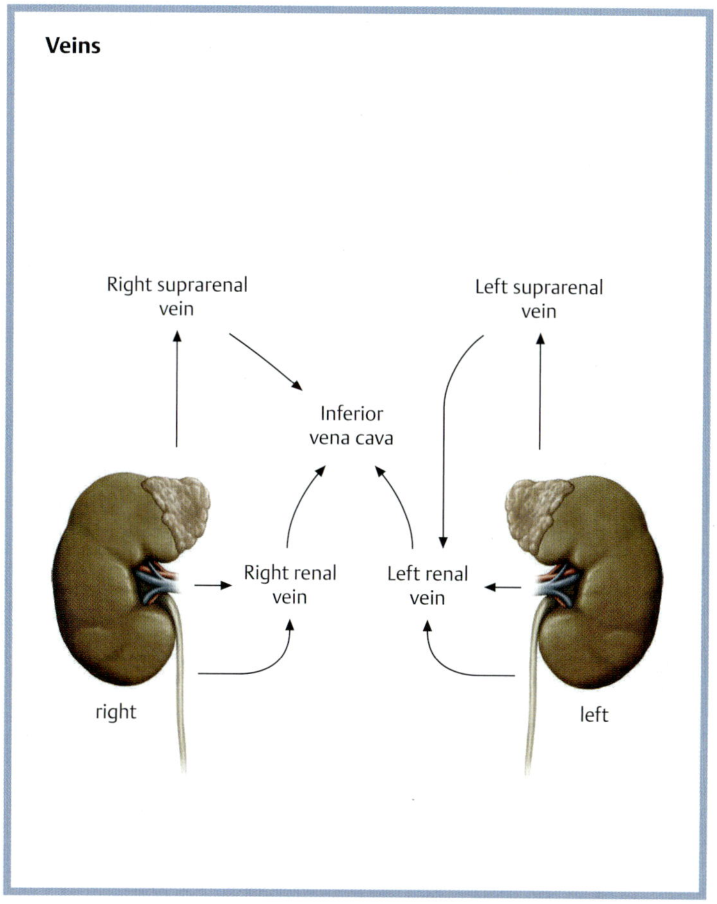

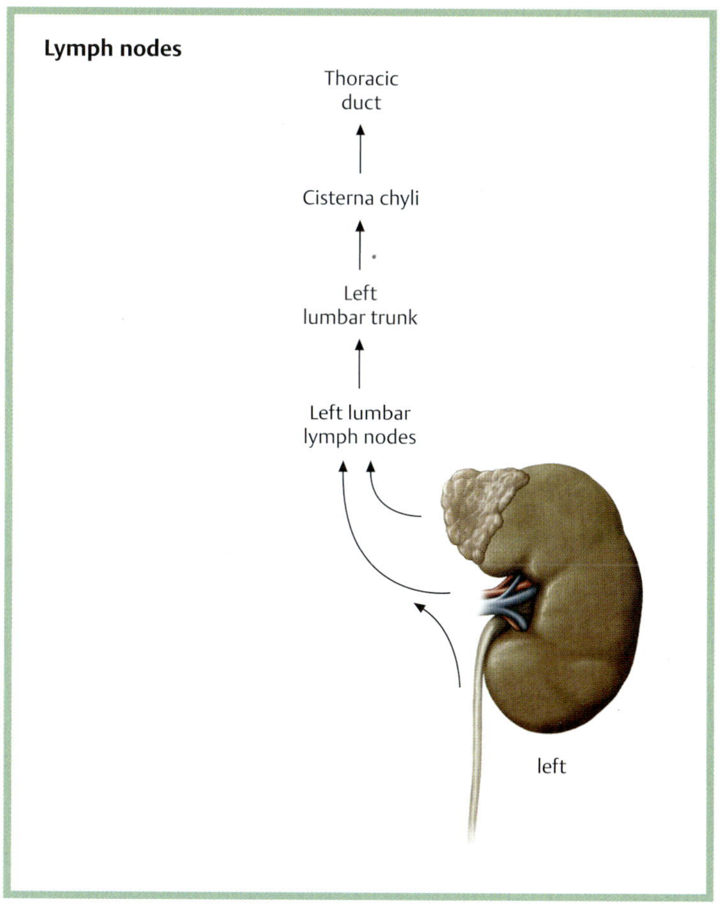

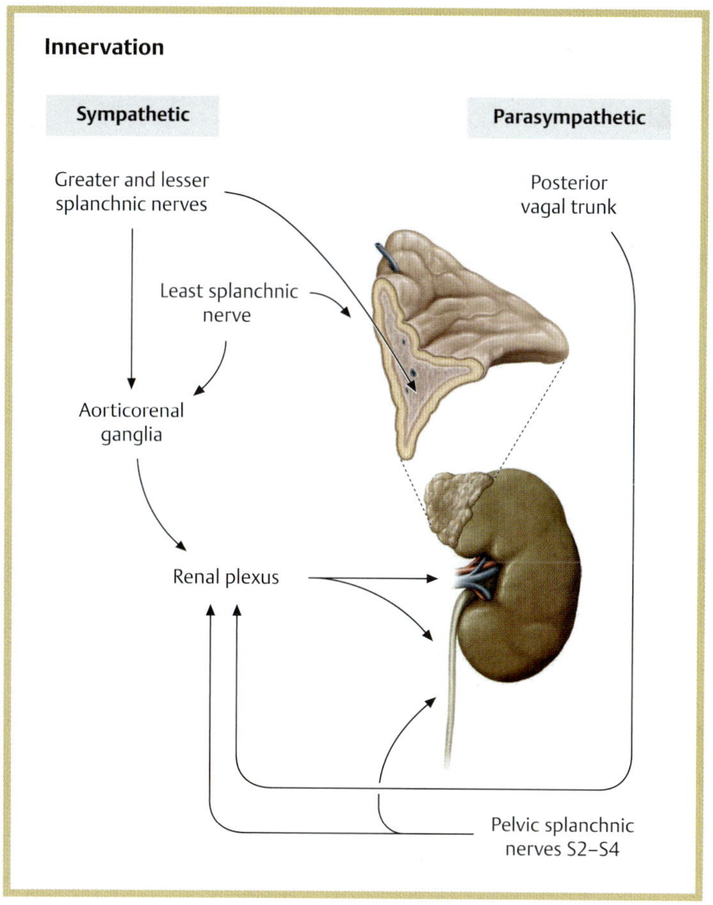

1.15 Urinary Bladder, Prostate, and Seminal Vesicle

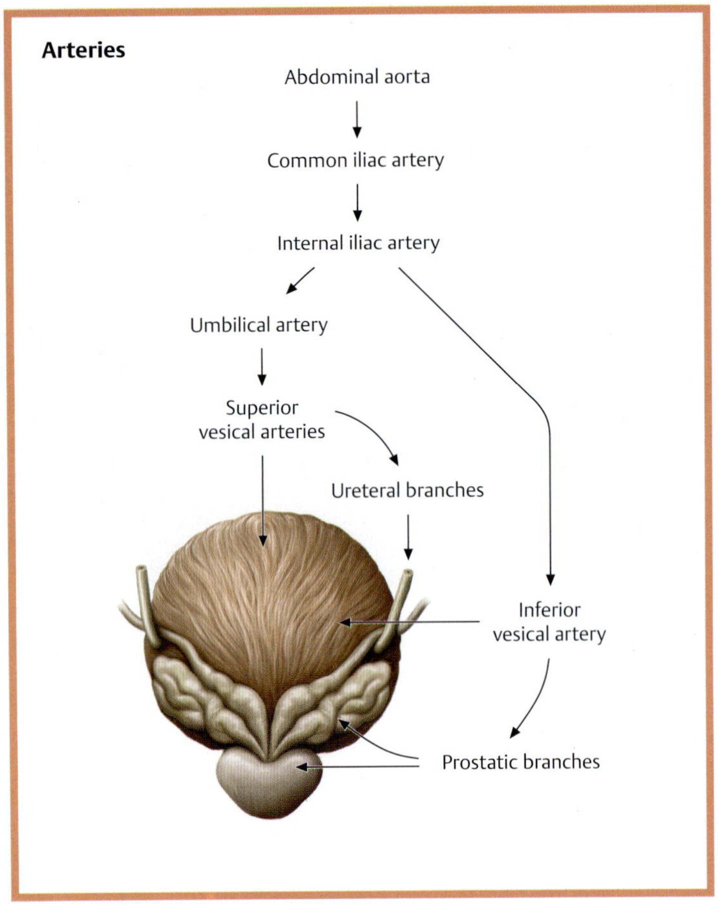

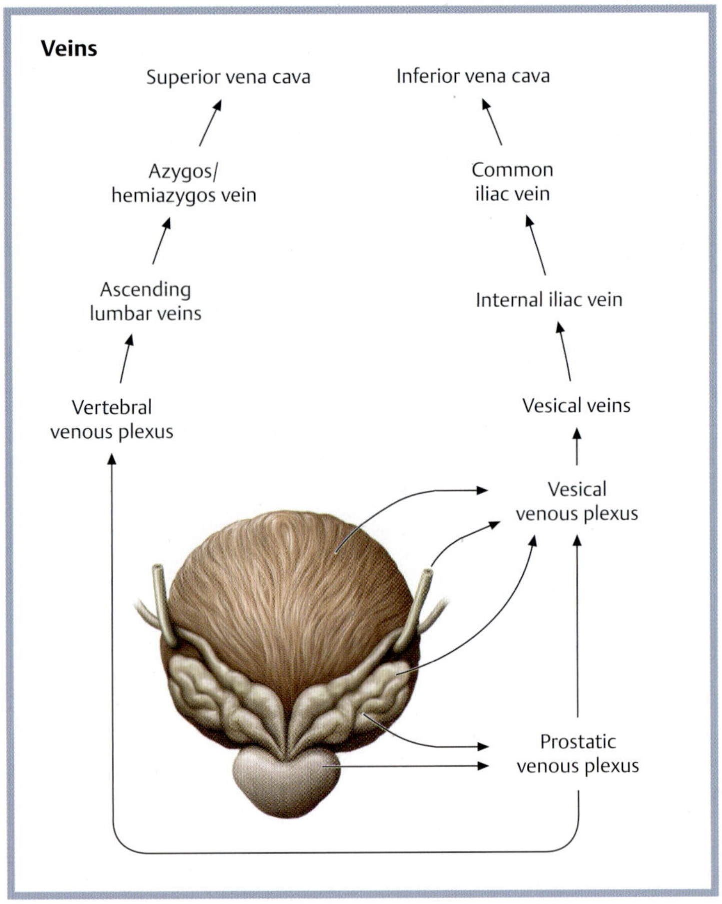

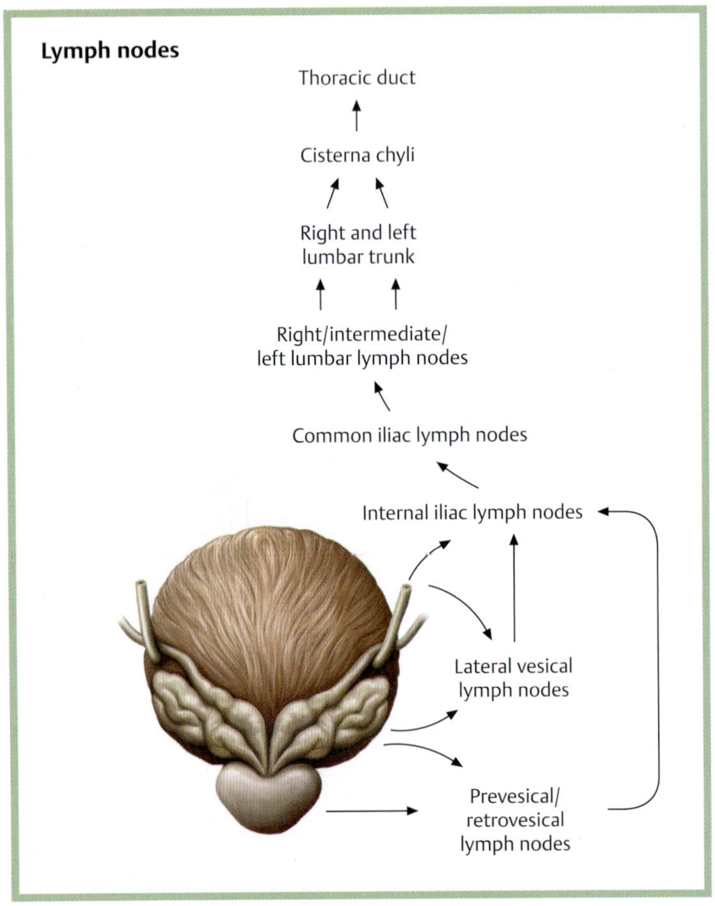

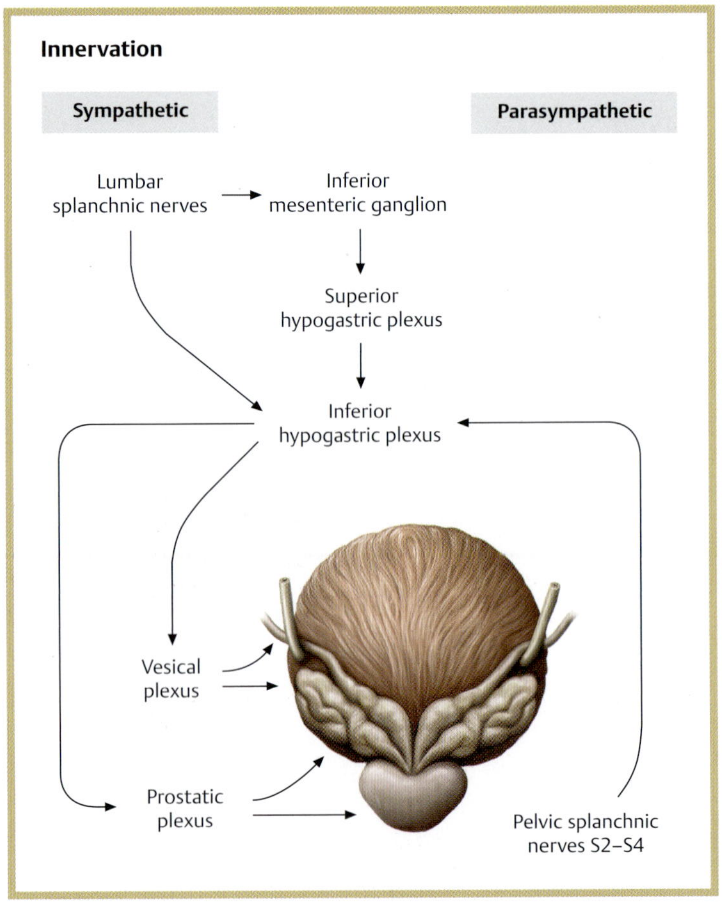

1.16 Testis, Epididymis, and Ductus Deferens

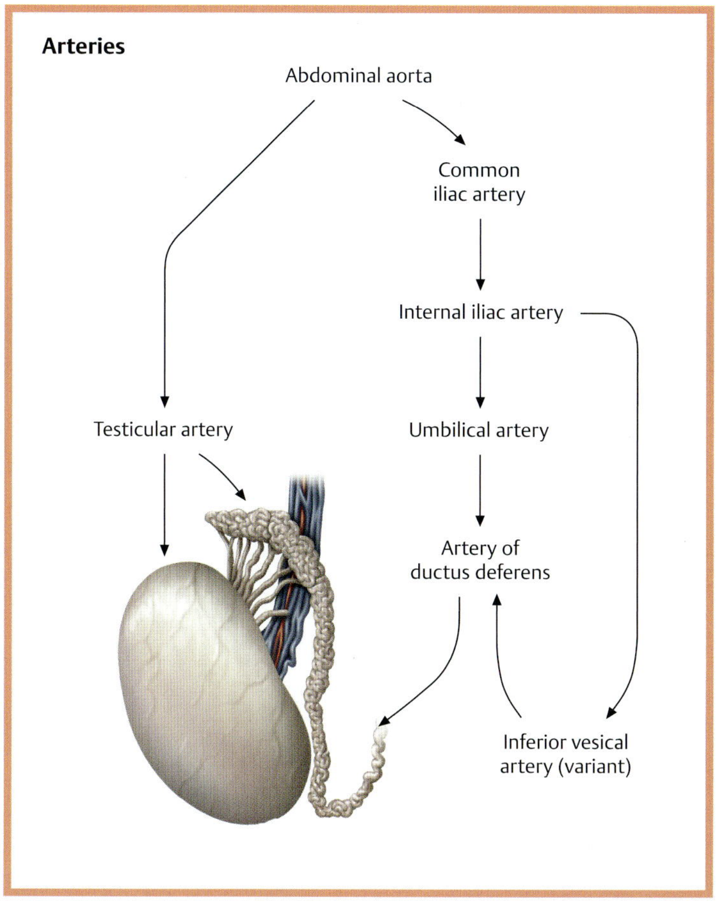

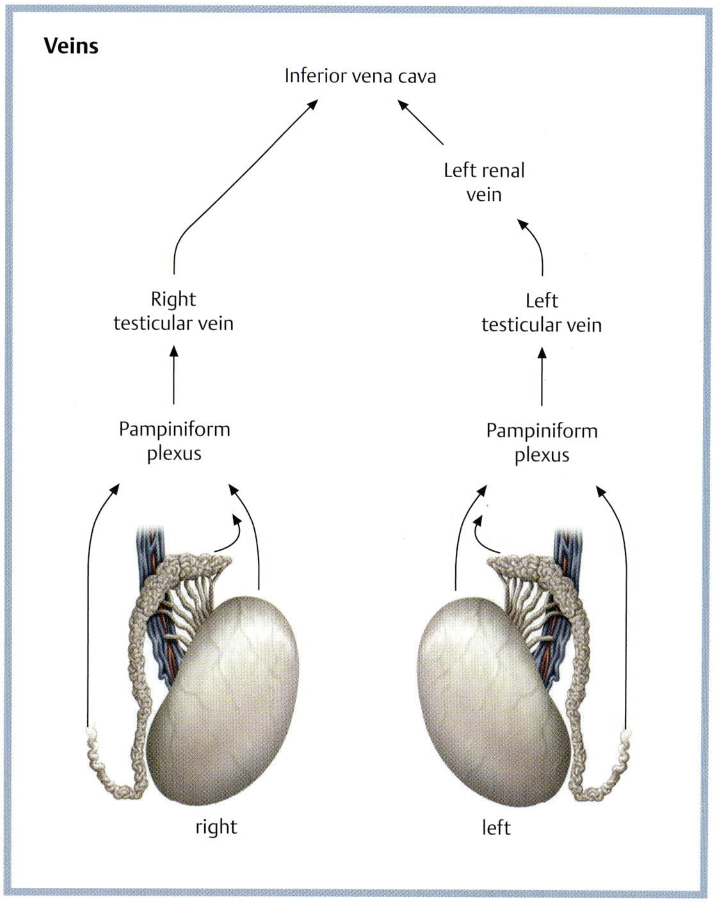

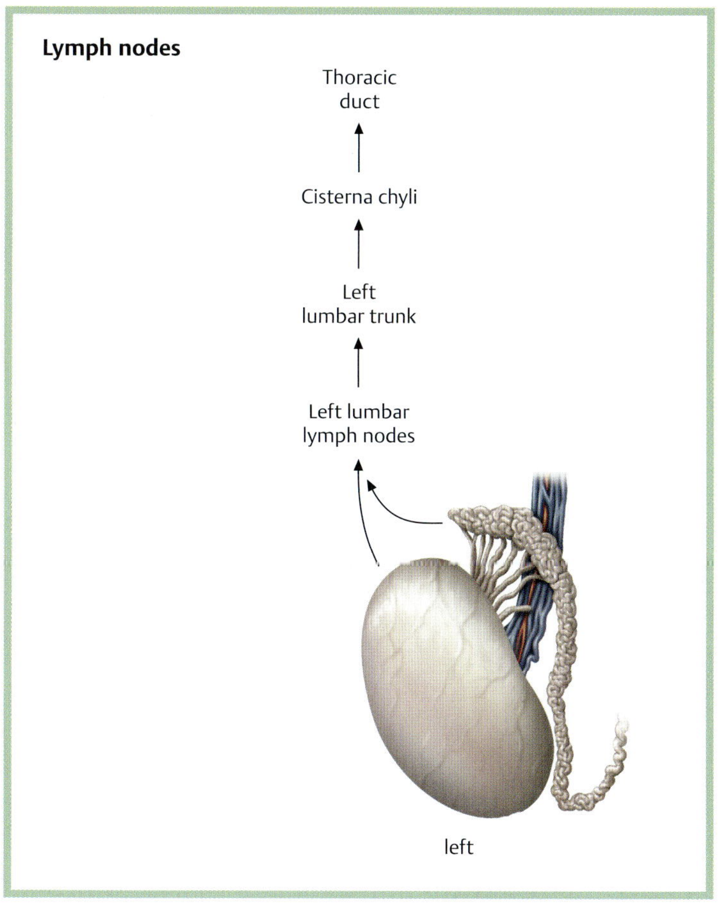

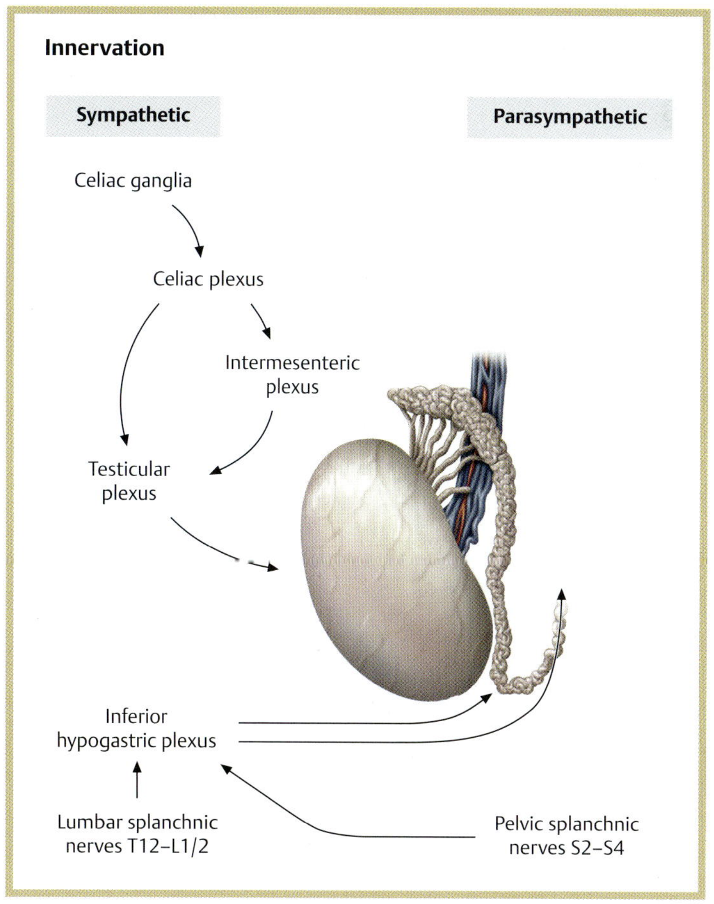

1.17 Uterus, Uterine Tube, and Vagina

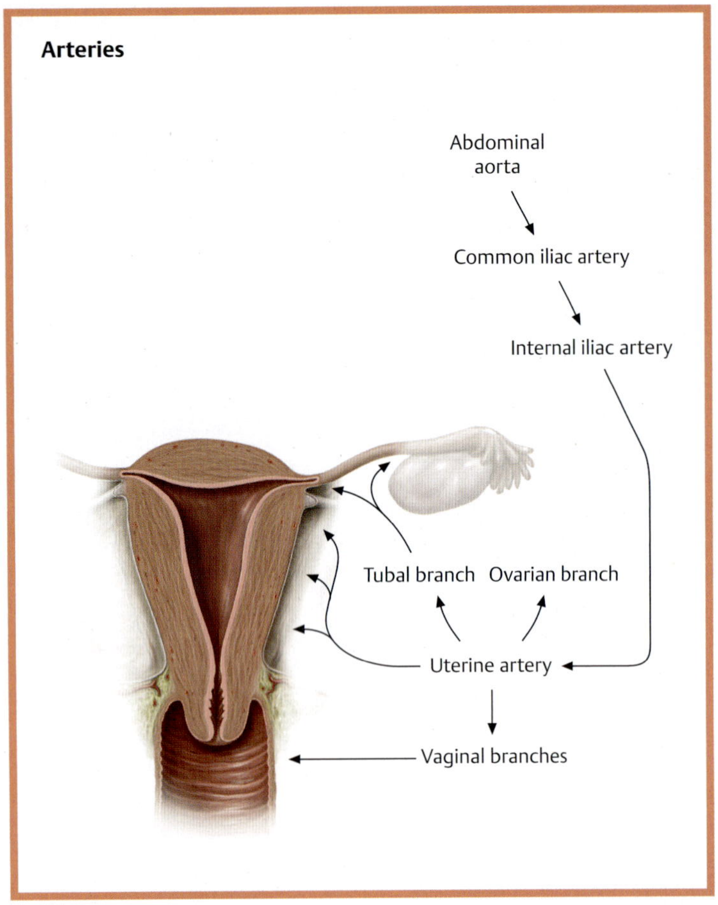

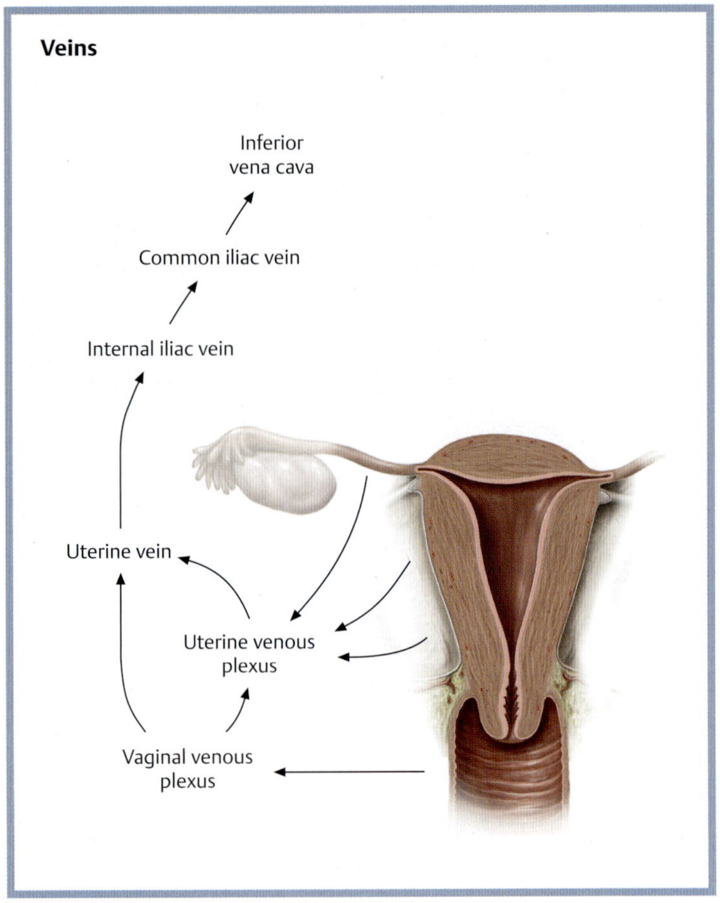

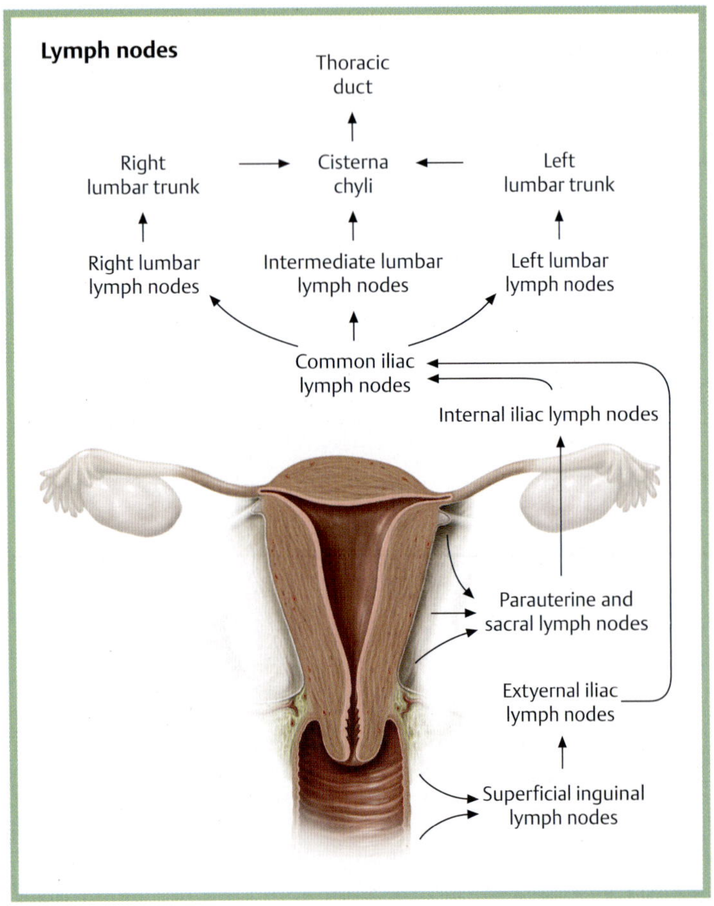

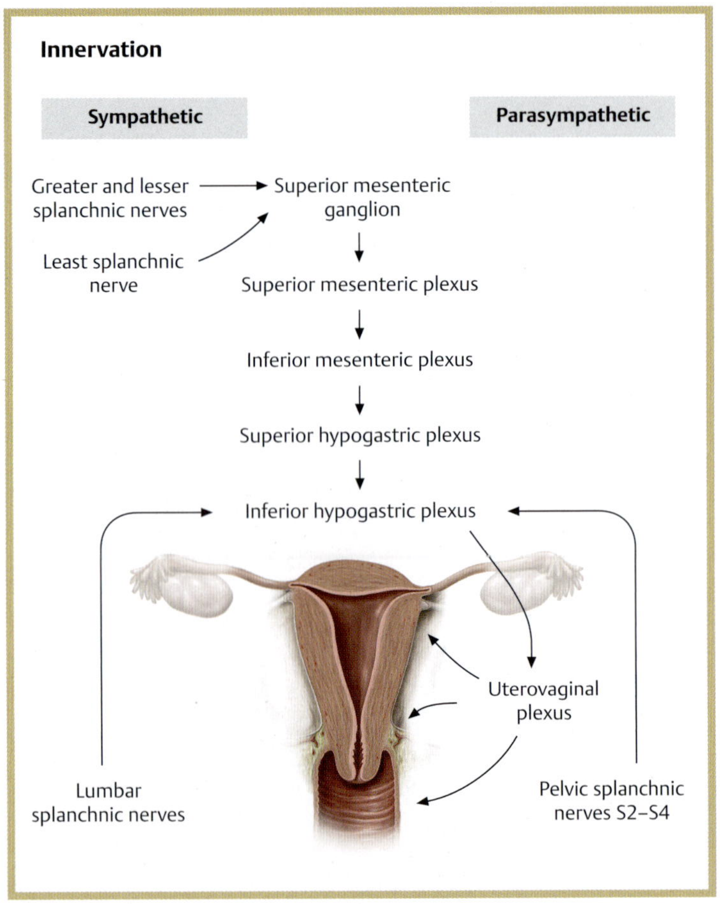

1.18 Uterine Tube and Ovary

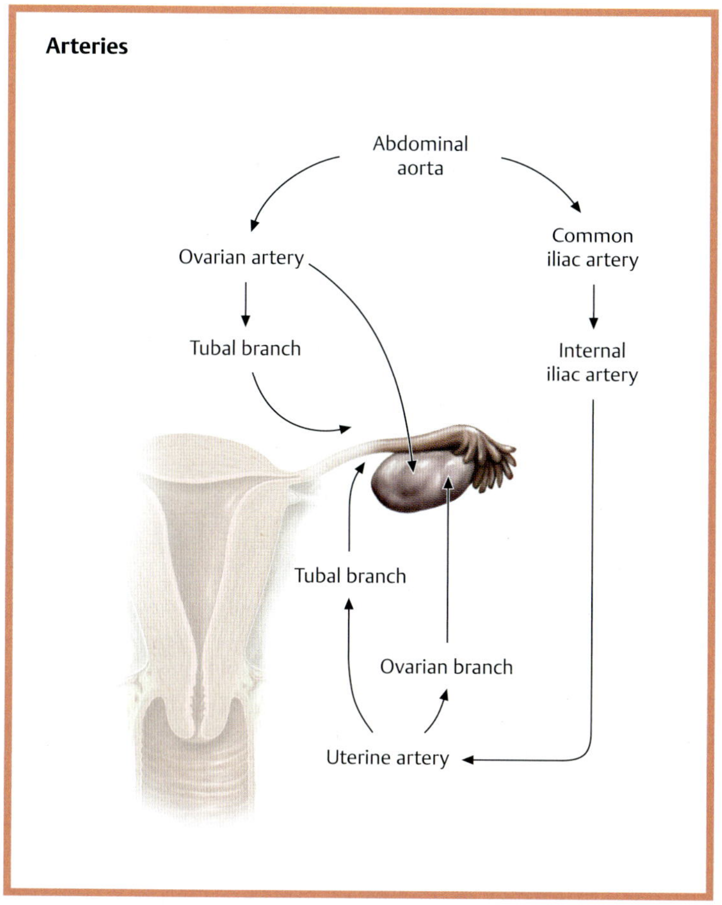

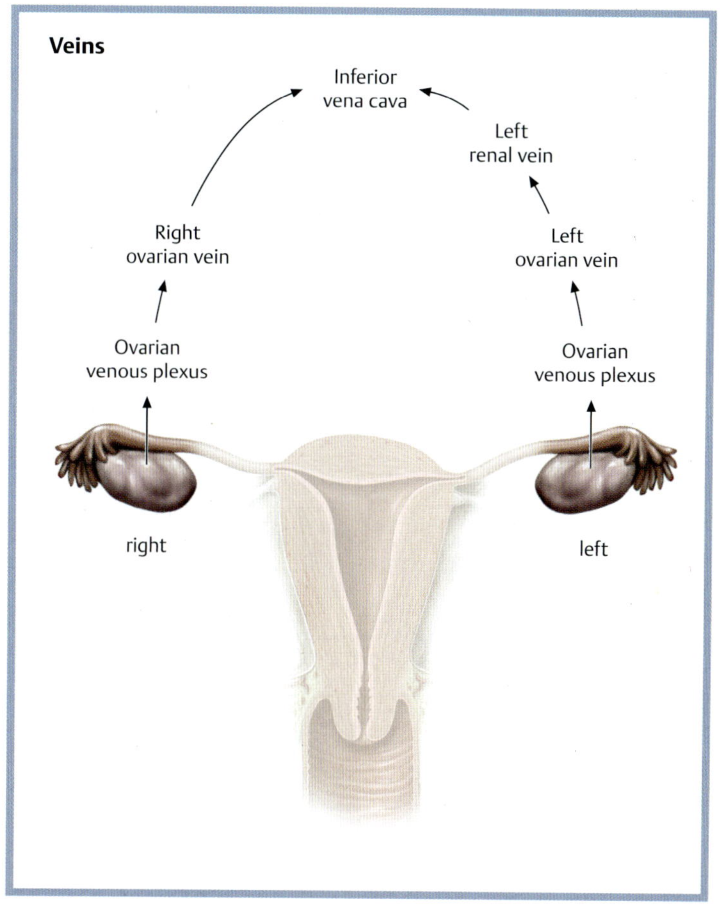

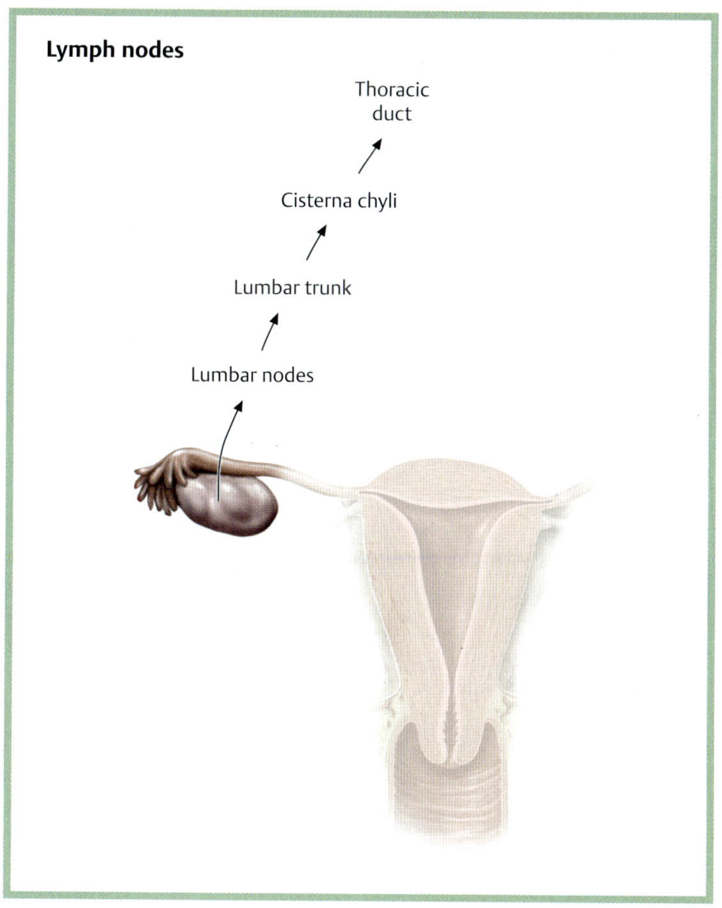

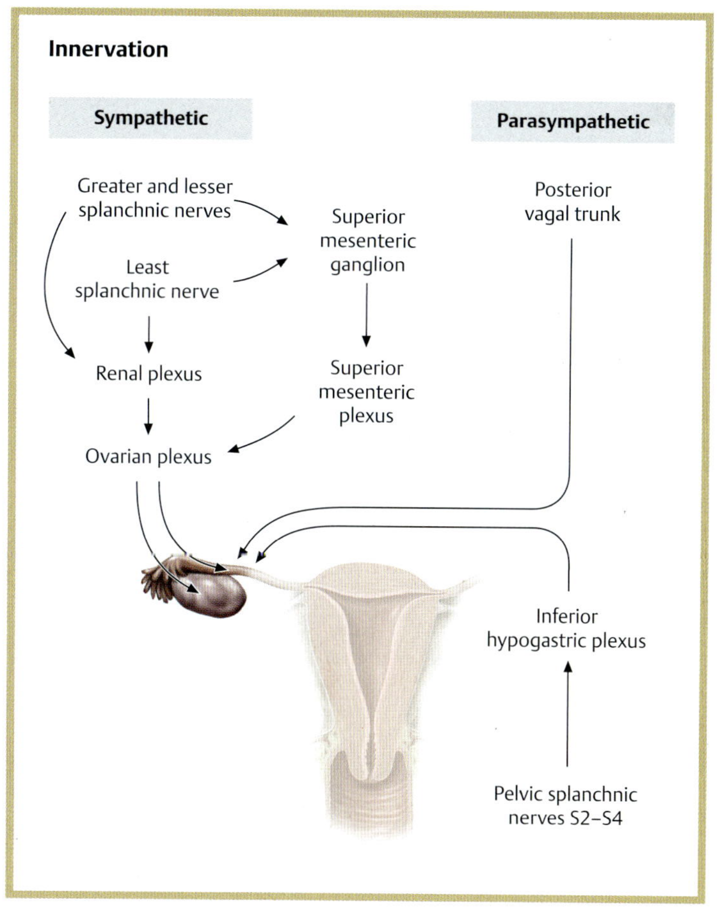

E Organ Fact Sheets

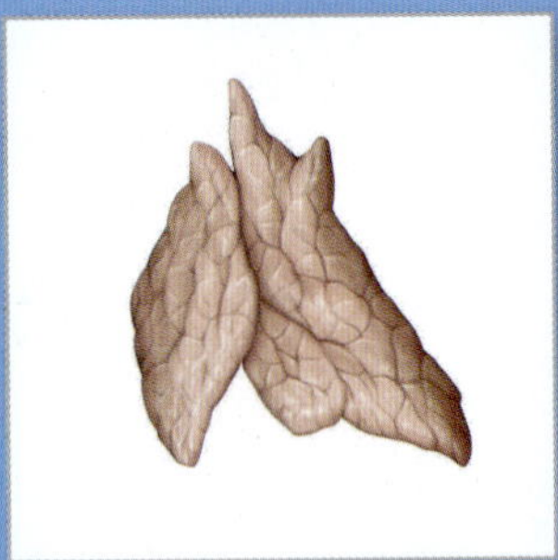
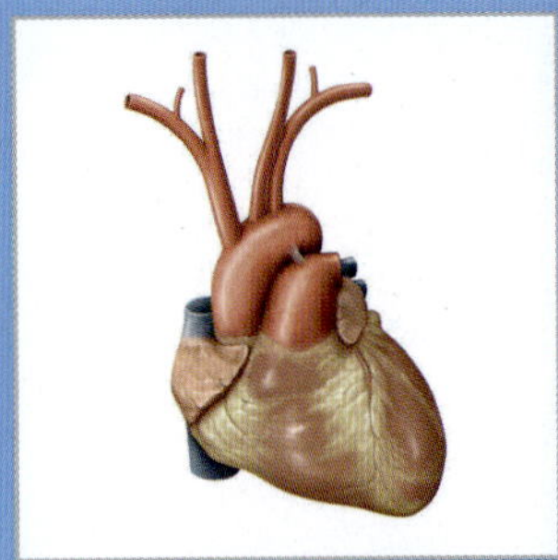
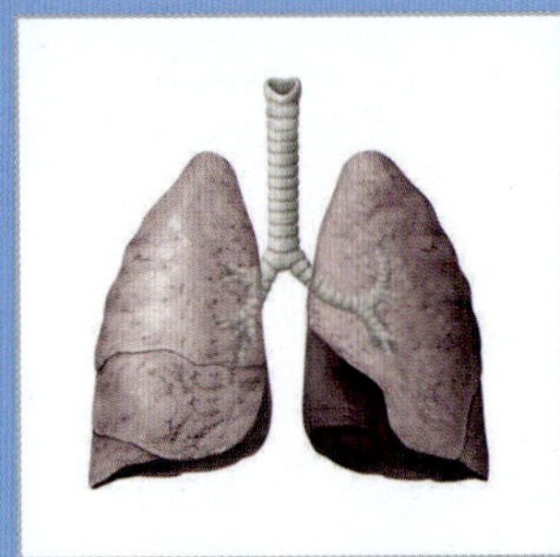
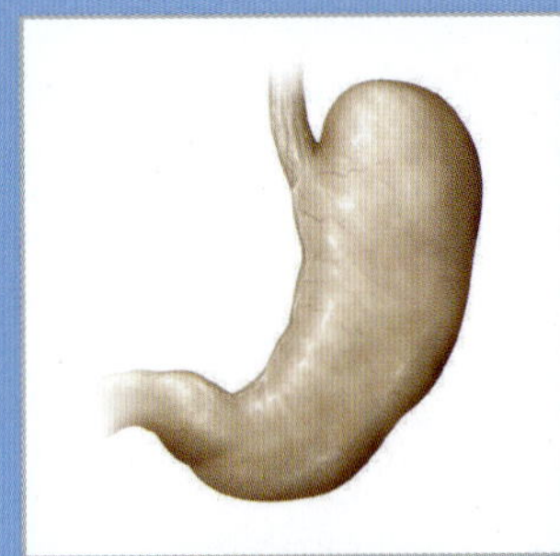
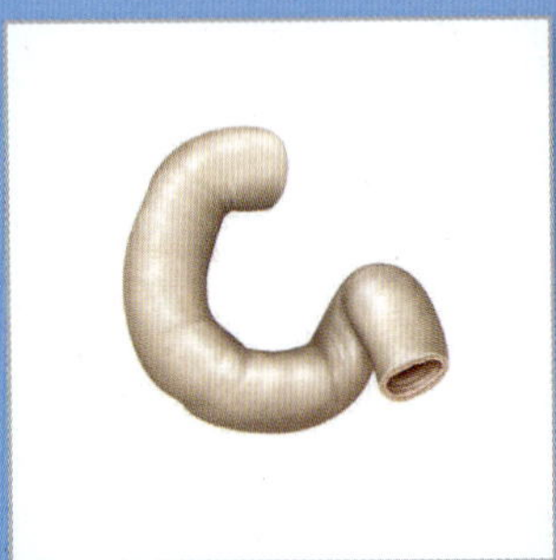
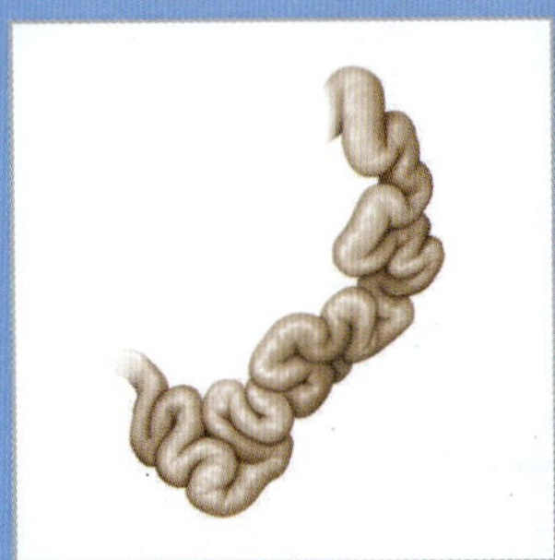
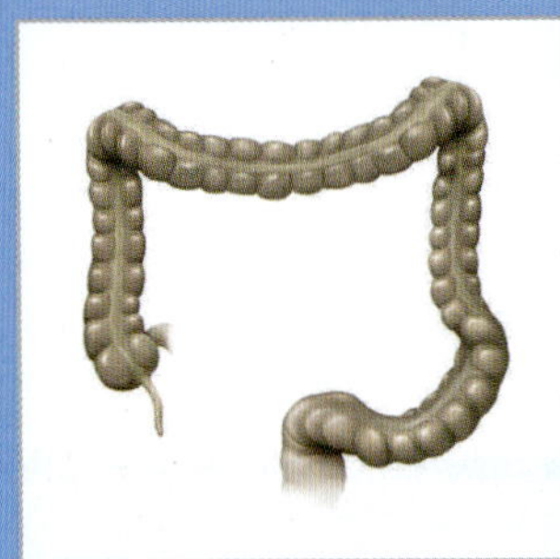
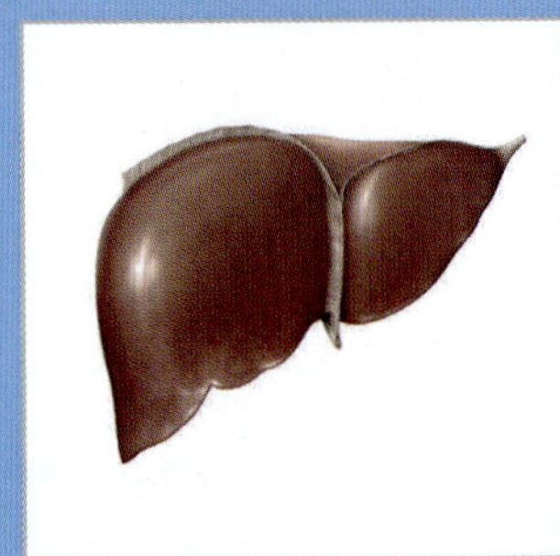
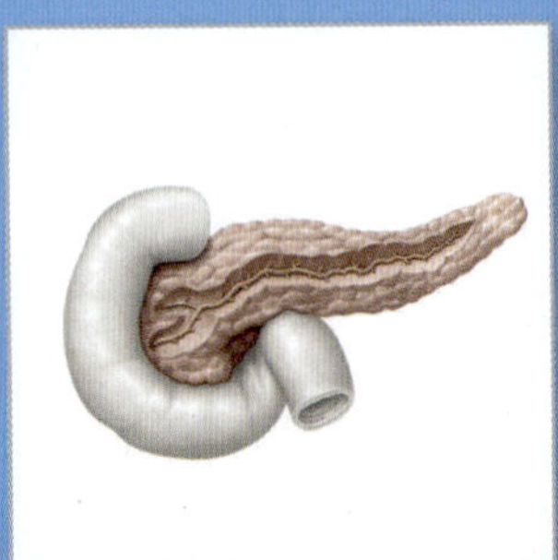
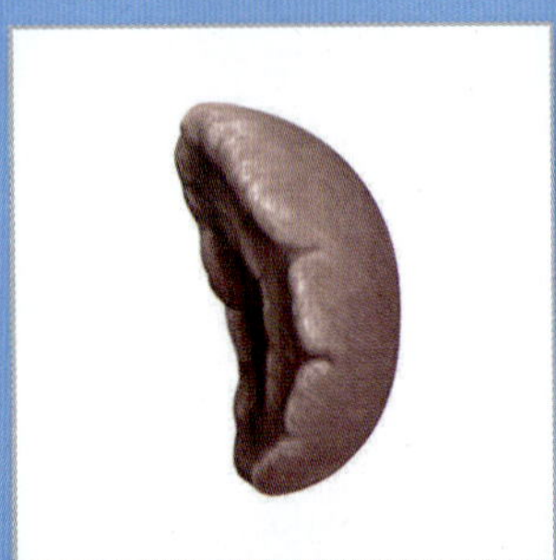
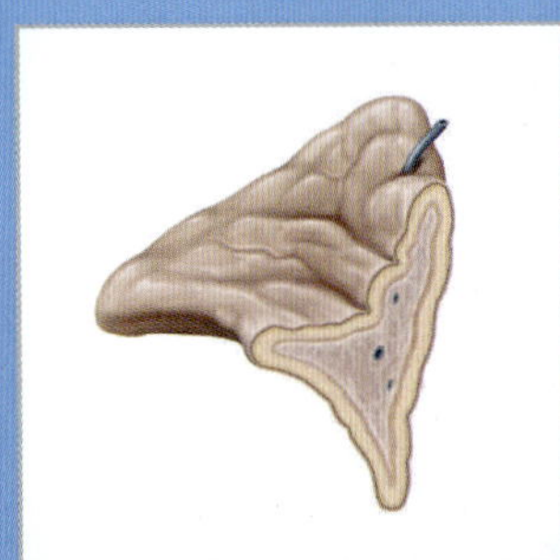
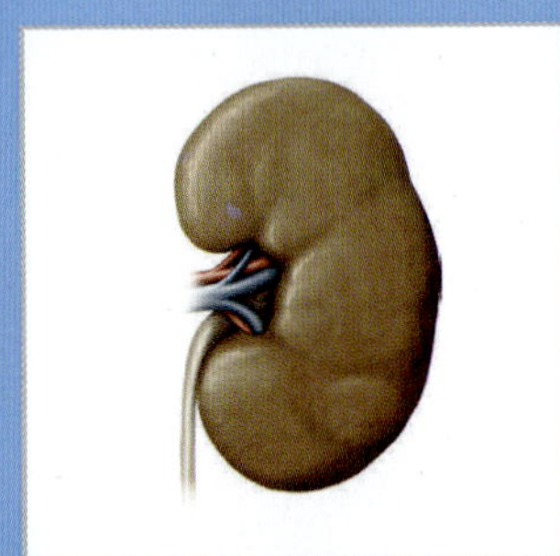
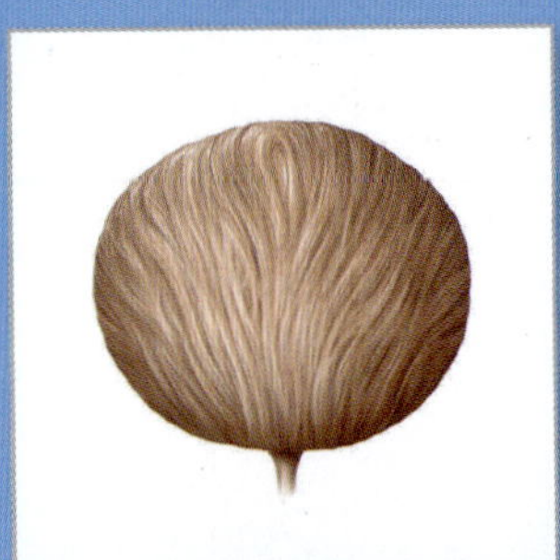
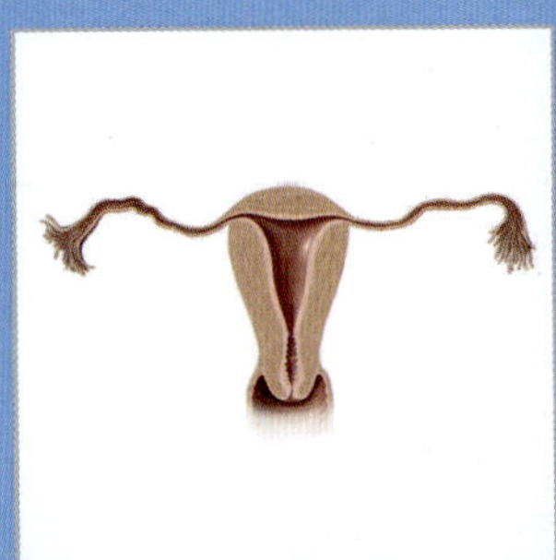
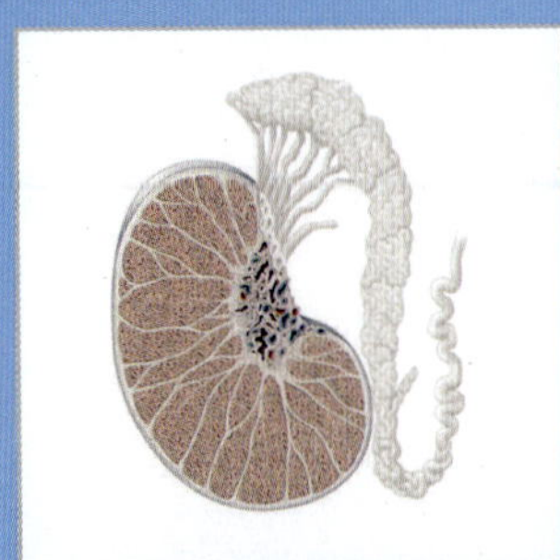
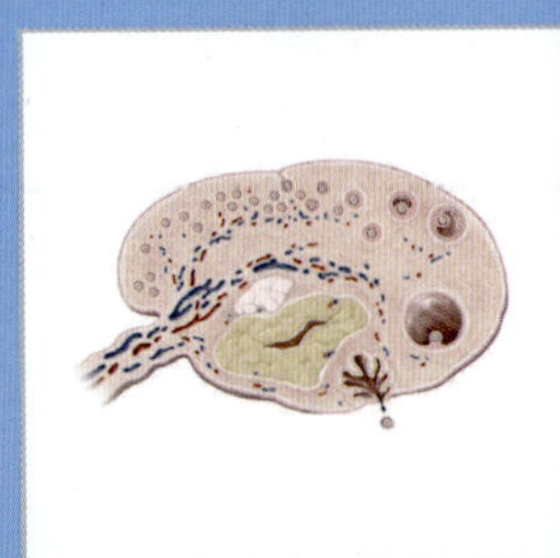

1.1 Thymus

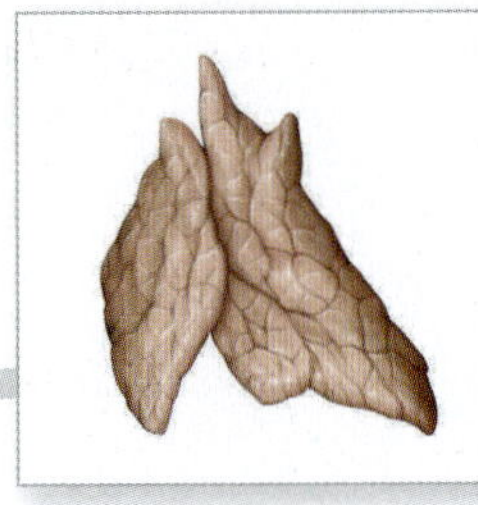

Location

- Situated in the superior mediastinum posterior to the sternum, and anterior to the pericardium and major vessels at the base of the heart
- Projection on the thorax is referred to as the thymic triangle.

Shape and structure

- Lymphoepithelial organ, usually consists of two lobes (left and right lobes).
- Delicate connective tissue capsule, and trabeculae that extend into the parenchyma subdividing the thymus into lobules
- Each lobule is divided into a (darker) cortex and (lighter) medulla. Epithelial cells form a densely packed subcapsular layer around the fibrous trabeculae (blood–thymus barrier) and join together inside the thymus to form a three-dimensional network that encloses the lymphocytes. Epithelial cells in the medulla aggregate to form Hassall's corpuscles.
- Other cell types: macrophages, myoid cells, dendritic cells

Neurovascular structures (see also p. 428)

Mediastinal circulation. Owing to its location in the superior mediastinum, the thymus is supplied by the neurovascular structures of the mediastinum (entering and exiting the head).

- *Arteries:* thymic branches arising from the internal thoracic artery (proximity to sternum);
- *Veins:* thymic veins drain into the brachiocephalic veins.
- *Lymphatic drainage:* through the brachiocephalic lymph nodes into the bronchomediastinal trunks
- *Autonomic innervation:*
  - parasympathetic through both vagus nerves, especially the recurrent laryngeal nerves
  - sympathetic through branches of the cervical ganglia (cervical cardiac nerves)

Function

- Maturation and differentiation (conferring immunological competence) of T-cells
- Induction of programmed cell death (apoptosis) in T-cells that respond to antigens: approximately 90% of immature T-cells die in the thymus.
- Production of immune-modulating hormones (thymosin, thymopoietin, thymulin)
- Primary lymphatic organ

Note: The thymus is an organ "of childhood and adolescence." It reaches its maximum size during puberty (approximately 30 grams). The degree of atrophy of thymic tissue in adults varies.

Embryonic development

- The thymic epithelium is derived from the epithelium of the third pharyngeal pouch (endodermal origin).
- The epithelial primordium is populated with lymphocytes (mesodermal origin).

Major diseases

- Disorders of the thymus are very rare
- Absence of the thymus may be life-threatening (thymic aplasia), resulting in lack of cellular immunity
- Lymphatic diseases (e.g., certain types of leukemia) may affect the thymus
- Thymomas: tumors that originate from the epithelial cells of the thymus, and because of the immunologic function of the thymus are often accompanied by autoimmune diseases: myasthenia gravis (muscle weakness).

1.2 Pericardium

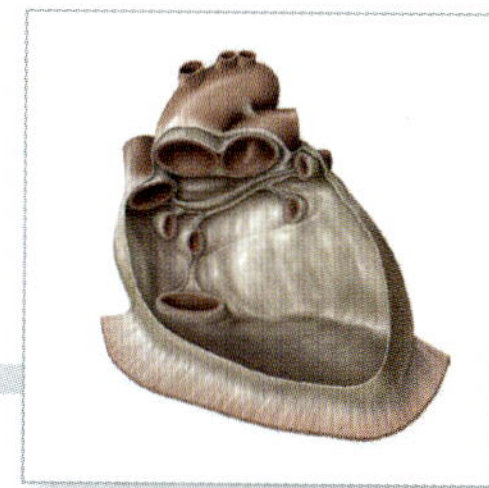

Location

Situated in the thorax (middle mediastinum).

Shape and structure

Fibrous sac that surrounds the heart consisting of

- Fibrous pericardium (outermost layer comprised of dense connective tissue; extends to the roots of the great vessels at the base of the heart);
- Serous pericardium (serous membrane) with
  - *parietal* layer (adhered to the fibrous pericardium),
  - *visceral* layer (epicardium, attached to the myocardium);
- Between parietal and visceral layer: pericardial cavity (narrow space);
- At the location where the visceral layer is folded back onto the parietal layer near the base of the heart, two sinuses are formed:
  - *transverse sinus* (between the arteries and veins)
  - *oblique sinus* (between the left and right pulmonary veins).

Openings

- One for the ascending aorta
- One for the pulmonary trunk
- Two for both caval veins
- Four for the four pulmonary veins.

Neurovascular structures (see also p. 431)

- Mediastinal circulation
- *Arteries:* pericardiacophrenic artery (from the internal thoracic artery)
- *Veins:* pericardiacophrenic vein (to the internal thoracic vein)
- *Lymphatic drainage:* prepericardial lymph nodes, lateral pericardial lymph nodes (also superior phrenic lymph nodes and tracheobronchial lymph nodes into the bronchomediastinal trunk)
- *Autonomic innervation:* negligible
- *Somatosensory innervation:* phrenic nerve (from the cervical plexus)

Function

Provides sliding-surface for the heart, however the pericardium is not essential for life.

Embryonic development

Derived from lateral plate mesoderm:

- Visceral parts derived from splanchnopleure
- Parietal parts derived from somatopleure

Major diseases

- Pericarditis: inflammation usually caused by viral or bacterial infection.
- Tuberculous pericarditis, which is rare nowadays, can lead to pericardial calcium deposits. As a result, the heart can no longer expand; it is constricted (also known as constrictive pericarditis).

1.3 Heart

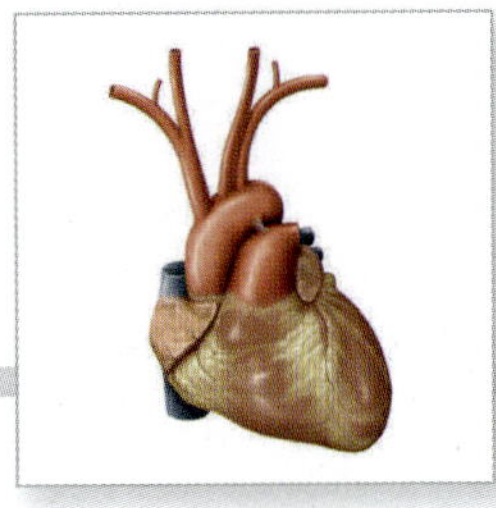

Location

- Located in the thorax within the pericardium.
- The base of heart is directed upward, backward, and to the right. The base of the heart is the location of the venous entry and arterial exit points (inferior and superior venae cavae, pulmonary veins, ascending aorta and pulmonary trunk).
- The apex of heart is directed downward, forward and to the left.
- The longitudinal axis of the heart (from the base to the apex, the anatomical axis of the heart) is at a 45-degree angle to all body planes.

Shape and structure

- Hollow organ, shaped like a cone: measures 12–14 cm in length, 9 cm in width at its broadest part.
- Weight: up to 300 g.

External structures of the heart

- **Surfaces:**
  - sternocostal surface (anterior)
  - right and left pulmonary surfaces
  - diaphragmatic surface (inferior)
- **Grooves on the outside of the heart:**
  - anterior/posterior interventricular sulci
  - coronary sulcus
- **Auricles:** (left/right): protrusions attached to the atria (analogous to the primitive atria; potential site for thrombus formation) produce atrial natriuretic peptide (ANP) for regulation of blood pressure.

Internal structures of the heart

Chambers and openings of the heart

- **Four contractile chambers:**
  - two atria: left and right atria separated by the interatrial septum (muscle);
  - two ventricles: left and right ventricles, separated by the interventricular septum (muscular part and membranous part, thus part muscle and part connective tissue); both ventricles have an inflow tract (with trabeculae carneae) and an outflow tract (smooth-walled) following the direction of blood flow.
- **Four openings** that connect the atria and ventricles, the right ventricle and pulmonary trunk, and the left ventricle and ascending aorta:
  - two openings in the right side of the heart: right atrioventricular orifice and pulmonary orifice;
  - two openings in the left side of the heart: left atrioventricular orifice and aortic orifice.
- Additionally, **openings for the two caval veins** (in the right atrium) and the four pulmonary veins (in the left atrium, see flow of blood below) as well as the opening of the coronary sinus (in the right atrium: opening of coronary sinus with the valve of the coronary sinus).

Flow of blood through the heart chambers

- Generally: from the right heart to the lungs (oxygen absorption), from there to the left heart and then to the aorta (oxygen is released to serially connected organs)
- More specifically: from the superior and inferior venae cavae into the right atrium, from there through the right atrioventricular orifice to the right ventricle and through the pulmonary orifice to the pulmonary trunk, through both of the pulmonary arteries, and into the lungs; from there to the four pulmonary veins, then to the left atrium and through the left atrioventricular orifice to the left ventricle and finally through the aortic orifice to the aorta.

Cardiac valves

- By closing and opening (papillary muscles, see below) **four valves** ensure that blood flows in only one direction through the heart:
  - two atrioventricular valves;
  - two semilunar valves (pulmonary valve and aortic valve).

  During ventricular contraction, the atrioventricular valves prevent backflow of blood from the ventricles into the atria; when the ventricles relax, the semilunar valves prevent the return of blood from the pulmonary trunk and ascending aorta back into the ventricles.
- **Valves of the right side of the heart:**
  - right atrioventricular valve at the right atrioventricular orifice = cuspid valve with three cusps: septal/anterior/posterior cusps = tricuspid valve;
  - pulmonary valve at the pulmonary orifice in the outflow tract of the right ventricle = semilunar valve with three cusps: anterior/left/right semilunar cusps;
- **Valves of the left side of the heart:**
  - left atrioventricular valve at the left atrioventricular orifice = cuspid valve with two cusps = bicuspid valve: anterior/posterior cusps;
  - aortic valve at the aortic orifice in the outflow tract of the left ventricle = semilunar valve also with three cusps: posterior/left/right semilunar cusps.

Grooves and crests on the inner walls of the chambers of the heart

Grooves (only in the atria):

- Right: fossa ovalis in the interatrial septum is the embryonic remnant of the foramen ovale.
- Left: valve of the foramen ovale is the counterpart of the fossa ovalis on the right side.

Crests (in atria and ventricles):

- Right and left *atria*: pectinate muscles: ridge-like muscle protrusions in the auricles, see above, correspond to the primitive atrium of the embryonic heart.
- Right and left *ventricles*:
  - trabeculae carneae (muscular columns that line the ventricles; more prominent in the right than the left ventricle)
  - papillary muscles: specialized extensions of the trabeculae carneae that project into the lumen of the ventricle; prevent the inversion or prolapse of valves during ventricular contraction
  - in the right ventricle: *three* papillary muscles for the *three* cusps of the tricuspid valve, see above, (anterior, posterior, and septal papillary muscles)
  - in the left ventricle: *two* papillary muscles for the *two* cusps of the bicuspid valve, see above (anterior and posterior papillary muscles)

Skeleton of the heart

The heart valves all lie in one plane (valve plane) and are covered by endocardium. The valve rings are composed of dense connective tissue. All fibrous rings, together with the collagenous bands through which they are connected, form the cardiac skeleton.

Layers of the heart wall

The wall of the heart consists of three layers. From the inside to the outside they are

- endocardium (simple squamous epithelium): lines the cavities of the heart and covers the heart valves;
- myocardium (muscle, the fibers of which are arranged in different directions): muscle fibers roughly arranged in three layers;
- epicardium (serous membrane of the pericardium, simple squamous epithelium): strictly speaking, it is part of the pericardium, although it is often referred to as part of the heart.

Neurovascular structures (see also p. 430)

- Mediastinal circulation
- *Arteries:* left coronary artery (with anterior interventricular branch and circumflex branch) and right coronary artery (with posterior interventricular branch), both arise from the ascending aorta where it exits the left ventricle.
- *Veins:* cardiac veins (great, middle, small), like the posterior vein of the left ventricle, the cardiac veins return blood to the right atrium through the coronary sinus.
- *Lymphatic drainage:* through the brachiocephalic lymph nodes and the tracheobronchial lymph nodes into the bronchomediastinal trunk
- *Autonomic innervation:* parasympathetic through the two vagus nerves (cervical and thoracic cardiac branches). The neuronal cell bodies are in the dorsal nuclei of the vagus nerves; sympathetic through branches of thoracic ganglia 2–5 (superior, middle and inferior cervical cardiac nerves) and thoracic cardiac nerves.

Function

The heart functions as a suction-pressure pump to distribute blood around the body (heart volume approximately 780 ml, ventricular stroke volume 70ml).

- The heartbeat can be felt as *pulse* (resting heart rate ~ 1 Hz).
- Cardiac activity is divided into two phases: *systole* (contraction of the myocardium) and *diastole* (relaxation of the myocardium).
- Contraction of the ventricular myocardium (closure of the AV valves) and closure of the aortic and pulmonary valves are audible as the *first* and *second* heart sounds.
- Cardiac excitation conduction system composed of specialized myocardial cells: impulses are generated by the *sinoatrial node* (SA node) in the right atrium adjacent to the opening of the superior vena cava. Excitation is spread to the ventricles through the *atrioventricular node* (AV node), at the junction of right atrium and right ventricle, and then through the *atrioventricular bundle* (bundle of His) with its right and left branches, which terminate in the Purkinje fibers.

Note: Because of its autonomous excitation, the heart can trigger the impulse that generates the heartbeat. Even an isolated heart beats. The autonomic innervation (see above) modifies only the activities of the autonomous excitation and conduction system. The parasympathetic nervous system reduces the heart rate and atrioventricular conduction. The sympathetic nervous system increases both and as well as the stroke volume.

Embryonic Development

Of mesodermal origin, derived from the primitive heart tube and subsequently formed cardiac loop.

Major diseases

- Heart diseases are important and are the leading cause of death in the industrialized world: *myocardial infarction* = occluded coronary arteries that lead to inadequate blood flow to distinct parts of the myocardium, which results in myocardial necrosis
- *Arrhythmia* and dysfunction of the conduction system
- *Valve defects* (congenital or caused by inflammation of the endocardium) = incomplete opening of the valve (valve stenosis) or incomplete valve closure (valve insufficiency)
- With *myocardial injuries* without damage to the pericardium, the heart continues to pump blood into the pericardial cavity until cardiac arrest occurs (*cardiac tamponade*).
- Generally: formation of pathological blood clots (thromboses) in the heart, which may travel through the blood stream, for example, to the brain.

1.4 Trachea, Bronchi, and Lungs

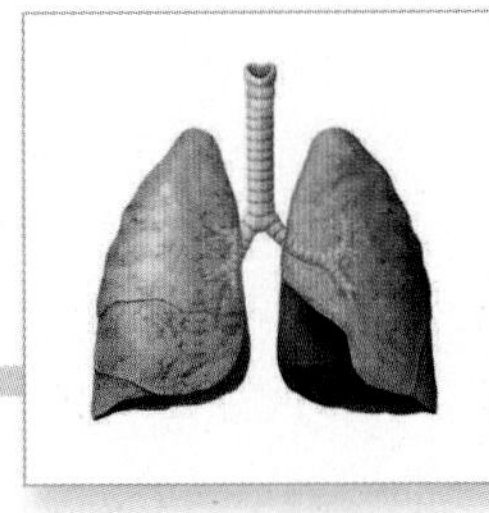

Location

- Cervical part of the trachea situated in the neck
- Thoracic part of the trachea and main bronchi situated in the mediastinum
- Lobar bronchi and all segments inferior: intrapulmonary location
- Lungs: situated on either side of the mediastinum
- Surface of the lung covered by visceral pleura (pulmonary pleura). On the mediastinal surface at the pulmonary ligament the parietal pleura is folded back onto the visceral pleura.

External structure of the lung

- Apex of lung
- Base of lung
- Lobes of the lung. Three lobes in the right lung: superior lobe, middle lobe, and inferior lobe; two in the left lung: superior lobe and inferior lobe
- Fissures, two in the right lung: horizontal fissure below the superior lobe; oblique fissure between the middle lobe and inferior lobe. In the left lung one oblique fissure between the superior and inferior lobes
- Two margins: anterior and inferior margins
- Four surfaces: costal surface (adjacent to the ribs), diaphragmatic surface (at the base, adjacent to the diaphragm), mediastinal surface (adjacent to the mediastinum), interlobar surface (in the fissures between lobes)

Note: A term for the posterior margin of the lung (where the costal and mediastinal surfaces meet) is not listed in the official Terminologia Anatomica.

Shape and structure of the airways

- Generally: tubes that divide by dichotomous branching with decreasing caliber
- The intrapulmonary airways, connective tissue, and neurovascular structures form a spongy organ—the paired lungs.

Structure of the trachea and bronchial tree:
- Trachea to terminal bronchioles = conducting (carrying air) portion.
- Terminal bronchioles to alveoli = respiratory (gas exchange) portion.

Components of the conducting portion:
- Cervical part of the trachea: first tracheal ring, see below, to superior thoracic aperture
- Thoracic part of the trachea: superior thoracic aperture to tracheal bifurcation
- At the tracheal bifurcation: division of the trachea into the right and left main bronchi
- Division of the right main bronchus into three lobar bronchi: superior, middle and inferior lobar bronchi
- Division of the left main bronchus into two lobar bronchi: superior and inferior lobar bronchi
- Division of the lobar bronchi into segmental bronchi: ten segmental bronchi in the right lung and 9 segmental bronchi in the left lung
- Division of the segmental bronchi into subsegmental bronchi

Components of the respiratory portion:
- Respiratory bronchioles: first to third order (where alveoli begin to appear)
- Alveolar ducts
- Alveolar sacs

Structure of the airway wall

Trachea:
- Hollow, tubular organ with 16–20 horseshoe-shaped cartilage rings
- Tracheal rings joined together by collagen and elastic fibers (annular ligaments)
- Mucosa of the trachea covered with respiratory epithelium, contains multiple glands (tracheal glands).
- Posterior tracheal wall: non-cartilaginous, composed of connective tissue (membranous wall of trachea), permeated by smooth-muscle cells (trachealis muscle).

Main, lobar, segmental and subsegmental bronchi:
- Generally similar in structure to the trachea.
- Concentric or spiral sheets of smooth-muscle cells in all bronchi (active changes in caliber)
- In segmental and subsegmental bronchi cartilaginous plates instead of cartilage rings
- Pseudostratified respiratory epithelium like tracheal mucosa

Terminal bronchioles:
- Non-cartilaginous walls
- Single-layer ciliated and non-ciliated columnar epithelium.

Respiratory bronchioles:
- Transition to alveoli generally non-ciliate columnar to cuboidal epithelium with occasional type II pneumocytes
- Alveoli (gas exchange): type I and type II pneumocytes

Internal structure of the lungs

Structure of the airways determines the structure of the lungs:

- Both lungs aerated by trachea.
- Main bronchi (left and right, respectively) each aerate one lung (left and right, respectively).
- Lobar bronchi each aerate one lobe (pulmonary lobe).
- Segmental bronchi each aerate one lung segment (bronchopulmonary segment).
- Lobular bronchioles each aerate one lobule (pulmonary lobule).
- Terminal bronchioles each aerate one acinus; a group of acini forms a lobule.

Neurovascular structures (see also p. 432)

Mediastinal circulation

- The intrapulmonary neurovascular structures in the lung either run along the divisions of the bronchial tree or within the connective tissue framework.
- Characteristic feature of the lungs: two circulation systems: bronchial arteries and veins to supply the lung itself, and pulmonary arteries and veins for gas exchange through the entire body.

Bronchial arteries and veins:
- *Arteries:* bronchial branches directly from the thoracic aorta or indirectly from posterior intercostal arteries
- *Veins:* on the right, bronchial veins to the azygos vein, on the left to the hemiazygos vein or accessory hemiazygos vein

Pulmonary arteries and veins:
- *Arteries:* the pulmonary arteries (left, right) carry deoxygenated blood from the pulmonary trunk. Segmental branches (segmental arteries) of the pulmonary arteries follow the segmental bronchi into the center of one of the 10 or 9 segments.
- *Veins:* drainage of oxygenated blood usually through four pulmonary veins into the left atrium of the heart
- *Lymphatic drainage:* through the intrapulmonary, bronchopulmonary, tracheobronchial, and paratracheal lymph nodes into the bronchomediastinal trunks
- *Autonomic innervation:*
  - parasympathetic through the two vagus nerves to the pulmonary plexus,
  - sympathetic through branches mainly from thoracic ganglia 2 or 3–4 (varies), also to the pulmonary plexus

Function

Generally, the exchange of oxygen and carbon dioxide between the atmosphere and blood circulation, more specifically:

- Trachea and bronchi as well as their divisions (bronchial tree) except for the finest terminal portions: air conduction
- Final divisions of the bronchial tree (alveoli): gas exchange between atmosphere and blood; thus the important role of the lungs for
  - energy production: oxygen is extracted from the atmosphere for oxidation processes.
  - regulation of acid-base balance (release of carbon dioxide in the air when exhaling and thus influencing bicarbonate levels in the blood)
- Changes in the volume of the thoracic cavity are passed on to the lungs through the pleural layers (capillary forces cause the visceral pleura to adhere to the parietal pleura); a change in lung volume leads to a change in intrapulmonary pressure, in turn resulting in drawing in or expelling air from the lungs.

Embryonic development

Of endodermal origin, derived from the cranial foregut:

- Lung buds or respiratory diverticulum develops from a small outpouching on the ventral surface of the embryonic esophagus.
- Lung buds undergo repeated dichotomous branching (total of 22) to give rise to the trachea along with the bronchial tree including the alveoli.

Note: The lungs are fully matured at approximately the age of 10.

Major diseases

The bronchial tree and lungs are the parts of the body most commonly affected by diseases (entry points for infectious pathogens):

- Acute inflammation of the bronchial tree (bronchitis, bronchial catarrh, cold) is usually caused by viral infections and is generally harmless.
- Chronic inflammation (chronic bronchitis) is much more common in smokers.
- Bronchial asthma (often triggered by allergies) is a result of insufficient expansion of small bronchi and bronchioles during expiration.
- Lung overexpansion and rupture of the alveoli (pulmonary emphysema)
- Chronic obstructive pulmonary disease (COPD): end-stage of the three previously mentioned diseases, with destruction of gas exchange tissue
- Malignant tumors (bronchial carcinoma) is among the leading causes of death for smokers.
- Pulmonary embolism: Acute occlusion of a pulmonary artery (or one of its branches) is caused by a blood clot that most commonly was formed in a vein and carried from the right heart to the lung. In that case it is crucial that the lungs possess a double circulation. Blood from the bronchial branches is sufficient to supply the tissue. Hence, blockage of the pulmonary artery does not result in tissue undersupply and subsequent destruction.

1.5 Esophagus

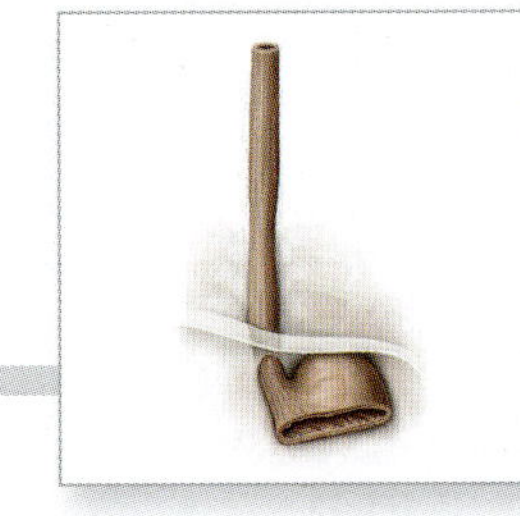

Location

Situated in the neck and thorax (mediastinum) between the trachea and spinal column, as well as in the abdomen

Shape, size and segments

- Tubular organ, measures about 23–27 cm in length from the entrance of the esophagus to its terminal portion.
- Measures about 20 mm in width (but see constrictions of the esophagus).

Divided into three parts corresponding to the regions of the body they are located in (see above)

- Cervical part (C 6–T 1): to the superior thoracic aperture
- Thoracic part (T 1–T 11): to the esophageal hiatus (site where the esophagus passes through the diaphragm)
- Abdominal part: to the cardiac orifice of the stomach (shortest segment, measures only 2–3 cm in length, lies intraperitoneally).

Esophageal constrictions (maximum width of 14 mm instead of the usual 20 mm)

- Upper constriction: pharyngoesophageal constriction at the C6 level; 14–16 cm from the incisors
- Middle constriction: thoracic constriction at the T 4/T 5 level; 25–27 cm from the incisors, esophagus passes to the right of the thoracic aorta.
- Lower constriction: phrenic constriction at the T 10/T 11 level; 36–38 cm from the incisors, site where the esophagus pierces the diaphragm; functional closure of the esophagus by muscles and venous cushions of the esophageal wall, and muscles of the diaphragm

Wall structure

- Basically the same as in the gastrointestinal tract: mucosa, submucosa, muscularis, and adventitia, or in the lower part in proximity to the stomach: subserous membrane and serous membrane.
- Mucosa with stratified non-keratinized squamous epithelium (has no digestive function but provides mechanical protection against passing food, lubricated by esophageal glands)
- Musculature in the upper esophagus (variable degree of expansion), striated (like the pharyngeal muscles), in the middle and lower part smooth muscle (like the stomach), the lower part contains numerous veins.
- Muscles also contain fibers that wind obliquely around the esophagus.
- Combination of circular and longitudinal muscle fibers allows for the expansion and constriction of the esophageal inlet and outlet (swallowing).

Neurovascular structures (see also p. 429)

- Primarily mediastinal circulation (thoracic part); to a lesser extent also cervical (cervical part) and upper abdominal circulation (abdominal part)
- *Arteries:* numerous esophageal branches of the inferior thyroid artery (cervical), thoracic aorta (thoracic), and left gastric artery (abdominal)
- *Veins:* numerous esophageal veins to the inferior thyroid vein (cervical), azygos veins and hemiazygos veins (thoracic), and left gastric vein (abdominal)
- *Lymphatic drainage* through the paraesophageal lymph nodes into the deep cervical lymph nodes (cervical), bronchomediastinal trunks (thoracic) and left gastric lymph nodes (abdominal)
- *Autonomic innervation:*
  - parasympathetic through the two vagus nerves (vagal trunks), in the neck region specifically through the recurrent laryngeal nerves. Neurons for the smooth esophageal muscles in the dorsal nucleus of the vagus nerve, neurons for the striated muscles in nucleus ambiguus
  - sympathetic through branches of thoracic ganglia 2–5.

The autonomic fibers form the esophageal plexus on the esophagus.

Function

During swallowing, active transport of solids and liquids from the pharynx to the stomach; when vomiting, transport of stomach contents from the stomach to the pharynx.

Embryonic development

- Derived from the endoderm of the cranial foregut.
- Lower part of the mesoesophagus may remain in the form of the hepatoesophageal ligament (connects liver to abdominal part of esophagus).

Note: As a result of the rotation of the stomach in the embryo, the esophagus also shifts slightly. Thus, the longitudinal layer of the smooth esophageal muscles is arranged in a rightward spiral pattern.

Major diseases

Diseases of the esophagus itself (rare except for esophageal reflux):

- Diverticulum (outpouchings of the wall), most common at the junction between the hypopharynx (laryngopharynx) and esophagus (also known as Zenker's diverticulum, which is not an esophageal but a hypopharyngeal diverticulum).
- Malignant tumors (esophageal carcinoma; relatively rare)
- Inflammation of the esophageal mucosa as a result of chronic alcohol consumption
- Esophageal reflux: inflammation of the esophageal epithelium caused by reflux of stomach acid; caused by insufficient closing mechanisms at the junction of the esophagus and stomach.
- Barrett's esophagus: as a result of chronic esophageal reflux, the columnar epithelium of the stomach may replace the squamous epithelium of the esophagus: increased risk of cancer.

In the case of liver cirrhosis, abnormally enlarged esophageal veins (esophageal varices: hemorrhagic risk) serve as a portacaval detour (drainage into the azygos system!).

1.6 Stomach

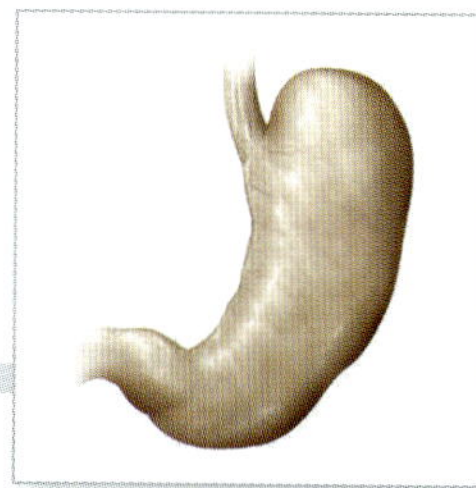

Location	Lies *intraperitoneally* in the left upper quadrant (=epigastrium).	
Shape and segments	• Sac-like hollow organ with anterior and posterior walls; different shapes may be encountered (hook-shaped stomach, bull-horn-shaped stomach, long stomach). • Four parts of the stomach in cranial to caudal direction: – top right: cardia = cardiac orifice = esophageal inlet – fundus of stomach (base or dome of the stomach; appears on radiographs as an air-filled space above a fluid level) – body of stomach – bottom right: pyloric part of stomach = pylorus with pyloric antrum and pyloric canal; stomach terminates at the pylorus, which closes the pyloric orifice (exit from the stomach into the duodenum)	• The body of stomach has two curvatures: – *lesser curvature*, faces right and upward, lesser omentum (connects the liver to the stomach) extends from it. – *greater curvature*, faces left and downward, greater omentum extends from it. • The stomach has two notches: – the cardiac notch at the junction between the cardia and the body of stomach – the angular notch at the junction between the body of the stomach and the pylorus
Wall structure	• Basically the same wall structure as the entire gastrointestinal tract: mucosa, submucosa, muscularis, and subserosa and serosa. • Exception: muscularis consists of three layers: oblique fibers, circular layer and longitudinal layer (important for peristaltic motion).	• Mucosa contains specialized glandular cells that produce HCl and intrinsic factor (parietal cells), pepsinogen (chief cells; protein digestion) and mucus (surface epithelial cells and accessory cells, mucin-producing; protection against self-digestion).
Neurovascular structures (see also p. 435)	Upper abdominal circulation. • *Arteries:* owing to the location in the upper abdomen, all gastric arteries arise directly (left gastric artery) or indirectly (through the common hepatic or splenic artery) from the celiac trunk: left and right gastric arteries supply the lesser curvature, left and right gastro-omental arteries supply the greater curvature; variably a posterior gastric artery for the posterior wall of the stomach. • *Veins:* left and right gastric veins, left and right gastro-omental veins, prepyloric vein and short gastric veins directly or indirectly (splenic or superior mesenteric vein) into the hepatic portal vein	• *Lymphatic drainage:* through groups of lymph nodes at the lesser curvature (left and right gastric lymph nodes), greater curvature (left and right gastro-omental lymph nodes), and at the pylorus (pyloric lymph nodes with prepyloric and retropyloric lymph nodes) into the celiac lymph nodes and from there into the cisterna chyli • *Autonomic innervation:* – parasympathetic through the two vagus nerves (vagal trunks) – sympathetic, primarily through the greater splanchnic nerves and partially through the lesser splanchnic nerves (through the celiac ganglia
Function	• Temporary reservoir for food, hence its large volume (1.2–1.8 l) and high elasticity. • Start of digestive process requirements: – production of gastric juice containing HCl (approximately 2 l per day, responsible for protein denaturation and sterilizing food, HCl concentration 5 M/L) and protein-digesting enzymes (pepsin)	– liquefaction and mechanical grinding (through peristaltic motion of the stomach wall) of food into chyme which is passed in small amounts through the pylorus to the duodenum. Peristaltic transport of chime – secretion of intrinsic factor for the intestinal resorption of vitamin B_{12}
Embryonic development	• Of endodermal origin, derived from the foregut. • The stomach has a dorsal and a ventral mesogastrium that develop into the greater and lesser omentum, respectively.	• As the stomach and the mesogastrium rotate, the liver and spleen shift to the right and left upper quadrants and the duodenum comes to lie retroperitoneally.
Major diseases	• Acute and chronic inflammation (gastritis) • Ulcer (often caused by a type of bacteria called Helicobacter pylori)	• Malignant gastric tumor (gastric carcinoma)

1.7 Small Intestine: Duodenum

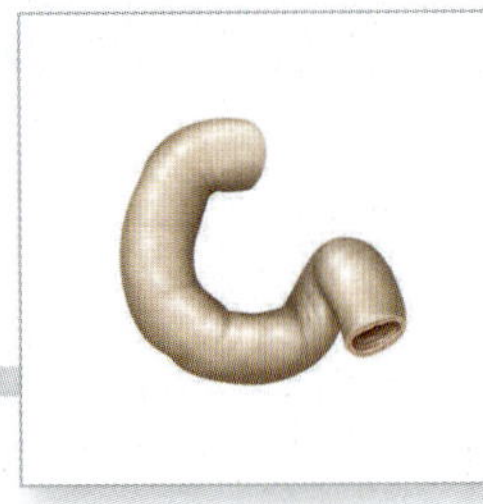

Location

- Largely secondarily *retroperitoneal* in the right upper quadrant just below the liver, with approximately 2 cm of the superior part in proximity to the stomach remaining *intraperitoneal*.
- As a result of the tilt and rotation of the stomach during embryonic development the duodenum shifts to the right, superior and posterior.

Shape and parts of the duodenum

- Hollow, tubular organ, in anterior view: c-shaped
- Shortest segment of the small intestine and has a length of approximately 12 finger-widths
- 4 parts from top to bottom:
  - superior part
  - descending part
  - inferior or horizontal part
  - ascending part

Wall structure

- Basically the same wall structure as the entire gastrointestinal tract: mucosa, submucosa, muscularis (with circular and longitudinal layers), subserosa, and serosa or adventitia, with the duodenal mucosal folds being the most distinct and diminishing in size toward the end of the small intestine.
- Mucosa with specialized circular folds (also known Kerckring's folds). Duodenal glands (also known as Brunner's glands) open into the intestinal lumen.

Neurovascular structures (see also p. 436)

Upper abdominal circulation and superior mesenteric circulation

- *Arteries:* indirect branches of the celiac trunk (duodenal branches of the gastroduodenal artery with anterior and posterior superior pancreaticoduodenal arteries) and the superior mesenteric artery (small branches of the inferior pancreaticoduodenal artery)
- *Veins:* drainage via the pancreaticoduodenal veins into the hepatic portal vein
- *Lymphatic drainage:* indirectly through the pancreaticoduodenal lymph nodes and pancreatic lymph nodes to the celiac lymph nodes or into the intestinal trunk
- *Autonomic innervation:*
  - parasympathetic primarily through the right vagus nerve (posterior vagal trunk)
  - sympathetic through the greater splanchnic nerves (celiac ganglia)

Function

- Digestion of food through enzymatic breakdown of carbohydrates, fat, and proteins. The enzymes are produced by the duodenal epithelium or are secreted by the pancreas and released through the major duodenal papilla (opening of the joined common bile duct and main pancreatic duct) and minor duodenal papilla (opening of the accessory pancreatic duct) into the duodenal lumen. The addition of the common bile duct serves to supply bile for emulsifying fat.
- Transport of absorbed nutrients in the bloodstream directly to the liver (with the exception of fats)
- Peristaltic transport of chyme

Note: Gallstones may obstruct the common opening for the common bile and pancreatic ducts, and reflux of pancreatic juice that contains highly active enzymes may cause an acute inflammation of the pancreas (pancreatitis).

Embryonic development

- Of endodermal origin, derived from the foregut and midgut
- A dorsal and a smaller ventral mesoduodenum

Note: The duodenal epithelium gives rise to the primordia for the liver, gallbladder, and pancreas.

Major diseases

- Duodenal ulcer
- Acute and chronic inflammation (duodenitis)
- Malignant tumors (very rare)

1.8 Small Intestine: Jejunum and Ileum

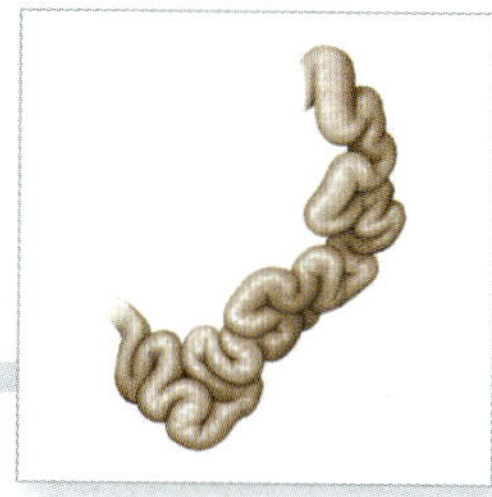

Location	• Lies *intraperitoneally* between the transverse mesocolon and the level of the pelvic inlet in the upper part of the peritoneal cavity. • Defining their location by reference to skeletal landmarks is not useful because the small bowel loops are very mobile, generally surrounded and framed by the large intestine.
Shape and parts	• Hollow, tubular organ with numerous loops • Longest single organ (measures up to 5 m), ensures long transit time of food: jejunum accounts for approximately ⅖ of the entire length; ileum (longest single segment) accounts for approximately ⅗. *Note:* The ileum is connected in an end-to-side fashion to the cecum.
Wall structure	• Basically the same wall structure as the entire gastrointestinal tract: mucosa, submucosa, muscularis (with circular and longitudinal layers), subserosa, and serosa. • Mucosa with numerous folds and villi. Mucosal fold height decreases from proximal to distal, thus from jejunum to ileum. • Submucosa (particularly in the terminal ileum) with distinct collections of lymphoid follicles for immune response to antigens present in intestinal contents (aggregated lymphoid nodules = Peyer's patches). Effect of oral inoculation is based on the stimulation of Peyer's patches.
Neurovascular structures (see also p. 437)	Superior mesenteric circulation. • *Arteries:* numerous jejunal and ileal arteries (branches of the superior mesenteric artery). Additionally, in the terminal ileum the ileocolic artery. Arteries extend in the mesentery to the intestinal segments and form arcades close to the bowel, thus forming anastomoses, hence impaired circulation in the intestine is very rare. • *Veins:* jejunal and ileal veins into the superior mesenteric vein and from there into the hepatic portal vein. The terminal ileum is also drained by the ileocolic vein. • *Lymphatic drainage:* through lymph nodes located in the mesentery (juxta-intestinal mesenteric lymph nodes) into the superior mesenteric lymph nodes • *Autonomic innervation:* – parasympathetic primarily through the right vagus nerve (posterior vagal trunk) – sympathetic through the greater and lesser splanchnic nerves (partially celiac ganglia, but mainly superior mesenteric ganglia)
Function	• Enzymatic breakdown and digestion of carbohydrates, proteins, and fats as well as absorption of their components; additionally, absorption of vitamins, trace elements and minerals • Slow (transit time 8–16 h) peristaltic transport of chyme through the jejunum and ileum, with mucosal lining in close contact with food • Absorbed nutrients are carried off in the bloodstream directly to the liver (via the hepatic portal vein) (with the exception of lipids: they are transported via lymphatic capillaries to the cisterna chyli).
Embryonic development	• Of endodermal origin, derived from the midgut • Jejunum and ileum with dorsal mesentery
Major diseases	• Acute and chronic inflammation (enteritis) • Ulcers primarily in the presence of chronic inflammation (Crohn's disease); malignant tumors (very rare) • At the three constrictions (pyloric orifice, duodenojejunal flexure, and ileal orifice) foreign bodies that have been swallowed may get stuck (risk of life-threatening *mechanical ileus*).

1.9 Large Intestine: Cecum with Vermiform Appendix and Colon

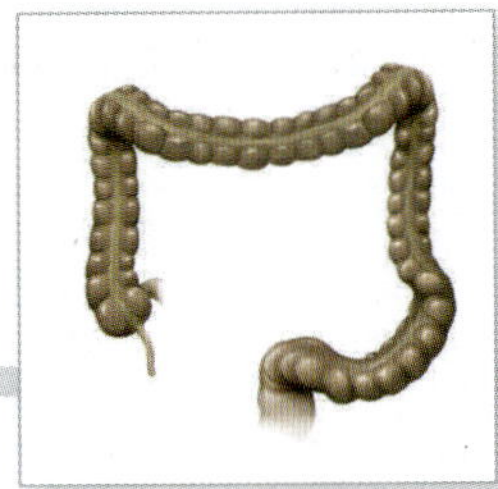

Location

Frame-like, primarily in the lower abdomen, transverse and lateral segments:

- Ascending and descending colon secondarily *retroperitoneal*
- Transverse and sigmoid colon *intraperitoneal*
- Cecum intraperitoneal or more or less fully secondarily retroperitoneal
- Vermiform appendix remains intraperitoneal.

Note: Only the intraperitoneal segments of the mature organism have a dorsal mesentery.

Shape and parts

Hollow, tubular organ, shaped like a frame that is partially open at its inferior aspect, with *cecum* and vermiform appendix; and *colon* with ascending, transverse, descending and sigmoid colon

Wall structure

- Basically the same wall structure as the entire gastrointestinal tract
- Deep mucosal depressions (crypts), but, unlike the small intestine, no folds or villi
- Numerous lymphoid follicles in the submucosa (recognize enteric antigens), unlike the sterile small intestine, the large intestine is always populated by bacteria.

Note: The longitudinal layers of the muscularis of the colon are in the form of three discontinuous longitudinal bands of muscle (free taenia, mesocolic taenia, omental taenia).

- The circular layers of the muscularis form constrictions (visible internally as semilunar folds) with sacculations located between the folds (haustra = haustrations of colon). Serosa with fat deposition (epiploic appendices).
- Taeniae, haustra, and epiploic appendices are distinctive morphological features of the colon and cecum, which are helpful in distinguishing the large intestine from the small intestine during surgery. Taeniae are not present in the rectum where the longitudinal muscle fibers again form a continuous layer. (The junction between the colon and rectum is visible externally.)

Neurovascular structures (see also p. 438f)

Proximal to the left colic flexure **superior mesenteric circulation**:

- *Arteries:* right and middle colic arteries and ileocolic artery (from the superior mesenteric artery) with anterior and posterior cecal arteries and appendicular artery
- *Veins:* right and middle colic veins and ileocolic vein with anterior and posterior cecal veins and appendicular vein into the superior mesenteric vein and from there into the hepatic portal vein
- *Lymphatic drainage:* through the pre- and retrocecal lymph nodes and appendicular lymph nodes, and right and middle colic lymph nodes, into the superior mesenteric lymph nodes
- *Autonomic innervation:*
  - parasympathetic primarily through the right vagus nerve (posterior vagal trunk)
  - sympathetic through the greater and lesser splanchnic nerves (superior mesenteric ganglia)

Distal to the left colic flexure, **inferior mesenteric circulation**:

- *Arteries:* left colic artery and sigmoid arteries arising from the inferior mesenteric artery
- *Veins:* left colic vein and sigmoid veins into the inferior mesenteric vein and from there into the hepatic portal vein
- *Lymphatic drainage:* through mesenteric lymph nodes (left colic lymph nodes and sigmoid lymph nodes) into the inferior mesenteric lymph nodes and from there via the intestinal trunks into the cisterna chyli
- *Autonomic innervation:*
  - parasympathetic through the pelvic splanchnic nerves (from S2–S4) via the inferior hypogastric plexus,
  - sympathetic through the lumbar splanchnic nerves (via the inferior hypogastric plexus), partially through the greater and lesser splanchnic nerves (superior mesenteric ganglia).

Note: Close to the left colic flexure distinct anastomoses between the middle colic artery and left colic artery (*Riolan anastomosis*) and convergence of autonomic fibers (*Cannon-Böhm point*) mark the boundary between the midgut and hindgut.

Function

- To some extent resorption of food components broken down by enzymes
- Primarily thickening of the chyme through salt and water absorption (colon), hence slow peristaltic transport of the chyme
- Immune recognition of antigens in the food (mainly cecum and vermiform appendix = "tonsil" of the gastrointestinal tract).

Embryonic development

Of endodermal origin, derived from the midgut (up to the left colic flexure) and hindgut (after the left colic flexure)

Major diseases

- Acute and chronic inflammation (enteritis)
- Benign tumors (polyps), which often become malignant (Large intestine carcinomas are one of the most common malignant tumors in the industrialized world.)
- Acute inflammation (mostly bacterial) of the vermiform appendix is very common (acute appendicitis, mistakenly referred to as typhlitis). Spreading of the inflammation to the peritoneum can lead to life-threatening peritonitis. Therapy: surgical removal of the appendix (appendectomy).

1.10 Large Intestine: Rectum

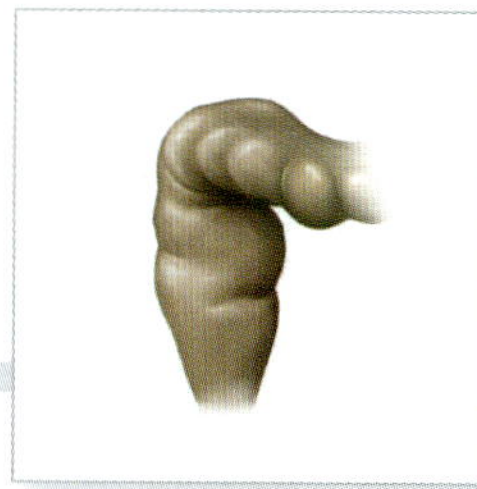

Location

Situated in the lesser pelvis, extends anterior to the sacrum to the pelvic floor, largely in the extraperitoneal space in the pelvis. The *proximal* end may be *intraperitoneal*, and the rest lies in the *extraperitoneal* space (retroperitoneal and subperitoneal spaces).

Shape and parts

Hollow, tubular organ with

- Rectal ampulla (ampulla = circumscribed dilation that serves as a stool reservoir; accumulation of a certain volume of stool triggers the defecation mechanism) and
- Anal canal.

Note: The rectum (straight) is by no means straight but has curves proximal to the sacrum (sacral flexure) and above the pelvic floor (perineal flexure).

Wall structure

Basically the same wall structure as the gastrointestinal tract with mucosa, submucosa, muscularis (with circular and longitudinal layers), subserosa, and serosa or adventitia.
Note the following characteristics in which the rectum differs from the rest of the large intestine: absence of taeniae and haustra, no epiploic appendices; three transverse folds instead of semilunar folds.

Neurovascular structures (see also p. 440)

Blood and lymphatic vessels (not the autonomic innervation) originate from **two sources**:

Hindgut derivatives of the rectum, primarily the rectal ampulla, **inferior mesenteric circulation**:
- *Arteries:* unpaired superior rectal artery from the inferior mesenteric artery
- *Veins:* superior rectal vein into the inferior mesenteric vein and from there into the hepatic portal vein to the liver
- *Lymphatic drainage:* 2 ways:
  - through superior rectal lymph nodes into the inferior mesenteric lymph nodes
  - through sacral and pararectal lymph nodes into the internal iliac lymph nodes

Pelvic floor derivatives, the anal canal and anus, **pelvic circulation (iliac circulation)**:
- *Arteries:* paired middle rectal arteries (not always present) from the internal iliac arteries, and inferior rectal arteries from the internal pudendal arteries
- *Veins:* (paired) middle rectal veins directly and (paired) inferior rectal veins via internal pudendal veins into the internal iliac veins
- *Lymphatic drainage:* through the pararectal lymph nodes and superficial inguinal lymph nodes into the internal iliac lymph nodes

Autonomic innervation (the same for both parts):
- Parasympathetic through the pelvic splanchnic nerves (S2–S4)
- Sympathetic through the lumbar and (to a lesser extent) sacral splanchnic nerves (via superior, middle, and inferior rectal plexuses)

Function

As part of the large intestine, temporary and controlled storage of fecal matter (continence) and its controlled elimination (defecation).
Note: Functional continence is ensured by gas-tight closure of the rectum. The rectal cavernous plexus (hemorrhoidal plexus), which is supplied by the superior rectal artery, remains filled up as part of the permanent contraction of the muscular sphincter apparatus.

Embryonic development

- Largely (mainly the rectal ampulla) derived from the hindgut with an endodermal lining.
- The distal part of the rectum, the anal canal, develops from the ectodermal cells of the pelvic floor.

Note: Terminologically, the anal canal is considered either part of the rectum (with the rectal ampulla as the part derived from the endoderm) or as a separate part of the intestine.

Major diseases

- Malignant tumors (rectal cancers) are one of the most common malignant tumors in industrialized nations.
- Hemorrhoidal disease (dilation of the hemorrhoidal plexus; when bleeding occurs: bright red arterial blood)
- Anal fistulas and anal abscesses

1.11 Liver

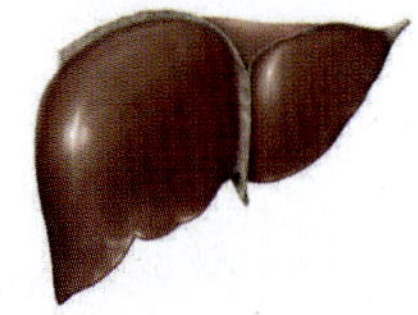

Location

- Lies intraperitoneally in the right upper quadrant.
- As a result of the rotation of the stomach and the ventral mesogastrium in the embryo, the liver moves under surface of the diaphragm where it becomes partially attached (the area of the liver devoid of peritoneum = bare area), moves with respiration.

Shape and parts

- Heaviest human parenchymal organ (weighs approximately 1.5 kg), in anterior view almost triangular in shape
- Morphologically divided into right and left lobes, with caudate and quadrate lobes included on the visceral surface.
- Based on vascular structures it is functionally and clinically divided into 8 segments; one segment = area supplied by one segmental branch of the hepatic artery.

Models to describe the microstructure of the hepatic parenchyma:

- *(central venous) hepatic lobule:* lobules measuring 1–2 mm in size. In their midst lies the central vein. Cube-shaped hepatocytes are arranged around the central vein in a star-like pattern. Venous drainage is of primary importance to this concept of liver organization.
- *(peri-) portal lobules:* where multiple lobules touch, they are connected through periportal areas (connective tissue with interlobular artery, vein, and bile duct = portal triad). At the center of the periportal lobule is the periportal area or portal (interlobular) triad; see p. 273 for a discussion of the concept of "triad." This classification system is based primarily on bile secretion (the liver as an exocrine gland).
- *Hepatic acinus:* in the shape of a rhombus, the outer angles of which are formed by two opposite periportal areas and two opposite central veins. This concept is based on arterial supply as the structural organization, most recent concept, important for pathophysiology.

Neurovascular structures (see also p. 434)

Upper abdominal circulation.

- *Arteries:* proper hepatic artery from the common hepatic artery (branch of the celiac trunk)
- *Portal vein:* venous inflow from most of the entire gastrointestinal tract via the hepatic portal vein
- *Veins:* hepatic veins (usually three) open into the inferior vena cava.
- *Lymphatic drainage:* primarily through the hepatic lymph nodes into the celiac lymph nodes, but also through the diaphragm into the mediastinal lymph nodes
- *Autonomic innervation:*
  - parasympathetic through the vagus nerves (vagal trunks)
  - sympathetic primarily through the greater splanchnic nerves, but also partially through the lesser splanchnic nerves (celiac ganglia)

Note: The liver has two sources of vascular inflow: the proper hepatic artery and the hepatic portal vein. Blood supplied by the proper hepatic artery is sufficient to sustain liver function. The hepatic veins transverse the bare area and open into the inferior vena cava. Liver segments can be resected individually, as the remaining parts of the liver have high regenerative potential.

Function

- Largest "metabolic laboratory" of the human body. The hepatic portal vein carries the nutrient-rich blood from the gastrointestinal tract to the liver.
- *Exocrine* gland: via intra- and extrahepatic bile ducts, bile is secreted into the duodenum discontinuously and as needed. In the duodenum, bile emulsifies dietary fat. Emulsified fat particles have enlarged surface areas making it easier for duodenal enzymes to further break them down.
- *Endocrine* gland: produces most of the blood proteins including coagulation factors and the prohormone angiotensinogen. The proteins are released into the hepatic veins.
- Detoxification (metabolism) of numerous pharmaceuticals. They become water-soluble through metabolism and can thus be excreted through bile or blood (kidney).

Embryonic development

Of endodermal origin, derived from the liver bud, sprouting of duodenal epithelium into the ventral mesogastrium and the very small ventral mesoduodenum.

Major diseases

- Acute and chronic inflammation (hepatitis), usually caused by alcohol or viral infection (hepatitis A, B, or C).
- Primary liver cell carcinoma is very rare in Europe; however, the liver is often the site of metastases of carcinoma of the large intestine (metastatic migration of tumor cells through the venous bloodstream via the hepatic portal vein).

1.12 Gallbladder and Bile Ducts

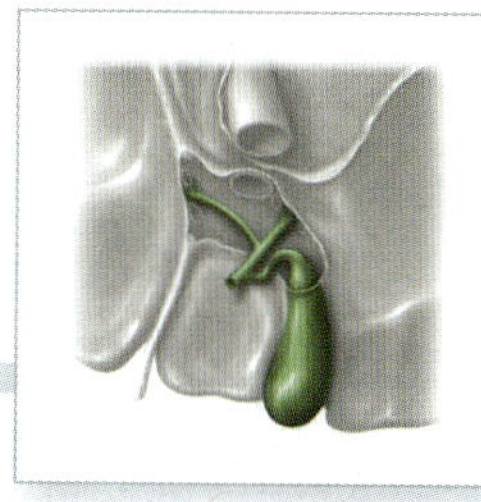

Location

- Gallbladder: lies *intraperitoneally* at the visceral surface of the liver. The neck of the gallbladder (exit point of the gallbladder) is oriented toward the portal fissure. The *fundus* of gallbladder is just visible below the sharp inferior border of the liver along the mid-clavicular line beneath the costal arch. (When the gallbladder is inflamed, tenderness to pressure may be noted at this location.)
- Extrahepatic bile ducts: lie *intraperitoneally* mainly in the hepatoduodenal ligament (part of the lesser omentum). The terminal portion of the common bile duct that traverses the pancreas and approaches the duodenum is secondarily *retroperitoneal*.

Note: By definition the gallbladder is part of the bile duct system. In order to provide a better overview and because it is a blind sac connecting to the duodenum, it is listed separately. The intrahepatic bile ducts (bile canaliculi and interlobular bile ducts), as intrinsic components of the liver structure (see liver), are not mentioned separately.

Shape, parts, and wall structure

- Gallbladder: small, pear-shaped pouch, measures up to 12 cm in length.
- Extrahepatic bile ducts are divided into
  - right and left hepatic ducts
  - common hepatic duct
  - cystic duct
  - common bile duct (formed by the merger of the common hepatic duct and cystic duct) opens into the duodenum.

Note: Right before opening into the duodenum, the bile duct and the pancreatic duct join.

The **walls** of the gallbladder and the extrahepatic bile ducts include a mucosa and a strong muscularis for transporting bile.

Neurovascular structures (see also p. 434)

- *Arteries:* because of its proximity to the liver, the arterial supply (cystic artery) is provided by the proper hepatic artery (from the right branch).
- *Veins:* cystic vein into the hepatic portal vein
- *Lymphatic drainage* (through the hepatic and cystic lymph nodes) primarily into the celiac lymph nodes
- *Autonomic innervation* same as for the liver:
  - parasympathetic through the vagus nerves (vagal trunks)
  - sympathetic through the greater splanchnic nerves (celiac ganglia)

Function

- Storage and thickening of the bile produced by the hepatic cells, and the controlled release of bile through the cystic duct and common bile duct into the duodenum (through contraction of the muscular wall)
- Reservoir function: the gallbladder can store up to 50ml of bile.

Embryonic development

Of endodermal origin. All parts of the bile ducts develop from the liver bud, from a sprouting of the duodenal epithelium into the ventral mesogastrium and the very small ventral mesoduodenum.

Major diseases

- Gallbladder stones (concrements, crystal-like, hard substances in the liquid bile) not painful per se, painful only when the gallbladder tries to push out the stones through rhythmic muscle contractions, causing sudden onset of severe pain (colic); Fat digestion is possible even after surgical removal of the gallbladder because the liver continues to produce bile; however, due to the absence of the bile reservoir, large amounts of fat can no longer be digested.
- Inflammation of the gallbladder (cholecystitis) and malignant tumors are rare.

1.13 Pancreas

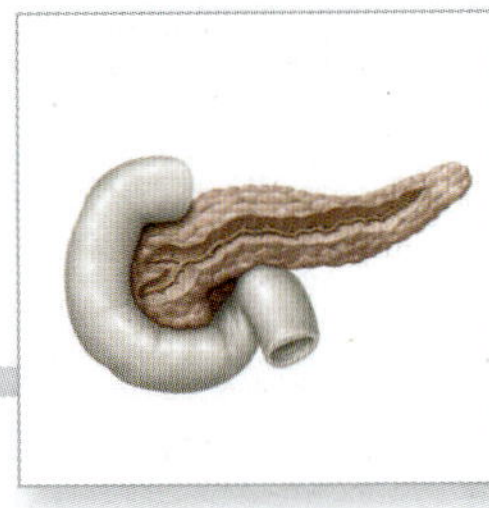

Location

Lies obliquely in the upper abdomen along the posterior wall of the omental bursa. Most of the body of the pancreas lies at the L1 level, the head of the pancreas extends to the L2 level.

Shape and parts

Elongated gland with little connective tissue composed of

- Head of pancreas
- Body of pancreas
- Pancreatic uncinate process
- Tail of pancreas

Structure

Histologically and functionally the pancreas can be divided into

- *Exocrine pancreas:* numerous small glands that secrete through an outflow duct (pancreatic duct)—mostly together with the bile duct—into the duodenum. Often, there is a second (accessory) pancreatic duct present.
- *Endocrine pancreas:* islets of epithelial cells scattered throughout the exocrine pancreas. The islet cells release hormones directly into the bloodstream.

Neurovascular structures (see also p. 436)

Upper abdominal and mediastinal circulation:

- *Arteries:* the arterial supply is from two directions via the pancreatic arcade:
  - superiorly from branches of the celiac trunk (branches of the splenic artery: great pancreatic artery; pancreatic branches; inferior pancreatic artery. Branches of the common hepatic artery: gastroduodenal artery with anterior and posterior superior pancreaticoduodenal arteries)
  - inferiorly from a branch of the superior mesenteric artery: the inferior pancreaticoduodenal artery
- *Veins:* pancreatic veins (via splenic vein) or pancreaticoduodenal veins (via superior mesenteric vein) or directly into the hepatic portal vein
- *Lymphatic drainage:* through superior and inferior pancreatic lymph nodes and pancreaticoduodenal lymph nodes into the celiac lymph nodes and superior mesenteric lymph nodes
- *Autonomic innervation:*
  - parasympathetic through vagus nerves (primarily right vagus nerve as posterior vagal trunk)
  - sympathetic through greater and lesser splanchnic nerves (celiac ganglia and superior mesenteric ganglia)

Function

- *Endocrine part* (pancreatic islet cells): predominantly production of insulin and glucagon (two antagonistic hormones of glucose metabolism)
- *Exocrine part:* production of numerous enzymes for the digestion of carbohydrates, fats, proteins and nucleic acids in the small intestine

Embryonic development

- Exocrine pancreas of endodermal origin, derived from two epithelial buds of the duodenum (ventral and dorsal pancreatic buds) that later merge
- Endocrine pancreas from endoderm derived primitive islets

Major diseases

- Inflammation of the pancreas (pancreatitis) can be caused by bile reflux due to blockage of the common duct from a gallstone, or from chronic alcohol consumption. Insufficient secretion from the exocrine pancreas leads to lack of digestive enzymes and maldigestion.
- The most common disease of the endocrine pancreas (and the pancreas in general) is insufficient insulin production from the islet cells that leads to *type 1 diabetes.*

Note: The superior mesenteric artery and vein pass adjacent to the pancreatic tissue in the area between head and body of the pancreas. Pancreatic tumors can lead to possible occlusion of these vessels. Cancer of the head of the pancreas can lead to occlusion of the common bile duct.

1.14 Spleen

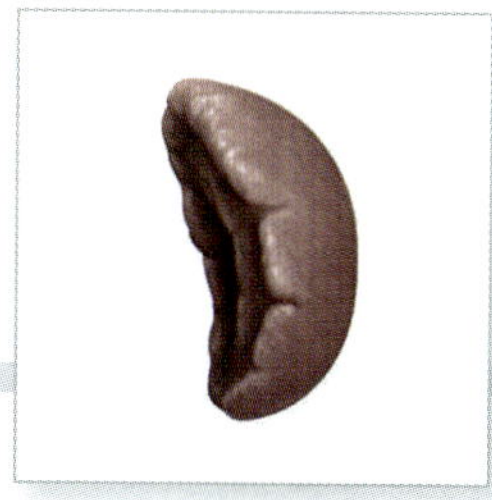

Location

Lies intraperitoneally in the left upper quadrant directly above the left colic flexure. Its longitudinal axis is oriented parallel to the 10th rib. Because of its location just below the diaphragm its position varies considerably with respiration.

Shape and parts

"Coffee bean shaped" with

- The splenic hilum, the entry and exit route for neurovascular structures, directed toward the stomach
- One pole directed forward and downward (anterior extremity) and one pole directed backward and upward (posterior extremity) as well as an inferior and a superior margin
- The diaphragmatic surface of the spleen is directed toward the diaphragm and ribs. The gastric, colic, and renal surfaces are directed toward the corresponding organs.
- Thickness × width × length approximately 4 × 7 × 11 cm (4711 rule), and reddish-brown color because of its abundance of red blood cells

Microstructure

- Blood from vessels located in strands of connective tissue (trabeculae) flows into the reticular meshwork through profusely branching vessels that are surrounded by aggregations of lymphocytes (*lymphoreticular* organ).
- The blood vessels empty into the meshwork (splenic sinuses) with low flow velocity (allowing for age verification of erythrocytes) and into the connective tissue itself (open circulation, a distinctive feature of the spleen). The blood then flows back from the sinuses into the trabecular veins.

Neurovascular structures (see also p. 434)

Upper abdominal circulation:

- *Arteries:* splenic artery from celiac trunk
- *Veins:* through the splenic vein to the hepatic portal vein
- *Lymphatic drainage:* through the splenic lymph nodes (some through the celiac lymph nodes) into the intestinal trunk
- *Autonomic innervation:*
  - parasympathetic: primarily through the right vagus nerve (posterior vagal trunk)
  - sympathetic through greater splanchnic nerves and partly through the lesser splanchnic nerves (celiac ganglia).

Function

- Largest lymphoid organ
- Monitors the blood immunologically.
- Destroys aged (80–100 days old) erythrocytes.

Embryonic development

- Derived from mesodermal tissue that sprouts into the dorsal mesogastrium
- As the stomach rotates, the spleen moves to the left upper quadrant.

Note: During physical exercise (running), blood flow to the spleen increases, and as a result the spleen swells. Stretching of the peritoneal connection between the spleen and colon (splenocolic ligament) is believed to be the cause of "side stitch" (a piercing sensation felt below the rib cage).

Major diseases

- Affected by dysfunction of the hemolymphatic system (e.g., leukemia)
- Painful swelling of the spleen resulting from mononucleosis (a common viral infection)
- Until recently, in cases of more severe upper abdominal injuries, a damaged spleen was often removed because it is very difficult to repair due to its soft consistency.

Today, because the immune function of the spleen is very important, surgical procedures where the spleen is preserved are increasingly common (using fibrin glue). 5% of patients who have undergone splenectomy are affected by overwhelming post-splenectomy infection (OPSI) syndrome, a condition in which encapsulated bacteria often cause fatal sepsis.

1.15 Suprarenal Glands

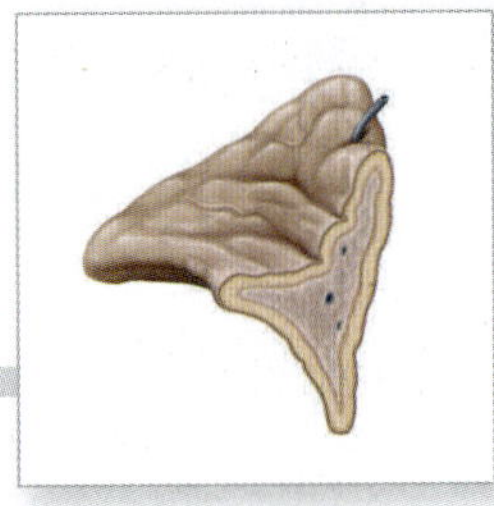

Location	• Primarily *retroperitoneal* (extraperitoneal) in the retroperitoneal space in the abdominal cavity, each of the glands lies on the superior pole of the associated kidney	• Located together with the kidneys in the perirenal fat capsules
Shape and structure	• Triangular-shaped (cocked hat of Napoleon; renal, anterior and posterior surfaces) • Larger (three-layered) outer cortex (with zona glomerulosa, zona fasciculata, and zona reticularis), the epithelial cells of the cortex form columns and conglomerates.	• Smaller inner medulla consists of sympathetic neurons that secrete into the blood: sympathetic paraneurons. • Suprarenal endothelial cells are active in phagocytosis—part of Aschoff's reticuloendothelial system.
Neurovascular structures (see also p. 441)	Retroperitoneal abdominal circulation: • *Arteries:* arterial supply provided by three tiers of arteries: – superior suprarenal arteries from the inferior phrenic arteries – middle suprarenal arteries from the abdominal aorta – inferior suprarenal arteries from the renal arteries • *Veins:* drainage through the suprarenal veins, on the right side into the inferior vena cava and on the left side into the renal vein • *Lymphatic drainage:* directly into the lumbar lymph nodes • *Autonomic innervation:* – parasympathetic: unclear.	– sympathetic: preganglionic sympathetic fibers from the greater splanchnic nerves supply innervation to the medulla. *Note:* The preganglionic sympathetic nerve fibers synapse with the postganglionic cells directly in the suprarenal medulla and not in the sympathetic trunk as is often the case in the sympathetic nervous system. Thus, the preganglionic transmitter of the first sympathetic neuron is acetylcholine as is generally the case in the sympathetic nervous system, whereas the second paraneuron secretes mainly epinephrine and some norepinephrine (10%).
Function	Each of the paired suprarenal glands consists of two endocrine parts, which have different embryonic origins: • *Suprarenal cortex:* production of steroid hormones (glucocorticoids, mineralocorticoids, and male sex hormones) affecting glucose, fat and protein metabolism, and mineral balance	• *Suprarenal medulla:* release of epinephrine and norepinephrine directly into the blood; functional component of the sympathetic nervous system ("two glands one organ") *Note:* Blood flows from the cortex to the medulla (downstream).
Embryonic development	• Suprarenal cortex: cells originate from the steroidogenic zone (mesodermal). • Suprarenal medulla: cells migrate from the neural crest (ectodermal).	
Major diseases	Dysfunction of the suprarenal cortex • Loss of suprarenal cortex (suprarenal hypofunction, *Addison's disease*; without hormone replacement it is life-threatening), for example, resulting from destruction of the suprarenal gland through tuberculosis or metastatic involvement (malignant melanoma) or	• Hyperfunction of the suprarenal cortex (*Cushing's syndrome*), which may occur as a result of ACTH producing tumors.

1.16 Kidneys

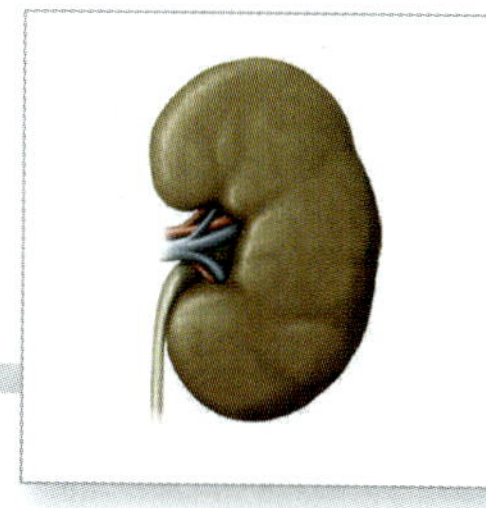

Location

- Lies primarily *retroperitoneally* (extraperitoneally) in the retroperitoneal space of the abdominal cavity at the L 1/L 2 level, together with the suprarenal glands within the perirenal fat capsule.
- Right kidney lower than the left kidney because it is pushed down by the larger liver.

Shape and structure

- Bean-shaped, measuring 12 × 6 × 3 cm (length × width × thickness)
- The renal hilum, directed medially, is the site of entry and exit for neurovascular structures and the ureter.
- Superior and inferior poles (extremities), and anterior and posterior surfaces
- Lateral and medial margins
- The entire renal tissue mass is enveloped by a tough fibrous renal capsule.

Microstructure

- The outer renal cortex contains numerous renal corpuscles for formation of primary urine by ultrafiltration.
- Toward the renal medulla are microscopically fine tubular systems (proximal and distal straight and convoluted tubules with loop of Henle) for concentration of primary urine.
- Urine is discharged via renal calyces into the renal pelvis adjacent to the hilum, and then into the ureter.

Neurovascular structures (see also p. 441)

Retroperitoneal abdominal circulation

- *Arteries:* left and right renal arteries directly from the abdominal aorta
- *Veins:* left and right renal veins directly into the inferior vena cava
- *Lymphatic drainage:* directly into the lumbar lymph nodes
- *Autonomic innervation:*
  - parasympathetic primarily through the vagus nerves (posterior vagal trunk), and partially through pelvic splanchnic nerves from S2–S4 (mainly to the renal pelvis)
  - sympathetic primarily through the lesser and least splanchnic nerves (celiac and aorticorenal ganglia), and partially through the inferior hypogastric plexus (mainly to the renal pelvis)

Note: On the left side the left renal vein receives the left testicular/ovarian vein and the left suprarenal vein. The left renal vein runs between the abdominal aorta and superior mesenteric artery and can become compressed ("nutcracker syndrome") as it courses right into the inferior vena cava.

Function

- Regulation of water-, acid-base- and sodium-balance
- Excretion of substances normally discharged with urine
- Regulation of blood pressure
- Stimulation of red blood cell production
- Influences metabolism of Vitamin D for regulation of calcium.

Embryonic development

Of mesodermal (intermediate mesoderm) origin, derived from the primitive metanephros (metanephrogenic blastema). The primitive metanephros develops in the pelvis and migrates upward until it is just inferior to the diaphragm (renal ascent).

Major diseases

- *Kidney stones:* when the solubility of compounds in the urine is exceeded, dissolved components may form crystallization nuclei. They may develop anywhere in the kidney (e.g., staghorn calculi in the renal pelvis). If they become lodged in the ureter, they may stimulate muscular contractions causing severe pain (colic).
- Inflammation of the kidney (*nephritis*) is possibly caused by bacterial involvement of the renal pelvis (*pyelonephritis*), or autoimmunological involvement of the renal corpuscles (glomerulonephritis).
- *Renal artery constriction* caused by atherosclerosis (with a drop in blood pressure) may lead to an increase in systemic blood pressure due to the kidney's compensatory ability in blood pressure regulation.
- Chronically elevated blood sugar (*diabetes*) may lead to renal dysfunction and increased blood pressure as a result of damage to the small renal arteries (microangiopathy).

1.17 Ureter

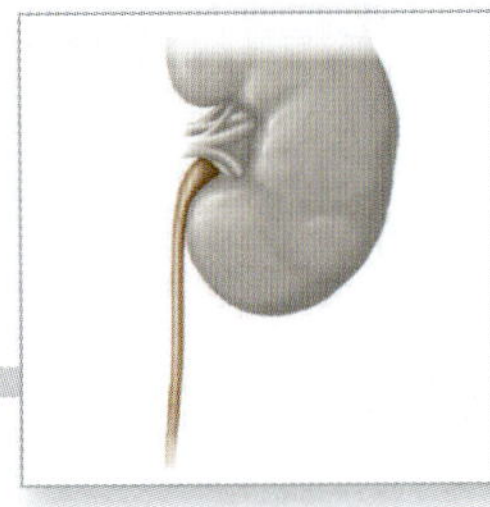

Location

Lies primarily *retroperitoneal* (extraperitoneal) in the abdomen and pelvis.

Shape and parts

Hollow tubular organ (pipeline) with narrow lumen; measures 24–31 cm in length, three parts:

- Abdominal part: in the retroperitoneal space of the abdominal cavity adjacent to the vertebral column, it runs from renal pelvis to linea terminalis of bony pelvis.
- Pelvic part: in front of the sacrum in the retroperitoneal space and subperitoneal pelvis; runs from linea terminalis to bladder wall.
- Intramural part: in the bladder wall.

Note: In the female, the ureter passes through the broad ligament and crosses below the uterine artery (risk of injury during surgery!).

Structure

- Mucosa with specialized urothelium (protection against hyperosmotic urine)
- Submucosa
- Muscularis with strong muscle fibers (active transport)
- Adventitia for integration into the connective tissue of the extraperitoneal space of the abdomen and pelvis

Neurovascular structures (see also p. 441f)

Retroperitoneal abdominal circulation and pelvic circulation (iliac circulation):

- *Arteries:* depending on which part of the ureter, ureteral branches of the neighboring arteries of abdomen (renal arteries) and pelvis (superior vesical arteries: possibly internal iliac arteries)
- *Veins:* depending on which part of the ureter, into the neighboring abdominal veins (renal veins) and pelvic veins (vesical venous plexus: possibly internal iliac veins)
- *Lymphatic drainage:* depending on which part of the ureter directly into the lumbar lymph nodes, lateral vesical lymph nodes or iliac lymph nodes
- *Autonomic innervation:*
  - parasympathetic through pelvic splanchnic nerves primarily from S2–S4
  - sympathetic through lesser or least splanchnic nerves via the celiac and aorticorenal ganglia, as well as lumbar splanchnic nerves via the inferior hypogastric plexus

Function

- Active peristaltic transport of urine in quanta from renal pelvis to bladder
- Preventing reflux of urine and thus ascending infection in cases of bladder infection

Embryonic development

Of mesodermal origin, in both the male and female the ureter is derived from the mesonephric duct. The ureter develops in the pelvis and moves upward with renal ascent.

Distinctive features

Clinically significant constrictions (3 ureteral constrictions) due to

- Proximity of the ureter to the inferior pole of the kidney
- The ureter being crossed by vessels (common iliac artery) at the level of the linea terminalis, as well as
- Passage of the ureter through the muscular bladder wall
- An additional fourth constriction may occur where the ureter crosses below the testicular or ovarian vessels.

The constrictions are potential sites where stones from the kidneys may lodge (ureteral stones).

Major diseases

- Ureteral stones, which may lodge at ureteral constrictions, may cause severe pain when the ureter contracts in order to push the stones toward the bladder (*ureteral colic*)
- Bacterial inflammation of the bladder may cause pathogens to pass through the ureters to the kidney, resulting in ureteral inflammation (*ureteritis*).

1.18 Urinary Bladder

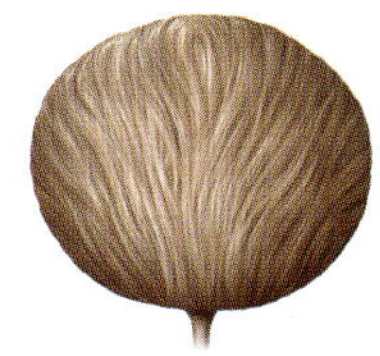

Location

Situated in the extraperitoneal space of the lesser pelvis posterior to the pubic symphysis; the bladder sits on top of the pelvic floor.

Peritoneal relations

The superior surface of the bladder is covered by urogenital (visceral) peritoneum. The peritoneum is reflected onto the anterior abdominal wall and behind the bladder onto the anterior wall of the adjacent organ located posteriorly (uterus or rectum) where it is continuous with the parietal peritoneum.

Note: A well-distended bladder pushes the peritoneum superiorly. When it rises above the pubic symphysis this provides an access route for puncture of the anterior wall of the bladder that is devoid of peritoneum (suprapubic bladder aspiration).

Shape

Hollow organ shaped like a tureen or ball depending on the degree of distention, can hold up to 500–1000 ml. Body with apex (upper portion) and fundus, and bladder neck (toward the pelvic floor).

The ureteral orifices and the internal urethral orifice (with uvula of bladder) form a triangle (trigone of the bladder) on the inside wall of the fundus.

Wall structure

- Mucosa with specialized urothelium (protection against osmotic effects of urine)
- Submucosa
- Distinct multilayered muscularis, responsible for closing (continence) and opening (micturition) the bladder
- Adventitial layer (visceral pelvic fascia), integrates the bladder into the surrounding connective tissue. The superior surface of the bladder is covered by urogenital peritoneum, a serosa.

Neurovascular structures (see also p. 442)

Pelvic circulation (iliac circulation).

- *Arteries:* via the visceral branches of the internal iliac arteries: Superior and inferior vesical arteries
- *Veins:* drainage into the visceral branches of the internal iliac veins via the vesical veins
- *Lymphatic drainage:* into the internal iliac lymph nodes
- *Autonomic innervation:*
  - *parasympathetic* through the pelvic splanchnic nerves from S2–S4
  - *sympathetic* through the lumbar and sacral splanchnic nerves (via the inferior hypogastric plexus)

Function

Temporary and controlled storage of final urine (continence) and controlled discharge of urine (micturition)

Embryonic development

Largely of endodermal origin, derived from the urogenital sinus, part of the cloaca; a small part (a portion of the posterior wall) of mesodermal origin, derived from both of the mesonephric ducts that are integrated into the bladder.
Note: An enlarged uterus, located posterior to the bladder (during pregnancy or resulting from muscular tumors in the wall of the uterus [myoma]), reduces the bladder capacity resulting in frequent urination. Descent of the muscular pelvic floor due to structural weakness caused by multiple vaginal deliveries may lead to failure of the closure mechanism and thus to urinary incontinence.

Major diseases

- Bacterial inflammation (cystitis) caused by germs that enter through the urethra, and is much more common in the female than the male due to the short urethra in the female.
- Bladder carcinoma as a malignant tumor
- Urinary incontinence resulting from pelvic floor descent (mechanical insufficiency of the pelvic floor, which may develop if the pelvic diaphragm slackens and descends after multiple vaginal deliveries).
- Trabeculated bladder: obstruction of the outlet of the bladder with hypertrophied muscle bundles due to benign prostatic hyperplasia (BPH)

1.19 Urethra

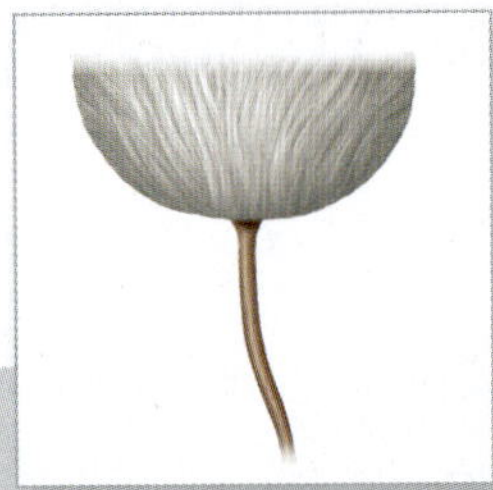

Note: Owing to gender differences regarding shape and function, the urethra is differentiated into

- Female urethra
- Male urethra

Location

In both the male and the female the urethra is directly below the bladder in the extraperitoneal space of the pelvic cavity. In the male it is also in the corpus spongiosum.

A portion of the male urethra below the bladder is surrounded by the prostate.

Shape

Hollow tubular organ with two orifices:

- *Internal* urethral orifice at the bladder outlet (in both the male and female)
- *External* urethral orifice on the body surface: in the female into the vestibule of the vagina, in the male on the glans penis

Parts

Female urethra (straight and approximately 3–5 cm long) divided into two parts:

- Intramural part (very short, in the bladder wall)
- Spongy part (longer portion, opens into the vestibule of the vagina)

Male urethra (20 cm long, has two curves) divided into four parts:

- Intramural part (very short, in the bladder wall, only for urine passage; with internal urethral sphincter)
- Prostatic part (3 cm long, urinary and seminal passage, surrounded by prostate; with urethral crest and seminal colliculus)
- Membranous part (1–2 cm long, passes through the urogenital hiatus in the pelvic diaphragm, distal portion with expandable urethral ampulla)
- Spongy part (15 cm long; in the corpus spongiosum, the dilated part known as the navicular fossa is right before the external orifice; the proximal portion of the spongy part is attached to the pelvic floor; the distal portion is suspended).

- *Two curves of the male urethra:*
  - infrapubic curve: at the junction between the membranous and spongy parts
  - prepubic curve: at the junction between the proximal and distal portions of the spongy part
- *Three constrictions of the male urethra:*
  - Pintramural part
  - membranous part (proximal portion)
  - external urethral orifice
- *Three dilated parts of the male urethra:*
  - prostatic part
  - urethral ampulla
  - navicular fossa

Wall structure

Mucosa (urothelium in proximal portion, stratified non-keratinized squamous epithelium in distal portion) with urethral glands, muscular coat and adventitial coat.

Neurovascular structures

Pelvic circulation.

- *Arteries:* urethral artery from the internal pudendal artery and smaller branches (in the male from the prostatic branches; in the female from the inferior vesical artery and middle rectal artery)
- *Veins:* drainage to the vesical plexus (in the female) or vesical plexus, prostatic plexus, and veins of the penis (in the male)
- *Lymphatic drainage:* lumbar lymph nodes (via internal iliac lymph nodes or inguinal lymph nodes)
- *Autonomic innervation* (sparse):
  - parasympathetic through the pelvic splanchnic nerves (S2–S4)
  - sympathetic through the sacral splanchnic nerves or inferior hypogastric plexus
  - somatic sensory innervation through the pudendal nerve

Function

Discharge of urine from the body (in both the male and the female); transport of semen during ejaculation (in the male)

Embryonic development

Derived from the urogenital sinus (males and females), and an ingrowth of ectodermal cells from the glans penis (males)

Major diseases

- Acute or chronic inflammation (urethritis, very common!) caused by bacteria (in most cases) or fungus (less common). Burning sensation while urinating. Women are much more frequently affected than men.
- Deformities during fetal development include urethrovaginal fistulas in young girls, or an atypical opening on the penis (mostly on the underside of the penis, known as hypospadias) in young boys.

1.20 Vagina

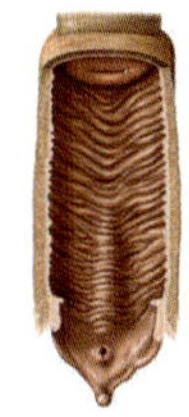

Location

Lies extraperitoneally in the extraperitoneal space of the pelvis. The vagina traverses the pelvic floor posterior to the urethra in the urogenital hiatus and opens into the vestibule between the labia minora.

Shape

Hollow, elongated tubular organ (measuring 8–10 cm in length).

Wall structure

- Specialized mucosa composed of stratified epithelium (mechanically resilient) where bacteria convert glycogen into lactic acid (acidic pH protects against ascending infections)
- Strong muscularis
- Adventitia integrates the vagina into the surrounding pelvic connective tissue.

Note: There are no glands in the vaginal wall. The wall is moistened by transudation.

Neurovascular structures (see also p. 444)

Pelvic circulation (iliac circulation)

- *Arteries:* vaginal arteries (not always present) as distinct branches of the internal iliac arteries, or vaginal branches of the uterine arteries
- *Veins:* vaginal venous plexus directly into the uterine veins or via the uterine venous plexus
- *Lymphatic drainage:* partially (only the superior portion) into the parauterine lymph nodes, mostly into the superficial inguinal lymph nodes (given that the vagina is a derivative of the pelvic floor) and then into the external iliac lymph nodes
- *Autonomic innervation:*
  - parasympathetic through the pelvic splanchnic nerves (S2–S4)
  - sympathetic through the lumbar and sacral splanchnic nerves (via the inferior hypogastric plexus)
- additional *somatosensory* innervation through the pudendal nerve

Function

Copulatory organ, birth canal

Embryonic development

Derived from epithelial evaginations in the pelvic floor (sinovaginal bulbs that fuse to form the vaginal plate). The vaginal plate develops initially as a solid structure that later undergoes secondary canalization.

Major diseases

- Infections caused by bacteria or fungi because of disruption of the normal vaginal milieu
- Malignant tumors (vaginal carcinoma) are rather rare.
- Rare, but explainable with regard to fetal development, are congenital fistulas to the urethra or rectum resulting in urine or feces being passed through the vagina (bacterial infections).
- Atrophy of the vaginal epithelium after menopause: strictly speaking this is not a disease given that menopause is a physiological process. It may however lead to subjective symptoms (vaginal dryness).

1.21 Uterus and Uterine Tubes

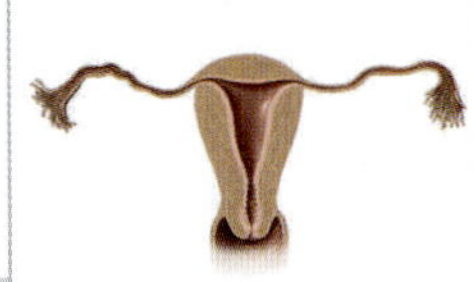

Location

Lies intraperitoneally in the lesser pelvis (covered by urogenital visceral peritoneum). Only a small portion of the uterine cervix lies extraperitoneally.

Uterus:
- Between the bladder and rectum
- The broad ligament attaches the uterus to the lateral pelvic walls; the uterus is tilted anteriorly (*anteverted*); the body of the uterus forms an angle with uterine cervix and is bent forward (*anteflexed*).

Note: The broad ligament of the uterus is a sheet of connective tissue in which courses the neurovascular structures to the uterus and uterine tubes, and partially also to the ovaries. That is why it is considered as "meso" (mesometrium/mesosalpinx/mesovarium = mesentery component of the uterus/uterine tube/ovary).

Uterine tubes: situated in the upper margin of the broad ligament

Shape and parts

- Hollow, muscular, pear-shaped organ (uterus)
- On the left and right sides arise a 7–10 cm long hollow tubular organ (right and left uterine tubes).
- The end of the uterine tube (ampulla of uterine tube) curves over a plum-sized and shaped organ (ovary) in order to receive the ovulated egg (see ovary).

Parts of the uterus:
- Body of the uterus (⅔) with posterior and anterior surfaces, and the blind-ended fundus of the uterus
- Uterine cervix (⅓) with uterine isthmus and cervical canal, vaginal and supravaginal parts of cervix
- External os of the uterus (opening in the vagina)

Note: A cervical mucus plug seals off the uterine cervix from the vagina and guards against the passage of bacteria ascending from the vagina.

Parts of the uterine tubes from lateral to medial:
- Abdominal ostium (fimbriated funnel-shaped end)
- Infundibulum of the uterine tube
- Ampulla of the uterine tube
- Isthmus of the uterine tube
- Uterine part (very narrow, passes through the wall of the uterus) with uterine ostium of uterine tubes

Wall structure

Uterus:
- Mucosa (endometrium with basal and functional layers), specialized to receive zygote. In sexually mature woman the endometrium undergoes cyclic changes with menstruation.
- Muscularis (myometrium): during pregnancy maintains uterine closure (cervical closure); expulsion of the fetus
- Serosa (perimetrium): allows for growth of the uterus in the peritoneal cavity during pregnancy.

Note: Contraction of the muscles in the uterine wall is controlled not only by nerves but also by hormones (oxytocin).

Uterine tubes:
- Mucosa specialized to generate fluid flow (kinocilia) towards uterus, helps to transport the immobile zygote and to move mobile sperm in the required direction (positive rheotaxis).
- Muscularis: responsible for movement of uterine tubes when sweeping the surface of the ovaries.
- Serosa (peritoneal covering) of the uterine tube is continuous with the mesosalpinx (see "location" above).

Neurovascular structures (see also p. 444f)

Pelvic circulation (iliac circulation)

Uterus:
- *Arteries:* uterine arteries from the internal iliac arteries
- *Veins:* drainage to the uterine venous plexus and to the internal iliac veins
- *Lymphatic drainage:* via parauterine and sacral lymph nodes to internal and common iliac lymph nodes (mainly from the body of the uterus) and inguinal lymph nodes (cervix, drainage same as external genitals)
- *Autonomic innervation:*
  - parasympathetic: pelvic splanchnic nerves (S2–S4)
  - sympathetic: mainly lumbar splanchnic nerves and partly sacral splanchnic nerves (via inferior hypogastric plexus)

Uterine tubes:
- *Arteries:* tubal branches from the uterine arteries and ovarian arteries
- *Veins:* drainage to uterine venous plexus or ovarian plexus
- *Lymphatic drainage:* directly or indirectly (via parauterine lymph nodes) into lumbar lymph nodes
- *Autonomic innervation:* see uterus

Note the uterus–uterine tube angle: In the female, the round ligament of the uterus traverses through the inguinal canal along with lymphatic vessels. Thus, metastatic tumor cells from the uterus–uterine tube angle may settle within the inguinal lymph nodes.

Function	**Uterus:** • Nurturing and sheltering of fetus during pregnancy • Expulsion of fetus	**Uterine tubes:** • Collection of ovulated egg • Passage-way for ascending sperm • Site for fertilization • Transport of zygote to uterus
Embryonic development	**The uterus and uterine tubes** are of mesodermal origin, derived from the paramesonephric ducts: • Uterus derived from the fused ducts • Uterine tubes derived from parts of the ducts that remain unfused	
Major diseases	**Uterus:** • Benign muscle tumors (myomas or fibroids), the growth of which may be influenced by sex hormones. They may put pressure on surrounding organs (bladder, rectum) or the uterine mucosa (possible disruption of menstrual cycle). • Malignant tumors may develop in the mucosa of the body of the uterus (endometrial carcinoma) or the uterine cervix (cervical carcinoma). • Descent of the pelvic floor may lead to descent of the uterus.	**Uterine tubes:** • Bacterial inflammation (adnexitis) generally ascends from the uterus. • Chronic inflammation may lead to occlusion of the tubal lumen (may inhibit conception). • Infections may spread from the abdominal ostium of the uterine tube to the peritoneal cavity.

1.22 Prostate and Seminal Vesicle

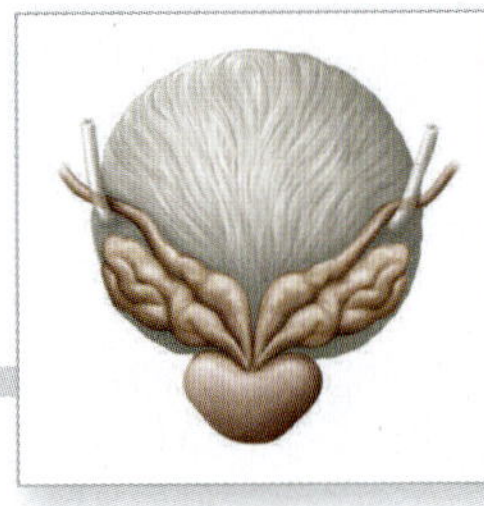

Location

Prostate: lies extraperitoneally just inferior to the bladder in the subperitoneal space of the pelvic cavity; lies upon the levator ani, surrounds the proximal portion of the urethra (prostatic part of urethra).

Seminal vesicle: lies largely extraperitoneally directly adjacent to the posterior bladder wall (the most posterosuperior tip is the only portion covered by peritoneum).

Shape and structure

Prostate:
- Unpaired gland that is enveloped by a fibrous capsule
- Numerous branched epithelial ducts that empty into the urethra by small ducts
- The outflow duct of each seminal vesicle merges with the adjacent ductus deferens to form the ejaculatory duct that passes through the prostate.

Seminal vesicle:
- Paired, elongated (5cm long) organs consisting of a tube that is coiled upon itself
- The glands are surrounded by a fine capsule.

Note: The histological division of the prostate into zones is done for clinical purposes. The term "seminal vesicle" is misleading: the gland does not store semen. Their secretions constitute approximately 70% of the ejaculate.

Neurovascular structures (see also p. 442)

Pelvic circulation (iliac circulation) for both organs

- *Arteries:* prostatic branches mainly from the inferior vesical arteries
- *Veins:* prostatic venous plexus with drainage into the vesical venous plexus (often described together as the vesicoprostatic venous plexus)
- *Lymphatic drainage:* partially into prevesical/retrovesical lymph nodes and then into the internal iliac, sacral and lumbar lymph nodes
- *Autonomic innervation:*
  - parasympathetic through the pelvic splanchnic nerves (S2–S4)
  - sympathetic through the lumbar splanchnic nerves and (to a lesser extent) the sacral splanchnic nerves (via the inferior hypogastric plexus)

Function

Produce secretions that, as components of the ejaculate, contains substances of functional importance for sperm motility. Secretions are alkaline and (particularly for the seminal vesicles) rich in fructose (energy source for sperm).

Embryonic development

Prostate: outgrowths of the urethral epithelium

Seminal vesicle: outgrowths of the mesonephric epithelium (mesonephric ducts)

Major diseases

Prostate: benign and malignant tumors:

- Benign hyperplasia of the epithelium and stroma with urethral stricture and urinary retention is particularly common in the transition zone of older men. As the prostate enlarges it causes the bladder wall to thicken (known as trabeculated bladder) as the bladder tries to force urine out. Treatment consists of urethral dilation.
- Prostatic carcinoma: develops in the peripheral zone in the epithelium below the capsule. Prostatic carcinoma is one of the most common malignant tumors in older men. Often, tumor cells spread to the bones, particularly to the spinal column, because the veins between the prostatic venous plexus and the venous plexus of the spinal cord lack valves (pain in the lower region of the spinal column in older men).

Seminal vesicle: rare cases of inflammation caused by genital infections.

1.23 Epididymis and Ductus Deferens

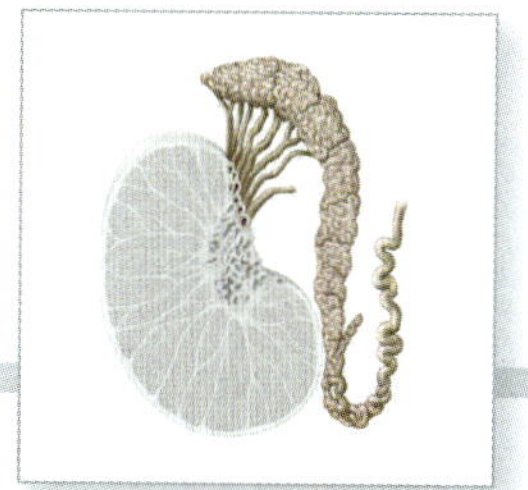

Location

Epididymis: lies adjacent and posterolateral to the testis, partially within the tunica vaginalis of the testis.

Ductus deferens: (continuous with epididymis) passes through the inguinal canal and runs along the superior and posterior surface of the bladder to the prostate. The part that is situated on the superior surface of the bladder is covered by urogenital peritoneum ("subperitoneal location").

Shape and structure

Epididymis: up to 12 m long, highly convoluted duct (epididymal duct), that is divided into the head, body and tail of the epididymis. The tail of the epididymis is continuous with the ductus deferens.

Ductus deferens: approximately 40 cm in length with strong muscle fibers that spiral around the very narrow lumen (often appears three-layered in histological section). The epithelium bears stereocilia. At the prostate gland the duct widens out to form the ampulla where it then continues as the ejaculatory duct (after joining with the duct of the seminal vesicle) through the prostate.

Note: Owing to its strong muscle fibers, the ductus deferens has the thickness of a pencil and is palpable in the inguinal canal.

Neurovascular structures (see also p. 443)

Epididymis: retroperitoneal abdominal circulation (with testicular vessels). Partially pelvic circulation as well (iliac circulation). Some of the epididymal neurovascular structures join the neurovascular structures of the testis.

- *Arteries:* branches of the testicular arteries
- *Veins:* drainage to the pampiniform plexus into the testicular veins
- *Lymphatic drainage:* lumbar lymph nodes
- *Autonomic innervation:*
  - pparasympathetic through pelvic splanchnic nerves (S2–S4)
  - sympathetic through lumbar splanchnic nerves and via the inferior hypogastric plexus

Ductus deferens: pelvic circulation (iliac circulation)

- *Arteries:* artery of the ductus deferens from the umbilical artery
- *Veins:* drainage partially to pampiniform plexus, partially to vesical venous plexus
- *Lymphatic drainage:* lumbar lymph nodes
- *Autonomic innervation:*
  - parasympathetic through pelvic splanchnic nerves (S2–S4)
  - sympathetic through lumbar splanchnic nerves and via the inferior hypogastric plexus

Function

Epididymis: storage and maturation of sperm produced in the testes

Ductus deferens: rapid transport of sperm into the urethra during ejaculation

Note: The formation and maturation of sperm in the testis and epididymis, the migration of sperm in the epididymis, and their final storage in the caudal part of the epididymal duct takes approximately 80 days.

Embryonic development

Both organs are of mesodermal origin, derived from the caudal portion of the mesonephric duct.

Major diseases

Inflammation of the epididymis (*epididymitis*) or ductus deferens is rare.

1.24 Testis

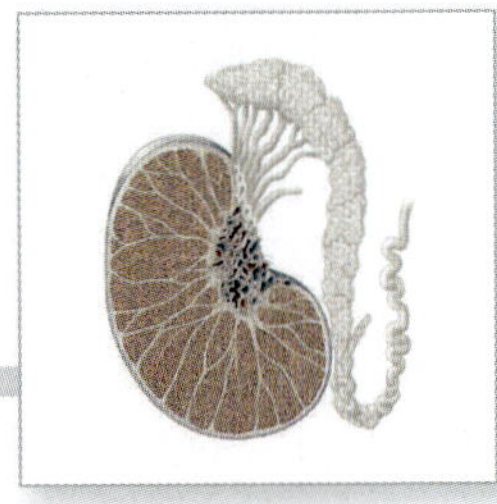

Location

Extracorporeal in the scrotum; largely surrounded by a closed peritoneal sac (tunica vaginalis). The position in the scrotum is the result of fetal testicular descent.

Shape and structure

Paired organ with the approximate size and shape of a plum, divided by fibrous septa into approximately 350 lobules. Each lobule containS2–4 convoluted seminiferous tubules lined by specialized epithelium where the spermatocytes develop (spermatogenesis). The tissue between the tubules contains Leydig cells, which produce testosterone.

Neurovascular structures (see also p. 443)

Retroperitoneal abdominal circulation (despite extracorporeal location)
During development, the testis together with its neurovascular structures descend from the upper abdomen into the scrotum. Thus, the neurovascular structures do not arise from structures in the pelvis (analogous to the ovary).

- *Arteries:* testicular arteries from the upper portion of the abdominal aorta
- *Veins:* drainage to the pampiniform plexus and then through the testicular veins on the right side directly into the inferior vena cava, and on the left side into the left renal vein
- *Lymphatic drainage:* lumbar lymph nodes
- *Autonomic innervation:*
  - from sacral nerves S2–S4 (pelvic splanchnic nerves)
  - sympathetic primarily through the lesser and least splanchnic nerves via the superior mesenteric and aorticorenal ganglia (via the testicular plexus)

Function

Produce gametes (sperm) and male sex hormones (testosterone).

Embryonic development

Of mesodermal origin, derived from the initially undifferentiated gonadal primordia in the urogenital ridge in the area of the upper lumbar spine. Sperm precursor cells migrate secondarily from the wall of the yolk sac.

Note: The testis are located in the scrotum (extracorporeal location) because the higher temperature within the abdominal cavity would inhibit spermatogenesis.

Major diseases

- Failure of normal testicular descent leads to *abdominal testes* (testis remains in the abdominal or pelvic cavity) or *inguinal testes* (testis remains in the inguinal canal). The higher temperature within the abdominal or pelvic cavity (as the testis is located closer to the core) inhibits the production of sperm and may lead to male infertility (with normal hormone production).
- Dilations of the pampiniform venous plexus (varicoceles, mainly left sided) may lead to overheating of the testis (due to the increased amount of warm blood) and reduced fertility.
- Malignant testicular carcinoma is one of the most common cancers in young men. The risk of malignant testicular cancer (seminoma, teratoma) increases with cryptorchidism (an undescended testis located within a body cavity).

1.25 Ovary

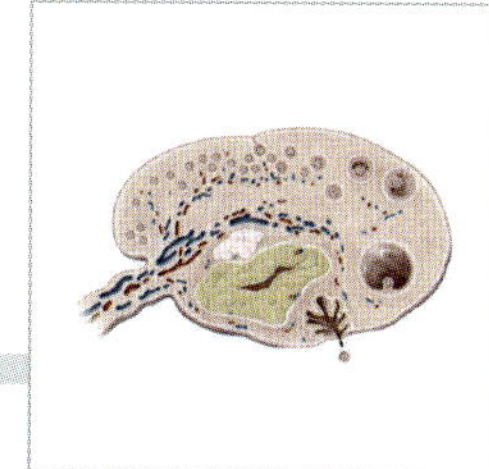

Location

Lies intraperitoneally in the lesser pelvis in the iliac fossa (after descent).
Note: The peritoneal covering of the ovary has mistakenly been referred to as germinal epithelium although it does not participate in egg production. The "germinal epithelium" of the testis, however, does not describe a peritoneal covering but rather the epithelium that produces sperm.

Shape and structure

- Paired organ with the approximate size and shape of a plum, presenting a tubal end (vascular pole) and a uterine end (uterine pole)
- Divided into
  - connective tissue capsule (tunica albuginea),
  - ovarian cortex and ovarian medulla.

The ovarian cortex consists of ovarian follicles at various stages of development. Each follicle contains a single oocyte surrounded by follicular epithelial cells and an envelope of connective tissue (theca folliculi).
Note: Female sex hormones are not produced by the ovum but by cells of the connective tissue surrounding it.

Neurovascular structures (see also p. 445)

Primarily retroperitoneal abdominal circulation, pelvic circulation (iliac circulation) plays a minor role.

- *Arteries:* ovarian arteries from the abdominal aorta, and ovarian branches of the uterine arteries (together they form the ovarian arcade)
  Note: When surgically removing the ovary two vascular systems need to be ligated due to the ovary's dual blood supply.
- *Veins:* on the right side the ovarian vein into the inferior vena cava, on the left side into the left renal vein; also ovarian venous plexus to uterine venous plexus
- *Lymphatic drainage:* into the lumbar lymph nodes
- *Autonomic innervation:*
  - parasympathetic primarily through the vagus nerves
  - sympathetic primarily through the lesser and least splanchnic nerves (via superior mesenteric and aorticorenal ganglia)

Function

- Production of female gametes (eggs)
- Cyclic production of female sex hormones

Embryonic development

Derived from the gonadal primordia in the intermediate mesoderm of the urogenital ridge in the area of the upper lumbar spine. From there, the ovary descends into the lesser pelvis (ovarian descent).
Note: The embryonic ovary is initially retroperitoneal in location, and moves intraperitoneal as the urogenital ridges fuse. As the ovary descends from the upper abdomen into the pelvis, it drags its neurovascular structures with it. Thus, the neurovascular structures course within a fold of the peritoneum (the suspensory ligament of the ovary).

Major diseases

- Ovarian cancer: particularly malignant because the tumor cells can easily spread within the entire abdominal cavity.
- Dysfunction of follicular development leading to reduced fertility or menstrual cycle disorder.

Appendix

References

Agur AMR. Grants Anatomie. Lehrbuch und Atlas. Stuttgart: Enke; 1999

Anschütz F. Die körperliche Untersuchung. 4th ed. Heidelberg: Springer; 1985

Aumüller G, Aust G, Engele J et al. Anatomie. Duale Reihe. 4th ed. Stuttgart: Thieme; 2017

Bähr M, Frotscher M. Neurologisch-topische Diagnostik. 10th ed. Stuttgart: Thieme; 2014

Becker C. CT-Diagnostik der koronaren Herzkrankheit. Teil I: Indikation, Durchführung und Normalbefundung der CT-Koronarographie. Radiologie up2date 2008; 1: 55-67; DOI 10.1055/s-2007-995498

Behrends JC, Bischofberger J, Deutzmann R et al. Physiologie. Duale Reihe. 3rd ed. Stuttgart: Thieme; 2016

Block B, Meier PN, Manns MP. Lehratlas der Gastroskopie. Stuttgart: Thieme; 1997

Block B, Schachschal G, Schmidt H. Der Gastroskopie-Trainer. 2nd ed. Stuttgart: Thieme; 2005

Brambs H-J. Pareto-Reihe Radiologie. Gastrointestinales System. Stuttgart: Thieme; 2007

Bücheler E. Einführung in die Radiologie. 11th ed. Stuttgart: Thieme; 2005

Claussen CD, Miller S, Fenchel M et al. Pareto-Reihe Radiologie. Herz. Stuttgart: Thieme; 2006

Dauber W. Bild-Lexikon der Anatomie. 10th ed. Stuttgart: Thieme; 2008

Dietrich Ch, Hrsg. Endosonographie. Lehrbuch und Atlas des endoskopischen Ultraschalls. Stuttgart: Thieme; 2008

Dorschner W, Stolzenburg J-U, Neuhaus J. Structure and Function of the Bladder Neck. Advances in Anatomy, Embryology and Cell Biology Vol. 159. Berlin: Springer; 2001

Faller A, Schünke M. Der Körper des Menschen – Einführung in Bau und Funktion. 18th ed. Stuttgart: Thieme; 2020

Fanghänel J, Pera F, Anderhuber F, Nitsch R, Hrsg. Waldeyer – Anatomie des Menschen. 24th ed. Berlin: De Gruyter; 2009

Flachskampf F. Kursbuch Echokardiografie. 6th ed. Stuttgart: Thieme; 2017

Földi M, Földi E, Kubik S. Lehrbuch Lymphologie. 7th ed. Stuttgart: Urban & Fischer, Elsevier; 2010

Frick H, Leonhardt H, Starck D. Allgemeine und spezielle Anatomie. Taschenlehrbuch der gesamten Anatomie, Bd. 1 and 2. 4th ed. Stuttgart: Thieme; 1992

Fritsch H, Kühnel W. Taschenatlas der Anatomie. Bd. 2. 11th ed. Stuttgart: Thieme; 2013

Gonska BD, Heinecker R. EKG in Klinik und Praxis. 14th ed. Stuttgart: Thieme; 1999

Graumann W, von Keyserlingk D, Sasse D. Taschenbuch der Anatomie. Stuttgart: Gustav Fischer; 1994

Greten H, Hrsg. Innere Medizin. 13th ed. Stuttgart: Thieme; 2010

Hamm B, Krestin GP, Laniado M, Paul G, Volkmar N, Taupitz M, Hrsg. MRT von Abdomen und Becken. 2nd ed. Stuttgart: Thieme; 2010

Haferlach T. Taschenatlas Hämatologie. 7th ed. Stuttgart: Thieme; 2018

Hegglin J. Chirurgische Untersuchung. 4th ed. Stuttgart: Thieme; 1988

Ignjatovic D et al. Can the gastrocolic trunk of Henle serve as an anatomical landmark in laparoscopic right colectomy? A postmortem anatomical study. The American Journal of Surgery 2010; 199: 249–254

Jin G, Tuo H, Sugiyama M et. al. Anatomic study of the superior right colic vein: its relevance to pancreatic and colonic surgery. The American Journal of Surgery 2006; 191: 100–103

Kacprzyk A, Droś J, Stefura T et al. Variations and Morphometric Features of the Vermiform Appendix: A Systematic Review and Meta-Analysis of 114,080 Subjects with Clinical Implications. Clinical Anatomy 2020; 33: 85–98)

Kuzu MA, Ismail E, Çelik S et al. Variations in the Vascular Anatomy of the Right Colon and Implications for Right-Sided Colon Surgery. Diseases of the Colon & Rectum Volume 60: 3 (2017): 290–298

Lange S. Radiologische Diagnostik der Thoraxerkrankungen. 4th ed. Stuttgart: Thieme; 2010

von Lanz T, Wachsmuth W. Praktische Anatomie. Bd. II/6 Bauch. Berlin: Springer; 1993

Lippert H, Pabst R. Arterial Variations in Man. München: Bergmann; 1985

Loeweneck H. Diagnostische Anatomie. Berlin: Springer; 1981

Lüllmann-Rauch R. Taschenlehrbuch Histologie. 5th ed. Stuttgart: Thieme; 2015

Masuhr KF, Neumann M. Neurologie. Duale Reihe. 7th ed. Stuttgart: Thieme; 2013

McNeal JE. Regional morphology and pathology of the prostate. Am J Clin Pathol 1968; 49: 347–357

Messmann H, Hrsg. Lehratlas der Koloskopie. 2., revised edition. Stuttgart: Thieme; 2014

Möller T, Reif E. Taschenatlas der Röntgenanatomie. 7th ed. Stuttgart: Thieme; 2021

Möller T, Reif E. Taschenatlas der Schnittbildanatomie. Bd. 2: Thorax, Abdomen, Becken. 4th ed. Stuttgart: Thieme; 2019

Moore KL, Persaud TVN. Embryologie. 5th ed. München: Urban & Fischer bei Elsevier; 2007

Nauth HF. Gynäkologische Zytodiagnostik. 2nd ed. Stuttgart: Thieme; 2013

Netter FH. Farbatlanten der Medizin. Stuttgart: Thieme; 2000

Pape HC, Kurtz A, Silbernagl S. Physiologie. 8th ed. Stuttgart: Thieme; 2018

Platzer W. Taschenatlas der Anatomie. Bd. 1. 11th ed. Stuttgart: Thieme; 2013

Platzer W. Atlas der topographischen Anatomie. Stuttgart: Thieme; 1982

Rauber A, Kopsch F. Anatomie des Menschen. Bd. 1–4. Stuttgart: Thieme; Bd 1. 2nd ed. 1997; Bde. 2 and 3 1987; Bd. 4 1988

Reiser M, Kuhn FP, Debus J. Radiologie. Duale Reihe. 4th ed. Stuttgart: Thieme; 2017

Rohde H. Lehratlas der Proktologie. Stuttgart: Thieme; 2006

Rohen JW. Topographische Anatomie. 10th ed. Stuttgart: Schattauer; 2007

Romer AS, Parson TS. Vergleichende Anatomie der Wirbeltiere. 5th ed. Hamburg und Berlin: Parey; 1983

Schneider H, Ince H, Kische S, Rehders TC et al. Management der Aortenisthmusstenose im Erwachsenenalter: Diagnostik, Prognose und Behandlung. Kardiologie up2date 2008; 4: 85–99; DOI: 10.1055/s-2007-995625

Schünke M. Topografie und Funktion des Bewegungssystems – Funktionelle Anatomie. 3rd ed. Stuttgart: Thieme; 2018

Schumacher GH, Aumüller G. Topographische Anatomie des Menschen. 7th ed. Stuttgart: Urban & Fischer, Elsevier; 2004

Schumpelick V, Bleese N, Mommsen U. Kurzlehrbuch Chirurgie. 8th ed. Stuttgart: Thieme; 2010

Schwalenberg T, Neuhaus J, Dartsch M et al. Funktionelle Anatomie des männlichen Kontinenzmechanismus. Der Urologe 2010; 49: 472–480

Seitz K, Braun B, Hrsg. Sonografie kompetent. Stuttgart: Thieme; 2016

Siegenthaler W, Blum HE, Hrsg. Klinische Pathophysiologie. 9th ed. Stuttgart: Thieme; 2006

Silbernagl S. Taschenatlas der Physiologie. 8th ed. Stuttgart: Thieme; 2012

Stelzner F. Chirurgie an viszeralen Abschlußsystemen. Stuttgart: Thieme; 1998. Unter Benutzung der Ergebnisse von Widmer O. Die Rektalarterien des Menschen. Z Anat Entwickl-Gesch 1955; 118

Stelzner F. Der Verschluß der terminalen Speiseröhre. Deutsch Med Wochensch 1968; 93: 1679–1685

Strohmeyer G, Dölle W. Ösophagusvarizen: Bedeutung, Ursachen und Behandlung. Med Klein 1963; 58: 1649–1653

Thelen M, Erbel R, Kreitner KF, Barkhausen J, Hrsg. Bildgebende Kardiodiagnostik. Stuttgart: Thieme; 2010

Tillmann B. Farbatlas der Anatomie. Zahnmedizin – Humanmedizin. Stuttgart: Thieme; 1997

Wallner C, Dabhoiwala NF, DeRuiter MC et al. The Anatomical Components of Urinary Continence. European Urology 2009; 55/4: 932–944

Wedel T. Funktionelle Anatomie – Voraussetzung zum Verständnis von Defäkationsstörungen. In: Chir Gastroenterol 2007; 23: 220–227

Wedel T, Stelzner S. Persönliche Mitteilung

Index

M

T

U